D1383464

TEXTBOOK OF SURGERY

Pocket Companion

Edited by

DAVID C. SABISTON, Jr., M.D.
James B. Duke Professor and Chairman
Department of Surgery
Duke University Medical Center
Durham, North Carolina

H. KIM LYERLY, M.D.
Assistant Professor of Surgery and Pathology
and Member of the Cancer Center
Department of Surgery
Duke University Medical Center
Durham, North Carolina

W.B. SAUNDERS COMPANY
Harcourt Brace Jovanovich, Inc.
Philadelphia London Toronto Montreal Sydney Tokyo

W. B. SAUNDERS COMPANY
Harcourt Brace Jovanovich, Inc.

The Curtis Center
Independence Square West
Philadelphia, Pennsylvania 19106

Library of Congress Cataloging-in-Publication Data

Textbook of surgery pocket companion / [edited by] David C.
Sabiston, Jr., H. Kim Lyerly.
  p. cm.

Pocket companion to: Textbook of surgery / edited by David
C. Sabiston, Jr. 14th ed. 1991.
ISBN 0–7216–3535–0

1. Surgery—Handbooks, Manuals, etc.   I. Sabiston, David
C.   II. Lyerly, H. Kim.   III. Textbook of surgery.

[DNLM: 1. Surgery, Operative—handbooks. WO 100 T3552
1991 Suppl.]

RD31.T4732   1992
617—dc20
DNLM/DLC   91–38830

Editor: W. B. Saunders Staff
Designer: Ellen Bodner-Zanolle
Production Manager: Carolyn Naylor
Manuscript Editor: Rose Marie Klimowicz
Indexer: Julie Figures

Textbook of Surgery Pocket Companion   ISBN 0–7216–3535–0

Last digit is the print number: 9 8 7 6 5 4 3 2 1

CONTRIBUTORS

ONYE E. AKWARI, M.D., F.R.C.S.(C)
Duke University

EBEN ALEXANDER III, M.D.
Harvard Medical School

J. WESLEY ALEXANDER, M.D., Sc.D.
University of Cincinnati College of Medicine

JAMES A. ALEXANDER, M.D.
University of Florida

D. BERNARD AMOS, M.D.
Duke University Medical Center

ROBERT W. ANDERSON, M.D.
Northwestern University Medical School

MICHAEL F. ANGEL, M.D.
University of Virginia

STANLEY W. ASHLEY, M.D.
Washington University School of Medicine

ROBERT W. BAILEY, M.D.
University of Maryland School of Medicine

WILLIAM H. BAKER, M.D.
Stritch School of Medicine, Loyola University

CLYDE F. BARKER, M.D.
University of Pennsylvania School of Medicine

ROBERT H. BARTLETT, M.D.
University of Michigan

JAMES M. BECKER, M.D.
Harvard Medical School

FOLKERT O. BELZER, M.D.
University of Wisconsin Medical School

HARVEY W. BENDER, Jr., M.D.
Vanderbilt University School of Medicine

JOHN J. BERGAN, M.D., F.A.C.A., HON. F.R.C.S. (Eng)
Northwestern University Medical School

F. WILLIAM BLAISDELL, M.D.
University of California, Davis, School of Medicine

R. RANDAL BOLLINGER, M.D., Ph.D.
Duke University School of Medicine

R. MORTON BOLMAN III, M.D.
University of Minnesota

TERENCE BOYLE, M.R., B.Ch.
Duke University Medical Center

GENE D. BRANUM, M.D.
Duke University Medical Center

GERT H. BRIEGER, M.D., Ph.D.
Johns Hopkins University School of Medicine

LOUIS A. BRUNSTING, M.D.
University of Michigan

CHRISTOPHER E. H. BULLER, M.D.
Duke University Medical Center

JOHN H. CALHOON, M.D.
University of Texas Health Science Center

JOHN J. CALLAGHAN, M.D.
University of Iowa Hospital and Clinics

JOHN L. CAMERON, M.D.
Johns Hopkins University School of Medicine

ENRICO M. CAMPORESI, M.D.
State University of New York Health Science Center

PETER C. CANIZARO, M.D.
Texas Tech University Health Sciences Center

C. JAMES CARRICO, M.D.
University of Texas Southwestern Medical School

ALDO R. CASTANEDA, M.D.
Harvard Medical School

JAMES CERILLI, M.D.
University of Rochester Medical Center

LAURENCE Y. CHEUNG, M.D.
University of Kansas School of Medicine

W. RANDOLPH CHITWOOD, Jr., M.D.
East Carolina University School of Medicine

FRANK W. CLIPPINGER, M.D.
Duke University Medical Center

JOHN A. COLLINS, M.D.
Stanford University School of Medicine

ROBERT E. CONDON, M.D.
Medical College of Wisconsin

REX B. CONN, M.D.
Jefferson Medical College of Thomas Jefferson University

JOEL D. COOPER, M.D., F.R.C.S.(C)
Washington University School of Medicine

JAMES L. COX, M.D.
Washington University School of Medicine

FRED A. CRAWFORD, Jr., M.D.
Medical University of South Carolina

ROBERT D. CROOM III, M.D.
University of North Carolina School of Medicine

DONALD C. DAFOE, M.D.
University of Pennsylvania School of Medicine

THOMAS A. D'AMICO, M.D.
Duke University Medical Center

R. DUANE DAVIS, Jr., M.D.
Duke University Medical Center

RICHARD H. DEAN, M.D.
Bowman Gray School of Medicine of Wake Forest University

HAILE T. DEBAS, M.D., F.R.C.S.(C)
University of California, San Francisco

JEROME J. DeCOSSE, M.D., Ph.D.
Cornell University Medical College

E. PATCHEN DELLINGER, M.D.
University of Washington School of Medicine

RALPH G. DePALMA, M.D.
George Washington University School of Medicine

ARNOLD G. DIETHELM, M.D.
University of Alabama School of Medicine

JAMES M. DOUGLAS, Jr., M.D.
Duke University School of Medicine

MILTON T. EDGERTON, M.D.
University of Virginia Health Sciences Center

JAMES M. EDWARDS, M.D.
University of Washington School of Medicine

JOHN A FEAGIN, Jr., M.D.
Duke University Medical Center

AARON S. FINK, M.D.
University of Cincinnati School of Medicine

JOSEF E. FISCHER, M.D.
University of Cincinnati College of Medicine

ROBERT D. FITCH, M.D.
Duke University Medical Center

J. LAWRENCE FITZPATRICK, M.D.
University of Maryland School of Medicine

M. WAYNE FLYE, M.D., Ph.D.
Washington University School of Medicine

THOMAS J. FOGARTY, M.D.
Sequoia Hospital, Redwood City, California

DOUGLAS L. FRAKER, M.D.
University of California, San Francisco

ROBERT J. FREEARK, M.D.
Stritch School of Medicine of Loyola University

ALLAN H. FRIEDMAN, M.D.
Duke University Medical Center

DAVID FROMM, M.D.
Wayne State University School of Medicine

WILLIAM J. FRY, M.D.
Medical School, University of Michigan

WILLIAM E. GARRETT, Jr., M.D., Ph.D.
Duke University Medical Center

WILLIAM A. GAY, Jr., M.D.
University of Utah School of Medicine

J. WILLIAM GAYNOR, M.D.
Duke University Medical Center

GREGORY S. GEORGIADE, M.D.
Duke University Medical Center

DONALD D. GLOWER, M.D.
Duke University Medical Center

J. LEONARD GOLDNER, M.D.
Duke University Medical Center

RICHARD D. GOLDNER, M.D.
Duke University Medical Center

CLEON W. GOODWIN, Jr., M.D.
Cornell University Medical College

ROBERT D. GORDON, M.D.
University of Pittsburgh

JOHN P. GRANT, M.D.
Duke University Medical Center

PAUL D. GREIG, M.D., F.R.C.S.(C)
University of Toronto

WARD O. GRIFFEN, Jr., M.D., Ph.D.
Temple University School of Medicine

HERMES C. GRILLO, M.D.
Harvard Medical School

JAY L. GROSFELD, M.D.
Indiana University School of Medicine

FREDERICK L. GROVER, M.D.
University of Colorado Health Sciences Center

J. CAULIE GUNNELLS, Jr., M.D.
Duke University School of Medicine

CARL E. HAISCH, M.D.
University of Vermont College of Medicine

JOHN D. HAMILTON, M.D.
Duke University School of Medicine

CHARLES B. HAMMOND, M.D.
Duke University Medical Center

WILLIAM T. HARDAKER, Jr., M.D.
Duke University Medical Center

ALFRED HARDING, M.D.
University of Missouri Hospital and Clinics

ALDEN H. HARKEN, M.D.
University of Colorado School of Medicine

JOHN M. HARRELSON, M.D.
Duke University Medical Center

JULIO HOCHBERG, M.D.
West Virginia University School of Medicine

JAMES W. HOLCROFT, M.D.
University of California, Davis, School of Medicine

WILLIAM L. HOLMAN, M.D.
University of Alabama at Birmingham

RICHARD A. HOPKINS, M.D.
Georgetown University Medical School

ROBERT P. IACONO, M.D.
University of Arizona Health Sciences Center

J. DIRK IGLEHART, M.D.
Duke University School of Medicine

SUZANNE T. ILDSTAD, M.D.
University of Pittsburgh

ANTHONY L. IMBEMBO, M.D.
University of Maryland School of Medicine

BERNARD M. JAFFE, M.D.
State University of New York Health Science Center
at Brooklyn

RICHARD A. JONAS, M.D.
Harvard Medical School

OLGA JONASSON, M.D.
Ohio State University College of Medicine

R. SCOTT JONES, M.D.
University of Virginia Health Sciences Center

ROBERT H. JONES, M.D.
Duke University School of Medicine

GREGORY J. JURKOVICH, M.D.
University of Washington

A. A. KASSIR, M.B., F.R.C.S.I.
University of California, San Diego

KEITH A. KELLY, M.D.
Mayo Medical School

JAMES K. KIRKLIN, M.D.
University of Alabama at Birmingham

JOHN W. KIRKLIN, M.D.
University of Alabama at Birmingham

MICHAEL S. KLEIN, M.D.
University of Illinois College of Medicine

JOHN J. KLOSAK, M.D.
Loyola University Medical Center

THOMAS J. KRIZEK, M.D.
University of Chicago

TERRY C. LAIRMORE, M.D.
Washington University School of Medicine

BERNARD LANGER, M.D., F.R.C.S.(C)
University of Toronto

JOHN G. LEASE, M.D.
University of Chicago

LASALLE D. LEFFALL, Jr., M.D.
Howard University College of Medicine

ALAN T. LEFOR, M.D.
University of Maryland School of Medicine

GEORGE S. LEIGHT, Jr., M.D.
Duke University School of Medicine

L. SCOTT LEVIN, M.D.
Duke University Medical Center

GARY K. LOFLAND, M.D.
Medical College of Virginia, Virginia Commonwealth University

WILLIAM P. LONGMIRE, Jr., M.D.
University of California, Los Angeles, Medical Center

DONALD E. LOW, M.D., F.R.C.S.(C)
Virginia Mason Medical Center

JAMES E. LOWE, M.D.
Duke University Medical Center

H. KIM LYERLY, M.D.
Duke University Medical Center

JAMES W. MacKENZIE, M.D.
University of Medicine and Dentistry of New Jersey, Robert Wood Johnson Medical School

JOHN A. MANNICK, M.D.
Harvard Medical School

G. ROBERT MASON, M.D., Ph.D.
Loyola University Medical Center

DOUGLAS J. MATHISEN, M.D.
Harvard Medical School

RICHARD L. McCANN, M.D.
Duke University Medical Center

DONALD E. McCOLLUM, M.D.
Duke University Medical Center

JOHN C. McDONALD, M.D.
Louisiana State University Medical Center

WILLIAM J. MEISLER, M.D.
Duke University Medical Center

ANTHONY A. MEYER, Ph.D., M.D.
University of North Carolina

WILLIAM C. MEYERS, M.D.
Duke University Medical Center

GREGORY L. MONETA, M.D.
Oregon Health Sciences University

FRANK G. MOODY, M.D.
The University of Texas Medical School at Houston

A. R. MOOSSA, M.D.
University of California, San Diego

JON F. MORAN, M.D.
University of Kansas Medical Center

RAYMOND F. MORGAN, M.D., D.M.D.
University of Virginia Health Sciences Center

JOSEPH A. MOYLAN, M.D.
Duke University Medical Center

GORDON F. MURRAY, M.D.
West Virginia University School of Medicine

DAVID L. NAHRWOLD, M.D.
Northwestern University Medical School

JOHN S. NAJARIAN, M.D.
University of Minnesota

ALI NAJI, M.D., Ph.D.
University of Pennsylvania

BLAINE S. NASHOLD, Jr., M.D.
Duke University Medical Center

JEFFREY A. NORTON, M.D.
National Cancer Institute, National Institutes of Health

WILLIAM I. NORWOOD, M.D., Ph.D.
University of Pennsylvania

LLOYD M. NYHUS, M.D.
University of Illinois College of Medicine

W. JERRY OAKES, M.D.
Duke University Medical Center

DANIEL J. O'BRIEN, Ph.D.
University of Florida

C. WARREN OLANOW, M.D., F.R.C.P.(C)
University of South Florida

H. NEWLAND OLDHAM, Jr., M.D.
Duke University Medical Center

DON B. OLSEN, D.V.M.
University of Utah

SUSAN L. ORLOFF, M.D.
University of California, San Francisco

MARK B. ORRINGER, M.D.
University of Michigan Medical Center

ALBERT D. PACIFICO, M.D.
University of Alabama at Birmingham

THEODORE N. PAPPAS, M.D.
Duke University Medical Center

DAVID F. PAULSON, M.D.
Duke University Medical School

MARY C. PAWLINGA, M.D.
State University of New York Health Science Center

LEONARD J. PERLOFF, M.D.
University of Pennsylvania

HIRAM C. POLK, Jr., M.D.
University of Louisville School of Medicine

WALTER J. PORIES, M.D.
East Carolina University School of Medicine

JOHN M. PORTER, M.D.
Oregon Health Sciences University

BASIL A. PRUITT, Jr., M.D.
U.S. Army Institute of Surgical Research

SCOTT K. PRUITT, M.D.
Duke University Medical Center

KENNETH P. RAMMING, M.D.
University of California, Los Angeles, School of Medicine

J. SCOTT RANKIN, M.D.
University of California, San Francisco

NORMAN M. RICH, M.D.
F. Edward Hebert School of Medicine, Uniformed Services
University of the Health Sciences

WILLIAM J. RICHARDSON, M.D.
Duke University Medical Center

WAYNE E. RICHENBACHER, M.D.
University of Utah

LAYTON F. RIKKERS, M.D.
University of Nebraska Medical Center

WILLIAM C. ROBERTS, M.D.
Georgetown University

MICHAEL S. ROHR, M.D., Ph.D.
Bowman Gray School of Medicine of Wake Forest University

FRANCIS E. ROSATO, M.D.
Jefferson Medical College

JOEL J. ROSLYN, M.D.
University of California, Los Angeles, School of Medicine

DAVID C. SABISTON, Jr., M.D.
Duke University Medical Center

FRED SANFILIPPO, M.D., Ph.D.
Duke University Medical Center

BRUCE D. SCHIRMER, M.D.
University of Viriginia

STEVE J. SCHWAB, M.D.
Duke University Medical Center

STEWART M. SCOTT, M.D.
Duke University Medical Center

H. F. SEIGLER, M.D.
Duke University Medical Center

DONALD SERAFIN, M.D.
Duke University Medical Center

GEORGE F. SHELDON, M.D.
University of North Carolina at Chapel Hill School of
Medicine

DONALD SILVER, M.D.
University of Missouri Health Sciences Center

NORMAN A. SILVERMAN, M.D.
University of Michigan School of Medicine

RICHARD L. SIMMONS, M.D.
University of Pittsburgh School of Medicine

JAMES D. SINK, M.D.
University of Pennsylvania School of Medicine

KEVIN M. SITTIG, M.D.
Louisiana State University Medical Center

DAVID B. SKINNER, M.D.
Cornell University College of Medicine

PETER K. SMITH, M.D.
Duke University Medical Center

JAMES B. SNOW, Jr., M.D.
National Institute on Deafness and Other Communication
Disorders, National Institutes of Health

HANS W. SOLLINGER, M.D., Ph.D.
University of Wisconsin School of Medicine

JAMES H. SOUTHARD, Ph.D.
University of Wisconsin

DAVID I. SOYBEL, M.D.
Yale University School of Medicine

THOMAS L. SPRAY, M.D.
Washington University School of Medicine

RICHARD S. STACK, M.D.
Duke University Medical Center

ROBERT J. STANLEY, M.D.
University of Alabama School of Medicine

THOMAS E. STARZL, M.D., Ph.D.
University of Pittsburgh School of Medicine

DELFORD L. STICKEL, M.D.
Duke University Medical Center

JAMES L. TALBERT, M.D.
University of Florida College of Medicine

GORDON L. TELFORD, M.D.
Medical College of Wisconsin

JAMES C. THOMPSON, M.D., M.A.
The University of Texas Medical Branch

SATORU TODO, M.D.
University of Pittsburgh School of Medicine

DOUGLAS S. TYLER, M.D.
Duke University Medical Center

ANDREAS G. TZAKIS, M.D.
University of Pittsburgh School of Medicine

ROSS M. UNGERLEIDER, M.D.
Duke University School of Medicine

A. K. UPADHYAY, M.B., F.R.C.S.
University of California, San Diego

JAMES R. URBANIAK, M.D.
Duke University Medical Center

PETER VAN TRIGT, M.D.
Duke University Medical Center

ROBERT B. WALLACE, M.D.
Georgetown University School of Medicine

ANDREW S. WECHSLER, M.D.
Medical College of Virginia, Virginia Commonwealth
University

RONALD J. WEIGEL, M.D.
Duke University Medical Center

JOHN L. WEINERTH, M.D.
Duke University Medical Center

SAMUEL A. WELLS, Jr., M.D.
Washington University School of Medicine

H. BROWNELL WHEELER, M.D.
University of Massachusetts Medical School

GLENN J. R. WHITMAN, M.D.
Medical College of Pennsylvania

ROBERT H. WILKINS, M.D.
Duke University Medical Center

DOUGLAS W. WILMORE, M.D.
Harvard Medical School

WALTER G. WOLFE, M.D.
Duke University Medical Center

BRUCE G. WOLFF, M.D.
Mayo Medical School

CHARLES J. YEO, M.D.
Johns Hopkins University School of Medicine

MICHAEL J. ZINNER, M.D.
University of California, Los Angeles, School of Medicine

KARL A. ZUCKER, M.D.
University of Maryland School of Medicine

PREFACE

The rapid strides in medical science have made possible more accurate diagnosis and improved methods of treatment for a variety of clinical disorders. Simultaneously, the quantity of medical data available has become enormous and at times overwhelming. For these reasons, medical students, residents, and practicing surgeons have recognized the need for a compact text to serve as an *introduction* to the more complete descriptions of medical illnesses. This *Companion* has been written to accompany the recently published Sabiston, *Textbook of Surgery: The Biological Basis of Modern Surgical Practice* (14th edition). A *key* feature of this companion text is that each of its chapters corresponds to the same chapter in *complete* form in the *Textbook of Surgery*. Moreover, the authors of the comprehensive text were selected for their national and international reputations and knowledge in each specific field, and these same authors have contributed the identical chapters in the *Companion*. Therefore, the major text can be considered a *definitive* reference source for each topic discussed. In every instance this *handbook* should be used as a preliminary step to the main text, since it is not sufficiently complete to be read alone.

The *Companion* is designed to conveniently fit in a coat pocket, especially those of medical students and residents, as an immediate and instantly available source of information often needed on an urgent basis. Moreover, it is often helpful to have a condensed version that summarizes the major points prior to reading the complete description in the major text. It should be emphasized that in all situations the reader is referred to the *Textbook of Surgery* as the complete source of information, as the *Companion* represents only the first step in the reading process.

The editors are most grateful to each of the contributors for their careful condensation of much material and will be pleased to receive comments from the readers.

DAVID C. SABISTON, JR., M.D.
H. KIM LYERLY, M.D.

CONTENTS

THE DEVELOPMENT OF SURGERY:
Historical Aspects Important in the Origin and Development of Modern Surgical Science

Gert H. Brieger, M.D., Ph.D.

The history of disease is at least as old as the history of mankind. It can be assumed that surgical disease, or the surgical response to disease, is of similar antiquity. The basic forms of disease—tumors, infections, trauma, and congenital abnormalities—have existed unchanged. Surgeons today obviously manage them differently from their colleagues of prehistoric time, yet some aspects of the surgeon's work are timeless.

In Greek and Roman antiquity, surgeons existed as specialists, but only when diet and drugs were of no avail did they resort to surgery. In cases of injury, of course, the surgeon might be called upon immediately. In the great Greek medical works that are ascribed to Hippocrates, but certainly not all written by him, there are books on fractures, dislocations, and other surgical disorders. One of the most interesting is simply entitled *On the Surgery*, in which the author described what the surgeon should know, how he should proceed with treatment, and what general qualifications he should possess. Much of the work concerns bandaging of various types of injuries.

In the later Middle Ages, when medicine was in a stagnant state except for the contributions of the Arabs, surgery was the branch that again began to show progress. Surgery was separated from medicine during the time of Galen, or before, and the two branches of medicine followed quite different paths during the next 1500 years. There were probably many reasons why surgeons were accorded less prestige and became a much less learned group than their medical colleagues, but the separation of surgery from medicine was not decreed by the church, as history books stated for years.

By the thirteenth and fourteenth centuries surgery was condemned and avoided by physicians, who had received their education in the universities that were now arising all over Europe. Along with theology and law, medicine was usually one of the basic faculties. Surgeons, however, were often unlettered, lower-class individuals who were scorned in clerical circles. The surgeons were taught the ways of their craft by apprenticeship.

See the corresponding chapter or part in the *Textbook of Surgery*, 14th edition, pp. 1–18, for a more detailed discussion of this topic, including a comprehensive list of references.

The barbers and surgeons of England had belonged to separate guilds since the fourteenth century. In 1540, a compromise as to the rights and duties of each was achieved, and a single company of Barbers and Surgeons was formed. Surgeons agreed to do no barbering, and the barbers restricted their surgery to dentistry. The union lasted 200 years; it was dissolved in 1745, and the surgeons' company again existed independently, jealously guarding its prerogatives and protecting its interests. In 1800, George III chartered the Royal College of Surgeons of London, which by charter from Queen Victoria in 1843 became the Royal College of Surgeons of England.

Anatomic dissection became more common again at the end of the thirteenth century. With the first manual for dissection written by Mondino de Luzzi in 1316, students had some guidance. The early dissections were still often confined to the bodies of animals and sometimes were autopsies performed to ascertain the cause of death, especially if foul play was suspected. These dissections were usually the responsibility of the surgeon. Only by the middle of the fifteenth century did anatomic dissection become so common that a special theater for it was built in Padua.

By the end of the fifteenth and early in the sixteenth century, occasional illustrated medical works began to appear. Johannes de Ketham's *Fasiculus medicinae*, Venice, 1491, and Berengario da Carpi's *Commentari . . . Super Anatomia Mundini* are two of the best known. Others appeared, but the best and most prevailing proved to be the *De humani corporis fabrica* of Andreas Vesalius. The publication of the *Fabrica* in 1543 coincided with the publication of another great book in the history of science, the *De revolutionibus orbium coelestium* of Nicolaus Copernicus.

The importance of Vesalius is that by his work and example he set forth a program. The famous frontispiece depicting him at the dissecting table, knife in hand, is itself programmatic. This young man, born in Louvain in 1514 and educated in Brussels and Paris, went to Padua to complete his medical studies. At the age of 23, upon receiving his degree, he was appointed professor of anatomy and surgery, an important academic combination for centuries to come.

There were numerous obstacles to the advancement of surgery. Pain, infection, hemorrhage, and shock were four of the most difficult to overcome. As each was mastered, the bounds of surgery enlarged. As the limits of surgery were extended, the field of individual surgeons appears to have become more and more restricted.

Since the fundamental aim of all medical art and science has always been to alleviate human pain and suffering, the development of anesthesia for use during surgical operations ranks as one of the most dramatic discoveries in the annals of medicine. The use of alcohol, mandrake root, opium, and even bleeding or reduction of blood flow to the brain to reduce sensibility was known to the ancients in a crude sense, but the really effective use of general anesthesia can be very precisely dated to the 1840s. In 1842, a rural Georgia practitioner, Crawford W. Long, used ether to remove small skin tumors, but he did not report his results until 3 years after William Morton successfully etherized a patient for John Collins Warren on October 16, 1846, at the Massachusetts General Hospital. James Young Simpson of Edinburgh introduced chloroform in the next year, and a new age in surgery emerged. Speed of operation would now no longer be the hallmark of the great surgeons.

Although the mid-nineteenth century English physician John Snow, famous for his writing about cholera and the Broad Street pump, was one of the first to present himself as an anesthesiologist, not until the years just before World War II did the specialty of anesthesiology develop. No longer was it sufficient for a surgical house officer or even a medical student to be delegated the task of administering the anesthetic and monitoring the patient, who often was neglected as the student eagerly watched the surgeon operate.

Anesthesia found speedy acceptance. The same, unfortunately, cannot be said of the attempts at control of infection. Wound healing in the days before Lister was a confused and depressing aspect of surgery. Wounding, either accidental or iatrogenic, was often followed by what was termed irritative fever, usually continuing a few days with accumulation of pus in the wound. Sometimes the pus was creamy white; this thick exudate was often termed "laudable pus." If the patient was fortunate, there was a slow healing process to recovery. This was the state of surgery from the patient's view, and it had existed for centuries.

In his earlier Edinburgh and Glasgow years, Lister investigated a number of problems closely related to surgery, such as inflammation, wound healing, and the role of blood coagulation in both. His approach to the problems of surgery was distinctly modern in the sense that it was scientific and physiologic. Despite Lister's attempts to sterilize his wards and to perform surgery as cleanly as possible, there was still an appalling rate of the common surgical complications of hospital gangrene, pyemia, and erysipelas among his patients.

In the years just prior to 1865, through the efforts of the French scientist Louis Pasteur, a germ theory of disease evolved. Pasteur clearly demonstrated that fermentation and putrefaction, observed since ancient days, were caused by living, multiplying matter. He reasoned that pus formation, wound infection, and some fevers must also be caused by minute organisms from the environment.

Lister's first papers describing his method and its success appeared in 1867. In the following years he changed the technical details of his method, added the steam-powered spray for the operating environment, and continued to battle for his principles in many publications. Subsequently, he was able to perform operations safely that previously no capable surgeon would have dared attempt. The successful wiring of a fractured patella in 1877, which converted a closed fracture to an open one, brought much scorn upon him, but patience, determination, and scrupulous attention to detail eventually led to success. Lister admitted in the 1880s that the spray was not necessary and indeed may have been harmful to operators and patients alike. He gracefully accepted the development of aseptic surgery by the Germans and acknowledged that it was but a step beyond his own work and a logical extension of it.

The acceptance of listerism, as already indicated, was not universal and, retrospectively, was quite slow. There were many reasons for this, most of them not tied to simple conservatism or resistance to change. Lister's method was complicated; the carbolic acid was an unpleasant nuisance and could actually be harmful, and the method was time-consuming and expensive and required assistance. Some surgeons and physicians believed the germ theory to be mere speculation; therefore, acceptance of the underlying theory or the rationale for Lister's technique was also slow. Also, it must be remembered that many leading surgeons simply could not duplicate Lister's good results, hard as they might try. Theodor Billroth was one who tried the method, wanted to accept it, but found it somewhat frustrating. By the late 1870s he had adopted listerism fully, but not without much discouragement.

Among the many difficult technical problems confronting nineteenth century surgeons was that of reconnecting the divided ends of hollow tubes, especially blood vessels and intestine. Just as cardiovascular surgery has captured both public and professional attention in the past 2 or 3 decades, 90 to 100 years ago it was abdominal surgery that had the same role. The successful removal of an inflamed appendix prior to rupture, the Billroth operations for esophageal and gastric cancer causing obstruction, the improved hernia operations of Bassini and Halsted, and abdominal operations for such other reasons as diseases of the ovary all caused great excitement in the medical world of the late nineteenth century.

In America, one of the important contributions to the advance of surgery stemmed from the work of a pathologist, Reginald H. Fitz of Boston, and the surgeons Charles McBurney and Henry B. Sands of New York and John B. Murphy of Chicago. In 1886, Fitz published his classic paper on appendicitis, a term he created. Known for centuries under a variety of names such as perityphlitis and iliac passion, acute inflammation of the *vermiform* appendix was a surgical disease according to Fitz.

Charles McBurney, professor of surgery at the College of Physicians and Surgeons, working mainly at Roosevelt Hospital in New York, in 1889 described the point of maximal tenderness now bearing his name and 5 years later proposed a new incision for appendectomy. It is important to note that the understanding of this common disease and the operative concept for it was determined by the cooperative efforts of physicians of several specialties.

Much has been written in the past 100 years about the training of the surgeon, the proper qualifications, and what it means to be a surgeon. Between the simple apprenticeship or even the transfer of knowledge from father to son that held sway until the nineteenth century and the thorough grounding in pathology, research, and operative and postoperative management required of today's surgeon, much surgical history has passed.

The subject of surgical training in America invariably brings to mind the name of William S. Halsted, no doubt partly because of his famous address entitled "The Training of the Surgeon" delivered at Yale in 1904. Halsted, who was born in New York City in 1852 and died in Baltimore 70 years later, made numerous important contributions to surgical technique and teaching.

Halsted developed improved methods for operating on hernias and cancer of the breast; he introduced the use of rubber gloves in surgery; and he constantly stressed the relationship of surgery to physiology. Careful handling of tissues and the minimization of blood loss were concepts he passed on to the many fine surgeons he trained during 30 years. Justifiable as has been his fame, Halsted was not solely responsible for establishing the surgical residency system as it is known. He would have been the first to note that the great German teachers of surgery, especially von Langenbeck and his pupils including Billroth, were his models. Moreover, Halsted's colleague William Osler deserves equal credit for instituting the system at Hopkins.

Late twentieth-century surgery has increasingly become a part of human biology. It is not only skill with surgical instruments, which for so long was the hallmark of the leading surgeons; a knowledge of the body's physiologic processes and their control has assumed equal if not even greater importance. Such knowledge has facilitated the development of techniques such as hypothermia, safer anesthesia, and the heart-lung machine. The great expansion of the surgeon's ability to have a role in an increasing number of afflictions has been materially influenced by the ability to regulate the body's fluids and electrolytes and especially by the advent of better means to control postoperative infections.

Perhaps nothing is more indicative of the great changes that have occurred, even in just the past 100 years, than to emphasize again that surgery has moved from the theatricality and the drama of the operating theater to the privacy and the relative sterility of the operating room. No longer is the drama of the operation or the technical skill or virtuosity of the surgeon on center stage. In the old surgery it was the *art* that predominated. In the new surgery it is *science*. The focus has thus shifted increasingly from the operation itself to the results that now provide the drama.

2

HOMEOSTASIS:
Bodily Changes in Trauma and Surgery
Douglas W. Wilmore, M.D.

Surgeons care for patients who experience sudden, rapid, and intense changes in normal physiology and metabolism. Such alterations occur following an elective operative procedure, but more dramatic perturbations arise following major accidental injury. Both of these events interrupt normal fluid and electrolyte homeostasis, alter food intake, change tissue perfusion, and often disrupt vital organ function.

The human body responds to these stresses with dramatic resilience. Mechanisms are initiated for the restoration of blood volume and the redistribution of blood flow to ensure perfusion of vital organs. Substrate is mobilized to provide a constant energy supply, and inflammatory responses are stimulated to initiate tissue repair and enhance host resistance. These biologic alterations that occur following injury and other stresses are a reflection of a unique and indelible program that is genetically encoded in higher species. In strict Darwinian terms, these responses are the result of an evolutionary process that favors survival of the fittest in the struggle for existence. In teleologic terms, these responses have a purpose: to benefit the organism and aid recovery. Knowledge of homeostatic adjustments that occur in critically ill patients is essential for optimal patient care and necessary for rehabilitation and recovery from a life-threatening illness.

BODY COMPOSITION AND ITS RESPONSE TO SURGICAL STRESS

The body is composed of two major components: a non-aqueous and an aqueous phase. *Body fat and extracellular solids* such as bone compose the *anhydrous portion of the body*. The aqueous phase supports a heterogeneous mass of cells generally referred to as the *lean body mass*. These cells represent the functioning components of the body that actively exchange oxygen, glucose, and other metabolites.

These components of the body change with disease. For example, with congestive heart failure, total body water and exchangeable sodium increase. With starvation, there is a decrease in skeletal muscle mass (a component of the lean body mass) and loss of adipose tissue (Table 1). Whereas body fat provides an excellent fuel source for the individual during stress, *loss of lean body mass represents loss of body protein*

See the corresponding chapter or part in the *Textbook of Surgery*, 14th edition, pp. 19–33, for a more detailed discussion of this topic, including a comprehensive list of references.

TABLE 1. Body Composition in Normal Individuals and Catabolic Surgical Patients

	Normal Individuals (% Total Body)	Catabolic Patients (% Total Body)
Body weight (kg.)	70.4	58.9
Extracellular fluid (L.)	25.6 (36)	31.9 (54)
Body cell mass (kg.)	24.7 (35)	14.7 (25)
Estimated fat mass (kg.)	20.1 (29)	12.3 (21)

Data from Shizgal, H. M.: Body composition. *In* Fischer, J. E. (Ed.): Surgical Nutrition. Boston, Little, Brown & Company, 1983, pp. 1–17.

(i.e., nitrogen), and this is associated with *loss of body structure and function*. The erosion of body protein is not without consequences, and if moderately severe it delays wound healing, impairs immunologic responses to infection, and prolongs recovery.

HOMEOSTATIC RESPONSES TO SPECIFIC COMPONENTS OF INJURY

Clinical illness causes a number of complex interacting homeostatic responses. The clinical features observed are the sum of changes known to occur following a single perturbation. These initiating factors include *volume loss, underperfusion, simple starvation, tissue damage, and invasive infection*. Each single alteration has been studied in detail, and it is well known that each perturbation stimulates a number of hormonal and chemical reactions that initiate the appropriate homeostatic adjustments. However, tissue damage and infection markedly accelerate catabolic responses. Following tissue injury, inflammatory cells soon appear in and around the wound. These cells release a number of mediator substances including *cytokines,* soluble biochemical signals that influence the local proliferation, development, and function of specific cells, most of which are immunologically active, which aid host resistance and wound repair. Although cytokines may function locally through paracrine and endocrine activities, they may also reach the bloodstream to exert systemic effects such as mediating *fever,* stimulating the elaboration of *acute-phase proteins and leukocytes,* and causing the *redistribution of trace elements* (such as iron and zinc). In addition, cytokines such as interleukin-1 (IL-1) and tumor necrosis factor (TNF) may *stimulate elaboration of pituitary hormones,* which also initiate and mediate metabolic responses.

A frequent complication of simple injury is invasive infection. Infection alone initiates catabolic responses that are similar to (but not necessarily the same as) those described following injury in noninfected patients. Both processes cause *fever, tachypnea, tachycardia, accelerated gluconeogenesis, increased proteolysis, and lipolysis.* If infection is sudden and severe, hypotension and septic shock may result. It has recently been found that the mediators of these events are cytokines, those products of the host's own cells. In most cases, the signal initiating these alterations is *bacterial endotoxin* released by gram-negative organisms. However, antigen-antibody reactions may also trigger these events. One cytokine elaborated following endotoxin exposure is TNF, and systemic responses that mimic disease occur in a dose-dependent manner following infusion of TNF into patients (Table 2). Other cytokines have been identified as postinflammatory circulating signals, and these include IL-1, IL-2, IL-6, and interferon-gamma.

RESPONSES FOLLOWING AN ELECTIVE OPERATION

The earliest response following a major operation is the stimulation of the *pituitary-adrenal axis*. Cortisol remains two to five times normal levels for approximately 24 hours after a major operation. In addition, urinary catecholamines are elevated for 24 to 48 hours after operation and then return to normal. Insulin is low, and glucagon is elevated; this hormonal environment stimulates hepatic glycogenolysis and gluconeogenesis. In addition, diminished food intake and elevated cortisol favor net skeletal muscle proteolysis. These amino acids are processed in the liver to urea, which is excreted in the urine. The operative stress also stimulates the secretion of aldosterone and antidiuretic hormone, which diminishes the excretion of free water. This retained fluid eventually returns to the circulation as the wound edema subsides, and diuresis commences 2 to 4 days following operation.

RESPONSES FOLLOWING ACCIDENTAL INJURY

The events that occur following injury are generally graded responses: the more severe the injury, the greater the response. The events also change with time. Initially following injury there is a decrease in metabolic functions and in core temperature. With restoration of blood flow, the patient's metabolic rate rises, body temperature becomes elevated, and blood insulin levels normalize (Table 3). During this period, the counterregulatory hormones glucagon, cortisol, and catecholamines are elevated, and insulin is normal or slightly increased. In addition, cytokines have been detected in tissues and the bloodstream, and these substances undoubtedly mediate many of the responses.

The *characteristic responses to injury* include *hypermetabolism* or increase in the resting metabolic rate, *increased nitrogen loss*, and *accelerated gluconeogenesis*. The rise in resting metabolic rate is related in part to the elevation in body temperature, referred to as posttraumatic fever. However, the increased oxygen consumption is also related to heightened activity of a number of metabolic cycles. The hormonal environment favors accelerated breakdown of skeletal muscle protein, and this is reflected in the increased loss of nitrogen

TABLE 2. Host Responses to Various Doses of Tumor Necrosis Factor (TNF)

Dose of TNF Infused (µg./sq. m.²/24 hr.)	Response	Clinical Correlate
1	Hypoferremia	Subclinical infection
20	Myalgia and headache, anorexia, fever, tachycardia, elevated acute-phase proteins	Influenza, acute appendicitis
>500	Rigors, elevated stress hormones, fluid retention, lymphopenia, hypotension	Intra-abdominal abscess, major thermal injury
>620	Decreased consciousness, profound hypotension, pulmonary edema, oliguria	Septicemia, severe acute pancreatitis, infected massive burns

TABLE 3. Alterations That Occur Following Injury

"Ebb" Phase	"Flow" Phase
Blood glucose elevated	Glucose normal or slightly elevated
Normal glucose production	Increased glucose production
Free fatty acids elevated	Free fatty acids normal or slightly elevated—flux increased
Insulin concentration low	Insulin concentration normal or elevated
Catecholamines and glucagon elevated	Catecholamines high-normal or elevated; glucagon elevated
Blood lactate elevated	Blood lactate normal
Oxygen consumption depressed	Oxygen consumption elevated
Cardiac output below normal	Cardiac output increased
Core temperature below normal	Core temperature elevated

in the urine. Skeletal muscle amino acids, primarily alanine and glutamine, contribute their carbon skeletons to the synthesis of new glucose. In addition, glutamine serves to buffer the acid load generated during this accelerated catabolism and also provides a specific fuel for rapidly growing cells, such as fibroblast, enterocytes of the intestine, and stimulated macrophages and lymphocytes. The glucose is utilized by the injured tissue but is incompletely oxidized and generates lactate. The lactate is recycled to the liver and reconverted to glucose. Glucose is also utilized by the kidney and the central nervous system, but not by skeletal muscle, which utilizes fat.

SUMMARY

Homeostatic adjustments constantly occur in surgical patients in an effort to maintain the *milieu intérieur* and ensure wound healing. Multiple factors, including diminished blood volume, tissue underperfusion, reduced food intake, extensive tissue damage, and invasive infection, initiate these responses via the neuroendocrine system. As a result of these physiologic adjustments, tissue perfusion is maintained, which supports the increased metabolic demands accompanying critical illness. Increased skeletal muscle proteolysis and accelerated gluconeogenesis are coupled responses that also occur; these biochemical alterations provide essential nutrients for the support of vital organ function and wound repair.

3

SHOCK: Causes and Management of Circulatory Collapse

James W. Holcroft, M.D., and F. William Blaisdell, M.D.

DEFINITION AND CLASSIFICATION OF SHOCK

Shock can be defined as a condition in which the metabolic needs of the body are not met because of an inadequate cardiac output. It can be classified as hypovolemic, traumatic, septic, neurogenic, cardiac compressive, cardiogenic, or cardiac obstructive and can arise from any of three primary causes: inadequate circulatory blood volume, loss of autonomic control of the vasculature, or impaired cardiac function (Table 1).

HYPOVOLEMIC SHOCK

DIAGNOSIS. The symptoms and signs of hypovolemic shock depend on the degree of blood volume depletion, the duration of shock, and the body's compensatory reactions to the shock itself. These compensatory reactions begin with cardiovascular adrenergic discharge. The systemic venules and small veins constrict. Residual blood is displaced to the heart, ventricular end-diastolic volumes are partially restored, and stroke volumes and cardiac output are partially reestablished. The arterioles in the skin, fat, skeletal muscle, and, eventually, splanchnic organs and kidneys constrict to maintain blood flow to the heart and brain. Angiotensin and vasopressin are generated to add to the constriction of the noncardiac and noncerebral arterioles. Release of vasopressin and aldosterone augments reabsorption of water and sodium from the glomerular filtrate for preservation of the remaining blood volume.

The symptoms and signs of hypovolemic shock are manifested progressively by (1) signs of adrenergic discharge to the skin, (2) oliguria, (3) hypotension and electrocardiographic signs of myocardial ischemia, and (4) neurologic signs and symptoms. The findings in shock correlate with the organs that are compromised, that is, the findings correlate with the severity of the shock. Flow to the skin is sacrificed first, then flow to the kidneys and viscera, and finally flow to the heart and brain (Table 2).

Moderately severe and severe shock are usually easy to recognize, but early or mild hypovolemic shock can pose a problem in diagnosis—the signs of adrenergic discharge to the skin can be subtle and difficult to detect. Yet recognition

---

See the corresponding chapter or part in the *Textbook of Surgery*, 14th edition, pp. 34–56, for a more detailed discussion of this topic, including a comprehensive list of references.

TABLE 1. Classification and Causes of Shock

Primary Cause of Shock	Type of Shock	Mechanisms Underlying the Primary Cause	Associated Clinical Conditions
Inadequate circulating blood volume	Hypovolemic shock	Hemorrhage (hemorrhagic shock) Loss of fluid into gut or dehydration (nonhemorrhagic hypovolemic shock)	Hemorrhage Vomiting Diarrhea Bowel obstruction
	Traumatic shock (including burn shock)	External blood or plasma loss combined with internal losses Loss of plasma into tissues and sequestration of blood in the cutaneous vasculature	Trauma Burns
	Septic shock		Systemic sepsis
Loss of autonomic control of the vasculature	Neurogenic shock	Pooling of blood in denervated venous beds and excess perfusion of relatively unessential vascular beds	Spinal cord injury Regional anesthetic

Impaired cardiac function			
	Cardiac compressive shock	Compression of great veins or cardiac chambers or both	Pericardial tamponade
			Tension pneumothorax
			Ascites
			Hemoperitoneum
			Inflation of abdominal portion of pneumatic anti-shock garment
			Diaphragmatic rupture
			Mechanical ventilation
	Cardiogenic shock	Intrinsic abnormality of the heart	Congenital abnormalities
			Arrhythmias
			Myocardial ischemia
			Valvular or septal defects
			Cardiomyopathies
			Coronary air embolism
	Cardiac obstructive shock	Obstruction of either the pulmonary or systemic circulation	Pulmonary embolism
			Mechanical ventilation
			Pulmonary vascular disease
			Engorgement of pulmonary vasculature
			Mechanical obstruction of aorta
			Systemic arteriolar constriction
			Polycythemia

TABLE 2. Characteristics of Shock States

| | Hypovolemic or Traumatic Shock | | | Early Septic Shock | Late Septic Shock | Neurogenic Shock | Cardiac Compressive Shock | Cardiogenic Shock | Cardiac Obstructive Shock |
	Mild	Moderate	Severe						
Skin perfusion	Pale	Pale	Pale	Pink	Pale	Pink*	Pale	Pale	Pale
Urine output	Normal	Low	Low	Low	Low	Low	Low	Low	Low
Blood pressure	Normal	Normal	Low	Low	Low	Low	Low	Low	Normal
Mental status	Thirsty	Restless	Obtunded	Abnormal	Abnormal	Normal†	Normal†	Normal†	Normal†
ECG	Normal	Normal	Abnormal	Normal	Normal†	Normal†	Normal†	Abnormal	Abnormal
Neck veins	Flat	Flat	Flat	Flat	Flat	Flat	Distended	Distended	Distended
Cardiac output	Low	High	Low	High	Low	Low	Low	Low	Low
Systemic vascular resistance	High	High	High	Low	High	Low	High	High	High
Mixed venous oxygen content	Low	Low	Low	High	Low	Low	Low	Low	Low
Oxygen consumption	Low	Low	Low	Low	Low	Low	Low	Low	Low

*In denervated areas.
†Will be abnormal if shock is severe.
‡In relation to oxygen needs.

of early or mild shock can be critical, not because mild shock in itself threatens the patient, but because the pathologic process that is causing the mild shock now might go on to produce severe shock later. For help in the detection of mild or progressing hypovolemic shock, the urinary output should be monitored, and serial hematocrits should be measured. In addition, in selected patients, postural changes in blood pressure should be elicited.

Assessment of urinary output is almost as sensitive as detection of the signs of cutaneous adrenergic discharge in diagnosing early and progressing hypovolemic shock. A Foley catheter should be placed for monitoring purposes in any patient who manifests mild shock and whose future status is uncertain. Such a catheter can be placed safely in all patients, except in those with a torn urethra and those with pathologic lesions in the urethra or bladder. A fall in the hematocrit with intravenous administration of asanguineous fluid is another easily interpretable sign of hypovolemia. The initial hematocrit obtained immediately after hemorrhage is normal, and the hematocrit in a patient with a bowel obstruction or major burn might even be high. Asanguineous fluid resuscitation that restores peripheral perfusion, urinary output, and blood pressure, however, decreases the hematocrit. Generally, in an adult patient, a fall in the hematocrit of three or four points with fluid resuscitation indicates that the patient's blood volume before resuscitation was depleted by 500 ml. Failure of the hematocrit to reach equilibration implies continuing volume loss. Postural changes in blood pressure, if they can be obtained, are a simple and sensitive indicator of early shock. A fall in the systolic pressure of 10 mm. Hg that persists for more than 30 seconds suggests hypovolemia.

Contrary to tradition and to experiments in anesthetized animals, the pulse rate does not consistently increase in response to graded volume loss. Hypovolemic patients frequently have heart rates within the normal range, and severely hypovolemic patients can even develop a bradycardia as a preterminal event. A rapid heart rate can be assumed to be an indicator of possible hypovolemia; a normal or slow heart rate indicates very little or, on occasion, might even reflect myocardial ischemia and impending cardiac arrest.

Signs of adrenergic discharge to the skin and oliguria are not reliable indicators of hypovolemia in the inebriated patient. High blood alcohol levels induce a generalized vasodilation that can override the effects of discharge of the adrenergic nervous system. Alcohol also inhibits the secretion of vasopressin from the pituitary so that hypovolemic patients may still have adequate urinary outputs. The generalized vasodilation of alcohol intoxication, however, causes systemic arterial hypotension, even in mild to moderate shock. Hypotension in the noninebriated patient is a late sign of hypovolemia, whereas in the inebriated patient it can be an early sign.

Blood flow to both the heart and the brain is decreased in severe shock. Hypovolemia should be excluded with absolute certainty in any patient who presents with cerebral symptoms after any injury, even if the patient has an obvious head injury. Correction of hypovolemia sometimes completely corrects all abnormalities in mental status. As a corollary, cardiovascular instability should never be ascribed to a head injury.

Hypoglycemic shock may present with signs and symptoms similar to those of hypovolemic shock. Any patient in shock who is suspected of being an insulin-dependent diabetic should have the blood glucose measured by a Dextrostix and should be given an infusion of 25 gm. of glucose for treatment of the possibility of hypoglycemia. Although the patient may have been in an accident, the accident may have been caused by the lethargy of a hypoglycemic reaction.

TREATMENT

Initial Resuscitation and Venous Access. The principles of treatment for hemorrhagic and nonhemorrhagic forms of hypovolemic shock are similar. Resuscitation should begin with ensuring adequate ventilation and oxygenation. If the patient is unconscious, lowering the head with support of the jaw for prevention of airway obstruction and administering supplemental oxygen may be all that are needed. In those patients with obtundation or airway obstruction, the trachea should be intubated and mechanical ventilation initiated.

Hypovolemic shock caused by hemorrhage is best treated by prompt identification of the source followed by immediate control of bleeding. External hemorrhage should be tamponaded by compression; internal hemorrhage caused by trauma should be surgically exposed and controlled; that from the gastrointestinal tract should have the source identified and specific treatment initiated. Intravenous fluid should be administered simultaneously or as preparations are being made to control bleeding. If the patient's only sign of hypovolemia is cutaneous vasoconstriction, percutaneously placed venous cannulas in the upper extremities should be used initially. If the hypovolemia is severe, to the point that urinary output is diminished, two or three large-bore intravenous catheters should be inserted. The best large-bore catheters are a cutoff length of intravenous tubing or a large-bore (12-gauge or larger) catheter, ideally placed into a surgically exposed saphenous vein at the ankle.

Crystalloid Infusion. A nonsugar, nonprotein crystalloid solution with an electrolyte composition approximating that of plasma is preferable in the initial resuscitation of patients with all forms of shock, except cardiogenic shock, assuming that large-bore vascular access has been obtained and that large volumes of fluid can be administered rapidly. The authors prefer lactated Ringer's, but the solution can be acetated Ringer's or normal saline supplemented with administration of an ampule of sodium bicarbonate for each liter of fluid. The lactated Ringer's or other crystalloid solution should not be given in glucose solution unless the patient is thought to be in hypoglycemic shock from an insulin reaction. Rapid administration of glucose, even as a 5 per cent solution, can induce an osmotic diuresis. Administration of fluid not only helps in resuscitating patients in hemorrhagic shock but also serves as a diagnostic test for detecting continuing bleeding. Two to three liters of fluid given over 5 to 15 minutes resuscitate any patient with arrested hemorrhage. The need for administration of more fluid indicates continuing bleeding. Such hemorrhage usually requires surgical control.

Blood Administration. If the patient can be operated on promptly, it is best to withhold administration of blood until surgical control of the bleeding is obtained or at least until just before induction of anesthesia. A young patient with a normal heart can tolerate hematocrit values as low as 15 per cent even when the anemia is induced rapidly, as long as the blood volume is kept normal by administering adequate volumes of asanguineous solutions. At times, however, blood has to be administered before surgical control of hemorrhage is obtained (see Chapter 6, Blood Transfusions and Disorders of Surgical Bleeding). Type-specific blood, which can be obtained within 10 minutes from most blood banks, should be given if crossmatched units are not available. If type-specific blood is not available, O-negative blood can be transfused.

The amount of blood given depends on the presumed status of the patient's coronary arteries and on the circumstances that indicate the need for transfusion. Hematocrit values of 20 per cent after resuscitation are usually adequate if control of hemorrhage is assured, but the generally accepted desired hematocrit is 25 per cent. Lower levels might be dangerous if the patient unexpectedly starts to bleed again. Patients with coronary artery disease should be transfused to a hematocrit of approximately 30 to 35 per cent, since their hearts do not have the reserve to tolerate even transient episodes of ischemia.

Nonhemorrhagic hypovolemic shock is treated with the same goals in mind as those used for hemorrhagic shock except that blood is not necessary. In shock caused by loss of fluid into the gut lumen, asanguineous fluids should be given to establish a normal urinary output and to bring the hematocrit down into the mid-30 per cent range. The fluid used for replenishment of the vascular volume should have an electrolyte composition similar to that which was lost.

TRAUMATIC SHOCK

DIAGNOSIS. Traumatic shock, including shock caused by burns, is caused by both internal and external volume losses—from loss of blood or plasma externally, from the wound or burn surface, and from loss of blood or plasma into the damaged tissues. These volume losses are worsened by plasma extravasation into tissues and organs distal from the injured areas. This extravasation arises from a generalized systemic intravascular inflammatory response, which is generated by the release of inflammatory mediators from the damaged tissues when they are reperfused during resuscitation. Resuscitation from traumatic shock is associated with remote organ failure syndromes, whereas pure hemorrhagic shock is not.

The major consequences of traumatic shock are not manifested fully until 24 to 48 hours following the initial injury as the inflammation-mediated vascular permeability develops gradually over many hours. Initially right-sided venous pressure provides a guide to the adequacy of volume therapy. As the pulmonary microvasculature becomes occluded with particulate matter generated by intravascular coagulation, however, and as the vasculature constricts in response to vasoactive inflammatory mediators from white cells and platelets, the right ventricle can fail. Left-sided and right-sided filling pressures can diverge, and measurement of left-sided pressures with a Swan-Ganz catheter can become essential for guiding fluid administration.

TREATMENT. The primary treatment of traumatic shock is immediate correction of hypovolemia and prompt débridement of ischemic or devitalized tissue and immobilization of fractures to prevent further tissue damage. If the respiratory rate exceeds 30 to 35 per minute or if the P_{O_2} cannot be maintained above 70 mm. Hg, intubation and ventilatory support are indicated. The urinary output should be maintained between 0.5 and 1.0 ml. $\cdot$ kg.$^{-1}$ $\cdot$ hr.$^{-1}$ Urinary output below this indicates circulatory inadequacy and the need for more volume. If fluid requirements appear excessive, a Swan-Ganz catheter should be placed to determine left-sided filling pressures. If low, the pulmonary artery wedge pressure should be raised gradually by balanced salt crystalloid infusion to 12 to 15 mm. Hg and the effect on cardiac output and urinary output determined. The lowest wedge pressure consistent with a hyperdynamic cardiac output and an adequate urine volume should be used. An additional 5 to 10 mm. Hg filling pressure on a rare occasion may be necessary if the patient requires high positive end-expiratory pressures (150 mm. H_2O or above).

SEPTIC SHOCK

DIAGNOSIS. The initial clinical manifestations of sepsis are those that arise from the development of a hypermetabolic state (Table 2). Heat production increases, and heat loss is accomplished by the diversion of blood flow to the skin through the opening of cutaneous arteriovenous shunts. The capacitance of the cutaneous vascular bed expands so that unless fluid volume is provided simultaneously, other areas of the body become deprived of blood flow. As systemic sepsis develops, an intravascular inflammatory process is activated similar to that observed in traumatic shock, causing a vigorous reaction within the vascular system with damage to the endothelial cells. The end result is a diffuse increase in microvascular permeability.

The first cardiovascular manifestation of systemic sepsis is usually an increased fluid requirement for maintenance of urinary output and peripheral perfusion. At this stage, two factors—hypovolemia and increased metabolism—work in opposition to one another. Sepsis-induced hypermetabolism causes a fever, which activates the hypothalamic temperature control center. Cutaneous arteriovenous shunts open to dissipate heat externally. The cutaneous vasodilation, however, causes pooling of blood in the cutaneous venous capacitance bed. Perfusion of vital organs becomes compromised. This stage constitutes early septic shock or "red shock."

Eventually, hypoperfusion of vital organs activates cutaneous pressor mechanisms, diverting blood away from the less essential skin and subcutaneous tissue and transiently restoring vital organ perfusion. Decreased skin perfusion causes a fall in skin temperature and a cold sensation perceived by the patient, which progresses to shaking chills. The cutaneous vasoconstriction compromises the body's ability to dissipate heat and initiates another rapid rise in body temperature. The increased temperature once again activates the hypothalamic temperature control center, which reinitiates a cycle of cutaneous vasodilation, hypotension, and splanchnic and renal hypoperfusion.

TREATMENT. Septic shock is best treated by prevention, with the early recognition of sepsis and definitive treatment of the infection. This prevention requires identifying the source of infection, administering specific antibiotics, and instituting surgical drainage if possible. Circulatory resuscitation must be prompt, and large volumes of fluid may be required to correct the hypovolemia that is responsible for the shock. In almost all instances a Swan-Ganz catheter should be passed to facilitate the prompt optimization of the circulation without overinfusion of fluids. Fluid administration should begin with 2 liters of a balanced salt solution, which can be administered over 10 to 15 minutes to most adult patients with safety, but as much as 10 to 15 liters of fluid may be required in the first 24 hours of resuscitation. If the circulation does not respond to the first few boluses of fluid, a Starling curve of cardiac function should be obtained by determining the optimal filling pressures that generate an adequate cardiac output. Because of the presence of wide open skin shunts, adequate organ flow requires cardiac outputs far in excess of normal. The patient's pulmonary function should be monitored because the increases in permeability generated by severe sepsis cause pulmonary dysfunction. Almost all patients in septic shock require endotracheal intubation and mechanical ventilation so that adequate arterial oxygenation is ensured. Cultures of all suspicious sources should be obtained immediately. Unless the organism has been previously identified, broad-spectrum antibiotics should be administered. Most commonly the bacteria responsible for septic shock are gram-negative, and therapy should be directed to include the spectrum of enteric organisms.

NEUROGENIC SHOCK

DIAGNOSIS. Diagnosis of neurogenic shock is usually based on the neurologic examination or on the knowledge that the patient has had a regional anesthetic or has received an autonomic blocker. The degree of shock directly relates to the level and duration of the denervation. The shock pattern resembles that seen in patients with warm septic shock (Table 2).

TREATMENT. Filling of the heart should be corrected by administering a balanced salt solution in a volume of several liters (in an adult). If the blood pressure does not respond promptly, a vasoconstrictor should be given to restore venous tone. Vasoconstrictor-induced constriction of the systemic arterioles also increases arterial blood pressure, but this effect is less important than the effect on the venous capacitance bed and on cardiac filling. Elevation of the legs is effective in the initial treatment of patients in neurogenic shock while fluid therapy is being initiated. Body temperature should be monitored and excessive heat loss prevented by appropriate cover.

CARDIAC COMPRESSIVE SHOCK

DIAGNOSIS. The key to the diagnosis of cardiac compressive shock in acutely injured patients is observing distended neck veins or an elevated central venous pressure in a patient who presents with a history and findings that are otherwise consistent with hypovolemic or traumatic shock (Table 2). The absence of distended neck veins, however, does not exclude cardiac compressive shock in the hypovolemic injured patient. Distention of the neck veins may become evident only after the patient's blood volume is replenished.

The conditions that produce cardiac compressive shock have distinctive clinical characteristics (see Table 1). These include positive-pressure ventilation with large tidal volumes causing compressive shock in hypovolemic patients (1) by compressing the cavae, right atrium, and right ventricle to limit right ventricular filling, (2) by compressing the pulmonary microvasculature between inflated alveoli to hinder right ventricular emptying, and (3) by compressing the large pulmonary veins, left atrium, and left ventricle to limit left ventricular filling. Definitive diagnosis usually requires measurements from a Swan-Ganz catheter, which document a low cardiac output with modestly elevated right atrial and pulmonary artery wedge pressures. The right atrial and wedge pressures are usually within a few millimeters Hg of each other. Cardiac compression can be assumed to be present in patients without a Swan-Ganz catheter if they are oliguric and if they are receiving tidal volumes in excess of 12 ml. per kg. or positive end-expiratory pressure greater than 100 mm. H_2O, assuming that other causes of shock and oliguria have been excluded.

TREATMENT. Treatment of cardiac compressive shock consists of fluid administration to increase ventricular filling pressures and correction of the underlying mechanical cause of the shock. Treatment of cardiac compression caused by mechanical ventilation usually requires volume expansion combined with adjustment of the ventilator. In the acute situation, when Swan-Ganz catheterization is not available, the tidal volumes should be kept small (10 ml. per kg.), the inspiratory to expiratory ratios short (I:E ratios of 1:3), and end-expiratory pressures zero. High inspiratory oxygen con-

centrations are usually necessary to ensure adequate oxygenation.

CARDIOGENIC SHOCK

DIAGNOSIS. Patients with cardiogenic shock on the basis of either right or left ventricular dysfunction present with the clinical findings associated with discharge of the adrenergic nervous system and with release of angiotensin and vasopressin (Table 2). In shock caused by right ventricular dysfunction, the neck veins are distended. In shock caused by left ventricular dysfunction, the patient has rales and a third heart sound or gallop rhythm. If the dysfunction is chronic or severe, the heart may be enlarged, and signs of right ventricular dysfunction, such as distended neck veins, may be present as well.

TREATMENT

Optimization of Heart Rate. The initial treatment of cardiogenic shock begins with administration of oxygen by nasal prongs or mask. Treatment beyond that depends on the cause of myocardial failure but can usually be approached sequentially by (1) correcting arrhythmias and optimizing the heart rate, (2) optimizing ventricular end-diastolic volumes, (3) providing adequate peripheral vasodilation, (4) maximizing myocardial contractility, (5) preserving marginal myocardium with the use of beta-blocking agents, (6) assuring adequate perfusion of the coronary vasculature with the use of vasoconstrictors, (7) providing mechanical assistance to the heart, and (8) surgical correction of cardiac lesions.

The optimal heart rate varies with age and with the status of the coronary arteries. A patient with normal coronary arteries can mount a pulse rate equal to the difference of 220 and age in years multiplied by three fourths. In the presence of coronary disease, the rate should not exceed this number minus 30. The definitive test for determining if a heart rate is excessively rapid is to observe the patient for signs of myocardial ischemia, the heart being the first organ to show the ill effects of an inappropriately rapid rate. Anginal chest pain and electrocardiographic signs of ischemia are the most sensitive indicators.

Life-threatening bradycardias in unstable patients should be cardioverted. More stable patients with a bradyarrhythmia can be treated with a chronotropic agent. Atropine is the drug of first choice. External pacing, followed if necessary by transvenous pacing, is the second choice if atropine fails.

With the exception of asystole, all tachyarrhythmias that create hemodynamic instability should be cardioverted. In the case of asystole, the patient should be treated first with epinephrine and atropine for the production of ventricular fibrillation, which should then be cardioverted. If the patient with a tachyarrhythmia is relatively stable, a full 12-lead electrocardiogram should be obtained. If the QRS complex is longer than 0.08 seconds, the patient should be cardioverted. If the complex is shorter than 0.08 seconds, the electrocardiogram should be searched for P waves. If no P waves are

apparent and the QRS complexes are irregular, verapamil should be given to slow the ventricular rate. If P waves are present, the carotid bulb should be compressed. In response to the compression, the ventricular rate slows, reverts, or remains unchanged. If compression reverts or has no influence on the arrhythmia, verapamil should be given; if the rate slows, the patient has a sinus tachycardia—treatment should be directed toward the underlying cause.

Adjustment of Ventricular End-Diastolic Volumes. Optimization of ventricular end-diastolic volumes, by either augmentation or diminution, is next considered. If the patient is thought to be hypovolemic, a fluid bolus of 250 ml. should be given over a period of 10 minutes to see if the cardiac status improves with augmentation of end-diastolic volumes. If the patient's condition worsens with the bolus or if, at initial evaluation, the patient is thought to be hypervolemic, a single intravenous dose of furosemide, 40 mg., should be given. A prompt diuresis with resolution of shock supports the diagnosis of cardiac failure and volume overload. Minimal or no response should prompt reconsideration of the diagnosis. The decision to use volume expansion or reduction is simplified if a Swan-Ganz catheter is in place. The goal is to produce the highest cardiac output with the lowest filling pressures. The pitfalls of measuring atrial pressures with the Swan-Ganz catheter should also be borne in mind.

Vasodilators. Vasodilators have several attractive features and very few drawbacks if they are used carefully. They can decrease the systemic and pulmonary vascular resistances and ease ventricular emptying. Nitroglycerin and, to a lesser extent, nitroprusside dilate the systemic venules and small veins and thus decrease filling of the right heart, pulmonary vasculature, and left heart. Decreased right atrial and coronary sinus pressures and reduced tension in the ventricular wall increase coronary blood flow as well. Myocardial oxygen demands decrease.

Inotropic Agents. Inotropic agents are next to be considered but have to be used with caution. Dopamine and dobutamine, the two most useful inotropes, both increase myocardial oxygen needs (Table 3) and can produce excessive vasoconstriction and ischemia in the extremities. In most surgical patients, the goal of any therapeutic intervention on the cardiovascular system should be to increase cardiac index to a slightly hyperdynamic state (5.0 liters $\cdot$ min.$^{-1}$ $\cdot$ m.$^{-2}$ for young patients and 3.5 liters $\cdot$ min.$^{-1}$ $\cdot$ m.$^{-2}$ for old patients) while maintaining pulmonary artery wedge pressures at low levels (7 mm. Hg for patients breathing spontaneously and 12 mm. Hg for those on positive-pressure ventilation). Effects on systemic arterial blood pressure and urinary output are usually secondary. Dopamine and dobutamine should be used to increase flow in the cardiovascular system; they should not be used as vasoconstrictors or as diuretics.

Beta-Blocking Agents. An occasional patient in cardiogenic shock with an ischemic myocardium and a rapid heart rate benefits from administration of a beta-blocker, such as propranolol, although such agents usually decrease the cardiac output. Decreasing myocardial contractility, decreasing the

TABLE 3. Effects of Same Therapeutic Interventions on Circulatory Derangements in Cardiogenic Shock

Intervention	Cardiac Output	Atrial Pressures	Myocardial Oxygen Needs
Trendelenburg's position	↓ ↑	↑	↑
Correction of bradycardia	↑	↓	↑
Correction of tachyarrhythmia	↑	↓	↓
Administration of fluid	↑ ↑	↑	↑
Administration of diuretic	↓ ↑	↓	↓
Administration of vasodilator	↑	↓	↓
Administration of inotrope	↑	↓	↑
Administration of beta-blocker	↓	↓ ↑	↓
Administration of vasoconstrictor	↓ ↑	↑	↑
Use of intra-aortic balloon pump	↑	↓	↓

heart rate, and dilating the peripheral vasculature all decrease myocardial oxygen requirements, as do smaller stroke volumes and diminished stroke work (Table 3). This state of myocardial hibernation can be beneficial for a patient with a recent myocardial infarction and surrounding marginal tissue.

Vasoconstrictors. Vasoconstrictors including norepinephrine, phenylephrine, and metaraminol are sometimes of value in treating patients with cardiogenic shock by increasing aortic diastolic blood pressure and perfusion of the coronary circulation. They may also increase myocardial contractility. The beneficial effects of increased coronary artery pressure and increased contractility, however, are frequently offset by increased myocardial work. On balance, vasoconstrictors usually do more harm than good (Table 3).

Intra-aortic Balloon Pump. Mechanical circulatory assistance with an intra-aortic balloon pump can be of substantial value in selected patients with severe left ventricular dysfunction. It can be highly effective in treating cardiogenic shock and is usually preferable to long-term use of inotropic agents and generally preferable to vasoconstrictors (Table 3). It should be used only in patients with Swan-Ganz catheters in place.

Reconstructive Surgery. Although last in this discussion of shock treatment, reconstructive surgery should be an early option for some patients in cardiogenic shock. It can be particularly effective in selected cases of coronary insufficiency, ventricular septal rupture, papillary muscle rupture, and mitral valve dysfunction (see Chapter 57, The Heart).

CARDIAC OBSTRUCTIVE SHOCK

DIAGNOSIS AND TREATMENT. The conditions that produce cardiac obstructive shock usually affect one ventricle more than the other, and the diagnosis frequently arises from the findings of single ventricle dysfunction combined with the clinical characteristics of the condition causing the dysfunction. Treatment of cardiac obstructive shock should be directed to the cause of shock. Anticoagulation with large-dose heparin can sometimes dramatically reverse obstruction to right ventricular output. Adjustment of the ventilator along with fluid administration usually overcomes the ill effects of mechanical ventilation on a compromised right heart. Treatment of pulmonary vascular disease may require surgical correction of a congenital defect or medical treatment of a superimposed pulmonary infection. Engorgement of the pulmonary vasculature from left-sided failure usually responds well to diuresis. Vasodilators can sometimes reverse the failure produced by an aortic cross-clamp. Vasodilators generally reverse the failure of extreme arteriolar constriction unless the heart has become irretrievably damaged by long-standing hypertension. Polycythemia is effectively treated by phlebotomy.

4

FLUID AND ELECTROLYTE MANAGEMENT OF THE SURGICAL PATIENT

Peter C. Canizaro, M.D.

BODY FLUID COMPARTMENTS

Water constitutes between 50 and 70 per cent of total body weight; the average normal value for young adult males is 60 per cent, and for young adult females 50 per cent. The actual figure for a healthy individual is remarkably constant and is a function of several variables, including lean body mass (lower percentage with obesity) and age (percentage decreases with age).

Intracellular fluid (ICF) represents approximately 40 per cent of body weight with the largest proportion in the skeletal muscle mass; potassium and magnesium are the principal cations, and phosphates and proteins the major anions. The extracellular fluid (ECF) represents approximately 20 per cent of body weight and has two major subdivisions: plasma volume (5 per cent of body weight) and the interstitial or extravascular, extracellular fluid volume (15 per cent of body weight). Sodium is the predominant cation, and chloride and bicarbonate the major anions.

The differences in ionic composition between the ICF and the ECF are maintained by the cell membrane, a semipermeable barrier that is freely permeable only to water. The *effective* osmotic pressure is generated by those substances that fail to pass freely through the cell membrane (i.e., the electrolytes). Any condition that alters the effective osmotic pressure (changes the concentration of electrolytes or any nondiffusible substance such as glucose) causes redistribution of water between the two compartments until equilibrium is regained. Loss of ECF alone, not accompanied by changes in the concentration of nondiffusible substances, does not cause transfer of free water from the ICF. Thus, isotonic losses of ECF are not generally shared by the ICF, and for practical consideration, most losses and gains of body fluid are directly from the ECF compartment.

Effective osmotic pressure between the plasma and interstitial compartments of the ECF (designated the *colloid osmotic pressure*) is due primarily to plasma proteins, since they do not diffuse freely across the capillary membrane.

See the corresponding chapter or part in the *Textbook of Surgery*, 14th edition, pp. 57–76, for a more detailed discussion of this topic, including a comprehensive list of references.

CLASSIFICATION OF BODY FLUID CHANGES

The disorders in fluid balance may be classified in three general categories: disturbances of (1) volume, (2) concentration, and (3) composition. Of importance is the concept that although these disturbances are interrelated in clinical settings, each is best considered as a separate entity.

If an isotonic salt solution is added to or lost from the body, only the *volume* of the ECF changes. For example, loss of intestinal fluid causes a decrease in ECF volume but little or no change in the ICF. Fluid is not transferred from cells to refill the depleted ECF as long as osmolality remains the same in the two compartments.

An internal loss of ECF, such as sequestration of fluid in a burn wound, peritonitis, ascites, or muscle trauma, is termed a *distributional* change. This transfer or functional loss of ECF internally may be into the ECF interstitium (e.g., peritonitis) or intracellular (e.g., hemorrhagic shock). In any event, the distributional shift causes a contraction of the *functional* ECF space.

If the *concentration* of osmotically active particles changes in one compartment (e.g., if water alone is added to or lost from the ECF), an appropriate transfer of water between the two spaces does occur until equilibrium is restored. Such changes in concentration (or osmolality) are reflected by changes in the level of serum sodium; even though this ion is largely confined to the ECF space, its level reflects total body fluid osmolality. Concentration disturbances of most other ions within the ECF compartment (e.g., K^+, Ca^{++}, Mg^{++}) are referred to as *compositional* changes (for want of a better term).

Volume Changes

An ECF excess or deficit must be diagnosed by clinical examination because direct measurement of this space is not feasible clinically. There are several laboratory tests, however, that indirectly reflect changes in ECF volume. The blood urea nitrogen rises with an ECF deficit of sufficient magnitude to reduce glomerular filtration. The serum creatinine may not increase proportionally in young individuals with healthy kidneys, and this discrepancy is often used as one test to differentiate prerenal and renal azotemia; more important, the rise in serum creatinine often parallels the increase of blood urea nitrogen in elderly patients and those with chronic renal disease. The concentrations of formed elements in the blood (erythrocytes, leukocytes, platelets, plasma proteins) increase with ECF deficit and decrease with ECF excess. The concentration of serum sodium, however, is not related to the volume status of the ECF: a severe ECF deficit may exist with a normal, low, or high sodium level.

VOLUME DEFICIT. Extracellular fluid volume deficit is by far the most common fluid disorder in surgical patients; it often occurs without a significant change in concentration (i.e., serum sodium normal). Common causes include (1) external losses of gastrointestinal fluids due to vomiting, nasogastric suction, diarrhea, and intestinal fistulas; and (2) internal losses (sequestrations) due to soft tissue injuries and infections, intra-abdominal and retroperitoneal inflammatory processes, burns, and intestinal obstruction.

Central nervous system (CNS) signs are similar to barbiturate intoxication and may be overlooked by the casual observer if the volume deficit is mild. Cardiovascular signs are secondary to the decrease in plasma volume, and hypotension may occur if it is severe. Assessment of skin turgor may be difficult in elderly patients or in patients with recent weight loss, and skin turgor is not diagnostic in the absence of other confirmatory signs. Severe volume depletion depresses all body systems (in addition to the CNS) and may interfere with clinical evaluation of a patient. For example, a volume-depleted patient with severe sepsis from peritonitis may have a normal temperature and white blood cell count, complain of little pain, and have unimpressive findings on abdominal examination. The clinical presentation changes dramatically, however, as the ECF volume is restored. Oliguria is secondary to renal hypoperfusion (prerenal azotemia) and occasionally may be difficult to distinguish from oliguria caused by intrinsic renal disease (renal azotemia). The diagnostic urinary tests are useful, but some may be misleading in elderly patients because of the diminished ability to concentrate urine generally associated with aging; many, however, retain the ability to conserve sodium. In this group, the *renal failure index* and the *fractional excretion of filtered sodium* are the most accurate tests.

Exact quantification of ECF deficits is not possible, but they can be estimated on the basis of the severity of clinical signs. A mild deficit represents a loss of approximately 4 per cent of body weight (e.g., 70 kg. $\times$ 0.04 = 2.8 liter deficit), a moderate loss 6 to 8 per cent, and a severe deficit 10 per cent or greater. Fluid replacement should be initiated and changes made according to the clinical response of the patient. Reliance on a formula or single clinical sign for determining the adequacy of resuscitation is unwise. Rather, reversal of the signs and symptoms of the volume deficit combined with stabilization of blood pressure and pulse and an hourly urine volume of 30 to 50 ml. are used as general guidelines. The type of fluid for replacement depends on the presence of concomitant concentration or compositional abnormalities. A balanced salt solution is used for a pure ECF volume loss or when there is only minimal concentration or compositional abnormalities. In a patient who also has mild hyponatremia, hypochloremia, and metabolic alkalosis, however, normal saline would be more appropriate. The rate of fluid administration depends on factors such as the severity and type of fluid disturbance, the presence of continuing losses, the cardiac status, and the urgency of a needed operative procedure. The most severe deficits may be safely replaced initially at a rate of 500 to 1000 ml. per hour, reducing the rate as the fluid status improves. Constant observation is mandatory when fluids are given at this high rate. Associated cardiovascular disorders do not preclude replacement of existing volume deficits; they require slower, more careful correction and appropriate monitoring, including the central venous pressure or pulmonary artery wedge pressure.

VOLUME EXCESS. Extracellular fluid volume excess is generally iatrogenic or secondary to renal insufficiency. Both the plasma and the interstitial fluid volumes are increased. The signs are generally those of circulatory overload and excessive tissue fluid. In elderly patients, congestive heart failure with pulmonary edema may develop quickly with only a moderate volume excess.

Concentration Changes

Hypo- and hypernatremia can be diagnosed by clinical manifestations, but discernible signs and symptoms are not usually present until the changes in osmolality are severe. Therefore, the cause of an abnormal sodium concentration should be determined early and corrected promptly. More important, knowledge of the blood glucose concentration is necessary to evaluate the significance of an altered sodium level. Since glucose does not enter cells by passive diffusion, it exerts an osmotic force in the ECF compartment. With an elevated glucose level, increased osmotic pressure causes transfer of cell water into the ECF, causing dilutional hyponatremia. Hyponatremia, therefore, may be observed when the effective osmotic pressure of the ECF is normal or even above normal. For clinical purposes, the effect of an elevated glucose on serum sodium can be estimated by the following: the serum sodium falls approximately 2 mEq. per liter for each 100 mg. per 100 ml. rise of serum glucose above normal. A rise in blood urea nitrogen concentration has similar effects; the serum sodium falls 2 mEq. per liter for each 30 mg. per 100 ml. rise in blood urea nitrogen.

HYPONATREMIA. Acute *symptomatic* hyponatremia is characterized by CNS signs of increased intracranial pressure (usually seizures) and tissue signs of excessive intracellular water. There are no cardiovascular signs *per se*; the accompanying hypertension is induced by the rise in intracranial pressure and returns to normal after correction of the sodium level. Of importance with severe hyponatremia is the relatively rapid development of oliguric renal failure if therapy is delayed. Many hyponatremic states are asymptomatic until the serum sodium level falls well below 120 mEq. per liter. An important exception is the patient with increased cerebrospinal fluid pressure (e.g., closed head injury) in whom mild hyponatremia may be deleterious, even fatal. This is due to the progressive increase in cell water (further increasing intracranial pressure) as ECF osmolality falls.

Correction involves considerations of both the severity of hyponatremia and status of the ECF volume. (Whereas ECF volume changes occur frequently without changes in concentration, the reverse is not true; disease states that cause alterations in osmolality often produce changes in ECF volume.) If severe, symptomatic hyponatremia complicates an

ECF volume loss, prompt correction of the concentration abnormality to the extent that symptoms are relieved is first necessary. Volume replacement can then be accomplished with slower correction of the remaining concentration abnormality. Initial correction of severe symptomatic hyponatremia usually requires use of a 5 per cent sodium chloride solution. The sodium deficit is estimated by multiplying the decrease in serum sodium concentration below normal (in mEq. per liter) times liters of total body water. The estimate is based on total body water, since ECF osmolality cannot be increased without increasing osmolality proportionally in the ICF. Generally, only a portion of the total deficit is replaced initially for relief of acute symptoms; further correction is facilitated when renal function is restored by correction of any associated volume deficit. Of importance, central pontine and extrapontine myelinolysis may occur during rapid correction of hyponatremia and cause irreversible CNS damage or death. It is recommended, therefore, that serum sodium not be increased more than 12 mEq. per liter during the first 24 hours and even less during each subsequent 24-hour period. In practice, the infusion of small, successive increments of hypertonic saline solution with frequent evaluations of the clinical response and sodium concentration is recommended. For treatment of moderate hyponatremia (asymptomatic) with an associated ECF volume deficit, volume replacement can be initiated immediately with concomitant correction of the sodium deficit. Normal saline is usually appropriate for this purpose, but only a few liters may be necessary for correction of sodium concentration; the remainder of the volume deficit can then be replaced with a balanced salt solution.

Treatment of moderate hyponatremia associated with ECF volume *excess* is accomplished by fluid restriction. If hyponatremia is symptomatic, a small amount of hypertonic salt solution may be infused cautiously for alleviation of symptoms. This causes additional ECF volume expansion and is contraindicated in patients with limited cardiac reserve; peritoneal dialysis or hemodialysis is preferred in this situation.

HYPERNATREMIA. Hypernatremia, although uncommon, is a dangerous abnormality and is easily produced when renal function is normal. In surgical patients, it arises most often from excessive or unexpected hypotonic volume losses, including evaporative water losses from large burn wounds, diabetes insipidus following head injury, use of osmotic diuretics, uncontrolled hyperglycemia during total parenteral nutrition, and high-output renal failure.

CNS signs of restlessness progressing to delirium, dry mucous membranes, flushed skin, oliguria, and high fever characterize symptomatic hypernatremia. A profound ECF volume deficit is often present.

Management consists of correction of hypernatremia concomitant with repletion of the volume deficit using half-strength sodium chloride or half-strength balanced salt solution. ECF osmolality should not be reduced too rapidly, however, since convulsions and coma may result. The problem is somewhat simplified when a sufficient quantity of fluid has been given to permit renal excretion of the solute load.

Compositional Changes

Compositional abnormalities of importance include changes in acid-base balance and concentration changes in potassium, calcium, and magnesium.

ACID-BASE BALANCE. For maintenance of pH between 7.38 and 7.42, the body neutralizes and eliminates impressive quantities of both volatile acids (from cellular combustion of carbohydrates and fats) and nonvolatile acids (a product of protein metabolism). The acids are buffered immediately following production, which prevents sudden changes in pH. The principal buffer systems of the body are proteins and phosphates in the ICF, the bicarbonate–carbonic acid system in the ECF, and hemoglobin in the red blood cells. The buffering effect is the result of the formation of an amount of weak acid or base equivalent to the amount of strong acid or base added to the system. The resultant change in pH is considerably less than if the substance were added to water alone.

In clinical practice, the bicarbonate–carbonic acid system is the one chosen for analysis because of the ease with which its component parts can be measured. After a reasonable equilibration time, changes in this system accurately reflect changes in other body buffers. Their function is expressed in the Henderson-Hasselbalch equation, which defines the pH in terms of the ratio of the salt and acid.

The diagnosis of most acid-base disorders can be made with a minimum of laboratory data, including pH, P_{CO_2}, bicarbonate concentration, urine chloride, and the calculated anion gap. For an accurate diagnosis, however, these laboratory values *must be correlated with the clinical situation*. The respiratory component of the disorder can be determined with certainty by measuring the arterial P_{CO_2}; a value below 40 mm. Hg indicates excessive pulmonary ventilation, and a value above 40 mm. Hg indicates hypoventilation. Whether a change in ventilation represents a primary disorder (respiratory acidosis or alkalosis) or compensation for a primary metabolic problem (metabolic acidosis or alkalosis) is a matter of clinical judgment. The metabolic component is evaluated by measuring the "CO_2 content" or "CO_2-combining power." A change in bicarbonate concentration may reflect a primary metabolic disorder or a compensatory change for a respiratory-induced disorder. Again, the differentiation can be made only by matching the data to the clinical situation. Use of the calculated "standard bicarbonate" and the "delta base" adds little to the diagnosis.

In general, treatment of an acid-base disorder is directed toward correction of the cause, not the pH. Treatment of the pH itself with an acid or alkaline solution is rarely indicated; at best, such measures offer only temporary control.

Respiratory Acidosis. The underlying cause of respiratory-induced disorders is usually apparent from the history and physical examination. A number of conditions causing inadequate ventilation, including airway obstruction, pulmonary disease (e.g., pneumonia and chronic obstructive pulmonary disease), CNS injury or disease causing respiratory depression, and various thoracic injuries, may exist singly or in combination to produce respiratory acidosis. A not infrequent problem in the postoperative period is restlessness, hypertension, and tachycardia; this may be due to pain but may also reflect inadequate ventilation and hypercarbia, which may be compounded by the mistaken use of narcotics for control of the restlessness. Management involves prompt correction of the pulmonary defect, when feasible, and measures to ensure adequate ventilation. This is particularly important in trauma patients with closed head injury or hypoxic brain damage; acute hypercarbia aggravates existing cerebral edema owing to cerebral vasodilation and increased cerebral blood flow.

Respiratory Alkalosis. Hyperventilation due to apprehension, pain, hypoxia, CNS injury, and assisted ventilation are common causes of respiratory alkalosis. Any of these conditions may cause rapid depression of arterial P_{CO_2} and elevation of pH.

The dangers of a severe respiratory alkalosis are related to potassium depletion (entry of potassium ions into cells in exchange for hydrogen, and excessive urinary potassium loss in exchange for sodium) and include the development of ventricular arrhythmias and fibrillation, particularly in patients who are digitalized or have hypokalemia. Cerebral ischemia and acidosis due to cerebral vasoconstriction may also occur and cause irreparable damage in patients with impaired cerebral blood flow from obstructive arterial disease or during performance of a carotid endarterectomy. Other complications include a shift of the oxygen dissociation curve to the left, which limits the ability of hemoglobin to unload oxygen at the tissue level, and depression of ionized calcium, which may cause tetany, convulsions, and the potentiation of cardiac arrhythmias.

Severe and persistent respiratory alkalosis is often difficult to correct and may be associated with a poor prognosis owing to the cause of hyperventilation (e.g., intracranial injury). Treatment is directed toward the cause of the disorder when possible. Additionally, proper use of mechanical ventilators and correction of any existing potassium deficits are important.

Metabolic Acidosis. Metabolic acidosis follows retention or production of acids (azotemia, diabetic ketoacidosis, lactic acidosis) or loss of bicarbonate (diarrhea, pancreatic or small bowel fistula). Pulmonary compensation for this disorder is mediated through the medullary respiratory center to increase the rate and depth of respiration, causing an approximate 1.1 mm. Hg compensatory reduction in P_{CO_2} for each 1 mEq. per liter fall in bicarbonate concentration. More definitive control is subsequently effected by the kidneys.

The causes of metabolic acidosis can be approximately divided into two groups by estimating the level of unmeasured serum anions ("the anion gap"). The normal value is

10 to 12 mEq. per liter and is calculated by subtracting the sum of serum chloride and bicarbonate from the sodium concentration. The unmeasured anions that constitute the gap are sulfate and phosphate plus lactate and other organic acid anions. If acidosis is due to loss of bicarbonate (e.g., pancreatic fistula) or gain of a chloride acid (e.g., administration of ammonium chloride), the anion gap is *normal*. Conversely, if the acidosis is due to increased production of an organic acid (e.g., lactic acid in circulatory shock) or the retention of sulfuric or phosphoric acid (e.g., renal failure), the concentration of unmeasured anions (anion gap) is *increased*.

Treatment of metabolic acidosis is always directed toward correction of the cause. One of the most common in surgical patients is acute circulatory failure with accumulation of lactic acid. Acute hemorrhagic shock causes a rapid and profound drop in pH, and attempts at correction of the acidosis by infusion of large quantities of sodium bicarbonate without restoration of flow are futile. Following the restoration of volume, lactic acid production ceases, and the remaining lactic acid is cleared rapidly. The routine use of sodium bicarbonate during resuscitation of patients in hypovolemic shock is discouraged. A mild metabolic *alkalosis* is a common finding following resuscitation, which is in part due to the alkalinizing effects of blood transfusions and other resuscitation fluids (e.g., lactated Ringer's solution).

Metabolic Alkalosis. For diagnostic and therapeutic purposes, states of metabolic alkalosis can be divided into *chloride-responsive* and *chloride-resistant types*, depending on the amount of chloride in the urine in the untreated state. States of chloride-resistant metabolic alkalosis are associated with a slightly increased ECF volume and most are secondary to adrenal disorders. The high level of steroid secretion causes maximal tubular resorption of sodium and bicarbonate and excessive loss of chloride in the urine; this causes metabolic alkalosis and expansion of the ECF volume. Management involves correction of the adrenal disorder.

Chloride-responsive types are considerably more common and often associated with marked ECF volume depletion. The prototype for this type of alkalosis is that which occurs from persistent vomiting or prolonged nasogastric suction with an obstructed pylorus. Unlike losses from vomiting with an open pylorus (loss of gastric, pancreatic, biliary, and intestinal secretions), these losses are almost exclusively hydrogen, chloride, and potassium. The expected renal response to the loss of acid would be retention of hydrogen and resorption of less bicarbonate. The progressive ECF deficit, however, stimulates maximal renal resorption of sodium; in the distal tubule, this requires exchange for hydrogen or potassium and the generation of a bicarbonate ion. To compound the problem, the developing hypochloremia mandates increased distal tubular resorption of sodium (less chloride available for resorption with sodium in the proximal tubule), and potassium depletion causes more hydrogen to be exchanged for sodium. These changes produce the characteristic findings of a severe systemic alkalosis and an acid urine (paradoxical aciduria).

Management involves replacing the ECF deficit with isotonic sodium chloride solution and potassium (when adequate urinary output is established). The provision of chloride allows increased sodium resorption in the proximal tubule; the alkalosis begins to resolve, therefore, as less hydrogen ion is secreted and less bicarbonate is generated in the distal tubule. Additionally, hydrogen ion secretion is decreased further as hypokalemia is corrected, since more potassium is now available for exchange with sodium.

It is emphasized that alkalosis (regardless of the type or cause) increases potassium loss, and potassium depletion itself may induce metabolic alkalosis. In the latter, potassium lost from body cells is replaced in part by hydrogen, which causes ECF alkalosis. The same process occurs in the distal renal tubular cells, so there is less potassium to exchange for sodium, and more hydrogen must be excreted in the urine in exchange for sodium. Conversely, alkalosis increases potassium loss. As hydrogen leaves the cell, it is replaced in part by potassium. In the renal tubular cell, more potassium than hydrogen is available for exchange with sodium, causing a rise in urinary potassium.

POTASSIUM ABNORMALITIES. Ninety-eight per cent of body potassium is intracellular; the small amount of potassium in the ECF (62 to 65 mEq. in adults) is critical for cardiac and neuromuscular function. The distribution of potassium between the two spaces is influenced by many factors. For example, large amounts of cellular potassium are released into the ECF in response to severe injury, surgical stress, and acidosis. If this occurs in patients with renal disease or injury, the rise in potassium may be impressive, although dangerous hyperkalemia is rarely encountered if renal function is normal.

Hyperkalemia. Signs and symptoms of hyperkalemia are limited to the cardiovascular and gastrointestinal systems; those in the gastrointestinal system include nausea, vomiting, intermittent intestinal colic, and diarrhea. Cardiovascular signs are apparent on the electrocardiogram (ECG) initially with high peaked T waves, widened QRS complex, and depressed ST segments. Disappearance of T waves, heart block, and diastolic cardiac arrest may develop with increasing levels of potassium.

Management consists of immediate measures for reduction of the serum potassium level, withholding of exogenously administered potassium, and correction of the underlying cause if possible. Temporary suppression of the myocardial effects can be obtained by the intravenous administration of 1 gm. of 10 per cent calcium gluconate with ECG monitoring. This does not affect serum potassium concentration but does counteract the effects of hyperkalemia on cardiac cells by restoring a more normal differential between threshold and resting cellular transmembrane potential. Thereafter, serum potassium levels may be lowered by administration of bicarbonate and glucose with insulin (45 mEq. $NaHCO_3$ in 1000 ml. of 10 per cent dextrose in water with 20 units regular insulin). These maneuvers are temporary and allow time for definitive removal of excess potassium by cation exchange resins, peritoneal dialysis, or hemodialysis.

Hypokalemia. Hypokalemia is a more common problem in surgical patients and may occur as a result of excessive renal excretion, movement of potassium into cells, prolonged administration of potassium-free parenteral fluids with continued obligatory renal loss of potassium (20 mEq. per day or more), parenteral hyperalimentation with inadequate potassium replacement, and loss in gastrointestinal secretions.

The signs of potassium deficit are related to failure of normal contractility of skeletal, smooth, and cardiac muscle and include weakness that may progress to flaccid paralysis, diminished to absent tendon reflexes, and paralytic ileus. Sensitivity to digitalis with cardiac arrhythmias and ECG signs of low voltage, flattening of T waves, and depression of ST segments are characteristic. The signs may be masked by a severe ECF volume deficit.

Treatment involves, first, prevention of the state. During replacement of gastrointestinal fluids, it is safe to replace the upper limits of loss, since an excess is readily handled by the patient with normal renal function. No more than 40 mEq. of potassium should be added to a liter of intravenous fluid, and the rate of administration should not exceed 40 mEq. per hour unless the ECG is being monitored. In the absence of specific indications, potassium should not be given to an oliguric patient or during the first 24 hours following severe surgical stress or trauma. In the presence of severe ECF volume depletion and hypokalemia, adequate volume replacement for restoration of a normal urinary output should be accomplished before potassium is given.

CALCIUM ABNORMALITIES. The normal serum calcium level is between 9 and 11 mg. per 100 ml. (depending on the individual laboratory). Fifty per cent is not ionized and is bound to plasma proteins, whereas another 5 per cent is bound to other substances in the plasma and interstitial fluid. The remaining 45 per cent is the ionized portion that is responsible for neuromuscular stability. Knowledge of the plasma protein level, therefore, is essential for proper analysis of the serum calcium level. The ratio of ionized to nonionized calcium is also related to pH; acidosis causes an increase in the ionized fraction, and alkalosis causes a decrease.

Hypocalcemia. The symptoms of hypocalcemia are numbness and tingling of the circumoral region and the tips of the fingers and toes. The signs are of neuromuscular origin and include hyperactive tendon reflexes, positive Chvostek's sign, muscle and abdominal cramps, tetany with carpopedal spasm, convulsions (with severe deficit), and prolongation of the Q-T interval on the ECG.

Common causes include acute pancreatitis, massive soft tissue infections (necrotizing fasciitis), acute and chronic renal failure, pancreatic and small intestinal fistulas, and hypoparathyroidism. Transient hypocalcemia may occur in a hyperparathyroid patient following removal of a parathyroid adenoma as a result of inactivity of the remaining glands. Asymptomatic hypocalcemia may occur with hypoproteinemia (normal ionized fraction), whereas symptoms may appear with a normal serum calcium level in a patient with severe alkalosis (low ionized fraction).

Treatment is directed toward correction of the cause with concomitant repletion of the deficit. Acute symptoms may be relieved by the intravenous administration of calcium gluconate or chloride. Calcium lactate may be given orally, with or without supplemental vitamin D, in the patient requiring prolonged replacement.

Hypercalcemia. The symptoms of hypercalcemia are rather vague and of gastrointestinal, renal, musculoskeletal, and CNS origin. Early manifestations include easy fatigue, lassitude, weakness of varying degree, anorexia, nausea, vomiting, and weight loss. With higher serum calcium levels, lassitude gives way to somnambulism, stupor, and finally coma. Other symptoms include severe headaches, pains in the back and extremities, polydipsia, and polyuria. The two major causes of hypercalcemia are hyperparathyroidism and cancer metastatic to bone.

Treatment of acute hypercalcemic crisis is an emergency. The critical level of serum calcium is between 16 and 20 mg. per 100 ml., and unless treatment is instituted promptly, the symptoms may rapidly progress to death. Rapid repletion of the associated ECF volume deficit immediately lowers the calcium level by dilution. A loop diuretic (furosemide) in doses of 20 to 40 mg. every 6 hours greatly enhances urinary excretion of calcium. The large losses of fluid must be replaced, however, and close monitoring of fluid status and electrolyte balance is mandatory. Intravenous sulfates and phosphates have also been recommended, although use of the latter may be associated with severe complications. Intravenous mithramycin has proved to be a safe and effective drug. Reduction in the serum calcium level is apparent in 24 hours, with a peak effect at 3 days and a duration of action of 5 to 7 days.

Definitive treatment of acute hypercalcemic crisis in patients with hyperparathyroidism is surgical therapy. Treatment of hypercalcemia in patients with metastatic cancer is primarily that of prevention. The serum calcium level is assessed frequently; if it is elevated, the patient is placed on a low-calcium diet, and measures ensuring adequate hydration are instituted.

MAGNESIUM DEFICIENCY. Magnesium deficiency is known to occur with starvation, malabsorption syndromes, protracted losses of gastrointestinal fluids, prolonged parenteral fluid therapy with magnesium-free solutions, and hyperalimentation. Other causes include acute pancreatitis, diabetic ketoacidosis during treatment, primary aldosteronism, and chronic alcoholism.

The magnesium ion is essential for proper function of most enzyme systems, and depletion is characterized by neuromuscular and CNS hyperactivity. The signs and symptoms are similar to those of calcium deficiency, including hyperactive tendon reflexes, muscle tremors, and tetany with a positive Chvostek's sign. Progression to delirium and convulsions may occur with a severe deficit. A concomitant calcium deficiency may be present. The diagnosis of magnesium deficiency depends on an awareness of the syndrome and clinical recognition of the symptoms. Laboratory confirmation is available but not always reliable, since the syndrome may exist in the presence of a normal serum magnesium level. The possibility of magnesium deficiency should always be entertained in a surgical patient who exhibits disturbed neuromuscular or cerebral activity.

Treatment is by parenteral administration of magnesium sulfate or magnesium chloride solution. If renal function is normal, as much as 2 mEq. of magnesium per kg. of body weight can be administered in a day in the presence of severe depletion. Magnesium sulfate (50 per cent solution contains approximately 4 mEq. of magnesium ion per milliliter) may be given intravenously or intramuscularly. The intravenous route is preferable for the initial treatment of a severe symptomatic deficit. The solution is prepared by the addition of 80 mEq. of magnesium sulfate (20 ml. of 50 per cent solution) to a liter of intravenous fluid and administered over a 4- to 6-hour period. The heart rate, blood pressure, respiration, and ECG should be monitored closely for signs of magnesium intoxication, which can cause cardiac arrest. Calcium chloride should be available to counteract any adverse cardiac effects of a rapidly rising plasma magnesium level.

Partial or complete relief of symptoms may follow this infusion, although continued replacement over a 1- to 3-week period is necessary for adequate replenishment of the ICF compartment. For this purpose and for the asymptomatic patient who is likely to have significant magnesium depletion, 10 to 20 mEq. of 50 per cent magnesium sulfate solution is given daily mixed in maintenance intravenous fluids. Following complete repletion of intracellular magnesium and in the absence of abnormal loss, balance may be maintained by the administration of as little as 4 mEq. of magnesium ion per day.

INTRAOPERATIVE FLUID MANAGEMENT

If preoperative replacement of ECF volume has been incomplete, hypotension may develop promptly with the induction of anesthesia. This can be insidious, since the ability of the awake patient to compensate for a mild volume deficit is revealed only when compensatory mechanisms are abolished with anesthesia.

Blood loss is replaced as necessary during the operative procedure, bearing in mind that a hematocrit of 30 per cent is adequate for most patients. In addition to blood losses, functional ECF volume depletion is common during major intra-abdominal operative procedures owing to the accumulation of interstitial fluid into the peritoneum and peritoneal cavity, in the lumen and the wall of the small bowel, and in the retracted muscle of the operative wound itself. These losses should be replaced with a balanced salt solution as they are incurred. The amount of fluid needed depends principally on the extent and degree of tissue trauma and averages 500 to 1000 ml. per hour in adults. The actual amount given varies widely and is guided by signs such as the stability of the patient's vital signs and urinary output. The addition of albumin solutions is not necessary.

POSTOPERATIVE FLUID MANAGEMENT

Immediate postoperative evaluation should include a review of preoperative fluid status, the amount of fluid lost and gained during operation, and clinical examination of the patient with assessment of vital signs and urinary output. Initial fluid orders are written for correction of any existing deficit followed by maintenance fluids for the remainder of the day. For patients who have received or lost large amounts of fluid or who were hypotensive during a part of the operative procedure, it may be difficult to estimate fluid requirements for the ensuing 24 hours. Fluids may be ordered 1 liter at a time, and the patient examined frequently until the situation is clarified.

Daily maintenance fluids thereafter begin with an assessment of the patient's volume status and any concentration or compositional disorders as reflected by serum electrolytes. All sensible (measured) and insensible (estimated) losses are replaced with fluids of appropriate composition, allowing for any existing volume or electrolyte abnormality. Additionally, 40 mEq. of potassium is given daily for baseline renal excretion in addition to approximately 20 mEq. per liter for replacement of gastrointestinal losses.

Insensible losses (from skin and lungs) are relatively constant in an individual and average 500 to 1000 ml. per day depending on the size of the patient. This loss is replaced with 5 per cent dextrose in water (D5W). In an adult, approximately 1 liter of fluid should be given to replace that volume of urine required to excrete the catabolic end products of metabolism. This may be given as D5W, since normal kidneys are able to conserve sodium quite well. It is unnecessary to stress the kidneys to this degree, however, and a small amount of salt solution may be given in addition to water to cover urinary loss. Elderly patients may not be able to conserve sodium as well, and a gradual hyponatremia may develop if these losses are replaced with D5W. Sensible losses, by definition, can be measured and replaced on a milliliter for milliliter basis. Most are gastrointestinal losses and are appropriately replaced with an isotonic salt solution.

Serum electrolytes are determined as needed; they are often unnecessary during an uncomplicated 2- to 3-day postoperative course but may be required daily in patients with excessive fluid losses. If concentration or compositional abnormalities develop, adjustments can be made in the type of intravenous fluid given for maintenance. For example, gastrointestinal losses should be replaced with normal saline solution in a patient with hyponatremia, hypochloremia, and mild metabolic alkalosis, and this should be continued until the abnormalities are corrected. In a hyponatremic patient with obvious volume overload, the total amount of maintenance fluid given is restricted. In the presence of hyponatremia and mild metabolic acidosis, lactated Ringer's solution is ideal. With use of this approach, severe concentration and compositional changes can be avoided or corrected while an adequate ECF volume is maintained.

5

PRINCIPLES OF PREOPERATIVE PREPARATION OF THE SURGICAL PATIENT

Hiram C. Polk, Jr., M.D.

The modern preparation of the patient for operation characterizes the emergence of all the surgical disciplines from art to science.

ASSESSMENT OF OPERATIVE RISK

Calculation of operative risk is a major component of the relative rewards and risks of treatment of a specific illness (Table 1). The overt nature of the surgical method magnifies the significance of adverse results and permits clear understanding of this expression in the therapeutic ratio, that is, the relative harm (risk) and the relative good (benefit) that are *likely* to follow a specific operation for a specific illness in a specific patient. The *natural history* of a given illness is the course of the disease and its ultimate outcome if untreated, a factor of particular significance in times of therapeutic chauvinism.

The *stages* of disease being considered must be *clinically* comparable. Errors in clinical staging produce the greatest number of controversies regarding medical or surgical therapy or both. Differences between treatments are attributable more often to differences in clinical staging of the patient populations under comparison and less to different results of the putative therapies. The therapeutic ratio of appendectomy for *suspected* appendicitis is clearly in favor of intervention. Treating appendicitis by excision—even with a 20 per cent incidence of normal appendices—is much better than allowing a single appendix to perforate, in view of the exaggerated morbidity and geometric effect on mortality if

See the corresponding chapter or part in the *Textbook of Surgery*, 14th edition, pp. 77–84, for a more detailed discussion of this topic, including a comprehensive list of references.

TABLE 1. Basic Factors Affecting Operative Risk*

Age over 70 years
Overall physical status
Elective versus emergency operation
Physiologic extent of procedure
Number of associated illnesses

*30-day hospital deaths.

perforation occurs. This potential for an adverse effect has been redefined in a current analysis of managed care trends in current medical practice.

The urgency of an operation may determine the period of time for and indirectly limit the measures taken for preparation of the patient. Although chronic malnutrition cannot be corrected in 2 to 3 hours, it is possible to begin correction of concentration and volume deficiencies. Thus, the nature of the disease being treated influences outcome (e.g., the patient with advanced cancer with anemia, weight loss, and metastases that alter hepatic, pulmonary, or cerebral function). No definitive correction of all the manifestations of cancer can be achieved, preoperatively or even postoperatively. By contrast, the systemic effects of an inflammatory process that has led to contamination of the entire peritoneal cavity may be treated vigorously with parenteral fluids, antibiotics, and intestinal decompression with full knowledge that surgical correction of the offending focus is definitive.

The elderly often require concurrent management of multiple-organ degenerative disease. When one disease produces a complication that can be controlled only by operation, particular attention should be given to the often subtle but physiologically important alterations of the other organs essential for life support. Among the specific considerations that markedly influence operative risk are age and cardiovascular, respiratory, renal, and gastrointestinal disease. Significant impairment of more than one organ system profoundly influences operative risk.

The capacity for sound clinical *judgment* is the ultimate characteristic of the mature physician. A quantitative approach to clinical judgment may be unnecessary; despite general agreement as to principles of *intra*operative decisions in a common major operation, practicing surgeons often deviate from accepted standards, those deviations being associated with significant increases in death after operation and in decreased cure of some colorectal cancers.

PERSONAL RELATIONSHIPS

When an operation is being considered, a genuine bond of communication and personal responsibility must be established between the surgeon and the patient. The patient's confidence is based on real understanding, allowing him to participate, when appropriate, in judgments affecting risks, future life-style, and the process of postoperative recovery.

The patient in a teaching institution finds his or her illness and operation a focal point for the education of trainees at several levels. Properly conducted, this can be a positive influence for the patient psychologically, as many enjoy such attention, provided it involves the patient personally and considers the medical problems in a tactful manner.

The *specific permission* for conduct of an operative procedure is a focal point of medical, legal, and sociologic discussion. Local custom and recent legal practice often determine which of these is most appropriate.

GENERAL PREPARATION OF THE PATIENT
Psychological Preparation

A frank but optimistic discussion of the possibilities ahead is valuable to the patient undergoing a major surgical procedure. The preoperative steps, as well as drainage devices and various forms of intubation, should be enumerated, justified, and explained in detail. The surgeon must not equivocate in discussing possible disfiguring operations, such as upon the head and neck, breasts, or genital organs, and most especially with respect to methods of urinary or fecal elimination. When an illness is apt to have a clinically significant course beyond the duration of the early posthospital follow-up, it is usually very reassuring for the surgeon to explain his or her continuing commitment to the patient.

Often it is useful to allow the patient to spontaneously ask about the status of the disease process. However, if this has not occurred within a period of several days, the surgeon should take the initiative and review with the patient the operative finding and the probable prognosis. Such gentle frankness guarantees that the patient, who may reach even more difficult stages of the illness, will again turn to the surgeon as a person who has been honest about future prospects.

Physiologic Preparation

BLOOD VOLUME CONSIDERATIONS. A number of chronic disease processes are associated with anemia. In some instances, these represent visible external losses, as in carcinoma of the cecum. Other instances are far less clear and are associated with chronic infection or with chronic inflammatory processes of the bowel. These patients all fit a pattern in which there is substantial blood loss producing reduction of red cell mass. Indeed, such patients have a normal *total blood volume.* They have compensated for a significantly decreased red blood cell volume by expansion of the plasma volume to supernormal levels. Whereas *acute* intravascular volume deficiencies are manifested by an increased pulse rate or decreased blood pressure, chronic volume deficiency is restored by expanding the plasma volume, often at the expense of the extracellular fluid, to compensate for the loss of or nonproduction of red cell mass. Correction of these concentration deficits before an elective operation requires recognition that even large deficits in red cell mass occurring over a long period are well tolerated. The key issue is tissue oxygen delivery. Enhanced oxygen delivery can be achieved in the following ways: (1) increase in heart rate, (2) increase in stroke volume, and (3) increase in oxygen extraction. The last may be least amenable to improvement, and to increase stroke volume or pulse rate places a definite physiologic stress on the heart, which often is diseased in the elderly patients who acquire such chronic illnesses. Therefore, there is a reasonable limit to the hemoglobin concentrations that are safe for a major operation.

OTHER FLUID DEFICITS. Whereas blood deficits are

primarily concentrational, plasma and extracellular fluid deficits are significant in both volume and concentration in terms of the preparation of most patients preoperatively. Special problems are presented when the volume deficiencies are *pre-existing* or *concealed*. For example, *pre-existing* losses may represent vomitus and/or diarrhea occurring before hospitalization. Some losses occur more visibly, as in a fracture of the femur or in a major third-degree burn of an extremity, and are manifested by visible swelling; more often such fluid losses are concealed and thus inadequately estimated.

The problem of *concealed* loss is particularly difficult. These "third space losses" in which blood, plasma, or extracellular fluid is extravasated are often associated with fractures, and it is only by careful comparison of the fractured and unfractured limb for circumference that one can appreciate the magnitude of such losses. Objective estimation of pre-existing and continuing fluid deficits is most usefully obtained by hourly urinary output through a urinary catheter. As difficult as estimation of pre-existing or concealed losses may be, this first step in assessment of continuing losses is essential to reconstruction of that deficit. Hemoglobin concentration, appearance of the mucous membranes, and skin turgor assist in such judgment. A common error in quantitating concentrational deficits is to assume that the normal serum concentration of a specific electrolyte assures that there has been no loss. Isotonic losses of water, salt, chloride, and potassium may produce profound volume deficiencies with maintenance of normal concentrations of the commonly measured serum electrolytes. When concentrational abnormalities exist, they imply only that the loss of electrolyte concentration has been relatively greater than the loss of water or vice versa.

TIMING AND PARAMETERS. Urgency of the operation is the major determinant in the time available for correction of fluid and electrolyte balance. Not all volume and concentrational deficits need be corrected before operation is undertaken. In general, the longer a patient has been ill, the more time one can take to correct the deficiencies. In other words, the patient has adjusted physiologically to the deficiency induced by the illness. One must be certain that the rapid replenishment of those deficits does not impose a risk greater than the illness itself.

Nutrition

Nutritional replenishment and supplementation has become a common (and expensive) worldwide surgical practice; its specific role in improved survival from certain illnesses or after certain operations continues to defy documentation and certainly defies cost-benefit analysis. As a skeptic, the author recommends accepting the tide of surgical opinion concerning the value of aggressive nutrition in certain situations, perhaps assuming that such supportive measures are providing the basis for prolonged in-hospital survival and that some future advance will be required to convert longer in-hospital courses to ultimate improvement in hospital discharge data.

Prevention of Infection

Infection continues to be a major source of morbidity and a disconcerting source of mortality in the surgical patient. The patient who is badly injured or who undergoes a major operation and survives despite the development of secondary shock and electrolyte disturbances is at very high risk for serious infection. Therefore, control of infection is a major consideration before, during, and after every operation (Table 2). During preoperative evaluation, the patient should be protected from any patient with extramural or hospital-acquired infections. The proposed operative site should be cleansed with an appropriate antiseptic agent on several occasions before operation, and shaving should be done either as close to the time of operation as is feasible or not at all, with substitution of either clipping or depilatory agents where removal of hair is desired.

A primary factor to be considered is antibiotic prophylaxis. Explicit laboratory studies were confirmed by a now seemingly endless flow of randomized clinical trials that showed *systemic* antibiotics to be highly effective when used just before, during, and immediately after an operation. However, one must always balance the risk of an adverse effect of an antibiotic with its potential benefit (Table 3). The agent selected should have sustained antibiotic activity in the surgical wound itself. Declining wound antibiotic activity is an indication to readminister the agent or to seek a drug producing more sustained wound levels. With regard to delivery of antimicrobial protection to the wound itself, one may administer systemic antibiotics or choose topical antibiotics in the wound. A method of wound management that has stood the test of time in badly contaminated cases is *delayed* primary closure of the wound.

SPECIFIC ORGANS AND SYSTEMS

CARDIOVASCULAR. Every patient scheduled for any operation should have specific, careful cardiovascular evaluation. In the young, previously overlooked congenital lesions

TABLE 2. Factors Influencing Likelihood of Infection After Operation

Definite Decreased Host Resistance	Possible Decreased Host Resistance	Minimal, If Any, Effect on Host Resistance
Increasing age	Cancer (some forms)	Patient's gender
Obesity/malnutrition	Radiation therapy	Patient's race
Diabetic ketoacidosis	Adrenocortical deficiency	Controlled diabetes mellitus
Acute/chronic steroid therapy	Percutaneous foreign bodies	Acute nutritional deprivation
Immunosuppressive drugs	Early shaving of operative site	
Remote, synchronous infection		

TABLE 3. Operations Benefiting from Systemic Antibiotic Prophylaxis

Head and neck, which open upper aerodigestive tract
Esophageal, excluding hiatal hernia repair
Gastroduodenal, except for complications of uncorrected
    hyperacidity
Biliary tract for patients
    over 70 years old
    with acute cholecystitis, and/or
    requiring choledochostomy
Small and large bowel resections
Gangrenous or perforated appendicitis
Hysterectomy
Abdominal and lower extremity revascularizations, including a
    prosthetic graft
Other clean operations implanting a high-risk prosthesis, e.g., hip,
    knee, aortic valve

may be discovered; in the elderly, prevalent atherosclerosis must be sought. Initial efforts to quantitate what appeared to be subjective impressions were enhanced by the work of Mauney and co-workers. Goldman and associates advanced this concept toward precise determination of operative risk. The capacity of the patient to increase cardiac output in response to intra- and postoperative challenges is perhaps the most fundamental determinant of survival following complex operations. The risk factors that predict fatal and nonfatal, but life-threatening, complications of cardiac origin after *noncardiac* operations are listed in Tables 4 and 5. Also significant in detecting the unsuspected high-risk patient is the work of Del Guercio and Cohn on preoperative pulmonary wedge pressure monitoring with and without challenge. More important, their method has revealed some patients

TABLE 4. Preoperative Factors Associated with Postoperative Cardiac Complications in Order of Discovery Significance

Jugular vein distention or S_3 gallop
Myocardial infarct in previous 6 months
Premature atrial contractions or rhythm other than sinus on
    electrocardiogram
Three to five premature ventricular contractions per minute
Age over 70 years
Significant aortic valvular stenosis
Poor general medical condition
    $Pao_2 < 60$ mm. Hg; $Paco_2 > 50$ mm. Hg
    $K^+ < 3.0$ mEq./L.; $HCO_3 < 20$ mEq./L.
    Blood urea nitrogen > 50 mg./100 ml.; creatinine > 3.0 mg./100
    ml.
    Elevated transaminase
    Signs of chronic liver disease
    Patient bedridden from noncardiac causes

Modified from Goldman, L., Caldera, D. L., Nussbaum, S. R., et al.: Multifactorial index of cardiac risk in noncardiac surgical procedures. N. Engl. J. Med., 297:845, 1977.

TABLE 5. Weighting of Cardiac Risk Factors

Criteria	Points
Historical	
Age over 70 years	5
Myocardial infarction previous 6 months	10
Examination	
S_3 gallop/jugular venous distention	11
Significant aortic valvular stenosis	3
Electrocardiogram	
Premature atrial contractions or rhythm other than sinus	7
More than 5 premature ventricular contractions per minute	7
General Status	3
Abnormal blood gases	
K^+/HCO_3^- abnormalities	
Abnormal renal function	
Liver disease/bedridden	
Operation	
Emergency	4
Intraperitoneal/intrathoracic/aortic	3
Total possible	53

Modified from Goldman, L., Caldera, D. L., Nussbaum, S. R., et al.: Multifactorial index of cardiac risk in noncardiac surgical procedures. N. Engl. J. Med., *297*:845, 1977.

with prohibitive cardiac risk and allowed others to be improved prior to operation.

Thromboembolism is a generally infrequent clinical event; the value of brief or mini-anticoagulation for some patients is widely debated and is discussed in detail elsewhere in this text. Patients at increased risk include (1) those with a clear history or clinical signs of prior thrombosis or embolism; (2) those likely to have prolonged operations, with special emphasis on procedures that temporarily interfere with lower extremity blood flow, such as some aortic reconstructions or perineal operations requiring the use of stirrups; and (3) those with certain reconstructive operations upon the hip. The clinician may then employ a number of methods for reducing the risk of thromboembolism, including elastic stockings, exercises, early ambulation, and variable degrees of anticoagulation.

RESPIRATORY. Respiratory complications of operations occur in two major groups: (1) patients with grossly normal lungs who develop respiratory abnormalities secondary to anesthetic agents and operation; and (2) the increasing number of patients with overt chronic lung disease who require operation, thus with superimposition of the problems of anesthesia and operation on intrinsically diseased pulmonary tissue. Risk factors are outlined in Table 6. One test of proven value is preoperative documentation of the normal resting *arterial blood gases*. There is no "normal" blood gas profile for all patients. Although consideration of standard age-related changes in $P(A-a)O_2$ may be the only resource in an emer-

**TABLE 6. Risk Factors for Postoperative
Pulmonary Complications**

Thoracic and upper abdominal surgery
Preoperative history of chronic obstructive pulmonary disease
  (COPD)
Preoperative purulent productive cough
Anesthesia time greater than 3 hours
History of cigarette smoking
Age greater than 60 years
Obesity
Poor preoperative state of nutrition
Symptoms of respiratory disease
Abnormal findings on physical examination
Abnormal chest film findings

From Houston, M. C., Ratcliff, D. G., Hays, J. T., and Gluck, F.
W.: Preoperative medical consultation and evaluation of surgical risk.
South. Med. J., *80*:1385, 1987.

gency, determination of a patient's normal range of blood
gases is mandatory before an elective operation when the
procedure is of great magnitude or when other clear factors,
including age, suggest the possibility of respiratory complications.

RENAL. With appropriate perioperative hydration, renal
complications of major surgical endeavors have become relatively uncommon. A normal blood urea nitrogen determination may, however, be misleading. Conversely, the most
common erroneous consideration in the surgical patient is
the fear that renal disease exists. Renal disease is not nearly
so frequent in the apparently asymptomatic population as
are cardiovascular and respiratory diseases. With the screening procedures of blood urea nitrogen, creatinine determination, and urinalysis, one may proceed to an operation and
subsequent fluid therapy reasonably confident that the pa-

TABLE 7. A Sample Preoperative Checklist

Operative permit—appropriately signed and witnessed
Dietary considerations
  For abdominal operation, liquid diet and laxatives to ensure clean
    collapsed bowel
  Nothing by mouth at least 6 hours before operation
Review of life-support systems
  Vital signs recorded often enough to establish "normal"
  Pulmonary system—chest films; other studies as indicated
  Cardiac function—electrocardiogram; other studies as indicated
  Renal function—urinalysis; blood urea nitrogen and creatinine
    determinations
Adequate hydration up to time of operation—especially to
  compensate for laxatives and fasting
Area of operation cleansed with appropriate germicidal detergent
  and shaved, clipped, or cleansed with depilatory agent
Blood transfusions prepared as anticipated
Order that patient should void on call to operating room
Preoperative medications—vagolytic and sedative drugs
Special medications—digitalis, insulin, etc.

---

tient will tolerate judiciously managed fluid loads with ease. The most common cause of oliguria on surgical services continues to be *hypo*volemia rather than incipient renal failure.

HEPATIC. The signs and symptoms of significant liver impairment are detectable in a number of standard examinations. The overwhelming risk of cirrhosis in nonshunting operations has identified factors that preclude all but absolute immediate lifesaving operations.

NEUROLOGIC. Maintenance of cerebral function via appropriate oxygenation and circulation is of vital concern to the anesthesiologist and the surgeon. Of special concern is the prevalence of occult cerebrovascular disease in the elderly, who constitute a major proportion of patients requiring surgical attention.

SPECIAL PROBLEMS

A number of special problems demand preoperative correction. Foremost among these is incomplete cleansing of the alimentary tract. Pulmonary aspiration is a dreaded surgical complication, the treatment of which remains inadequate, whereas prevention is simple. There are almost no circumstances in which general anesthesia should be induced without specific attention to evacuation of the patient's stomach, ascertained in any questionable case by the surgeon. Although so simple to prevent, aspiration remains one of the more common causes of surgical mortality. A useful checklist of preoperative considerations that should be reviewed at the time of writing preoperative hospital orders is depicted in Table 7.

6

BLOOD TRANSFUSIONS AND DISORDERS OF SURGICAL BLEEDING

John A. Collins, M.D.

Adequate hemostasis is fundamental in surgery. If the patient has a faulty hemostatic mechanism, the surgeon must have sufficient understanding of hemostasis to be able to estimate the risks of the proposed procedures, to modify surgical technique as necessary, and to help direct the correction of the hemostatic defects.

NORMAL HEMOSTASIS

Current views of normal hemostasis focus on four major components: the vascular endothelium, platelets, coagulation, and inhibition of coagulation and lysis of its products.

Vascular endothelium is nonthrombogenic because of several physicochemical properties. It also synthesizes and releases an impressive array of vasoactive, thrombogenic, and antithrombotic materials. It interacts significantly with platelets, the coagulation cascade, and the fibrinolytic system. Endothelium contains abundant contractile proteins, so even muscle-less capillaries can constrict.

Platelets adhere to exposed collagen and interact with signals released by injured vascular endothelium. Even when the exposed collagen is covered by a layer of platelets, more platelets accumulate, forming a substantial mass. This aggregation reaction can be caused by a wide number of substances, the most physiologically relevant of which are epinephrine, collagen, thrombin, and adenosine diphosphate. These agonists can also cause synthesis and/or release of certain vasoactive and thrombogenic substances and the expression (exposure) of certain membrane receptors. Platelet aggregation and activation may be largely modulated by 3',5'-adenosine monophosphate, which counteracts the effects of platelet agonists.

The formation of a fibrin clot is the next important step in hemostasis. The mechanisms by which this occurs, termed *coagulation*, are a series of linked reactions involving circulating proteins. Most steps involve enzymatic conversion of inactive precursors to active forms, which then cause the activation of the next step in the sequence. There is a general increase in effect from step to step, so that the overall sequence forms a biologic amplification device. Various control mechanisms are active at most steps, and there are

---

See the corresponding chapter or part in the *Textbook of Surgery,* 14th edition, pp. 85–102, for a more detailed discussion of this topic, including a comprehensive list of references.

substantial feedback loops and crossover effects of both amplification and inhibition. The coagulation sequence leads to the formation of thrombin, which splits fibrinogen to form soluble fibrin monomers. The monomers polymerize to form insoluble fibrin, which is acted upon by factor XIII to increase cross-linking, forming a firmer clot more resistant to lysis. The reactions requiring phospholipid occur largely on the membranes of activated platelets, further linking platelets and coagulation and positioning the ensuing clot where it is needed. The fibrin mesh helps seal the breaks in the blood vessels and stop the loss of blood through its immediate physical effect, through its strengthening of the platelet plug and aiding the recruitment of more platelets, and through the improved binding of the entire hemostatic plug via its interaction with platelets, vessel wall and collagen, and other adhesive proteins such as von Willebrand factor, fibronectin, and thrombospondin.

Producing clots is necessary in order to stop bleeding; controlling clots is necessary in order to preserve circulation and control healing. When a fibrin clot is formed, it contains within itself the seeds of its own destruction in the form of adsorbed plasminogen, which has its greatest efficacy against fresh clots. In addition to the controlling mechanisms that act locally at the site of the injury, it is essential to prevent systemic activation of the coagulation cascade. This is accomplished by two approaches: inhibiting various activated components of the coagulation cascade, and activating fibrinolytic enzymes. The primary mechanism for removing fibrin is lysis by plasmin. Plasmin circulates in the inactive form of plasminogen, which can be activated by a variety of stimuli and which is adsorbed to the surfaces of a forming fibrin plug. The most important action of plasmin is the dissolution of fibrin clots, but it is far from a specific enzyme. In addition to fibrin, plasmin attacks fibrinogen and factors II, V, and VIII, and possibly IX and XI. It can digest adrenocorticotropic hormone, growth hormone, insulin, and complement. It activates factor XII and via factor XIIa amplifies coagulation and activates the kinin and complement systems. It even acts on plasminogen, making it more susceptible to activation. Clearly, something with this power must be carefully controlled. The primary circulating inhibitor is alpha$_2$-plasmin inhibitor, which is rapid and effective. Congenital deficiencies of plasminogen cause a thrombotic tendency, whereas defects in alpha$_2$-plasmin inhibitor cause a hemorrhagic disorder.

One of the most important and fundamental questions in hemostasis remains unanswered: how are beneficial clots maintained while harmful or rogue clots are usually lysed? Intricate antagonistic controlling mechanisms have been identified, but it is not clear how they are so precisely orchestrated.

DISORDERS OF HEMOSTASIS

The most common congenital abnormality of hemostasis is classic hemophilia (hemophilia A), a sex-linked inherited disorder that also occurs spontaneously in approximately 1 in every 25,000 births. In this disorder, the blood is almost totally lacking in factor VIII activity. Bleeding, both spontaneous and after even slight trauma, is the main problem. Treatment consists of maintenance of factor VIII levels by periodic infusion of factor VIII. Higher levels of infused factor VIII are needed for surgical procedures or if the patient is bleeding.

Hemophilia B (Christmas disease) is a congenital deficiency of factor IX and is the second most common congenital disorder of coagulation. Some patients require maintenance therapy for prevention of spontaneous bleeding. Although hemophilia B is easily confused with hemophilia A on screening tests and may resemble it clinically, it does not respond to the administration of factor VIII. Accurate diagnosis is therefore essential.

Von Willebrand's disease, which is lack of the factor of the same name, is the third most common inherited disorder of coagulation. It is easily mistaken for one of the hemophilias. Clinically, it has the added problem of platelet dysfunction. It varies in severity, but the bleeding tends to be more from mucous membranes than from the musculoskeletal system. The platelet disorder responds to the infusion of material containing factor VIII and von Willebrand factor.

Among the acquired disorders of coagulation, probably the most common in the United States today are those related to drugs. Vitamin K antagonists (warfarin-like drugs) inhibit the production by the liver of factors II, VII, IX, and X and proteins C and S. Deficiency of vitamin K can occur in normal neonates and can follow obstructive jaundice, use of antibiotics that suppress gut flora, prolonged inanition, short gut syndrome, malabsorption of fat, and others. Some antibiotics (e.g., moxalactam and cefamandole) contain a moiety, *N*-methylthiotetrazole, that may interfere with the utilization of vitamin K by the liver, thereby greatly augmenting and accelerating the effect of antibiotics on production of vitamin K–dependent factors.

Heparin exerts its effects by combining with antithrombin III (AT-III) to inhibit thrombin, plasmin, kallikrein, and the activated forms of factors IX, X, XI, and XII. The effects against plasmin, kallikrein, and factor XIIa are responsible for the anti-inflammatory activity of heparin. The effects of heparin are therefore dependent on the circulating levels of AT-III, which are decreased after trauma or operation, with active clotting, during prolonged treatment with heparin, and during episodes of disseminated intravascular coagulation (DIC). The effective dose of heparin is uncertain and may vary with time in the same patient as the level of AT-III changes. Thrombocytopenia occurs in about 1 to 2 per cent of patients receiving heparin, sometimes associated with arterial thromboses.

Hepatic insufficiency can be devastating in its impact on hemostasis. The liver is the sole site of production of fibrinogen and of the vitamin K–dependent coagulation factors; it is the main site of production of circulating factor V and probably of prekallikrein and high-molecular-weight kininogen, and of plasminogen, AT-III, antiplasmin, alpha$_1$-anti-trypsin, and perhaps alpha$_2$-macroglobulin. In addition, the liver is normally the primary site for clearance from the circulation of activated coagulation components, plasminogen activators, and fibrin degradation products (some of which act as anticoagulants). Moreover, many forms of chronic liver disease cause portal hypertension and secondary hypersplenism with its thrombocytopenia. When the patient with hepatic insufficiency is bleeding actively, it is usually necessary to liberally administer both platelets and coagulation factors in the form of fresh frozen plasma (to include factor V), but this is often relatively futile. Lack of synthesis is often compounded by accelerated consumption in the form of DIC. The management of bleeding in such patients can be extremely difficult.

Uremia is often accompanied by a prominent bleeding tendency. The main hemostatic defect in uremia relates to platelets. Almost all tests of platelet function are markedly abnormal in some patients, and the prolonged bleeding times do not correlate with platelet counts, which are usually normal. Infused platelets quickly become as dysfunctional as the patient's platelets. Many of these platelet defects improve with dialysis, but the clinical bleeding tendency does not always respond. The duration of an episode of bleeding in uremic patients can also be shortened by administration of conjugated estrogens or desmopressin (DDAVP), reinforcing speculation that the interaction between platelets and factor VIII and von Willebrand factor is the primary hemostatic defect in uremia.

Some systemic diseases are accompanied by the formation of paraproteins or immunoglobulins that interfere with various aspects of hemostasis. Probably the best studied is the "lupus anticoagulant," an immunoglobulin produced by some patients with systemic lupus erythematosus.

Acquired disorders of platelet function are most commonly related to drugs, many of which interfere with the synthesis of arachidonic acid metabolites. Aspirin is the prototype, but there are many others. Accelerated destruction of platelets occurs in many disorders that cause enlargement of the spleen (secondary hypersplenism) and in idiopathic thrombocytopenic purpura. The distinction between thrombocytopenia due to accelerated destruction and that due to impaired production is clinically significant because the younger platelets associated with accelerated destruction are functionally superior. Disseminated intravascular coagulation (DIC, also called consumption coagulopathy or defibrination syndromes) is perhaps the most troublesome of the acquired disorders of hemostasis. The mechanisms, causes, incidence, and even definition are still subject to disagreement. There are at least two forms. In one, coagulation and its sequel, fibrinolysis, are activated diffusely throughout the circulation by the introduction of potent thrombogenic materials into the circulation. The other type of DIC is less well understood and much more resistant to treatment. Often the antecedent event is (1) severe infection, (2) severe and sustained hypoperfusion, or (3) severe liver disease.

Therapeutic use of fibrinolytic drugs is becoming more common. Such drugs induce activation of plasmin, with the aim of lysing recently formed clots. Such agents are particularly hazardous in patients who have had operations within a week to 10 days, especially in deep body cavities where bleeding cannot be easily detected or controlled by direct pressure.

EVALUATING THE PATIENT

The tests relating to coagulation are the most familiar. Whole blood clotting time measures the intrinsic and common pathways, but the test is too variable, too insensitive to important changes, and too sensitive to unimportant changes. The recalcification time is more reproducible but shares the same problems of sensitivity. The one-stage prothrombin time measures the extrinsic and common pathways, factors I, II, V, VII, and X, but is most sensitive to deficiencies in VII. The partial thromboplastin time is similar to the prothrombin time, but a phospholipid similar to platelet factor III instead of a tissue thromboplastin is used. The intrinsic and common pathways are measured. The results are very reproducible, but the greatest sensitivity is to the early intrinsic pathway factors, which may correlate poorly with clinical events. The thrombin time measures the time required for plasma to form a gross clot after addition of a standard solution of thrombin. This is primarily sensitive to the conversion of fibrinogen to fibrin and the polymerization of the latter. Factor VIII can now be measured readily in most centers. The other coagulation components can be measured individually with varying degrees of difficulty. The template bleeding time may be the most useful screening test for platelet function, but it is very sensitive to variations in technique. More sophisticated and specific tests are available. Most of the major circulating coagulation inhibitors can now be measured independently, including protein C. Measurements of fibrinolytic components are still largely indirect. The measurement of specific products of the activity of plasmin and of thrombin is being developed.

It has long been known that the best screening test for hemostasis in surgical patients is a carefully obtained *history* soliciting evidence of hemostatic defects in the patient and in close relatives. The history is so valuable a screen that it makes laboratory screening of hemostasis unnecessary in most prospective surgical patients who can provide an adequate history. For the actively bleeding patient or for the patient with a suggestive history, laboratory testing is mandatory. Treatment should be chosen in conjunction with the results of appropriate tests and guided by serial changes in those tests. The significantly bleeding patient should be treated by empiricism only when appropriate tests are not available in a timely manner or no clear pattern to guide treatment can be discerned. Poor mechanical hemostasis remains the most common cause of significant bleeding in a postoperative or injured patient.

PRODUCTS THAT AID HEMOSTASIS

Fresh frozen plasma (FFP) is the plasma component of whole blood separated soon after collection and immediately frozen and stored in the frozen state. Most of the coagulation factors approach the concentration in normal plasma, but none of the factors is in a concentration greater than normal. FFP has an important role in the urgent management of patients with multiple coagulation defects following hepatic insufficiency or various drugs, of patients with DIC who need replacement of consumed and lysed factors, and rarely (and doubtfully) of the patient in whom the labile coagulation components have been depleted by the transfusion of very large amounts of old stored blood. The use of FFP in the United States has risen dramatically in the past decade, seemingly far out of proportion to reasonable estimates of need. The recent consensus conference of the National Institutes of Health confirmed these indications for use and questioned the safety of its use in other circumstances. FFP is a single-donor product with the same risk of transmitting viral diseases as that of whole blood. It contains the major anti-A, anti-B, and Rh antibodies, so type- and Rh-specific plasma should be used.

Cryoprecipitate is a source of factor VIII and von Willebrand factor in concentrated form. It also contains about one third the amount of fibrinogen found in a unit of whole blood and is a source of fibronectin. The major advantages of cryoprecipitate are its small volume and its single-donor status. There are various commercially prepared factor VIII concentrates. Recent methods of controlled heating appear to have eliminated the risk of transmitting human immunodeficiency virus (HIV), a very major problem for hemophiliacs in the last decade.

The other category of commercially prepared coagulation factor concentrate involves the prothrombin complex factors: II, VII, IX, and X. This product was designed for use in patients with factor IX deficiency (hemophilia B), for whom there is no other product that has factor IX in concentrated form. It is obviously also suited to patients who need rapid reversal of the effects of vitamin K antagonists. Its detrimental effects are the high risk of transmitting hepatitis and HIV infection, but the latter has probably also been eliminated by production methods using controlled heating. This product had an unusual additional problem; some lots caused a high incidence of serious thromboembolic events, especially with rapid infusion after injury.

Platelets are prepared in each blood bank or regional blood center as needed because platelets cannot be stored for more than a few days. Most of the time, platelets are used in "packs" containing the platelets from a single donor in 30 to 50 ml. plasma. The number of platelets recovered varies with the techniques used, and it is well to contact periodically the local source as to the average concentration of platelets in their products. It is highly advisable to measure the platelet concentration in the recipient's blood several times after infusion (1 and 24 hours are useful) to determine the immediate response to the infused platelets and their persistence after infusion. The effect of infusing platelets varies with the hemostatic status of the patient. Infection, fever, previous infusion of platelets, an enlarged spleen, active bleeding, and large wounds are all associated with a less-than-expected response to infused platelets. The prophylactic use of platelets, that is, giving platelets to prevent possible bleeding, is a very uncertain area.

RED BLOOD CELLS

The most common indication for transfusing red cells is to increase the recipient's mass of red cells. Transfused red cells are removed from the circulation in two ways: rapid (within 24 hours) removal of dead or damaged red cells (should be less than 25 per cent of transfused cells), and removal of the remainder at the normal rate as they reach senescence. Transfused red cells are thus only a temporary supplement to the recipient's supply. The oxygen-carrying capacity of the blood is an important, but not the only, component of the oxygen-delivering system, and it is not the only one altered by transfusion. The relationship between hematocrit and oxygen delivery is complex. The oxygen content of blood varies directly and linearly with changes in the hematocrit, but the resistance of blood to flow varies inversely and complexly with changes in the hematocrit. There is, moreover, a marvelously efficient compensatory mechanism within the red cells themselves, the alteration of the affinity of hemoglobin for oxygen by the synthesis of 2,3-diphosphoglyceric acid (2,3-DPG). At maximal production of 2,3-DPG, human red cells can nearly double their efficiency as oxygen-delivering agents under physiologic conditions at the cost of consumption of a bit more glucose.

Anemic patients who are stable and doing well should be allowed to replace their own red cell mass. The key should be individualization, with emphasis on how the patient is tolerating the anemia and what challenges are confronted before endogenous correction can occur. The too common practice of using a single trigger for transfusing all patients, commonly a hematocrit of 30 per cent, is to be firmly condemned. There is no good evidence supporting such a practice, and by its very nature it is unscientific and clinically harmful.

HAZARDS OF TRANSFUSION

Infusing red cells of blood group A or B into a recipient lacking that blood group antigen is likely to produce acute intravascular hemolysis, which, then, often causes DIC and acute renal failure and death. The reverse problem also exists: if enough plasma products containing anti-A or anti-B are infused into a recipient whose red cells contain A or B, hemolysis also occurs although perhaps less explosively. In the United States, most hemolytic reactions caused by transfusion follow misidentification that occurs outside the blood bank. It is because of the gravity of such an error that most hospitals have somewhat elaborate and rigid requirements for identification of the recipient and confirmation of the product before infusion, usually by at least two individuals. These safeguards should not be bypassed. The other blood group antigens, including those of the Rh system, are usually clinically important only in patients who have been transfused previously or who have had multiple pregnancies, or who may become pregnant subsequent to transfusion.

The most frequent serious complication directly attributable to transfusion is the transmission of disease. Although many diseases have been transmitted by transfusion, the most important is hepatitis. The recent development of a method of identifying the most common form of transfusion-transmitted hepatitis should improve, but not eliminate, the hazards of transfusion. There is now a test for anti-HIV antibody that is applied to all blood donors at each donation. This has certainly lowered the incidence of transmission by transfusion but has not eliminated it. The problem here is that infectivity precedes the appearance of circulating antibodies.

Massive transfusion means the continuous rapid infusion of large amounts of blood. The term generally implies a total at least equal to the recipient's normal blood volume continuously infused over no more than 6 to 8 hours. Consideration of the degree of exchange that actually occurs during transfusion is pertinent to many of the potential metabolic and related problems that can arise after transfusion, especially to the problem of hemostatic breakdown.

Autologous transfusion, the return of the patient's own blood, occurs in two ways. Electively, the patient can be bled several days to weeks before operation and the blood stored for use then if needed. Several units of blood may safely be collected in most patients. Blood shed at operation or recovered from a variety of closed, sterile drainage systems can be processed by a variety of devices and reinfused as needed. The safest method involves washing the shed red cells and reinfusing them in a simple electrolyte solution, with avoidance of the potential problems from tissue factors or other contaminants.

7

METABOLISM IN SURGICAL PATIENTS: Protein, Carbohydrate, and Fat Utilization by Oral and Parenteral Routes
Josef E. Fischer, M.D.

Nutritional support is an important therapeutic adjunct to surgery. It has recently evolved from the first phase of unabashed enthusiasm to the second phase of critical evaluation. A third phase—nutritional pharmacology, in which specific nutrients may be used almost as drugs—is now making its appearance. In order to understand nutritional support, it is first essential to understand the requirements.

REQUIREMENTS

The requirements for protein and calories are, in general, well known, both at rest and corrected for activity and in certain disease states. Although it is possible to measure energy requirements by the use of various metabolic carts, that is, indirect bedside calorimetry, studies comparing estimations of caloric requirements by use of the Harris-Benedict equation* and various corrections with estimations by metabolic cart determinations and corrections for activity have revealed that the two are equally efficacious and similarly inaccurate. At baseline, most patients require 55 mg. of nitrogen per kg., or, as translated into amino acid equivalent, 1.75 gm. of protein equivalent per kg. per day, as a "safe" requirement. The conversion factor from milligrams of nitrogen to grams of protein is that for each 1 gm. of nitrogen there are 6.25 gm. of mixed protein. Caloric requirement is generally estimated at 30 to 35 calories per kg. per 24 hours. At rest, approximately 75 per cent of the caloric requirement is derived from fat, including much of the fuel upon which the viscera, such as liver and kidney, depend. Protein is responsible for approximately 15 per cent of the requirement for energy, and carbohydrate for an additional 10 per cent. In disease, particularly in sepsis, this changes. The percentage of calories derived from protein increases to between 15 and 20 per cent, but because the caloric requirement increases anywhere from 10 to 30 per cent in trauma, from 30 to 50 per cent in sepsis, and up to 100 per cent with severe burns, the absolute amount of protein subjected to proteolysis for

---

*Basal energy expenditure (BEE) = $66.5 + 13.7 W + 5.0 H - 6.8 A$ (male); $65.6 + 9.6 W + 1.7 H - 4.7 A$ (female); W is weight in kg., H is height in cm., and A is age in years.

See the corresponding chapter or part in the *Textbook of Surgery*, 14th edition, pp. 103–140, for a more detailed discussion of this topic, including a comprehensive list of references.

providing energy increases dramatically. The caloric requirement increases to at least 45 to 50 calories per kg. per 24 hours. There is controversy as to the equivalence of carbohydrate and fat in sepsis. Whereas it is generally agreed that carbohydrate and fat are equally efficacious as caloric sources in baseline conditions, it is still not clear whether fat is utilized under conditions of severe stress and/or sepsis, although fat is cleared normally in sepsis. In practice, given the available caloric sources in the United States, approximately 70 per cent of nonprotein calories will be derived from carbohydrate and the remainder from fat, usually in the form of a lipid emulsion if given parenterally, or long-chain and/or medium-chain triglycerides if given enterally. This differs from normal dietary practices in which approximately 50 per cent of the caloric intake is derived from fat.

THE NEED FOR NUTRITIONAL INTERVENTION: IDENTIFYING THE PATIENT AT RISK

This has long been a controversial area of nutritional support. Nutritional assessment, in which a host of parameters are measured, many of which are static and not functional, and many of which have little or nothing to do with risk, is being increasingly focused so that it is possible to identify the population at risk. This is complicated by the fact that malnutrition, in and of itself, does not place the patient at risk; indeed, in a severely malnourished population, there will be patients who will be at risk for sepsis or death (following operation, for example) and patients who will be otherwise perfectly normal. The defect is clearly immunologic, but one that has not yet been identified with certainty as to what the efferent arm is. However, over the past several years a number of studies have accumulated to enable identification of the patient at risk:

1. Those who have lost more than 15 per cent of their body weight over a 3- to 4-month period, or patients who are losing weight and who weigh less than 85 per cent of their ideal body weight.

2. Stable, well-hydrated patients with a serum albumin of less than 3 gm. per 100 ml.

Additional tests for identifying such patients include a true transferrin of less than 220 mg. per 100 ml. and anergy to injected (not applied as in commercially available skin test devices) cutaneous recall antigens. These two tests are confirmatory; they are not primary determinants of patients at risk.

If one includes all patients who have lost more than 15 per cent of their body weight, with a serum albumin of less than 3 gm. per 100 ml., about 60 per cent of these patients will be at risk for severe sepsis following operation. The other 40 per cent, however, will be perfectly normal. It is not yet possible to specifically identify all of such patients, but it is now possible to at least identify the group at risk. Two logit functions have been proposed:

From Mullen and co-workers:

$$PNI = 158 - 16.6\ ALB - 0.78\ \text{triceps skinfold} - 0.20\ TFN - 5.8\ DTH$$

where ALB = albumin (usually serum), PNI = prognostic nutritional index, and TFN = transferrin.

From Christou's work:

$$P\ |\ \text{death}\ | = 1/\{1 + e^{(-23.45 + 1.75*(ALB) + 0.3*(\ln[DTH\ score])}\}$$

where DTH = delayed cutaneous hypersensitivity (asterisk = multiplication).

NUTRITIONAL SUPPLEMENTATION

Over the past 5 to 10 years, there has been increased emphasis on the use of the gut as the route for nutritional supplementation, if it is available. There are a number of reasons for this. The first is that the gut is the natural portal of entry of nutrients, and the relationship of the gut and its portal circulation to the liver is critical in the liver's continued function, but more important is appreciation of the liver's role in continual uptake, processing, and storage, with release upon a hormonal or neural stimulation of nutrition. In addition, numerous recent studies have made clear that even in the postoperative state, it is only the stomach and the colon that are subject to ileus, but the small bowel is perfectly functional from the first postoperative day. New technology in terms of tubes that are easy to pass *per os* or *per naris* into stomach, duodenum, and small bowel, as well as the technique of percutaneous endoscopic gastrostomy and the frequent use of needle catheter and other jejunostomies at the time of operation, makes access to the gut much easier and safer.

Another reason for the increased use of the gut is the rediscovery of the gut mucosal barrier and the possible role of the breakdown of this barrier in advanced disease. In the absence of gut enteral intake, an atrophy of the gut wall occurs, and it may be that total parenteral nutrition (TPN) produces atrophy of the gut wall over and above that of the atrophy of disuse. This may be nutrient-related, or it may be secondary to the absence of putative gut peptide hormones released by specific nutrients or specific routes. The hypothesis that translocation of bacteria, or more likely their products, is causative of nonlocalized sepsis or contributory to multiple organ failure has excited a great deal of experimental work. It is appropriate to express a note of caution and to emphasize that at the present, translocation of bacteria has been implicated only in the hypermetabolism of burns and perhaps in some of the deleterious effects that follow shock. Malnutrition is not, in and of itself, an etiologic agent for increased translocation of bacteria or their products, and no study has shown any difference in outcome between identical feedings given enterally or parenterally. It remains a challenging hypothesis, but it is by no means proven.

Nutrition may be given in the stomach, small bowel, or

duodenum. For safety's sake, duodenal or direct enteral supplementation is preferred. Indeed, most of the mortality of a well-run enteral support program relates to intragastric feeding and sudden changes in gastric motility, with vomiting and aspiration as the cause of mortality. It is more convenient to give the nutrient material into the stomach, as the stomach can dilute hyperosmolar material by inhibiting gastric motility and delaying pyloric emptying until the material administered becomes iso-osmotic when transfer across the pylorus in the normal 2- to 4-ml. aliquots begins. The stomach, by nature of the larger tubes used for gastrostomy, lends itself more easily to a variety of feedings. If one is to utilize the duodenum or small bowel, the tubes are usually of necessity smaller, and a thinner, less viscous material is usually administered. Here one must be careful with osmolality. Administration of hyperosmolar material into the small bowel may cause diarrhea, which at times may cause serious complications such as dehydration, hypernatremia, and hyperosmolar nonketotic coma, since the small bowel cannot as easily render feedings iso-osmolar.

PARENTERAL NUTRITION

If the gut is not available or if, because of an intercurrent disease state such as peritonitis, the gut simply does not work, it is necessary to provide nutritional support by parenteral means. Although there are a few units that still practice the lipid system, that is, a form of parenteral nutrition in which the catheter(s) is placed in the arm and a 5 per cent dextrose/5 per cent amino acid solution is given with lipid in a Y connection, a limiting factor in experience has been the need for central access because of lack of veins. Central parenteral nutrition (or TPN, as it is known in the United States) has been the mainstay of nutritional support for the past 20 years. It is usually based on a hypertonic dextrose/amino acid mixture. The dextrose usually comprises 70 to 75 per cent of the patient's total caloric needs, the remainder being provided by lipid, usually in the form of a phosphatide emulsion. The theoretic limit for lipid administration in adults is 2 gm. per kg. per day, and in children it is higher, approximately 4 gm. per kg. per day. In practice, most units supply 25 to 50 per cent of the patient's caloric requirements as a lipid emulsion. Caution is required in the management of septic patients because it is not clear that lipid is utilized. Likewise, in patients with liver disease, there are some studies suggesting that use of lipid, although probably metabolized quite well, may cause increased hepatic encephalopathy.

Indications for parenteral nutrition are usually categorized as (1) those with proven efficacy as primary therapy, that is, the disease state is positively affected, altering the outcome; (2) those in which nutritional support is established, but efficacy not proved; and (3) those that are controversial or under intense study.

Parenteral Nutrition as Primary Therapy: Efficacy Shown

GASTROINTESTINAL-CUTANEOUS FISTULAS. By providing a means of nutritional support as well as bowel rest, the use of parenteral nutrition has increased the rate of spontaneous closure to 10 and 32 per cent in two large series. However, mortality, at least in these two institutions, did not decrease, but it is likely that mortality has decreased overall in institutions not accustomed to treating large numbers of fistulas; also, the surgeon is able to operate at his convenience and when the patient is ready.

RENAL FAILURE. TPN has decreased mortality in patients with renal failure. The solution utilized, whether essential amino acids alone with hypertonic dextrose or a more complete mixture, is a matter of controversy. It is the author's practice to use essential amino acids and hypertonic dextrose in patients in whom the need for dialysis, particularly hemodialysis, is not clear. Others may disagree.

THE SHORT BOWEL SYNDROME. Repeated small bowel resections for Crohn's disease and major enterectomy following mesenteric thrombosis are the two major causes of the short bowel syndrome. Since there is little alternative, there are no prospective randomized trials to emphasize what appears logical, that this is an efficacious form of therapy. Recent interest has focused on glutamine and other specific enterocyte fuels as perhaps aiding hypertrophy. Epidermal growth factor and other peptide hormones may also prove useful.

BURNS. The sharp decrease in mortality from burns from 1965 to the present is likely due at least in part to aggressive nutritional support. This is now performed largely through the gut, with the intravenous approach being used in patients who cannot tolerate gastrointestinal feedings.

HEPATIC FAILURE. It is now clear from a number of reviews that in patients with acute hepatic decompensation superimposed on chronic liver disease, decreased hepatic encephalopathy as well as (in some series) increased survival follows aggressive nutritional support with a modified amino acid solution. The solution generally used is a high branched chain amino acid–modified solution with 36 per cent of the amino acids being present as the branched chain amino acids—leucine, isoleucine, and valine—in equimolar amounts and with decreased aromatic amino acids. Improved outcome has been limited to those series in which the calories were supplied by glucose.

Parenteral Nutrition as Primary Therapy: Efficacy Not Shown

INFLAMMATORY BOWEL DISEASE. Parenteral nutrition is indicated in inflammatory bowel disease when the patient is unlikely to survive operation or does not wish to be operated upon. Approximately 75 per cent of patients subjected to parenteral nutrition for the purpose of forestalling operation will undergo surgical therapy within the next 15 months.

ANOREXIA NERVOSA. Restoration of lean body mass as well as repletion of protein in the central nervous system enables the patient to participate in psychotherapy.

Parenteral Nutrition as Supportive Therapy: Efficacy Shown

ACUTE RADIATION ENTERITIS OR CHEMOTHERAPY TOXICITY. There is no alternative but to support the patient with TPN while the gut heals.

Parenteral Nutrition as Supportive Therapy: Efficacy Probably Present

WEIGHT LOSS PRELIMINARY TO MAJOR SURGICAL THERAPY. The three questions that need to be asked concerning such perioperative therapy are now well established: (1) Can the group at risk be identified? This group (previously referred to) has lost 15 per cent or greater of their body weight, with a serum albumin of less than 3 gm. per 100 ml. (2) If so, can short-term parenteral nutrition alter the outcome? (3) If so, for how long should it be administered? A period of perioperative parenteral nutrition that is efficacious is thought to be between 5 and 7 days, probably tending closer to 7 days. If the patient is only moderately malnourished and parenteral nutrition is used, the incidence of non–catheter-related, presumably nosocomial infections is increased.

MALIGNANT DISEASE. This is an area of profound controversy dependent on whether one can block the use by the tumor of nutrients supplied. All agree that overfeeding probably is deleterious and probably increases tumor growth.

CARDIAC SURGERY. Patients with cardiac cachexia often have impaired cardiac function on a nutritional basis that is extraordinarily difficult to reverse; in the laboratory, reversal of cardiac cachexia requires approximately 4 to 6 weeks. No prospective randomized studies have suggested that TPN is useful in cardiac surgery.

RESPIRATORY FAILURE. Prolonged nutritional as well as respiratory support is logical. Nutritional needs must also be maintained in a vigorous treatment situation. Excessive glucose may contribute to excess carbon dioxide production, but this is rare.

Parenteral Nutrition as Supportive Therapy: Controversial Areas

CANCER. These patients may benefit from parenteral nutrition in a perioperative situation provided they are severely malnourished, as was previously suggested. There is little question that current formulations, and especially overfeeding, probably contribute to tumor growth. The challenge is to provide a more appropriate means of nutritional support, with respect to source, route, and the like, to make certain that the patient is nourished and not the tumor. At present, it is impossible to guarantee this.

SEPSIS. It is clear that preservation of lean body mass in sepsis is extraordinarily difficult owing to some recently described cytokines. However, the energy needs of the organism must be met. Branched chain amino acids, having been proposed as a source of energy, not going through glucose, and which may be efficacious when the oxidation of either fat or glucose is severely impaired, show a tendency of improving nutritional, but not clinical outcome in most seriously ill patients.

COMPLICATIONS OF PARENTERAL NUTRITION

Technical complications largely follow an attempt to pass a catheter through a crowded thoracic inlet. These complications decrease with experience, but even the most talented operator may have a complication. Sepsis is the most feared of catheter complications. It can be minimized to its present rate of less than 0.6 per cent with strict attention to catheter care.

Metabolic complications include hyperglycemia, which may be potentially lethal. The appearance of hyperglycemia in a patient who has been previously stable suggests that within 24 hours, sepsis will occur.

8

SURGICAL ASPECTS OF DIABETES MELLITUS

Olga Jonasson, M.D.

Diabetes mellitus is the result of a deficiency of insulin or resistance to the action of insulin, causing hyperglycemia. The major aim of therapy is consistent normoglycemia through diet, oral hypoglycemic agents, and exogenous insulin. Strict control of the blood glucose level is required for successful management of the diabetic surgical patient.

Insulin is produced in the beta cells of islets of Langerhans as proinsulin and a connecting peptide (C peptide). Glucose is the main stimulus for insulin release. Insulin acts through binding to insulin receptors followed by intracellular processes leading to peripheral glucose utilization. Glucagon, produced by the pancreatic alpha islet cells, is a counter-regulatory hormone that acts to promote glycogenolysis and hepatic gluconeogenesis. Diabetes is the result of failure of insulin production, deficiencies in binding of insulin, or intracellular defects in insulin action.

Diabetics have fasting blood glucose levels greater than 140 mg. per 100 ml. on at least two occasions or have abnormal glucose tolerance tests. Hyperglycemic patients must be appropriately treated for normalization of their blood glucose levels during any acute illness, stress, or operation. The classification of diabetes mellitus is given in Table 1. Hypoglycemia is a frequent complication of insulin administration especially in patients who do not eat properly. Hypoglycemic episodes must be suspected in all obtunded or neurologically impaired diabetic patients receiving insulin.

COMPLICATIONS

Diabetic patients are all at risk for the development of complications caused by hyperglycemia. The long-term complications of diabetes include blindness, neuropathy, renal failure, and accelerated advanced atherosclerosis.

METABOLIC COMPLICATIONS. The immediate effect of hyperglycemia is glucosuria and osmotic diuresis with dehydration. Absence of insulin promotes release of free fatty acids, which are metabolized in the liver to ketone bodies and appear in the plasma and urine. Electrolyte losses occur in the urine to buffer the ketone body acids. If uncorrected, the condition of diabetic ketoacidosis occurs—extreme hyperglycemia, ketosis, and acidosis (Table 2).

INFECTIONS. The most common site of infection in diabetics is the urinary tract. Pulmonary infections with common

See the corresponding chapter or part in the *Textbook of Surgery*, 14th edition, pp. 141–147, for a more detailed discussion of this topic, including a comprehensive list of references.

TABLE 1. Classification of Diabetes Mellitus

Type I	Insulin-dependent diabetes mellitus (also termed IDDM, previously termed juvenile onset diabetes)
	20 per cent of all diabetes mellitus
	Onset in childhood or adolescence
	Not obese
	Entirely dependent on exogenous insulin
	Prone to develop ketosis and acidosis
Type II	Non-insulin-dependent diabetes (also termed NIDDM, previously termed adult onset diabetes)
	Onset after age 30; patients are usually obese
	Not dependent on insulin; insulin levels may be normal or high; insulin resistance is common
	Not prone to ketosis or acidosis
Secondary Diabetes	
Pancreatic diabetes	Occurs with pancreatic insufficiency such as in chronic pancreatitis or hemochromatosis or after pancreatectomy
	Entirely insulin-dependent
	"Brittle"—no glucagon, exocrine insufficiency, poor food absorption
Hormonal excess diabetes	Increased insulin resistance due to excess corticosteroids or drugs such as thiazide diuretics
Drug-induced diabetes	

TABLE 2. Hyperglycemic Crises in the Surgical Patient

Symptoms	Signs	Laboratory Values
Diabetic Ketoacidosis		
Type I diabetic	Hypotension	Blood glucose >350 mg./100 ml.
Missed insulin doses	Hypothermia	
Vomiting	Kussmaul breathing	Arterial pH <7.3
Polyuria, polydipsia	Fruity odor	Elevated plasma ketones
Weakness	Mental status changes	
Blurred vision	Abdominal rigidity	NaHCO$_3$ <15 mEq./L.
Abdominal pain		Leukocytosis
		Osmols >300
Nonketotic Hyperosmolar Syndrome		
Type II diabetic	Obtundation or coma	Blood glucose >600 mg./100 ml.
Complicating medical illness	Severe dehydration	
	Oliguria	Osmols >330
Mental status changes	Urosepsis, pneumonia, congestive heart failure, or myocardial infarction	Arterial pH >7.3
		Elevated blood urea nitrogen, creatinine

organisms occur frequently and are associated with high mortality. Necrotizing cellulitis and fasciitis can occur especially in the perineal region of elderly male diabetics with urethral catheters (Fournier's gangrene). These polymicrobial infections with aerobic and anaerobic organisms must be treated with aggressive surgical débridement, colostomy, and systemic antibiotics.

NEUROPATHY AND THE DIABETIC FOOT. Peripheral neuropathy develops in both Type I and Type II patients (see Table 1) with long-standing diabetes and can affect autonomic as well as peripheral nerves. Most common is peripheral neuropathy of the feet and distal lower extremity with loss of sensation in the foot. Minor trauma and pressure points may develop into ulcers and deep infections in the foot. Infections with anaerobic organisms are especially virulent and must be treated with aggressive surgical débridement and drainage.

GASTROINTESTINAL AND CARDIAC NEUROPATHY. Autonomic neuropathy is associated with gastroparesis. Hypoglycemic episodes and poor diabetic control are common. Bethanecol, erythromycin, and metoclopramide are used to increase gastric motility, but surgical procedures have been ineffective. A neurogenic bladder is often present in diabetic patients. Intractable diarrhea and steatorrhea are advanced manifestations. Dysmotility may also occur in the esophagus. In diabetic patients with dysphagia, fiberoptic esophagoscopy is indicated for determining if candidiasis is present. Cardiac autonomic neuropathy is associated with postural hypoten-

---

TABLE 3. Preoperative Work-up of the Diabetic Patient

History
  Duration of diabetes; insulin, diet, or oral hypoglycemic therapy; episodes of diabetic ketoacidosis or hypoglycemia
  Complications; visual impairment, neuropathy, symptoms of renal or peripheral vascular disease
  History of heart disease; angina, congestive failure, myocardial infarction
  Drug history; antihypertensive drugs, calcium channel blockers, beta blockade, coronary vasodilators, diuretics
  Symptoms of infection at any site—urinary tract, lungs, skin and subcutaneous tissues, gums, feet, intra-abdominal

Physical Examination
  Ophthalmoscopy—the eye is the window to the kidney
  Blood pressure—often elevated
  Circulation—evidence of congestive failure or peripheral vascular insufficiency
  Neurologic examination—evidence of peripheral neuropathy, mental status evaluation
  Status of feet—ulcers, infection, sensation

Laboratory Evaluation
  Blood glucose, serum Na, K, and $NaHCO_3$ levels
  Renal function—proteinuria, blood urea nitrogen and creatinine
  Cardiac evaluation—electrocardiogram, radioisotope myocardial stress studies, possible coronary angiogram

TABLE 4. Insulin Preparations and Regimens

Preparation*	Peak	Duration
Rapid-acting—regular†	0.5–4 hours	5–7 hours
Semilente	4–6 hours	12–16 hours
Intermediate—NPH, Lente	4–12 hours	18–24 hours
Long-acting—PZI, Ultralente	18–24 hours	>36 hours

Regimens
1. Intermediate + regular (⅔ + ⅓) in A.M., 0.5 unit/kg. ideal body weight. Check blood glucose at 4–5 P.M. to regulate next day's dose.
2. Intermediate ⅔ in A.M. and ⅓ in P.M. plus supplemental regular for late A.M. or bedtime hyperglycemia. *Regular is never given at bedtime.*
3. Single small dose of intermediate in A.M. and 5–10 units subcutaneously before each meal.
4. CSII‡ with an open loop pump set at basal infusion of 1 unit per hour with 5–10 units bolus 15 minutes before each meal.

*Available as pork or beef extract, semisynthetic, or human recombinant.
†Only regular insulin can be administered intravenously.
‡CSII, continuous subcutaneous insulin infusion.

sion or hemodynamic instability during hemodialysis and a mild tachycardia.

DIABETIC NEPHROPATHY. Diabetic nephropathy occurs in approximately 40 per cent of Type I diabetics and many Type II diabetics. More than 15 years after the onset of diabetes, overt proteinuria appears (greater than 0.5 gm. per 24 hours, positive dipstick test). When overt proteinuria appears, median survival is reduced to 7 to 8 years. Poorly controlled diabetic patients are highly susceptible to the nephrotoxic effects of iodinated radiologic contrast agents.

ATHEROSCLEROSIS AND CORONARY ARTERY DISEASE. Vascular insufficiency is more prevalent in diabetic patients and together with a high frequency of foot infections

TABLE 5. Perioperative Management

Discontinue oral hypoglycemic agents 24 hours before operation.

Give no intermediate or long-acting insulin on the day of operation.

Nothing by mouth after midnight.

Start IV infusion of 5% dextrose in water or 5% dextrose in normal saline with 20 mEq. KCl/liter at 6 A.M. Run at 100–200 ml./hour.

Start second IV infusion of insulin, 25 units/250 ml. normal saline. Run 75 ml. through the IV tubing, then discard (to occupy protein-binding sites on tubing). Run at 1–2 units/hour via infusion pump.

Monitor blood glucose at 30-minute intervals until stable at 150–200 mg./100 ml.; then monitor hourly until patient is awake, every 4 hours until diet is resumed.

Convert to maintenance regimen when diet has resumed by giving 80% of previous day's total insulin, ⅔ as intermediate and ⅓ as regular. Adjust daily using blood glucose values (see Table 4).

and ulcers is responsible for a high rate of amputation of the lower extremity. In addition to large vessel occlusion, small arteries are diseased.

The principal threat to life of the diabetic patient is coronary artery disease. Mortality from an acute myocardial infarction is twice that in nondiabetics. The strong likelihood of significant coronary artery occlusive disease must be considered when surgical treatment of any diabetic patient is undertaken (see Table 3).

MANAGEMENT

The basic goal of management of diabetes is the consistent maintenance of a normal blood glucose. Most Type II diabetics respond well to dietary management alone. Type I and other insulin-dependent patients require daily insulin (Tables 4 and 5).

HYPOGLYCEMIA. Ten per cent of insulin-dependent (Type I) patients have one or more episodes of severe hypoglycemia each year, and hypoglycemia contributes to 3 to 6 per cent of premature deaths. Severe hypoglycemia should be treated by oral carbohydrates, but an unconscious patient requires an intravenous bolus of 20 ml. of 50 per cent glucose, repeated as necessary, and an intravenous infusion of 5 or 10 per cent dextrose until the blood sugar is above 100 mg. per 100 ml. and the patient is conscious.

HYPERGLYCEMIA. Diabetic patients who have infections

TABLE 6. Treatment of Hyperglycemic Crises in the Surgical Patient

Admit to intensive care unit.
Insert nasogastric tube.
Consider endotracheal intubation.
Institute cardiac monitoring including central venous pressure measurement or placement of a Swan-Ganz pulmonary artery catheter for hemodynamic monitoring.

Begin IV infusion of NS solution through large-bore catheter.
Base fluid requirements on hemodynamic and biochemical parameters. Plan on 5–10 liters of fluid for resuscitation.

Through a separate IV line begin insulin infusion using solution of 1 unit insulin/10 ml. NS. Discard first 75 ml. after running through the tubing. Give loading dose of 1–2 units/kg. and then infuse at 0.1 unit/kg./hour. Rate can be doubled if necessary.

Monitor blood glucose hourly. Goal is to reduce hyperglycemia by 100 mg./100 ml./hour. More rapid reduction is likely to cause cerebral edema.
When serum Na is ≥150 mEq./L., change IV fluids to 0.45% saline with 20 mEq. KCl/L. Monitor serum K closely.

When blood glucose is ≤250 mg./100 ml., reduce insulin infusion to 1–2 units/hour and change IV fluids to 5% dextrose in water with 20 mEq. KCl, at 50–100/hour.
Monitor serial 1:2 dilutions of patient's plasma for ketones, and continue to resuscitate with glucose-potassium-insulin solutions until reaction is negative (Acetest tablets).

or other acute illnesses and stress and insulin-dependent diabetics who have not had sufficient insulin may present with diabetic ketoacidosis. Non-insulin-dependent (Type II) diabetics develop nonketotic hyperosmolar hyperglycemia associated with coma. Since these patients are elderly and there is usually a serious underlying condition, the mortality for the nonketotic hyperosmolar syndrome is 50 per cent. Aggressive treatment with insulin is required (Table 6).

Replacement of the pancreatic beta cells by transplantation of the vascularized pancreas or isolated islets of Langerhans in Type I (insulin-dependent) patients is currently achieving an excellent patient survival (95 per cent in some centers) and fair graft success.

9

ANESTHESIA

Enrico M. Camporesi, M.D., and Mary Pawlinga, M.D.

HISTORICAL ASPECTS

The first public demonstration of a general anesthetic was on October 16, 1846, by Morton, a medical student and a practicing dentist, who anesthetized a young man with vapors of ether (sulfuric ether). The surgeon, J. Warren at the Massachusetts General Hospital, continued to use ether successfully in the next few days, and within 2 months ether anesthesia was provided in Paris and in London. The timing of the discovery was fortunate, since the surgical techniques had matured and the invasiveness of the procedures was increasing rapidly. The early days of research in anesthesiology were marked by a quest for an "ideal" anesthetic agent, with the hope of discovering an agent with high pharmacologic potency, total inertness, and high therapeutic safety. Whereas no single agent was ever discovered that approached these ideal properties, it was soon appreciated that other adjunctive therapeutic drugs such as narcotics, barbiturates, and tranquilizers, and later supplementation with muscle relaxants, would be very useful in combination with general anesthetics. Anesthetic requirements—analgesia, unconsciousness, muscle relaxation, and rapid emergence—are being approached today with a better understanding of the pharmacologic principles underlying quantitative pharmacology in man.

Pharmacokinetics of an active pharmacologic compound involves the study of transfer of drugs from the administration site into the blood, through the distribution in tissues, and ending in the elimination phase by metabolism or excretion. *Pharmacodynamics*, however, relates to drug concentration at the level of the active receptor where the drug is effective. Compartmental analyses were stimulated in the last 20 years from advances in analytical chemistry that were able to assign specific parametric values to components of drugs in different compartments. This development hallmarks a more rational administration of drugs in order to maximize their potency and minimize side effects.

CHOICE OF ANESTHETIC TECHNIQUE

Anesthetic techniques utilized today include general anesthesia, regional anesthesia, intravenous sedation, or a combination of general and regional techniques. Factors relating to the patient and the type of surgical therapy influence these choices. Patient factors include patient preference and prior

See the corresponding chapter or part in the *Textbook of Surgery*, 14th edition, pp. 148–163, for a more detailed discussion of this topic, including a comprehensive list of references.

anesthetic experience, age, coexisting diseases, pre-existing pathophysiologic changes, airway management, and probability of a "full stomach." Surgical factors include location and duration of the proposed surgical procedure, patient positioning during operation, elective versus emergency surgical procedures, and the skill and preference of the surgeon.

General Anesthesia

The objectives of general anesthesia are to render the patient unconscious and pain-free, to provide muscle relaxation, and to reduce or abolish autonomic reflexes during operation. This reversible process must be accomplished while respiratory and cardiovascular functions are preserved. Induction of general anesthesia rapidly is achieved by the use of inhalational or intravenous agents, which produce a selective depression of the central nervous system. Maintenance of general anesthesia is traditionally accomplished by the continuous use of inhalation agents. These include nitrous oxide (N_2O) and the halogenated agents: halothane, enflurane, and isoflurane.

NITROUS OXIDE. Nitrous oxide, the most widely used inhalation agent, is an odorless gas. It is relatively insoluble in blood, and this property causes it to produce rapid induction and recovery. It has low potency as an anesthetic agent and produces analgesia and amnesia at 50 and 80 per cent concentrations, respectively, but it requires higher concentrations for achieving a true anesthetic state. Such concentrations would produce hypoxic mixtures unless administered at higher than normal pressures. In fact, full anesthetic potency is displayed at environmental pressures greater than one atmosphere (1 ATA), when partial pressure of N_2O is raised to 1.05 ATA. Nevertheless, nitrous oxide is still popular because it enhances uptake of other inhalational agents while reducing dosage of coadministered inhalational and intravenous drugs. Fifty per cent nitrous oxide intrinsically depresses myocardial contractility. Activation of the sympathetic nervous system causes an increase in systemic vascular resistance. Nitrous oxide must be used with caution or not at all in the presence of pneumothorax, closed-loop intestinal obstructions, and operations with potential for air embolism because of the tendency of this gas to diffuse into and rapidly expand closed gas-filled spaces. Nitrous oxide indirectly interferes with the synthesis of DNA by inactivating the vitamin B_{12}–dependent enzyme methionine synthetase. Prolonged use of nitrous oxide may also cause bone marrow depression and neuropathies.

VOLATILE HALOGENATED VAPORS. In general, the volatile inhalational agents (halothane, enflurane, isoflurane) produce dose-dependent decreases in alveolar ventilation and ventilatory responses to hypercarbia and hypoxia. Volatile anesthetics produce bronchial smooth muscle relaxation and depression of airway reflexes. All three agents produce dose-dependent depression in central nervous system function as well as increases in cerebral blood flow (halothane > enflurane > isoflurane). High inspired concentrations of enflurane, especially when accompanied by low $Paco_2$, may produce epileptiform patterns by electroencephalography. Halothane and enflurane produce dose-dependent reductions in cardiac output; isoflurane produces only small decreases at concentrations greater than 1 minimum alveolar concentration (MAC). This relative maintenance of cardiac output may be due to a vagolytic effect of isoflurane as well as to its potent vasodilator ability. Halothane "sensitizes" the myocardium to epinephrine-induced ventricular dysrhythmias. All the volatile agents produce direct skeletal muscle relaxation, and they potentiate the action of nondepolarizing muscle relaxants.

Biotransformation of all volatile anesthetics occurs in the liver by the action of cytochrome P-450 enzymes. Twenty per cent of an administered dose of halothane is metabolized through this enzymatic pathway. It has been hypothesized that the reductive metabolites of halothane may be responsible for postoperative elevation of liver transaminases, or "halothane hepatitis," a syndrome that may rarely progress to overt symptoms, probably in association with marked reduction in hepatic blood flow. Two per cent of enflurane is biotransformed into fluoride ions, which have a potential for nephrotoxicity. Isoflurane, however, is very stable and undergoes only minimum biotransformation (0.17 per cent).

MAC, a qualitative parameter that measures anesthetic potency, is the minimal alveolar concentration of anesthetic, in percentage of one atmosphere pressure, that prevents skeletal muscle movement in response to a noxious stimulus in 50 per cent of patients. This index of anesthetic potency correlates well with lipid solubility. The MAC of nitrous oxide, halothane, enflurane, and isoflurane is, respectively, 104, 0.75, 1.68, and 1.15.

INTRAVENOUS AGENTS. Intravenous agents used for induction of anesthesia include ultra–short-acting barbiturates (thiopental, thiamylal, methohexital), ketamine, benzodiazepines (diazepam, midazolam), propofol, and narcotics (morphine, meperidine, fentanyl, sufentanil, alfentanyl).

Barbiturates are highly lipid-soluble and produce a rapid onset of hypnosis in less than 1 minute, which is of short duration (several minutes). The rapid emergence from a single intravenous induction dose (3 to 5 mg. per kg. in the adult) is attributed to redistribution of the drug from the "vessel-rich" group of organs (e.g., brain and heart) to other body compartments (e.g., skeletal muscle and fat). Elimination half-life of thiopental via biotransformation and excretion requires several hours. Barbiturates do not produce analgesia or skeletal muscle relaxation. They are potent cerebral vasoconstrictors and may produce brain protection by lowering intracranial pressure and by reducing the oxygen consumption of the brain. Respiration is depressed. Myocardial depression, vasodilation, and a reflex increase in heart rate occur as a result of thiopental administration.

Ketamine is a phencyclidine derivative that produces "dissociative anesthesia," i.e., a dissociation of the state of consciousness. This is similar to a cataleptic state with profound analgesia and increased skeletal muscle tone. Ketamine increases heart rate and blood pressure by stimulation of the sympathetic nervous system. It is therefore a favored induction technique in hypovolemic patients or children with congenital heart defects. Ketamine intrinsically depresses the myocardium; therefore, caution must be taken in the hypovolemic patient if sympathetic reserves are exhausted because profound hypotension results. Caution should also be taken in using ketamine in patients with coronary artery disease or cerebral aneurysm in whom an increase in heart rate and blood pressure is not desired. Ketamine may also be used as an induction agent in patients with asthma because of its potent bronchodilator effects.

Benzodiazepines produce anxiolysis, skeletal muscle relaxation, anterograde amnesia, and anticonvulsant effects. In larger doses, they induce anesthesia. Benzodiazepines produce minimal reductions in blood pressure and cardiac output. Respiratory depression may occur when large doses are used. Metabolism of the benzodiazepines occurs in the liver. Midazolam is a water-soluble agent with a relatively short duration of action (elimination half-life less than 3 hours). This is in contrast to diazepam, which is water-insoluble, is available as an oily solution, and may be painful on injection. The duration of diazepam action is longer, since its elimination half-life may be as long as 40 hours, especially in the elderly, and since some of its metabolites are pharmacologically active.

Propofol, a di-ortho-substituted phenol, is an intravenous hypnotic agent that may be used for the induction and maintenance of anesthesia. Hypnosis is produced within 40 seconds of an intravenous dose of propofol, with recovery within 8 minutes owing to rapid distribution from the brain to less well perfused tissues. The most significant hemodynamic effect of propofol is a 20 per cent decrease in blood pressure. Respiratory depression is also produced with propofol. Because it has a faster recovery time than thiopental, benzodiazepines, and ketamine, propofol may be the induction agent of choice in healthy patients, especially in the setting of outpatient surgical procedures.

Narcotics may be used as adjuvant agents in anesthesia, or, when administered in large doses, as primary anesthetics. Narcotics produce their analgesic effect by interacting with opioid receptors in the spinal cord and brain. With the exception of meperidine, narcotics by themselves do not produce direct myocardial depression. Addition of a benzodiazepine or nitrous oxide may cause decreases in blood pressure and cardiac output. Narcotics are able to suppress the "stress response" to anesthesia and surgical procedures by decreasing central sympathetic outflow of catecholamines. Histamine-induced decreases in systemic vascular resistance are seen with rapid injection of morphine and meperidine but not with the newer synthetic opioids (fentanyl, sufentanil, alfentanil). Bradycardia is produced by central vagal stimulation in all the narcotics with the exception of meperidine.

Dose-dependent respiratory depression occurs secondary

to narcotic depression of the medullary ventilatory center. Rapid intravenous injection of large doses of narcotics may produce skeletal muscle rigidity, especially chest wall rigidity, which may impair ventilation. Rigidity is treated intraoperatively with a muscle relaxant. Other effects of narcotics include nausea and vomiting through the stimulation of the medullary chemoreceptor trigger zone, biliary tract spasm, urinary retention, and constipation. High-dose narcotics have become the mainstay of cardiac anesthesia as well as being part of a "balanced" anesthetic when used in smaller doses. Fentanyl is 80 to 100 times as potent as morphine, with an elimination half-life of about 220 minutes. Sufentanil is more receptor-specific and is 5 to 10 times as potent as fentanyl with an elimination half-life of about 150 minutes. Alfentanyl is one third as potent as fentanyl with an extremely short duration of action secondary to its short elimination half-life of 70 to 90 minutes. Because the effects of these drugs on the body are similar, the choice of one narcotic over the other is based on their onset and duration of action.

When the induction is completed, patency of the airway must be managed by mask ventilation or by endotracheal intubation. General anesthesia can now be maintained in one of several ways. Inhalational agents can be continued with their concentrations adjusted according to the degree of surgical stimulation. A nitrous oxide/oxygen/relaxant/narcotic, or "balanced" technique, utilizes individual agents to provide separately for the objectives of general anesthesia (hypnosis, muscle relaxation, analgesia, and blunting of sympathetic responses to operative procedures). More commonly, a combination of these techniques is used for maintenance of general anesthesia. For example, a baseline concentration of volatile inhalational agent can be added to a "balanced" technique.

MUSCLE RELAXATION. Muscle relaxation is accomplished by the use of agents that exert their effect on the neuromuscular junction through either a depolarizing or nondepolarizing blockade. Succinylcholine, which is structurally similar to two molecules of acetylcholine (ACh), is an example of a depolarizing agent that binds to ACh receptors located on the muscle end plate of a neuromuscular synapse, causing depolarization of the end plate and accommodation (inexcitability) of the adjacent muscle membrane. This blockade ends when succinylcholine diffuses away from the receptor and is hydrolyzed by pseudocholinesterase, an enzyme commonly found in liver and plasma.

Nondepolarizing muscle relaxants competitively bind to ACh receptors and block them from interacting with ACh. Thus, the neuromuscular blockade can be reversed by increasing the concentration of ACh at the receptor sites and thereby displacing the muscle relaxant. This reversal is accomplished by intravenous administration of an anticholinesterase (neostigmine, pyridostigmine, or edrophonium) to increase the concentration of ACh, usually combined with an anticholinergic (atropine or glycopyrrolate) to block the muscarinic effects of ACh.

Examples of nondepolarizing agents are d-tubocurarine

(dTC) metocurine, atracurium, vecuronium, and pancuronium. Nondepolarizing agents also redistribute away from the synapse and, with the exception of atracurium, which is mainly catabolized via spontaneous breakdown of the molecule (Hoffman elimination) and ester hydrolysis, are all excreted by the kidneys and/or bile. Over 70 per cent elimination of a dose of pancuronium and metocurine, and over 50 per cent of dTC is through the kidneys. These agents also undergo some hepatic metabolism and excretion through the bile. Conversely, 80 per cent of a dose of vecuronium is dependent on the biliary tract for excretion. It is therefore obvious that the choice of muscle relaxant is tempered by the desired onset and duration of action and the presence of coexisting renal or hepatic diseases. The degree of neuromuscular blockade should be monitored by a peripheral nerve stimulator.

Emergence from general anesthesia is produced by a resolution of activity of the agents used for induction and maintenance of anesthesia. Inhalational agents are exhaled out of the body or metabolized as discussed in the preceding text; the fixed intravenous agents are redistributed or metabolized; and nondepolarizing muscular blockade usually requires pharmacologic reversal. Extubation of the trachea is usually accomplished when the patient is awake and responsive and able to protect the airway while supporting adequate ventilation. Supplemental oxygen is commonly administered in the early recovery period for support of oxygenation during awakening.

Regional Anesthesia

Regional anesthesia involves blockade of afferent nerve impulses in selected regions of the body and consists of major conduction blockade (spinal and epidural anesthesia) and peripheral nerve blockade (plexus, individual nerves). Local anesthetics are the agents used for reversibly binding to sodium channels of the nerve membranes, thereby inhibiting sodium conductance and development of action potential propagation across the nerve membrane. Because local anesthetics are weak bases and are available as hydrochloride salts, they are able to exist in an un-ionized (free base) or ionized (cationic) form. Both forms are necessary to block conduction. The uncharged form penetrates the nerve membrane so that the charged form may bind internally to the sodium receptor for achieving impulse blockade. Structurally, the local anesthetic consists of a lipophilic unsaturated benzene ring separated from a hydrophilic amine group by an intermediate chain. This intermediate chain confers anesthetic potency and contains either an ester or amide link. Thus, local anesthetics are divided into two categories, the amino-esters (procaine, tetracaine, chloroprocaine) or the amino-amides (lidocaine, mepivacaine, bupivacaine, etidocaine). The difference between ester and amide anesthetics lies in the way they are metabolized and in their potential for an allergic-type reaction. Ester agents are hydrolyzed by plasma cholinesterases, with a principal metabolite, para-aminobenzoic acid (PABA), being capable of eliciting an allergic reaction in selected individuals. Allergic reactions to amide agents, which are metabolized by hepatic microsomal enzymes, are extremely rare.

Spinal anesthesia is achieved by injection of a local anesthetic into the intrathecal space. The onset, duration, and spread of spinal anesthesia is directly related to the dosage of the agent. Duration also depends on the particular agent used. Vasoconstrictors prolong the duration of a local agent. Cardiovascular toxicity may be treated with intravenous fluid boluses, atropine for bradycardia, and vasopressors (ephedrine, phenylephrine, epinephrine), depending on the degree of circulatory collapse. Extracorporeal bypass has been used for support of patients in cardiac arrest from bupivacaine toxicity who were unresponsive to cardiopulmonary resuscitation.

Absolute contraindications for regional anesthesia include lack of patient consent, known allergy to the anesthetic agent, and infection at the site of needle insertion. Anticoagulation is a relative contraindication for spinal and epidural anesthesia because of the possibility of an epidural hematoma compressing and compromising the spinal cord perfusion.

Intravenous sedation, including benzodiazepines, barbiturates, or narcotics, can be utilized to complement a regional technique or a local anesthetic infiltration by the surgeon. Significantly, a combination of narcotics and benzodiazepines may cause hypotension, complicating an otherwise successful analgesic block.

MONITORING OF THE ANESTHETIZED PATIENT

The high potency of modern anesthetic agents requires periodic or continuous assessment of physiologic parameters. The primary intent of monitoring was linked historically to the measurement of depth of surgical anesthesia, whereby the respiratory rate, cardiac rate, and pupillary reflexes were utilized to establish the depth of anesthesia with powerful inhalational agents. Currently, with the increasing custom of controlling cardiac rate with drugs and ventilation with the aid of a mechanical ventilator, the emphasis of monitoring has shifted to maintenance of a physiologic range of values from the preoperative time, through the operation, toward the postoperative recovery period.

Physiologic monitoring is today becoming a standard of medical practice during general anesthesia. In addition to inspection of the patient's color and assessment of pulse, it is customary to use a continuous electrocardiographic display, a blood pressure measurement, usually indirectly with a cuff device, automatic temperature probes, and a precordial or esophageal stethoscope through which the anesthesiologist is constantly in contact with cardiac sounds and respiratory sounds. Also becoming universal is the use of an oxygen analyzer in the inspired limb of the anesthesia machine for assurance that patients are not exposed to hypoxic gas mixtures, together with finger pulse oximetry for verification of a satisfactory saturation of peripheral blood. Additional specialized monitoring may be required in various conditions, which have been rapidly defined from the experience obtained in the critical care area. Ventilation is usually assessed with the supplemental help of specialized monitoring, including serial arterial blood gas measurements, end-tidal carbon dioxide monitoring, spirometry, and/or mass-spectrometry of inspired and exhaled gases. This provides a satisfactory quantitation of anesthetic vapors, which are often used in concentrations well below 1 per cent.

The *cardiovascular system* of the symptomatic patient is monitored with specialized equipment to record the electrocardiogram, often with analysis of the ST segment for signs of myocardial ischemia, as well as a continuing indwelling catheter for peripheral arterial and pulmonary arterial pressures. These measures can often provide periodic or continuous assessment of cardiac output during anesthesia. *Central nervous system activity* is often monitored by electroencephalographic analysis, which is compressed and displayed in rapidly readable frequency domains. Additionally, evoked potential and muscular relaxation depth can be measured by nerve stimulators. *Renal function* is usually monitored through urine collection from a bladder catheter in order to quantify urinary flow and osmolarity. Temperature can be monitored at a variety of sites, usually in the esophagus or rectum, but occasionally in other cavities.

In recent years, careful analysis of major anesthetic mishaps has revealed that in about half of major anesthetic catastrophes, human error constitutes a significant component of the problem. This has originated increasing utilization of simulators for anesthetic administration in the training of anesthesiologists, similar to flight-simulators utilized in the training of pilots.

PREOPERATIVE ASSESSMENT

The American Society of Anesthesiologists (ASA) has provided a graded scale into which all patients are assessed before anesthesia. This scale summarizes the significance of the patient's illness before anesthesia and, in addition, describes the level of emergency assessed before operation. In general, this simplified algorithm correlates well with complications and patient outcome.

- ASA I are healthy individuals with no systemic disease undergoing elective surgery. This comprises all patients not at extremes of age, usually less than 1 year and over 70 years of age.
- ASA II are individuals with one systemic disease, well controlled to the level of not affecting daily activities. Other anesthetic risk factors, such as mild obesity and smoking, can be incorporated at this level.
- ASA III comprises individuals with multiple system disease or well-controlled major systemic diseases. In

this group, the physical status limits daily activity; however, there is no immediate danger of death from any individual disease.

- ASA IV comprises individuals with severe incapacitating disease, normally poorly controlled or at end stage. The danger of death due to organ failure is always present.
- ASA V comprises patients in imminent danger of death and in whom operation may be a last resorted attempt at preserving life. All ASA grade patients might in addition be defined by the emergency (E) of the procedure, although it has been argued that ASA V patients can never undergo elective surgery by definition.

When an appreciation of the anesthetic risk for each patient is reached, a preoperative assessment requires a brief general physical examination, including

1. neurologic function, from cranial nerves to peripheral reflexes, especially in patients in whom regional anesthesia is contemplated;

2. airways—this is an essential area that can prevent the difficulty of management in subsequent times; in this category, poor dentition, loose teeth, short neck, abnormality of neck and mandibular motion, trismus, deviated trachea, neck masses, and macroglossia are added;

3. pulmonary examination comprising a smoking history, the presence of asthma, productive cough, chronic chest disease, acute dyspnea, and determination of blood gases at rest and pulmonary function tests if indicated;

4. cardiovascular assessment, with presence of symptoms of cardiac or peripheral vascular disease, hypertension, recent myocardial infarction, and angina;

5. renal examination, with an assessment of chronic renal disease and acute problems; this should guide in the management of intraoperative fluid balance;

6. pharmacologic history comprising a full list of current medication and all known allergies; this should extend to a medication plan for continuance of essential drugs during the perioperative period.

Preoperative evaluation provides an important opportunity for physicians to gain the patient's confidence and to reduce perioperative morbidity. This is accomplished by optimizing preoperative status and by planning the anesthetic management in the recovery period. With the present changing practice of anesthesia, new constraints are imposed on surgical practice by the limited time available for assessment of patients for operative procedures. The attempt to maximize the preoperative diagnostic screening of the patient by ordering a battery of laboratory tests, however, has proved inefficient when a proper history and rational assessment are not elicited. It has been demonstrated that unnecessary testing causes additional risk to the patient, inefficiency in operating room scheduling, and unnecessary costs to society.

History and physical examination remain the best measures for screening for disease. An additional measure of proven efficacy is the utilization of patient questionnaires. This usually allows selection of appropriate laboratory tests and requests for consultation from other specialist physicians.

POSTOPERATIVE CARE

After emergence from general anesthesia, the postoperative period is characterized by multiple physiologic and pharmacologic changes. These include re-establishment of function for the renal, hepatic, and neurologic systems, and the return of protective reflexes. Postoperative surveillance has been developed from the establishment of procedures and protocols for the prevention of vomiting, aspiration, dysrhythmias, and sudden cardiac death; today it is extended to obtain complete self-protection such that the patient can be discharged to a general ward situation. The most stringent observation is necessary at this time for the avoidance of anesthetic and surgical complications.

Anesthetic Complications

The major difficulty in assessing the patient's postoperative recovery resides in attempting to define an adequate scale for assessment of recovery progress. No absolute scales exist, but a postanesthesia recovery score (PARS) introduced by Aldrete has provided impetus to analyze this period. Based on motor performance, respiratory and hemodynamic stability, and level of consciousness in a manner similar to the Apgar score of the neonate, the PARS system enables recovery room staff nurses to qualify recovery for an individual patient; in some instances, the system enables comparison of anesthetic techniques and recovery, both in quality and in duration of the process. In addition, patient temperature, which is often subtly abnormal, must be monitored, especially after long surgical procedures with peripheral attending vasoconstriction.

Surgical Complications

Postsurgical care may comprise assessment of complications, like potential hemorrhage in key areas such as following thyroidectomy and after major vascular surgery; surveillance for intra-abdominal hemorrhage; and acute pain management.

SURGICAL INTENSIVE CARE UNIT. Initially an extension of the postanesthesia recovery room, surgical intensive care units have acquired responsibility distinct from the recovery room. Although the operating room provides most admissions to this area, the unit also is utilized for preoperative stabilization and as a diagnostic and resuscitative area following trauma and sepsis. The postcardiac surgical intensive care unit provides an example of further development, as do postneurosurgical intensive care and pediatric intensive care units. The common denominator characterizing all intensive care areas is specialized nursing service with highly motivated and continually updated nursing staff, continuous in-unit physician surveillance, ready access to all hospital services including respiratory therapy, diagnostic radiology, and a designated medical director who provides continuity of care and coordination of resident instruction among different hospital services.

OUTPATIENT ANESTHESIA

The progress provided in recovery management by the increasing field of outpatient anesthesia is represented by the requirement for a rapid recovery and the criterion for street-fitness to be reached by patients before discharge. A variety of anesthetic agents and techniques have been recommended for outpatient anesthesia, demonstrating that no uniform anesthetic for this type of operation is prescribed. Surgical procedures requiring frequent utilization of powerful narcotics or major intravenous fluid administration are by definition inappropriate for outpatient surgery. Discharge criteria often include verification by a physician of the present status of the patient, stable vital signs, return of protective reflexes including cough and swallow, ability to ambulate, absence of airway or respiratory problems and of major cardiac arrhythmias, and status of consciousness such that the patient is fully awake and oriented in time and place with minimal nausea and vomiting and absence of acute pain. This comprises a well-planned program for continuing analgesic care at home. The most frequent complications following outpatient anesthesia and operative procedures are sore throat, headache, nausea and vomiting, pain, bleeding, croup, and slow emergence. Although life-threatening complications are rare, hospital admission criteria should be formulated to address these complications. Maintenance of high standards of safety in this setting will be the mainstay for its continuing success.

10

WOUND HEALING: Biologic and Clinical Features
Ronald J. Weigel, M.D.

Surgical techniques are based on the response of living tissues to injury, and familiarity with the healing process forms the primary basis for surgical decisions. Decisions concerning the type of suture used, when to place a drain, and when to remove sutures are not arbitrary but are based on a thorough knowledge of normal and abnormal healing processes.

BIOLOGIC CONSIDERATIONS

When living tissue is injured, the organism responds with a complex system of cellular and physiologic processes termed wound healing. Humans for the most part have lost the ability to regenerate tissue architecture following injury. Except for a few circumstances (e.g., liver regeneration), injured tissue heals by a process of scar formation, which is remarkably similar for a variety of tissue injuries. The cellular response to a surgical incision or to a myocardial infarction is replacement of necrotic tissue with a scar. For illustrative purposes it is best to consider the healing response to a surgical incision. Clinically, incisions can be simple closed wounds or open wounds with or without tissue loss.

Closed Wounds

Wound healing is a dynamic process that begins at the time of injury and persists for months to years after injury. Although the response to injury is an integrated process, wound healing will be approached in several components.

INFLAMMATION. The inflammatory phase initiates the process of wound healing. After initial vasoconstriction, vessels dilate, capillaries become permeable to plasma proteins, and white cells adhere to the endothelium of small venules and migrate through the vessel wall. Within several hours, the wound becomes filled with an inflammatory exudate composed of white cells, red cells, plasma proteins, and fibrin strands.

Substances released by tissue injury serve as mediators of the inflammatory process. Histamine liberated from mast cells, granulocytes, and platelets causes vasodilation and increased vessel permeability. The effects of histamine, however, are limited to short periods of time (less than 30

See the corresponding chapter or part in the *Textbook of Surgery*, 14th edition, pp. 164–177, for a more detailed discussion of this topic, including a comprehensive list of references.

minutes). More recent work indicates that the *kinins* and *prostaglandins*, especially PGE_1 and PGE_2, are mediators of the inflammatory response. Kallidin and bradykinin are released from alpha$_2$-globulin of plasma by the enzymatic action of kallikrein found in plasma and granulocytes. The kinins and components of the complement system induce local cells to release prostaglandins. The kinins, prostaglandins, and components of the complement system act as mediators of the inflammatory response to increase vessel permeability and as chemotactic factors for inflammatory cells.

Leukocytes invade the wound and begin to engulf cell debris and bacteria. Initially, polymorphonuclear leukocytes predominate, but these short-lived cells are replaced by monocytes, which can continue their scavenging activity for weeks. Monocytes are also needed for a normal fibroblast response. The duration of the inflammatory phase depends on the extent of tissue injury. For a clean incision, the inflammatory phase lasts a few days. Extensive tissue necrosis, infection, or foreign bodies can prolong the inflammatory phase for months.

EPITHELIALIZATION. At the edge of epithelial wounds, basal epithelial cells begin to divide and migrate across the defect. Fibrin strands serve as a scaffold upon which the epithelial cells migrate. Within 48 hours of injury, the wound surface is re-epithelialized. After covering the wound surface, epithelial cells differentiate, and the surface cells keratinize. The epithelial-mesenchymal interface does not regain a normal architecture, and the re-epithelialized skin is *void of sweat glands and hair follicles.*

CELLULAR PHASE. On approximately the third day following injury, fibroblasts begin to appear and capillary proliferation is evident. Monocytes present during the inflammatory phase aid in causing the appearance of fibroblasts. Most wound fibroblasts are derived from the adventitia of blood vessels. Fibroblasts migrate into the wound, using fibrin strands as a scaffold. Endothelial cells from blood vessels undergo rapid mitosis, lose their attachments to the basement membrane, and migrate into the area of injury. These migratory endothelial cells establish a network of small vessels. Endothelial cells synthesize many enzymes, including collagenases, plasmin, and plasminogen activator, which lyse the fibrin network.

Fibroblasts synthesize collagen fibers, which begin to appear in the wound by 4 days. Initially, collagen is present as randomly oriented protein fiber bundles, but these enlarge to produce a dense collagenous structure (scar). The rate at which a wound gains strength is directly related to the rate of collagen formation. Wound strength is measured as either tensile strength (force per cross-sectional area at rupture) or burst strength (force required to break a wound). Although the burst strength of wounds of eyelid skin and back skin are different because of their thickness, their tensile strengths are comparable. Two days after injury, the burst strength of rat skin reaches 50 to 100 gm. per linear centimeter. After the appearance of collagen on the third day, strength increases rapidly, reaching over a kilogram per linear centimeter by 3 weeks. Wounds gain strength at a relatively constant rate for approximately 4 months; however, strength continues to increase at a slower rate for over a year.

Open Wounds

Although open wounds heal by a process identical to that of closed wounds, certain clinically important differences exist. Open wounds heal by secondary intention in which epithelialization and wound contraction have a greater role than for closed wounds (primary intention healing). The *major* differences between primary and secondary intention healing are shown in Table 1. After several days, an open wound fills with granulation tissue composed of inflammatory cells, ground substance, fibroblasts, and budding capillaries, which give granulation tissue its reddish appearance. Open wounds close by a process of wound contraction. Even impressive abdominal wounds can contract to a thin linear scar. The ultimate appearance of an open wound can be estimated by reapproximating the wound edges. Sutures used to close a wound perform the role of normal wound contraction.

The force of wound contraction is derived from living cells. Although some debate has existed, the force of wound contraction has now been established to be generated by a modified fibroblast (myofibroblast) that has characteristics of fibroblasts and smooth muscle cells. Contraction can be minimized by replacing missing skin immediately with thick skin grafts or pedicle flaps. Thin split-thickness skin grafts partially inhibit contraction. In areas of fixed tissues, maximal contraction may not be able to close large defects. Epithelialization can close defects of 1 to 2 cm., but larger defects may become a chronic open ulcer. Over long periods of time, these areas can develop a highly malignant form of squamous cell carcinoma, probably owing to the chronic proliferative stimulus of epithelial cells. Adequate coverage with a graft can prevent malignant transformation.

Factors Affecting Wound Healing

Patients who are malnourished heal wounds poorly, although the mechanism for this remains obscure. Protein

TABLE 1. Comparison of Primary and Secondary Intention

Primary Intention Healing	Secondary Intention Healing
Minimal tissue loss or necrosis	Tissue necrosis present
Usually sterile	Often infected
Rapid healing	Slow healing
Maintenance of normal tissue architecture	Healing by granulation and scar formation
Minimal wound contraction (performed by sutures)	Wound closes by wound contraction
Minimal re-epithelialization	Re-epithelialization of areas not able to close by contraction

depletion delays wound healing in animal studies; however, this effect appears unrelated to collagen synthesis. Vitamin C deficiency has profound effects on collagen synthesis, especially when rapid synthesis is required. Relatively small amounts of vitamin C correct this abnormality. Vitamin A deficiency also has been implicated in delayed wound healing, but again the mechanism is unclear. Experimental studies have shown that supplemental vitamin A can prevent radiation-induced defects in wound healing. Zinc is a cofactor in many metabolic enzymes, and a deficiency retards epithelialization and gains in strength.

Poor tissue oxygenation has clearly been shown to delay wound healing. Wounds occurring in the presence of peripheral vascular disease and wounds in poorly vascularized areas heal more slowly. Decreased oxygen delivery has been used for explaining delayed wound healing in the presence of anemia, but this has been more difficult to prove conclusively. Hemodialysis has been shown to decrease subcutaneous oxygen tension, and this probably is responsible for increased wound morbidity seen in hemodialysis patients.

Steroids *markedly* delay the rate of wound healing, cortisone decreases the rate of protein synthesis, stabilizes lysosomal membranes, and inhibits the normal inflammatory response. In large doses, it also inhibits neovascularization, fibroblast proliferation, and the rate of epithelialization.

Radiation therapy can delay wound healing in the area of irradiation. Most antimetabolic chemotherapeutic agents (e.g., 5-fluorouracil, thio-TEPA) do not delay wound healing when given in standard clinical doses. Doxorubicin (Adriamycin) has been shown to decrease the rate of healing, and its use should be delayed until approximately 4 weeks postoperatively.

WOUND CARE

Because normal wound healing requires cellular metabolism, healing tissue must be provided adequate perfusion. Gross changes in tissue perfusion may be due to shock (hypovolemia, vasoconstriction, reduced flow states). More subtle decreases in perfusion to healing tissue may be due to drying of exposed tissue, which can kill surface cells and alter normal blood flow in small vessels. Sutures placed under tension can cause ischemia at wound edges.

Alcohol, iodine, and povidone are commonly used for skin preparation with little effect on intact skin. However, these substances kill cells on contact in an open wound. Necrotic tissue, foreign bodies, and fluid collections prevent normal fibroblast penetration and can also increase the incidence of wound infections. Débridement of dead tissue and prevention of fluid collections are part of good wound management.

The type of suture material used depends on the amount of strength needed and the amount of time the suture needs to supply strength. For example, plain gut retains its strength for approximately 3 weeks. By 3 weeks, most wounds have obtained 15 per cent of their ultimate strength. If this degree of strength is sufficient, then absorbable suture is appropriate. Additionally, pain in the surgical site often limits the amount of stress a patient applies to a wound. Special care should be taken when a patient is extubated from general anesthesia, since the patient may exert uninhibited maximal strain, which can disrupt a fascial closure.

Because permanent sutures can serve as a nidus for infection, absorbable sutures have an advantage in contaminated or potentially contaminated wounds. If a permanent suture is required, monofilament suture is preferable, especially in a contaminated field.

Skin sutures present for extended periods of time can injure skin, causing increased scarring. When cosmesis is important, skin sutures should be removed early. The exact timing of suture removal varies in different areas of the body and in different individuals.

Operations performed in the presence of bacterial contamination have an increased rate of wound infection. Wound infections can cause secondary fascial dehiscence and other postoperative complications. For avoidance of wound infection, wounds are often left open and allowed to heal by granulation and wound contraction (secondary intention). Since epithelial cells do not migrate on a surface composed of dead or infected tissue, careful débridement with sharp instruments or wet to dry dressings is often necessary for an open wound to heal. If an open wound has good granulation and no evidence of infection, it can be closed with the use of skin tapes, thereby reducing the time required for wound contraction. Normally the wound can be closed on the fifth postoperative day, at which time bacterial contamination is at a nadir. This technique, known as delayed primary closure, has become more popular in recent years.

In some instances, normal wound contraction can have undesirable consequences. Functional impairment can follow contraction of large wounds in areas of normal body movement such as the hand and neck. The most effective method of preventing contraction is early coverage with flaps or full-thickness skin grafts. Treating a fully contracted and epithelialized wound requires excision with recreation of the original defect and immediate grafting.

Wound remodeling is a normal process in which wounds change in color and size. The remodeling process can continue for months or even a year after injury. For this reason, reconstruction or cosmetic procedures should be delayed until scar remodeling has reached completion.

CONTROLLING THE HEALING PROCESS

Control of the healing process would be clinically useful especially when fibrosis and scarring are the cause of morbidity (e.g., pulmonary fibrosis). Increasing the rate of wound healing would also have obvious advantages. Experiments have demonstrated that dried powdered cartilage and elevated oxygen tension can produce minor increases in the rate of wound healing with a 15 to 20 per cent increase in wound strength by 1 week. Although these results are interesting for their prospective value, such minor increases lack clinical significance.

In an attempt at alteration of undesirable scar formation, for example, esophageal stricture or valvular deformity following endocarditis, experimental methods for control of collagen formation have been investigated. Ferrous iron chelators and proline analogs have been used experimentally to specifically inhibit collagen formation. Beta-aminopropionitrile (BAPN) is an osteolathyrogen that acts to inhibit collagen crosslinking. Penicillamine is also lathyrogenic but produces its effect through a different mechanism. Lathyrogenic collagen lacks the tensile strength of normal collagen and can be disrupted easily. Animal studies using lathyrogenic compounds have produced some interesting results, including improved tendon gliding after tendon injury and prevention of esophageal stenosis after lye burn. However, these compounds have not yet attained clinical usefulness. It may be that in the future it will be possible to specifically alter collagen formation in scar tissue for control of the healing process in a clinically useful way.

11

BURNS: Including Cold, Chemical, and Electric Injuries

Scott K. Pruitt, M.D., Basil A. Pruitt, Jr., M.D., and Cleon W. Goodwin, Jr., M.D.

More than two million people are burned in the United States each year, with 6500 burn- and fire-related deaths. Whereas most burn injuries are of limited extent and can be cared for on an outpatient basis, 3 to 5 per cent are sufficiently severe to require in-hospital care. Those with major burn injury, defined as (1) burns of more than 10 per cent total body surface area (BSA) in patients younger than 10 years and older than 50 years, (2) burns of more than 20 per cent BSA in patients of intervening age, (3) significant burns of the face, hands, feet, genitalia, perineum, or major joints, (4) full-thickness burns of more than 5 per cent BSA, (5) significant electric injury, (6) significant chemical injury, and (7) lesser burns with inhalation injury, concomitant mechanical trauma, or significant pre-existing medical disorders, are best cared for in a specialized burn center.

PREHOSPITAL AND EMERGENCY CARE OF BURNS

Initial on-scene care includes removing the patient from the heat source, copiously irrigating any chemically injured tissues, and administering standard cardiopulmonary resuscitation as indicated. A peripheral intravenous line should be placed if the patient is more than 30 to 45 minutes from the treatment center, has cardiac irregularities, or has sustained significant blood loss. One hundred per cent oxygen should be administered to patients suspected of having carbon monoxide poisoning, which is common in those who sustained burns in a closed space.

In the emergency room, fluid resuscitation should be initiated by infusing a balanced salt solution through a large-caliber intravenous cannula. Patency of the airway should be assessed, with endotracheal intubation utilized as needed, and an adequate history and physical examination should be performed. An arterial blood sample should be obtained for determination of pH, blood gases, carboxyhemoglobin, electrolytes, blood urea nitrogen, glucose, and hematocrit. The depth of the burn should be assessed and the extent of the

See the corresponding chapter or part in the *Textbook of Surgery*, 14th edition, pp. 178–209, for a more detailed discussion of this topic, including a comprehensive list of references.

The opinions or assertions contained herein are the private views of the authors and are not to be construed as official or as reflecting the views of the Department of the Army or the Department of Defense.

burn should be estimated by use of a burn chart or the rule of nines. Fluid needs are then estimated on the basis of the total extent of second- and third-degree burns and total body weight. A Foley catheter should be placed in all burn patients requiring intravenous fluid therapy to permit measurement of hourly urinary output.

FLUID RESUSCITATION AND EARLY CARE

Intravenous fluid resuscitation should be initiated as soon as possible in all patients with burns involving 15 per cent or more of the body surface. Various formulas for fluid administration have been developed, all of which are clinically effective, but those that avoid administration of colloid during the first 24 hours post burn are recommended. Fluid requirements may be greater than estimated in patients with high-voltage electric injury, inhalation injury, delayed resuscitation, or alcohol intoxication. During the second 24 hours post burn, when capillary permeability has returned to normal, plasma volume deficits are replaced with colloid-containing fluids.

Sufficient fluid should be administered to maintain an hourly urinary output of 30 to 50 ml. in the adult (1 ml. per kg. per hour in children who weigh less than 30 kg.) throughout the resuscitation period. Invasive monitoring of cardiac function and central venous pressures should be reserved for patients who fail to respond to fluid administration as anticipated.

Oliguria during the first 48 hours post burn is generally due to inadequate resuscitation and should be treated by increased fluid administration. Diuretic therapy is indicated in patients with extensive burns who remain oliguric despite infusion of fluids in excess of twice estimated needs. If heavy loads of heme pigments appear in the urine of patients with high-voltage electric injury, mechanical soft tissue injury, or particularly deep burns involving muscle, the fluid infusion rate should be increased to maintain urinary output at 75 to 100 ml. per hour to promote clearance of the hemochromogens. If infusion of additional fluid does not clear the pigment from the urine, diuretic therapy with mannitol is indicated.

Fluid management after the resuscitation period should permit excretion of the water and salt loads infused during resuscitation and permit the patient to return to preburn weight by the eighth to tenth postburn day. Thermal destruction of the water vapor barrier of the skin results in marked elevation of evaporative loss of electrolyte-free water from the burn surface. A variable fraction of that loss must be replaced with electrolyte-free fluid to prevent dehydration and hypernatremia. Insensible water loss (after resuscitation) can be estimated as water loss (ml. per hour) = (25 + percentage of body surface burned) × total body surface area (sq. m.). Potassium supplements, proscribed by cell destruction–related hyperkalemia during resuscitation, may be needed thereafter.

Edema formation beneath circumferential burns of the

extremities or thorax may compromise the peripheral circulation or ventilation, respectively. The amount of edema that forms in a burned limb may be reduced by limb elevation and active motion, but if circulation is compromised, escharotomy is indicated. Signs of compromised blood flow include cyanosis, impaired capillary refilling, paresthesias, and relentless deep tissue pain. More reliable than those signs, as an indication of the need for escharotomy, is the progressive diminution of pulsatile flow as detected by serial ultrasonic flowmeter examinations or absence of flow as detected by a single ultrasonic examination.

Escharotomy is performed as a ward procedure and does not require anesthesia. The eschar of the limb is incised down through the superficial fascia in either the midlateral or midmedial line, extending the entire length of the burned area. When ventilation is impaired by restriction of chest wall motion, anterior axillary line escharotomies should be performed.

Usually escharotomy produces rapid return of blood flow, but fasciotomy may be required to restore circulation. A muscle compartment requiring fasciotomy is characteristically stony hard to palpation, a finding most frequently present in patients with electric injury and in burn patients with associated soft tissue trauma. Fasciotomy should be performed in the operating room under general anesthesia, and the fascia of all involved compartments must be adequately released. Topical antimicrobial agents should be applied to all fasciotomy and escharotomy incisions to minimize the risk of infection.

INHALATION INJURY

Inhalation injury should be suspected in any patient burned in a closed space or during a period of impaired mentation due to inebriation, drug overdose, or head trauma. Clinical findings that should alert one to the possibility that inhalation injury is present include (1) head and neck burns, (2) singed nasal hair, (3) inflammation of the oropharyngeal mucosa, (4) brassy cough, (5) hoarseness and wheezing, (6) bronchorrhea, (7) unexplained hypoxemia, and (8) most specifically, carbonaceous sputum production. Chest films obtained on the day of admission are insensitive in detecting inhalation injury. Conversely, fiberoptic bronchoscopy, performed at the bedside in patients suspected of having inhalation injury, is very reliable. Mucosal inflammation and ulceration as well as deposition of carbon particles on the endobronchial mucosa on bronchoscopic examination indicate inhalation injury. Treatment of inhalation injury includes (1) administration of warm, humidified oxygen; (2) frequent scheduled pulmonary toilet, which may require repeat therapeutic bronchoscopy; and, if indicated, (3) endotracheal intubation and mechanical ventilation. Prophylaxis with steroids is not indicated and increases septic complications.

BURN WOUND CARE

The burn wound should be cleansed using a surgical detergent, all loose nonviable skin trimmed away, and all hair shaved from the burned area and a generous margin of unburned skin. Following daily cleansing and débridement, the topical antimicrobial agent of choice is applied. Mafenide acetate (Sulfamylon) is bacteriostatic, is freely soluble, readily diffuses through eschar, and has the broadest spectrum of activity against *Pseudomonas* organisms in particular and gram-negative organisms in general, making it the best agent for treating patients with a dense bacterial population in the eschar or in whom other topical agents have failed. Limitations of Sulfamylon include carbonic anhydrase inhibition, which leads to bicarbonate wasting and hyperventilation, and pain. Silver sulfadiazine 1 per cent (Silvadene) is bacteriostatic but diffuses poorly and penetrates eschar less well than does Sulfamylon. It produces no pain or acid-base disturbances. Limitations include the development of neutropenia and ineffectiveness against certain gram-negative organisms. One half per cent silver nitrate solution has a broad spectrum of antimicrobial activity and causes no pain but must be applied in multilayered dressings that impede motion of involved joints. Other limitations of the 0.5 per cent silver nitrate soak treatment include leaching of sodium, potassium, chloride, and calcium through the eschar and transeschar absorption of water.

BURN WOUND EXCISION

Excision of the burned tissue in full-thickness and most deep partial-thickness burns should be performed as soon as possible after resuscitation is complete. Adverse effects of excision include anesthesia risk; operative stress associated with prodigious blood loss, which can occur when excision of more than 20 per cent BSA is performed during a single procedure; susceptibility of the excised wound to infection from adjacent unexcised burn; sacrifice of viable skin intermixed with areas of full-thickness burn; and the immunosuppressive effects of transfusions needed for replacement of excision-related blood loss. Advantages of burn wound excision include decreased hospital stay, early return to work, fewer complications, and a reduction of the time during which the wound is at risk of invasive infection. Wounds not requiring excision should be cleansed daily, with repeat application of topical antimicrobial agents.

Excised wounds or those treated simply by daily débridement that have adequate granulation tissue, a surface bacterial count of less than 10^5 organisms per sq. cm. of wound surface, and absence of beta-hemolytic streptococci are ready for split-thickness autograft closure. Autografts 0.012 to 0.015 inch in thickness are generally used for initial skin coverage in patients with extensive burns. The mesh dermatome can be utilized to increase, by up to ninefold, the extent of wound covered by skin from a given donor site. Expansion ratios of more than 4:1 result in excessive time for closure and increased scar formation.

Wounds unable to be autografted, but with little nonviable tissue and good granulation tissue, can be closed temporarily with a biologic dressing. Biologic dressings in order of preference include viable cutaneous allograft, lyophilized allograft, cutaneous xenograft, amnion, and various synthetic membranes. Skin allografts reduce wound desiccation, promote maturation of granulation tissue, limit bacterial proliferation in the wound, prevent exudative protein and red blood cell loss, decrease wound pain, and diminish evaporative water loss.

ELECTRIC INJURY

High-voltage electric injury not only causes tissue damage at the contact sites, where the injury is most severe, but also damages underlying tissues and organs along the route taken by the current. Thus, small cutaneous lesions may overlie extensive areas of devitalized muscle that may liberate large quantities of myoglobin and cause acute renal failure. The infusion of resuscitation fluids should be increased as necessary because estimates based on the extent of visible burn underestimate requirements and further predispose the patient to acute renal failure. High-voltage electric and lightning injury may produce cardiac arrhythmias, and thus those patients who have lost consciousness or have an abnormal electrocardiogram should be monitored for at least 48 hours. Since neurologic changes, including peripheral nerve deficits and spinal cord functional deficits, may occur at variable times after high-voltage electric injury, a full neurologic examination should be performed on admission and at selected intervals thereafter in such patients.

Following adequate resuscitation and patient stabilization, limbs having sustained electric injuries should be surgically explored. All muscles must be thoroughly explored and necrotic tissue debrided. If amputation is necessary, the amputation wound is left open, and 24 to 48 hours later the patient is returned to the operating room for further débridement or closure as necessary.

CHEMICAL INJURIES

In contrast to other burn patients, immediate wound care takes priority over resuscitation in those with chemical injuries in order to limit the duration of chemical agent contact with the skin and other tissues. Thus, all contaminated clothing should be immediately removed; simultaneously, copious water lavage should be immediately initiated and continued for at least 30 minutes. Chemicals that require more specific therapy include hydrofluoric acid, treated by irrigation with benzalkonium chloride or topical calcium gluconate gel, and phenol, which requires washing with a lipophilic solvent such as polyethylene glycol after water lavage.

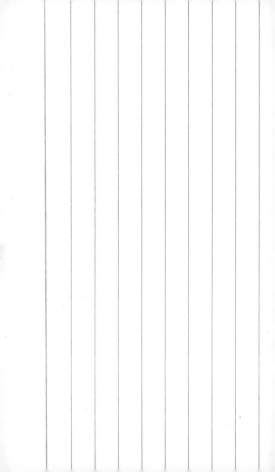

METABOLIC ALTERATIONS AND NUTRITIONAL SUPPORT

Postburn hypermetabolism, related to burn size, is manifested by increased oxygen consumption, elevated cardiac output and minute ventilation, increased core temperature, wasting of lean body mass, and increased urinary nitrogen excretion. These changes appear to be mediated by increased catecholamines and other counterregulatory hormones.

Nutritional needs of the extensively burned patient can be estimated as being 2000 to 2200 kcal. per sq. m. BSA per day and 12 to 18 gm. of nitrogen per sq. m. BSA per day. In practice, enteral feedings are initiated on postburn day 3 and increased to predicted requirements by day 5. Any commercially available formula with a nitrogen-to-calorie ratio between 100:1 and 150:1 can be used. In patients unable to tolerate feeding by the enteral route by day 5, parenteral nutrition is initiated by infusing standard hypertonic glucose–amino acid solutions, with use of lipid emulsions only to prevent essential fatty acid deficiencies.

COMPLICATIONS IN BURN PATIENTS

None of the available topical agents sterilize the burn wound, and consequently the protection they afford may be inadequate for preventing the development of invasive burn wound infection. The entirety of the burn wound must be examined at the time of daily wound cleansing for identification of any changes indicative of burn wound infection, such as conversion of an area of partial-thickness burn to full-thickness necrosis and/or the appearance of focal areas of black or dark hemorrhagic discoloration. The diagnosis of burn wound infection can be confirmed most rapidly and reliably by histologic examination of a burn wound biopsy. The presence of microorganisms in unburned viable tissue confirms invasive burn wound infection. Treatment of bacterial infection includes immediate change to Sulfamylon topical therapy, the administration of systemic antibiotics, and excision of the infected tissue. Treatment of invasive fungal infection consists of topical antifungal therapy, systemic amphotericin B, and prompt wide excision of the infected tissue. Other infectious complications include airborne or hematogenous pneumonia (the most common infection in burn patients), suppurative thrombophlebitis, which can occur in any previously cannulated vein, acute endocarditis, suppurative sinusitis, and systemic sepsis.

Gastrointestinal complications in burn patients include acalculous cholecystitis, pancreatitis, and acute ulceration. Acute ulceration of the stomach and duodenum, Curling's ulcer, is effectively controlled by prophylactic antacid or histamine H_2-receptor antagonist therapy.

Burn scar carcinoma, also known as Marjolin's ulcer, is a rare neoplasm occurring in the unstable scar of a full-thickness burn. Because these tumors are highly invasive, all ulcerative lesions in burn scars should be biopsied; if carcinoma is found, all tumor must be completely excised.

COLD INJURY

Frostbite results in the freezing of tissue and produces damage by ice crystallization in tissue, cellular dehydration, and microvascular occlusion. Clinical signs range from hyperemia, edema, and superficial freezing of the epidermis in first-degree frostbite to full-thickness necrosis of the skin extending into muscle and bone in fourth-degree frostbite. Rapid rewarming of the frozen part is the single most effective therapeutic maneuver for preserving potentially viable tissue and can be accomplished by immersion in a 40° C. water bath. Surgical intervention is delayed until clear demarcation between viable and nonviable tissue has occurred, which may require many weeks, if not months.

12

PRINCIPLES OF OPERATIVE SURGERY: Antisepsis, Technique, Sutures, and Drains

Julio Hochberg, M.D., and Gordon F. Murray, M.D

ANTISEPSIS AND ASEPSIS

Antisepsis refers to the use of antimicrobial chemicals on human tissue; disinfection applies to the employment of these agents on inanimate objects. Hygienic hand-washing, preoperative preparation of the patient's skin, gloving and sterile draping during operation, isolation precautions, autoclaving of instruments, and proper waste disposal are all examples of the aseptic technique.

Aseptic Procedures

THE OPERATING ROOM. The operating room should provide an environment that is as free of bacterial contamination as possible. Appropriate ventilation rapidly clears bacteria from the air. However, organisms recovered from air often are not those that cause wound infection. The most important source of contamination is the patient, and the secondary source is the operating team.

THE PATIENT. Infections that develop from operations classified as clean-contaminated, contaminated, or dirty are primarily caused by bacteria already present in the operative field. Preparation of the patient's skin before an incision is one of the most important methods of decreasing infection in clean operations. The most commonly used antimicrobial agents for intact skin antisepsis are iodophors (Betadine). Intact skin can withstand very strong disinfecting agents, whereas cells of a fresh surgical wound are very susceptible to further damage. In heavily contaminated wounds, high-pressure irrigation can be of benefit in decreasing the number of bacteria. The patient has another role in the bacteria versus host relationship. Age, obesity, diabetes, cirrhosis, uremia, and connective tissue disorders, as well as hereditary or induced immune deficiency states, have all been associated with increased infection rates.

THE OPERATING TEAM. The operating team should scrub 3 to 5 minutes with an antiseptic before each operation. Agents such as iodophors or chlorhexidine combined with a detergent have proved effective. During the operation, a face mask should cover the mouth and nose. Gloves perform a dual function: they protect the patient from the hands of the surgeon and protect the surgeon from potentially contaminated blood. A sterile gown functions as a barrier for the prevention of the transmission of bacteria to the patient. The

See the corresponding chapter or part in the *Textbook of Surgery*, 14th edition, pp. 210–220, for a more detailed discussion of this topic, including a comprehensive list of references.

primary function of the sterile drapes is to define and preserve the sterile field during operative procedures. Drapes should be nearly impermeable to bacteria, even when wet. The sterile field should be constantly monitored and maintained. Instruments and equipment to be used at the operating table can be sterilized by steam heat, chemical solutions, dry heat, or gas methods.

SURGICAL TECHNIQUE

INCISIONS. An incision should be properly planned with regard to shape, direction, and size. In general, incisions are made along the normal skin lines. In reoperations, every attempt should be made to use the original incision. Skin incisions should be made with the stainless steel surgical scalpel. Incision of the skin should be perpendicular to the epidermal surface. Skin margins should be handled gently to minimize necrosis that may promote infection or delay healing.

DISSECTION. The least amount of trauma is accomplished by dissecting natural tissue planes. The surgeon's index finger readily dissects many lightly adherent normal tissue planes. Sometimes the tissue density and adherence require the use of a dampened gauze sponge. A blunt-tipped scissors is excellent for opening tissue planes that are too dense for finger or sponge dissection. A sharp knife is needed for dissection where tissue is heavily scarred.

DÉBRIDEMENT. The most important single factor in the management of the contaminated wound is the débridement. It removes tissue heavily contaminated by bacteria or foreign bodies and protects the patient from the threat of invasive infection.

HEMOSTASIS. The objectives of hemostasis are the minimization of blood loss during and after operation and the prevention of hematoma formation. It is also imperative to maintain a clear, bloodless field during incision and dissection. If digital pressure is maintained for 15 to 20 seconds, small clots usually form in the ends of smaller vessels, and no further bleeding occurs. Definitive hemostasis of larger vessels is obtained by ligatures, suture ligatures, or metal clips.

WOUND CLOSURE. Wounds containing less than 10^5 bacterial organisms per gram of tissue nearly always heal primarily following closure. A wound containing greater than 10^5 bacterial organisms per gram of tissue cannot be reliably closed, since the incidence of wound infection that follows is 50 to 100 per cent. When the wound is contaminated by exceedingly large numbers of organisms, delayed primary closure should be considered. Closure of dead space by sutures potentiates the development of infection. The collapse of such spaces should be achieved by relaxing incisions, rotation of flaps, and splinting. When wounds involve vital structures that may be destroyed by exposure, flaps must be transposed immediately.

SUTURING. Simple interrupted sutures coapt the wound

edges and correct any intervening gaps or discrepancies in height. Subcuticular sutures are an excellent choice when good cosmetic results are desired. Running cuticular suture is an easy and rapid method of skin closure and is readily removed postoperatively. Vertical mattress sutures are intended to gain both a secure grasp of tissue and a good approximation of the skin margins. Unfortunately, permanent hatchmark scars may result. Retention sutures are utilized for closing wounds under tension.

DRESSING. During the early postoperative period (48 hours), the fresh incision should be protected by dry dressings until epithelization is completed. Draining and infected wounds require dressings that can absorb exudate and remove necrotic tissue remnants after surgical débridement. When skin loss is extensive, biologic dressings are helpful in achieving wound coverage and protection against bacterial invasion and evaporative loss. Immobilized tissue demonstrates resistance to the growth of bacteria superior to nonimmobilized tissue. When the site of any injury is immobilized, lymphatic flow is reduced, thereby minimizing the spread of the wound microflora.

SUTURE REMOVAL. An important factor that influences the timing of suture removal is the eventual cosmetic result. Percutaneous sutures create a sinus tract, and a typical railroad track appearance can be the final result. Other factors that determine the timing of suture removal include the amount of tension on the wound edges, nutritional status, prior radiation therapy, concurrent chemotherapy, exogenous steroid administration, and the presence of sepsis.

PROPHYLACTIC ANTIBIOTICS. Prophylactic antibiotics are defined as those administered in the absence of or before infection and are distinguished from therapeutic antibiotics used to treat an established infection. Prophylactic antibiotics are recommended for operations that are associated with a high risk of infection, or operations associated with life-threatening consequences if infection occurs. Parenteral antibiotic prophylaxis should be started within 2 hours before the operation.

ELECTROCAUTERY. A unipolar electrosurgical unit is used both for surgical dissection and for hemostasis. The cutting cautery may be of significant value in saving operative time and diminishing the blood loss during massive excisional surgery. However, compared with cold knife dissection, there is an increased susceptibility to infection and seromas. A bipolar cautery is more precise and confines the damage to the tissues between the tips of the cauterizing forceps. It is indicated for control of bleeding in microvascular and microneural surgery.

MEDICAL LASERS. Surgeons can now employ energy from light as a scalpel. The light is monochromatic, which permits selective optical absorption and consequent selective tissue heating, thereby providing a new approach to the damage or removal of tissue. Forward penetration of the laser beam is least with the argon laser, intermediate with the CO_2 laser, and deepest with the neodymium:yttrium-aluminum-garnet (Nd:YAG) laser. The Nd:YAG laser is capable of directing light energy via a flexible quartz fiber, which permits the use of fiberoptic endoscopes.

CUSA KNIFE. The Cavitron ultrasonic surgical aspirator (CUSA) functions as an acoustic vibrator and selectively fragments and aspirates tissue of high water and low collagen content, that is, tumors, sparing other tissues such as blood vessels and nerves. Advantages of reduced blood loss, reduced tissue injury, and improved visibility, compared with the scalpel or cautery, have been demonstrated for hepatic, splenic, and renal resection.

SUTURES

SELECTION OF SUTURE MATERIAL. The choice of suture for a particular procedure should logically be based on the known physical and biologic characteristics of the suture material and the healing properties of the sutured tissues. Adequate suture tensile strength is required for wound closure, but the finest suture that will hold the tissues together safely should be used. All sutures should be avoided in dirty, contaminated, or infected wounds whenever possible.

ABSORBABLE SUTURES. Selecting a specific absorbable suture requires assessment of the length of time the material will be present and the strength it will have over that time.

Catgut. Catgut is made from the intestines of cattle or sheep. The absorption rate of plain catgut is about 10 days. Chromic catgut has been treated with a chromium salt to retard its absorption to 20 days. Plain catgut usually evokes a greater inflammatory reaction than does chromic catgut.

Polyglycolic Acid. An absorbable, braided, synthetic suture material, polyglycolic acid (Dexon) has a higher tensile strength than that of catgut. Total reabsorption by hydrolysis during wound healing occurs at 60 to 90 days postoperatively. Dexon is useful in muscle, fascia, capsule, tendon, and subcuticular skin closure. Generally, braided suture, absorbable or nonabsorbable, adversely influences bacterial growth.

Polyglactic Acid. Polyglactic acid (Vicryl) is a braided synthetic suture. The tensile strength is very high (second to that of Dexon), and it is completely absorbed in 60 days. It is extremely useful as a completely buried suture to approximate wound edges.

Polydioxanone. The synthetic polymer of poly-*para*-dioxanone (PDS) is a monofilament absorbable suture with a long duration of absorbability and an extremely high tensile strength. This low reactive suture is capable of maintaining its integrity in the presence of bacterial infection.

NONABSORBABLE SUTURES

Silk. Silk is a protein filament obtained from the silkworm larva. The suture has good tensile strength, is easy to handle, and has excellent knot characteristics.

Cotton. Processed from braided cotton fibers, cotton is a strong, pliable suture material. Cotton should not be used in wounds known or suspected to be contaminated.

Polyester. Constructed of polyester fibers (Dacron), these braided sutures have superior strength and durability. The uncoated suture (Mersilene) tends to cut slightly when pulled through tissue; thus, Teflon (Tevdek), silicone (Tri-Cron), and polybutilate (Ethibond) have all been employed in its manufacture.

Nylon. A synthetic polyamide polymer, nylon is available in both monofilament and multifilament forms. It is very strong and smooth, but extra care must be taken when tying to prevent knot slippage. Its smooth monofilament composition ensures facile passage through tissue and minimal reaction. Nylon sutures are the most commonly used sutures in cutaneous surgery.

Polypropylene. A monofilament suture material, polypropylene (Prolene) provides smooth passage through tissues and minimal tissue reaction. Easy removability renders it an ideal suture for a running intradermal stitch, and it is a superior suture for fascial closure in the presence of contamination or infection. In fine-caliber sizes, Prolene is invaluable for microvascular surgery.

Stainless Steel. Stainless steel wire can be monofilament or multifilament. Wire is the strongest and least reactive suture. However, its handling characteristics are very poor. Wire is used mainly in surgery of ligaments, tendons, and bones.

STAPLES. Stapling is faster than a traditional hand-sewn effort, resulting in reduced operation and anesthesia time, tissue trauma, blood loss, and overall hospital stay. Contemporary devices include a great number of skin and internal stapling instruments.

SKIN TAPES. Skin tapes are impervious to sweat, maintain the integrity of the epidermis, lessen the likelihood of wound infection, and avoid suture marks. In children, selection of skin tapes avoids the ordeal of suture placement and removal.

SURGICAL ADHESIVES. Autologous fibrin glue is a biologic adhesive consisting of fibrinogen, factor XIII, fibronectin, thrombin, apoprotinin, and calcium chloride. It is effective in stabilizing esophagogastric, small intestinal, and nerve anastomoses. It is also effective in obtaining hemostasis at skin graft donor sites and in the fixation of skin grafts. The autologous fibrin glue is prepared from single-donor human plasma, eliminating the danger of multi-donor pools.

DRAINS

It is probable that in the abdominal cavity drains can serve only two purposes. The first is the provision of egress for loculated pus or intestinal contents. Second is the prophylactic removal of any fluids within the peritoneal cavity, such as bile and pancreatic juices, before their presence can cause complications. On the contrary, the use of prophylactic drains for peritoneal contamination has been abandoned. Abdominal drains are quickly surrounded by omentum and bowel, which isolate the drains as ineffective sinus tracts. Soft tissue drains may help coapt tissue and prevent the collection of serum or blood underneath large undermined areas. However, drains must not be considered a substitute for hemostasis or as a replacement for meticulous technique. For either prophylactic or therapeutic indications, the surgeon should select the form of drainage, either passive or active, that is best suited for the purpose intended. The drain must be appropriate to the demands of the viscosity or the volume of the expected drainage. In general, prophylactic drainage may be best accomplished by the use of closed wound suction drainage. As the volume or complexity of drainage increases and therapeutic drainage is indicated, passive and sump drains are more efficacious. Decreased drainage or the absence of drainage usually indicates that the drain may be withdrawn. The material of which the drain is made is of utmost concern: it should be soft to avoid injury, nonirritating to the tissue, firm to remain in its intended place, resistant to decomposure, and smooth to allow easy removal. Three types of drains are used primarily: (1) the Penrose drain, (2) the closed suction drain, and (3) the sump drain. Percutaneous catheter drainage represents a new method that is proving to be exceedingly valuable.

CONTROVERSY. Drains left *in situ* are not innocuous: they may erode into the intestine or the blood vessels and thus promote the development of adhesions, which cause intestinal obstruction. Sutures can be inadvertently placed around or through drains, and drains may break off inside the body. For the benefit of wound drainage, the surgeon must consider the risk of contaminating the wound and increasing the incidence of infection. To drain or not, which drain, and for how long all remain unanswered questions; but the diversity of answers suggests that no single policy is necessarily correct.

13

SURGICAL INFECTIONS

I

Surgical Infections and Choice of Antibiotics

J. Wesley Alexander, M.D., Sc.D. and
E. Patchen Dellinger, M.D.

More than 1,000,000 wound infections occur in the United States each year, causing an economic loss of several billion dollars. Both medicolegal and humanitarian considerations demand that surgeons make every effort to prevent this complication.

CAUSES OF WOUND INFECTION

Wound infections occur whenever the microbial inoculum in the wound is sufficiently large to overcome local host defense mechanisms. In normal individuals, surprisingly large numbers of organisms are necessary. Studies in traumatic and surgical wounds in healthy humans have shown that bacterial contamination with less than 100,000 organisms per sq. cm. of wound or gram of tissue seldom produces an infection. In small clean wounds, more than 1,000,000 *Staphylococcus aureus* are required. However, certain organisms such as *Streptococcus pyogenes* are more virulent, whereas others such as *Pseudomonas aeruginosa* and *Escherichia coli* are usually less virulent. In the immunocompromised host, it is easy to understand that reduced mechanisms for antimicrobial clearance increase infection rates with a specific bacterial inoculum. In addition, nearly anything that reduces blood flow or cell deposition to the surgical incision increases infection rates. These include vascular occlusive states, hypovolemic shock, the use of vasopressors or vasoconstrictors either locally or systemically, uremia, old age, or use of large doses of steroids. More complex problems such as cancer or trauma that are associated with complement activation and the generation of tissue-derived inhibitors of cellular function adversely influence both T cell and phagocytic cell processes. In addition, local wound factors profoundly influence the development of infection. Such factors can influence the infectibility of organisms by more than 10,000-fold and include insertion of foreign bodies such as sutures or prosthetic devices, lack of accurate approximation of tissues, strangu-

---

See the corresponding chapter or part in the *Textbook of Surgery*, 14th edition, pp. 221–236, for a more detailed discussion of this topic, including a comprehensive list of references.

lation of tissues with sutures that are too tight, and the presence of any dead tissue, hematomas, or seromas.

PREVENTION OF WOUND INFECTION

Prevention of wound infection is a multifaceted ongoing process that requires continuous attention to details of surgical technique and behavior of the operating team as well as the application of adjunctive therapy. By using discharge of any pus from the wound within the first 30 days as the definition of wound infection, wound infection rates for clean wounds should be less than 1.5 per cent, for clean-contaminated wounds less than 3 per cent, and for contaminated wounds less than 5 per cent. Deviations above these values are indicative of failure of the preventive systems, and intensified efforts must be made to determine the cause of the failure. In this regard, a continuing program for the surveillance of surgical wound infections with feedback to the individual surgeon has been found to be an effective means for maintaining surgical infection rates at a low level.

Avoidance of Bacterial Contamination

In many hospitalized and ill patients, there are increased numbers of resident pathogenic organisms on the skin. Because of this, it is important to require preoperative showers, with use of antimicrobial soaps such as chlorhexidine or povidone iodine the night before operation whenever possible. Removal of hair from the skin should be done by clippers immediately before operations, since shaving of the hair causes damage to the skin and approximately doubles the incidence of wound infection. Preparation of the skin with an antimicrobial soap and the use of drapes on the incision is a time-honored technique. However, an alternative method of protection of the wound from skin surface organisms is the use of antimicrobial incise drapes after the skin has been prepped with a solution of alcohol or tincture of iodine to kill surface bacteria and degrease the skin. Antimicrobial soaps should not be used with incise drapes because this prevents adherence of the drape and can actually increase the incidence of infection. Contamination from the operating team is frequent and is, perhaps, the most important source of organisms causing infection in clean operations. Vigilance for breaks in sterile technique, changes of gloves whenever punctures arise, and the use of water-impermeable drapes and gowns are important factors that the operating team can control.

Endogenous Contamination

At the time of transection of the gastrointestinal, respiratory, or genitourinary tracts, careful draping with change of instruments, gowns, and gloves can minimize contamination from endogenous organisms. When contamination of the operative site has occurred, liberal irrigation of the wound with a saline solution containing 1.0 gm. of kanamycin or 2.0 gm. of cephalothin per liter has been shown to be an effective adjuvant for preventing infection.

Importance of Surgical Technique

The amount of damaged tissues that remain in the surgical wound is directly related to the number of infections. Repeated studies have shown that sharp dissection is less damaging to tissues than is dissection with electrocautery or laser. However, electrocautery for the control of small bleeding points may be less harmful than is the use of ligatures because less foreign material is introduced into the wound. All devitalized tissues and foreign bodies should be removed from traumatic wounds whenever possible. When complete débridement is not possible, the wound should not be closed primarily. In contaminated wounds, experimental and clinical studies show that monofilament, nonabsorbable polypropylene or nylon sutures are preferable to multifilament or absorbable sutures. Also, running sutures are associated with less infection than are interrupted sutures when used for closure. The presence of hematomas, seromas, or dead spaces favors bacterial localization and growth and prevents the delivery of phagocytic cells to bacterial foci. Where a potentially contaminated but not infected dead space occurs in an operative wound, the best method for preventing fluid collection is to provide a system of closed suction drainage. In contrast, open drainage of such wounds increases rather than decreases the degree of contamination and the incidence of infection. In very heavily contaminated wounds, delayed primary closure is a useful technique, but it has also been shown that skin closure with placement of a closed suction catheter in subcutaneous tissue with subsequent irrigation of topical antibiotics sufficient to fill the wound cavity may provide an alternative solution.

Systemic Factors

Extraordinary precaution should be taken to prevent the development of wound infections in surgical patients who are immunodepressed by disease or drug therapy. This includes correction or control of the underlying defect whenever possible. Severely malnourished subjects should be fed for correction of the malnutrition, preferably by the oral route. Disturbances of circulation during the intraoperative and immediate postoperative period should be avoided, and a high inspired oxygen for improving oxygen delivery to the incision is also an important factor in preventing wound infection.

Preventing Wound Infections by Prophylactic Chemotherapy

Prophylactic antibiotics are usually recommended in the following circumstances:

1. Accidental wounds with heavy contamination and tissue damage when treatment is unavoidably delayed or when adequate débridement cannot be accomplished. In such instances, the antibiotic should be administered by the intravenous route as soon as possible after injury.

2. All operative wounds classified as "contaminated."

3. Most operative procedures categorized as "clean-contaminated." The decision for the use of antibiotic therapy must be based on an estimate of the degree of contamination, the length and severity of the operation, the status of non-specific host resistance, and the potential consequence of infection. Examples of "clean-contaminated" operations for which prophylactic systemic antibiotics should be used regularly include common bile duct exploration, gastrectomy for carcinoma or bleeding, small bowel resection for obstruction, and hysterectomy.

4. Operative procedures classified as "clean" whenever there is insertion of a prosthesis.

5. When emergency operation is indicated in patients with pre-existing or recently active infection.

6. When pre-existing valvular heart damage is present in a patient, in order to prevent the development of bacterial endocarditis.

Prophylactic antibiotic therapy is clearly more effective when initiated preoperatively and continued through the intraoperative period with the aim of achieving therapeutic blood levels throughout the operative period. This produces therapeutic levels of the antibiotic agent in any seromas and hematomas that may develop at the operative site. Antibiotics initiated as late as 1 to 2 hours after bacterial contamination are markedly less effective, and it is completely without value to start prophylactic antibiotics after wound closure. Failure of the effectiveness of prophylactic antibiotics has resulted in part from a lack of appreciation of the importance of the timing and dosage of these agents, which are critical determinants. For most patients with elective surgery, the first dose of prophylactic antibiotics should be given intravenously at the time of induction of anesthesia. It is unnecessary to start them more than 1 hour preoperatively, and it is rarely beneficial to give them after the patient leaves the operating room.

Prophylactic antibiotic therapy is generally ineffective in those clinical situations in which continuing contamination is apt to occur, such as for tracheostomies or tracheal intubation, indwelling urinary catheters, indwelling central venous lines, most open wounds including burn wounds, and immunologically deficient patients or those receiving immunosuppressive therapy unless there are other indications for systemic antibiotic therapy.

Topical antibiotics should be considered an alternative to systemic prophylactic antibiotics when it is desirable to avoid systemic use, and as a complement to systemic use when heavy contamination has occurred.

THE NATURE, DIAGNOSIS, AND TREATMENT OF SURGICAL INFECTIONS

Surgical infections are distinguished from medical infections by the presence of an anatomic or mechanical problem that must be resolved by an operation such as incision and drainage of abscess, opening an infected wound, removing an infected foreign body, repairing or diverting a bowel leak, or draining an intra-abdominal abscess with a percutaneous catheter. Antibiotic treatment of a surgical infection without this mechanical solution does not resolve the infection. The most important aspect of the initial approach to a surgical infection is the recognition that operative intervention is required.

Soft Tissue Infections

The most important distinction between surgical and medical infections in superficial tissues is the presence of dead tissue in surgical infections. An abscess with its necrotic center must be distinguished from cellulitis, which is a soft tissue infection with intact blood supply and viable tissue. Cellulitis resolves with appropriate antibiotic therapy alone if treatment is initiated before tissue death occurs. An abscess may be mistaken for cellulitis when it is located deeply beneath overlying tissue layers and cannot be readily detected by physical examination or is located where fibrous septa join skin and fascia, dividing subcutaneous tissue into compartments that limit the local expression of fluctuance, such as with perirectal abscesses, breast abscesses, and infections in the distal phalanx of the finger (felon). Superficial abscesses on the trunk and head and neck are most commonly caused by *Staphylococcus aureus*, often combined with streptococci. Abscesses in the axillae often have a prominent gram-negative component. Abscesses below the waist, especially on the perineum, are frequently found to harbor a mixed aerobic and anaerobic gram-negative flora.

Necrotizing Soft Tissue Infections

Necrotizing soft tissue infections, both clostridial and nonclostridial, are less common than subcutaneous abscesses and cellulitis but much more serious conditions whose severity initially may be unrecognized. These infections lack clear local boundaries or palpable limits, which may be responsible for the frequent delay in recognizing their surgical nature. Anatomically, these infections are marked by a layer of necrotic tissue, which is not walled off by a surrounding inflammatory reaction. In addition, the overlying skin has a relatively normal appearance, and the visible degree of involvement is substantially less than that of the underlying tissues. A clostridial infection classically involves underlying muscle and is termed clostridial myonecrosis or gas gangrene. Most nonclostridial and some clostridial necrotizing infections spread in the subcutaneous fascia, between the skin and the deep muscular fascia. These infections have been described under a number of labels but are most commonly termed necrotizing fasciitis.

An apparent cellulitis with ecchymoses, bullae, any dermal gangrene, or crepitus suggests an underlying necrotizing infection and mandates operative exploration for confirming the diagnosis and ensuring definitive treatment. This is more important than applying a very specific diagnostic label to the process. Operative treatment requires excision of involved tissues for clostridial myonecrosis. On an extremity this may mean amputation. Nonclostridial infections can often be managed by wide incision and débridement and do not usually require amputation. In either case, all areas of necrotic tissue must be unroofed and debrided, and this often produces large disfiguring wounds.

Intra-abdominal and Retroperitoneal Infections

The majority of serious intra-abdominal infections require surgical intervention for resolution. Specific exceptions to this include pyelonephritis, salpingitis, amebic liver abscess, enteritis (*Shigella, Yersinia,* and so on), spontaneous bacterial peritonitis, some cases of diverticulitis, and some cases of cholangitis. If the diagnosis of one of these exceptions cannot be made, a patient with fever and abdominal pain should not be given antibiotics without a plan for operation or other drainage procedure. The administration of antibiotics in this setting before diagnosis may obscure subsequent findings and delay diagnosis and certainly delay definitive operative management. If the patient is too sick to go without antibiotic therapy, he is also too sick to avoid operative intervention and definitive diagnosis and treatment.

Despite modern antibiotics and intensive care, mortality from serious intra-abdominal or retroperitoneal infection remains high (5 to 50 per cent), and morbidity is substantial. Outcome is improved by early diagnosis and treatment. The risk of death and of complications increases with increased age, pre-existing serious underlying diseases, and malnutrition. Initial treatment of a patient with intra-abdominal infection consists of cardiorespiratory support, antibiotic therapy, and operative intervention. In most cases, the responsible bacteria and sensitivity information are not available for 48 to 72 hours after cultures are obtained. Since most intra-abdominal infections yield three to five different aerobic and anaerobic pathogens, specific, targeted antibiotic therapy is not possible and the initial choice must be empiric, designed to cover a range of possible organisms.

The antibiotic combination with the greatest experience and published information is an aminoglycoside combined with clindamycin or metronidazole. For infections acquired in the community with a small likelihood of resistant gram-negative rods and for a patient who is not severely ill, empiric therapy can be initiated with cefoxitin or cefotetan. For a more severely ill patient or a patient who has been in the hospital, more comprehensive treatment is needed. This could be imipenem alone or a combination of two drugs, one antibiotic with broad activity against aerobes and one active against anaerobes. Empiric antibiotic choice for other serious infections with a similar spectrum of pathogens, such as the necrotizing soft tissue infections, is the same.

OPERATIVE INTERVENTION FOR INTRA-ABDOMINAL OR RETROPERITONEAL INFECTION. The goal of operative intervention in patients with intra-abdominal infection is correction of the underlying pathologic problem. Recently, computed tomography scans have provided precise localization of intra-abdominal abscesses, permitting selected abscesses to be drained percutaneously under radiologic or ultrasound guidance. This is accomplished by needle puncture with aspiration of a small sample of pus to confirm the location, diagnosis, and type of organism and subsequent placement of a drainage catheter over a guidewire. If a patient has multiple abscesses or abscesses combined with an underlying pathologic process that requires operative correction, or if a safe percutaneous route to the abscess is not present, then open, operative drainage may be required.

Postoperative Fever

Postoperative fever occurs frequently; however, the majority of febrile postoperative patients are not infected, and indeed a significant proportion of infected patients may not be febrile, depending on the definition of "fever." Because fever is common in the absence of infection, it is important to consider causes of postoperative fever other than infection and to make a presumptive diagnosis before the institution of antibiotic treatment. The most common nonsurgical causes of postoperative infection and fever, urinary tract infection, respiratory tract infection, and intravenous catheter-associated infection, are all readily diagnosed. The other important causes of postoperative infection and fever, wound infection and intra-abdominal infection, require operative treatment and are not properly managed with antibiotics in the absence of operative treatment. Neither the prolongation of perioperative prophylactic antibiotics nor the initiation of empiric therapeutic antibiotics is indicated without a presumptive clinical diagnosis and a plan for operative intervention when indicated. Fever in the first 3 days following operation is most likely to have a noninfectious cause. However, when the fever begins 5 or more days postoperatively, the incidence of wound infections exceeds the incidence of undiagnosed fevers.

Etiologic Agents

GRAM-POSITIVE COCCI. Whereas coagulase-positive staphylococci are the most common pathogen associated with infections in wounds and incisions not subject to endogenous contamination, it has become increasingly clear that in the correct clinical setting, coagulase-negative staphylococci can also cause serious disease. They are the most common organisms recovered in nosocomial bacteremia and are frequently associated with clinically significant infections of intravascular devices. The precise significance of enterococci in surgical infections is controversial. Enterococci are commonly recovered as part of a mixed flora in intra-abdominal infections but are rarely recovered alone from a surgical infection. Enterococcal bacteremia in association with a surgical infection has a grave prognosis. The most effective antibiotic combination for treating enterococcal infections is gentamicin combined with ampicillin.

AEROBIC AND FACULTATIVE GRAM-NEGATIVE RODS. A great variety of gram-negative rods are associated with surgical infections. The greatest number of these are facultative anaerobic bacteria (*Enterobacteriaceae*). *Pseudomonas* species and *Acinetobacter* species (aerobes) are most commonly found in hospital-associated pneumonias in surgical patients but may also be recovered from the peritoneal cavity or severe soft tissue infections. These species are often antibiotic-resistant and require treatment with specific antipseudomonal antibiotics such as ceftazidime, aztreonam, imipenem, ciprofloxacin, an acylureido-penicillin, or an aminoglycoside.

ANAEROBES. The most common anaerobic isolate from surgical infections is *Bacteroides fragilis*. *B. fragilis* and *B. thetaiotaomicron* are two common anaerobic species with significant resistance to many beta-lactam antibiotics. The most effective antibiotics against these species are metronidazole, clindamycin, chloramphenicol, imipenem, and the combination ticarcillin/clavulanate.

The other important genus of anaerobic bacteria found in surgical infections is *Clostridium*. Although clostridia can survive for variable periods of time exposed to oxygen, they require an anaerobic environment for elaboration of the toxins that are responsible for their dramatic virulence in soft tissue infections. *C. tetani* is the member of this genus responsible for tetanus. The prevention of tetanus is accomplished solely through active and passive immunization and not through antibiotic administration.

The recovery of anaerobes from a soft tissue infection or even from the blood implies a focus of dead tissue or a defect in the anatomic integrity of the gastrointestinal tract. Both of these conditions require surgical correction, and thus the great majority of anaerobic infections require surgical intervention. Certainly an anaerobic bacteremia should always prompt a search for an abscess or for an enteric lesion that requires surgical intervention.

FUNGI. Fungi are infrequently the primary pathogens in deep-seated surgical infections. Pathogens from the *Candida* genus, however, may be seen frequently as an opportunistic invader in patients with serious surgical infections who have received broad-spectrum antibiotic treatment, which suppresses normal endogenous flora.

Antibiotics

Several handy pocket-sized references exist that provide detailed information regarding all commercially available antibiotics, such as doses and dose ranges, pharmacokinetic data, sensitivity patterns, incompatibilities, and excretion data. The reader is referred to standard references for this information. This section focuses on principles of antibiotic use.

When antibiotics are employed, the goal of therapy is achieving levels of antibiotics at the site of infection that exceed the minimal inhibitory concentration for the pathogens present. Mild infections, including most outpatient infections, may be treated with oral antibiotics when appropriate choices are available. For severe surgical infections, however, the systemic response to infection makes absorption of oral antibiotics unpredictable and serum levels unreliable. Thus, most initial antibiotic therapy of surgical infections is intravenous.

Each patient with a serious infection should be evaluated daily or more frequently for assessment of response to treatment. If obvious improvement is not seen within 2 to 3 days, the following question should be addressed: Why is the patient failing to improve? Likely answers include the following:

1. The initial operative procedure was not adequate.
2. The initial procedure was adequate but a complication has occurred.
3. A superinfection has developed at a new site.
4. The drug choice is correct, but not enough is being given.
5. Another drug or a different drug is needed.

The choice of antibiotics is not the most common cause for failure unless the original choice was clearly inappropriate, such as failing to provide coverage for anaerobes in an intra-abdominal infection.

As the patient improves, one must decide when to discontinue antibiotics. A good guideline is to continue antibiotics until the patient has shown an obvious clinical improvement based on clinical examination and has had a normal temperature for 48 hours or more. Signs of improvement include such things as improved mental status, return of bowel function, and spontaneous diuresis.

II

Surgical Aspects of the Acquired Immunodeficiency Syndrome

Terence Boyle, M.B., B.Ch., Douglas Tyler, M.D., and H. Kim Lyerly, M.D.

The acquired immunodeficiency syndrome (AIDS) is characterized by profound defects in cellular immunity leading to opportunistic infections and unusual neoplasms. AIDS was first recognized in 1981 and is caused by a human retrovirus termed human immunodeficiency virus Type 1 (HIV-1). HIV-1 has a unique tropism for the CD4 molecule found on T helper-inducer cells and monocytes-macrophages. Following infection of such cells, intracellular replication of HIV-1 leads to the production of infectious progeny and to the destruction or dysfunction of the infected cell. It is the quantitative or qualitative deficiency in T-helper/inducer lymphocytes that produces the immune defects in AIDS, because these cells control the proliferation of natural killer cells and cytotoxic T cells.

Acute infection with HIV-1 may cause a mononucleosis-like syndrome, but after the acute infection, a variable asymptomatic period may occur that may last for as long as 7 to 10 years. This asymptomatic period may be followed by a period of symptomatic disease consisting of constitutional signs including weight loss, fever and night sweats, or infections that do not meet the criteria for the complete syndrome of AIDS (Table 1). These features comprise the AIDS-related complex. Other manifestations of progressive HIV-1 infection include immune thrombocytopenia and neurologic disease. AIDS represents the most severe manifestation of infection with HIV-1; most, if not all, of those infected develop AIDS within a mean period of 8 years. AIDS is characterized by a progressive lymphopenia, predominantly of T-helper/inducer cells, that is clinically manifested by susceptibility to life-threatening opportunistic infections and malignancies. Such infections and/or neoplasms are typically recurrent, and life expectancy is estimated to be 1 to 2 years without specific anti–HIV-1 therapy but has increased with improved management of opportunistic infections.

Zidovudine (AZT) is a thymidine analog that acts as a chain terminator for the reverse transcriptase–driven elongation of HIV-1 DNA. The use of AZT has led to an improvement in the quality and length of life for patients with AIDS and has been demonstrated to decrease the number and severity of opportunistic infections in these patients. There is currently no curative therapy available for AIDS. The standard method of testing for HIV-1 infection is by the identification of anti–HIV-1 specific antibodies. After infec-

---

See the corresponding chapter or part in the *Textbook of Surgery*, 14th edition, pp. 237–248, for a more detailed discussion of this topic, including a comprehensive list of references.

TABLE 1. AIDS-Surveillance Definition of the Centers for Disease Control

AIDS: The occurrence of a disease that is at least moderately predictive of a defect in cell-mediated immunity, occurring in a person with no known cause for diminished resistance to that disease. These diseases include:

Kaposi's sarcoma (in patients less than 60 years of age)

Primary lymphoma of the central nervous system

Cryptosporidium enterocolitis of more than 4 weeks' duration

Pneumocystis carinii pneumonia

Esophagitis due to *Candida albicans*, cytomegalovirus, or herpes simplex virus

Extensive mucocutaneous herpes simplex of more than 5 weeks' duration

Progressive multifocal leukoencephalopathy

Pneumonia, meningitis, encephalitis, or disseminated disease due to one or more of the following: *Aspergillus, C. albicans, Cryptococcus neoformans,* cytomegalovirus, *Nocardia, Strongyloides, Toxoplasma gondii,* zygomycosis, atypical *Mycobacterium* species (not tuberculosis or lepra)

In the absence of the above opportunistic infections, any of the following diseases if the patient has a positive serologic or virologic test for HTLV-III/LAV:

Disseminated histoplasmosis

Isosporiasis causing diarrhea for more than 1 month

Non-Hodgkin's lymphoma of high-grade pathologic type, and of B-cell or unknown phenotype

Kaposi's sarcoma (in patients less than 60 years of age)

---

tion, such antibodies are usually present within 6 to 8 weeks and can be detected by using an enzyme-linked immunosorbent assay or western blot analysis. After infection with HIV-1, a number of individuals may remain seronegative for weeks to years. Confirmation of infection in these individuals relies on the direct detection of HIV-1 by viral culture, the demonstration of HIV-1–specific proteins in body fluids, or the detection of HIV-1–specific nucleic acid sequences in cellular material.

EPIDEMIOLOGY

Risk groups for the development of AIDS include homosexual or bisexual males, intravenous drug abusers, hemophiliacs receiving factor VIII concentrates, recipients of blood or blood products, heterosexual partners of infected individuals, and children of a parent with AIDS or at risk for AIDS. Transmission of HIV-1 is through sexual contact with infected partners, direct exposure to contaminated blood or blood products, and perinatal transmission from infected mothers to their offspring.

OCCUPATIONAL RISK OF HEALTH CARE WORKERS

HIV-1 can be transmitted to health care workers through occupational exposure; however, it is difficult to assess the magnitude of risk for such exposure. Combined data from 10 prospective studies indicate that the risk for HIV-1 transmission from a single parenteral exposure is 0.37 per cent. There is no evidence at present of HIV-1 transmission following a single mucous membrane exposure. Occupational exposure is minimized by implementation of universal blood and body fluid precautions, but the continued risk of accidental exposure has led to the development of strategies for reducing the risk of HIV-1 infection after such exposure. Postexposure prophylaxis with AZT is advocated for health care workers accidentally exposed to HIV-1. AZT is recommended for massive exposure (injections or transfusions of HIV-1–containing blood), is endorsed for serious parenteral exposures (deep needlesticks), and is available but not encouraged for less severe exposures. The National Institutes of Health recommend 200 mg. of AZT orally every 4 hours for 42 days. At the San Francisco General Hospital the same dose is administered, but the 4 A.M. dose is omitted, and the duration of therapy is 28 days. Administration of AZT is based on the serologic status of the source. Toxic effects following administration of AZT are primarily hematologic and dose-related. Severe toxic effect rarely occurs during the first 4 weeks of therapy.

TRANSFUSION-ASSOCIATED AIDS

Transmission of HIV-1 has been documented after transfusion of whole blood, packed red blood cells, fresh frozen plasma, cryoprecipitate, and platelets (single-donor blood products). Blood products derived from pooled plasma can also transmit HIV-1. Transmission of HIV-1 by transfusion has become rare since the introduction of voluntary deferral of donors at risk for HIV-1 infection and the routine testing of all donations. The estimated risk of acquiring HIV-1 ranges from 1 in 36,000 to 1 in 100,000 per unit of blood transfused. The current risk of HIV-1 infection from organ transplantation is unknown but is thought to be comparable to the risk from blood transfusion.

CLINICAL FEATURES

The majority of the morbidity observed in AIDS patients is related to overwhelming infections. Clinical syndromes that occur frequently include diffuse pneumonia, fever, diarrhea, central nervous system disorders, generalized lymphadenopathy, and esophagitis. Although infectious complications are a prominent feature in AIDS, unusual neoplasms are also encountered in large number. These include Kaposi's sarcoma (KS) and non-Hodgkin's lymphoma. KS encountered in AIDS patients is characterized by the sudden onset and often widespread appearance of lesions involving not only skin but oral mucosa, lymph nodes, and visceral organs. The *average survival* of patients is 18 months; however, visceral involvement implies a poor prognosis. Small localized lesions may be treated by electrodesiccation and curettage or by surgical excision, and KS tumors are generally responsive to local radiation; however, it has not been demonstrated that local or systemic therapy for KS alters the ultimate course of the disease.

Most AIDS-related lymphomas are B-cell tumors of high-grade pathologic type, and as many as 63 per cent may present with Stage IV disease. The therapy of choice for AIDS-related lymphomas is unknown because multiagent chemotherapy may worsen the patient's immune dysfunction and susceptibility to infection. Median survival of patients with AIDS-related lymphoma is less than 1 year but has improved. The incidence of non-Hodgkin's lymphoma appears to be increasing, especially in those treated with AZT.

SURGICAL CONSIDERATIONS IN HIV-1 INFECTED INDIVIDUALS

HIV-1 infected individuals not only are susceptible to standard medical problems and surgical disorders but also may tolerate surgical interventions differently from nonimmunosuppressed individuals as well as being susceptible to a variety of unique conditions that frequently require surgical intervention.

EVALUATION BY ORGAN SYSTEM

ESOPHAGUS. Diffuse esophagitis secondary to *Candida albicans* (most frequently), herpes simplex virus, or cytomegalovirus (CMV) is the most common lesion observed. Empiric therapy with ketoconazole *(Candida)* or acyclovir (herpesvirus) may be successful; however, endoscopy and biopsy may be required to differentiate these lesions. Esophageal ulceration, thought to be secondary to an as yet undefined virus, may occur. KS lesions of the esophagus may bleed or rarely cause pharyngeal obstruction and thus require excision.

STOMACH AND DUODENUM. Commonly encountered lesions include KS, non-Hodgkin's lymphoma, and CMV infections. KS lesions are usually asymptomatic but are the most common cause of upper gastrointestinal bleeding in HIV-1 infected individuals and can occasionally cause gastric outlet obstruction. Surgical excision is required if radiotherapy, chemotherapy, or immunotherapy fails to control the tumor. Non-Hodgkin's lymphoma may cause hemorrhage, obstruction, or perforation. Surgical excision is preferable to chemotherapy initially because intestinal perforation secondary to extensive tumor lysis after chemotherapy may occur. CMV infections of the stomach and duodenum cause ulceration, which may perforate and require surgical intervention. Despite operation, morbidity and mortality following perforation secondary to CMV are high.

LIVER. The majority of HIV-1–related opportunistic infections and the neoplastic complications of HIV-1 infection, KS and non-Hodgkin's lymphoma may affect the liver, but operative intervention is rarely required for therapy. Liver biopsy is occasionally indicated, and liver abscesses may occasionally require surgical intervention for drainage. Constitutional symptoms and abnormal liver function tests are indicative of liver involvement. Most patients with AIDS have serologic evidence of previous hepatitis B infection. Other types of viral hepatitis are also common.

GALLBLADDER AND BILIARY TRACT. Numerous cases of acute acalculous cholecystitis have been documented in HIV-1 infected individuals. Inciting organisms include *Cryptosporidium* and CMV (most commonly), *Campylobacter*, and *Candida*. Diagnosis is by ultrasonography, and cholecystectomy is the treatment of choice. This operation is usually well tolerated in asymptomatic HIV-1 infected individuals but has a high morbidity and mortality in patients with AIDS.

Papillary stenosis and sclerosing cholangitis are observed with surprising frequency in HIV-1 infected individuals. Cryptosporidiosis and CMV infection are the likely cause. Extrinsic compression of the bile ducts secondary to KS lesions, lymphadenopathy, or lymphoma should be excluded by ultrasonography and/or computed tomographic scanning. Papillary stenosis can be relieved by endoscopic sphincterotomy; sclerosing cholangitis by balloon dilation and stenting. Surgical intervention may be required for relief of extrinsic compression or when endoscopic sphincterotomy fails.

INTESTINE. HIV-1–related neoplastic lesions affecting the intestine include non-Hodgkin's lymphoma and KS. Lymphomas are usually symptomatic, presenting with signs of pain, fever, night sweats, weight loss, jaundice, ascites, obstruction, bleeding, and/or perforation. Diagnosis is by computed tomographic scan. Surgical intervention is frequently indicated and is advised before chemotherapy for the prevention of intestinal perforation secondary to post-chemotherapy tumor lysis. Intestinal KS lesions are present in 40 to 50 per cent of patients with cutaneous KS lesions but are usually asymptomatic. Lesions causing bleeding or obstruction may require surgical excision.

CMV infection may cause intestinal perforation, necessitating surgical exploration and segmental bowel resection. Morbidity and mortality after such a procedure remain high (40 per cent) because of the lack of appropriate systemic antiviral therapy. Several organisms can cause an inflammatory response in the terminal ileum that mimics regional enteritis or appendicitis, leading to surgical exploration. These include *Yersinia, Campylobacter, Shigella, Salmonella,* and *Mycobacterium avium-intracellulare.*

APPENDIX. Whereas appendicitis occurs in HIV-1 infected individuals via the same mechanisms through which it occurs in seronegative individuals, appendiceal obstruction may also follow AIDS-related neoplasms such as KS and lymphoma. Appendicitis is often more difficult to diagnose in patients with AIDS, since they frequently have chronic abdominal complaints.

COLON. Lesions affecting the colon in HIV-1 infected individuals are predominantly infectious in nature. CMV infection can lead to perforation requiring surgical intervention. A number of bacterial and parasitic organisms can cause a severe colitis, which usually presents with abdominal pain and diarrhea.

ANUS AND RECTUM. Anorectal complaints are common in HIV-1 infected individuals, especially homosexuals and AIDS patients. Symptoms include pain, discharge, incontinence, bleeding, mass, and/or tenesmus. Such symptoms may be caused by a wide variety of viral, bacterial, fungal, protozoal, and helminthic infections; lesions such as anal fissures, anal fistulas, and perirectal abscess; or tumors such as KS, lymphoma, or squamous cell carcinoma. The frequency of these lesions in AIDS patients appears to increase their risk of developing anal and rectal carcinoma. Treatment of the various anorectal lesions should be as conservative as possible because patients appear to heal poorly after attempted surgical therapy.

EVALUATION BY CLINICAL SIGNS OR SYMPTOMS

ABDOMINAL PAIN. Three broad categories of abdominal pain have been defined in AIDS patients: abdominal pain secondary to standard surgical problems, abdominal pain secondary to AIDS-related surgical problems, and nonsurgical abdominal pain. It appears that abdominal pain requiring surgical intervention in this patient population is uncommon. Abdominal pain may occur secondary to standard surgical conditions such as appendicitis, cholecystitis, perforated gastric or duodenal ulcer, diverticulitis, adhesive small bowel obstruction, or incarcerated hernias. Some of these conditions may, however, have AIDS-related inciting factors. In general, the more immunocompromised the HIV-1 infected individual, the more often an atypical presentation and poor outcome can be expected. AIDS-related conditions leading to abdominal pain and surgical intervention include KS and non-Hodgkin's lymphoma. Such lesions may cause gastrointestinal bleeding, obstruction, or perforation. CMV infection may lead to enteritis or colitis causing abdominal pain, bleeding, and diarrhea. Surgical intervention is required when free perforation, uncontrolled hemorrhage, or toxic megacolon occurs. The majority of HIV-1 infected patients who have abdominal pain *do not require* surgical intervention. Most often the etiology is related to some infectious agent that can be treated medically. Evaluation of such patients involves a number of diagnostic studies including endoscopy with biopsy and culture, stool examination, and computed tomographic scan.

GASTROINTESTINAL BLEEDING. Gastrointestinal bleeding is an unusual occurrence in HIV-1 infected individuals. Most lesions causing gastrointestinal bleeding are directly related to HIV-1 infection. Such lesions include KS and non-Hodgkin's lymphoma. Because these lesions are frequently treatable, gastrointestinal bleeding should be treated aggressively in HIV-1 individuals who are not terminally ill.

LYMPHADENOPATHY. Generalized lymphadenopathy is a relatively common finding in patients with HIV-1 infection.

The recognition of HIV-1 as the etiologic agent in AIDS and the development of accurate serologic tests for antibodies to HIV-1 have rendered routine diagnostic lymph node biopsy unnecessary. Selective use of lymph node biopsy may assist in the diagnosis of a specific infection, lymphoma, or disease process and thus alter the clinical management of the patient.

OTHER CONSIDERATIONS

POSTOPERATIVE COURSE. Postoperative morbidity and mortality in HIV-1 infected individuals appear to be related to the patient's underlying immunocompetence and the nature of the underlying illness requiring surgery. Asymptomatic HIV-1 infected individuals undergoing elective surgical procedures have no more problems with wound healing and postoperative infection than does the normal population. There is debate regarding the healing ability of patients with AIDS after elective procedures. Surgical intervention in this patient population, however, has been reported to occasionally exacerbate underlying HIV-1 infection. Extremely high morbidity and mortality are reported following emergent surgery in AIDS patients.

TRAUMA. Trauma surgeons must always consider the risk of occupational exposure to HIV-1 while dealing with severely injured patients, patients who are often actively bleeding at the time of presentation and who may require multiple invasive procedures in the emergency room. In one study, approximately 3 per cent of such patients were seropositive for HIV-1 at presentation. The highest prevalence was among black males and in patients aged between 25 and 34 years. Penetrating trauma was associated with an increased seroprevalence (13.6 per cent). A policy of universal blood and body fluid precautions should be followed by all health care workers regardless of whether the HIV-1 status is known.

14

SNAKE AND INSECT BITES AND RABIES

Kenneth P. Ramming, M.D.

SNAKEBITE

BIOLOGY. The fangs of pit vipers are long, hollow tubes set forward in the maxilla, ideal for deep delivery of venom. Pit vipers can control the position of the fangs and the amount of venom injected, and this may explain variability in the toxic effects of different bites. The fangs of the coral snake are fixed. Large snakes produce more venom than do small ones.

CLINICAL MANIFESTATIONS. In *Crotalus* (pit viper) bites there is an almost immediate, intense destruction of local tissue. Edema and erythema result, provoking a subjective sensation of intense pain. Permeability of blood vessels is altered, and extravasation of plasma and blood into tissues produces ecchymosis and bulla formation. Sloughing of tissue often occurs at the wound site.

When large amounts of venom are injected, severe systemic effects ensue. Often massive tissue necrosis and edema of an entire extremity result. Red blood cells respond by swelling and becoming spherical, and some are lysed. The hematocrit falls, and the number of platelets can be markedly reduced. Bleeding, coagulation, and prothrombin times are increased. Hematuria, melena, hematemesis, epistaxis, and hemoptysis may result. Blood vessel walls are altered, and there is increased resistance in postcapillary veins, causing pooling of blood in the lungs and chest. Pulmonary edema may result, and bleeding may occur in the peritoneum or pericardium. All these, together with direct toxic effects on the myocardial cells, contribute to the clinical pattern of peripheral vascular collapse.

The renal lesion of crotalid envenomation is glomerulonephritis, often accompanied by progressive, proliferative endarteritis and cortical necrosis. Necrosis of the tubular epithelium appears to be a direct local effect of the toxin. This, along with profound circulatory collapse and intravascular hemolysis, is responsible for the acute renal failure that frequently occurs in rattlesnake bites. A systemic anaphylaxis has also been described.

Elapidae (coral snake) venoms cause less tissue damage and far greater neuromuscular changes. Reaction around the bite is frequently absent, pain is minimal, and symptoms are systemic, such as numbness, nausea, vomiting, euphoria, salivation, paresthesia, ptosis, weakness, abnormal reflexes, depression, dyspnea, and respiratory arrest. In most experi-

---

See the corresponding chapter or part in the *Textbook of Surgery*, 14th edition, pp. 249–257, for a more detailed discussion of this topic, including a comprehensive list of references.

mental preparations, the first changes in electrical conduction induced by crude venom occur at the neuromuscular junction, but with small doses, changes of varying degree occur. The ultimate clinical catastrophe, which can occur with acute suddenness, is total respiratory paralysis.

The management of snakebite should follow a rational sequence. Avoid panic or overtreatment, since the majority of bites exhibit little toxicity. The following are suggested guidelines.

1. Retard absorption of the venom. A tourniquet can be left in place for up to 2 hours. However, it must occlude only venous and lymphatic return and not arterial flow. The ingestion of alcohol or application of ice is absolutely contraindicated.

2. Remove as much venom as possible from the wound. Excision of the bitten area is excellent early treatment if the patient is seen at a hospital emergency room. Incisions over the fang marks and suction of the venom has long been advised and as emergency field therapy in remote areas probably is still useful.

3. Neutralize the venom. Administration of polyvalent antivenin for neutralizing the venom has traditionally been advocated in the past. However, there are recent series that question the advisability of using antivenin. With the exception of its use in patients with heavy envenomation from large rattlesnakes who are seen early after envenomation, its routine use is not encouraged.

4. Prevent or reduce the effects of the venom. When indicated, appropriate infusions of saline, plasma, blood, and vasopressor drugs should be instituted for preventing shock. Blood coagulation studies should be obtained, and fibrinogen replacement may be required. Fasciotomy may become necessary for prevention of ischemic necrosis in a grossly edematous limb. Massive dosage of hydrocortisone, coupled with early wide wound incision and fasciotomy, has achieved good functional limb salvage in patients with heavy envenomation, particularly in patients with known sensitivity to antivenin. However, the routine use of massive corticosteroids has not gained universal acceptance.

5. Prevent complications. Broad-spectrum antibiotics are given to combat infection, and tetanus toxoid or tetanus immune globulin is administered. Vomiting, excessive salivation, and convulsions are treated symptomatically. Assisted ventilation may be necessary, and renal function must be monitored.

Patients bitten by coral snakes should be admitted to the hospital for careful observation for at least 48 hours, since the effects of this venom are characteristically slow to develop. The wound should be carefully washed because small amounts of the highly toxic venom may remain on the skin. The only commercially available coral snake antivenin is Soro Anticlapidico manufactured by the Instituto Butantan, São Paulo, Brazil, and is available from most zoos and reptile houses in the United States. If respiratory paralysis occurs, intubation and assisted respiration are required.

RABIES

The incidence of rabies in the United States has varied from 0 to 5 cases per year since 1960. This low incidence is because of the effectiveness of animal immunization programs. However, the disease in wildlife—especially skunks, foxes, raccoons, and bats—has become more prevalent in recent years, representing approximately 85 per cent of all reported cases of animal rabies every year since 1976. Wild animals now constitute the most important potential source of infection for both humans and domestic animals in the United States.

THERAPY. The management of dog and other animal bites embodies the application of the usual surgical principles in the care of soft tissue injury (cleansing, antisepsis, and, if necessary in severe bites, débridement of necrotic tissue). The most pressing medical decision is whether to treat the patient for rabies. In cases in which the biting animal is known and confined, this problem is resolved, since therapy can be deferred during an observation period in which the animal will or will not die from rabies. Rabies virus must be demonstrated in the animal's saliva or glands during this time. However, when the biting animal is not captured, this decision must be made on the basis of the incidence of rabies in that species in the locale, and especially on the behavior of the biting animal.

SYSTEMIC TREATMENT. Rabies virus is poorly antigenic. In clinical infections, it appears that the virus must reach the brain before high antirabies antibody levels are achieved. Although the virus may be eliminated ("autosterilization") by this immune response, the course of the disease is unfortunately not altered. The rationale for postexposure prophylaxis is therefore to give vaccine for inducing an immune response against rabies and to administer antiserum (passive transfer) for effecting elevated antibody levels immediately while the body mounts its own immune response to the vaccine.

Before 1980, duck embryo vaccine was the only licensed vaccine available in the United States. However, human diploid cell rabies vaccine is now approved and widely available. This vaccine, derived from human cells in culture, has the significant advantages of being more immunogenic and not causing the toxic effects (pain, fever, erythema, allergic reactions, anaphylaxis) associated with duck embryo vaccine. In addition, the dreaded intraperitoneal injections are no longer necessary, as this can be given intramuscularly.

A complete summary of postexposure antirabies treatment is contained in Table 1.

HUMAN BITES

Human bites are relatively rare but can constitute serious problems. The three types are (1) a genuine bite in which the assailant sinks his teeth into the victim, producing puncture wounds, lacerations, or avulsion of tissue (particularly of the tip of the nose, the earlobe, or the tongue); (2) abrasion and

TABLE 1. Postexposure Antirabies Treatment Guide

Animal Species	Condition of Animal at Time of Attack	Treatment of Exposed Person[1]
Domestic		
Dog and cat	Healthy and available for 10 days of observation	None, unless animal develops rabies[2]
	Rabid or suspected rabid	RIG and HDCV[3]
	Unknown (escaped)	Consult public health officials; if treatment is indicated, give RIG and HDCV[3]
Wild		
Skunk, bat, fox, coyote, raccoon, bobcat, and other carnivores	Regard as rabid unless proven negative by laboratory tests[4]	RIG and HDCV[3]
Other		
Livestock, rodents, and lagomorphs (rabbits and hares)	Consider individually. Local and state public health officials should be consulted on questions about the need for rabies prophylaxis. Bites of squirrels, hamsters, guinea pigs, gerbils, chipmunks, rats, mice, other rodents, rabbits, and hares almost never call for antirabies prophylaxis.	

Adapted from Morbidity and Mortality Weekly Report, Vol. 33, No. 28. Centers for Disease Control, United States Public Health Service, Atlanta, July 1984.

[1]All bites and wounds should immediately be thoroughly cleansed with soap and water. If antirabies treatment is indicated, both rabies immune globulin (RIG) and human diploid cell rabies vaccine (HDCV) should be given as soon as possible, regardless of the interval from exposure. Local reactions to vaccines are common and do not contraindicate continuing treatment.

[2]Begin human rabies immune globulin and human diploid cell rabies vaccine at first sign of rabies in biting dog or cat during holding period (10 days).

[3]Vaccine antibody, human rabies immune globulin, is administered only once, at the beginning of antirabies therapy. The recommended dose is 20 IU per kg. Up to half the dose should be infiltrated around the wound and the rest administered intramuscularly in the buttocks. Five 1-ml. doses of human diploid cell rabies vaccine are given, one as soon as possible after exposure along with human rabies immune globulin; subsequent injections are given at 3, 7, 14, and 28 days after the first dose. Discontinue vaccine if fluorescent antibody tests of animal killed at time of attack are negative.

[4]The animal should be killed and tested as soon as possible. Holding for observation is not recommended.

laceration of the knuckles and hand, which occur from the clenched fist's striking the victim's mouth and teeth; and (3) a self-inflicted wound, usually of the tongue or lip, occurring often after falls or seizures.

BACTERIOLOGY. Infection is the most severe complication of human bites. The human mouth contains many more pathogenic organisms than those of most animals and can be a reservoir for *Staphylococcus, Streptococcus,* anaerobic streptococcus, gonococcus, Vincent's bacillus, fusiform bacillus, spirochetes, tetanus bacillus, gas gangrene bacillus, *Treponema pallidum,* and others. Heavy contamination of the wound should be assumed and treatment directed toward its eradication.

THERAPY. All wounds should be cultured, thoroughly scrubbed with bacteriostatic soap, and liberally irrigated with sterile saline. Examination of damage to deep structures should be made and tendon injury noted. Damaged tissues should be débrided. Severed tendons and nerves should not be sutured primarily.

Despite the potential for infection, following immediate administration of antibiotic therapy, soft tissue wounds of the head and face area that are properly cleansed and débrided can usually be sutured primarily when seen within 6 hours of injury. This applies even when cartilage of the nose or ear is exposed. Good cosmetic effects usually result. All other wounds should be left open. Broad-spectrum antibiotics in therapeutic dosage are routinely given systemically and are modified subsequently on the basis of the organism cultured. Tetanus toxoid is administered.

All patients should be observed carefully for signs of cellulitis or gangrene, especially in bites of the fingers. Wounds seen late with cellulitis and secondary infections require hospitalization for massive antibiotic therapy, immobilization, and débridement. Avulsed wound defects require plastic surgery repair after infection subsides.

BITES OF BEES, WASPS, HORNETS, AND OTHER INSECTS

INCIDENCE. Arthropods of the order Hymenoptera include the honeybee, bumblebee, wasp, yellow jacket, yellow and black hornet, ant, and sawfly. Probably more than 100,000 species of this order exist, and more bites and stings are inflicted upon humans by these creatures than by any other venomous group. Their venom is just as toxic as that of the rattlesnake, and more deaths follow insect bites in the United States yearly than from all snakebites. Less venom is injected in insect bites, and severe allergic reactions rather than direct toxic effects of the venom are responsible for most fatalities. Bees, wasps, hornets, and ants represent 65 per cent of deaths, spiders 31 per cent, and scorpions 4 per cent.

THERAPY. In 50 cases of fatal anaphylaxis produced by insect bites over a 10-year period, 62 per cent of the patients were dead in the first hour. Inadequate or no treatment was the practice. In a similar survey of 100 nonfatal cases of severe anaphylaxis, 87 per cent of the patients received treatment in the first hour after the bite. The most frequent types of systemic reactions in these survivors were general urticaria (74 per cent), syncope (65 per cent), and respiratory tract obstruction (38 per cent).

LOCAL CARE. The retained sting shaft, if present, should be scraped off with a blade. The wound is washed with soap and water. Cellulitis or gangrene may require débridement. Local injection of lidocaine (Xylocaine) in uncomplicated cases has relieved persistent pain.

TOXIC REACTIONS. In multiple bites, the total amount of injected toxin may be sufficient to cause severe systemic symptoms, principally diarrhea, vomiting, faintness, edema, muscle spasms, or convulsions. Supportive therapy such as sedation, intravenous fluids, antibiotics, and antihistamines may be necessary. The toxic effects of the venom can be counteracted by calcium gluconate infusion.

ALLERGIC REACTIONS. Immediate treatment is the key to success. Epinephrine 1:1000, 0.3 to 0.5 ml. for adults, is given subcutaneously. This is short-acting, and the dose may have to be repeated at 15- to 20-minute intervals. An antihistamine is also injected immediately. In severe cases, intravenous fluids, pressor agents, plasma expanders, and respiratory assistance may be required.

PREVENTION. All patients with a history of severe reaction to insect bites should be desensitized according to the directives of the Insect Allergy Committee of the American Academy of Allergy. The use of specific venom skin tests is probably the most accurate way for determining insect hypersensitivity. Desensitization should be instituted 14 days after a severe bite. Sensitive patients should wear long-sleeved clothing, avoid obvious hazards, and carry a kit containing 10-mg. isoproterenol tablets for sublingual use, epinephrine aerosol for inhalation, and tweezers for removal of the sting shaft.

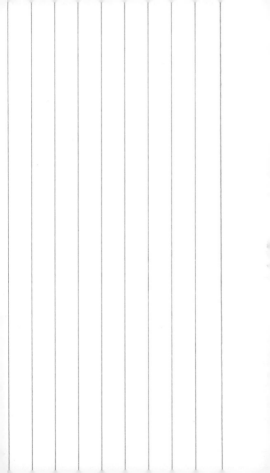

15

TRAUMA: Management of Acute Injuries

Gregory J. Jurkovich, M.D., and C. James Carrico, M.D.

The pivotal role of the trauma surgeon mandates a working knowledge of prevention, prehospital care, emergency room care, and rehabilitation in addition to the direction and provision of acute surgical care. This chapter will focus on the acute management of specific injuries. The important issues in trauma care systems are discussed in the main text.

INITIAL RESUSCITATION OF THE ACUTELY INJURED PATIENT

Initial care of the injured patient necessitates two assumptions. The first is that the patient may have more than one injury; the second is that the obvious injury is not necessarily the most important one. The key to initial care is an approach predicated on prioritizing injuries by their life-threatening potential. The priorities of initial trauma care are often referred to as the ABCs of trauma resuscitation.

AIRWAY. The crucial first step in the management of the injured patient is securing an adequate airway. In the majority of severely injured patients, this involves endotracheal intubation. The potential for cervical spine injury should always be considered, and injudicious movement of the neck in the process of *endotracheal* intubation must be avoided. *Nasotracheal* intubation is an option in the spontaneously breathing patient without midface injury. In rare patients, a surgical airway (tracheostomy) may be required.

BREATHING. When an adequate airway is secured, ventilation must be assured. The three most common reasons for ineffective ventilation following successful placement of an airway are malposition of the endotracheal tube, pneumothorax, and hemothorax. There is generally time to perform a chest radiograph before invasive therapeutic procedures. However, with a high suspicion of tension pneumothorax in the patient with profound hemodynamic instability, urgent needle catheter decompression before chest radiography can be both diagnostic and therapeutic.

CIRCULATION. Control of obvious hemorrhage, placement of an intravenous line, and fluid resuscitation are the next priority. Intravenous cannulas are usually placed percutaneously in the arm or groin. They should be large bore, and a minimum of two should be placed. Lines should not be inserted distal to extremity wounds with potential vascular injury. Alternative access sites are the saphenous cutdown

See the corresponding chapter or part in the *Textbook of Surgery*, 14th edition, pp. 258–298, for a more detailed discussion of this topic, including a comprehensive list of references.

route or intraosseous infusion in children under the age of 6 years. With the exception of the use of the large (8-Fr.) introducer catheter, subclavian venipuncture is not a rapid route for fluid administration and is best reserved for monitoring response to fluid therapy. Fluid resuscitation begins with a 1000-ml. bolus of lactated Ringer's solution for an adult, or 20 ml. per kg. for a child.

DISABILITY/NEUROLOGIC ASSESSMENT. At this juncture, a brief examination to determine the severity of neurologic injury is indicated. This includes calculation of the Glasgow Coma Scale, which is a method of following both the evolution of neurologic disability and prognosticating future recovery.

EXPOSURE FOR COMPLETE EXAMINATION. The next step is to completely, but expeditiously, re-examine the patient for diagnosis of other injuries. Appropriate laboratory and radiologic tests are obtained. Additional lines, catheters (nasogastric, Foley), and monitoring devices are now placed as needed. A priority treatment plan based on these initial findings should be established.

The following section considers the management of specific injuries. It is organized to reflect, in general, the probability that these specific injuries will impact negatively on airway, breathing, and circulation. Thus, thoracic and abdominal injuries are first, followed by the head and central nervous system, the neck, the face, and finally the extremities.

MANAGEMENT OF SPECIFIC INJURIES

Thoracic Injuries

One quarter of civilian trauma deaths are caused by thoracic trauma, and two thirds of these deaths occur after the patient reaches the hospital. Despite this high mortality, only 10 to 15 per cent of thoracic injuries require a thoracotomy. The simple lifesaving maneuvers of airway control and tube thoracostomy effectively treat the majority of chest trauma victims. The treatment of specific thoracic injuries is outlined below.

CHEST WALL AND LUNGS

RIB FRACTURES. Rib fractures are the most common thoracic injury. With simple fractures, pain on inspiration is the principal symptom. Localized pain, tenderness, and occasionally crepitus confirm the diagnosis. A chest film should be obtained for exclusion of other intrathoracic injuries and not necessarily for identification of the rib fracture. Narcotics, intercostal nerve blocks, and muscle relaxants are usually adequate treatment. For more severe injuries, hospital admission for pain relief, cough assistance, and endotracheal suction may be necessary for several days, particularly in elderly patients. Rib belts and adhesive taping, although formerly popular, should be avoided because the resultant limitation in motion increases the incidence of retained secretions and atelectasis. Fracture of the upper ribs (1–3), clavicle, or scapula implies significant trauma, and associated major vascular injury must be suspected, although angiography may be selectively employed.

FLAIL CHEST. With segmental fractures of multiple ribs, chest wall instability may be so severe as to limit the effectiveness of spontaneous respirations. This is known as flail chest. Endotracheal intubation and mechanical ventilation may be required. Tachypnea, hypoxia, and hypercarbia are indications for intubation and mechanical ventilation.

PULMONARY CONTUSION. Respiratory difficulty in flail chest injury is invariably aggravated by an underlying pulmonary contusion, although pulmonary contusion can also appear without any evidence of rib fracture, particularly in children. Fluid and blood from ruptured vessels enter the alveoli, interstitial spaces, and bronchi and produce localized airway obstruction. Pulmonary compliance decreases, and ventilation becomes more difficult. Positive end-expiratory pressure ventilation may be helpful in restoring functional residual capacity and reducing intrapulmonary shunts. Excessive fluid administration should be avoided.

PNEUMOTHORAX. Pneumothorax is the accumulation of air in the potential space between the visceral and parietal pleura following either a full-thickness violation of the chest wall or laceration of the visceral pleura. Accumulation of air in this space under pressure is known as a *tension pneumothorax.* Sufficient accumulation of air in this space will collapse the lung and shift the mediastinum into the contralateral thorax, causing hypoxia and a diminished venous return to the heart. Prompt venting of a tension pneumothorax can be lifesaving, and virtually all traumatic pneumothoraces should be treated with a tube thoracostomy to water-seal drainage. An *open pneumothorax* is a defect in the chest wall that provides a direct communication between the pleural space and the environment. A large wound provides an alternative air pathway of less resistance than the normal tracheobronchial tree. Inability to generate negative intrathoracic pressure causes lung collapse and marked paroxysmal shifting of the mediastinum with each respiratory effort. Diagnosis is usually apparent, as each inspiration draws air into the interpleural space, causing the characteristic "sucking chest wound." Treatment consists of prompt closure of the defect with a sterile dressing followed by venting of the chest with either a flutter valve or chest tube for treatment of the possible resultant tension pneumothorax.

HEMOTHORAX. Hemothorax occurs in some quantity in almost every patient with a diagnosable chest injury. Although an upright chest film can reveal an intrathoracic accumulation of as little as 200 ml. of blood, a supine film may miss collections of up to 1 liter. Since the lung itself is a low-pressure system, spontaneous hemostasis occurs for all but central hilar injuries or injury to the intercostal or internal mammary arteries. Tube thoracostomy with a 32- to 36-French chest tube placed in the sixth or seventh intercostal space at the midaxillary line should be promptly performed. When massive hemothorax is present, preparation for collection of the blood for autotransfusion should be made before tube insertion.

In 85 per cent of patients, tube thoracostomy is the only treatment required. However, an initial thoracic blood loss greater than 1500 ml. (30 per cent blood volume) or an ongoing loss of 250 ml. (5 per cent blood volume) for 3 consecutive hours is generally an indication for exploratory thoracotomy. This is only a guideline, however, and the clinical situation and overall condition of the patient should be the most influential factors.

TRACHEAL AND BRONCHIAL INJURIES. Tracheal and bronchial injuries are unusual but may be caused by blunt or penetrating trauma. Presenting signs are generally dramatic, with significant hemoptysis, hemopneumothorax, subcutaneous crepitance, and respiratory distress; mediastinal and deep cervical emphysema; or pneumothorax with a massive air leak. Emergency treatment usually consists of inserting the endotracheal tube (via endoscopic control) beyond the injury to facilitate ventilation and prevent aspiration of blood. Tube thoracostomy is required for hemo- or pneumothorax. Primary surgical repair is generally indicated.

HEART AND AORTA

MYOCARDIAL CONTUSION. A direct blow to the sternum with subsequent cardiac bruising is known as a myocardial contusion. The cardiac injury may vary from superficial epicardial petechiae to transmural damage. Dysrhythmia is the most common presenting finding, although right ventricular dysfunction and decreased cardiac output may occur. The major difficulty in treatment is early recognition. Although cardiac CPK isoenzymes are widely employed, they have not been shown to be adequately sensitive or specific diagnostic tests. Electrocardiograms may show nonspecific ST-T wave changes or dysrhythmias. Cardiac monitoring for 24 hours is indicated if electrocardiographic abnormalities are present or if a major contusion is suspected. Echocardiography is helpful in diagnosing ventricular dysfunction and in detecting blood in the pericardium. The management of myocardial contusion is supportive.

CARDIAC TAMPONADE. Most frequently caused by penetrating thoracic injuries, cardiac tamponade is occasionally observed in blunt thoracic trauma from superior vena caval or atrial rupture, coronary artery laceration, or descending dissection of an aortic tear. Accumulation of as little as 150 ml. of blood in the pericardial sac may significantly impair diastolic filling. Beck's classic triad of distended neck veins, muffled heart sounds, and hypotension is present in only one third of patients with tamponade. Pulsus paradoxus is even less frequently discernible. Pericardiocentesis can be both diagnostic and temporarily therapeutic. However, approximately 15 per cent of pericardiocenteses give false-negative results because of a clotted hemopericardium. Therefore, echocardiography before open pericardiotomy is advisable if it can be obtained promptly. If the patient is *in extremis,* emergency thoracotomy with pericardiotomy and cardiac repair should be performed.

AORTA. Rupture of the thoracic aorta is the most lethal

injury following blunt chest trauma. The exact mechanism of injury is not fully understood, but it is thought that the descending portion of the aortic arch undergoes flexion or torsion, disrupting the aortic wall at the ligamentum arteriosum immediately distal to the left subclavian artery. Most patients with aortic rupture die immediately from exsanguination, but in approximately 20 per cent the periaortic tissue temporarily contains the hematoma. Survival depends on prompt diagnosis and treatment. A suggestive mechanism of injury and a widening of the mediastinal shadow should prompt angiography, even though only 20 to 43 per cent of patients with a widened mediastinum have aortic injury. Other radiographic signs suggestive of aortic injury include loss of aortic knob contour, right shift of trachea and nasogastric tube, apical capping, and left hemothorax.

DIAPHRAGM AND ESOPHAGUS

Penetrating lacerations of the diaphragm outnumber blunt ruptures at least four to one. Both may produce herniation through the diaphragm and both require repair, even small stab wounds. With isolated diaphragm injuries, diagnosis may be difficult. The initial chest film may be normal in 30 per cent of patients with right-sided diaphragmatic rupture. Herniation of the viscera may not occur immediately, and the patient may present months or years later with incarceration of abdominal contents in the hernia. Fortunately, the diagnosis is often incidentally made at the time of laparotomy, since most patients have concomitant intra-abdominal injuries.

Blunt injury to the esophagus is rare, and penetrating injuries are rarely isolated. The most common symptom of esophageal perforation is extreme chest pain with the slow evolution of fever several hours later. Regurgitation of blood, hoarseness, dysphagia, or respiratory distress may also be present. Suspicious radiographic findings are mediastinal air and widening, presence of a foreign body, pleural effusion, or hydropneumothorax. All gunshot wounds traversing the mediastinum should be evaluated for possible esophageal injury. Both endoscopy and esophagography have reported sensitivities that vary from 50 to 90 per cent and should be considered complementary studies. Esophageal injury requires immediate débridement, suture closure, and drainage. Delays of 12 to 24 hours may preclude primary repair and mandate proximal diversion and distal feeding access.

Abdomen: Mechanisms and Diagnosis of Injury

In the awake, alert, responsive patient with *isolated* abdominal injury, the physical examination and history are quite accurate in predicting the presence of significant visceral injury. However, in the patient with altered level of consciousness or multiple injuries, an impaired ability to recognize abdominal pain makes diagnosis more difficult. The overall sensitivity (95 per cent), specificity (98 to 99 per cent), and accuracy (97 per cent) of diagnostic peritoneal lavage make this technique the mainstay for diagnosis of intraperitoneal injury in the multiple-injury trauma patient. Computed tomography (CT) is useful in assessing the abdomen of the *hemodynamically stable* patient and is particularly useful in assessing the retroperitoneum, an anatomical area of injury for which diagnostic peritoneal lavage is not helpful. Peitzman and colleagues have listed five indications for abdominal CT scans in *hemodynamically stable* trauma victims: (1) an equivocal abdominal examination, (2) closed head injury, (3) spinal cord injury, (4) hematuria, and (5) patients with pelvic fractures and significant bleeding.

The diagnosis of intraperitoneal injury in penetrating abdominal trauma remains controversial. In general, gunshot wounds require laparotomy; stab wounds can be more selectively managed. It should be emphasized that if there is any doubt regarding the potential for intra-abdominal injury, exploratory laparotomy remains the best method of evaluation and treatment.

Abdomen: Intraperitoneal Injuries

SPLEEN

The spleen is the most commonly injured intra-abdominal organ. Splenectomy is no longer the only management option for splenic injuries. Trauma surgeons must also consider splenic repair or nonoperative management as viable options in select patients, with recognition of the rare but highly lethal syndrome of overwhelming postsplenectomy sepsis (see main text). Splenorrhaphy (repair) can be considered for injuries to all areas of the spleen except the central hilar area. Although the reported success rate of splenic repair varies, most large trauma centers report splenic salvage rates to be between 40 and 60 per cent of all splenic injuries. In patients with multiple intra-abdominal injuries or extensive peritoneal contamination from visceral perforation, it is good surgical judgment to weigh the benefits of splenic salvage against the safer and more expedient course of splenectomy. In addition, splenic salvage is probably not warranted if only 50 per cent or less of the splenic substance is to be preserved.

The safety and effectiveness of nonoperative management of selected pediatric patients with isolated splenic injuries is acceptable, but similar management in adults is controversial. The unknown incidence of delayed splenic rupture and the incidence of associated injuries are reasons often given for avoiding nonoperative management. An additional factor considered in weighing the risk of nonoperative management versus splenorrhaphy or splenectomy is the risk of blood transfusion.

LIVER

The liver is the second most commonly injured organ following blunt trauma and is the most commonly injured abdominal organ following penetrating trauma. Over 50 per cent of all liver injuries are nonbleeding at the time of initial exploration, and an additional 20 per cent can be managed by direct suture ligation, cautery, or hemostatic agents. The remaining severe liver injuries can be difficult to manage and are responsible for the high overall liver injury mortality of 11 per cent and morbidity of 22 per cent.

With deeper lacerations, bleeding may initially be so significant as to prevent adequate exposure. Direct compression and inflow occlusion (Pringle maneuver) are effective maneuvers for providing exposure and allowing direct ligation of vessels and biliary radicals. Although the exact length of warm ischemia time tolerated by the human liver is not known, inflow occlusion for at least 20 minutes, and perhaps up to 1 hour, appears to be well tolerated. Liver lacerations should not be sutured closed. This predisposes to liver abscesses and hemobilia. Closed suction drainage should be provided in all cases.

Selective ligation of the right or left hepatic artery is necessary in less than 1 per cent of all liver injuries; injudicious hepatic artery ligation may cause liver infarction. The proper hepatic artery must never be ligated. Resection of hepatic parenchyma is also unusual following liver injuries. In one large review consisting of over 1300 liver trauma patients, hepatic resectional débridement was performed in only 36 patients (2.6 per cent), hepatotomy and vessel ligation in 50 patients (3.7 per cent), and segmentectomy in 18 patients (1.3 per cent). Formal hepatic lobectomy was performed in only 12 patients (0.9 per cent). Perihepatic packing with delayed reoperation is of benefit in a selected group of patients in whom packing controls the hemorrhage, and associated injuries, coagulopathy, or hemodynamic status make attempts at direct repair unwise.

If inflow occlusion is unsuccessful, it is presumed that the patient has a retrohepatic inferior vena cava injury, hepatic vein injury, or juxtacaval intraparenchymal hepatic vein injury. In this rare circumstance, atrial-caval shunting may be considered. The liver injury is tightly packed, extended exposure is obtained, and both hepatic vascular inflow and outflow are controlled. Despite this technique, mortality for retrohepatic caval and intraparenchymal hepatic vein injuries exceeds 50 per cent.

STOMACH

Most full-thickness gastric injury is due to penetrating trauma. Gastric rupture secondary to blunt trauma is rare, but vigorous ventilation with an endotracheal tube misplaced in the esophagus can cause iatrogenic gastric rupture in the trauma patient. If there is any reason to suspect a gastric injury, the gastrocolic omentum must be widely opened so that the entire posterior surface of the stomach may be completely inspected. If there is any blood in the gastrohepatic ligament, the lesser curvature of the stomach must be closely examined. Most gastric injuries can be treated simply with débridement and closure in layers.

SMALL INTESTINE

The incidence of small bowel injury approaches 50 per cent for all penetrating abdominal injuries and ranges from 5 to 15 per cent following blunt abdominal trauma. During any laparotomy for trauma, the entire small bowel should be meticulously examined. Abdominal wall entrance and exit wounds cannot be used to predict the likely site of a small bowel injury. Each tear, as it is encountered, should be controlled in order to prevent further leakage and contamination. Simple lacerations of the small bowel are generally sutured with a single layer of interrupted nonabsorbable Lembert sutures after removal of any devitalized tissue. Where damage to the bowel wall is extensive or where multiple tears are situated fairly close to one another, resection of the involved segment rather than repair of the individual perforations is preferred.

COLON AND RECTUM

Because of a concern for anastomotic breakdown following primary repair, it has long been thought that the safest way of managing most colon injuries is by colostomy. This concept has dominated modern management of colon wounds and can be traced to the surgical experience of World War II, when colostomy was credited with reducing mortality from colonic injury to 37 per cent, down from the World War I mortality of 60 per cent for colon injuries treated by primary repair. However, the need for uniform colostomy in civilian colon trauma has been challenged, the premise being that unlike war injuries, most civilian colon wounds are due to low-velocity handguns or stab wounds. As a consequence, many trauma surgeons maintain that more than half of all civilian colon injuries can be treated by primary repair instead of exteriorization or colostomy.

Primary repair is generally applicable only to the stable patient without a history of hypotension, minimal soilage or contamination, intact colon blood supply and minimal colon tissue loss, and few or no associated injuries. In addition, most surgeons treat the various anatomic components of the colon with some unique distinction. There is a general trend to repair *right* colon injuries and *stab* wounds or *low-velocity* gunshot wounds primarily. More significant penetrating injuries and most blunt injuries to the right colon are managed by right colectomy; primary reconstruction via ileotransverse colostomy may be performed in a stable patient in whom there is an isolated injury with no evidence of shock or gross fecal contamination. Otherwise, a right colectomy is accompanied by the creation of an ileostomy and mucous fistula. The same guiding principles for primary repair of minor wounds can be followed for the left colon, although resection with primary anastomosis is generally not recommended owing to the different vascularity, fecal consistency, and bacterial load. More extensive left colon injuries are generally treated by resection with proximal end colostomy and distal mucous fistula or Hartmann's pouch. Stab wounds and low-velocity gunshot wounds of the transverse colon can also be considered for primary repair or exteriorized as loop colostomies.

RECTUM. Primary closure is *not* used *without colostomy* if the wound is full thickness and occurs above the dentate line. Presacral drains and rectal stump washout are employed. For wounds below the dentate line, débridement, repair, and drainage without colon diversion are appropriate.

Abdomen: Retroperitoneal Injuries

DUODENUM

Whereas the diagnosis of penetrating duodenal injuries is generally made during laparotomy immediately following injury, the insidious nature of many blunt duodenal injuries makes the initial diagnosis difficult. This delay may be lethal. One report documents a fourfold increase in mortality (11 per cent versus 40 per cent) if the diagnosis was delayed longer than 24 hours.

Early diagnosis requires a high index of suspicion in patients with appropriate injury mechanisms. Serum amylase should be initially obtained and, if elevated, repeated at 6-hour intervals. An early suspicion of retroperitoneal duodenal rupture is best confirmed (or excluded) by a Gastrografin upper gastrointestinal series or abdominal CT scan with oral and intravenous contrast enhancement. Diagnostic peritoneal lavage is unreliable in detecting duodenal injuries, but approximately 40 per cent of patients with duodenal injury have associated intra-abdominal injuries that cause a positive diagnostic peritoneal lavage and subsequent surgical exploration.

Most (80 to 85 per cent) duodenal wounds can be safely repaired primarily. Approximately 15 to 20 per cent require more complex procedures. Protection of a tenuous duodenal repair may be aided by lateral tube duodenostomy or duodenal drainage via a retrograde jejunostomy, or by complete diversion of gastric contents away from the duodenum either by a Berne duodenal "diverticulization" (antrectomy and Billroth II gastrojejunostomy) or by "exclusion" of the pylorus and duodenal diversion via a loop gastrojejunostomy.

Duodenal hematomas do not usually require operative intervention. The initial diagnostic gastrografin examination (CT or upper gastrointestinal study) should be followed by barium to provide greater detail needed to detect the "coiled spring" or "stacked coin" sign. Continuous nasogastric suction should be employed and total parenteral nutrition begun. The patient should be re-evaluated with upper gastrointestinal contrast studies at 5- to 7-day intervals. Operative exploration and evacuation of the hematoma may be considered if resolution has not occurred after 2 weeks of conservative therapy.

PANCREAS

Combined morbidity and mortality of approximately 50 per cent emphasizes the significance of pancreatic injuries. Associated injuries are common because the pancreas is surrounded by major abdominal organs and blood vessels. Concomitant vascular injuries are responsible for half of all pancreatic trauma deaths and nearly all of the immediate deaths. Infection is responsible for the majority of the late deaths. The key determinant of long-term outcome is the presence or absence of pancreatic duct injury, since this determines the likelihood of postoperative complications. The implication of these observations is that the first priority in managing pancreatic trauma should be control of hemorrhage and repair of intestinal injuries to limit bacterial contamination. A diligent search for potential pancreatic duct injury should follow.

The preoperative evaluation of patients with penetrating abdominal wounds and possible pancreatic injury is relatively straightforward, as abdominal exploration is generally warranted. The evaluation of patients with blunt injury is more complex. Serum amylase determination has limited sensitivity or specificity for pancreatic injury. In one report, the serum amylase level was elevated in only 16 per cent of the patients with penetrating pancreatic injuries and in only 61 per cent of those who had blunt pancreatic trauma. Isoamylase differentiation does not increase the test's accuracy. Nonetheless, an elevated serum or peritoneal lavage effluent amylase raises concern about pancreatic injury and mandates further evaluation by either CT scan or surgical exploration.

At operation, the majority (95 per cent) of pancreatic injuries can be diagnosed by careful inspection following adequate exposure. The remaining 5 per cent of injuries may require more elaborate investigative techniques for diagnosis of ductal injury, such as contrast studies through the biliary tree, ampulla, or tail of the pancreas when there is major concern about the integrity of the main pancreatic duct. The routine performance of intraoperative pancreatography when proximal duct injury is strongly suspected decreased the postoperative morbidity rate from 55 to 15 per cent in the authors' institution.

The principles of managing pancreatic injuries are to control hemorrhage, débride devitalized pancreatic tissue, provide adequate external drainage of injuries or resections, and preserve as much functional pancreatic tissue as possible. The difficult decisions in managing pancreatic trauma involve patients with parenchymal disruption and major duct injury. In general, distal pancreatic duct injuries are treated by resectional débridement. Proximal duct injuries are treated by a combination of wide drainage, resection, or enteric drainage. A more detailed discussion of the management of pancreatic injuries is provided in the main text.

MAJOR ABDOMINAL VESSELS

The mortality from abdominal vascular trauma ranges from 15 to 80 per cent, highest for aortic wounds, followed by superior mesenteric vessels and iliac vessels, and lowest for vena caval wounds, although suprarenal wounds can be very difficult to repair. One third of abdominal vascular trauma patients present to the emergency room in shock. Rapid control of the injury is therefore the primary management goal, and since most injuries are due to penetrating wounds, immediate triage to the operating room is simplified and must be expedited.

Operative control of major vessel hemorrhage can be challenging. If active hemorrhage is encountered, it must be controlled immediately, initially by packing. Any retroperitoneal hematoma should suggest the possibility of associated vascular injury. Specific approaches to individual intraabdominal vessels depend on the location of the surrounding hematoma.

Midline suprarenal hemorrhage is perhaps the most difficult to control, since the aorta, celiac axis, mesenteric vessels, or vena cava may be responsible. In addition, with the usual penetrating wound, associated gastric, duodenal, or pancreatic injuries are likely. Proximal aortic control may be attempted via direct aortic compression through either the gastrohepatic ligament or a left anterolateral thoracotomy. Rotation of the descending colon, spleen, pancreas, and left kidney to the midline allows complete exposure of the aorta from the hiatus to the aortic bifurcation. The left diaphragmatic crux may be divided to provide even more proximal exposure. Suprarenal vena caval injuries are approached with an extended Kocher maneuver and retraction of the liver superiorly. Retrohepatic vena caval injuries (see Liver) are extremely difficult to control and are generally lethal.

Midline infrarenal hematomas can usually be approached directly through the retroperitoneum or the base of the mesentery, and direct control with vascular clamps can be accomplished. The maneuvers utilized are similar to those used in the approach to abdominal aortic aneurysms.

Lateral hematomas may be due to renal parenchymal or vascular injury. Preoperative evaluation with "one-shot" intravenous pyelography is often helpful. Following blunt trauma, if the kidney is well perfused, and the hematoma small and nonexpanding with no urine leak, no further exploration is required (see Urinary Tract). In penetrating trauma, however, all lateral hematomas should be explored and the path of injury meticulously followed. Renal vascular control should be obtained first before opening Gerota's fascia. This step, while often unnecessary, appears to decrease the incidence of nephrectomy.

The approach to *pelvic hematomas* again depends on mechanism of injury. A retroperitoneal pelvic hematoma following blunt trauma should *not* be explored (see Pelvic Injuries). Pelvic bone fixation and angiography with embolization have a role in managing these injuries. Penetrating pelvic wounds, however, require exploration of the projectile or stab pathway. Injuries to the common or external iliac artery should be repaired, if at all possible. In contrast, injuries to the internal iliac artery can be ligated with impunity, even if they occur bilaterally.

URINARY TRACT

There is no degree of hematuria that is diagnostic of major urinary tract injury, and the absence of major hematuria does not exclude significant injury. Therefore, a key tenet to be applied in diagnosing urologic trauma is to suspect injury by assessing the mechanism and forces involved. Signs of a lower urinary tract injury include blood at the urinary meatus, a "high riding" or misplaced prostate that cannot be palpated on rectal examination, urinary retention, bladder distention, or the desire to void but an inability to empty the bladder. In the presence of these signs, a retrograde urethrogram is indicated before attempts at inserting a Foley catheter. The presence of pelvic crush injury also suggests the need to obtain a retrograde cystourethrogram for evaluation of bladder or urethral injury, even in the absence of blood at the meatus.

Specific signs of upper urologic tract injury include either gross or microscopic hematuria. If upper urinary tract injury is suspected, the initial evaluation depends in part on the patient's associated injuries and hemodynamic stability. If the patient requires emergent surgical therapy for associated injuries, a limited "one-shot" intravenous pyelogram may be obtained in the emergency room or on the operating room table by the rapid intravenous injections of 60 ml. of high-density contrast medium followed by a flat plate radiograph of the abdomen and pelvis in 1 to 5 minutes. This study generally identifies the presence or absence of functioning kidneys but is an extremely limited study that may falsely fail to identify a renal outline in the presence of shock. In the hemodynamically stable patient, either intravenous pyelography or CT with intravenous contrast is an effective method of evaluating the urinary tract, although CT scans provide more detailed information about both the urologic injury and the potential associated intra-abdominal and retroperitoneal injuries. The degree of renal parenchymal injury identified on CT scans is also useful in classifying the injury and defining management plan. Demonstration by either CT scan or intravenous pyelography of the apparent presence of a solitary kidney or a lack of function of a segment of the kidney is an indication for immediate arteriography.

Pelvic Injuries

Pelvic fractures are the third most common injury sustained in motor vehicle accidents. The majority require straightforward skeletal management, but approximately 20 per cent are complex crush injuries and open pelvic fractures with mortality in excess of 50 per cent.

Examination begins by administering anteroposterior and lateral compression for assessment of instability and pain. A rectal and vaginal examination must be performed to assess blood, fragments, mucosal lacerations, and prostate location in the male. Blood at the urethral meatus requires retrograde urethrocystography before insertion of a Foley catheter. The initial radiographic examination should include an anteroposterior plain film of the pelvis. More select views, including CT, may be indicated as time and the patient's condition allow but must not take precedence over the search for associated injuries.

The management objectives in a patient with a pelvic fracture are control of hemorrhage, skeletal fixation, and treatment of associated injuries. Massive blood loss (up to 20 units) can occur into the retroperitoneal space from arterial or venous injuries or the fracture line itself. Extensive collateralization, difficult exposure, and release of the tamponade effect of the posterior peritoneum make surgical exploration of pelvic hematomas generally frustrating and fruitless. Application of the pneumatic anti-shock garment may be beneficial as a temporizing agent, pending either immediate skeletal fixation or angiographic evaluation and embolization. If pelvic hematoma-related blood requirements exceed 4 to 6 units, either angiographic intervention or emergent skeletal fixation may be indicated. There currently exist no comparative data for determining which method or approach is superior, nor are there exact indications for their use.

Approximately 25 per cent of pelvic fracture victims have associated intra-abdominal injury. Diagnostic peritoneal lavage should be performed in the supraumbilical location, since false-positive rates range from 16 to 50 per cent if it is performed in the standard infraumbilical location. A grossly positive peritoneal lavage is generally an indication for immediate exploratory celiotomy. Computed tomography is an alternative diagnostic modality in the hemodynamically stable patient.

Central Nervous System Injuries

CRANIUM AND BRAIN

The two guiding principles of initial care are (1) *assessment of injury severity* and (2) *protection of the brain from further injury* until definitive diagnosis and therapy can be achieved. The treatment plan depends on identifying the two fundamental head injuries: focal or diffuse. Focal injuries consist of mass lesions that cause neurologic dysfunction, largely by brain compression, and often require surgical evacuation. Diffuse brain injuries are equally frequent and cause prolonged coma without intracranial masses. These do not require surgical therapy but can be as devastating as focal injuries.

ASSESSMENT OF INJURY SEVERITY. The severity of brain injury can be estimated in less than 1 minute by evaluating three factors: *level of consciousness, pupillary function,* and *lateralized weakness* of the extremities.

Level of consciousness is best assessed by the Glasgow Coma Scale (GCS), a system that evaluates eye opening, best motor response, and verbal response. *Pupillary function* is assessed by the size, equality, and response to bright light. Whether or not there has been ocular injury, any pupillary asymmetry greater than 1 mm. must be attributed to intracranial injury unless proved otherwise. With few exceptions, the largest pupil is on the side of the mass lesion. The *lateralized extremity weakness* is detected by testing motor power in patients able to cooperate or by observing symmetry of movement in response to painful stimulus. As the severity of injury increases, lateralized weakness is more difficult to recognize, and small differences may be important.

The presence of any of the following criteria suggests serious injury: (1) a GCS score of less than 10, (2) a decrease in the GCS score by 3 or more regardless of the initial GCS score, (3) pupillary inequality greater than 1 mm. regardless of the GCS score, (4) lateralized extremity weakness regardless of the GCS score, (5) markedly depressed skull fractures, and (6) open cranial wounds with brain exposed.

PROTECTION FROM FURTHER INSULT. Delivering adequate oxygen to the brain is the primary goal in preventing further injury. Arterial oxygen content must be optimized. This often involves intubation, oxygen supplementation, and mechanical ventilation. If urgent intubation is required, paralytic agents, pharyngeal anesthesia, and barbiturate induction limit the massive elevation of intracranial pressure (ICP) that may occur. Brain injury *per se rarely* causes hypotension during the early period following trauma, but the brain is extremely susceptible to hypoxia and inadequate perfusion. Cerebral perfusion pressure (MAP − ICP) greater than 40 mm. Hg must be maintained by appropriate fluid and blood replacement while volume overload is avoided.

Even after relatively short periods of ischemia, the brain may respond to reperfusion in a pathologic manner with prompt and severe brain swelling and marked increases in ICP. Elevated ICP can best be managed in the early phases of injury by controlled hyperventilation to P_{CO_2} values in the low-mid 20s. Decreasing brain water with diuretics or hyperosmotic agents may also be helpful.

DEFINITIVE CARE. Definitive care begins with a definitive diagnosis, which is established exclusively by computed tomography. Cranial CT has a high priority in the evaluation of a patient with an altered level of consciousness or lateralizing neurologic signs. It should be performed as soon as cardiorespiratory stability has been achieved and a lateral cervical spine roentgenogram demonstrates no fracture or dislocation. Seriously injured patients who are intubated should receive neuromuscular blockage during the study. A good quality CT scan identifies focal mass lesions and allows the diagnosis of diffuse brain injury. *Focal injuries* with significant mass effect require surgical evacuation; patients with these injuries go directly to the operating room.

Patients with *diffuse brain injury* are managed in the intensive care unit. Monitoring devices for ICP are placed for on-line management of intracranial hypertension in both groups. Principal treatment efforts are directed toward controlling intracranial hypertension, providing adequate cerebral oxygenation, and preventing infectious complications of prolonged coma. Although both barbiturates and glucocorticoids have been advocated in the management of severe head injury, recent clinical evidence does not support their use.

VERTEBRAE AND SPINAL CORD

All patients with blunt trauma must initially be treated as if they have a spinal cord injury. Proper care of the potentially unstable spine begins at the scene of injury with proper immobilization of the head, neck, and spine on a backboard and continues until the spine has been proved stable. Careful follow-up examinations must be made during a traumatized patient's hospitalization if there are complaints of pain in the back or neck; if weakness, numbness, or loss of control of extremities or sphincters develops; or if only screening radiographs were obtained during admission evaluation.

The history and physical examination should specifically assess the presence of any spinal column pain or transient neurologic abnormalities. If a neurologic deficit is present, the examination focuses on defining the neurologic level of injury and on determining whether there is sparing of some spinal cord function across this level. A patient with a complete spinal cord injury has no distal motor or sensory function. Most incomplete spinal cord injuries exhibit mixed motor and sensory sparing rather than a classic pattern of partial injury. Sacral sparing may be the only evidence that paralysis may not be complete. The natural history of incomplete cord injuries is improvement. If deterioration is observed, emergency diagnostic and surgical treatment may be warranted. Since changes in the neurologic examination are so crucial, it is essential that neurologic function be accurately recorded in the prehospital and emergency room notes to allow later comparison.

Good quality roentgenograms are essential and must be accomplished before moving the neck of all blunt trauma patients, particularly those who are unconscious, obtunded, or complaining of neck pain. The initial screening view is a cross-table lateral of the supine patient. Formal anteroposterior, lateral, and odontoid views should be obtained before the cervical spine is "cleared," but flexion and extension radiograms are rarely indicated and only if the patient is conscious and cooperative. Computed tomography and magnetic resonance imaging have a role in defining in greater detail the spinal cord and bony column injury in the hemodynamically stable patient.

Neck Injuries

The neck is classically divided into anatomic triangles. Penetrating wounds that enter through the anterior triangle or sternocleidomastoid muscle have a high likelihood of significant vascular, airway, or esophageal injury. In contrast, wounds to the posterior triangle rarely involve the esophagus, airway, or major vascular structures, although if they are directed inferiorly, intrathoracic injury can occur. The other major anatomic landmark in the neck is the platysma muscle. Wounds that fail to penetrate the platysma are considered superficial and do not warrant extensive evaluation. Wounds that penetrate the platysma mandate hospital admission and either immediate operative exploration or further diagnostic evaluation.

The anterior neck is further divided into three zones defined by horizontal planes. Zone I injuries (low neck) have the highest mortality because of the risk of major vascular and intrathoracic injury. Zone II injuries (mid neck) are the most common but have the lowest mortality. Significant injury is generally apparent, and exposure of vital structures is readily accomplished. Zone III wounds (high neck) risk injury to the distal carotid artery, salivary glands, and pharynx. Operative exposure can be particularly difficult.

In general, all patients with platysma-penetrating wounds and clinical signs of vascular, airway, or esophageal injury (shock, hemorrhage, expanding hematoma, hemoptysis, hematemesis, subcutaneous emphysema, others) require prompt operative exploration. Patients with "clinically silent" platysma-penetrating wounds should at least be admitted to the hospital. At Harborview Medical Center in Seattle, the authors continue to explore the majority of neck wounds that penetrate the platysma. More specifically, injuries to the base of the skull and thoracic outlet (Zone III and Zone I) require angiography before, and occasionally in lieu of, exploration. Injuries to the midneck (Zone II) are generally managed by exploration without prior invasive diagnostic studies.

The signs of neck injury following blunt trauma can be subtle but the consequences of an overlooked injury can be devastating. A neurologic deficit unexplained by head CT findings in a patient with blunt neck trauma mandates four-vessel angiography. Hoarseness, dysphagia, hemoptysis, or hematemesis in such victims portends airway and/or esophageal injury. Patency of the airway must be assured. Panendoscopy and esophagography should be liberally employed. Computed tomography can be extremely helpful in delineating laryngeal injuries.

Maxillofacial Injuries

While preserving sight and speech and minimizing deformity are important goals, they occupy a relatively low priority in the care of the multiply injured patient. Rather, it is a fact that maxillofacial trauma is frequently associated with upper airway compromise and difficult hemorrhage that mandate attention in the initial resuscitation of the trauma victim. Definitive airway control can be difficult in the presence of facial injuries, and the physician must always be prepared and equipped to perform emergency tracheostomy.

Severe hemorrhage in conjunction with a facial fracture can be a particularly vexing problem. Hemorrhage typically occurs from the nasal or oral cavity and can usually be controlled by fracture reduction combined with anterior and posterior nasopharyngeal packing. Substantial hemorrhage in a patient with severe midface fractures that is not controlled by these techniques should arouse suspicion of laceration of one or both internal maxillary arteries, or basilar skull fracture with internal carotid artery involvement. If these maneuvers fail to control hemorrhage, immediate angiographic evaluation and embolization is indicated and generally preferred over operative attempts at external carotid artery or selective branch ligation.

The initial examination of the patient includes palpation of all external facial features, evaluation of ocular muscle activity, and visual acuity examination. A gloved hand should be used to intraorally assess maxillary stability, dentition, and the mandibular contour. However, the diagnosis of maxillofacial trauma has been revolutionized by CT. The accuracy of CT scanning is unsurpassed when compared with plain radiographs or tomography, particularly in the evaluation of certain soft tissue injuries and injuries to the paranasal sinuses, orbits, and mandibular condylar heads. This information can be extremely useful to the surgeon in directing a treatment plan. The management of specific maxillofacial injuries is discussed in greater detail in the main text.

Extremity and Peripheral Vascular Injuries

The management of most musculoskeletal injuries is discussed in other sections of this text. The following section highlights three key areas of trauma care involving the extremities: early fracture stabilization, soft tissue injury, and vascular trauma.

EARLY FRACTURE STABILIZATION

Hemorrhage due to massive disruption or transection of major blood vessels constitutes the only situation in which extremity injuries are immediately life-threatening. However, multiple long bone fractures have recently been recognized to have a strikingly adverse impact on survival following injury. Although specific treatment of fractures is not addressed in this chapter, the crucial role of early fracture fixation in the care of the multiply injured victim cannot be overlooked. Early fixation of long bone fractures decreases the incidence of adult respiratory distress syndrome, fat embolization syndrome, and subsequent development of sepsis and multiple organ failure. The exact mechanism of this beneficial effect remains unknown but appears to be related to the *early* fracture stabilization with subsequent diminished inflammatory response and an ability to rapidly mobilize the patient and begin early feedings. Early discharge of the patient from the intensive care unit undoubtedly has additive beneficial effects.

SOFT TISSUE INJURIES

The principles of management of soft tissue injuries are débridement of devitalized tissue, restoration of adequate blood supply, and adequate coverage of vital structures including nerves, blood vessels, tendons, and other soft tissues subject to desiccation. All lacerations and penetrating injuries of the extremities should be cleansed and meticulously débrided. No maneuver contributes as much to the prevention of tetanus or gas gangrene infection as *complete débridement of all devitalized tissue*. Patients with tetanus-prone wounds should be evaluated for immunization status and treated accordingly (see main text). Re-exploration under anesthesia should generally be planned within the next 24 hours, particularly if there is any question regarding the viability of residual tissues. Rapidly spreading cellulitis, crepitus, erythema, and unexplained pain in an extremity are indications for immediate surgical exploration and débridement.

Restoration of blood supply to an injured extremity receives high priority, since as little as a few hours of ischemia may cause tissue necrosis and subsequent amputation. The classic signs of vascular compromise include *pain, palor,* and *pulselessness,* although more subtle findings such as delayed capillary refill and venous congestion are signs of vascular compromise that jeopardize healing of soft tissue wounds and invite secondary infection.

Adequate soft tissue coverage of exposed vital structures is essential for preventing desiccation, secondary infection, and vascular suture disruption. Although primary closure of native soft tissue is ideal, this is often impossible owing to the presence of contaminated or ischemic tissue, infection, or large-area soft tissue defects. Early closure with auto-, allo-, or xenografts of skin can provide temporary coverage pending more elaborate soft tissue reconstructive maneuvers such as free muscle flaps or combined muscle and skin rotational flaps.

PERIPHERAL VASCULAR INJURIES

Penetration, perforation, transection, and lateral lacerations are the usual forms of injury among patients with penetrating wounds, whereas fracture of the intima with obstruction and thrombosis is the usual type of arterial injury following blunt trauma. Both mechanisms may also induce significant arterial spasm in the vicinity of the injury that diminishes extremity blood flow, but which will improve spontaneously. Because of the possibility of hidden lacerations or the delayed development of aneurysm or arteriovenous fistulas, injuries *near* all major blood vessels should be thoroughly explored or otherwise evaluated. Whereas some authors have advocated only observation of wounds in proximity to blood vessels without major signs of vascular injury, these very reports contain case studies of delayed diagnoses and overlooked injuries. Although this particular issue remains controversial, current consensus favors angiographic or noninvasive (Doppler ultrasonography) evaluation for wounds in proximity to major vessels.

Preoperative angiography is generally helpful in order to plan the operative approach and ascertain the extent of damage, especially if blunt trauma or multiple vascular injuries are involved. It is of less benefit in penetrating trauma with obvious vascular injury. An unstable patient should not undergo angiography. Spontaneous cessation of bleeding is often only temporary, and the sudden recurrence of severe hemorrhage is likely.

Vascular injuries are often associated with long bone fractures in the distal part of the leg. In particular, fracture dislocation at the level of the knee is often associated with combined popliteal artery and vein injury, and arteriography should be routinely considered with a "free floating" or posterior knee dislocation. Popliteal vascular trauma is particularly devastating, causing amputation more often than any other arterial injury. Complex combined vascular and orthopedic injuries demand coordination of operative approach and often require temporary vascular conduits while bony repair is performed.

The principles of operative treatment of vascular injuries of the extremity are identical to those described elsewhere for elective vascular repair. However, fasciotomy is perhaps more often used in the trauma setting and is usually necessary when there are combined popliteal artery and vein injuries, when the patient has extensive bony and muscular injury, or following prolonged shock or several hours of extremity ischemia time. Current techniques allow routine and frequent measurements of compartment pressures and accurately indicate those patients who require fasciotomy. The authors favor a double-incision, four-compartment fasciotomy with full incision of the skin.

Whether venous injuries are best treated by repair or by ligation is still controversial. Data compiled by the Vietnam Vascular Registry revealed a significant reduction in the morbid sequelae of lower extremity venous injuries treated by repair instead of ligation, especially when associated arterial injuries were present. Civilian trauma experience supports this observation, and most trauma surgeons perform simple venorrhaphy repair of major (unpaired) venous lacerations in the stable patient. However, the incidence of post-repair thrombosis following more complex repairs is high, and the extra time required may be ill-advised in the multiply injured or unstable patient. If ligation is performed, prolonged postoperative elevation and elastic extremity wrapping reduce edema and decrease late morbidity.

16

SURGICAL COMPLICATIONS

A. R. Moossa, M.D., A. A. Kassir, M.B., F.R.C.S.I.,
and A. K. Upadhyay, M.B., F.R.C.S.

Any deviation from normal recovery and return to regular function is a postoperative complication. Some complications may be unavoidable; others are preventable by careful preoperative anticipation and advice (cessation of smoking, correction of obesity, respiratory exercise, meticulous surgical technique intraoperatively, and early correction of abnormalities postoperatively).

POSTOPERATIVE FEVER AND INFECTION

Fever is a common response to an operation observed in nearly half of patients following major procedures. No infection is found in 80 per cent, and pyrexia resolves spontaneously within a few days. A careful clinical examination is essential initially with attention to the timing and pattern of the fever.

INFECTIOUS CAUSES OF PYREXIA. Most infections follow intraoperative contamination at the operative site via airways during general anesthesia or from cannulas and catheters. Hospital-acquired pathogens are often involved and are difficult to treat because of antibiotic resistance. Local factors predisposing to infection include ischemia, devitalized and necrotic tissues, hematoma formation, and the presence of foreign bodies. These provide an ideal environment for bacteria by protecting them from host defenses. Systemic factors include neonates, the elderly, diabetes mellitus, hepatic disease, disseminated malignancy, malnutrition, obesity, and drugs (i.e., steroids, alcohol, chemotherapeutic agents). Clinical manifestations include signs of a local inflammatory response (heat, pain, redness, mass). Systemic manifestations are chills, rigors, and elevated core body temperature. Fever beginning within 24 hours suggests atelectasis and urinary tract or wound infections. Abscesses usually become evident in the second week, with recurrent spiking pyrexia. Intravenous and urinary catheters should be examined. Pulmonary infections are common, since atelectasis often follows general anesthesia, aspiration, or the use of contaminated ventilation equipment. Patients who smoke and those with nasogastric tubes are more at risk. Urinary tract infections are associated with indwelling catheters, bladder outflow obstruction, and anorectal operations. Cellulitis and phlebitis, lymphangitis, and regional lymphadenopathy

---

See the corresponding chapter or part in the *Textbook of Surgery*, 14th edition, pp. 299–316, for a more detailed discussion of this topic, including a comprehensive list of references.

may be seen with infected venous cannulas. Central line sepsis is more occult and requires cultures of blood or the catheter tip.

NONINFECTIOUS PYREXIA. Postoperative fever may be a manifestation of disseminated malignancy, reaction to drugs or blood transfusion, formation of a hematoma, or inflammation around an intravenous catheter after administration of irritant fluids or drugs. Deep venous thrombosis may manifest as mild pyrexia after the fifth day. Acute pancreatitis after upper abdominal surgery, especially in mild cases, may not be evident from the amylase or lipase levels, and a computed tomographic scan may be required for diagnosis. Supportive care is usually adequate. Some conditions may be precipitated by surgical stress. Thyroid storm and pheochromocytoma are life-threatening. Beta-blockade and antithyroid therapy have to be instituted in the former, and both alpha- and beta-blockade along with nitroprusside for control of hypertension and catecholamine release are needed in the latter. Malignant hyperthermia manifests with fever, tachycardia, rigidity, skin mottling, and cyanosis in the susceptible individual shortly after induction of anesthesia, and is treated with dantrolene, bicarbonate, insulin, and active cooling of the patient; mortality is 30 per cent.

MISCELLANEOUS CAUSES

Thrombophlebitis. Usually a noninfective, inflammatory reaction at the site of the intravenous cannula, thrombophlebitis is a common cause of fever after the third postoperative day. Occasionally bacterial infection with suppurative phlebitis ensues, which requires excision of the vein.

Postoperative Parotitis. This complication is observed in the elderly and debilitated. Malignancy, dehydration, and poor oral hygiene are predisposing factors. The infection is usually staphylococcal and occurs within 2 weeks of operation. The parotid gland is swollen and tender, and a drop of pus may be seen at the intraoral opening of Stensen's duct. Cultures should be obtained and the appropriate antibiotic instituted. Incision and drainage may become necessary, care being taken to avoid facial nerve damage.

WOUND COMPLICATIONS

HEMATOMA. The formation of hematoma is due to the collection of blood in the wound, usually owing to imperfect hemostasis. Aspirin and low-dose heparin may increase risk slightly. Patients on anticoagulants or with coagulopathy have a higher risk. Hypotension at operation and hypertension postoperatively may contribute to wound hematoma formation. On examination, a fluctuant, discolored swelling in the wound is found. Small hematomas may resorb, but they increase the incidence of wound infection. Larger hematomas should be evacuated and any bleeding vessel ligated with wound closure. Neck hematomas are dangerous because they may expand rapidly and compress the trachea.

SEROMA. Seroma is a collection of fluid other than blood or pus. This usually follows liquefaction necrosis of fat or interruption of lymphatics (i.e., mastectomy, nodal dissection, groin operations). Treatment is aspiration and compression.

WOUND INFECTION. A collection of pus in the wound signifies infection. It may be primary or secondary to a hematoma or seroma. Treatment is incision and drainage. Skin sutures or staples must be removed along with any necrotic tissue. Irrigation, packing, or covering have the same efficacy provided free drainage is achieved.

WOUND FAILURE. A partial or total disruption of any or all layers of the wound indicates wound failure. It may be early (wound dehiscence) or late (incisional hernia). Chest wounds rarely dehisce; if they do, it is usually following median sternotomy. Laparotomy wounds have a 1 per cent incidence of "burst abdomen" with a 20 per cent mortality; it is largely preventable by secure mechanical closure of the wound. Infection is a major local factor. Predisposing systemic factors include sepsis, uremia, malnutrition, diabetes, liver failure, and corticosteroid therapy. Serosanguineous fluid discharge from the wound is a pathognomonic sign. Sudden evisceration following an episode of coughing or retching may be the presentation. Management begins with reassurance, analgesia, covering the wound with moist sterile towels, and surgical repair under general anesthesia with nonabsorbable, interrupted, nonreactive sutures employing healthy tissues and deep bites.

RESPIRATORY COMPLICATIONS

ATELECTASIS. Atelectasis is the most common complication following general anesthesia. It denotes loss of patency and collapse of small airways and alveoli. Stasis in the airways with accumulation of secretions predisposes to infection, especially at the lung bases. Clinical signs include rales, diminished breath sounds, and bronchial breathing accompanied by rapid pulse and fever with radiologic evidence of consolidation due to associated pneumonia. Cessation of smoking, avoidance of prolonged anesthesia, and physiotherapy in the bronchitic patient are important preventive measures. Postoperatively, management is rigorous physiotherapy, postural drainage, suction (via endotracheal tube, mini-tracheostomy, bronchoscopy), nebulized bronchodilators, mucolytic agents, and antibiotics as deemed necessary. Assisted mechanical ventilation may be required. Analgesia is important.

ASPIRATION PNEUMONITIS. Aspiration of the sterile acid contents of the stomach produces a chemical burn of the airway. The presence of food particles adds insult by encouraging an intense inflammatory reaction as well as blockage of distal airways by larger particles. Clinically the patient is dyspneic and cyanosed soon after the aspiration, with chest radiographs revealing interstitial pulmonary edema. Arterial blood gases show hypoxemia and hypercarbia. Rapid deterioration to respiratory failure may occur.

ASPIRATION PNEUMONIA. The oropharynx contains

bacteria, primarily anaerobes. Aspiration of the contents of the oropharynx is a common cause of pneumonia. Aspiration pneumonia may progress to pulmonary abscess, which is characterized by foul-smelling sputum and a fluid level in a cavity on chest film.

PULMONARY EDEMA. Pulmonary edema presents as orthopnea, hypoxia, and elevated jugular venous pulse. Confirmation is by clinical examination and chest film. Treatment is by upright positioning of the patient, oxygen administration, and restriction of intravenous fluids. An electrocardiogram is important for outlining any cardiac causes (infarction, arrhythmias). Drugs include diuretics, digoxin, and morphine. Mechanical ventilation and phlebotomy may be indicated.

IMMEDIATE POSTOPERATIVE RESPIRATORY DEPRESSION. This usually is due to narcotic agents and/or muscle relaxants used in anesthesia. It should be recognized and treated accordingly. Other conditions that may present similarly are aspiration, laryngeal edema, massive atelectasis, pneumothorax, and hypothermia. These may be exacerbated by mechanical ventilation and thus should be excluded.

ACUTE RESPIRATORY FAILURE. Respiratory failure is the inability to maintain adequate gas exchange in the lungs. In practical terms, it is Pa_{O_2} less than 60 mm. Hg or Pa_{CO_2} more than 60 mm. Hg (in the absence of metabolic alkalosis) on breathing room air. It may have an insidious onset with increasing respiratory rate and effort. Management is geared toward increasing oxygenation and reducing the work of breathing. It includes intermittent mandatory ventilation, which provides ventilatory support; positive end-expiratory pressure for reinflating the collapsed alveoli; or a combination of both. Continuous positive airway pressure may be an alternative to positive end-expiratory pressure in patients who require intervention for hypoxemia without hypercarbia or ventilatory insufficiency.

SHOCK

Acute circulatory failure, commonly termed shock, is a well-known surgical complication. Hypotension is the usual presenting feature of all types of shock. Occasionally, low blood pressure could be due to vasovagal reflex or orthostatic changes. Shock can be classified into three categories according to the etiology: (1) hypovolemic, (2) cardiogenic, and (3) septic. Hypovolemic shock is due to a fall in circulating blood volume and is the most frequent cause of postoperative shock. Cardiogenic shock is usually secondary to myocardial ischemia or infarction, arrhythmias, cardiac tamponade, pulmonary embolism, adrenal insufficiency, myocardial depression (as in sepsis), and fluid overload especially in the elderly with pre-existing myocardial disease. Septic shock occurs when infection from gram-negative or gram-positive organisms or a fungus produces septicemia. Clinically, this may present as either warm shock or cold shock. The final common pathway in shock is inadequate tissue perfusion for meeting metabolic demands. Any form of shock must be recognized and treated early before irreversible multiorgan damage ensues.

RENAL FAILURE

Acute renal failure must be considered in any patient with oliguria after an operation. When the hourly urinary output is less than 0.5 ml. per kg. per hour (35 ml. per hour for a 70-kg. man), renal failure is secondary to prerenal, renal, or postrenal causes. Prerenal failure implies an inadequate renal blood flow and usually is a direct result of diminished circulating blood volume. Acute parenchymal renal failure is caused by obstruction of the urinary tract and usually presents as anuria. It is important to exclude bladder outflow obstruction in such patients. Proper assessment of the patient and identification of the cause of renal failure is mandatory in management. An intravenous fluid challenge is usually helpful in evaluating the etiologic factor. Patients at risk may require a central venous or pulmonary artery catheter prior to administration of intravenous fluids. If urinary output remains low but blood volume is normal, an intravenous infusion of mannitol 25 gm., furosemide 25 mg. over 20 minutes, or a low-dose infusion of dopamine (2–5 mg./kg./min.) may be considered. The use of diuretics is controversial.

Lack of response to the measures outlined suggests acute or postrenal failure. At this stage, the possibility of postrenal failure must be excluded especially in patients following operations involving a retroperitoneal or pelvic dissection. This usually involves an imaging procedure such as intravenous pyelography, cystoscopic retrograde pyelography or technetium-labeled diethylene tetramine pentacetic acid (DTPA) scan. When renal failure is established, an acute renal failure regimen is instituted. This involves close attention to fluid balance, hemofiltration or dialysis, or peritoneal dialysis.

DEEP VEIN THROMBOSIS AND PULMONARY EMBOLISM

Thrombosis of lower limb and pelvic veins is an important cause of morbidity, both because of its frequency and because of the potentially fatal consequences related to pulmonary embolism.

Clinically, the classic features of deep vein thrombosis are calf swelling, tenderness, elevated temperature, and a positive Homans' sign. These may be absent, and the first manifestation may be a fatal pulmonary embolus. The risk factors include obesity, old age, oral contraception, malignancy, trauma, immobility, and certain specific surgical procedures involving the prostate, hip joint, and pelvis. Venography is the standard among diagnostic investigations, others being Doppler ultrasonography, ^{125}I-fibrinogen studies, and plethysmography. Prophylactic measures directed to prevention of deep vein thrombosis and pulmonary embolism may be divided into mechanical devices that prevent venous pooling and stasis and drugs that inhibit blood coagulation. Pneumatic calf compression is the only mechanical measure with proven efficacy. The use of various pharmacologic agents remains controversial. The most studied and frequently used method is a subcutaneous heparin regimen of 5000 units preoperatively and every 12 hours thereafter until the patient is mobile. It is doubtful whether these measures reduce the incidence of pulmonary embolism.

ALIMENTARY TRACT DYSFUNCTION

In the postoperative period, the normal propulsive activity of the gastrointestinal tract is temporarily depressed. The term *paralytic ileus* is a misnomer because small bowel motility rapidly returns.

Complications involving the alimentary tract include acute gastric dilation, gastroduodenal mucosal hemorrhage, intestinal obstruction, fecal impaction, colitis, anastomotic leak, and dysfunctions of the hepatobiliary-pancreatic system. Patients with acute dilation of the stomach usually present with severe pain and dyspnea, although sometimes it is insidious in nature. Treatment consists of gastric decompression with a nasogastric tube and fluid replacement. Gastroduodenal mucosal hemorrhage is a well-recognized complication in severely ill and septic postoperative patients. Histamine-receptor antagonists are recommended both as a prophylactic measure and for definitive therapy. Under extreme situations, an operation may be required. Intestinal obstruction may be the result of paralytic ileus or mechanical obstruction. Acute colonic pseudo-obstruction is a localized form of paralytic ileus affecting the large bowel. Mechanical obstruction is most often caused by postoperative adhesions or an internal hernia. The initial treatment is conservative, but if the obstruction persists or increasing abdominal signs develop, laparotomy should be performed. Fecal impaction is treated with laxatives and enema; occasionally, manual evacuation under general anesthesia is necessary. Postoperative diarrhea is occasionally due to *Shigella*, *Salmonella*, or *Campylobacter*. Patients treated with antibiotics are at risk of bacterial overgrowth with resistant staphylococci and occasionally a more serious condition termed pseudomembranous colitis. This is associated with *Clostridium difficile*, an anaerobic bacterium that releases a toxin.

Anastomotic leakage is usually a technical complication. The successful outcome of an anastomosis depends on many factors including good blood supply, impermeable mechanical apposition of serosa to serosa, avoidance of tension on the anastomotic line, and avoidance of gross contamination. Colonic anastomoses are more prone to leak. Pericolic abscess and enterocutaneous fistula may follow a leak. More seriously, a diffuse peritonitis may result, and it requires rapid resuscitation with intravenous fluids and nasogastric aspiration followed by laparotomy.

The incidence of hepatobiliary complications is greatest

after operations on the liver, biliary tract, and pancreas, but they may occur after any operation involving general anesthesia. Anesthetic agents, particularly halothane, have been implicated as a cause of potentially fatal postoperative hepatitis, especially after re-exposure to the same agent. Extrahepatic obstruction is caused by direct surgical injury to the bile ducts, retained common bile duct stones, tumors, or pancreatitis.

NEUROLOGIC AND PSYCHOLOGICAL COMPLICATIONS

Operations on the brain or spinal cord and spinal or epidural anesthesia are associated with occasional focal lesions. Septic emboli may cause a brain abscess. Peripheral nerves may be damaged during operative procedures. Stroke occurs in 1 to 3 per cent of patients after carotid endarterectomy or other reconstructive operations on the extracranial portion of the carotid system. Cerebral injuries are capable of producing convulsions. Epilepsy or metabolic derangements may also cause convulsions in the postoperative period.

Anxiety and fear are normal in patients who undergo surgical procedures. Confusion is common in the elderly, and sleep deprivation, which is especially common in patients in intensive care units, may cause disorientation and hallucinations. Patients requiring a stoma, mastectomy, or amputation may perceive an alteration in body image. Postoperative psychosis occurs in approximately 0.2 per cent of cases but is much higher following open heart surgery. Postoperative delirium could be due to factors such as drug dependency, dementia, brain lesions, or metabolic abnormalities including uremia and hepatic insufficiency.

17

ACUTE RENAL FAILURE IN SURGICAL PATIENTS:
Prevention and Treatment

R. Randal Bollinger, M.D., Ph.D.,
and Steve J. Schwab, M.D.

Acute renal failure (ARF) is a potentially lethal complication in the surgical patient. Despite recent advances in dialysis and intensive care support, almost half of the patients who develop ARF in the postoperative period die. The severity of the trauma, the magnitude of the surgical procedure, the gravity of underlying medical conditions that predispose to ARF, and the high incidence of sepsis all contribute to multiorgan failure with high mortality. Prompt and effective treatment of each component of the multifaceted etiology of ARF can prevent the syndrome and offers the surgical patient the best likelihood of survival.

Acute renal failure is defined as an abrupt decline in renal function sufficient to cause retention of nitrogenous waste. This definition of ARF does not depend on the urinary output of the patient. The emphasis is on the quality of the urine rather than the quantity, since nonoliguric forms of ARF occur quite frequently. Whether or not oliguria is present, a progressive rise in blood urea nitrogen and serum creatinine concentration in the posttrauma or postoperative period should suggest ARF.

CLASSIFICATION

When renal failure occurs abruptly, *acute* renal failure is present. When the azotemia develops gradually over many weeks or months, the renal failure is termed *chronic*. If a patient in renal failure presents with asymptomatic azotemia, the differentiation of acute from chronic disease may be difficult. Several aspects of the history and radiologic examination, particularly the presence of small, "end-stage" kidneys, provide the correct classification of the patient's disease. Renal failure is termed *oliguric* if less than 400 ml. of urine is produced in 24 hours. Patients with *nonoliguric* renal failure produce large volumes of isosthenuric urine but are unable to clear nitrogenous wastes.

Acute renal failure is conveniently classified according to

See the corresponding chapter or part in the *Textbook of Surgery*, 14th edition, pp. 317–337, for a more detailed discussion of this topic, including a comprehensive list of references.

its cause as prerenal, renal, or postrenal. Each of these may present in either the oliguric or nonoliguric form, and all are associated with a rising blood urea nitrogen and serum creatinine. The difficult problem posed by surgical patients is to distinguish a normal kidney that is attempting to correct an abnormal internal environment (prerenal failure) from a kidney that is no longer able to maintain the internal environment (renal failure).

Acute renal failure is most commonly initiated by a critical underperfusion of the kidney with consequent intense arteriolar vasoconstriction with resultant ischemic tubular injury. In other circumstances, direct tubular cell damage is sustained from a toxin such as aminoglycoside or amphotericin. Myoglobin or hemoglobin pigment may cause direct tubular injury with intratubular obstruction when proteins coagulate. Iodinated contrast and nonsteroidal anti-inflammatory drugs may also be cellular toxins but are also powerful mediators of intrarenal vasoconstriction. When tubular damage is sustained, a number of factors converge to maintain the renal failure. These include back-leak of filtrate across disrupted tubular barriers, intraluminal obstruction from cell swelling and sloughing, persistent vasoconstriction that serves to perpetuate cellular ischemia, and changes in glomerular capillary membrane permeability. Even in apparently intact renal tubular cells, the intracellular metabolism that supports the transport functions of the cell is severely disturbed from hypoxia, free oxygen radical accumulation, and high levels of free ionized cytoplasmic calcium. The result is failure in the homeostatic maintenance of the extracellular fluid and failure to excrete accumulating toxic metabolic wastes. Biochemical alterations in acute renal failure include retention of nitrogenous wastes, metabolic acidosis, hyperkalemia, hyponatremia, hyperphosphatemia, hypocalcemia, and hypermagnesemia.

CONDITIONS THAT PREDISPOSE TO ACUTE RENAL FAILURE

ARF is a frequent complication of surgical procedures. The most common cause of ARF is acute tubular necrosis. Of the approximately 30 patients annually per million population who require dialysis for ARF, 20 patients have acute tubular necrosis, three quarters of these as a complication of surgical procedures. Many factors cause this high incidence of ARF in the postoperative period. An important factor is the severity of any underlying diseases, both medical conditions existing in the patient before operation and the trauma or illness that necessitated the surgical procedure. Exposure to anesthetic agents and incompatible blood transfusion, both possible causes of ARF, are high-risk factors for the surgical group. The most important factor, however, is hypovolemia from preoperative fluid restriction, surgical fluid loss, surgical blood loss, and gastric tube drainage of fluids. The already ischemic kidney in the hypovolemic patient may be easily injured by nephrotoxic antibiotics and other drugs. The combination of toxic and ischemic damage to tubular epithelium is the direct cause of postoperative ARF.

PREVENTION OF ACUTE RENAL FAILURE

Any postrenal problem that is allowed to persist may cause acute tubular necrosis. Postoperative and posttrauma patients with a sudden onset of anuria should be considered to have mechanical obstruction of the ureters or lower urinary tract until this possibility has been excluded. Operative or traumatic injury of the urinary tract in the retroperitoneal or pelvic areas is suspected whenever absolute anuria develops, since total anuria is rarely seen in the intrinsic renal and prerenal forms of ARF. The diagnosis can be established by cystoscopy, retrograde catheterization of the ureters, and radiographic techniques including ultrasonography, intravenous pyelography, and computed tomographic scan of the abdomen. The cystogram and urethrogram demonstrate traumatic rupture of the bladder and disruption of the urethra, respectively. These causes of postrenal ARF should be suspected in cases of pelvic fracture, particularly if the rectal examination reveals displacement of the prostate gland.

Prerenal causes of ARF are prevented by optimizing volume status, cardiac function, and blood pressure while avoiding nephrotoxins and infections. Extracellular volume can be estimated by physical examination in many cases. When it cannot be judged accurately, central venous pressure or pulmonary capillary wedge pressure must be measured. An important means of evaluating the volume status in oliguric patients is by fluid challenge. The intravascular volume is increased by infusing crystalloid or colloid until the wedge pressure is raised to 15 to 18 cm. of water. A brisk diuresis suggests a prerenal cause for the oliguria. If oliguria persists, an intrinsic renal problem is suspected.

The mean arterial blood pressure must be restored to normal levels and vasoconstriction reversed for maintenance of the glomerular filtration rate above 60 ml. per minute and avoidance of activation of the renin-angiotensin system. In patients who are oliguric after hypotension, the blood pressure should be monitored by means of an intra-arterial cannula. Blood pressure should be restored to a mean pressure of 80 mm. Hg and maintained at that level by adequate volume replacement. The extracellular volume replacement is adequate if urinary output is 40 ml. or more per hour and the central venous pressure is normal.

Treatment with a loop diuretic such as furosemide or an osmotic agent such as mannitol may reverse early ARF by flushing the tubules and reducing their oxygen consumption. This treatment may convert oliguric renal failure to the nonoliguric form, but it does not alter the course of acute tubular necrosis. High-output renal failure is easier to manage clinically and may have a better prognosis for survival. Although loop diuretics are effective agents for increasing urinary flow in postoperative and posttrauma patients, they should not be used until the extracellular fluid volume has been restored to normal. Furosemide may convert homeo-static oliguria to ARF by inducing a large urine loss in a patient who is already volume depleted and whose oliguria is a normal response to the physiologic condition. For guarding against the indiscriminate and dangerous use of loop diuretics, measurement of central venous or left atrial pressure should be made before administration to an oliguric patient. When the extracellular fluid volume is proved normal, up to 200 mg. of furosemide or 12.5 gm. of mannitol may be given intravenously. Alternatively, 5 μg. per kg. per minute of dopamine, a nonpressor dose, may be administered to increase renal blood flow directly. If these measures fail to reverse the acute oliguria, further diuretic therapy is not helpful, and dialysis should be instituted as metabolic abnormalities or uremic symptoms develop. In cases of hemorrhagic or septic shock, diuretic therapy may be given as part of the resuscitation. If the pulmonary capillary wedge pressure is normal or low, mannitol is an appropriate agent. If the wedge pressure is high, furosemide is a better choice. Dopamine should be part of either regimen, but diuretic therapy is no substitute for adequate volume replacement. In fact, even dopamine given alone can dehydrate critically ill patients.

DIAGNOSIS OF ACUTE RENAL FAILURE

A systematic approach to the patient with oliguria and a rising creatinine concentration is of great importance. The physician must first consider prerenal and postrenal causes of the deteriorating renal function before concluding that intrinsic renal tubular damage has occurred. When the distinction between prerenal failure and ischemic tubular necrosis is unclear, the patient's response to careful volume expansion and optimization of cardiac performance is assessed. It is essential to consider the possibility that volume contraction, compromised cardiac output, or some toxic insult is superimposed upon pre-existing chronic renal insufficiency. The most important diagnostic test may be volume restitution and improving the cardiac performance. Critically ill patients with multiple clinical problems and recent tissue injury suggest not only acute ischemic tubular necrosis but the concomitant presence of prerenal and postrenal compromises. ARF in the postoperative setting is commonly associated with combinations of volume depletion, third-space body fluids, heart failure, and intrinsic tubular injury from ischemia and toxins and perhaps even an element of urinary tract obstruction. Failure to systematically consider each of these possible causes for a decline in renal function delays specific effective therapy and jeopardizes renal recovery.

Evaluation should begin with a careful *clinical assessment* including consideration of the clinical context, review of the clinical course, and physical examination with attention to blood pressure, heart rate, orthostatic changes, and serial changes in body weight. Detailed examination of intake and output is essential. Fluid intake should match fluid losses both in quantity and in quality.

Laboratory studies should include urinalysis, urine and plasma osmolality, urea, creatinine, and sodium. These values may be used to calculate urine diagnostic indices that are helpful in the differential diagnosis of acute renal failure. Each of these *diagnostic indices* is useful and should routinely be employed; together, they can provide highly accurate diagnostic information. However, each test has proven exceptions and should not be interpreted rigidly. Efforts should be directed toward improving circulatory hemodynamics, treating infection, relieving obstruction, and removing nephrotoxins. Following the clinical course while making these improvements may prove to be the most important diagnostic maneuver.

Sophisticated *radiographic studies* may be necessary when the diagnosis remains unclear. Radiologic techniques detect hydronephrosis, impairments in renal blood flow, abnormalities of size, shape, or location of the kidney, and certain abnormalities of the collecting system. Plain films show renal size and radiopaque stones. Ultrasonography demonstrates obstruction, morphologic changes, and stones. Radionuclide scans document perfusion, function, and urinary extravasation. Intravenous pyelography demonstrates the level of an obstruction. Computed tomographic scanning defines location, size, and morphologic change of the kidney and disease in adjacent organs. Arteriography is useful in patients with suspected arterial lesions.

Biopsy is reserved for those cases of ARF in which the diagnosis of acute tubular necrosis appears doubtful and one or more intrinsic renal etiologic factors may be present, such as acute glomerular nephritis, acute interstitial nephritis, or acute vasculitis. When postrenal and prerenal causes of ARF have been excluded in a surgical patient, the majority have acute tubular necrosis, so renal biopsy has a *very* limited role in management. An exception is the renal transplant patient with ARF in whom biopsy differentiates acute rejection from acute tubular necrosis, drug toxicity, and recurrent primary disease. Percutaneous needle biopsy of the native kidney has some risk (e.g., a 9 per cent complication rate in one series) and should be performed only for clear indications such as prolonged renal failure beyond 3 weeks. It is contraindicated in the presence of bleeding diathesis or uncontrolled hypertension.

MANAGEMENT OF THE PATIENT WITH ESTABLISHED ACUTE RENAL FAILURE

When oliguria and/or a rise in blood urea nitrogen and creatinine supervene in the postoperative patient, the clinician should be alert to the possibility of evolving ARF. Attention should be directed toward seeking and excluding specific reversible causes of the apparent deterioration of renal function. When the reversible factors have been corrected and the urinary indices have established tubular injury, a program of therapy should be undertaken immediately.

HYPERKALEMIA. Early attention must be given to fluid and electrolyte status of the patient with ARF, particularly hyperkalemia, which is the most serious electrolyte abnormality. The threat of hyperkalemia is cardiac arrest. The severity of hyperkalemia can be judged by the electrocardiographic changes, which include peaked T waves, prolongation of PR intervals, loss of P waves, and widening of the QRS complex. These changes indicate diminished cardiac excitability and imminent cardiac standstill. When significant electrocardiographic changes are apparent, emergent therapy is indicated. First, a calcium infusion with one to three ampules of 10 per cent calcium gluconate should be given over 5 to 15 minutes for stabilizing the cardiac membranes and reversing the toxic effects of hyperkalemia. This membrane-stabilizing action of calcium is immediate in onset but is relatively short-lived. It is often lifesaving, but other therapy must be instituted to actually lower the serum potassium and remove the excess potassium from the body. These therapies include the intravenous administration of concentrated glucose, insulin and sodium bicarbonate.

Glucose and insulin therapy is best administered as a 10 per cent glucose solution with 20 to 30 units of regular insulin per liter. The rate of intravenous administration should be titrated according to serial serum potassium values but may be administered as rapidly as 500 ml. per hour. Glucose-insulin therapy may be initiated with a bolus of 50 per cent glucose plus 10 units of regular insulin intravenously, followed by the drip infusion. The action of glucose and insulin begins within 10 minutes and persists for as long as the drip is continued. Sodium bicarbonate is either administered as a bolus over 5 to 10 minutes or diluted in 5 to 10 per cent glucose in water and infused slowly. Both forms of therapy lower the serum potassium by driving potassium into cells rather than removing it from the body. Ultimately, therefore, enteral administration of cation-exchange resins such as sodium polystyrene sulfonate (Kayexalate) or dialytic therapy must be employed to remove the potassium from the body. Each therapy has its limitations. With glucose-insulin infusion, water overload with progressive hyponatremia is a concern, and with large amounts of sodium bicarbonate, volume overload, pulmonary congestion, and hypernatremia are problems. Cation-exchange resins are most effective if they are administered orally with sorbitol. The presence of an ileus or intestinal injury precludes this mode of administration, and one must then rely on the less effective but still useful rectal route of administration. Precipitous reduction in serum potassium via hemodialysis can be associated with complex ventricular arrhythmias, particularly if other electrolyte disturbances coexist. Continuous electrocardiographic monitoring is mandatory.

FLUID VOLUME. Careful monitoring of fluid intake and output along with daily weights can prevent volume overload in the patient with ARF. If the patient is oliguric, excessive salt and water input cause hypertension and pulmonary edema. The clinician should restrict fluid intake to match actual fluid losses plus 500 to 700 ml. per day of insensible loss and 200 ml. per day per degree of fever. It is important that frequent regular quantitation of all fluid losses be performed because nasogastric drainage, wound drainages, stool losses, or urinary flow vary from hour to hour. It is best that standing orders for a fixed amount of fluid per day not be written because fluid administration must match fluctuating losses and determine necessary administration of blood products, antibiotics, nutrition, and so on. Volume overload in the oliguric patient can be treated with phlebotomy or some mode of dialysis.

HYPONATREMIA. Evolution of hyponatremia indicates that free water intake is exceeding free water elimination. Severe hyponatremia is often a contributing factor to the encephalopathy and propensity to convulsions that complicate ARF when administered intravenous fluid is excessive and hypotonic. When hyponatremia evolves, free water restriction must be prescribed. If the serum sodium concentration falls below 120 mEq. per liter, convulsions are imminent. Dialysis is the only maneuver that can correct hyponatremia in this situation; administration of hypertonic sodium chloride in the oliguric patient who is usually already fluid overloaded is avoided. Hyponatremia is best managed by an awareness of how it might evolve and preventing it.

METABOLIC ACIDOSIS. Metabolic acidosis often accompanies acute renal failure, especially in association with major surgical therapy, traumatic injury, or sepsis. In the hypercatabolic patient, acid production is substantially increased, and the markedly reduced renal function allows no means for excretion of the accumulating acid or the regeneration of consumed bicarbonate. Harmful effects from the progressive metabolic acidosis include nausea, vomiting, and cerebral dysfunction as well as cardiac depression, insulin resistance, impaired cellular metabolism, and hyperkalemia. Metabolic acidosis is treated with oral administration of Shohl's solution, intravenous or oral sodium bicarbonate, or dialysis. Enough alkali must be administered not only to repair the already existing acidosis but to maintain arterial pH and bicarbonate reserves at a level that will match the daily endogenous acid production from catabolism. In the average resting adult, daily acid production is approximately 1 mEq. per kg. per day. Therefore, 70 to 100 mEq. of alkali would suffice to maintain acid-base balance. However, in the hypercatabolic patient with tissue injury, recent surgical therapy, or sepsis, endogenous acid production can be two to three times this amount, which must be matched by alkali administration. Such large amounts of sodium bicarbonate expand extracellular volume, may precipitate pulmonary edema, and are often associated with hypernatremia. If large amounts of sodium bicarbonate are required to maintain arterial pH, dialytic therapy must be initiated.

HYPOCALCEMIA AND HYPERPHOSPHATEMIA. Hypocalcemia and hyperphosphatemia occur most commonly in the patient who has experienced tissue necrosis from crush injury or burn. When the serum phosphate exceeds 6 mg. per 100 ml., magnesium-free phosphate-binding antacids should be prescribed to minimize elevations in the calcium-phosphate product and attenuate soft tissue deposition of calcium-phosphate crystals. Ionized calcium in acute renal failure is usually near-normal owing to acidosis, uremia, and hypoalbuminemia. Infusion of calcium is therefore unnecessary unless carpopedal spasm or tetany develops. If phosphate is not lowered, infusion of calcium produces soft tissue precipitation of calcium-phosphate. Ultimately dialysis may be required to control phosphate and calcium balance.

USE OF DIALYSIS IN ACUTE RENAL FAILURE

Dialysis should be initiated when there is life-threatening hyperkalemia, severe acidosis, volume overload, uremic encephalopathy, or uremic pericarditis. Dialysis is best initiated prophylactically before the occurrence of any of these life-threatening complications of ARF rather than as an urgent procedure. The goals of dialysis are to (1) remove uremic nitrogenous metabolites and ameliorate the uremic state; (2) correct metabolic acidosis; (3) remove excess fluid; (4) normalize serum electrolyte concentrations; (5) improve platelet and leukocyte function; and (6) permit effective hyperalimentation. There are currently three forms of renal replacement therapy for use in patients suffering from ARF. Hemodialysis, peritoneal dialysis, and hemofiltration are each available in a series of modifications. Each mode of therapy has its own advantages and disadvantages. Consultation with a nephrologist for selecting and initiating renal replacement therapy is usually the best course of action.

MANAGEMENT OF THE LATE COMPLICATIONS OF ACUTE RENAL FAILURE

The one factor that determines patient survival in ARF more than any other single factor is the nature and severity of the associated illnesses. The evolution of complications during the course of renal failure dramatically impacts upon patient prognosis. More than 50 per cent of patients who die in the setting of ARF do so because of sepsis and pulmonary infections. Respiratory and cardiac failure represent another 25 per cent, and severe bleeding is responsible for 10 to 15 per cent of patient deaths. Malnutrition is a frequent concomitant and probably a primary permissive factor. When the postoperative patient with ARF is stabilized with regard to acute fluid and electrolyte complications and intensity of uremia is being controlled by an individualized dialysis prescription, attention must be directed toward preventing and managing these late complications.

PROGNOSIS OF ACUTE RENAL FAILURE

Untreated acute renal failure in surgical patients rapidly causes death from fluid overload or hyperkalemia. When early resuscitation efforts are successful, infection, which causes 50 to 80 per cent of deaths, becomes the overwhelming concern. In patients who have severe, multisystem trauma, ruptured abdominal aortic aneurysms, major surgical procedures for advanced cancer, abdominal catastrophies, or cardiovascular circulatory failure in addition to their ARF, mortality greater than 50 per cent is reported in nearly every series. With early, aggressive, repeated dialysis for prevention of the metabolic derangements associated with acute renal failure and successful management of the late complications of bleeding, sepsis, and drug intoxication, most patients recover renal function after postoperative ARF. A spectrum of outcomes was observed among survivors of acute tubular necrosis: 30 to 40 per cent of patients had normal renal function, 40 to 50 per cent of patients had complete clinical recovery but persistent defects in glomerular or tubular function, 10 per cent required medical management, and the remaining 10 to 20 per cent required dialysis. Even during the recovery phase, *prevention* of ARF by avoidance of insults that might reinjure the recovering kidneys is much easier, more cost effective, and more successful than is treatment of ARF.

18

TRANSPLANTATION

I

Historical Aspects of Transplantation

*R. Randal Bollinger, M.D., Ph.D.,
and Delford L. Stickel, M.D.*

ANCIENT ACCOUNTS OF TRANSPLANTATION

Transplantation, the removal or partial detachment of a part of the body and its implantation to the body of the same or a different individual, has fascinated mankind for centuries. Legends of transplantation are recorded in the early written histories of both Eastern and Western cultures. Homer in his *Iliad* describes the monstrous Chimaera, a remarkable creature of transplanted animal parts created by the gods. This mythical hybrid animal had parts of a goat, a lion, and a serpent. All three of its heads breathed fire. The term *chimera* is now used in transplantation to describe individuals who possess hybrid characteristics such as the circulating cells of both donor and recipient after bone marrow transplantation. The Christian legend of Cosmas and Damian describes transplantation of a black leg to the amputation stump of a white parishioner as one of the miraculous feats of these two medical martyrs. Tragically, in 1492 two boys were bled to death in a vain attempt to save the life of Pope Innocent VIII by means of transfusion of young blood. Ancient Hindu surgeons described methods for repairing defects of the nose and ears about 700 B.C., and a Chinese document written about 300 B.C. contained a legendary account of organ transplantation.

A new Western tradition of transplantation surgery arose during the Renaissance in Bologna. The sixteenth century anatomist and surgeon Gasparo Tagliacozzi developed his technique for reconstructing the nose by use of a flap of skin from the inner aspect of the upper arm. He carved the flap of skin in the shape of the patient's nose and then stitched it to the forehead and inner surface of the cheek, leaving a slender attachment to the arm for maintaining blood supply until circulation was re-established from the face. Following this painful procedure, the patient had to sit upright with the arm alongside the face and the head turned toward the arm for the next 3 weeks of healing, at which time the

See the corresponding chapter or part in the *Textbook of Surgery*, 14th edition, pp. 338–344, for a more detailed discussion of this topic, including a comprehensive list of references.

attachment to the arm was severed. The technique is still in use, known as the tagliacotian flap or the *Italian method*.

EARLY EXPERIMENTS IN TRANSPLANTATION

The Scottish surgeon John Hunter (1728–1793) is rightfully known as the father of experimental surgery because of his pioneering research. Several of his experimental procedures involved transplantation, including autografting a cock's claw to its comb and xenografting a human tooth to the comb of a cock. A number of connective tissue transplant procedures including skin and cornea were performed successfully for the first time during the eighteenth and nineteenth centuries.

The first well-documented report of successful free autografts of skin was in 1804 by Baronio, who experimented with sheep, although free autografts of human skin may have been used successfully centuries before. In 1822, Bunger reported successful use of a free full-thickness human skin autograft for repair of a nasal defect. In 1870, Reverdin reported that small grafts of epidermis on a granulating surface increased in size and grew out to coalesce with adjacent grafts. In 1886, Thiersch in Germany described the resurfacing of wounds with large sheets of split-thickness skin. Such grafts are still sometimes termed Thiersch's grafts, although essentially the same procedure was reported 14 years earlier by Ollier in France.

Corneal xenografts attempted early in the nineteenth century were unsuccessful. A corneal allograft between two gazelles was reported by Bigger in 1835, but the necessity of using a cornea from the same species was not recognized until 1872 to 1880, when successful corneal allografts were reported in animals and in man. Refinements of operative techniques, methods of preservation of grafts, and systems of graft procurement were subsequently developed. During the period 1925 to 1945, corneal transplantation emerged as a widespread and accepted therapeutic practice.

TRANSPLANTATION IN THE TWENTIETH CENTURY

The first long-functioning renal transplant was reported by Ullmann in March 1902. He transplanted kidneys in dogs with use of magnesium tube stents and ligatures for making the vascular anastomoses. That same year, the French surgeon Alexis Carrel reported his new technique of suturing blood vessels together by use of triangulation and fine silk suture material. His revolutionary technique was rapidly applied to the problems of organ transplantation. Between 1902 and 1912, Carrel and Guthrie of Chicago performed a large series of animal transplantation experiments, including the transfer of blood vessels, kidneys, hearts, spleens, ovaries, thyroids, extremities, and even the head and neck. In 1905, in his preliminary communication entitled "The Transplantation of Organs," Carrel stated, "This operation consists of extirpating an organ with its vessels, of putting it in another region, and of uniting its vessels to a neighboring artery and vein. If the organ is replaced in the same animal from which it was removed the operation is called an *auto-transplantation*. If it is placed in another animal of the same species it is called a *homotransplantation*, while if it is placed into an animal of a different species, the operation is called a *heterotransplantation*. The correct modern terminology is *syngeneic, allogeneic,* and *xenogeneic* transplantation as shown in Table 1. Depending on the site of implantation, grafts are termed *orthotopic* if surrounded by the same type of tissues or located in the same part of the body after transplantation. Otherwise, they are termed *heterotopic*.

PROBLEM OF REJECTION. Although the immunity theory of graft rejection was postulated by several authors during the first decade of the century, the theory was questioned largely because there was no direct evidence that circulating antibody—the traditional hallmark of immunity—was involved in the rejection process. Cellular immunity, histocompatibility antigens, and immunologic tolerance were important discoveries in the understanding of transplant rejection.

In 1914, Murphy reported lymphocytic infiltrates in host tissues surrounding rejecting transplanted tumors, and by 1954 certain forms of immunity were observed to be transferable to an unimmunized subject by lymphoid cells and not by serum, a phenomenon designated *adoptively acquired immunity*. Jensen observed that a second graft did not survive as long as the first when a mouse received two grafts of a tumor separated by an interval of several days, and he suggested that immunity was responsible for the difference. This *second-set phenomenon* was observed in human skin graft recipients by Holman while treating burn patients at the Johns Hopkins Hospital in the 1920s. In 1932, Shinoyi in Japan described the specificity of the second-set phenomenon. Gibson and Medawar, working in England in 1943, reported similar observations with burn patients, and use of the term *second-set* dates to this report. Medawar demonstrated the immunologic specificity of the phenomenon, which was observed uniformly only when the same donor was used for both the first- and the second-sets of grafts. Medawar also contrasted the histologic characteristics of first- and second-set rejections. First-set rejection was predominantly a cellular event, whereas both cellular and humoral mechanisms were involved in the rejection of the second-set of grafts.

HISTOCOMPATIBILITY ANTIGENS. When immunity, both cellular and humoral, had been established as the cause of graft rejection, study was focused on the antigens that both stimulated graft rejection and were the targets of the ensuing immune response. The antigens responsible for graft rejection and the genetic control of these antigens were extensively studied in the mouse by Jensen, Little, Gorer, and Snell. The serologic identification of human transplantation antigens began in 1952 when Dausset discovered a leukocyte antigen responsible for transfusion reactions. Payne found in 1958 that antileukocyte antibodies were

TABLE 1. Transplantation Terminology

Recent Nomenclature	Older Nomenclature	Relationship of Donor and Recipient of Graft
Syngeneic (isogeneic) graft	Autograft	Same individual
	Isograft	Same species and genetically identical
Allogeneic graft	Homograft	Same species but not genetically identical
Xenogeneic graft	Heterograft	Different species

TABLE 2. The Era of Organ Replacement

Organ	First Experimental Animal Success	First Extended Human Survival
Kidney	1902 Ullman	1954 Murray
Heart	1905 Carrel and Guthrie	1967 Barnard
Pancreas	1922 Banting and Best	1966 Lillehei
Liver	1955 Welch	1967 Starzl

frequent in the sera of multiparous women, thus establishing a rich source of reagents for tissue typing. The new system of tissue matching was first used for selection of appropriate donors and recipients by Hamburger of Paris. In 1964, Payne reported the first clear evidence that these leukocyte antigens segregated in families as a genetic system. Terasaki in 1964 introduced the sensitive and specific microlymphocytotoxicity test. Definition of the HLA system, the major histocompatibility gene complex of man, was the result of a series of international workshops begun in 1964 by Amos. A major advance that same year was the discovery that lymphocytes from potential donors and recipients, when mixed together in tissue culture, undergo a vigorous proliferative response. This reaction, termed a *mixed lymphocyte culture*, became, along with microlymphocytotoxicity, a major method for histocompatibility testing.

IMMUNOLOGIC TOLERANCE. Chimerism was found to occur naturally in dizygotic cattle twins by Owen in 1945. He reported that each of such twins carry two different types of erythrocytes, and he postulated that the marrow of each individual had become populated by cells of both *in utero* when the circulation of the two placentas was mixed. Owen successfully exchanged skin grafts between the cattle twins, and in 1955 Simonson reported that kidneys as well as skin could be readily transplanted between them. In 1953, Billingham, Brent, and Medawar reported their experiments on "actively acquired tolerance of foreign cells" with use of inbred strains of mice of various ages. It became clear that the barrier between self and non-self could be overcome if the exposure to alloantigens occurred in the neonatal period. Grafts established on the fetus survived permanently, and the host was tolerant to other grafts from the donor strain; grafts performed more than a day or two after birth were rejected, and the rejection of subsequent grafts from the donor strain was accelerated. Animals rendered tolerant prenatally or neonatally were normal except for being chimeras and for being specifically nonreactive to antigens of the donor. Many subsequent studies have been directed toward the objective of inducing tolerance in the adult by methods that would be applicable to therapeutic transplantation in man. Since an effective method of producing acquired tolerance to transplantation antigens in adult animals and humans has not yet been discovered, the progress of transplantation has depended on the development of methods of immunosuppression.

IMMUNOSUPPRESSION. Total body irradiation was used

extensively for preventing rejection of grafts in experimental animals before it was used in the first successful human allografts from living, related donors in Paris and in Boston. Although one allograft lived for 25 years, radiation therapy as an immunosuppressive agent was judged "too blunt, nonspecific and unpredictable." Schwartz and Dameshek reported in 1959 that the capacity of rabbits to form antibody was blocked by 6-mercaptopurine, which Calne and Zukoski used successfully in canine renal transplants. Hitchings and associates developed an imidazole derivative termed azathioprine in 1961 that could be administered conveniently and safely in an oral form. Murray, Hume, and Starzl reported clinical successes with azathioprine that same year, thus initiating the modern era of transplantation. With the advent of chemical immunosuppression, the brief but exciting history of clinical transplantation began. For the first time, several vascularized organs were transplanted with regular success as shown in Table 2.

II

The Immunology of Transplant Antigens

D. Bernard Amos, M.D., and
Fred Sanfilippo, M.D., Ph.D.

The groundwork for understanding the immunology and genetics of organ transplants in man was accomplished in experiments with inbred mice that established the "laws" of transplantation:

- A graft would succeed if transplanted to a member of the same (donor) inbred strain; it would be rejected by a mouse of a different (allogeneic) strain.
- Grafts to a hybrid between the donor strain and the allogeneic strain (F1) would be accepted.
- Grafts to a hybrid made by crossing two F1 animals (F2) or by crossing an F1 animal to an animal of the allogeneic strain (resistant back-cross) would succeed in a proportion of recipients.

The basis for these laws depended on the inheritance of histocompatibility (H) antigens. Although there were many H antigens, one called H-2 was the strongest, and it was termed the major histocompatibility antigen. All animals of

See the corresponding chapter or part in the *Textbook of Surgery,* 14th edition, pp. 345–356, for a more detailed discussion of this topic, including a comprehensive list of references.

the original inbred (donor) murine strain shared the same H-2 antigen. Animals of different (allogeneic) strains had different H-2 antigens; they became immune to the H-2 of tissues transplanted from the original strain. H-2 was codominantly expressed like the human A and B blood group antigens, so the F1 hybrid expressed the H-2 of both parents and did not react to the graft. Some F2 and back-cross animals inherited donor H-2 and others did not; those that inherited donor H-2 resembled the F1 and did not reject. H-2 was soon shown to be a set of two or more antigens controlled by several genes placed together on a short stretch of chromosome 17. These were known as closely linked loci, and the system of genes was termed the major histocompatibility complex (MHC). Many of the individual antigens encoded by the complex could be detected by antibodies. When organ transplantation became practicable in man, a search was made for the human equivalent of H-2 by use of antisera from multiparous women or from patients who rejected transplants of skin or kidneys for detection of these antigens. The antigens found are now known as HLA antigens.

HLA was shown to be governed by the same laws of transplantation by an exchange of experimental skin grafts between family members. Like H-2, the HLA antigens were codominantly expressed, and the genes formed a closely linked complex on the sixth chromosome. This gene complex is termed the HLA haplotype. The father and mother of a family each possess two HLA haplotypes; one or the other is passed to each child. The father's haplotypes are often designated a and b, the mother's c and d. The children must inherit the a and c, a and d, b and c, or b and d haplotypes; if there are five children, one must inherit the same two haplotypes as one of its siblings, for example, ac, ac. Skin grafted from one ac sib to another ac sib is known as an HLA-identical transplant. These grafts survive for an average of nearly 20 days. As in the mouse, grafts are ultimately rejected because of incompatibility for minor H loci. Skin from an ac sib to an ad sib, to a bc sib, or to the ab father or cd mother shares one haplotype; these grafts are called haploidentical and last for about 13 days. Skin from a sib sharing neither haplotype is rejected in 11 days. From these observations it is clear that the laws of transplantation apply to skin grafts in man. Long experience with kidney transplants has shown that the same laws apply; kidneys from HLA-identical sibs require less immunosuppression and with rare exceptions function better and longer than do other grafts.

Individual H-2 or HLA antigens can be serologically identified, and unrelated subjects can be H-2 or HLA typed and matched. In earlier studies with random bred mice, matching did not produce prolonged graft survival. This was because a pair of "matched" unrelated subjects do not inherit exactly identical haplotypes from common ancestors; they are not genotypically identical. For man, as for mice, subjects with similar antigenic profiles are termed phenotypically identical. It must be emphasized that although two unrelated individuals may appear similar in serologic typing, they are not truly identical, and T cells can usually recognize the difference. Phenotypically identical grafts often fare better than do unmatched grafts, but there are numerous exceptions. In man, the differences between matched sibling and matched unrelated graft have become more indistinct as immunosuppression has improved. HLA-identical sibling grafts are superior to "matched" grafts from unrelated donors.

THE HLA ANTIGENS OVERVIEW

The two major series of HLA antigens are referred to as Class I and Class II; they differ in their structure, function, and tissue distribution. Class I genes and their products include HLA-A, HLA-B, HLA-C, HLA-E, HLA-F, and HLA-G. Class I products are found on almost all the tissues. Incompatibility for Class I characteristically induces a cytotoxic T cell (CD8) response, and the Class I antigens are important in the presentation of intracellular (e.g., viral) antigens. HLA-A and HLA-B are highly polymorphic; they have many variant forms or alleles. Class II antigens are found on B lymphocytes, endothelial cells, some macrophages, and activated T cells and activated parenchyma cells. Class II differences are mainly associated with the activation of helper T cells (CD4) and the presentation of exogenous antigens. The Class II series includes HLA-DR, HLA-DQ, HLA-DP, and HLA-DO/DN. Although the polymorphism of HLA-DR is best known, new alleles of HLA-DQ and HLA-DP are being discovered. Like HLA-F, HLA-DO/DN has no known product or function.

The chromosomal segment carrying the HLA genes is termed the HLA haplotype. The haplotype also has genes coding for complement components C2, C4, and factor B, for two variants of the enzyme 21-hydroxylase, and for tumor necrosis factors α and β. The HLA antigens and the haplotype are vital for the induction of many forms of immune responsiveness. The T-cell receptor (TcR) recognizes the combination of an HLA Class I molecule and a nominal antigen such as the influenza antigen. Compatibility between the Class II antigens of B cell and T cell is required for antibody responses; the Class II genes are the immune response genes. Besides its action in antigen presentation, HLA also acts as a restricting element. Immunity to a particular HLA and to a nominal antigen can be recalled only when that antigen is presented again with the same HLA antigen.

HLA Class I Genes and Their Products

The Class I genes include flanking sequences and a number of exons and introns. The HLA protein is glycosylated in the Golgi stack and combines with an invariant light chain termed β_2-microglobulin before being inserted into the membrane as the Class I heterodimer. Sequence variability occurs at particular sites in the α_1 and α_2 domains. Radiologic crystallographic studies of an HLA-A2 molecule have provided a three-dimensional picture. The conserved α_3 domain and β_2-microglobulin form the bottom support of a platform consisting of a β pleated sheet structure with two α helices above. The α helices form a groove that is believed to contain antigenic peptide fragments. The variable sequences in the α_1 and α_2 domains localize around this groove and constitute individual binding sites or epitopes that are recognized by alloantibodies or by TcR. Similar but not identical sequences appear as extensive cross-reactive sets of antigens. The amino acid residues recognized by many of the antibodies have been identified through competitive binding and site-directed mutagenesis. The epitopes for T-cell binding are less well established. T cells, however, appear to bind to sites on the peptide as well as to the structures surrounding the groove. The specificity of T-cell binding is important for self versus non-self discrimination and for MHC-restricted immune recognition. Class I molecules are predominantly recognized by the CD8[+] subset of T cells.

HLA Class II Genes and Products

The Class II molecules consist of a heavier, acidic α chain non-covalently bound to a lighter basic β chain. Unlike the Class I molecule for which the light chain is encoded on a separate chromosome, the light and heavy chains of Class II are paired together in subregions of the HLA haplotype. The typical gene structure of a Class II heavy chain includes five exons; the light chain has six exons.

The structure of the Class II molecule is believed to be similar to that of the Class I protein, but an invariant chain is added during assembly of the molecule. Processing of the molecule through the Golgi is by a different pathway from Class I, and the invariant chain is lost when the molecule is inserted into the membrane. It is thought that antigen presentation is initiated within cytoplasmic vesicles during processing of the Class II molecules. The Class II molecules are recognized principally by the CD4[+] T cell (helper) subset.

The number of Class II genes on different haplotypes is variable, and clusters of these genes constitute a series of subregions. Each subregion contains at least one α chain gene with one or more β chain genes. The heavy chain from each subregion is glycosylated and paired with the light chain from the same subregion.

CLINICAL TYPING

General Considerations

Immune responses do not occur when donor and recipient are exactly alike, as in identical twins and in HLA-identical sibling pairs. The greater the divergence between the members of a transplant pair, the greater the probability of an immune response between them, but a single amino acid substitution can, on occasion, stimulate a strong cellular response that causes rapid graft rejection. HLA matching of unrelated recipient-donor pairs can therefore be regarded only as a guide. Immune response genes and the capacity of a recipient to respond cannot at present be measured. T cells do not necessarily detect the same epitopes recognized by antisera, and some epitopes recognized by T cells are not detected at all serologically. The converse is probably true, so HLA typing and matching *unrelated* pairs is no guarantee of identity. In families, the clinician is on firmer ground. The probability of rejection between an HLA-identical sibling pair who are also mixed lymphocyte reaction (MLR)-unreactive is extremely small. This is because HLA-identical siblings inherit exactly the same haplotypes from their parents. The very infrequent exceptions may be due to the summation of effects of independently segregating minor histocompatibility antigens or to mutation (recombination) in one sib involving an unrecognized exchange of part of the haplotype. The MLR can be invaluable in detecting such aberrations.

Cytotoxicity Testing

The microlymphocytotoxicity test is used by all clinical laboratories. Most antisera are obtained from multiparous women. Postpartum sera are screened against cells from a donor panel of known HLA types, and those that appear to recognize a given HLA specificity are tested against a larger cell panel that includes donors from different ethnic groups. The serum sets sold commercially may include monoclonal antibodies together with antibodies from transplant patients or transfusion recipients. In the basic test, a small volume, usually 1 microliter of serum, is mixed with cells, and rabbit complement is added. For reading the test, a vital dye, usually eosin, is added. Dead cells stain; live cells remain brightly refractile. There are numerous variants of the basic procedure. In one, a wash step is added. The sensitized cells are washed with buffer solution before the addition of complement; this increases the sensitivity and reduces the number of false-negative results. In another test, antiglobulin serum is added to the washed cells before the complement step. This antiglobulin test is extremely sensitive and is mainly reserved for the crossmatch procedure.

Tests for HLA-DR and other Class II antigens differ in several respects. A purified B cell suspension is used, the complement is selected, and the incubation times are often longer. Isoelectric focusing, cell-mediated lympholysis, restriction fragment length polymorphisms, and identification of sequences by use of oligonucleotide probes and DNA amplified by polymerase chain reaction (PCR) are sometimes used for the fine resolution of some antigens. Functional tests are used for testing for HLA-D and for other special purposes. Although HLA-D is treated as if it were a genetic locus, there is no HLA-D gene and consequently no gene product. HLA-D can be regarded as the sum of the D region genes, HLA-DR, DQ, and DP, and possibly also DO/DN; the resultant of these gene products is the functional activity known as HLA-D. The two-way MLR is used for detecting HLA-D differences. In one-way MLR, stimulator lymphocytes

TABLE 1. Listing of Recognized HLA Specificities (1987)

A	B	C	D	DR	DQ	DP
A1	B5	Cw1	Dw1	DR1	DQw1	DPw1
A2	B7	Cw2	Dw2	DR2	DQw2	DPw2
A3	B8	Cw3	Dw3	DR3	DQw3	DPw3
A9	B12	Cw4	Dw4	DR4	DQw4	DPw4
A10	B13	Cw5	Dw5	DR5		DPw5
A11	B14	Cw6	Dw6	DRw6		DPw6
Aw19	B15	Cw7	Dw7	DR7		
A28	B16	Cw8	Dw8	DRw8		
	B17		Dw9	DR9		
	B18		Dw10	DRw10		
	B21	Cw11				
	Bw22		Dw12			
	B27		Dw13			
	B35		Dw14			
	B37		Dw15			
			Dw16			
	B40					
Aw36	Bw41					
Aw43	Bw42		Dw20	DRw52		
			Dw21			
			Dw22	DRw53		
			Dw23			
	Bw46		Dw24			
	Bw47		Dw25			
	Bw48		Dw26			
	Bw53					
	Bw59					
	Bw67					
	Bw70					
	Bw73					
	Bw4					
	Bw6					

Specificities in parentheses after a narrow specificity, e.g., HLA-A23 (9), is optional. The following is a listing of these specificities that arose as clear-cut splits of the broad specificities.

Original Broad Specificities	Splits
A9	A23, A24
A10	A25, A26, Aw34, Aw66
Aw19	A29, A30, A31, A32, Aw33, Aw74
A28	Aw68, Aw69
B5	B51, Bw52
B12	B44, B45
B14	Bw64, Bw65
B15	Bw62, Bw63, Bw75, Bw76, Bw77
B16	B38, B39
B17	Bw57, Bw58
B21	B49, Bw50
Bw22	Bw54, Bw55, Bw56
B40	Bw60, Bw61
Bw70	Bw71, Bw72
Cw3	Cw9, Cw10
DR2	DRw15, DRw16
DR3	DRw17, DRw18
DR5	DRw11, DRw12
DRw6	DRw13, DRw14
DQw1	DQw5, DQw6
DQw3	DQw7, DQw8, DQw9
Dw6	Dw18, Dw19
Dw7	Dw11, Dw17
Bw4	
Bw6	

As adapted from the WHO report of 1987. Nomenclature for Factors of the HLA System. Vox. Sang., 55:119, 1988. See also Bodmer, J. G., et al.: Nomenclature for factors of the HLA system. Hum. Immunol., 28:236, 1990.

from the donor are inactivated by treatment with mitomycin C or irradiation. The MLR is not used for the identification of HLA-D types; for this, primed lymphocytes are used. In primed lymphocyte tests for assigning HLA-D specificities, the responding cells are prestimulated with lymphocytes from a donor of known HLA-D type. This test is more precise. The MLR is used for measuring the strength of differences at HLA-DR and DQ between a potential donor and recipient. This is particularly important clinically because many DR and DQ antigens are not identifiable serologically or can be identified only with great difficulty. In practice, haplotypes can often be established by simple HLA-A, B, and C typing of family members. However, HLA-DR and DQ typing or a negative MLC between potential donor-recipient pairs is also required for exclusion of recombination between HLA-B and HLA-DR and sometimes as an assessment of the validity of serologic testing.

A list of HLA antigens is given in Table 1. The antigens form two major categories called subtypic and supertypic specificities. The subtypic antigens have been "split" from the others. The first "split" separated HLA-A2 from HLA-A28. HLA-A28 is now further subdivided by special sera, and HLA-A2 is subdivided into no less than six variants on the basis of cellular and genomic typing. Nearly all of the earliest antigens recognized have been split, and the process is continuing. For some organs including cadaveric liver and heart, any matching is usually retrospective. Prospective typing and matching can be performed in transplants from living donors.

III

Mechanisms and Characteristics of Allograft Rejection

Fred Sanfilippo, M.D., Ph.D., and D. Bernard Amos, M.D.

Allograft rejection and complications of the immunosuppressive therapy required for prevention or treatment of rejection remain the major causes of morbidity and mortality for organ transplant recipients. This is despite the tremendous advances in knowledge of immune mechanisms and the improved outcome seen clinically over the past 10 years. The *major histocompatibility complex (MHC)* antigens (i.e., HLA

See the corresponding chapter or part in the *Textbook of Surgery*, 14th edition, pp. 357–374, for a more detailed discussion of this topic, including a comprehensive list of references.

in man) are the most important transplant antigens that stimulate and act as targets of graft rejection. The disparity of donor HLA antigens has a major impact in recipient selection and ultimate graft survival. For example, kidney grafts from HLA-identical siblings generally have the best outcome and require the least immunosuppression, whereas grafts expressing HLA antigens to which a recipient is pre-sensitized (i.e., has preformed anti-donor alloantibodies) usu-ally are rejected immediately. Increased understanding of the molecular and cellular aspects of host responsiveness to HLA and other alloantigens has had a significant impact on the development of new approaches used to characterize, diag-nose, and treat rejection reactions.

MECHANISMS OF REJECTION

There are three distinct components of host immune reac-tivity to any antigen: recognition, regulation, and response. The immune cells capable of specific *antigen recognition* are T and B lymphocytes. These cells recognize antigens usually after their processing and/or presentation by specialized cells termed *antigen presenting cells (APC)*. APC have the general characteristics of expressing Class II MHC antigens and secreting cytokines that can stimulate lymphocyte (and other cell) populations. In man, the major APC are monocyte/macrophages, dendritic cells, and some vascular endothelial cells. Following antigen breakdown and processing (usually by macrophages), the resulting peptide antigens are bound to the "antigen binding groove" of the MHC antigens on APC, which allows recognition by antigen-specific T cells.

The diversity of T-cell receptors (TcR) is as great as that of immunoglobulins, with more than a million clones of differ-ent specificity within each host. The repertoire of TcR in an individual is selected by interactions within the thymus that delete T cells that react with self-antigens and select those that are capable of recognizing peptide antigens associated with (restricted by) self-MHC determinants. T cells can be divided into two major subsets based on the class of MHC recognized in association with its bound antigen: Class I restricted T cells generally express the CD8 receptor, which binds to invariant portions of the Class I molecule; Class II restricted T cells generally express the CD4 molecule, which binds to invariant Class II determinants.

Only a small number of T cells generally recognize a specific antigen plus self-MHC combination. However, a very high percentage of T cells appear capable of directly recognizing intact allogeneic MHC molecules (allo-MHC) on donor cells. Thus, it appears that allogeneic tissue can stimulate host immunity by two distinct mechanisms: (1) direct activation of host clones that recognize intact allo-MHC on *donor* APC and (2) activation of host clones recognizing processed allo-MHC peptide fragments presented on *host* APC.

Recognition of processed alloantigen on host APC (or intact alloantigen on donor APC) typically causes stimulation of Class II restricted (CD4$^+$) T helper cells (T$_H$), which then promote and *regulate* the characteristics of the immune response. In mice, one subset of T helper cells (T_H1) secretes lymphokines (such as interleukin-1 [IL-1] and interferon-gamma [IFN-γ]) that preferentially stimulate effector T cell and macrophage (cellular immune) responses. Another subset (T_H2) preferentially promotes humoral (antibody) responses by secretion of IL-4, which stimulates B lymphocytes to differentiate into antibody-producing plasma cells. Antigen-specific responses may also be inhibited by cellular (T suppressor cell) and antibody (anti-idiotypic) mechanisms.

The *targets* of human allograft responses are predominantly disparate HLA and a few other (e.g., ABO blood group) antigens. Each disparate donor HLA molecule expresses antigenic determinants that can be recognized by alloantibody and/or alloreactive T cells. Most of the allogeneic class I (HLA-A, B) molecules are recognized by both antibody and T-cell receptors, whereas Class II molecules have some allogeneic determinants recognized by T cells but not antibody. The specificity of alloreactive T cells is most significantly affected by amino acid sequences of HLA molecules that affect their peptide binding, a concept consistent with the known dual recognition of antigen plus self-MHC by the T-cell receptor.

The specificity and expression of HLA molecules may impact on host rejection in a variety of ways. Different tissues vary in the number of APC with potentially stimulatory donor HLA, as well as in the expression of HLA antigens on parenchymal cells. It also appears that certain peptide-MHC combinations may be preferentially recognized (immunodominant) by T cells, thus provoking stronger responses. The particular MHC allele to which a given antigen binds may also qualitatively affect responsiveness by the preferential stimulation of T_H1 versus T_H2 regulatory cells. Thus, potential differences in rejection reactions may be based on the exact MHC specificities of the host and recipient.

CLASSIFICATION OF REJECTION

Allograft rejection can be categorized by immunologic, histopathologic, or clinical criteria (Table 1). From a mechanistic perspective, rejection can be classified as being mediated by humoral (antibody) versus cellular immune reactions. From a pathologic perspective, the major targets of allograft rejection are vessels (*vascular rejection*) and components in the interstitium (*interstitial rejection*) that can include donor dendritic cells, the microvasculature, or parenchymal cells. *Humoral rejection* typically presents as exudative inflammation following the deposition of alloantibody in vessels. Binding of alloantibody to HLA antigens on donor cells activates complement and attracts inflammatory cells with immunoglobulin and/or complement receptors (e.g., granulocytes, macrophages, and some lymphocyte populations). The predominant target of most humoral rejection reactions is the vasculature, where circulating alloantibodies first come in contact with donor alloantigens. *Cellular rejection* charac-

TABLE 1. General Criteria Used to Classify Allograft Rejection

Clinical		Immunopathologic		
Classification	Kinetics	Target	Response	Reactions
Hyperacute	Very rapid onset, minutes to hours posttransplantation	Vessels: Large, small	Humoral	Granulocytic infiltrates, vasculitis, hemorrhage
Acute	Rapid onset, usually early posttransplantation			
Interstitial		Parenchyma, small vessels	Cellular ≥ humoral	Interstitial edema, mononuclear mixed cell inflammation
Vascular		Vessels: large, intermediate	Humoral > cellular	Vasculitis, granulocyte mixed cell infiltrates
Chronic	Slow onset, usually late posttransplantation			
Interstitial		Parenchyma	Cellular > humoral	Interstitial fibrosis, mononuclear cell infiltrates
Vascular		Vessels: large, intermediate	Humoral ≥ cellular	Sclerotic vascular changes, secondary ischemic injury

teristically involves mononuclear cell infiltration predominantly by T cells and monocyte/macrophages, although in severe reactions neutrophils and eosinophils are seen.

The most commonly used classification system for describing rejection of any solid organ allograft was first established for renal transplantation in the mid-1960s. This system is based primarily on clinical characteristics related to the speed of onset and time posttransplant that graft dysfunction was observed, that is, hyperacute, acute, and chronic. *Hyperacute rejection* refers to those reactions occurring almost immediately after transplantation, causing overwhelming graft injury. Characteristically, these involve transplantation of a donor organ into a presensitized recipient with circulating anti-donor alloantibodies. Indeed, initial correlations between the risk of hyperacute rejection and preformed anti-donor HLA (or ABO) antibodies caused one of the major clinical applications of histocompatibility testing, that is, the crossmatch test (see later). Hyperacute rejection is best described as a humorally mediated–vascular rejection.

Acute rejection typically occurs several weeks to months after transplantation and is of rapid onset. It usually presents as a cellular mediated–interstitial reaction, not infrequently with a humoral and/or vascular component. Mechanistically, acute rejection may represent the development of a primary or secondary host alloimmune response. In some cases, an accelerated acute rejection can be seen that is more similar to hyperacute rejection and may represent an accelerated secondary antibody response against donor alloantigens. *Chronic rejection* generally describes a slow loss of function months to years posttransplantation. The typical pattern is one of low-grade interstitial and vascular inflammation with scarring. The immune mechanisms remain unclear.

HISTOCOMPATIBILITY TESTING

Histocompatibility testing remains an essential part of clinical organ transplantation, despite the improved graft survival seen with newer immunosuppressive therapies (Table 2). The three major procedures used are HLA typing, anti-HLA antibody screening, and donor-recipient crossmatching (Table 3). Although a range of procedures are available, the classic assays used for all these procedures involve variations of the *microlymphocytotoxicity* test. In this assay, serum is incubated with lymphocytes followed by complement, and positive reactions (cell injury) are identified by using a vital dye and microscope.

For *HLA typing*, well-categorized "reagent" sera of known HLA specificities are reacted with lymphocytes from the patient or donor for identification of the HLA antigens expressed by that individual. Some technical differences in typing for Class II (HLA-DR) versus Class I (HLA-A, B) antigens are necessary because the expression of Class II is limited to only certain cells (e.g., B cells, monocytes). In some cases of potential live-donor transplantation, serologic typing results may not provide enough information to determine the precise compatibility among family members, such that alternative procedures to identify cellular-defined HLA determinants may be needed. Traditionally, these have in-

TABLE 2. Results of Organ Transplantation in the U.S. 1987–1988

Organ	6-Month Actuarial Graft Survival (Number of Transplants)	
	First Transplants	*Repeat Transplants*
Kidney		
Cadaveric	82% (5828)	73% (1101)
Live donor		
2-Haplotype	96% (183)	90% (20)
1-Haplotype	93% (508)	95% (44)
0-Haplotype	94% (68)	100% (6)
Heart	85% (1473)	59% (54)
Heart and lung	75% (58)	— (4)
Lung	46% (19)	— (1)
Liver	74% (1267)	40% (273)
Pancreas	71% (137)	25% (61)

From the First Annual Report of the United Network for Organ Sharing, Richmond, Virginia, 1989.

TABLE 3. Histocompatibility Testing in Clinical Transplantation

Test	Purpose	Material	Methods
HLA typing (donor/recipient/family)	Donor selection	Patient lymphocytes; typing sera panel	Serologic (microlymphocytotoxicity) Cellular (mixed lymphocyte reaction, T cell clones) Genomic (restriction fragment length polymorphisms, specific probes)
Antibody screening (recipient)	Identify anti-HLA alloantibodies	Patient serum; HLA-typed cell panel	Microlymphocytotoxicity
Crossmatching (donor-recipient)	Identify donor-specific alloantibodies	Patient serum, donor cells	Microlymphocytotoxicity; flow cytometry

volved the *mixed lymphocyte reaction (MLR)* test, although more recently T cell clones of defined specificity have also been used. Alternatively, molecular genetic techniques have been used to compare and characterize donor and recipient HLA genes, such as by examining restriction fragment length polymorphisms, or binding with specific oligonucleotide probes. However, because of the time and cost, routine serologic typing methods suffice for almost all clinical transplant applications.

There are several reasons for HLA typing of donors and recipients. With potential family donors, it provides a means of identifying and comparing the extent of compatibility with the recipient. Fully HLA-identical siblings, who share both HLA chromosome segments *(haplotypes)*, have a very low risk of rejection and are typically placed on a low immunosuppressive therapy protocol. Likewise, there is an increased risk of rejection episodes for fully unmatched (0 haplotype) live-donor renal transplants compared with those sharing one or two haplotypes, although their ultimate graft survival is now becoming comparable (Table 2). For cadaveric-donor transplantation, HLA typing serves three potential purposes in donor selection. First, donor typing is necessary to identify HLA antigens to which a patient may have preformed antibody and thus should not receive. Second, donor typing can identify "acceptable" HLA antigens for presensitized patients to facilitate their transplantation. Third, the risk of rejection is associated with the degree of donor HLA disparity, especially with kidney allografts and for certain recipients at higher risk owing to prior graft rejection or presensitization.

For *antibody screening*, patient sera are routinely tested against a panel of 30 to 100 HLA-typed cells for identifying the degree of *panel-reactive antibody (PRA)*. This allows an approximate estimate of the risk of a positive crossmatch with a random donor and can often identify the specificity of alloantibodies that are present. However, many patients with a high panel-reactive antibody have alloantibodies against *cross-reactive* HLA antigens, multiple alloantibodies, or, in some cases, autoantibodies. Presensitization is most often caused by prior graft rejection, blood transfusion, or pregnancy and directly affects the time a patient must wait for a crossmatch-negative donor. Major approaches used to address the problem of transplanting highly sensitized patients include (1) sharing patient sera among many centers to permit testing of more potential donors, (2) prescreening patient sera against large extended panels to identify acceptable donor HLA antigens, and (3) removing alloantibodies from the patient by techniques such as immunoabsorption.

Recipient *crossmatching* is routinely performed before transplant for any patient with evidence of preformed alloantibodies. However, a negative antibody screen (PRA = 0) does not ensure a negative crossmatch with all potential donors, since an actual donor HLA antigen may not be represented on any of the panel cells tested. Moreover, a negative crossmatch does not ensure the absence of a biologically important anti-donor antibody, since some alloantigens (e.g., vascular endothelial cells) may not be expressed on lymphocytes, and some alloantibodies are not easily identified by complement-mediated cytotoxicity tests. The most detrimental alloantibodies appear to be IgG anti-Class I (HLA-A or B), although IgM alloantibodies and some anti-Class II HLA antibodies have been associated with early severe rejection. Recent studies have also suggested that the loss of certain donor-specific alloantibodies may allow successful transplantation of some patients with a crossmatch that is positive with old (historical) serum but negative with current serum. Autoantibodies and non-anti-HLA antibodies can give false-positive crossmatch results, which exclude potentially acceptable donors. However, alternative methods and modifications of standard assays can permit identification of the type and specificity of particular alloantibodies directed against donor antigens for improvement of the predictive value of the crossmatch test.

IV

Renal Transplantation

Clyde F. Barker, M.D., Ali Naji, M.D., Ph.D.,
Donald C. Dafoe, M.D., and Leonard J. Perloff, M.D.

RECIPIENT SELECTION AND MANAGEMENT

INDICATIONS. Transplantation should be seriously considered in all patients with end-stage renal disease, since both the quality of life and survival are superior to those of dialysis. The most common indications are glomerulonephritis, diabetes mellitus, hypertension, and pyelonephritis. Contraindications are infection or malignancy that cannot be eradicated and predictable noncompliance with immunosuppression. Advanced age or cardiovascular disease is a deterrent.

RECIPIENT EVALUATION AND PREPARATION. The evaluation of transplant candidates should include history and physical examination; complete blood count, urinalysis, urine cultures, and serum chemistries; assays for human immunodeficiency virus, cytomegalovirus, and hepatitis B virus; chest film; electrocardiogram; coagulation profile; Pap smear; and ABO typing. Regardless of the donor source, ABO compatibility and a negative complement-dependent cytotoxicity crossmatch are mandatory.

PRETRANSPLANT BLOOD TRANSFUSIONS. Traditionally, blood transfusions were avoided in prospective trans-

---

See the corresponding chapter or part in the *Textbook of Surgery*, 14th edition, pp. 374–393, for a more detailed discussion of this topic, including a comprehensive list of references.

plant recipients to avoid sensitization. In 1973, however, the surprising observation by Opelz and Terasaki that renal allograft survival was 10 to 15 per cent better in transfused than in nontransfused recipients led to a worldwide policy of deliberate pretransplant transfusion. Today, because of the improvement in graft survival in cyclosporine-treated patients and the fear of transmission of infection (HIV infection, hepatitis B), transfusions may still have benefit but are no longer widely recommended.

DONOR SELECTION AND MANAGEMENT

In addition to close histocompatibility, the use of a related-donor kidney has the advantage of decreasing waiting time on dialysis and of minimizing the likelihood of acute tubular necrosis related to organ recovery and transport. Since the advent of cyclosporine therapy in 1983, although short-term survivals of cadaveric allografts in some centers now approach those of related-donor kidneys, long-term results still favor related-donor transplantation, which represents about 25 per cent of kidney transplants in the United States.

Excellent long-term graft survival (greater than 90 per cent) can be expected when a related donor and recipient are HLA-identical. There is a progressively lower graft survival associated with one haplotype matching or mismatches for both haplotypes, which causes reluctance at some transplant centers to accept such donors. The operative mortality of about 0.05 per cent has led to a traditional policy of accepting only donors between the ages of 18 and 55 years and in perfect health. The fear of possible long-term deleterious effects of kidney donation, such as hypertension and renal dysfunction, have not been realized. Still, the shortage of cadaver donors may be the most compelling reason for use of totally mismatched related donors.

Cadaver donors should be previously healthy subjects between 3 and 65 years of age who have sustained fatal head injuries or cerebrovascular accidents. Factors that preclude organ donation are generalized infections (bacterial, viral, or fungal), malignancy other than nonmetastasizing brain tumors, renal disease, severe hypertension, and advanced arteriosclerosis.

Reports from European centers have generally indicated that HLA matching for cadaveric grafts has a beneficial effect, although this has not appeared so clear in reports from North America. This difference may be the greater genetic homogeneity of the European population and the uniformity of tissue typing that is performed only in the experienced laboratories of Eurotransplant.

The perception that cyclosporine overrides the effects of HLA mismatching has been used to support the concept that prompt local use of poorly matched kidneys is preferable to transplantation into better matched recipients at distant centers. Nevertheless, in comparing 9369 transplants done in the same center with 5553 exchanged between centers, Opelz found that HLA matching improved graft survival in both groups (85 per cent with local kidneys and 86 per cent with exchanged kidneys).

OPERATIVE TECHNIQUE FOR CADAVERIC DONORS. After declaration of brain death, the donor is brought to the operating room. Optimal respiration and circulation are maintained during the procedure, and it is often necessary to administer large volumes of intravenous fluids to restore blood volume. After removal of the extrarenal organs, the kidneys, ureters, aorta, and vena cava are excised *en bloc* and transferred to a basin of cold solution where careful dissection of the renal vessels is performed.

PRESERVATION OF CADAVERIC KIDNEYS. Two methods of preservation (simple cooling and continuous pulsatile perfusion) have become relatively standardized. Both allow sufficient time for transportation of kidneys to distant transplant centers. In 1987, Belzer introduced a solution (University of Wisconsin or UW solution, containing lactobionate, raffinose, and hydroxyethyl starch) that extended substantially the period of storage for livers and pancreases, and possibly kidneys.

THE RECIPIENT OPERATION. The iliac vessels are exposed retroperitoneally, and an end-to-side anastomosis of renal artery and vein to the external iliac artery and vein, respectively, is most often used. Urinary tract continuity is usually established by ureteroneocystostomy. Ureteropyelostomy is an alternative procedure that should be used in instances of ureteral devascularization or injury. Drains are avoided.

POSTTRANSPLANT MANAGEMENT

Unless the transplanted kidney has suffered ischemic damage, a brisk diuresis usually begins within minutes of revascularization. The transplant operation is relatively nondisruptive to intestinal function, and medications and fluids can usually be given by mouth within 12 to 24 hours.

Immunosuppression

AZATHIOPRINE AND STEROIDS. In the late 1950s, rejection of renal allografts was prevented by whole body irradiation, a profoundly immunodepressive procedure with a prohibitive risk of lethal infection. In the 1960s, the antimetabolite drug azathioprine was found to have a reversible and safer action than irradiation. Although adrenal corticosteroids were not sufficient to prevent rejection, they were found to be synergistic with azathioprine. In addition, brief courses of large-dose steroid therapy can often reverse acute rejection episodes.

ANTILYMPHOCYTIC ANTIBODIES. In the 1960s, a new immunosuppressive agent, antilymphocyte serum (ALS, a xenoantibody raised by repeated immunization of animals with human lymphoid cells), was found to be even more potent and somewhat more specific than azathioprine. Several problems diminished its usefulness. Even the purified globulin fraction (ALG) sometimes provoked allergic reactions, leukopenia, and thrombocytopenia. Antibody production to the heterologous protein limited its effectiveness, and repeated use and large doses or prolonged therapy often led to serious infections. Today, the most frequent indication for ALG is reversal of rejection crises, even those resistant to large-dose steroid therapy.

The effectiveness of ALS in reversing rejection led to the introduction by Cosimi and associates of monoclonal anti–T cell antibodies, which rapidly depleted T lymphocytes from peripheral blood while having little detrimental effect on red blood cells, platelets, or granulocytes. Because of greater availability, specificity, and ease of standardization, monoclonal pan–T cell antibodies such as OKT3 have largely replaced ALS and ALG.

CYCLOSPORINE. Since its release for general use in 1983, cyclosporine has been adopted by nearly all centers as the basis of contemporary immunosuppressive protocols. It is a fungal derivative first noted by Borel in 1974 to have immunosuppressive qualities. It appears to block production of the lymphokine IL-2 through inhibition of T-lymphocyte messenger RNA. Like azathioprine and unlike OKT3 and ALS, cyclosporine is most useful for prophylaxis rather than in the reversal of rejection. Cyclosporine has the major advantage over azathioprine of lacking bone marrow toxicity. Despite maintenance of blood levels in the therapeutic range, nephrotoxicity is its major side effect. Others include hypertension, hepatotoxicity, seizures, tremor, hypertrichosis, nausea, vomiting, and diarrhea. Because of uncertainty regarding the cumulative nephrotoxicity of long-term cyclosporine therapy, some centers use much lower initial doses in combination with azathioprine and prednisone (triple therapy) and/or discontinue cyclosporine completely and utilize only azathioprine and prednisone after stable graft function is established.

Patient survival has also been improved by the introduction of cyclosporine, probably because of a decreased incidence and severity of infections. Especially benefited are older patients, recipients of multiple transplants, and high immune responders. Disappointingly, there is little evidence that cyclosporine has the same favorable impact on long-term results as it does on early ones. Multicenter reports indicate a continuing attrition in late graft survival most likely due to chronic rejection, which apparently is not overcome by cyclosporine.

REJECTION

Although rejection is conveniently categorized into hyperacute, acute, and chronic forms, there are overlapping features and transitions between these categories.

HYPERACUTE REJECTION. Now rarely seen, hyperacute rejection occurs within minutes of kidney revascularization and is evidenced by bluish discoloration of the kidney, deterioration of perfusion, and irreversible sudden cessation of function. Extensive intravascular deposits of fibrin and platelets and intraglomerular accumulation of polymorpho-nuclear leukocytes, fibrin, platelets and red blood cells are seen histologically, along with accumulation of polymorpho-nuclear leukocytes in the peritubular and glomerular capillaries. Refractory to immunosuppressive or anticoagulant therapy, hyperacute rejection is usually correlated with the presence of preformed circulating antibodies against donor antigens, which now can be identified by a pretransplant leukocyte crossmatch.

ACUTE CELLULAR REJECTION. Acute cellular rejection most commonly occurs during the early weeks following transplantation. Prompt initiation of antirejection treatment can often prevent irreversible damage and reverse the entire process. Classic signs and symptoms are malaise, fever, tenderness and swelling of the wound, oliguria, and hypertension. Findings include weight gain, rising blood urea nitrogen and creatinine, and deterioration of flow and tubular function on radionuclide scans. Since, under the influence of cyclosporine, impaired renal function may be the only signal of rejection, transcutaneous allograft biopsy may be required.

Microscopic signs of acute rejection include the adherence of lymphocytes to the endothelium of peritubular capillaries and venules, progressing to disruption of these vessels, tubular necrosis, and interstitial infiltrates. Prompt institution of antirejection therapy (steroids, ALS, OKT3) is necessary to prevent permanent damage to the allograft. Steroid-resistant rejection, which occurs in 30 to 50 per cent of patients, responds to ALG or OKT3 in an additional 30 per cent of cases. During the 1970s (prior to the introduction of cyclosporine), a progressive improvement in patient survival occurred in most centers. This was the result of the realization that overly intense immunosuppression and repeated courses of antirejection therapy were dangerous. Recognition that eventual loss of some grafts could not be avoided allowed earlier transplant nephrectomy and reinstitution of dialysis. A later successful transplant and a live patient were found preferable to serious infection and even death from heavy immunosuppression given with little likelihood of forestalling eventual rejection.

CHRONIC REJECTION. Chronic rejection is the usual cause of late deterioration of renal allografts although other causes such as recurrent disease (glomerulonephritis, diabetes, oxalosis) and renal artery stenosis should always be considered. The typical course is gradual, progressive loss of renal function. It may begin after years of stable function but is more often seen in patients who have had multiple early and incompletely reversed episodes of acute rejection. Glomerular changes are also seen. Clinical manifestations include proteinuria, microscopic hematuria, hypertension, and fluid retention with progressive uremia. Histologic evidence of protracted humoral injury is marked by arterial intimal fibro-proliferative lesions. Also seen are increased mesangial matrix and mesangial proliferation. The glomerular basement membrane is thickened, and focal deposition of IgM, IgG, and complement may be identified.

Antirejection therapy is ineffective and large-dose steroid,

ALS, or OKT3 therapy should not be risked, since these may cause opportunistic infection or other serious sequelae. A prompt biopsy is warranted in cases of unexpected or precipitous deterioration in stable function, since episodes of late acute cellular rejection can sometimes be reversed. With judicious fluid and electrolyte control, patients with chronic rejection can often be maintained for months to years before returning to dialysis.

COMPLICATIONS OF RENAL TRANSPLANTATION

Complications occurring in the first few hours or days after transplantation are commonly related to technical mishaps.

VASCULAR COMPLICATIONS. Arterial obstruction, as a cause of early postoperative oliguria or anuria, should be considered if an established diuresis suddenly ceases. Although radioisotopic scanning and arteriography confirm the diagnosis, immediate reoperation without delay for diagnostic studies allows the best chance for the graft. Renal transplant artery stenosis may be confused with rejection, since both may cause hypertension and diminished renal function. Although renal transplant artery stenosis is a relatively unusual cause of decreased renal function, a high index of suspicion should be maintained, since it is correctable. The long-term results of percutaneous transluminal angioplasty and surgical therapy are probably approximately comparable, but because of simplicity and patient acceptability, most surgeons advocate percutaneous transluminal angioplasty as the initial approach.

URINARY TRACT COMPLICATIONS. The most common cause of sudden cessation of urinary output in the immediate postoperative period is presence of a blood clot in the bladder or urethral catheter. More serious causes of urinary obstruction (2 to 5 per cent in most series) should be investigated simultaneously with consideration of vascular occlusion, acute tubular necrosis, and rejection.

Devascularization of the ureter during donor nephrectomy is a serious problem and may cause ureteral necrosis and urinary fistula within the first few days or weeks following surgery. Analysis of fluid obtained from wound drains or needle aspiration, ultrasound, radioactive scans, cystograms, and antegrade pyeloureterography are other helpful studies. Treatment consists of reconstruction of the ureteroneocystostomy or ureteropyelostomy using the patient's own ureter.

ACUTE TUBULAR NECROSIS (ATN). In the absence of vascular or ureteral problems, initial nonfunction of cadaver kidneys may be attributed to ATN (incidence of 5 to 30 per cent). Oliguria in the early transplant period should be treated with boluses of fluid for exclusion of hypovolemia. Although mild ATN *per se* does not significantly worsen the prognosis for eventual transplant success, the overall impact of ATN is an adverse one, primarily because it may interfere with the early diagnosis of rejection and delay antirejection therapy. The nephrotoxic potential of cyclosporine is heightened with

ATN, which causes some surgeons to sharply lower the dose or avoid its use completely during ATN.

NONTECHNICAL COMPLICATIONS. *Infection,* the most common complication of immunosuppression, occurs in 30 to 60 per cent of patients during the first posttransplant year. Despite more cautious use of immunosuppression over the last decade, it is the major cause of death in half of the 5 to 10 per cent of patients who die during the first year.

Bacterial infections are the most common infections during the first month after transplantation, and the urinary tract, respiratory system, and wound are the most prevalent sites. These infections usually respond to prompt antibiotic therapy. It is important to exclude the possibility of infection before antirejection therapy, since immunosuppression should be decreased rather than intensified in this situation.

The period between the first and sixth months after transplantation, usually the time of most intense immunosuppression, is the most common time for *opportunistic infections.* Cytomegalovirus (CMV), a member of the herpes family, is an ubiquitous agent that infects most individuals at some time in their lives. It causes clinically silent or mild infection in healthy individuals, and the latent virus and seropositivity persist for life. Sixty-one per cent of seronegative recipients who receive a kidney from a seropositive donor develop symptomatic illness, which varies in severity from mild fever and malaise to a debilitating syndrome marked by leukopenia, hepatitis, interstitial pneumonia, arthritis, central nervous system changes, gastrointestinal ulceration and bleeding, renal insufficiency, bacterial or fungal infection, and even death. Distinguishing CMV disease, which has its usual onset 4 to 6 weeks after transplant, from rejection is especially difficult when renal manifestations are prominent and seroconversion may not occur for 3 to 6 weeks after the onset of fever. A biopsy is often helpful in making a decision for or against antirejection therapy. Fortunately, both the incidence and severity of CMV disease appear to be diminished in cyclosporine-treated patients. Prophylactic acyclovir decreases the incidence of CMV, and in established CMV disease, gancyclovir (DHPG) is quite effective.

Other opportunistic infections such as *Pneumocystis carinii* pneumonia, aspergillosis, blastomycosis, nocardiosis, toxoplasmosis, cryptococcosis, and tuberculosis are more likely to occur in transplant recipients than in nonimmunosuppressed patients.

GASTROINTESTINAL COMPLICATIONS. Ulceration and perforation of the gastrointestinal tract are not uncommon following transplantation, with the colon being especially vulnerable. Pancreatitis and infectious gastrointestinal complications such as *Candida* stomatitis and esophagitis, pseudomembranous colitis, and CMV ulceration are also common.

HYPERPARATHYROIDISM. Secondary hyperparathyroidism from chronic renal failure usually subsides after a successful transplant. However, it persists ("tertiary hyperparathyroidism") in 5 per cent of patients with normally functioning allografts. In cases in which significant hypercalcemia and elevated parathyroid hormone levels continue for more than 6 to 12 months despite normal renal function, the authors advocate total parathyroidectomy and autotransplantation of a portion of one gland.

TUMORS. Immune deficiency is associated with an increased risk of neoplasia. The incidence of cancer in dialysis patients is about twice that of the normal population. In transplant recipients, the 60 per cent incidence of *de novo* malignancy is approximately 100 times greater than that in normal age-matched populations. The most common neoplasms are squamous cell carcinomas of skin and lip. Transplant recipients have 350 times the normal incidence of lymphomas. Compelling evidence that *de novo* lymphomas may begin as lymphoproliferative lesions induced by viruses stems from the finding of Epstein-Barr virus in the genome of lymphoma cells. The patients often have a syndrome resembling infectious mononucleosis. During the stage of polyclonality, cessation of immunosuppression and the use of the antiviral agent acyclovir may cause regression of the lesions. Tumors that are initially polyclonal may develop the monoclonality characteristic of true B-cell lymphomas, which then do not regress following cessation of immunosuppression or acyclovir therapy.

RESULTS OF RENAL TRANSPLANTATION AND SOCIOECONOMIC CONSIDERATIONS

Between 1951 and 1966, renal allografts had a 63 per cent 1-year functional survival in sibling recipients and only 35 per cent with the use of cadaver donors. Since the advent of cyclosporine, 1- to 2-year graft survivals of 77 to 89 per cent have been reported both for related-donor and cadaveric grafts. The superior results with living-related compared with cadaver donors continues to justify their use, especially in the case of HLA-identical sibling recipients (95 to 100 per cent graft survival).

Patient survival after transplantation has improved even more dramatically than has graft survival. In 1967, the 1-year patient survival was only 56 per cent with cadaveric grafts, and by 1981 it was 90 per cent. For living-related donors it was 95 per cent. The improvement (which actually occurred before the use of cyclosporine) was mainly attributable to a striking fall in the incidence of severe infections related to a general policy of decreasing the intensity of immunosuppression. The release of cyclosporine further improved graft survival while lowering susceptibility to infection. One-year patient survivals of 95 to 98 per cent have been reported by some.

SOCIOECONOMIC CONSIDERATIONS IN TREATMENT OF END-STAGE RENAL DISEASE

Since the annual cost of end-stage renal disease in the United States is 3 billion dollars, it is pertinent that transplantation is more cost-effective than is chronic dialysis. Transplantation costs $36,000 to $38,000 for the first year and, if successful, about $4000 per year thereafter. Despite this high initial cost, the lower expenses of patients with functioning grafts compare so favorably with those of patients on maintenance hemodialysis ($20,000 per year for life) that the costs of transplantation (even including failed grafts) are recouped in about 3 years. Other important advantages of transplantation are better rehabilitation and quality of life.

The evolution of renal transplantation from an experimental approach to a highly successful clinical therapy represents one of the remarkable medical achievements of this century and has culminated in the award of the Nobel Prize to Dr. Joseph Murray, a pioneering transplant surgeon from Boston. End-stage renal disease, an entity that 40 years ago was uniformly fatal, can now be treated with greater success than can most malignancies. Since most victims of kidney disease are relatively young, the achievement of a successful transplant in this group is one of the most satisfying in medical practice.

V

Vascular Access Procedures for Renal Dialysis (Including Peritoneal Dialysis)

Carl E. Haisch, M.D., and James Cerilli, M.D.

Reliable vascular access is critical to dialysis. This access can be direct via access to the bloodstream as in hemodialysis, or indirect via the peritoneum. The most commonly used methods for hemoaccess are a double-lumen catheter into the subclavian or jugular vein, a fistula formed directly between an artery and vein, or a subcutaneously implanted polytetrafluoroethylene (PTFE) graft in an extremity. Peritoneal dialysis is performed by use of a catheter placed into the peritoneal cavity.

VASCULAR ACCESS

Types of Angioaccess

EXTERNAL ACCESS. The shunt, connecting an artery and vein via a plastic connection on the surface of the skin, is

---

See the corresponding chapter or part in the *Textbook of Surgery*, 14th edition, pp. 393–401, for a more detailed discussion of this topic, including a comprehensive list of references.

used infrequently. Its major use is in plasmapheresis and in rare instances for hemodialysis. The Scribner shunt was the first shunt successfully used long term and has continued to be the model for other shunts that have been developed. Presently, external access for dialysis is commonly obtained via the jugular, subclavian, or femoral vein through a dual-lumen catheter. The femoral catheter can be used for one or two dialysis runs and is then removed; however, the percutaneously inserted subclavian catheter can be used as long as a month in the absence of infection, clotting, or thrombosis. If longer access is required, a double-lumen catheter can be placed surgically through a cutdown into the internal or external jugular vein. This can be used for up to a year. Vascular access may be associated with complications of infection, thrombosis, and a short life span.

INTERNAL ACCESS. The ideal type of internal access is a natural fistula of which the Brescia-Cimino is considered the standard. This vascular anastomosis between the radial artery and cephalic vein causes increased flow and pressure in the forearm and can be accessed by needle puncture. Other natural fistulas can be formed between the brachial artery and adjacent basilic vein or between the brachial artery and the cephalic vein. These fistulas have a patency rate of between 55 and 90 per cent at 2 years. The most common complication of these fistulas is stenosis in the proximal venous limb, with aneurysms and thrombosis also occurring. A major advantage of these fistulas is that they become infected less frequently and have a higher patency rate than fistulas that use prosthetic material.

Prosthetic material is used in patients who do not have a vein and artery that can be brought into proximity. The material can be used to connect the radial artery to a vein in the antecubital fossa with a straight graft in the forearm, as a loop in the forearm between the brachial artery and the antecubital vein, or as a loop in the upper arm between the axillary artery and axillary vein. Some prefer to use a graft placed in the leg. The configurations may be a loop in the thigh between the saphenous vein and superficial femoral artery or between the popliteal artery and saphenous vein in a straight manner. These grafts have been reported to cause amputation and to be associated with a high mortality. Difficult access problems may require imaginative solutions, such as a loop on the anterior chest wall between the axillary vein and artery, or a cross chest placement between the axillary vein and axillary artery. While using this material, care must be taken not to twist the graft in the tunnel or there will not be adequate blood flow and clotting will result.

There are many complications of grafts that have been placed for dialysis. The major complication is thrombosis. This occurs with greater frequency in situations with low blood flow or in patients who develop venous end-intimal hyperplasia. Early thrombosis usually occurs for technical reasons; later thrombosis occurs secondary to venous intimal hyperplasia at or distal to the anastomosis. The outflow stenosis can be repaired with a patch graft, bypassed with a graft, or dilated with a balloon. Use of thrombolytic agents has been attempted but has met with mixed results largely dependent on the cause of the thrombosis. Dilation of the venous end with a balloon catheter after clot dissolution has been unsuccessful except in a few reports in which the dilation balloon has a very high pressure, over 10 atmospheres.

Infection is the second most common complication found with prosthetic grafts placed for dialysis. Local drainage may resolve the problem, but in some cases a small bypass around the infected area is necessary. If the suture line is involved or the graft is clotted, then the prosthesis must be removed. The salvage rate for infected grafts is between 25 and 50 per cent.

Patency. The patency rate of prosthetic grafts is less than that of autogenous fistulas. The patency rate for a PTFE graft in a forearm loop at 12 months is 80 per cent. One author has reported a patency rate of 93 per cent at 1 year and 77 per cent at 2 years. Fistulas placed in the leg have a patency rate of 80 per cent at 12 months, but it must be remembered that there can be disastrous complications of amputation and sepsis with the use of these fistulas.

PHYSIOLOGY

The size of the fistula is to be larger than the diameters of the artery and vein for avoidance of the problem of flow's being determined by the size of the fistula. A large functioning fistula may cause a fall in both systolic and diastolic blood pressure, an increase in cardiac output, and an increase in venous blood pressure both proximal and distal to the fistula. There can also be an increase in pulse rate and a slight increase in heart size. The lumen of a natural fistula gradually increases, and the artery elongates. Eventually smooth muscle atrophy develops and causes aneurysmal dilation with a tortuous vessel. The increased blood flow through the fistula causes an increase in blood flow around the fistula.

PERITONEAL DIALYSIS

The semipermeable nature of the peritoneum was discovered in the late 1800s and this knowledge was extended in the early 1900s. This has given rise to the use of the peritoneal cavity for dialysis. The most common use of the peritoneum is in chronic ambulatory peritoneal dialysis (CAPD). The exact surface across which dialysis occurs in the peritoneum is not known; however, it appears that the visceral peritoneum is more important than is the parietal peritoneum, although there are more capillary blood vessels in the parietal peritoneum.

Short-term peritoneal dialysis can be used (1) for acute renal failure, (2) during maturation of hemoaccess, (3) for a patient with chronic renal failure who has an acute exacerbation, or (4) for insertion of chemotherapeutic agents in abdominal or hepatic malignancy. CAPD is indicated in patients (1) desiring home dialysis, (2) with no available sites for vascular access, (3) with repeated infections of vascular access sites, (4) with an unstable cardiovascular system, (5) with diabetes who would benefit from a constant insulin infusion from the peritoneal cavity, (6) above 65 years of age, (7) with bleeding problems, (8) who want to avoid blood transfusion, (9) with AIDS, and (10) who are small children. An obliterated peritoneal space from surgical therapy or infection, poor peritoneal clearance, and lack of diaphragmatic integrity are some of the contraindications to CAPD use. Relative contraindications include respiratory insufficiency, a diffuse peritoneal malignancy, a large hernia, and low back pain caused by degenerative disc disease.

TECHNICAL CONSIDERATIONS. Catheters can be placed at the bedside for short-term peritoneal dialysis or in the operating room for CAPD. The catheters are designed to prevent omentum from obstructing inflow and outflow of dialysate. During placement, care must be taken to avoid bladder or bowel injury. After placement, patients are able to eat and leave the hospital within a day or two.

The dialysis fluids vary in dextrose concentration. The lowest concentration, 1.5 per cent, causes very little ultrafiltration of fluid (200 ml. per 2-liter exchange), whereas the greatest concentration, 4.5 per cent, treats or prevents fluid overload (800 ml. per 2-liter exchange).

Complications include those related to catheter placement and those occurring after placement. Those related to placement include (1) leakage of dialysate, (2) intraperitoneal bleeding, (3) bowel or bladder perforation, (4) subcutaneous bleeding with hematoma formation, and (5) ileus. After placement, the leading complication is peritoneal infection. Infection occurs approximately once every 16 to 18 months. The five routes of entrance for peritoneal infection include (1) infection of dialysis tubing and peritoneal catheter; (2) infection of tissues around the catheter; (3) fecal contamination, such as diverticulitis; (4) blood-borne infections; and (5) ascending infection through fallopian tubes in women.

Most of the infections are caused by gram-positive organisms, with gram-negative organisms responsible for a much smaller percentage. Rare causes include fungus and tuberculosis. Treatment with appropriate antibiotics usually cures the infection. Removal of the catheter is usually indicated if the Dacron cuff is infected.

The cost of CAPD and hemodialysis are at present almost identical. Both techniques require multiple hospitalizations, which also raises the cost. It is clear that the cost of either form of dialysis significantly exceeds that of successful renal transplantation.

VI

Principles of Immunosuppression

Suzanne T. Ildstad, M.D., Richard L. Simmons, M.D., and John S. Najarian, M.D.

Transplantation of solid organs has become an accepted therapy for end-stage renal, hepatic, cardiac, and pulmonary disease. After Alexis Carrel described the technique for vascular anastomosis in 1902, technical challenges for transplanting kidneys and other solid organ allografts were for the most part resolved. Subsequent advances that allowed solid organ transplantation to become clinically feasible were due to the development of immunosuppressive agents that could control or prevent rejection. Management of rejection requires an understanding of the complexity of the immune system and the cells and other factors involved in the rejection response.

APPROACHES TO IMMUNOSUPPRESSION

Lymphocytes and *macrophages* constitute the heart of the immune system. The rejection reaction begins when lymphocytes recognize foreign antigens present on cells of the transplanted tissue. The immunologic specificity for differentiating self from non-self resides in the lymphocytes, which are activated by recognition of major histocompatibility complex (MHC) locus or transplantation antigen differences.

Stimulation of the resting lymphocyte by the antigen causes it to transform into a large active cell that secretes signal substances called *lymphokines* effective across short distances that amplify the response and activate other cells. Manipulation of this complex of events offers many opportunities for immunosuppression in the attempt to halt or prevent the rejection response. Immunosuppression is less effective after the lymphocyte has responded to the foreign antigen, and the immune response is far more difficult to control after activation.

Current immunosuppressive agents act in a nonspecific manner to suppress the entire immune response. Because of their mechanism of action, they have associated toxic effects and side effects such as an increase in opportunistic infections and an increased occurrence of malignancy. Effective general immunosuppression may allow the graft to survive but may also cripple the host response to infections or prevent other proliferating cells, such as bone marrow and intestinal mucosal cells, from maintaining a safe population. Infections with cytomegalovirus and *Pneumocystis carinii*, which do not present a life-threatening problem to the normal patient, frequently become lethal to the transplant patient.

At present, clinical immunosuppression relies on two gen-

See the corresponding chapter or part in the *Textbook of Surgery*, 14th edition, pp. 401–417, for a more detailed discussion of this topic, including a comprehensive list of references.

eral approaches. The first is simply to reduce the number of peripheral lymphocytes by destroying them with corticosteroids or antiserum. The second uses a number of metabolic inhibitors to interrupt the antigen-induced lymphocyte proliferation and differentiation that are required for graft rejection. These agents are biochemically specific but do not distinguish between dividing lymphocytes and other proliferating cells.

THE BIOLOGY OF GRAFT IMMUNITY

The development of the lymphoid system begins with a pluripotent stem cell in the liver and bone marrow in the fetus. With maturation of the fetus toward term, the bone marrow becomes the primary site for lymphopoiesis. The marrow produces T lymphocytes, B lymphocytes, and macrophages, cells critical to the immune response. The thymus is the *primary lymphoid organ* in which the *T lymphocyte* (CD3+) is matured, or "educated," and released to stock the *peripheral lymphoid tissues* such as lymph nodes, the spleen, and the gut. It is in the thymus that T lymphocytes acquire their subset differentiation markers (CD4+, CD8+, and so on), which influence their ultimate functional role in the immune system. Another subpopulation that descends from the stem cell is the *B cell* line. The primary lymphoid organ that produces B cells in mammals is unknown, whereas in birds it is the bursa of Fabricius. Interleukin (IL)-4, IL-5, and IL-6 have been recently identified as lymphokines that stimulate the proliferation and maturation of activated B cells. Both T and B lymphocytes acquire their immune specificity during early development. Fully competent clones of small lymphocytes are waiting to respond to foreign antigens. An individual lymphocyte can recognize only one of a few closely related antigens. *Macrophages*, which also have an integral role in the immune response, are derived from the same pluripotent stem cells as the intraepithelial cells such as keratinocytes and tissue macrophages. They function to process antigen and present it to lymphocytes and to produce *cytokines*, soluble factors that amplify the immune response (Table 1).

The T cells, B cells, and macrophages have unique roles in orchestrating the immune response. It is a very tightly controlled network with the majority of communication mediated by *cytokines*. *B cells* synthesize antibody, and the subpopulations of *T cells* have several different activities. Certain T-effector cells can directly lyse a foreign cell, whereas others become killer (cytotoxic CD8+) cells. In addition, there are T-helper (CD4+) and T-suppressor (CD8+) cells that function to activate or suppress, respectively, the response to a specific antigen. Because each of these T-cell subpopulations expresses both the T-cell receptor (CD3+) plus their own unique receptor antigen (CD4+ or CD8+), individual subpopulations can be depleted, enriched, or modulated by use of antiserum or monoclonal antibody immunotherapy. OKT3, a monoclo-

TABLE 1. Properties of Some Human Cytokines*

Cytokine	Alternative Name	Source	Target Cell Type	Action
IFN-α- and IFN-β	—	Activated T cells, endothelial cells, macrophages, fibroblasts	Activated T and B, NK, LAK	Induces antiviral state; antitumor activity; induces fever; increases Class I and II MHC expression; stimulates activated B-cell differentiation and proliferation and NK activity; inhibits T and LAK cell activity
IFN-γ	—	Activated T cells, LAK cells	Activated and resting B, plasma, NK, endothelial, LAK, macrophage	Induces antiviral state; antitumor activity; induces fever; increases Class I and II MHC expression; stimulates activated B-cell differentiation and proliferation and NK and LAK activity; activates macrophages and endothelial cells; stimulates IgG2a isotype switch
TNF	—	Activated T cells, LAK cells, macrophages	Resting T, activated T and B, plasma, stem, endothelial, eosinophil, fibroblast, macrophage	Induces antiviral state; antitumor activity; induces fever; increases Class I MHC expression; activates macrophages, granulocytes, eosinophils, endothelial cells; chemotactic and angiogenic activity
IL-1	Endogenous pyrogen	Activated T and B cells, LAK cells, endothelial cells, macrophages, fibroblasts	Resting T and B, activated T and B, plasma, stem, endothelial, eosinophil, fibroblast, macrophage	Induces antiviral state; antitumor activity; induces fever; stimulates activated B-cell differentiation and proliferation; activates and stimulates proliferation of T cells; activates granulocytes and endothelial cells; stimulates hematopoiesis

IL-2	T-cell growth factor	Activated T cells, LAK cells	Activated T, activated and resting B, NK, LAK, macrophage	Activates macrophages, T, NK, and LAK cells; stimulates differentiation of activated B cells; stimulates proliferation of activated B and T cells; induces fever
IL-3	Multi-CSF	Activated T cells	Stem, activated B, eosinophil	Stimulates hematopoiesis, activated B cell proliferation, and eosinophil activity
IL-4	B-cell stimulating factor 1	Activated T cells	Activated T, activated and resting B, plasma, LAK, macrophage	Activates macrophages, T and B cells; stimulates differentiation of activated B cells; stimulates proliferation of activated B and T cells; induces IgE receptors on B cells; stimulates IgE and IgG1 isotype switch
IL-5	B-cell growth factor 2	Activated T cells	Activated and resting B, plasma, eosinophil	Stimulates IgA isotype switch and eosinophil activity
IL-6	B-cell stimulating factor 2, B-cell differentiating factor, interferon-β_2	Activated T cells, endothelial cells, fibroblasts, macrophages	Activated T, resting B, stem	Activates T cells; stimulates activated B-cell differentiation, activated T- and B-cell proliferation

Table continued on following page

189

TABLE 1. Properties of Some Human Cytokines* *Continued*

Cytokine	Alternative Name	Source	Target Cell Type	Action
IL-7	–	Activated T cells	Activated T and resting B	Stimulates activated T- and resting B-cell proliferation
IL-8	–	Activated B cells	Granulocytes	Stimulates granulocyte activity, chemotactic activity
G-CSF	–	Endothelial cells, fibroblasts, macrophages	Granulocytes	Stimulates granulocyte activity, hematopoiesis
M-CSF	–	Macrophages	Macrophages	Activates macrophages
GM-CSF	–	Endothelial cells, fibroblasts, activated T cells	Stem, granulocyte, macrophage, eosinophil	Activates macrophages; stimulates granulocyte and eosinophil activity, hematopoiesis

Cytokines are secreted polypeptides that mediate autocrine and paracrine cellular communication but do not bind antigen. They include those compounds previously termed interleukins and lymphokines. IFN, interferon; TNF, tumor necrosis factor; IL, interleukin; G, granulocyte; M, macrophage; CSF, colony-stimulating factor; NK, natural killer; LAK, lymphokine-activated killer.

*Based on the consensus cytokine chart of the British Cytokine Group.

From Balkwill, F. R., Burke, F.: The cytokine network. Immunol. Today, *10*:299, 1989.

nal antibody directed against the T-cell receptor, is used clinically in episodes of acute solid organ graft rejection.

Cell-to-Cell Interactions

When the lymphocytes are confronted with an antigen, the response is complex. Multiple cell-to-cell interactions are required to produce the final immune response. T cells, B cells, macrophages, and cytokines all have a role. Critical to this response are macrophages, which act in a nonspecific manner to bind antigen and "present" it to T and B cells. Certain complex antigens may need first to be partially digested by phagocytic cells before the antigenic information can be presented to the lymphocyte for self and non-self recognition. In addition, the activated macrophages produce and secrete *IL-1*, a cytokine that functions to further amplify the response and stimulate T-lymphocyte and B-lymphocyte activation.

The recognition of foreign cells is a complex process. One class of antigens on the surface of the graft cells stimulates certain T cells (T-helper cells; $CD4^+$) to divide. The proliferating cells do not destroy the graft; rather, they activate another group of T cells (cytotoxic), which damage the graft. T-helper cells are necessary for the development of the cell-mediated and antibody-mediated cytolytic activity of cytotoxic ($CD8^+$) T cells. T-helper cell proliferation is an important site of amplification of the immune response, and these actively dividing cells are particularly vulnerable to antimetabolites. The activities of the helper T cells are one of the major targets of clinical immunosuppression.

Whereas $CD4^+$ helper T cells function to augment the response of other T cells, another type is able to suppress the immune response. This type of T cell, the *suppressor cell* ($CD8^+$), probably helps to regulate the immune response and prevent an overreaction to a specific immunologic stimulus. If suppressor cells are able to inhibit the development of the immune response, it may open an avenue for clinical application in transplantation. Stimulating an abundance of specific suppressor lymphocytes would theoretically be a way to produce effective immunosuppression without toxicity.

Although the T and B cell systems have been presented as independent of each other, they cooperate to enhance immunity against a specific antigen. T cells develop "cellular immunity" in response to transplantation antigens, and in addition, helper T cells assist clones of B cells to produce specific antibody against the graft antigens. Finally, some T cells act as suppressors for antibody formation. After immunity has been acquired, additional cellular cooperation contributes to the destruction of the graft during the rejection episode.

As lymphocytes transform from resting to dividing cells, they pass through distinct phases common to all cells. Susceptibility to the commonly used immunosuppressive agents varies over the different cell phases. The small lymphocyte is in a resting (G_0) phase. Antigenic stimulation activates the cell and moves it into the first gap phase (G_1) of the proliferative cycle. After the cell becomes committed to divide, DNA synthesis (S phase) occurs. The gap (G_2) between S phase and the final mitosis (M phase) is relatively short. After mitosis has occurred, the cells enter into the G_1 phase again, and the cell cycle is complete.

Differentiation appears to progress with cell division, and, with each successive cycle, the cells become more and more capable of eliminating the activating antigen. After successive divisions, B cells become *plasma cells*, which are the most efficient producers of specific antibody. A similar progression occurs among T cells. T cell activation occurs through the T-cell receptor complex (CD3), IL-2, and the IL-2 receptor (IL-2R). Activated T cells secrete IL-2, a cytokine that functions as a T-cell growth factor. The IL-2 then binds to the IL-2R on resting T cells and stimulates cell mitosis and DNA synthesis via activation of the inositol phosphate pathway with protein kinase C. When the antigenic stimulus is no longer present, IL-2 is no longer produced, and T cell activation and proliferation cease. Continued presence of antigen causes an amplification of the T cell response through the cytokine IL-2. The presence of the IL-2R for activation suggests a hormone-receptor system with negative feedback control. An understanding of the process of the activation of the T cell via its receptor pathway will allow a more focused approach to immunosuppression.

Much of the susceptibility of lymphocytes to immunosuppression is due to the vast cellular changes that follow immune stimulation. The many biosynthetic events that occur make the lymphocytes vulnerable to inhibitions caused by structural analogs, *antimetabolites*. *Alkylating agents* and *radiation* produce cross linkages and breaks in DNA strands that interfere with cell differentiation and division.

GRAFT REJECTION

Graft rejection follows participation of various combinations of immunologically specific and nonspecific cells. T cells have the major role in most graft rejection. Three types of graft rejection are encountered. *Acute rejection* is the most common. It is mediated primarily by T lymphocytes and first occurs between 1 and 3 weeks following transplantation of a solid organ. *Hyperacute rejection* occurs during the first 1 to 2 days following transplantation and is primarily mediated by preformed cytotoxic antibody. *Chronic rejection* occurs over months and is probably a result of both T cell– and B cell–mediated responses.

CLINICAL IMMUNOSUPPRESSION

Until recently, clinical immunosuppression relied primarily on agents or procedures with antiproliferative activity. This includes the *antimetabolites, alkylating agents, toxic antibiotics,* and *irradiation,* all of which were borrowed from cancer chemotherapy. Recently, the introduction of agents that specifically influence T lymphocytes (cyclosporine and OKT3) has radically changed both the principles of immunosuppression in the organ allograft recipient and the outcome after transplantation.

Antiproliferative Agents

Antiproliferative agents inhibit the full expression of the immune response by preventing the differentiation and division of the immunocompetent lymphocyte after it encounters antigen. They act in one of two ways: either they structurally resemble needed metabolites, or they combine with certain cellular components, such as DNA, and thereby interfere with function. Alkylating agents and certain antibiotics include those compounds that combine with DNA and other cellular components. Because of their toxic effects, their use has been limited to bone marrow transplantation and as occasional substitutes for azathioprine.

ANTIMETABOLITES. The antimetabolites have a structural similarity to cell metabolites and either inhibit enzymes of that metabolic pathway or are incorporated during synthesis to produce faulty molecules. The antimetabolites include *purine, pyrimidine,* and *folic acid* analogs that are most effective against proliferating and differentiating cells. They are given at the time of transplantation when the immunocompetent cells are first stimulated and continued for the life of the graft.

Purine Analogs. Until recently, the purine analog *azathioprine* (Imuran) was the immunosuppressive drug most widely used in clinical organ transplantation. Azathioprine is 6-mercaptopurine (6-MP) plus a side chain to protect the labile sulfhydryl group. In the liver, the side chain is split off to form the active compound 6-MP. Full metabolic activity comes in the cell with the addition of ribose-5-phosphate from phosphoribosyl pyrophosphate to form 6-MP ribonucleotide. The structural resemblance of this molecule to inosine monophosphate is obvious, and 6-MP ribonucleotide inhibits the enzymes that begin to convert inosine nucleotide to adenosine and guanosine monophosphate, thereby interfering with nucleic acid synthesis. The biologic activity of azathioprine and 6-MP is greatest when nucleic acid synthesis is most active (S phase). They inhibit the development of both humoral and cellular primary immunity by interfering with the differentiation and proliferation of the responding lymphocytes. The toxicity of azathioprine follows the same mechanisms and includes bone marrow suppression, causing leukopenia. Toxic effects in the liver can also result.

CYCLOSPORINE. The discovery of cyclosporine in 1972 contributed significantly to the field of transplantation. It represents a completely new class of clinically important immunosuppressive agents. Many of its suppressive effects on T cells appear to be related to the inhibition of T-cell receptor–mediated activation events. It also inhibits lymphokine production by helper T cells *in vitro* and arrests development of mature CD8$^+$ and CD4$^+$ single-positive T cells in the thymus. Cyclosporine is a cyclic peptide produced by a fungus. It is nearly insoluble in aqueous solutions, and absorption from the gastrointestinal tract is slow and incomplete. There is a well-characterized enterohepatic cycle, and the excretion of the drug is primarily through the bile. The mechanism of action of cyclosporine is relatively specific for T lymphocytes. Other inflammatory cells are much less sensitive to its immunosuppressive effects.

Cyclosporine selectively inhibits activated T lymphocytes and prevents these cells from manufacturing and/or releasing IL-2. In addition, resting T lymphocyte activation by IL-2 is blocked by cyclosporine. Since IL-2 is necessary for the expansion of activated clones of T cells, cyclosporine effectively inhibits the immune responses to grafted antigens without eliminating any of the clonal repertoire. A number of kidney and other solid organ transplantation trials have shown that cyclosporine induces potent immunosuppression without myelosuppression. The adverse effects of cyclosporine include hirsutism, tremor and other neurotoxic effects, hypertension, hyperkalemia, nephrotoxicity, and hepatotoxicity. The principal toxic effect is nephrotoxicity.

FK 506. FK 506 is a potent new immunosuppressive agent that is also produced by a fungus. Its immunosuppressive effects are approximately 500 times greater than those of cyclosporin A. FK 506 functions to (1) inhibit IL-2 production; (2) inhibit mouse mixed lymphocyte culture cellular proliferation, which is mediated by helper T cells; (3) inhibit the generation of murine cytotoxic T cells; and (4) inhibit the appearance of IL-2 receptors on human lymphocytes. *In vivo,* FK 506 has been demonstrated to prolong the survival of MHC-disparate skin, cardiac, renal, hepatic, and small bowel allografts. It is currently in use in clinical trials as an immunosuppressive agent for liver, bowel, and renal allograft recipients.

Lymphocyte Depletion Measures

A number of clinically important agents for immunosuppression are effective because they deplete the host of lymphocytes. The most commonly used agents, *antilymphocyte globulin, radiation,* and *monoclonal antibody therapy,* appear to act by a relatively nonselective lymphocyte depletion or inactivation.

ANTILYMPHOCYTE GLOBULIN. Antilymphocyte globulins (ALGs) are antibodies produced when lymphocytes are injected into animals of a different species. ALG administration interferes most with the cell-mediated reactions, allograft rejection, tuberculin sensitivity, and the graft-versus-host reaction. ALG has a definite, but lesser, effect on T cell–dependent antibody production. Lymphocytes coated with ALG share the fate of erythrocytes coated with antibody; they are cleared from the blood by reticuloendothelial cells in the liver and spleen. ALG is widely used in clinical transplantation. It can be given prophylactically during the early posttransplant period and is also effective in reversing rejection. Allergic reactions to the antiserum itself are the most common clinical toxic effect. Urticaria, anaphylactoid reactions, and serum sickness, including joint pain, fever, and malaise, all follow immunity developed by the patient to the heterologous globulin. These reactions are reduced in the presence of the other immunosuppressive drugs used in renal transplantation.

MONOCLONAL ANTIBODY THERAPY. In 1975 Kohler and Milstein developed the technology for somatic cell hybridization *(hybridoma)* that could establish immortalized cultures of cell lines, each of which secretes a single or *monoclonal antibody* in limitless supply. Subsequently, a number of monoclonal antibodies have been generated that react with T cells in general (OKT3: anti-CD3) and various T-cell subsets (OKT4: anti-CD4; OKT8: anti-CD8). OKT3 has become the most useful clinically. It is used to halt episodes of acute graft rejection in kidney, liver, heart, and heart-lung transplantation. OKT3 binds to a site associated with the T-cell receptor (CD3) and functions to modulate the receptor and inactivate T-cell function.

RADIATION. Radiation was probably the first agent used clinically to produce immunosuppression. Most of the immunosuppressive effects of irradiation are caused by changes produced in nucleic acids. DNA is particularly vulnerable and, therefore, so is cellular replication. The effectiveness of radiation is dependent on the phase of the cell cycle in which the cell is found. Cells in the M or G_2 phase are most sensitive to irradiation. The timing of radiation therefore must be carefully planned for the greatest immunosuppressive effect.

Adrenal Corticosteroids

Adrenal corticosteroids are the immunosuppressive agents most commonly used in clinical practice. Glucocorticoids have many anti-inflammatory actions, which make them potent immunosuppressants. A profound decrease in the blood lymphocyte count occurs within the first 6 hours of steroid administration. Glucocorticoids cause emigration of recirculating T cells from the intravascular compartment to the lymphoid tissues with less effect on the distribution of B cells. Steroids also inhibit the production and the effect of T-cell cytokines, which amplify the responses of the lymphocytes and macrophages. In addition, the ability of macrophages to respond to lymphocyte-derived signals such as migration inhibition factor and macrophage activation factor is also blocked by steroids.

Toxic effects associated with the use of steroids include hypertension, weight gain, peptic ulcers, and gastrointestinal bleeding, euphoric personality changes, cataract formation, hyperglycemia, pancreatitis, and osteoporosis with avascular necrosis of the femoral head and other bones.

Other Immunosuppressive Approaches

BLOOD TRANSFUSION. Many studies have shown an improved kidney graft survival with the use of blood transfusions before kidney transplantation, and some form of transfusion protocol has become part of the preparative regimen for most patients in renal failure who are awaiting a graft. For circumventing sensitization, azathioprine administered at the time of transfusion reduces the rate of sensitization to 5 per cent. The exact mechanism by which transfusions exert a beneficial effect is unknown, but evidence suggests a possible suppressor cell phenomenon.

CONSEQUENCES OF IMMUNOSUPPRESSION

INFECTION. An increased incidence of bacterial, fungal, and viral infections is observed in patients who receive nonspecific immunosuppressive agents. Because of its nonspecific method of action, immunosuppression understandably increases the risk of infection. Infection is the most common complication of immunosuppression, and overall it is the most common cause of death in transplant recipients. Most of the deaths early in the history of kidney transplantation occurred in the first few posttransplant months as a result of highly pathogenic bacterial infections. More recently, improved antibiotics and greater skill in immunosuppression therapy have shifted the spectrum of organisms. There has been a relative increase in lethal infection caused by opportunistic organisms that are normally weakly pathogenic. Antibiotics eradicate the more aggressive bacteria, but opportunistic fungal, protozoal, and viral organisms remain free to colonize the susceptible transplant patient.

Fungal and Protozoal. The opportunistic organisms, which are normally eliminated by cellular mechanisms, can now proliferate with the relative T-cell depression. Fungi are prominent opportunists. *Candida albicans* infections are probably the most common. *Aspergillus* species are probably the second most common cause of fungal infection and typically produce upper lobe pulmonary cavities. *Rhizopus oryzae, Histoplasma capsulatum,* and *Cryptococcus neoformans* also invade the lung, and *C. neoformans* occasionally causes meningitis. *Pneumocystis carinii,* more commonly seen in patients undergoing cancer chemotherapy, usually causes an alveolar infiltrate with disproportionate dyspnea and cyanosis.

Viral. Viral infections appear to be almost ubiquitous in kidney transplant recipients. The herpes group of DNA viruses is most commonly present. Cytomegalovirus infection has also become a serious clinical problem with potentially lethal consequences.

MALIGNANCY. The incidence of malignancy is increased in recipients of transplants, but the rate is not sufficiently high to contraindicate the transplant procedure. The rate of development of malignancy in patients surviving renal transplantation may be as high as 30 times that in a similar normal population. The most frequent cancers include lymphomas, reticulum cell sarcomas, and squamous and basal cell carcinomas.

EXPERIMENTAL IMMUNOSUPPRESSION

The currently available immunosuppressive agents have revolutionized the field of transplantation. However, because they act in a nonspecific manner to suppress all aspects of immune function, associated toxic effects result. Consequently, investigative efforts have been directed at finding an improved, more specific method of immunosuppression. The complexity of the immune response gives rise to the hope that many potential points of vulnerability in activation and deployment of the cells responsible for the rejection reaction exist. Potential approaches include (1) immunosuppression by specific antigens, (2) donor-specific transplantation tolerance, (3) immunosuppression by specific antibodies, and (4) generation of specific suppressor cells to halt the rejection reaction. The goal is to induce donor-specific transplantation tolerance yet maintain host immunocompetence.

VII

Organ Preservation
Folkert O. Belzer, M.D., and James H. Southard, Ph.D.

Methods developed over the past 20 years for preservation of the kidney, liver, heart, and pancreas have contributed greatly to the use of organ transplantation for treatment of patients with various end-stage organ diseases. Successful methods of preserving these organs contribute greatly to the number of cadaveric organs available for transplantation, yield excellent quality preservation of the viability of organ function, allow transportation of organs on a national (and international) basis, and provide sufficient time for tissue matching for certain organs (kidney); they can make the surgical procedure an elective (scheduled) rather than an emergency procedure.

MECHANISM OF ACTION OF ORGAN PRESERVATION METHODS

Two methods of organ preservation are used: continuous machine perfusion, used primarily for kidney preservation; and simple cold storage, used for all transplantable organs. Machine perfusion uses a pump to perfuse the organ constantly with a perfusion solution at 5° C. The perfusate is delivered at a low flow rate and pressure and continually

See the corresponding chapter or part in the *Textbook of Surgery*, 14th edition, pp. 418–423, for a more detailed discussion of this topic, including a comprehensive list of references.

delivers nutrients and removes end products of metabolism from the organ. Even at cold temperatures metabolism continues, and the support of that metabolism provides long-term preservation of organs. Currently, canine kidneys have been successfully preserved by these methods for 5 days and livers for 3 days. The perfusion solution that allows this duration of preservation contains agents that suppress hypothermia-induced cell swelling (large-molecular-mass anions, lactobionic acid, and gluconic acid), a colloid that is nontoxic to the vascular endothelium (hydroxyethyl starch, molecular weight 250,000), adenosine to stimulate ATP synthesis, glutathione as an antioxidant, sodium, potassium, calcium, magnesium, and other agents. This method of organ preservation is superior to simple cold storage and yields less delayed graft function (kidney) and longer preservation times.

Simple cold storage is performed by flushing the blood from the organ with a cold (5° C.) solution containing agents that suppress cell swelling. Collins' solution contains a high concentration of potassium (115 mmol.) and glucose (140 mmol.), which effectively suppresses cell swelling in the kidney. With this solution, preservation times of 48 hours (dog kidneys) and 24 to 40 hours (human kidneys) can be readily obtained. This solution has been used most often for clinical kidney preservation. The EuroCollins' solution is a modification of the original Collins' solution and omits magnesium from the solution. This solution is not particularly effective for long-term preservation of other organs (6 to 8 hours). The University of Wisconsin cold storage solution uses lactobionic acid as an impermeant that suppresses hypothermia-induced cell swelling not only in the kidney but also in the liver, pancreas, and heart. This solution is similar to the perfusion solution and contains adenosine, glutathione, hydroxyethyl starch, a large-molecular-mass trisaccharide, raffinose, allopurinol, and other agents. With this solution, livers can be preserved for up to 48 hours (dog), pancreas for 72 hours (dog), and kidneys for 72 hours (dog). This solution has been used effectively in human liver, kidney, and pancreas preservation.

There appear to be at least three key requirements for successful long-term preservation of organs. The first is hypothermia (0 to 5° C.). Hypothermia suppresses the rate of catabolic reactions in the cell that degrade tissue nutrients and biologic structures (membranes). The second is the presence of agents for suppression of hypothermia-induced cell swelling. In the cold, the sodium pump is suppressed and water enters the cell. This swelling of cells is lethal, and prevention can be obtained by impermeants such as glucose, mannitol, raffinose, sucrose, phosphate, lactobionate, gluconate, and citrate. The third is the presence of metabolites that facilitate the restoration of normal metabolism upon transplantation. Agents that stimulate the rapid resynthesis of ATP (adenosine, adenine) contribute to better organ function and allow the organ to regenerate a normal distribution of cellular water and repair preservation-induced injury. Antioxidants are helpful in suppressing oxygen free radical injury during reperfusion, including glutathione and allopurinol.

The long-range goal of organ preservation is unlimited preservation time. This may require actual freezing of the organ, which is a method that is not well developed for organ storage at this time. However, improved preservation solution could contribute to preservation of organs for at least 1 week. These new solutions will probably require the presence of many agents, metabolites, and drugs. The basis of which agents are required will depend on gaining knowledge concerning the mechanism of injury to organs during preservation.

VIII

Liver Transplantation
Thomas E. Starzl, M.D., Ph.D.,
Robert D. Gordon, M.D., Andreas G. Tzakis, M.D.,
and Satoru Todo, M.D.

The therapeutic power and appeal of liver transplantation has had a pervasive impact on hepatology and liver surgery. Almost all patients with non-neoplastic chronic liver disease can now be considered for liver transplantation, and at least some of those with malignant hepatic tumors may benefit as well.

IMMUNOLOGIC CONSIDERATIONS

The liver is relatively resistant to antibody-mediated (humoral) rejection. Whereas kidneys and hearts are usually destroyed and hyperacutely rejected in patients whose serum contains anti-donor cytotoxic antibodies of the IgG class, the liver is usually spared this fate. Thus, a negative cytotoxic crossmatch is not required for liver transplantation. When liver transplantation is performed across an ABO incompatibility, there is a high risk of hemorrhagic necrosis and deposition of antibody and complement in the liver. HLA matching has not had a role in liver transplantation.

Acute cellular rejection of the liver is usually reversible with increased corticosteroids or treatment with antilymphoid globulin. However, reversal of histologic signs of rejection has been observed without change in treatment, and long-term survival of allografts may be possible without complete

---

See the corresponding chapter or part in the *Textbook of Surgery*, 14th edition, pp. 423–433, for a more detailed discussion of this topic, including a comprehensive list of references.

control of rejection. Chronic rejection may follow in which bile ducts and blood vessels become selective targets of injury. Intrahepatic biliary obstruction with jaundice, arteriopathy, and even cirrhosis may result with relatively good retention of synthetic and other hepatocyte function. Such patients become candidates for late retransplantation.

In many patients the need for chronic immunosuppression diminishes, although complete withdrawal of immunosuppression has been too dangerous to attempt deliberately. Some patients, for religious, noncompliance, or other reasons, have completely discontinued their medications for years without a subsequent severe rejection.

PROCUREMENT AND PRESERVATION

Techniques have been developed for removal of multiple organs from a single donor by carefully timed and controlled *in situ* infusion of cold preservation solutions into anatomic regions, the limits of which are defined by preliminary dissection of the regional blood supply. An improved preservation solution developed at the University of Wisconsin has extended the safe limits of static liver refrigeration to 18 to 24 hours. Two important constituents of this new solution are the sugars lactobionate and raffinose, which are impermeants and prevent water imbibition by cells.

SURGICAL TECHNIQUE

In removing the diseased liver, the inferior vena cava and the portal vein must be occluded. Routine use of a pump-driven venovenous bypass in adults and larger children relieves the resulting venous hypertension and has significantly reduced the incidence of heavy blood loss, renal failure, protracted ileus, and fluid sequestration in the gut that can result. Management of intraoperative coagulation by the anesthesiologist is greatly assisted by careful monitoring with the thromboelastogram, which can differentiate platelet deficiency, factor deficiencies, fibrinolysis, and hypercoagulability. Intraoperative air emboli can be avoided by flushing the liver graft, especially before completion of the last vena caval anastomosis.

Variations in hepatic arterial supply are frequently encountered in both donors and recipients. Multiple arteries to the donor liver are carefully preserved during procurement and can be reconstructed on the back bench into a single vessel for eventual anastomosis. If a suitable recipient artery cannot be found, donor iliac artery grafts can be inserted as conduits from the recipient aorta to the graft vessel(s). Similarly, donor iliac vein grafts can be used to bridge defects in the portal vein or to act as jump grafts from the recipient superior mesenteric vein if the host portal vein is thrombosed.

Biliary reconstruction is performed when feasible with end-to-end duct-to-duct anastomosis over a T-tube stent or, alternatively, with Roux-en-Y choledochojejunostomy.

IMMUNOSUPPRESSION

The use of cyclosporine with steroids, with or without azathioprine and antilymphoid globulins, has improved results with transplantation of all organs and especially the liver. Cyclosporine inhibits the activation of T lymphocytes by depressing the production of multiple cytokines, of which interleukin-2 and interferon-gamma have been the most extensively studied. Nephrotoxicity, often with hypertension, is the principal side effect of cyclosporine. Other undesirable effects include gingival hyperplasia, hirsutism, depression of insulin secretion by pancreatic islets, hypercholesterolemia, hyperuricacidemia, and neurotoxicity. Neurotoxic manifestations include tremors, increased sensitivity to light, paresthesias, mood changes, and insomnia. FK 506, which also affects T-lymphocyte function and is more potent than cyclosporine, has a different chemical structure and binding site (receptor). FK 506 has a similar but probably less severe toxicity profile. The usefulness of FK 506 is under clinical evaluation.

Increased vulnerability to opportunistic infections is a major risk of high immunosuppressive therapy. Prophylaxis with sulfamethoxazole-trimethoprim (Bactrim) can prevent *Pneumocystis carinii* pneumonia. Intravenous gancyclovir has significantly reduced the morbidity and mortality of systemic infections with cytomegalovirus. Lethal hepatitis from adenovirus, cytomegalovirus, or herpes simplex can occur after liver transplantation. The interposition of the liver between the heart and the intestinal tract exposes it to enteric organisms, especially if there is a flawed biliary reconstruction. Septic complications remain a major cause of mortality, but these have been easier to control under immunosuppression with cyclosporine and small-dose prednisone than with earlier regimens.

INDICATIONS FOR LIVER REPLACEMENT

In children, the most common indication for liver replacement is congenital biliary atresia. Portoenterostomy (the Kasai procedure) performed within 90 days after birth may relieve jaundice in the minority of patients, but these operations complicate eventual candidacy for transplantation, and their role is being re-examined. Many liver-based inborn errors of metabolism are now being treated by liver transplantation, such as alpha$_1$-antitrypsin deficiency, Wilson's disease, tyrosinemia, glycogen storage disease, Type II familial hypercholesterolemia, protein C deficiency, and even some forms of hemophilia. Other indications include neonatal (giant cell) hepatitis, familial cholestasis, chronic aggressive hepatitis, secondary biliary cirrhosis, Budd-Chiari syndrome, and primary hepatobiliary cancer. For most of these conditions, patient survival at 5 years is about 70 per cent, but small infants with biliary atresia have 10 per cent lower survival because of technical complications from previous operations and a higher incidence of hepatic arterial thrombosis. There is a high recurrence rate of malignant tumors after transplantation, but encouraging survival has been seen after combined transplantation and chemotherapy for hepatoblastoma.

In adults, liver replacement for chronic aggressive hepatitis not due to the hepatitis B virus (HBV), alcoholic cirrhosis, and cholestatic liver disease (primary biliary cirrhosis and primary sclerosing cholangitis) has been rewarded with a 5-year patient survival of nearly 70 per cent. Survival is about 15 to 20 per cent less with HBV hepatitis, primarily because of recurrent disease. Fulminant hepatic failure has become an accepted reason for liver transplantation but must be done before renal failure, deterioration of the central nervous system, and metabolic acidosis signal irreversible metabolic and neurologic changes.

Other indications for liver transplantation in adults include, but are not limited to, Budd-Chiari syndrome, secondary biliary cirrhosis, cystic fibrosis, inborn errors of metabolism, secondary biliary cirrhosis, and polycystic liver disease. Results after transplantation for malignant tumors have been poor, and efforts to improve the outlook with extended resections (such as cluster operations) and more aggressive chemotherapy are under evaluation.

AUXILIARY TRANSPLANTATION

Auxiliary liver transplantation in which the native liver is left in place and an extra liver is placed in an ectopic site offers the theoretic advantages of not leaving the patient totally at the mercy of an allograft and avoiding the need for a total hepatectomy. There has been a recent renewal of interest in auxiliary transplantation, and cautious further trials will undoubtedly be forthcoming.

IX

Pancreas and Islet Cell Transplantation
Hans W. Sollinger, M.D.

HISTORICAL ASPECTS

1959	Brooks and Gifford: Pancreas transplantation in a large animal model.
1960–1970	Dejode, Howard, Reemtsma, Merkel, Lillehei, Largiader, Bergan: Technical development of pancreas transplantation in animals.

See the corresponding chapter or part in the *Textbook of Surgery*, 14th edition, pp. 433–437, for a more detailed discussion of this topic, including a comprehensive list of references.

1966	Kelly, Lillehei: First pancreas transplant in man.
1973	Gliedman: Exocrine drainage to ureter.
1974	Groth: Exocrine drainage to small bowel.
1977	Dubernard: Duct injection with polymers.
1982	Sollinger: Bladder drainage.

INDICATIONS FOR PANCREAS TRANSPLANTATION

Pancreas transplantation is performed in three groups of patients with insulin-dependent diabetes mellitus.

Pancreas Transplantation Alone

The procedure is performed in patients who do not have renal failure.

ADVANTAGES: (1) None or few secondary diabetic complications; (2) good surgical risk; (3) early diabetic complications potentially reversible.

DISADVANTAGES: (1) Major surgical procedure; (2) side effects of immunosuppressive therapy; (3) poor results.

Pancreas Transplantation After a Successful Kidney Transplant

ADVANTAGES: Same immunosuppression as kidney transplant.

DISADVANTAGES: (1) Major surgical procedure; (2) diabetic complications already advanced; (3) poor results.

Simultaneous Pancreas-Kidney Transplantation

ADVANTAGES: (1) One surgical procedure; (2) same immunosuppression; (3) good results.

DISADVANTAGES: Already advanced diabetic complications.

ORGAN PROCUREMENT AND PRESERVATION

The pancreas can be procured alone or in combination with the liver. In the United States, combined pancreas-liver procurement has become increasingly frequent for meeting the demand for both liver and pancreas grafts. After *in situ* flushing with Belzer-UW (University of Wisconsin) solution, both organs are removed *en bloc* and divided *ex vivo*. The portal vein is divided midway between the pancreas and the liver, and the arterial blood supply of the pancreas is reconstructed with an iliac artery Y-graft. Belzer-UW solution is the best preservation solution, as demonstrated by a low rate of vascular thrombosis and graft pancreatitis. Three-year graft survival is 10 to 20 per cent better in grafts preserved with

UW solution, compared with other solutions. The maximal preservation time with the use of UW solution is approximately 30 hours.

SURGICAL TECHNIQUE

The pancreas may be transplanted as a whole organ (currently preferred technique) or as a segment (body and tail). Three surgical techniques are most commonly used. They differ in the way exocrine pancreas secretions are managed.

Enteric Drainage: Anastomosis of Pancreatic Duct to Bowel

ADVANTAGES: (1) No metabolic problems; (2) no urinary problems.
DISADVANTAGES: (1) High rate of septic intra-abdominal complications; (2) difficult to make diagnosis of rejection.

Duct Occlusion: The Pancreatic Duct Is Injected with Polymers

ADVANTAGES: (1) Surgically simple; (2) low infection rate.
DISADVANTAGES: (1) High thrombosis rate; (2) high fistula rate; (3) difficult to make diagnosis of rejection.

Bladder Drainage and Anastomosis of Pancreatic Duct to Bladder

ADVANTAGES: (1) Safe, low infection rate; (2) urinary amylase used to make diagnosis of rejection; (3) best results.
DISADVANTAGES: (1) Metabolic acidosis; (2) urinary problems: hematuria, urinary tract infection, urethritis.
Currently, bladder drainage is the most popular technique. Worldwide more than 85 per cent of all pancreas transplants are performed with bladder drainage.

DIAGNOSIS OF REJECTION

The early diagnosis of pancreas allograft rejection is difficult. Methods and laboratory tests for the diagnosis of rejection are as follows:

	Comments
Serum glucose	Specific but late marker
Urinary amylase	Early marker; specific; large fluctuations difficult to interpret
	Only possible with bladder drainage
Serum anodal trypsinogen	Specific early marker; not widely available; difficult test
Pancreas biopsy (percutaneous)	Technically difficult; yield is only 50 per cent; possible complications

	Comments *Continued*
Pancreas biopsy (transcystoscopic)	Requires general anesthesia; special expertise necessary; 85 per cent specificity
Nuclear perfusion scan	Useful confirmatory test when used in conjunction with other tests
Ultrasonography, computed tomography, magnetic resonance imaging	Not proven to be useful in diagnosis of rejection

INFLUENCE ON METABOLIC AND SECONDARY DIABETIC COMPLICATIONS

Benefits that may be provided by a well-functioning pancreas transplant are (1) insulin independence; (2) nearly normal blood glucose tolerance test result; (3) normalization of HgA₁ C; (4) prevention of progression of diabetic nephropathy; (5) improvement of peripheral and autonomic neuropathy; and (6) improvement in microcirculation.

Not all of these beneficial effects of pancreas transplantation on secondary diabetic complications have been proved. No study has conclusively demonstrated a beneficial effect of pancreas transplantation on diabetic retinopathy.

X

Cardiac and Cardiopulmonary Homotransplantation
R. Morton Bolman III, M.D.

CLINICAL CARDIAC TRANSPLANTATION

Originally introduced in 1967 by Barnard, clinical cardiac transplantation has recently enjoyed a great increase in popularity owing to the availability of the immunosuppressive agent cyclosporine. Approximately 1500 procedures have been performed each year from 1986 through 1989 as a result of this growth.

Recipient Selection

Individuals from newborn age up to the age of 60 years can be considered candidates for cardiac transplantation. They must be experiencing symptoms of Class IV congestive

---

See the corresponding chapter or part in the *Textbook of Surgery*, 14th edition, pp. 438–446, for a more detailed discussion of this topic, including a comprehensive list of references.

**TABLE 1. Recipient Selection Criteria
for Heart Transplantation**

Age newborn to 60 years
Irremediable cardiac disease—Class IV NYHA
Normal function or reversible dysfunction of kidneys, liver, lungs,
  central nervous system
Pulmonary vascular resistance less than 6–8 Wood units or
  pharmacologically reversible
Absence of:
  Active malignancy or infection
  Recent pulmonary infarction
  Severe peripheral or cerebrovascular disease

heart failure (NYHA). These individuals must have exhausted
all conventional medical and surgical options. Fixed, irreversible deficits in extracardiac organ function contraindicate
transplantation, since they would not be expected to be
corrected by improved cardiac function. Psychosocial screening is important for ensuring proper compliance with prescribed medical regimens after transplantation. From a hemodynamic standpoint, the most critical determinant of
operative risk is the pulmonary vascular resistance. If the
pulmonary vascular resistance is greater than 5 to 6 Wood
units and cannot be pharmacologically reversed with manipulations in the catheterization laboratory that could be dupli-
cated at the time of transplantation, then orthotopic transplantation would pose a substantial operative risk. Patients
must harbor no active malignancy or infection, and active
peptic ulceration is a contraindication as well (Table 1).

Donor Selection

Criteria for cardiac donor selection are outlined in Table 2.
Individuals up to the age of 55 and occasionally 60 years with
demonstrable normal function of the heart and absence of
severe coronary artery disease can be suitable donors. Useful
on-site screening tests include electrocardiography and echocardiography. Donor and recipient must be ABO-compatible,
and a prospective crossmatch is not necessary provided the
recipient is reactive to 10 per cent or less of a panel of

**TABLE 2. Donor Selection Criteria
for Heart Transplantation**

Age less than 60 years
Minimal pressor support
Negative cardiac history
Normal electrocardiogram
Normal echocardiogram
ABO compatibility
Size within 20%–50% of recipient
Negative T-cell crossmatch if panel-reactive antibodies
  10% or greater
Negative serologic tests for hepatitis, HIV infection

randomly selected HLA types (panel-reactive antibodies less than 10 per cent). Donor and recipient weight should be matched to within 20 to 50 per cent. Cardiac allografts can be procured at a distance, provided the period of graft ischemia is 4 hours or less between cross-clamping the aorta in the donor and restoring perfusion in the recipient. Donor hearts are preserved with 1 liter of crystalloid cardioplegia coupled with copious topical cooling.

The Operation

The recipient operation is not initiated until the donor heart has been visualized by the procurement team and found to be suitable for transplantation. At that point, the recipient is placed under anesthesia and made ready for cardiectomy and transplantation. The recipient heart is removed as the donor heart arrives at the transplant hospital; implantation ensues with left and right atrium, pulmonary artery, and aorta being anastomosed between donor and recipient. Careful hemostasis is mandatory because the complications attending excessive bleeding are potentially severe in the immunosuppressed host.

Immunosuppression

Prophylaxis against allograft rejection in most centers consists of "triple therapy," the combination of cyclosporine, azathioprine, and prednisone. This regimen has been associated with the lowest reported incidence of cardiac rejection and has yielded excellent rates of survival and a low incidence of infection.

Another approach being employed at some centers is that of "induction therapy" utilizing the murine monoclonal antibody OKT3, followed by administration of cyclosporine, azathioprine, and prednisone. Prednisone can then be discontinued in a certain number of these individuals.

Complications

ACUTE ALLOGRAFT REJECTION. Diagnosis of cardiac rejection rests on the judicious application of the endomyocardial biopsy guided by clinical indicators such as cardiac arrhythmia, hypotension, and fever. The endomyocardial biopsy remains the standard despite the proposal of numerous noninvasive methods. Rejection is treated with 3 days of pulse methylprednisolone followed by rebiopsy.

INFECTION. All patients who are cytomegalovirus seronegative before transplantation receive exclusively cytomegalovirus-negative blood and blood products. All patients receive Mycostatin and high-dose acyclovir for 3 months and trimethoprim-sulfamethoxazole indefinitely following their transplant procedure. Perioperative wound prophylaxis consists of a second-generation cephalosporin and vancomycin coupled with copious intraoperative vancomycin irrigation.

This regimen, coupled with a low incidence of rejection experienced as the result of triple therapy, has yielded a very low incidence of serious infection, and none of the author's patients has had mediastinitis or a sternal wound infection.

TRANSPLANT CORONARY DISEASE. A dreaded sequela of cardiac transplantation is that of transplant coronary artery disease. This entity continues to plague cardiac transplant recipients and will become an increasing problem with the passage of time. Olivari has reported the University of Minnesota's experience in this regard. Defined as any decrease in luminal coronary artery diameter, transplant coronary artery disease findings were demonstrated in 8 per cent of patients at 1 year, 24 per cent at 2 years, and 29 per cent at 3 years. This phenomenon is thought to represent a manifestation of chronic rejection, and close surveillance is required in the form of yearly coronary angiography. Treatment consists of percutaneous transluminal coronary angioplasty or, if severe, retransplantation.

Clinical Outcomes

In 163 patients transplanted at the University of Minnesota since the introduction of triple therapy in 1983, actuarial patient survival of 78 per cent at 5 years has been observed. Eighty-six per cent of patients are free of rejection at 1 year after transplantation, by far the lowest reported incidence in the literature.

Cardiac Transplantation Summary

Since its inception in 1967, cardiac transplantation has progressed steadily, and today this procedure has earned its rightful place in the treatment of end-stage heart disease. Improved patient selection, coupled with effective and safe immunosuppressive strategies, has restored health to patients formerly doomed to a premature death. Serious problems remain, which include a shortage of donor organs and the problem of transplant coronary artery disease, currently the number one factor limiting long-term survival.

CARDIOPULMONARY TRANSPLANTATION

Recipient Selection

Certain individuals have diseases of the heart and lungs that require replacement of these organs. Recipient selection criteria are outlined in Table 3. The most common indications for this procedure are primary pulmonary hypertension and Eisenmenger's syndrome. Patients should be severely limited by their disease and unable to work or attend school, and most are on supplemental oxygen therapy. These individuals must fulfill all the other criteria for transplantation as outlined in the section on heart transplantation.

**TABLE 3. Recipient Selection Criteria
for Cardiopulmonary Transplantation**

Age less than 50 years
End-stage pulmonary vascular or parenchymal disease associated
   with severe right ventricular compromise and/or severe tricuspid
   regurgitation
Absence of:
   Other nonreversible organ dysfunction or disease
   Major prior thoracotomy or sternotomy
   High-dose steroid therapy

Donor Selection

A small percentage of donors suitable for transplantation (10 to 20 per cent) also have lungs that can be transplanted. Criteria for suitable cardiopulmonary donors are listed in Table 4. In addition to normal heart function, the heart-lung donor must have normal gas exchange with low airway pressures. The chest radiograph should be normal and pulmonary secretions minimal. Donor and recipient are matched according to ABO type as well as on the basis of results of an HLA antibody screen. Size matching is also important. Current techniques of preservation allow successful transplantation following up to 4 hours of *ex vivo* preservation. Most programs employ the technique of cardioplegic arrest of the heart coupled with pulmonary artery flushing with a modified EuroCollins' solution, supplemented by copious topical cooling.

The Operation

The recipient is placed on cardiopulmonary bypass when word is received that the donor is stable and the organs are satisfactory. Cardiopulmonary bypass is then instituted and the heart removed. Pedicles of pericardium containing the phrenic nerves are isolated, and windows are created bilaterally through the posterior pericardium to allow passage of the donor lungs to their respective pleural cavities. The diseased lungs are then removed individually, and hemostasis is secured in the posterior mediastinum. The trachea is isolated and transected just above the carina. The donor heart-lung block is then passed into the chest, and implan-

**TABLE 4. Donor Selection Criteria
for Cardiopulmonary Transplantation**

Close size match—donor smaller than or same size as recipient
Satisfactory gas exchange—arterial $Po_2 > 400$ mm. Hg on Fio_2
   of 1.0
Normal lung compliance—peak airway pressure of 30 mm. Hg
   with normal tidal volume
Clear chest radiograph
Absence of purulent pulmonary secretions

tation proceeds with anastomoses of trachea, right atrium, and aorta.

Immunosuppression

Recipients of cardiopulmonary allografts receive triple therapy similar to that of heart transplant recipients with a few modifications. Corticosteroid therapy is administered perioperatively for 24 hours and then withheld for the ensuing 14 days for optimization of airway healing. Antilymphocyte globulin is administered for 3 to 5 days, during which cyclosporine levels are maintained deliberately at subtherapeutic levels for maintenance of normal renal function. After 14 days, prednisone is begun at a low dose, and maintenance therapy consists of triple-drug immunosuppression as outlined previously.

Complications

REJECTION. Most recipients experience an episode of rejection within the first 2 weeks. Heart and lungs do not necessarily reject synchronously; therefore, the heart biopsy is not a reliable means of monitoring lung rejection. Diagnosis of lung rejection rests on clinical grounds supplemented by transbronchial biopsy. Symptoms may include fever, breathlessness, malaise, and signs of decreased oxygenation, radiographic infiltrates, and so on. Treatment is with pulse corticosteroid therapy for a period of 3 days followed by reassessment.

INFECTION. Infection prophylaxis in the heart-lung recipient is identical to that described for the heart transplant recipient. Most infections following cardiopulmonary transplantation are, in fact, pulmonary, and any evidence of infection warrants urgent evaluation and treatment.

BRONCHIOLITIS OBLITERANS. The most serious complication that occurs in recipients of cardiopulmonary transplantation is bronchiolitis obliterans. Thought to represent a form of chronic rejection analogous to transplant coronary artery disease, this entity can occur a few months following transplant. It occurs in 30 to 50 per cent of cardiopulmonary recipients, and attempts to reverse its course in most cases have proved futile.

Clinical Outcomes

Since the pioneering work of Reitz, investigators at Stanford have continued to develop the techniques of cardiopulmonary transplantation, including refined patient selection and improved postoperative management. Comparing patients transplanted between March 1981 and February 1986 with patients transplanted subsequent to that period, one notes that improvements have been demonstrated in short-term and long-term survival, with decreased incidence of bronchiolitis obliterans in the later group as well. Improved results are attributed to the routine employment of triple-drug immunosuppression and more aggressive surveillance for rejection and infection, including routine application of bronchoscopy with bronchoalveolar lavage and transbronchial biopsy.

Cardiopulmonary Transplantation Summary

Owing to severe restrictions in donor availability, small numbers of these procedures have been performed in the United States each year. Despite this, gratifying results in individuals who do well have inspired further efforts in the field. Cardiopulmonary transplantation remains a therapeutic option for selected individuals for whom no other conventional or transplant alternative is available. Intensive research continues in the area of chronic rejection of the heart-lung allograft. This remains the single greatest impediment to long-term survival in these patients.

XI

Lung Transplantation
Donald E. Low, M.D., and Joel D. Cooper, M.D.

Since the successful clinical introduction of lung transplantation in 1983, the indications and techniques associated with both single and double lung transplantation have undergone significant revision. Single lung transplants were initially performed in patients with pulmonary fibrosis. However, the indications have gradually broadened for inclusion of patients with obstructive disorders such as emphysema, lymphangioleiomyomatosis, and eosinophilic granuloma as well as of patients with primary pulmonary hypertension and Eisenmenger's syndrome.

Double lung replacement was initially performed with an *en bloc* technique, but the technical difficulty of this procedure in addition to the relatively high incidence of complications has caused it to be gradually replaced by the bilateral "sequential single" transplant procedure. Bilateral lung transplantation is utilized in all patients with bilateral pulmonary sepsis such as cystic fibrosis and bronchiectasis because of the high risk of cross-infection of the transplanted lung from the remaining infected lung. It is also offered to younger patients with emphysema who have a greater opportunity to

See the corresponding chapter or part in the *Textbook of Surgery*, 14th edition, pp. 446–455, for a more detailed discussion of this topic, including a comprehensive list of references.

benefit from any increased functional improvement associated with bilateral lung replacement.

DONOR SELECTION AND LUNG RETRIEVAL

Suitable lungs for transplantation are generally less available than are other organs owing to their susceptibility to infection and edema, especially in the presence of brain death. Potential donors must have a chest film that is entirely clear and a documented arterial oxygen tension exceeding 300 mm. Hg with an FiO$_2$ of 100 per cent and 5 cm. of positive end-expiratory pressure. In addition, bronchoscopy before donor lung extraction must demonstrate no gross purulent secretions or suggestion of aspiration. Size matching of the lung is performed on the basis of vertical and transverse dimensions of the donor and potential recipient chest films. Sex, body weight, height, and overall chest circumference of the donor and recipient are also compared.

In patients undergoing single lung transplantation, the side with the poorest overall function determined by quantitative ventilation-perfusion scans is usually selected. Donor matching is currently performed on the basis of ABO compatibility and body size. An attempt is also made to provide all cytomegalovirus-negative recipients with organs from cytomegalovirus-negative donors.

Lung retrieval is almost always performed in conjunction with multiple organ removal for transplantation. The heart is removed before the lungs, leaving a cuff of left atrium containing the four pulmonary veins. Before extraction, 500 μg. of prostaglandin E$_1$ is injected into the pulmonary artery, and then the pulmonary vascular system is flushed with 3 liters of cold EuroCollins' solution. After removal of the heart, the trachea is doubly stapled at its midpoint and divided, the esophagus is divided high in the chest as well as at the level of the esophageal hiatus, and the lungs are removed *en bloc* along with the entire contents of the mediastinum. The lungs are transported immersed in a bag containing ice cold modified EuroCollins' solution, and separation of the lungs before transplantation is performed at the home institution, either for transplant into separate recipients or for bilateral lung transplantation.

TRANSPLANTATION TECHNIQUE AND IMMUNOSUPPRESSION

Single lung transplant is performed through a standard posterolateral thoracotomy incision following removal of the native lung. A small upper midline incision is utilized to mobilize the omentum, which is wrapped around the bronchial anastomosis to provide early neovascularization and protection should a bronchial anastomotic defect occur.

The donor lung is inserted with the sequential completion of the anastomoses of the main bronchus, main pulmonary artery, and pulmonary veins to the recipient left atrium. The technique for bilateral transplant is similar except that both lungs are sequentially inserted through bilateral anterolateral thoracotomies joined by a transverse sternotomy.

Postoperative immunosuppression comprises cyclosporine, azathioprine, and ALG (antilymphocyte globulin, Minnesota equine) for the first 5 to 7 days. After this time, the ALG is discontinued, and oral prednisone therapy is initiated and increased to a maximal dosage of 0.5 mg. per kg. per day. Over the next 12 months, both prednisone and cyclosporine dosages can be tapered. However, triple therapy with cyclosporine, azathioprine, and prednisone continues for life.

RESULTS

Between July 1989 and June 1990, 36 lung transplants were performed in 35 patients (mean age 44 years, range 21 to 60 years). Twelve patients underwent double lung replacement, whereas 23 single lung transplants were performed in 22 patients. Stay of this population in the intensive care unit ranged from 1 to 36 days, with a median of 4 days. Hospital stay ranged from 15 to 66 days, with a median of 24 days. No patient currently requires supplemental oxygen for maintenance of a room air PaO_2 greater than 60 mm. Hg. Currently, with a median follow-up of 8 months, the absolute survival rate in this population is 94.3 per cent.

These results compare favorably with the results surveyed from the International Lung Transplant Registry, which demonstrate a current survival rate of approximately 64 per cent in both single and double lung transplantation. Results will continue to improve as greater experience is gained with the technical aspects of the procedure and with continued improvements in the methods of lung preservation and immunosuppression.

XII

Autotransplantation
R. Randal Bollinger, M.D., Ph.D.

Autotransplantation is the transfer of an organ, a part of an organ, a tissue, or cells from one site to another in the same individual. Autotransplantation has several practical advantages over *allotransplantation* (transfer between individuals of the same species) or *xenotransplantation* (transfer between individuals of different species). Immunologic rejection does

---

See the corresponding chapter or part in the *Textbook of Surgery*, 14th edition, pp. 456–464, for a more detailed discussion of this topic, including a comprehensive list of references.

not occur, the donor is at all times readily available, and prolonged preservation is usually unnecessary in the case of autotransplants. Because of these advantages, autotransplantation was used earlier, more successfully, and more widely by all surgical specialties than were other forms of transplantation.

SKIN AUTOGRAFTS

Skin grafts are used to cover wounds where insufficient skin is available to permit immediate (primary) or delayed (secondary) suture closure. A *pedicle graft* is never separated from its blood supply, since revascularization at the recipient site is allowed to develop before the original blood supply is finally severed. A *free graft* is completely separated from its vascular, nervous, and lymphatic connections during the transplantation procedure. A *full-thickness* skin graft is a free graft including the entire epidermis and dermis, whereas a *partial* or *split-thickness* graft includes all of the epidermis and a variable part of the dermis. *Anastomosed free grafts*, in which the small arteries and veins supplying a graft are reanastomosed to small vessels at the recipient site, have gained popularity as microsurgical techniques have improved. Full-thickness skin grafts are used when pigment matching, resistance to contraction, or growth of a child are important considerations in wound healing. Split-thickness skin grafts survive better than do full-thickness grafts on compromised surfaces, such as granulating wounds contaminated with bacteria, because split-thickness skin is more richly supplied with open blood vessels on its underside. Since only a part of the dermis is taken, the donor site heals spontaneously by epithelial outgrowth from the remaining epithelial islands, sweat glands, and hair follicles. The wound to be skin grafted must be clean and well-vascularized but free from bleeding. Meshing or perforation of the graft prevents serum accumulation beneath it. If the recipient site is free of debris, if bleeding is controlled, and if motion between the graft and its bed is prevented by a pressure dressing or plaster splint, the approximation necessary for fibrin adhesion and subsequent capillary invasion will be achieved.

NERVE AUTOGRAFTS

Nerve autografts are used to repair unsuturable defects in major peripheral nerves. Wallerian degeneration occurs in the distal damaged nerve and the donor graft before reinnervation can occur. The Schwann cells, endoneural tubes, and connective tissue survive in the form of conduits through which the axons may regenerate to reach viable end organs at a rate of 1 mm. per day in free grafts and 1.5 mm. per day in revascularized nerve grafts.

MUSCULOSKELETAL AUTOGRAFTS

MUSCLE. Nonvascularized muscle transplants rapidly undergo ischemic necrosis, resorption, and replacement by fibrous tissue. Transfer of an entire muscle group without division of its neurovascular supply has been used to restore function in the distribution of an adjacent damaged nerve, for example, radial nerve and muscle transfer for ulnar palsy. Transplanted whole muscle can survive and be reinnervated 5 months after microneurovascular anastomosis.

BONE. The bulk of the bone implanted as a conventional free autograft does not survive transplantation. All but the most superficial cells of cortical grafts die of ischemia leading to bone resorption and replacement in a process termed *creeping substitution*. More cells survive in the case of cancellous bone, which has an open structure that facilitates diffusion of nutrients and ingrowth of osteoclasts and osteoblasts. Excellent local blood supply, broad contact with recipient bone, and complete immobilization contribute to success. Infection, scarring, and irradiation of the tissues usually are responsible for failure. Cancellous bone for the reconstruction of major skeletal defects is obtained from the iliac crest or the metaphyseal ends of long bones. Cortical grafts are derived from the ribs, the central and proximal portions of the fibula, and the diaphysis of long bones.

CARTILAGE. Autotransplantation of cartilage from the costochondral junctions is used primarily in facial reconstruction. Cartilage heals to adjacent tissue by formation of a fibrous or fibrocartilaginous scar. Grafts from adults do not grow, and portions frequently undergo slow resorption.

TENDON. Autografts of tendon are used to replace damaged or destroyed tendons in the hands and feet in order to restore motion and strength. Free tendon grafts are taken from the palmaris longus, the flexor digitorum superficialis of the ring finger, the triceps, the plantaris, or the extensor digitorum communis tendons of the toes.

COMPOSITE TISSUE AUTOGRAFTS. Transfers of entire functional units rather than individual components of the musculoskeletal system include toe-digital transfers and the iliac, rib, or fibular osteocutaneous neurosensory flaps. Osteocutaneous transplantation allows simultaneous reconstruction of both bone and skin defects with provision of sensation in the transplanted skin.

VASCULAR AUTOGRAFTS

Both autogenous arteries and veins are used to replace destroyed or obstructed sections of major arteries. Although femoral, popliteal, upper extremity, and neck veins have been used, the greater saphenous vein has proved to be the most satisfactory arterial replacement. The wall is strong yet is flexible and easily sutured. The diameter is sufficiently great (minimum of 4 mm.) for avoidance of thrombosis, and nourishment is provided by the intraluminal blood flow. The smooth, natural endothelial lining is less thrombogenic than is any known synthetic surface, particularly when placed across joints. Moreover, the lining surface heals itself and may sequester white cells to fight infection. Autografts heal even when placed into the infected bed of a previous synthetic graft. Saphenous vein is ordinarily harvested from the same leg for femoropopliteal bypass and from the opposite leg for repair of vascular trauma to the lower extremity. The vein is reversed to prevent obstruction by the valves. In cases of *in situ* saphenous vein bypass, the vein may be left in its bed, all branches ligated, all valves internally disrupted, and flow reversed by suturing the vein proximally to the femoral artery and distally to a tibial or peroneal artery.

The internal mammary artery is a preferred source of blood for partially occluded coronary arteries, and the splenic artery may be rotated down to the left renal artery to bypass proximal renal artery stenosis. Infected prostheses, mycotic aneurysms, and infected arterial repairs can be successfully managed by excision and replacement with autografts from the iliac arteries. Autografting for repair of diseased or damaged veins has been much less successful than is arterial replacement, primarily because of early graft thrombosis in low-pressure, low-flow venous systems.

ENDOCRINE AUTOGRAFTS

Every endocrine gland has been experimentally autotransplanted, providing identification of several technical requirements for success: delicate handling of the tissues, prevention of ischemia by cooling or placement in an appropriate medium, and implantation of small fragments. The oxygen and nutrients in interstitial fluid around a subcutaneous, intramuscular, or renal capsular implant will maintain an endocrine graft until revascularization occurs if the fragments are no more than 1 mm. thick. Although thyroid, pituitary, ovary, adrenal, testis, pancreas, and parathyroid have all been autografted in humans, only the last four are often transplanted therapeutically today.

Autotransplantation in the form of orchidopexy is the treatment of choice for an undescended testis. Autotransplantation of segmental pancreas grafts or of isolated islet cells may prevent diabetes after pancreatectomy in more than half of cases. Since parathyroid hormone replacement is not available and medical therapy for hypoparathyroidism is complicated, preservation and autografting of excised parathyroid tissue is essential for preventing the deficiency symptoms of tetany, psychologic disturbances, convulsions, coma, and death. Parathyroid glands are cut into 1-mm. pieces and reimplanted into pockets in the sternocleidomastoid muscle. When all glands are removed for diffuse parathyroid hyperplasia, implantation of fragments into the forearm muscles facilitates subsequent removal of more tissue under local anesthesia if hyperparathyroidism persists. Cryopreserved parathyroid tissue functions normally when autografted for treatment of hypoparathyroidism. Hyperplastic adrenal tissue may be autotransplanted for treatment of Cushing's disease, but autotransplantation of adrenal medulla for treatment of intractable Parkinson's disease has been abandoned because of postoperative morbidity.

URINARY AUTOGRAFTS

KIDNEY. Renal autotransplantation and extracorporeal reconstruction permit salvage of some kidneys that cannot be repaired *in situ*. Hypothermic pulsatile perfusion improves preservation and permits *ex vivo* microvascular surgery on the kidney before reimplantation. The kidney may be returned to its original site or grafted to the iliac vessels with use of allotransplantation techniques. The ureter may be reimplanted into the bladder or preserved intact during the autografting. Renal autografting has been employed for extensive renovascular disease from fibrous dysplasia, atherosclerosis, or abdominal aortic aneurysms; for repair of traumatic arterial injuries; for excision of renal cell carcinoma involving both kidneys or a solitary kidney; and for kidneys with diseased or damaged ureters too short for reimplantation.

URETER AND BLADDER. Autotransplantation of the bladder in the form of a vesicopsoas hitch or a bladder flap is the treatment of choice for injury or disease in the distal third of the ureter. Up to 18 cm. of distal ureter can be replaced with bladder by combining a tubular pedicle graft of bladder and the superior suturing (hitch) of posterior bladder to psoas tendon. Autotransplantation of a segment of ileum currently provides the most successful replacement conduit for proximal ureter or excised bladder. Alternative reconstructions include suturing one ureter to the other ureter (transureteroureterostomy), the skin (cutaneous ureterostomy), or the sigmoid colon (ureterosigmoidostomy). A contracted bladder can be enlarged successfully by autotransplantation of a segment of ileum and cecum, an augmentation ileocecocystoplasty.

GASTROINTESTINAL AUTOGRAFTS

The gastrointestinal tract is ideally suited for autotransplantation. The mesentery provides a long, natural vascular pedicle for attached grafts, and the vascular arcades provide easily anastomosed arteries and veins for free grafts. Small intestinal autografts are widely used to replace the colon after proctocolectomy for inflammatory bowel disease. Stomach, jejunum, colon, or free intestinal segments are used to replace the hypopharynx and esophagus following extirpation of carcinomas of the larynx, pharynx, or esophagus; ingestion of caustic substances; or severe head and neck trauma. Stomach remains the most frequently used autograft for esophageal reconstruction and may be transposed into the neck and sutured to the base of the tongue after pharyngolaryngectomy.

Many other tissues have found limited but effective use as autotransplants, including the greater omentum, hair, tongue, teeth, fascia lata, whole joints, and even the entire heart. Experimental autotransplantation studies have preceded and supported the ultimate feasibility of many allotransplantation procedures currently in clinical use.

19

THE ROLE OF PROSTAGLANDINS, THROMBOXANE, AND LEUKOTRIENES IN SURGERY

Bernard M. Jaffe, M.D.

PROSTAGLANDIN BIOSYNTHESIS

Prostaglandins are nearly ubiquitous; therefore, the biosynthetic components are common to an enormous spectrum of cells and cell types. Because of the ready availability of precursors and inducible enzymes, the synthesis of these compounds is extremely rapid. The synthesis of all prostaglandins is a three-step process: in response to appropriate stimuli, phospholipase is activated, permitting the cleavage from phospholipids of the major precursor fatty acid, arachidonic acid; as the final step, arachidonate is cyclized to form biologically active prostaglandins. Both glucocorticosteroids and nonsteroidal anti-inflammatory agents have been recognized as potent inhibitors of prostaglandin synthesis, but they act on different steps. Glucocorticosteroids induce an enzyme, lipocortin, which interferes with activation of phospholipase and thus prevents the release of precursor fatty acids. In contrast, the nonsteroidal anti-inflammatory agents inhibit the oxidative cyclization step.

CHARACTERISTICS OF THE NATURAL PROSTAGLANDINS

The prostaglandins constitute a substantial family of related compounds that share a number of general characteristics. They are all rapidly synthesized. The action of each prostaglandin counteracts the stimulus, and thus this action is controlled by feedback inhibition. Each of the compounds acts locally, and when large amounts are synthesized, they have access to the bloodstream and function as hormones. Finally, these agents are extremely rapidly inactivated, with biologic half-lives of less than 20 seconds. An overall assessment would support the contention that the prostaglandins are delicate modulators of host defense mechanisms.

See the corresponding chapter or part in the *Textbook of Surgery*, 14th edition, pp. 465–470, for a more detailed discussion of this topic, including a comprehensive list of references.

PROSTAGLANDIN ANALOGS AND THEIR FUNCTION

For most prostaglandins, the 15 position is critical to biologic function. Oxidation of the hydroxyl at this position to a keto group causes total inactivation; conversely, protection or substitution at this position drastically curtails pulmonary and renal metabolism. As a result, a number of methylated analogs have been synthesized and utilized clinically. These analogs have actions nearly identical to those of the native prostaglandins, have half-lives of up to 6 to 8 hours, are active at extremely small doses, and are absorbable from the gastrointestinal tract (whereas natural prostaglandins are inactivated by gastric acid). They thus offer the clinician effective and available pharmaceuticals for reproducing the biologic actions of the natural prostaglandins.

SELECTIVE CLINICAL USES OF PROSTAGLANDINS AND INHIBITORS OF PROSTAGLANDIN BIOSYNTHESIS

CARDIOVASCULAR USES. The ductus arteriosus is quite sensitive to the vasodilatory effects of prostaglandin compounds. This action has been exploited in the treatment of neonates with ductus-dependent cyanotic congenital heart disease. Infants with pulmonary valvular atresia or severe stenosis are totally dependent on pulmonary blood flow from the ductus, and dilation of the ductus causes dramatic improvement in oxygenation and hemodynamics. Prostaglandin E_1 (PGE_1) is an effective ductus vasodilator that increases oxygen saturation during its infusion. A number of cyanotic newborns have been treated with PGE_1 with great success, with mean oxygen saturation levels raised from 50 per cent to an average of 80 per cent or higher without deleterious effects. These infusions have enabled the survival of such critically ill babies long enough to prepare them for surgical creation of aortopulmonary shunts.

In a small but substantial number of infants with otherwise normal hearts, the ductus arteriosus remains patent after birth. In this circumstance, indomethacin-induced inhibition of prostaglandin biosynthesis has produced ductal closure in more than 85 per cent of treated babies.

The low incidence of atherosclerosis in Greenland Eskimos has been correlated with the high concentration of Ω-3 polyunsaturated fatty acids, eicosapentaenoic acid (EPA) and docosahexaenoic acid, in their diet. Supplementation of Western diets with these two fatty acids (in cod liver oil) produces a pronounced shift from doubly to triply unsaturated prostaglandins. In terms of their antiaggregatory and vasodilatory actions, PGI_3 and PGE_3 are at least as potent as PGI_2 and PGE_2. However, thromboxane A_3 is far less proaggregatory than is thromboxane A_2. Thus, a diet rich in Ω-3 fatty acids lowers blood pressure, inhibits platelet aggregability, prolongs the bleeding time, causes a more favorable fatty acid profile, and protects against induction of myocardial and cerebral infarction. These simple dietary alterations may provide an important new approach to the prevention and/or treatment of atherosclerosis.

CONTROL OF PLATELET FUNCTION. The platelet abnormality induced by aspirin attests to the importance of prostaglandins in the normal coagulation scheme. The specific prostaglandin responsible for normal clotting is thromboxane A_2. Thromboxane A_2 is synthesized by platelets and serves to counteract the effects of injury by causing vasoconstriction and inducing platelet aggregation (mediated by calcium fluxes). The effects of thromboxane are opposed by those of prostacyclin. This prostaglandin, synthesized by endothelial cells, is the most potent vasodilator known and, in addition, is a very effective inhibitor of platelet aggregation. PGI_2 thus serves to maintain vascular homeostasis. The balance between these two agents, thromboxane A_2 and PGI_2, is responsible for the moment-to-moment control of blood flow.

The recent innovation in the use of aspirin, small-dose therapy (325 mg. per day), is based on the presumption that thromboxane synthesis is significantly more sensitive to the effects of acetylsalicylic acid than is the synthesis of PGI_2. If this is correct, use of aspirin in this manner would inhibit thromboxane A_2 synthesis but would not affect the production of the antiaggregating and vasodilatory PGI_2. Unfortunately, it appears that aspirin may be equally effective in inhibiting the biosynthesis of both thromboxane A_2 and prostacyclin.

On the basis of their antiaggregatory effects, both PGE_1 and PGI_2 have been utilized in extracorporeal circulations experimentally and clinically. In cardiopulmonary bypass, these prostaglandins (with or without heparin) prevent platelet aggregation, which is manifested by the prevention of thrombocytopenia, absence of microaggregates on the filters, and appropriate anticoagulation. PGE_1 has one substantial advantage over PGI_2: as a result of pulmonary inactivation of PGE_1, at the conclusion of bypass when pulmonary blood flow is restored, coagulation parameters spontaneously return to normal.

GASTROINTESTINAL USES. The methyl analogs of PGE and PGA have been used extensively as inhibitors of acid secretion in patients with peptic ulceration. They have been shown to hasten the healing of both duodenal and gastric ulcers. In hypersecreting patients with duodenal ulceration, this effect is presumably due to the ability of PGE and PGA compounds to inhibit gastric secretion of acid and pepsin and stimulate gastric mucus secretion. Since most individuals with gastric ulcers are hyposecretors, another action must be responsible for the improvement in these patients. In this case, the effect is "cytoprotection," which implies that the gastric mucosa requires substantial amounts of prostaglandins for maintenance of its functional integrity. Cytoprotection may be mediated by secretion of bicarbonate ion, stimulation of mucus production, increased gastric mucosal blood flow, strengthening of the mucosal barrier, or accentuation of the sodium pump.

Prostaglandins have been implicated in the pathogenesis of cholesterol gallstone formation. Animals fed a diet high in cholesterol routinely develop cholelithiasis. Increasing biliary concentrations of cholesterol stimulate the secretion of PGE_2 and PGI_2, which then augment mucus secretion by the gallbladder epithelium. The intraluminal mucin serves as a nidus for the formation of gallstones. Inhibitors of prostaglandin synthetase both curtail the secretion of mucus and prevent the development of stones. Prostaglandins have also been implicated in the pathogenesis of cholecystitis.

Patients with inflammatory bowel disease are known to have elevated mucosal and luminal concentrations of prostaglandins. Since the prostaglandins increase intestinal motility, they may contribute to the diarrhea in these syndromes. Mucosa from patients with inflammatory bowel disease synthesize excessive amounts of the lipoxygenase derivative leukotriene B_4. Inhibition of leukotriene synthesis by steroids and sulfasalazine may explain the beneficial effect of these drugs in inflammatory bowel disease.

RENAL USES. Infusion of PGE_1 and PGE_2 into the renal artery decreases renal vascular resistance, increases renal blood flow, augments sodium and water excretion, contracts the extracellular fluid volume, and produces a hypotensive effect. The primary effect is on intrarenal resistance. It is not necessary to use PGE compounds directly in order to achieve these effects, since furosemide (Lasix) induces diuresis by stimulating endogenous prostaglandin synthesis. Consequently, addition of aspirin to a regimen including furosemide markedly diminishes the diuretic effect of this drug.

A prostaglandin deficiency may have some role in the development of essential hypertension. Decreased renal synthesis of PGE_2 would allow unopposed vasoconstrictor mechanisms and systemic hypertension. Although there is no firm substantiation of this hypothesis, it is clear that kidneys from patients with essential hypertension have lower levels of PGE and that the same tissues have an impaired ability to convert precursor arachidonic acid to the native prostaglandins.

IMPLICATIONS IN TUMOR BIOLOGY. Prostaglandins have been implicated in the pathogenesis of tumor-induced hypercalcemia. In one third of patients harboring malignancies, hypercalcemia and hypophosphatemia follow hyperprostaglandinemia, owing to excessive production of PGE_2 by the tumors. In patients with hyperprostaglandinemia without bone metastases, indomethacin consistently normalizes the serum calcium level. In contrast, in similar patients with bone metastases, indomethacin is relatively ineffective. This difference suggests that prostaglandins may have a role in the genesis of osseous metastases by mobilizing osteoclasts and preparing a site in bone for implantation of tumor.

INFLAMMATION. Prostaglandins have long been recognized as mediators of inflammation. The recent identification of the leukotriene derivatives of arachidonate via the lipoxygenase pathway has increased understanding of the inflammatory process. Leukotrienes induce chemotaxis, produce edema, cause local vasoconstriction, and stimulate broncho-constriction. A second more recently recognized group of lipoxygenase products, the lipoxins, are also proinflamma-tory. They activate protein kinase C, activate leukocytes, release thromboxane A_2, contract the bronchus, release su-peroxides, and cause local vasodilation. These lipoxygenase-mediated effects are sensitive to steroids that prevent the release of the arachidonic acid precursor of these derivatives.

20

IMMUNOBIOLOGY OF NEOPLASTIC DISEASE; MELANOMA; SOFT TISSUE SARCOMAS

I

Immunobiology and Immunotherapy of Neoplastic Disease

H. F. Seigler, M.D.

TUMOR-ASSOCIATED ANTIGENS

Human tumor cells express both Class I and Class II major histocompatibility antigens on their surfaces. Additionally, oncofetal antigens are also expressed on tumor cell membranes. The immunogenicity of tumor-associated antigens is undergoing intense study. Animals immunized with intact tumor cells or tumor antigen preparations demonstrate either a protection against subsequent tumor challenge or delay in growth of the tumor. These data suggest that tumor-associated antigens are somewhat immunogenic. Glycoprotein, glycolipid, and gangliosides have all been demonstrated to be present on the cell membrane of neoplastic cells and can serve as distinguishing cell markers. Human subjects serially immunized with human tumor cells have demonstrated an immune response to tumor-associated antigens.

MONOCLONAL ANTIBODY

In 1975 Koehler and Milstein reported a procedure for production of monoclonal antibodies to single antigen epitopes. Monoclonal antibodies recognize single antigenic determinants in a complex mixture of molecules. At present, monoclonal antibodies are used in immunopathology, immunochemistry, immunoscintigraphy, and immunotherapy. Cell markers present on the surface of leukemia and lymphoma cells serve as distinctive targets for monoclonal antibodies, and cell marker analyses have become standard in most pathology departments. Immunoperoxidase staining of tissue sections by use of a panel of monoclonal antibodies permits the surgical pathologist to more specifically diagnose

---

See the corresponding chapter or part in the *Textbook of Surgery*, 14th edition, pp. 471–477, for a more detailed discussion of this topic, including a comprehensive list of references.

tumors with difficult histopathologic features. Circulating tumor antigen or antigen-antibody complexes in body fluids have been detected with the use of monoclonal antibodies by radioimmunoassay or immunoabsorbent assay. Imaging studies using isotopes conjugated to monoclonal antibodies permit specific radionuclide scanning. In a therapeutic sense, monoclonal antibodies have been used both for serotherapy alone and as immunoconjugates with the monoclonal antibody being conjugated to chemotherapeutic agents, toxins, or isotopes.

THE IMMUNE RESPONSE TO TUMOR CELLS

Animal studies as well as early human data would suggest that regulation of the immune response to tumor cells is dependent on T cell interactions as well as the host response to idiotypes and lymphokines. Suppressor T cells can interfere with the host response to both spontaneous and induced tumors. Experimental animal data have indicated that if suppressor T cells are preferentially destroyed with cytotoxic drugs and the animal is specifically immunized against the tumor, host immunity can be provoked. Oncofetal antigens present on the surface of tumor cells have been shown to induce tumor transplantation resistance in experimental rodent models. The use of serial immunization as a potential for therapy was suggested following reports of host antitumor immune reactivity and the demonstration of effectiveness of such therapy in selected animal models. Critical for this approach is the expression of tumor-associated antigens against which the host is able to respond immunologically for producing tumor cell destruction.

IMMUNOTHERAPY

Scientists continue to search for ways to enhance the host response against malignant cells. Efforts have included immunologic techniques designed to enhance the cancer patient's immune response against target tumor cells. The advent of monoclonal antibody technology has led to numerous attempts utilizing passive serotherapy. Hybridoma cells can now be maintained in culture with the capability of producing large volumes of monoclonal antibodies that can be used for serotherapy or conjugated to cytotoxic drugs, toxins, or isotopes.

A number of animal studies have shown that specific active immunotherapy, using intact tumor cells as the immunizing antigen, viral oncolysates of tumor cells, or purified tumor-associated antigen preparations, will cause decreased tumor take and subsequent tumor growth. Specific active immunotherapy trials in man have shown significant promise in patients with both melanoma and colorectal carcinoma. Melanoma patients have been immunized with intact autochthonous or allogeneic cells or with a viral oncolysate prepared from such cells. The results of these studies suggest that a statistically significant therapeutic benefit can be realized in high-risk Stage I and Stage II patients treated in the adjuvant mode. Human subjects with high-risk colorectal carcinoma have also been immunized with irradiated autochthonous tumor cells. The data suggest that both improvement of the disease-free interval and ultimate survival are realized in immunized patients when compared with controls.

Adoptive cellular immunotherapy requires transfer of immune T cells. Both primary tumor and metastatic disease in animal models have suggested a significant antitumor response when the cells are transferred in conjunction with lymphokines. Preclinical studies demonstrated that lymphokine-activated killer cells administered with interleukin-2 produced a profound antitumor effect. These studies were followed by clinical trials that demonstrated both complete and partial responses in patients with a number of solid tumors. T cells obtained from growing tumors and expanded in interleukin-2 have shown more effective tumor cell killing when passively transferred to animals bearing significant tumor burdens. A Phase I clinical trial in patients with metastatic melanoma receiving adoptively transferred tumor-infiltrating lymphocytes and interleukin-2 has shown objective regression of the cancer in approximately 60 per cent of the patients under study.

CYTOKINES

Cytokines are a broad class of cell regulators that are important in the human immune response. They regulate cell growth and function. Interferons, tumor necrosis factor, interleukins, colony-stimulating factors, and transforming B-cell growth factors are well characterized lymphokines and can now be produced in pure forms by use of recombinant DNA technology. The interferons include subtypes alpha, beta, and gamma. The interferons appear to promote both monocyte and macrophage function as well as to promote HLA Class II antigen expression on both lymphocytes and target tumor cells. The interferons also appear to have an antiproliferative effect. Early clinical trials have been associated with an approximate 15 to 20 per cent patient response rate.

Tumor necrosis factor and four well-characterized colony-stimulating factors have been identified, and all are glycoproteins. When used alone, these cytokines do not appear to have an antitumor effect, but when used in combination they are capable of producing tumor regression.

The interleukins are part of a complex cytokine network and are produced by more than one cell type. The interleukins can stimulate or inhibit production of other cytokines. The interleukins are named according to their biologic properties, and six have been sequenced. Interleukin-2 (IL-2) has been extensively studied and evaluated as a useful substance for immunotherapeutic trial. IL-2 is a T-cell growth factor and is capable of activating natural killer cells to become highly cytotoxic but nonspecific in their action. IL-2 is coded for by a single gene and is not related to the interferons or other interleukins. Resting T lymphocytes do not respond to IL-2, because they do not express IL-2 receptors. When the T cells have been antigen activated, they initiate secretion of IL-2 and express IL-2 receptors.

ONCOGENIC VIRUSES AND ONCOGENES

Both DNA and RNA viruses can cause neoplasms in animals. RNA viruses that are oncogenic are termed *retroviruses*. By utilizing the enzyme reverse transcriptase, these RNA viruses are copied into DNA. These viruses are incorporated into the cell genome and code for a cell membrane–associated antigen that is immunogenic to the host. There are increasing data that suggest that neoplasia can follow heritable changes that permit unrestrained growth of cells that are associated with altered expression of oncogenes. These genes have normal cellular counterparts that regulate both normal cell proliferation and differentiation. These genes are referred to as proto-oncogenes. If genetic alterations including point mutations, chromosomal translocation, or gene amplification occur, this produces activation of cellular oncogenes that then contribute to cell neoplastic transformation. Approximately 20 oncogenes carried by acute transforming retroviruses have been described. Both human T-cell leukemia and B-cell lymphoma appear to have retroviral changes. Specific protein products of viral oncogenes have been identified. The expression of these proteins should permit specific immunization for both immunoprophylaxis and immunotherapy of these virally produced tumors.

II

Melanoma
H. F. Seigler, M.D.

Melanoma is a neoplastic disorder arising from the skin, mucous membranes, meninges, and ciliary body of the eye. This tumor is increasing in incidence more rapidly than any other malignant neoplasm.

PRECURSOR FACTORS

The one environmental factor that is associated with the development of this disease is ultraviolet irradiation. A ge-

See the corresponding chapter or part in the *Textbook of Surgery*, 14th edition, pp. 477–485, for a more detailed discussion of this topic, including a comprehensive list of references.

netic predisposition appears to be an important component of this disease process. Individuals with fair skin, red or blonde hair, and blue or green eyes are at greater risk for the development of melanoma than are individuals with dark skin, brown eyes, and brown or black hair.

CLINICOPATHOLOGIC FEATURES

The four histopathologic types of mucocutaneous melanoma include lentigo maligna melanoma, superficial spreading melanoma, acral lentiginous melanoma, and nodular melanoma. Lentigo maligna melanoma most commonly occurs in older individuals and on sun-exposed areas of the body. Superficial spreading melanoma usually grows for a period of time in a horizontal direction and does not have a metastatic potential. When vertical growth has been realized, a systemic potential exists. Acral lentiginous melanoma presents on the glabrous skin, subungual areas, and mucous membranes. Nodular melanoma demonstrates vertical growth from its inception and is associated with a less favorable prognosis.

PROGNOSTIC FACTORS

The three most predictive prognostic indicators for mucocutaneous melanoma include the level of invasion, tumor thickness, and ulceration. Patients with tumor thickness of less than 1 mm. have a less than 10 per cent metastatic potential and can usually be cured by simple excision alone. Patients with intermediate thickness melanoma from 1 to 4 mm. have an approximate 30 to 45 per cent risk of spread and are best managed by excision of the primary with adequate tissue borders and, in selected cases, elective lymph node dissection. Patients with tumor thicknesses exceeding 4 mm. have a high risk of a systemic element of their disease and are best managed by excision and careful follow-up. The likelihood that these patients will develop metastatic disease is approximately 70 per cent.

CHOICE OF BIOPSY

If the lesion is small and in a nonstrategic area, the preferred biopsy is excision of the pigmented area with subcutaneous fat submitted with the cutaneous elements. This permits the pathologist to accurately assess ulceration, tumor thickness, and level of invasion. If the primary lesion is large and on a strategic area, incisional biopsy including the area of greatest vertical growth should be selected. Shave biopsies, curettage, and electrocoagulation should not be performed.

SURGICAL MANAGEMENT OF THE PRIMARY LESION

When the histopathologic type has been confirmed by adequate biopsy, surgical management of the primary lesion can be accurately planned. For those lesions with Level I and Level II invasion and tumor thickness less than 1 mm., excision with 1- to 2-cm. margins is adequate. In most areas, this permits primary wound closure. Patients with invasive melanoma with intermediate or thick tumor measurements can adequately be managed by excision with 2 cm. of normal tissue around the primary site and primary closure when possible. The ultimate disease-free interval and patient survival are not predicted by the surgical margins. Clinical outcome is predicted by the prognostic variables rather than the margin of excision.

SURGICAL MANAGEMENT OF REGIONAL DISEASE

Lymphadenectomy is usually recommended for patients with clinically involved lymph nodes and without evidence of distant disease. The major controversy centers on the topic of the benefit of elective lymph node dissection. When the histopathologic type of the primary has been determined, univariate and multivariate analyses permit identification of the subset of patients who have the most to benefit from elective node dissection. There is a consensus that patients with intermediate tumor thicknesses between 1.5 and 4 mm. have the most to gain from the removal of their first-order lymph nodes on an elective basis. If the primary tumor is on an ambiguous area of the body, lymphoscintigraphy permits accurate determination of the lymph node group at risk.

SURGICAL CONSIDERATIONS FOR DISTANT DISEASE

Generally, only those patients with documented solitary metastases to distant sites benefit from surgical removal of the metastatic deposit. The common areas of distant metastatic disease include the lung, brain, adrenal gland, and small intestine. Surgical removal of the solitary metastasis coupled with systemic therapy is associated with increased disease-free interval as well as improved quality of life. Patients with multiple metastatic lesions are best managed by systemic therapy with little benefit gained from surgical intervention.

HORMONAL ASPECTS OF MELANOMA

The presence of estrogen receptors on malignant melanocytes has been extensively evaluated. At present, it appears that pigmented lesions have a false-positive estrogen receptor as determined by biochemical analysis. It appears that the estradiol-binding component in melanoma most probably represents an artifact and that true estrogen receptors are absent with this tumor. If the patient is diagnosed with melanoma during pregnancy, there is a greater likelihood that first-order lymph nodes will be involved than if pregnancy is not included at the time of initial diagnosis. Additionally, the disease-free interval is shorter for patients with pregnancy and melanoma occurring simultaneously. Ultimate patient survival is essentially the same between the pregnant and nonpregnant patient populations. Patients with a past history of melanoma do not appear to have increased risk if they become pregnant at a later date.

COMBINED MODALITY TREATMENT FOR MELANOMA

Conventional systemic chemotherapy for melanoma is associated with an approximate 40 per cent response rate. Only 10 per cent of patients experience complete resolution of their disease. More recently, high-dose chemotherapy with autologous bone marrow reconstitution has increased the drug response rate; however, defined disease-free interval and ultimate patient survival are yet to be determined. Both prophylactic and therapeutic isolated limb perfusion are associated with a prolonged disease-free interval and increased patient survival. The addition of hyperthermia also appears to improve the effectiveness of this therapeutic modality. Interferon, tumor necrosis factor, and monoclonal antibodies have yet to show clear therapeutic potential. Recombinant interleukin-2 administered in association with either lymphokine-activated lymphocytes or expanded tumor-infiltrating lymphocytes has been shown to be associated with a 25 to 60 per cent response rate. This new therapeutic modality must be considered experimental, and ultimate disease-free interval and improved patient survival are not yet defined. Specific active immunotherapy using melanoma vaccines has its greatest effect either in patients with small tumor burdens or in the adjuvant mode.

III

Soft Tissue Sarcomas
LaSalle D. Leffall, Jr., M.D.

Soft tissue sarcomas are relatively uncommon neoplasms, constituting only approximately 1 per cent of malignant tumors. There are more than 20 types of soft tissue sarcomas, each with distinguishing histologic and biologic behavior and varying tendencies for local infiltration and distant metas-

See the corresponding chapter or part in the *Textbook of Surgery*, 14th edition, pp. 485–491, for a more detailed discussion of this topic, including a comprehensive list of references.

tases. Liposarcomas, malignant fibrous histiocytomas, leio-myosarcomas, fibrosarcomas, and rhabdomyosarcomas occur most commonly, with other types presenting less frequently. They are not encapsulated but possess a pseudocapsule of compressed malignant and normal cells. Distant metastases occur most frequently to the lungs by the hematogenous route. Some of these tumors, especially synovial sarcoma, embryonal rhabdomyosarcoma, epithelioid sarcoma, and malignant fibrous histiocytoma, may metastasize to regional lymph nodes in 10 to 20 per cent of patients, with the histiocytoma having the highest incidence of lymphatic spread in adults.

TYPES

Liposarcomas can become the largest of all soft tissue sarcomas, are among the most common neoplasms noted in most series, and are the most frequent sarcomas of the retroperitoneum. Malignant fibrous histiocytomas are among the most common soft tissue sarcomas of adults, occurring with almost the same frequency as liposarcomas.

Fibrosarcomas are seen less frequently now because new histologic criteria classify some of them as malignant fibrous histiocytoma. Fibromatoses are connective tissue hyperplasias that infiltrate locally, do not metastasize, and tend to recur if not adequately excised. Both abdominal and extra-abdominal desmoids are benign, do not metastasize to distant organs, and have a great tendency for local recurrence. Wide excision is the treatment of choice.

Dermatofibrosarcoma protuberans (storiform fibrous histiocytoma) is considered to be a very low grade fibrosarcoma. It tends to recur locally but rarely metastasizes. Rhabdomyosarcoma is divided into four groups: (1) pleomorphic, (2) embryonal, (3) botryoidal, and (4) alveolar. Embryonal rhabdomyosarcoma is the most common soft tissue sarcoma in infants and children.

Synovial sarcomas are the most common soft tissue sarcomas of the hands and feet, affect primarily young adults, and occur in the vicinity of joints. Kaposi's sarcoma is a malignant blood vessel tumor and is thought to be multicentric in origin. It occurs predominantly in adult males and is greatly increased among homosexual males.

CLINICAL MANIFESTATIONS

The most common presenting symptom is a painless mass that gradually enlarges until it becomes painful or interferes with function. Pain alone may be the earliest symptom without a palpable mass. The pain usually persists despite rest. These neoplasms occur most often in the lower extremities, especially in the medial upper thigh, but may occur in other locations such as the upper extremities, trunk, retroperitoneum, head, and neck.

DIAGNOSIS

Biopsy is essential to establish the diagnosis and institute proper therapy. Biopsy incisions should be made along the longitudinal axis of the extremity in order that the biopsy site may be included in the subsequent wide excision, if indicated without sacrificing unnecessary overlying skin. Accurate histologic diagnosis is mandatory before proper therapy can be given. The American Joint Commission has developed a staging system for soft tissue sarcoma that utilizes histologic grading as the primary determinant of stage and thus of prognosis.

Chest films and/or computed tomographic scans are necessary for excluding pulmonary metastases. Computed tomography is of great value in ascertaining spatial relationships of the sarcoma to normal structures. Magnetic resonance imaging, which does not use ionizing radiation, generally produces images superior to those of computed tomographic scanning.

MANAGEMENT

The treatment of choice for soft tissue sarcomas is adequate surgical resection in order to eradicate the disease and decrease the incidence of distant spread and local recurrence. Simple enucleation must be avoided because this increases the opportunity for spread and decreases the likelihood for cure. Wide excision is essential because these sarcomas spread by infiltration along muscle and fascial planes. The surgical modalities are wide local excision, muscle group excision, and amputation.

Limb-sparing procedures should be considered in practically all patients with extremity sarcomas. If limited surgical therapy and radical dose irradiation are used, amputation may be reserved for irradiation failures. The combination of selected surgical therapy, irradiation, and chemotherapy has produced marked improvement in the treatment of embryonal rhabdomyosarcoma in children. With this regimen, amputations are rarely indicated for tumors of the extremities.

IV

Tumor Markers
Jeffrey A. Norton, M.D., and Douglas L. Fraker, M.D.

IDEAL TUMOR MARKER

The potential utility of tumor markers includes screening, diagnosis, prognosis, assessment of therapeutic efficacy, and detection of residual or recurrent disease. A successful screening test for the detection of cancer in the general population or at-risk individuals must possess a high sensitivity for early lesions for the detection of disease in asymptomatic patients with small curable tumor burdens. The best example of a marker for screening is the use of plasma levels of calcitonin following provocative testing with calcium and/or pentagastrin for detecting surgically curable C-cell carcinoma or medullary thyroid carcinoma *in situ* in patients from kindreds with familial multiple endocrine neoplasia Type IIa.

A second application for tumor markers is as an unequivocal diagnostic modality. Again, the best examples of this application are the hormone markers of endocrine tumors in which the diagnosis is dependent on the measurement of the marker in serum or the staining of the tumor for the marker by immunohistochemistry. A third application for measurement of tumor markers at the time of diagnosis is the yield of prognostic as well as diagnostic information by some markers. For example, in patients with colorectal cancer, the prognosis worsens with greater serum levels of carcinoembryonic antigen at the time of initial diagnosis. The final application for measurement of circulating tumor markers is a reflection of treatment efficacy and in follow-up for recurrent disease. In these settings, measurement of marker levels may influence management decisions such as continuing or discontinuing therapy or performing imaging studies or surgical therapy to detect recurrent disease.

Unfortunately, at present no ideal tumor markers exist. The characteristics of individual tumor markers such as specificity, sensitivity, and correlation of marker level with tumor burden and type of disease define the actual clinical utility for each marker in individual patients with specific tumors.

TYPES OF TUMOR MARKERS

Circulating tumor markers can be categorized by functional and biochemical characteristics into tumor antigens, enzymes, hormones, and other markers of tumor or host origin. Tumor antigens are defined by immunogenic structural characteristics and can be subcategorized by historical, biochemical, and distributional features as oncofetal antigens and polyclonal- or monoclonal-defined antigens. Oncofetal anti-

See the corresponding chapter or part in the *Textbook of Surgery*, 14th edition, pp. 491–509, for a more detailed discussion of this topic, including a comprehensive list of references.

gens are compounds produced during normal development by the placental-fetal complex and are also produced by neoplastic tissue. This group contains the original and most prevalent tumor markers including carcinoembryonic antigen, alpha-fetoprotein, and beta-human chorionic gonadotropin. A second and rapidly enlarging group of tumor markers are tumor-associated antigens that are detected by polyclonal or monoclonal antibodies directed against tumor extracts or cell lines. Tumor-associated antigens include carcinoma antigen (CA) CA 125, CA 19–9, and CA 15–3.

Enzymes and hormones were initially identified by bioactivity as catalysts of specific chemical reactions or biologic effects from binding specific receptors, respectively. Although they were formerly measured by cumbersome biologic assay techniques, currently immunoassay techniques exist for the quantitation of minute amounts of essentially all enzymes and hormones used as tumor markers. Enzymes produced in excess amount by the tumor or the tumor-bearing host can be used as circulating markers and include neuron-specific enolase and acid phosphatase. Hormones and hormone degradation products are specific and sensitive serum markers for a wide number of endocrine tumors. A miscellaneous group of tumor markers, host products that increase in response to the presence of tumor, includes serum levels of ferritin, lipid, and cytokines.

Carcinoembryonic Antigen and Colorectal Cancer

Carcinoembryonic antigen (CEA) is a glycoprotein (molecular weight 180 kd.) consisting of a single polypeptide chain with a variable carbohydrate content. In general, serum levels less than 2.5 ng. per ml. are normal, and concentrations greater than 5 ng. per ml. are elevated. CEA is a classic example of a tumor marker that, although widely used, is not an ideal marker because of low specificity and sensitivity. Both malignant and nonmalignant diseases may elevate serum levels of CEA (Tables 1 and 2). Although CEA is primarily associated with colorectal cancer, serum levels may also be elevated in cancer of the pancreas, stomach, lung, breast, thyroid, and ovary (Table 2). The lack of specificity is further proven by nonmalignant conditions that also may elevate serum CEA levels (Table 1): gastrointestinal disorders (including peptic ulcer disease, gastritis, pancreatitis, and inflammatory bowel disease), hepatobiliary diseases (including cirrhosis, hepatitis, and obstructive jaundice), and nonmalignant pulmonary disease (bronchitis and emphysema), as well as benign prostatic hypertrophy and renal failure.

Carcinoembryonic antigen has been studied as a marker of colorectal tumors for the past 2 decades. Although CEA is not colorectal tumor–specific, the highest concentrations in tissue and serum are found in patients with colorectal carcinoma. Serum CEA determinations are not useful in screening normal populations of adults for colorectal cancer. Elevated CEA levels occur in only 5 per cent of patients with localized,

TABLE 1. Serum Levels of Markers in Healthy Normal Controls and Other Nonmalignant Conditions

Marker	Mean Level	Upper Limit Normal	Percentage of Controls with Abnormal Levels at Upper Limit Normal	Nonmalignant Conditions Associated with Elevated Levels
CEA	1.9 ng./ml. nonsmokers	<2.5 ng./ml.	9–16	Hepatitis, cirrhosis, jaundice, chronic obstructive pulmonary disease, peptic ulcer, pancreatitis, inflammatory bowel disease, renal failure
	3.1 ng./ml. smokers	<5.0 ng./ml.	1–5	
AFP	1–10 ng./ml.	<10 ng./ml.	0–1	Chronic and active hepatitis, cirrhosis, pregnancy
		<40 ng./ml.	1–3	
beta-HCG	<1 unit/ml. men	<3 units/ml.	0	Pregnancy
	<3 units/ml. premenopausal women		<1	
	3–4 units/ml. postmenopausal women			
Prostate-specific antigen	1.1 ± 0.7 ng./ml.	<2.5 ng./ml.	<1	Benign prostatic hypertrophy, prostatic massage or biopsy
			1–3	
Tissue polypeptide antigen	66 ± 16 units/L.	<100 units/L.	5	
		<200 units/L.	<1	
CA 15-3	13.3 ± 6 units/ml.	<22 units/ml.	9	Acute and chronic hepatitis, cirrhosis, benign breast disease
		<25 units/ml.	5	
		<30 units/ml.	1.3	
CA 19-9	10.8 ± 7 units/ml.	<25 units/ml.	0–1	Acute and chronic pancreatitis, cirrhosis, sclerosing cholangitis, other extrahepatic cholestatic diseases
		<37 units/ml.		
CA 50		<17 units/ml.	0–1	Pancreatitis, cirrhosis, ulcerative colitis, sclerosing cholangitis

CA 125	10–16 units/ml. (greater in women)	<35 units/ml. <65 units/ml.	1	Pancreatitis, jaundice, pregnancy, menstruation, endometriosis, pelvic inflammatory disease, renal failure
Neuron-specific enolase	4.7–9.3 ng./ml.	<13 ng./ml.		
Prostatic acid phosphatase	Enzymatic assay: 0.1–0.5 unit/L. Immunoassay: 1.2 ± 0.5 ng./ml.	<0.8 unit/L. <2.1 ng./ml.	<1 1–3	Benign prostatic hypertrophy, hematologic disorders
Ferritin	27–96 ng./ml.	<300 ng./ml.	0–1	Alcoholism, hepatocellular disease, hematologic diseases, chronic inflammation

TABLE 2. Markers in Malignant Conditions

Marker	Malignant Condition in which Marker Is Useful	Maximal Percentage of Patients with Abnormal Levels	Other Cancers in which Marker May Be Elevated
CEA	Colon cancer	90	Breast, gastric, gynecologic, lung, pancreas, medullary thyroid
AFP	Hepatocellular carcinoma	80	Testicular, gastric, pancreatic, colorectal, lung
β-HCG	Testicular cancer	70	Trophoblastic, bladder, gynecologic
Prostate-specific antigen	Prostatic cancer	100	None
CA 15–3	Breast cancer	91	Gastrointestinal, lung, ovarian
CA 19–9	Pancreatic cancer	78	Colorectal, stomach, bile ducts, hepatoma, lung, ovary
CA 50	Pancreatic cancer	81	Colorectal, gastric, liver, biliary, prostatic, lung, breast
CA 125	Ovarian cancer	85	Fallopian, endometrial, endocervical
Neuron-specific enolase	Small cell lung cancer	80	Neuroendocrine, adrenal, islet cell, carcinoid, neuroblastoma, medullary thyroid, seminoma
Ferritin	Hepatoma	97	Lymphoma, leukemia, colorectal, breast, lung, pancreatic

surgically curable colon cancer and 65 to 90 per cent of patients with either distant or locally advanced disease. Screening of patients with conditions such as ulcerative colitis or polyposis coli that predispose to colorectal cancer has also been unsuccessful because these diseases may produce elevated serum levels of CEA.

Several reports have indicated that the preoperative serum CEA concentration before definitive resection of primary colorectal cancer is an independent prognostic parameter of subsequent survival; that is, the higher the serum CEA level, the poorer the prognosis of an individual colorectal cancer.

Elevated serum levels of CEA indicate recurrent colorectal cancer usually 4 to 6 months before it is clinically evident. In general, serum CEA levels will be elevated in approximately two of three patients before any other evidence of recurrent colon or rectal cancer. Serum CEA levels need not have been raised preoperatively to be elevated postoperatively as a marker of tumor recurrence following resection. Because there is no dramatic effective therapy for nonimageable colorectal carcinoma, a second-look exploratory procedure with resection of recurrent disease has been used by many groups. Results of CEA-initiated second-look procedures vary among different groups with one group reporting being able to remove all tumor in 70 per cent of patients and others finding no benefit. This strategy of reoperation can provide cure for a small percentage of patients (10 to 20 per cent) and can document recurrent colorectal carcinoma in a majority of patients (80 per cent) who can then graduate to other therapies.

Potential improvement in selection of patients and results for CEA-initiated second-look operative procedures may be achieved through better preoperative demonstration of the location and extent of disease. A new method is the use of radiolabeled antibody to CEA and external scintigraphy for detecting the exact location and extent of recurrent tumor. Patients with localized, resectable, locally recurrent disease or liver disease can then be selected for a second-look operation.

Serum levels of CEA appear to correlate fairly well with disease extent in patients with colorectal cancer. Serum levels usually rise with progression and fall with disease regression, but once markedly elevated they do not always correlate directly with tumor burden. Serum CEA levels have been used to follow the response to chemotherapy in patients with metastatic colorectal cancer. In patients with metastatic colorectal carcinoma who had elevated serum CEA levels and responded to chemotherapy, 89 per cent showed a decrease in serum CEA level. In patients who had progressive disease despite chemotherapy, 90 per cent had an increase in serum CEA level compared with pretreatment level.

Alpha-Fetoprotein and Hepatocellular Carcinoma

Alpha-fetoprotein (AFP) was the first oncofetal antigen discovered and is currently a useful tumor marker for primary hepatocellular carcinoma (HCC) and nonseminomatous germ cell tumors of the testis. Abnormal serum levels of AFP usually occur in malignant neoplasms but may occur in benign diseases of endodermally derived organs including hepatitis, inflammatory bowel disease, ataxia telangiectasia, and hereditary tyrosinemia (Table 1). However, highly elevated serum levels of AFP (greater than 500 ng. per ml.) are present almost exclusively in primary HCC and nonseminomatous testicular tumors (Table 2). Eighty per cent of patients with HCC have elevated serum levels of AFP. Patients with other malignant tumors may also have elevated serum levels of AFP. Twenty per cent of patients with gastric or pancreatic cancer and 5 per cent of patients with colorectal or lung cancer have significant elevations (greater than 5 ng. per ml.) of serum AFP levels (Table 2).

In 1983 a case report was published in the journal *Lancet* demonstrating the feasibility of screening a population at high risk for development of HCC with serial serum levels of alpha-fetoprotein. Other investigators have tried to use serum AFP levels to detect HCC in at-risk populations with disappointing results. Serum AFP levels may be normal in 35 to 50 per cent of patients with biopsy-proven HCC. In a minority of patients with HCC, serum levels of AFP fall despite continued tumor growth, and other patients have elevated levels of AFP and nonmalignant diseases of the liver (Table 1). However, in the presence of cirrhosis, a serum AFP level greater than 500 ng. per ml. is diagnostic of HCC.

Serum levels of AFP in patients with HCC may be of prognostic value. The subgroup of patients who have HCC and normal serum levels of AFP appear to have a relatively good prognosis. In these patients, the primary factor predicting better prognosis may be the absence of cirrhosis. Normal serum AFP levels are more common in patients without underlying cirrhosis. A rapid AFP doubling time is also associated with a poorer prognosis.

Serial measurement of serum AFP level can be helpful before and after presumably curative surgical therapy in patients with HCC. However, the serum levels of this tumor marker do not always show the presence of recurrent HCC. HCC may be recurrent despite normal serum AFP levels. There is variation in AFP synthesis in different parts of the same tumor. The ability of the tumor to secrete AFP may change with growth. It may be that tumor recurrences within the liver are really new primary tumors with different characteristics.

If specific chemotherapy is effective, serum AFP levels fall continuously, indicating tumor regression and effective treatment. If serum AFP levels demonstrate a continued rise despite antitumor treatment, the tumor is resistant to the treatment and an alternative regimen should be used. Monitoring of serum AFP levels in patients with HCC can avoid prolonged ineffective use of potentially toxic chemotherapy.

Alpha-Fetoprotein and Human Chorionic Gonadotropin in Testicular and Gynecologic Cancer

The characteristics of AFP have been described in the previous section. Human chorionic gonadotropin (HCG) is a placental hormone that is also a tumor marker for gestational trophoblastic neoplasms and nonseminomatous testicular cancer. It is a glycoprotein consisting of two distinct noncovalently bound subunits. Currently, there are many commercially available immunoassay kits for the measurement of HCG. The sensitivity of these assays is in the range of 1 unit per ml. or 0.2 ng. per ml. The upper limit of normal for circulating HCG is less than 5 to 8 units per ml. for women and less than 3 units per ml. for men.

The application of HCG as a circulating tumor marker ranges from the prototype of an ideal tumor marker for gestational trophoblastic neoplasia and a valuable tool in testicular cancer to a less well defined role in other gynecologic malignancies, uroepithelial tumors, and a spectrum of other solid tumors (Table 2). HCG is highly sensitive for the diagnosis of choriocarcinoma and the diagnosis of a trophoblastic neoplasm following evacuation of a molar pregnancy (Tables 1 and 2). In testicular cancer, 70 to 75 per cent of nonseminomatous tumors and 10 per cent of pure seminomas are associated with elevated serum HCG levels. If both serum HCG and AFP levels are measured, 89 per cent of patients with nonseminomatous testicular cancer have an elevation of one or both markers. Serum HCG and AFP levels are very useful as markers for detecting the response to therapy and for detecting persistent or recurrent testicular cancer. In addition, the serum levels of both AFP and HCG are inversely proportional to outcome in patients with testicular cancer.

Serum HCG elevations have been detected in a small proportion of patients with nontrophoblastic, nontesticular neoplasms (60 of 828, 7.2 per cent) (Table 2). Specifically, 20 per cent of patients with bladder cancer and between 13 and 36 per cent of patients with gynecologic cancers including cervical, endometrial, and vulvar cancer and 5 per cent of patients with ovarian cancer have elevated serum HCG levels. In addition, with newer techniques used to detect the free beta-subunit of HCG and the beta core fragment of HCG, 77 per cent of patients with ovarian and other gynecologic neoplasms have elevated serum HCG levels.

CA 125 and Ovarian Cancer

CA 125 is a carbohydrate epitope on a glycoprotein carcinoma antigen that is useful as a serum marker for ovarian cancer (Table 2). A murine monoclonal antibody was raised against a cultured cell line established from a patient with a serous papillary adenocarcinoma of the ovary. Immunoassay kits are available for measurement of CA 125; normal serum levels are less than 35 units per ml. since only 1 per cent of normal subjects have a value greater than 35 units per ml. (Table 1).

CA 125 antigen is abnormally elevated in the serum of 80 per cent of patients with nonmucinous epithelial ovarian carcinoma (Table 2). Serum levels of CA 125 correlate directly with tumor bulk. Elevated levels of CA 125 in the serum of patients with occult recurrent disease precede other clinical signs of recurrent ovarian carcinoma. Serum levels of CA 125 are also elevated in a high percentage of patients with fallopian, endometrial, and endocervical carcinoma (Table 2).

CA 19–9 and CA 50 in Gastrointestinal Cancer

CA 19–9 is a carbohydrate antigen that is identified by a monoclonal antibody raised versus a colorectal cancer cell line. Serum from patients with colorectal, pancreas, and gastric cancer can neutralize binding of this monoclonal antibody to its specific cell extracts, suggesting that CA 19–9 is present in the serum of these patients with cancer (Table 2). The antigen is present in normal fetal tissues, including salivary and lacrimal glands, conjunctivae, bronchi, pancreas, esophagus, stomach, small intestine, and gallbladder, but is absent in the fetal colon. The carbohydrate epitope may be present in the pancreas, salivary gland, endocervix, and gallbladder of normal adults.

Sensitive immunoassay kits are currently available for measurement of CA 19–9. A study of healthy subjects indicated normal serum levels of CA 19–9 were less than 35 units per ml. (Table 1). CA 19–9 is a serum marker for the management of patients with gastric, pancreatic, and colorectal cancer (Table 2). Patients with pancreatitis may also have an elevation of serum CA 19–9 levels (Table 1). However, in patients with pancreatitis, the serum levels of CA 19–9 seldom exceed 100 units per ml., and patients with pancreatic cancer have higher levels of this marker (73 per cent greater than 100 units per ml.). In the management of patients with gastric and colorectal cancer, serum CA 19–9 levels appear to offer no advantage over serum CEA levels.

CA 50 is a carbohydrate antigen closely related to CA 19–9 defined by monoclonal antibodies to a colorectal cancer cell line. CA 50 has the same determinants as does CA 19–9, but it also has a unique carbohydrate moiety that lacks a fucose residue and is not associated with CA 19–9 activity. Serum levels of CA 50 can be detected in approximately 5 per cent of the population who are Lewis antigen negative. Serum levels of CA 50 less than 17 units per ml. are normal (Table 1).

The utility of CA 50 parallels that of CA 19–9. CA 50 antigen is not detectable in normal tissue except the pancreas. CA 50 levels are not elevated in normal serum, but levels are increased in a few patients (less than 12 per cent) with benign liver disease and inflammatory bowel disease and in patients with sclerosing cholangitis (Table 1). Circulating CA 50 is elevated in a significant proportion of patients with colorectal, gastric, liver, biliary, prostatic, lung, and breast cancer (Table 2). The clinical utility of CA 50 and its comparison to other markers such as AFP, CEA, and CA 19–9 need further study.

CA 15–3 and Breast Cancer

CA 15–3 is a glycoprotein antigen that serves as a marker for breast cancer. It is identified by two specific monoclonal antibodies that recognize different epitopes on an identical antigen. CA 15–3 is both a differentiation antigen and a milk-related antigen because its production is increased during cell differentiation and it is present in breast milk. The mean value of CA 15–3 in the serum of normal subjects is 13.3 ± 6 units per ml., and over 90 per cent of normals have levels less than 22 units per ml. (Table 1).

Initial clinical studies suggest that CA 15–3 serum levels

may help in the management of patients with breast cancer (Table 2). The percentage of patients who have elevated serum levels of CA 15–3 increases with more advanced stage breast cancer. In addition, 66 per cent of patients with breast cancer who have normal serum levels of CEA have elevated serum levels of CA 15–3. CA 15–3 may be elevated in some patients with cancer besides breast cancer (Table 2).

Prostate-Specific Antigen, Prostatic Acid Phosphatase, and Prostate Cancer

Prostate-specific antigen (PSA) is a glycoprotein specific for prostatic tissue with utility as a tumor marker for prostatic cancer. Greater than 90 per cent of normal men have detectable serum levels of PSA (1.1 ± 0.7 ng. per ml.), and the normal range for men is less than 2.5 ng. per ml. (Table 1).

PSA is a very sensitive marker for prostatic cancer; 96 per cent of patients with very early stage lesions (Stage A) and 100 per cent of patients with more advanced disease have elevated serum levels of PSA (Table 2). However, 86 per cent of patients with benign prostatic hypertrophy have moderate elevations of serum PSA levels, limiting its ability as a screening test for prostate cancer. The level of the serum marker may also increase following prostatic massage, prostatic biopsy, and transurethral resection (Table 1).

Prostatic acid phosphatase is not a useful circulating tumor marker in patients with prostatic cancer (Table 1). Specifically, serum prostatic acid phosphatase level is not useful as a screening test because elevations frequently occur in patients with benign prostatic hypertrophy, and serum levels are not usually elevated in patients with early prostatic cancer or small amounts of residual disease.

Neuron-Specific Enolase and APUDomas

Neuron-specific enolase (NSE) is an acidic isoenzyme of enolase. NSE was initially isolated from bovine brain and reported to be found exclusively in neural tissue. Subsequent studies indicated a high level of NSE in neuroendocrine tissues, the amine precursor uptake and decarboxylation (APUD) cells.

The development of a specific radioimmunoassay enabled measurement of NSE in the serum of normal subjects and patients with malignant disease originating from neuroendocrine tissues. Normals have serum levels between 5 and 10 ng. per ml. (Table 1). Study of patients with different neuroendocrine tumors demonstrated elevated serum levels of NSE in patients with pancreatic islet cell tumors, gut carcinoids, adrenal tumors, neuroblastomas, medullary cancer of the thyroid, and small cell lung cancer (Table 2). Because additional, more specific and sensitive tumor markers exist for most patients with endocrine tumors, serum NSE levels do not help in the management of these patients.

However, recent studies suggest that circulating NSE levels may be a valuable marker for patients with small cell lung cancer, since other good alternative markers are not available. Another potential application of serum NSE levels is for management of patients with seminomas, since 73 per cent of patients have elevated levels.

21

THE BREAST

J. Dirk Iglehart, M.D.

Breast diseases may be disorders of function and normal physiology or benign or malignant neoplasms. Benign tumors are common and also the cause of much concern; they include cysts, fibroadenomas, and other neoplasms. Malignant tumors are generally neoplasms of the ductal epithelium within the breast. Modern treatment of breast carcinoma requires accurate diagnosis, knowledge of the extent of disease (stage), and knowledge of additional information such as hormone receptor content as well as measures of biologic behavior. Treatment has dramatically changed during the last several decades and continues to change today.

MICROSCOPIC ANATOMY

The mature breast is composed of an array of successively branching ducts connecting the milk-producing lobules to the nipple and areola. Under the areola, large subareolar (lactiferous) sinuses open onto the surface of the nipple through 15 to 20 orifices. At the lobular end of the ductal system are small ductules. These ductules enter clusters of blindly ending epithelium-lined spaces known as breast lobules. This entire system of epithelium-lined ducts and acini is surrounded by connective tissue and supported in a variable amount of fat.

ABNORMAL PHYSIOLOGY AND DEVELOPMENT

GYNECOMASTIA. Hypertrophy of the male breast is a common condition that tends to occur in young males *(puberal hypertrophy)* and in older men *(senescent hypertrophy)*. Hypertrophy in older men is very common, is frequently unilateral, and may be associated with systemic illnesses such as hepatic or renal disease. On examination, senescent hypertrophy is smooth, firm, sometimes tender, and symmetrically distributed beneath the areola. Carcinoma of the male breast is usually not tender, is asymmetrically located beneath or beside the areola, and may be fixed to the overlying skin or underlying pectoral fascia. Gynecomastia in young males and senescent gynecomastia are rarely treated by surgical therapy except for the occasional need to establish a diagnosis or for cosmetic reasons.

NIPPLE DISCHARGE. Nipple discharge is usually functional. It is important to establish the following historic points

---

See the corresponding chapter or part in the *Textbook of Surgery,* 14th edition, pp. 510–550, for a more detailed discussion of this topic, including a comprehensive list of references.

and physical findings: (1) Does the discharge come from one or both breasts? (2) Does the discharge come from one or multiple nipple orifices? (3) Is blood present within the discharge? (4) Is there a palpable mass present under the involved nipple and areola? Significant discharges are those that are unilateral, come from one nipple orifice, and may contain blood. In these cases, surgical biopsy is recommended. The most common finding is intraductal papilloma (a benign proliferation), and carcinoma is unusual.

FIBROCYSTIC CHANGE (DISEASE), CYSTIC MASTITIS. The term *fibrocystic disease* refers clinically to the firm, fibrous breast with or without cyst formation. On histologic examination, the fibrocystic complex contains cysts, fibrosis, and a variable amount of epithelial hyperplasia and adenosis. It has been questioned whether *fibrocystic disease* is a term that should be abandoned, since there is not consistent association between fibrocystic complex and breast cancer. Fibrocystic complex represents a health risk only in a very small group of patients.

DIAGNOSIS OF BREAST DISEASE

RISK FACTORS FOR BREAST CANCER. The incidence of breast cancer increases with age, and cancer is quite uncommon in women under the age of 30 years. Family history is most important when primary relatives (mothers, sisters, and daughters) have breast cancer, particularly if these primary relatives had cancer when they were young or if it was bilateral. *In situ* carcinoma, both ductal and lobular, increases the likelihood of development of mammary cancer, as does the presence of atypical epithelial hyperplasia within a breast biopsy specimen. Fibrocystic "disease" is not a predisposing factor unless it is associated with atypical hyperplasia.

PHYSICAL EXAMINATION. Visual inspection of the breast may disclose edema and erythema, termed *peau d'orange*, which is the hallmark of inflammatory carcinoma. Visible skin changes involving the nipple and areola may be a sign of Paget's disease. In this condition, intraductal carcinoma within subareolar ducts invades across the epidermal-epithelial junction and enters the epidermal layer of the skin on the nipple, producing a dermatitis that originates on the nipple and secondarily encompasses the areola. Masses are characterized by their size, shape, consistency, location, and fixation to the surrounding breast tissue, skin, or chest wall. Fine-needle aspiration can be performed to determine whether it is solid or cystic (fluid-containing). Cyst fluid is commonly turbid and dark green or amber in color. If the mass disappears after withdrawal and the fluid is not bloody, the diagnosis of a functional cyst is made. If the mass is solid, breast biopsy must be performed to exclude a carcinoma.

BREAST IMAGING (MAMMOGRAPHY AND ULTRASONOGRAPHY). The mammogram is the most sensitive and specific test that can be used in addition to physical examination. Mammographic features of malignancy are density abnormalities (including masses, asymmetries, and architectural distortions) and microcalcifications. Densities with indistinct margins, stellate borders, or significant architectural distortion of the surrounding parenchyma are most likely to be malignant. Microcalcifications are very small and never palpable unless associated with a density abnormality palpable on physical examination.

Screening mammography is probably beneficial if the studies are obtained annually after the age of 50 years. Benefit may extend to those between the ages of 40 and 50 years, but increased survival has been difficult to demonstrate for women in this group. In women with a personal or family history of breast cancer, the benefits of early and continued screening are likely to be greater.

Ultrasonography is indicated as a complement to mammography or physical examination but has no proven benefit in screening. The principal utility of ultrasonography is to distinguish solid from cystic masses.

BENIGN BREAST MASSES

BREAST CYSTS. Cysts are fluid-filled epithelial cavities that vary in size from microscopic to large and palpable masses. Formation, enlargement, and regression of cysts are influenced by ovarian hormones. The incidence of large cysts peaks after the age of 35 years, is rare in women before the age of 25 years, and sharply declines after menopause. The diagnosis of a cyst is made by needle aspiration or by ultrasonography. The relationship of cysts to carcinoma is not great, and the finding of a gross cyst should not be the subject of great concern to the patient or physician. Biopsy is reserved for those lesions that do not disappear completely after aspiration, for those that recur multiple times after aspiration, or when the fluid withdrawn is clearly bloody.

FIBROADENOMA AND RELATED TUMORS. Fibroadenoma is the most common benign solid tumor in the female breast and the most common breast tumor in young women. It is a solid tumor containing a proliferation of fibrous stroma and a variable proliferation of epithelium-lined ducts or spaces. In young women (under the age of 30 years), the differential diagnosis of a breast mass is usually between cyst and fibroadenoma. The two entities are distinguished by needle aspiration, which yields no fluid in the case of fibroadenoma. In older women, cancer must be added to the list of possibilities if aspiration reveals a solid mass.

Fibroadenomas have no malignant potential although they may be related to a group of tumors of stromal elements termed *cystosarcoma phyllodes* or phyllodes tumor. Phyllodes tumors are commonly benign but may be malignant, behaving much like soft tissue sarcomas elsewhere in the body. The treatment for fibroadenoma is excision of the tumor without the necessity for much margin of normal breast tissue.

BREAST ABSCESS AND INFECTIONS. Infections and

abscesses usually occur around the nipple and areola, presumably originating in large subareolar lactiferous sinuses. The treatment is usually conservative and consists of administration of antibiotics. Incision and drainage are reserved for the unusual case that cannot be controlled with antibiotics. Chronic, recurrent subareolar mastitis may respond to excision of the subareolar ductal tissue when the process is quiescent.

PAPILLOMA. Solitary intraductal papillomas are true benign polyps of the breast ducts. They are usually located in the large ductal spaces underneath the nipple and are the most common cause of a bloody nipple discharge. Papillomatosis is a term in common usage but refers to epithelial hyperplasia and not to true polyp formation as in solitary or multiple papilloma.

MALIGNANT TUMORS OF THE BREAST

Pathology of Breast Cancer

Malignancies of the breast are broadly divided into epithelial tumors of cells lining breast ducts and lobules and nonepithelial malignancies of the supporting breast stroma. A second important division of the epithelial malignancies is between noninvasive and invasive cancer. The noninvasive malignancies are of ductal origin (intraductal carcinoma) or arise in lobules (lobular carcinoma *in situ*). These are true carcinomas *in situ* and are distinguished by the fact that they do not invade the basement membrane of the ductal or lobular structures. As with carcinoma *in situ* elsewhere in the body, these lesions may coexist with invasive disease in the same malignant tumor. Most pathologists utilize the classification proposed by the World Health Organization and outlined in the fascicles of the Armed Forces Institute of Pathology.

DUCTAL CARCINOMA *IN SITU*, INTRADUCTAL CARCINOMA. In health, the breast ducts are lined by two or three cell layers of epithelium. In ductal carcinoma *in situ*, the ducts become swollen with malignant cells, which may grow in solid sheets or in a cribriform or papillary manner. Because they are confined to the basement membrane, angiogenesis is retarded, and the center may undergo necrosis with production of the "comedo" appearance. This necrotic debris may calcify, which produces the fine stippled or branching calcifications seen on high-quality mammography.

LOBULAR CARCINOMA *IN SITU*, LOBULAR NEOPLASIA. This *in situ* proliferation is confined to the breast lobules and causes their expansion. Central necrosis is not a feature of this malignancy, and calcifications do not occur. Because of this, lobular carcinoma *in situ* does not form a recognizable abnormality on mammography. Lobular carcinoma *in situ* is found incidentally during evaluation of biopsy material performed for unrelated masses or mammographic findings. This disease may not invariably progress to invasive cancer and is frequently multicentric and bilateral. Because of its low malignant potential, some refer to lobular carcinoma *in* *situ* as *lobular neoplasia* in order to distinguish it from more malignant proliferations.

INFILTRATING DUCTAL CARCINOMA. This is the most common malignant tumor in the breast recognized after biopsy. The term *ductal* refers to its origin from ductal epithelium, and it is commonly found coexisting with intraductal carcinoma. The term *infiltrating* refers to the fact that it has invaded beyond the basement membrane of the breast duct and is found in the surrounding stroma. This tumor accounts for at least 70 per cent of the invasive carcinomas of the breast.

INVASIVE LOBULAR CARCINOMA. As the name implies, the origin of the infiltrating cell is probably from the epithelium lining of the breast lobules. Invasive lobular carcinoma constitutes between 3 and 15 per cent of all invasive breast cancers. Clinically, lobular carcinoma behaves very similarly to its ductal counterpart.

LESS COMMON FORMS OF DUCTAL CARCINOMA. These tumors are a heterogeneous group and display different morphologic patterns. In general, these variants appear more differentiated and have an improved prognosis. An exception is medullary carcinoma of the breast, which is probably a ductal carcinoma characterized by bizarre and anaplastic tumor cells surrounded by an intense infiltrate of lymphocytes. Tubular carcinoma, characterized by small, well-formed ductal structures, and colloid or mucinous carcinoma, which produces lakes of mucin surrounding islands of tumor cells, both impart a better prognosis to their host than does the average ductal carcinoma.

Staging Breast Cancer

The most widely used method for staging breast carcinoma is the TNM (Tumor, Nodes, Metastasis) system proposed by the American Joint Committee on Cancer and the International Union Against Cancer (Table 1).

Current Surgical Therapy for Invasive Breast Cancer

The goal of surgical treatment is the eradication of local and regional malignant disease within the breast and axillary lymph nodes. The majority of patients with mammary cancer do not have detectable metastatic disease at presentation. However, many have a recurrence of breast cancer, and the majority of these recurrences are at sites outside the scope of the initial treatment field. During the past 2 decades, radical mastectomy has been replaced by the modified radical mastectomy. In this procedure, the breast is removed, leaving the underlying pectoralis major muscle. Removal of the pectoralis minor muscle is a modification that can provide better access to the axillary nodes. The axillary nodal dissection is variable but generally less extensive than in the radical mastectomy. The modified radical mastectomy has been the

TABLE 1. 1986 TNM Classification

Measuring the Size of the Primary Cancer
The tumor size is a measure of the invasive component. If there is a large *in situ* component (e.g., 4.0 cm.) and a small invasive component (e.g., 0.5 cm.), the tumor is coded T.

Multiple, Simultaneous Cancers
The following guidelines should be used when staging multiple, simultaneous primary (grossly measurable, infiltrating) cancers within the same breast. These criteria do not apply to multiple microscopic lesions (since they may represent intramammary spread).

Use the largest primary cancer to stage the case.
Enter on the record that the case is one of simultaneous, multiple primary cancers in one breast. These cases should be analyzed separately.
Include in breast checklist (pathology) simultaneous, multiple, primary infiltrating cancers.
Simultaneous *bilateral* breast cancers: Each should be staged independently.

Inflammatory Carcinoma
Inflammatory carcinoma of the breast is characterized by diffuse, brawny induration of the skin, with an erysipeloid edge, usually with no underlying palpable mass. This clinical presentation is due to tumor embolization of dermal lymphatics. The tumor of inflammatory carcinoma is coded T.

Primary Tumor (T)
The size of the intact tumor should be measured before any tissue is removed for special studies, such as estrogen-binding studies.

T	The primary tumor cannot be assessed.
T_0	No evidence of primary tumor.
TIS	Carcinoma *in situ*: intraductal carcinoma, lobular carcinoma *in situ*, or Paget's disease of the nipple with no tumor. Paget's disease associated with a tumor is classified according to the size of the tumor
T_1	Tumor is 2.0 cm. or smaller in greatest dimension.

T_{1a} 0.5 cm. or smaller
T_{1b} Larger than 0.5 cm. but not larger than 1.0 cm.
T_{1c} Larger than 1.0 cm. but not larger than 2.0 cm.

T_2	Tumor is larger than 2.0 cm. but not larger than 5.0 cm. in greatest dimension.
T_3	Tumor is larger than 5.0 cm. in greatest dimension.
T_4	Tumor of any size with direct extension to chest wall or skin. (Chest wall includes ribs, intercostal muscles, and serratus anterior muscle, but not pectoral muscle.)
T_{4a}	Extension to chest wall
T_{4b}	Edema (including peau d'orange), ulceration of the skin of the breast, or satellite skin nodules confined to the same breast.
T_{4c}	Both a and b, above.
T_{4d}^*	Inflammatory carcinoma (as defined above).

Note: Dimpling of the skin, nipple retraction, or other skin changes, except those in T_4, may occur in T_1, T_2, and T_3 without affecting the classification.

---

*If the skin biopsy is negative and there is no localized, measurable primary cancer, the T category is pT; when pathologically staging a clinical inflammatory carcinoma, cT_{4d}.

TABLE 1. 1986 TNM Classification *Continued*

Regional Lymph Node Stations (N)

Axillary (ipsilateral) and interpectoral (Rotter's nodes): lymph nodes along the axillary vein and its tributaries, which may be divided into the following levels:

Level I (low axilla): lymph nodes located lateral to the lateral border of the pectoralis major muscle.

Level II (mid axilla): lymph nodes located between the medial and lateral borders of the pectoralis minor muscle and the interpectoral (Rotter's) lymph nodes.

Level III (apical axilla): lymph nodes medial to the medial margin of the pectoralis minor, including those designated as the subclavicular, infraclavicular, or apical lymph nodes.

Intramammary lymph nodes are coded as axillary lymph nodes.

Internal mammary (ipsilateral): lymph nodes located in the intercostal spaces along the edge of the sternum in the endothoracic fascia.

All other lymph node metastases are coded as distant metastases (M_1), including supraclavicular, cervical, or contralateral internal mammary lymph nodes.

N—REGIONAL LYMPH NODES

N	The regional lymph nodes cannot be assessed (e.g., clinical staging: previously removed; pathologic staging: previously removed, or not removed for pathologic study).
N_0	No regional lymph node metastases.
N_1	Metastases in four or fewer ipsilateral axillary lymph nodes, none larger than 3.0 cm. in greatest dimension.
N_{1a}	Only micrometastases (none larger than 0.2 cm.)
N_{1b}	Metastases in one to three axillary lymph nodes, any one larger than 0.2 cm., but none larger than 3.0 cm.
N_2	Metastases in four or more ipsilateral axillary lymph nodes, and/or in any axillary lymph node larger than 3.0 cm., or in any ipsilateral internal mammary lymph node(s).
N_{2a}	Metastasis in five or more axillary lymph nodes, or any ipsilateral axillary metastasis larger than 3.0 cm.
N_{2b}	Metastasis in any ipsilateral internal lymph node(s).

Table continued on following page

standard procedure used in the past decade for treatment of operable breast cancer.

CONSERVATIVE SURGERY FOR OPERABLE BREAST CANCER. Pioneering work by radiotherapists demonstrated that removal of the primary breast tumor, a large dose of radiation to the remaining breast, and either removal or radiation of axillary lymph nodes produced survival rates that were equal to those achieved by the radical and modified radical mastectomy. In the United States, conservative procedures for operable breast cancer refers to wide local excision of the primary tumor with clear surgical margins, radiation using at least 4500 rads to the breast with a variable increase to the tumor bed, and removal of axillary lymph nodes through a separate incision. Currently, patients who are candidates for modified radical mastectomy should be considered for conservative breast surgery, and this alternative should be carefully discussed. Exactly which group of patients should be offered radiation and which are better treated by mastectomy is an important question for the coming decade.

TABLE 1. 1986 TNM Classification *Continued*

Distant Metastasis (M)

M	Distant metastasis cannot be assessed
M_0	No distant metastasis
M_1	Distant metastasis

Clinical Staging

Clinical staging includes the following: physical examination, including careful inspection and palpation of the skin, the mammary glands, and the lymph nodes (axillary, supraclavicular, and cervical); pathologic examination of the breast or other tissues to establish the diagnosis of breast cancer. The extent of tissues examined pathologically for clinical staging is less than that required for pathologic staging (see Pathologic Staging below). Appropriate operative findings are elements of clinical staging, including size and chest wall invasion of the primary cancer and the presence or absence of regional or distant metastasis.

Pathologic Staging

Pathologic staging includes the following:

All data used for clinical staging.

Surgical resection and pathologic examination of the primary cancer, including not less than excision of the primary carcinoma with no tumor in any margin of resection by *gross* pathologic examination. A case can be included in the pathologic stage if there is only microscopic, but not gross, involvement in a margin. If there is tumor in the margin of resection by gross examination, it is coded T.

Resection of at least five ipsilateral axillary lymph nodes.

Stage Groupings

Stage	0	TIS	N_0	M_0
Stage	I	T_1	N_0	M_0
Stage	II			
	II_a	T_0	N_1	M_0
		T_1	N_1†	M_0
		T_2	N_0	M_0
	II_b	T_2	N_1	M_0
		T_3	N_0	M_0
Stage	III			
	III_a T_3		N_1	M_0
		T_1,T_2,T_3	N_2	M_0
	III_b T_4		Any N	M_0
Stage	IV	Any T	Any N	M_1

†The prognosis of patients with N_{1a} is similar to that of patients with N_0.

From Lippman, M. E., Lichter, A. S., and Danforth, D. N., Jr. (Eds.): Diagnosis and Management of Breast Cancer. Philadelphia, W. B. Saunders Company, 1988, pp. 55–56.

Management of Noninvasive *In Situ* Breast Cancer

Special attention to the subject of noninvasive carcinoma is necessary because of the increasing frequency of its recognition and the controversy surrounding the proper treatment of ductal and lobular carcinoma *in situ*. With the current emphasis on screening mammography, the incidence of these malignancies is increasing, and their treatment should be curative.

DUCTAL CARCINOMA *IN SITU* OR INTRADUCTAL CARCINOMA. The proper treatment of ductal carcinoma *in situ* is based on several issues including (1) coexistence of occult invasive cancer with the *in situ* lesion, (2) multicentricity of intraductal carcinoma, (3) occurrence of disease in the contralateral breast, and (4) natural history following diagnosis by biopsy.

The following recommendation for treatment summarizes the current approach to intraductal carcinoma. If the tumor is small and totally removed with clear surgical margins, the patient may be a candidate for conservative surgery either with or without radiotherapy after excision. For patients with extensive ductal carcinoma *in situ* (greater than 2 cm.), with multifocal disease within the biopsy material, or in whom a clear surgical margin cannot be achieved, total mastectomy should be considered. Dissection of ipsilateral lymph nodes should be considered for those patients with very extensive *in situ* disease. The outlook for patients with pure intraductal carcinoma after adequate treatment should be quite good.

LOBULAR CARCINOMA *IN SITU*. Lobular carcinoma *in situ* is a relatively rare lesion that is detected in younger, premenopausal women. Haagensen introduced the term *lobular neoplasia* to emphasize that this entity predisposes to subsequent carcinoma after a long latency period and determined the actuarial probability of developing carcinoma at the end of 35 years to be 21 per cent. Significantly, 40 per cent of subsequent carcinomas that developed were purely *in situ* lesions, and one half were present in the contralateral breast. Although no complete survey of surgical practice has been performed, a conservative approach to lobular carcinoma *in situ* is probably more commonly practiced than is mastectomy. However, patients must be informed that the diagnosis of lobular carcinoma *in situ* predisposes to subsequent carcinoma and that their risk is life-long and applied to both breasts. Bilateral total mastectomy is a radical procedure, but it is a safe and reasonable choice for some patients.

Adjuvant Therapy for Operable Breast Cancer

Adjuvant chemotherapy of breast cancer is being intensely investigated and is rapidly changing. Many women with operable breast cancer are now offered additional therapy, either chemotherapy or hormonal therapy, after curative excision or radiotherapy. The recommendations made by the 1985 Consensus Development Conference on Adjuvant Therapy and Endocrine Therapy for Breast Cancer have generally been accepted as standards of care. (See *Textbook of Surgery*, 14th ed.) Two trials influencing the NIH-sponsored consensus panel were the National Surgical Adjuvant Breast and Bowel Project (NSABP) Protocol B–05 comparison of L-phenylalanine mustard (L-PAM) and a placebo and the National Cancer Institute (NCI)-Milan trial of combination cyclophosphamide, methotrexate, and 5-fluorouracil (CMF) versus no treatment. The design of these two trials was similar, and the results are convincingly positive for women treated with chemotherapy who are less than 50 years of age (premenopausal) with one to three lymph nodes positive for metastatic cancer. In both studies, the administration of chemotherapy produced at least a 50 per cent reduction in the likelihood of tumor recurrence for premenopausal patients with positive lymph nodes when the treated patients were compared with controls. Subsequent trials have confirmed the results of the NSABP and Milan trials. Most authorities now believe that combination chemotherapy for node-positive premenopausal women is the standard of care. For postmenopausal women with positive lymph nodes, the results of trials are more variable. However, the benefit of chemotherapy given as a postoperative adjuvant to women over the age of 50 years was statistically significant in an overview analysis of many trials.

ADJUVANT CHEMOTHERAPY IN NODE-NEGATIVE PATIENTS. At least one quarter of patients with negative axillary lymph nodes suffer relapse of breast cancer. Selective application of chemotherapy in high-risk women with node-negative breast cancer may improve their survival. The useful prognostic factors that mark tumors at higher risk for recurrence include (1) tumor size greater than 2 cm., (2) poor histologic and nuclear grade, (3) absent hormone receptors for estrogen (ER) and for progesterone (PgR), and (4) high proliferative rates, or S-phase, and aneuploid DNA content. Most studies of adjuvant chemotherapy in node-negative women specifically address subgroups of women whose tumors possess some of these markers of poor prognosis.

The results of published randomized trials of adjuvant chemotherapy in node-negative patients do not yet allow a definite conclusion to be drawn. A small study from Milan of 90 ER-negative, node-negative patients showed a significant improvement in the survival of those patients receiving CMF chemotherapy compared with a surgical control group. Two large cooperative studies in the United States are under way for evaluating adjuvant chemotherapy in node-negative women who are either receptor-negative or who have large primary tumor masses. Early results favor the treatment arms in these studies, but no long-term survival data are available. Application of therapy to groups of node-negative women whose prognosis is particularly poor appears justifiable outside of clinical protocols.

Hormonal Therapy of Breast Cancer

Many breast cancers retain sensitivity to ovarian steroid hormones. The biochemical basis of sensitivity is the presence of specific protein receptors for estrogen and progesterone within the tumor cells. These receptor proteins can be quantitated, and their levels within tissue accurately predict responsiveness to hormone therapy. The quantity of receptor is expressed as a binding capacity in femtomoles (10^{-15} moles) of radiolabeled steroid bound per milligram of protein within the tumor extract. Levels of either ER or PgR less than

3 fmol. per mg. are considered negative and indicate only a slight likelihood that the tumor will respond to hormone therapy. Levels of greater than 10 fmol. per mg. in the tumor indicate hormone sensitivity and a high probability of response to hormone treatment. Newer assay methods for ER and PgR use immunohistochemistry for measuring the content of the receptors in tissue sections of breast cancer.

Current first-line therapy for hormone-sensitive breast cancer is the use of the antiestrogen drug tamoxifen. Tamoxifen is an inactive ligand for the estrogen receptor and competes with the active ligand, estrogen, for binding. The result of treatment with tamoxifen is slowing or stopping of the growth of cells that contain ER and are normally responsive to estrogen. Tamoxifen is as effective as other hormonal manipulations to which it has been compared and is usually the first drug used in the treatment of advanced, hormone receptor–positive breast cancer.

ADJUVANT HORMONAL THERAPY FOR OPERABLE BREAST CANCER. Because of its effectiveness in metastatic disease, tamoxifen has been tested as an adjuvant after surgical therapy or radiotherapy for operable breast cancer. Two large trials in the British Isles have received considerable attention. Significant prolongation of survival was noted in all treatment groups in the Nolvadex Adjuvant Treatment Organization (NATO). The Scottish Cancer Trials Office conducted a similar trial in which all groups of patients received benefit from 5 years of postoperative tamoxifen compared with a control group who were observed without therapy. The NSABP has recently reported the results of a placebo-controlled trial in the United States and Canada of tamoxifen in node-negative women, both pre- and postmenopausal. Early results show significant prolongation of relapse-free survival in both groups of patients under 49 years of age and in those patients over 50 years of age. An overview analysis recently summarized the results of many of these tamoxifen trials.

Summary of Adjuvant Chemotherapy and Hormonal Therapy

The current approach to the treatment of patients with operable breast cancer is summarized in Table 2. The recommendations are not a consensus statement but are a series of reasonable options for guiding physicians in counseling

TABLE 2. Recommendations for Adjuvant Treatment Outside Clinical Trials

Menopausal Status	Axillary Nodes	Tumor Characteristics*	Recommended Treatment
Pre-	Positive	Favorable or unfavorable	Combination chemotherapy†
Pre-	Negative	Favorable	No data to support adjuvant therapy
Pre-	Negative	Unfavorable	Combination chemotherapy acceptable
Post-	Positive	Favorable	Tamoxifen ± chemotherapy
Post-	Positive	Unfavorable	Chemotherapy ± tamoxifen
Post-	Negative	Favorable	No data to support adjuvant therapy
Post-	Negative	Unfavorable	No data to support adjuvant therapy

*Favorable tumor characteristics include size <2 cm., ER- or PgR-positive, nuclear and histologic grade good (1 or 2). Unfavorable tumor characteristics include size >2 cm., ER- or PgR-negative, nuclear and histologic grade poor (3).

†Combination chemotherapy is usually CMF × 6 months (9 cycles).

patients and for providing a framework for students of breast cancer. These recommendations are changing, and clinicians caring for patients with breast cancer must continue to seek new information and utilize consultants with specialized knowledge in breast cancer management.

22

RECONSTRUCTIVE AND AESTHETIC BREAST SURGERY

Gregory S. Georgiade, M.D.

Reconstructive and aesthetic breast surgery have an increasingly important role for the female patient. Aesthetic surgery of the breast consists of a number of procedures.

Augmentation mammaplasty is the most common aesthetic breast operation. This procedure for enlarging the volume of the breast mound can be accomplished by insertion of a Silastic prosthesis in the submammary or subpectoral area with use of an inframammary, circumareolar, transareolar, or axillary surgical approach. The Silastic prostheses can be single- or double-lumen, filled with silicone gel, or inflated with saline solution. The outer surface of the Silastic prostheses can be smooth-walled or microtextured to produce a roughened exterior wall, or polyurethane can be bound to the outer wall of the Silastic prostheses. These last two types have become quite popular, since there are indications that there is a considerable decrease in scar contracture around the prostheses with these irregular configurations of the outer shell, which disrupt the linear contractures that occur with the smooth-walled prostheses. However, the polyurethane-covered prostheses have been shown to disintegrate with time, disseminating small fragments of polyurethane into the tissues that are gradually absorbed.

Reduction mammaplasty is the second most common procedure. Breast hypertrophy with associated ptosis creates a severe functional deformity with associated mastodynia, shoulder and back pain, and skin excoriations. Reduction mammaplasty can be performed by use of a number of techniques. A vertical, superior, or inferior-based dermal pedicle can be utilized to move the nipple-areola complex and reduce the amount of breast tissue from the base of the breast. The contour of the basic breast mound that contains the nipple-areola can be maintained and the reduction of the breast volume achieved by excision of measured quantities of breast tissue in a semicircular manner around the central core of breast tissue. This procedure can be performed with or without the use of an inferior dermal pedicle.

Ptosis of the breast is recognizable as an aesthetic problem with varying degrees of deformity depending on the position of the nipple on the breast mound. Mild ptosis can be improved many times by an augmentation mammaplasty. In the more severe cases, if there is sufficient volume of breast tissue, the nipple-areola complex can be elevated on a dermal pedicle, and the excess tissues are then excised in the infra-areola area.

See the corresponding chapter or part in the *Textbook of Surgery*, 14th edition, pp. 551–555, for a more detailed discussion of this topic, including a comprehensive list of references.

Reconstruction of the breast following ablative surgery can be accomplished at the time of the initial modified radical mastectomy or simple mastectomy, or reconstruction can be performed at a later date. Patients undergoing radiation therapy or chemotherapy should not undergo reconstruction until therapy has been completed.

The usual type of reconstruction is similar, whether immediate or delayed. The standard procedure involves the creation of a pocket beneath the pectoralis major and serratus anterior muscles with extension of the undermining beneath the rectus fascia. A standard gel-filled Silastic implant or an inflatable prosthesis with a reservoir is inserted at the initial stage. When an acceptable breast mound has been attained, the final prosthesis is inserted and the nipple-areola is reconstructed by use of a full-thickness skin graft from the groin for the areola and nipple sharing, or a local chest flap is created for the nipple reconstruction with subsequent tattooing as needed on the nipple. Extensive loss of breast skin or underlying pectoralis musculature necessitates use of a latissimus dorsi musculocutaneous flap based on the thoracodorsal artery. The second alternative for larger defects is a rectus abdominis musculocutaneous flap based on the superior epigastric artery. A free microvascular rectus abdominis musculocutaneous flap should also be considered when simpler types of reconstruction are not available and in situations in which a large amount of breast coverage is needed and can be supplied only with large abdominal flaps. The management of the opposite breast in patients with unilateral carcinoma of the breast is a problem that should be dealt with during reconstruction of the patient's breast. A simple mastectomy or subcutaneous mastectomy should be considered in the overall treatment plan in selected patients. The use of the subcutaneous mastectomy is favored, when practical, and it is favored by most women who would like to have their nipple-areola preserved. This allows excision of approximately 95 per cent of the breast tissue, with a small amount of breast tissue left in the infra-areolar area for preserving the blood supply to the nipple-areola complex.

In summary, during the last decade a number of highly reliable techniques have been developed that allow correction of many different types of breast abnormalities. This allows improvement in many aesthetic abnormalities of breasts and reconstruction of extensive breast deformities after ablative surgery for breast malignancies. As these techniques have improved, the satisfaction of the patient and the aesthetic results have also improved.

23

THE THYROID GLAND

I

Historical Aspects and Anatomy
H. Kim Lyerly, M.D.

HISTORICAL ASPECTS

The first thyroidectomy was reportedly performed in A.D. 952 by Abul Casem Kahalaf Ebn Agbbas, a Moorish surgeon. However, only occasionally was successful extirpation of the thyroid performed because intraoperative death due to hemorrhage was common. Lister's discovery of antisepsis in 1867 and the development and use of hemostatic forceps around 1870 heralded a new era of thyroid surgery. In Switzerland, long known for its high incidence of goiter, Theodor Kocher performed his first thyroidectomy in 1872. His operative mortality was originally 13 per cent, but by 1898, Kocher reported a series of 600 patients with only a single death. At the end of his career, Kocher had performed more than 5000 thyroidectomies for goiter with the amazingly low mortality of only 1 per cent.

Kocher recognized that after thyroidectomy, one third of his patients developed signs and symptoms of what was later to be described as thyroid insufficiency. In 1891, Murray, Gley, and Vassale demonstrated improvement in a myxedematous patient after the administration of a sheep thyroid extract. Baumann established the presence of a high iodine content in thyroid tissue in 1896. Oswald prepared iodothyroglobulin in 1904. In 1915, Kendall isolated thyroxin, and in 1927, Harrington and Barger synthesized it. Antithyroid medication made preoperative control of hyperthyroidism possible, thus greatly reducing the risks of thyroid operations for hyperthyroidism.

ANATOMY

EMBRYOLOGY. The bulk of the thyroid gland develops in approximately the third to fourth week from the entoderm of the floor of the pharynx, evaginating, then descending to emerge as a bilobed diverticulum connected to the pharynx by a narrow stalk known as the thyroglossal duct. Usually obliterated when the fetus is 8 weeks old, it can be identified in the normal adult at its two ends: its origin in the tongue, found as the foramen cecum, which is located in the midline of the tongue at the junction of its anterior two thirds and

---

See the corresponding chapter or part in the *Textbook of Surgery*, 14th edition, pp. 556–560, for a more detailed discussion of this topic, including a comprehensive list of references.

posterior one third; and the thyroid end as a pyramidal lobe of the thyroid, found in 75 per cent of the population. The developing thyroid meets and accommodates tissue from the ultimobranchial bodies, which develop from branchial pouches at the fifth to sixth week to form C cells.

GROSS ANATOMY. The normal adult thyroid weighs approximately 15 to 20 gm. and has two lateral lobes, 4 cm. long and 2 cm. wide, found along the lower half of the lateral margins of the thyroid cartilage. The isthmus joins the two lobes just below the cricoid cartilage and usually obscures the second, third, and fourth tracheal rings anteriorly. A pyramidal lobe may arise from the isthmus. The immediate anterior relations of the gland are the sternothyroid muscles and sternohyoid muscles. More superficial is the investing fascia of the neck, encasing the sternocleidomastoid muscles laterally, with the anterior jugular veins in between. The sternothyroids lie on the thyroid capsule, meeting in the midline, and are innervated at their cranial ends by the descendens hypoglossi nerves and at the caudal end by the ansa hypoglossi.

Laterally and posteriorly the lobes of the thyroid are related to the carotid artery, the internal jugular vein, the cervical sympathetic trunk, and the inferior thyroid artery. Posteriorly and medially are the parathyroid glands, the recurrent laryngeal nerves, and the esophagus. The esophagus lies behind the trachea and larynx, and the recurrent laryngeal nerve ascends in the tracheoesophageal sulcus.

HISTOLOGY. The microscopic appearance of the thyroid demonstrates numerous follicles (acini) filled with proteinaceous colloid. The acini are arranged in subunits of 20 to 40 and demarcated by connective tissue to form lobules, each supplied by an individual artery. The height of the epithelial cells lining the follicles varies with the state of functional activity. The most prominent component of the cytoplasm is the rough endoplasmic reticulum. This organelle occupies most of the space in the basal and paranuclear parts of the cell and gives the follicle cell a strong resemblance to exocrine glandular cells. The follicular lumen is completely filled with a fine granular substance that appears homogeneous and moderately dense.

BLOOD SUPPLY AND LYMPH NODE DRAINAGE. The blood flow to the thyroid is 4 to 6 ml. per gm. per minute, primarily through the paired inferior thyroid arteries and the paired superior thyroid arteries. The recurrent laryngeal nerve lies in front of the inferior thyroid artery, among its branches, or behind it. The superior arteries, usually arising as the first branches from the external carotid arteries, are closely related to the superior laryngeal nerves; they enter the superior poles of the thyroid to divide into anterior and posterior branches. The thyroidea ima artery, a vestige of the embryonic aortic sac, varies from a minute vessel to one the size of the inferior thyroid artery and may originate from the innominate artery, the internal mammary artery, or the aortic arch; it may be present in up to 12 per cent of the population.

The superior thyroid veins drain to the internal jugular or common facial veins, the middle thyroid veins to the internal jugular veins, and the inferior thyroid veins to the brachio-cephalic veins. The thyroid has a lymphatic capillary network that drains to lymph nodes on the larynx above the isthmus (Delphian node), paratracheal nodes near the recurrent laryngeal nerve, and nodes on the anterior surface of the trachea. From these nodes, lymph drains to the cervical lymph node chains.

VARIANT ANATOMY. Complete or almost complete absence of the thyroid is said to occur in 1 of 10,000 live births and causes the infant to become a cretin. Most other variant anatomy involves the abnormal location of thyroid tissue. Thyroid tissue may be present in the anterior mediastinum. Substernal goiter may develop in this location and is often continuous with the cervical thyroid. The thyroid remains within its capsule, and the arterial supply and venous drainage of such a gland are by the normal routes. Rarely, posterior mediastinal thyroid tissue is found, and from it may arise large goiters that are usually not continuous with the cervical thyroid gland. Other abnormalities include thyroid tissue in the thyroglossal duct between the tongue and the root of the neck and a lingual thyroid gland, a very rare abnormality in which the thyroid gland develops in the tongue and may represent the only thyroid tissue.

Thyroglossal duct cysts and fistulas are conditions associated with a persistent thyroglossal duct. Thyroglossal duct cysts are most common in children at approximately the age of 5 years and usually present as painless cystic swellings in the midline in the region of the hyoid bone. Cysts frequently present with infection and are treated by incision and drainage of the cyst and subsequent excision of the fistula. The middle of the hyoid bone must be excised with the fistula because of its intimate relationship with the fistula.

An important anatomic anomaly of the recurrent laryngeal nerve is the so-called nonrecurrent laryngeal nerve on the right side. The nerve runs directly to the larynx and does not pass beneath the right subclavian artery.

II

Physiology
H. Kim Lyerly, M.D.

The thyroid gland functions primarily to produce thyroid hormone for development and regulation of metabolism. Thyroid hormone production is regulated by the anterior

---

See the corresponding chapter or part in the *Textbook of Surgery*, 14th edition, pp. 560–568, for a more detailed discussion of this topic, including a comprehensive list of references.

pituitary hormone thyrotropin, or thyroid-stimulating hormone (TSH), and by a system of autoregulation within the thyroid gland.

Iodine is necessary for the synthesis of thyroid hormones, and 200 to 500 μg. of iodine is ingested daily. The inorganic iodine is reduced to iodide ion in the intestine and absorbed and cleared from the bloodstream. The thyroid actively transports and concentrates iodide in the thyroid follicular cell at a rate of about 2 μg. per hour. Iodide is rapidly oxidized by thyroid peroxidase to bind tyrosine residues in thyroglobulin. After its synthesis and intracellular transport, thyroglobulin accumulates in the follicle lumen. The colloid that fills the follicle lumen is almost exclusively composed of iodinated thyroglobulin. After being bound to thyroglobulin, iodide proceeds to be part of thyroxin (T_4) and triiodothyronine (T_3) via monoiodotyrosine (MIT) and diiodotyrosine (DIT). By a complex coupling mechanism, two molecules of DIT combine to form T_4, and one molecule of DIT plus one molecule of MIT forms T_3.

Thyroglobulin breakdown and thyroid hormone release occur when colloid is engulfed and forms endocytotic vesicles that fuse with lysosomes. Proteases within these vesicles hydrolyze the thyroglobulin to iodothyronines, which are secreted. Approximately 1 per cent of the thyroid's hormone store is released into the circulation each day. The thyroid gland has a storage reserve of approximately 3 weeks. Although T_4 is the principal secretory product of the thyroid gland, the principal active hormone in metabolic regulation is T_3. Under normal circumstances, most T_3 is produced in the liver, heart, and kidneys by peripheral conversion of T_4. The concentration of total thyroxin is 30 to 50 times the concentration of T_3. However, only 0.03 per cent of the total serum T_4 and 0.3 per cent of the total serum T_3 is present in the unbound or biologically active form.

The major serum thyroid hormone–binding proteins are thyronine-binding globulin, (TBG), thyroxin-binding prealbumin, and albumin. Hormone-binding proteins are the principal intravascular factors influencing total hormone concentration. Because alterations in TBG may alter the total hormone concentration independently of the metabolic status of the body, free hormone, rather than the total hormone, is a more accurate indicator of the thyroid hormone–dependent metabolic state.

Thyroid hormones have numerous metabolic effects. Enhancement of the basal metabolic rate as reflected by increased oxygen consumption is one of the classic actions of thyroid hormone. An optimal amount is necessary for balanced growth and maturation. Many of the effects of thyroid hormones on carbohydrate metabolism appear permissive with respect to the effects of other hormones. They characteristically lower the level of serum cholesterol by enhanced excretion in the feces and conversion of cholesterol to bile acids. The generalized metabolic response increases the demand for vitamins and cofactors, and there is a magnified catecholamine effect produced by excess thyroid hormone.

The principal regulatory mechanisms of the thyroid gland are the hypothalamic-pituitary-thyroid control system and the intrathyroidal autoregulatory system.

THYROID-STIMULATING HORMONE (TSH). TSH is a glycoprotein hormone with alpha- and beta-subunits. The beta-subunit is responsible for its biologic and immunologic specificities. The normal serum concentration of TSH is 0.5 to 4.5 μunits per ml. TSH is required for the normal production and secretion of thyroid hormone and has a major role in thyroid growth. Iodide deficiency and blockers of iodide binding to thyroglobulin cause increased TSH secretion and thyroid enlargement.

THYROTROPIN-RELEASING HORMONE (TRH). TRH is a tripeptide (pyroglutamyl-histidylprolineamide) produced by the supraoptic and paraventricular nuclei of the hypothalamus that passes down their axons to the median eminence, where it is stored. Secretion into the pituicytes stimulates TSH secretion and synthesis, as well as prolactin release and synthesis. The primary role of TRH appears to be tonic stimulation of TSH-producing cells within the pituitary because the normal secretion of TSH and thyroid hormone is dependent on hypothalamic stimulation.

AUTOREGULATION OF THYROID FUNCTION. The thyroid gland has the intrinsic ability to alter the production and release of thyroid hormone. As iodide levels in plasma increase, there is an increase in the amount taken up and bound by the thyroid gland. After a critical amount of iodide accumulates, there is a progressive inhibition of iodide binding. The Wolff-Chaikoff block (acute block of iodide binding) is induced by an elevation of the plasma iodide concentration to approximately 25 μg. per 100 ml.

Monovalent anions including thiocyanate, perchlorate, and nitrate inhibit iodide uptake. Thiocyanate and perchlorate both stimulate discharge of free iodide from the thyroid gland, and thiocyanate also inhibits iodide binding and iodotyrosine coupling. Thionamides such as methimazole and propylthiouracil are commonly used antithyroid medications. They impair the covalent binding of iodine to thyroglobulin and iodide peroxidase.

THYROID FUNCTION TESTS

The fundamental issues in the evaluation of thyroid disease are the metabolic status of the patient, the etiology of the disease process responsible for the hormonal imbalance, and the etiology of the thyroid gland abnormality in the euthyroid patient.

THYROIDAL RADIOIODIDE UPTAKE (RAIU). After oral ingestion of ^{123}I (which has a short half-life and is associated with minimal radiation, compared with ^{131}I), the thyroid uptake as counted with a gamma counter is near its peak at 24 hours. Normal values for 24-hour RAIU in most parts of North America are approximately 15 to 30 per cent.

TOTAL THYROXIN AND TOTAL TRIIODOTHYRO-NINE (T_4 AND T_3). Measurement of T_4 and T_3 in serum and the estimation of their free concentration have become the most commonly used tests for the evaluation of thyroid hormone–dependent metabolic status. The usual concentration of T_4 in adults ranges from 5 to 11.5 μg. per 100 ml. Normal serum T_3 concentration in the adult is 80 to 190 ng. per 100 ml. Although total levels do not reflect the metabolic state of the patient, the free T_4 index remains a popular indirect measure of free T_4. Free T_3 and T_4 can be measured most specifically and easily by radioimmunoassay.

RESIN TRIIODOTHYRONINE UPTAKE (RT$_3$U). RT$_3$U measures the unoccupied thyroid hormone binding sites on TBG by measuring the competitive binding for radioactive T_3 between TBG and a resin and provides an indirect measure of T_4. The radioactive T_3 added to the system is bound preferentially by the resin if the thyroid hormone binding sites on TBG are occupied by T_4. The resin uptake of T_3 is directly proportional to the fraction of free T_4 in the serum and inversely related to the TBG binding sites. RT$_3$U is high in thyrotoxicosis. Normal values of RT$_3$U are 25 to 35 per cent. The test serves as an indirect measurement of the unbound fraction of T_4 and is valuable because it is simpler to perform than are other measurements of T_4. The free T_4 index is total T_4 multiplied by the ratio of the patient's RT$_3$U to the normal RT$_3$U:

$$FT_4I = TT_4 \times \frac{RT_3 U \text{ (Patient)}}{RT_3 U \text{ (Normal)}}$$

SERUM THYROGLOBULIN. Elevated serum levels are present in patients with goiter, hyperthyroidism, thyroiditis, and thyroid tumors. Serum thyroglobulin is suppressed in factitious thyrotoxicosis, a feature that helps differentiate this condition from subacute thyroiditis. The major clinical application of serum thyroglobulin levels is in the management of thyroid carcinoma, in which elevation may suggest recurrent disease.

SERUM CALCITONIN. Serum calcitonin is elevated in association with a number of conditions. Clinically, the most important is medullary thyroid carcinoma.

THYROTROPIN (TSH). Concentrations of TSH become elevated before there is any measurable reduction in serum T_4 and T_3, so the elevated TSH levels observed in primary hypothyroidism help confirm this diagnosis. Since reliable detection of low levels of TSH is difficult, a true absence of the hormone is difficult to distinguish from a nondetectable level that may be observed in some normal individuals. However, a low or undetected TSH level in association with a low thyroxin concentration is indicative of pituitary or hypothalamic disease.

THYROTROPIN STIMULATION TEST. This test is employed to differentiate primary thyroid failure from thyroid hypofunction caused by inadequate TSH stimulation. If an increase in radioactive iodine uptake of 10 per cent or more or a rise in T_4 of at least 2 μg. per 100 ml. can be demonstrated, it is likely that the thyroid can respond to exogenous TSH stimulation.

THYROID-RELEASING HORMONE (TRH) STIMULA- TION TEST. The TRH stimulation test measures the increase of pituitary TSH in serum in response to the administration of synthetic TRH. The magnitude of the TSH response to TRH is modulated by the thyrotrope response to active thyroid hormone and is thus inversely proportional to the concentration of free thyroid hormone in serum. The test provides a unique method of distinguishing between secondary and tertiary hypothyroidism. A TSH response is indicative of a hypothalamic disorder, and a failure to respond is compatible with intrinsic pituitary dysfunction.

THYROID SUPPRESSION TEST. This test is based on the principle that the administration of thyroid hormone suppresses the patient's thyroid function unless normal homeostatic mechanisms are disrupted. RAIU is performed after administration of thyroid hormone. Autonomously functioning thyroid tissue will continue to take up ^{123}I.

ANTITHYROID ANTIBODIES. The primary indications for measuring antithyroid antibodies include diagnosis of Hashimoto's disease and identification of those patients with Graves' disease who, by having antibodies, are particularly susceptible to hypothyroidism after subtotal thyroidectomy.

RADIOACTIVE SCANNING. Radioactive scanning is very useful in distinguishing a solitary nodule from a multinodular goiter. It is also helpful in localizing aberrant thyroid tissue in the tongue and in the line of the thyroid's descent in the midline of the neck.

ULTRASOUND SCANNING. Ultrasonography can be used to distinguish between solid and cystic lesions, which is a distinction that cannot be made by radioactive scanning.

BIOPSY AND FINE-NEEDLE ASPIRATION. Closed biopsy can be made by the Vim-Silverman or Tru-cut needle, which provides a core of tissue for histologic study. Another technique is fine-needle aspiration, in which cells are aspirated into a syringe barrel and then smeared onto a glass slide. These techniques can be helpful in diagnosing thyroiditis, anaplastic carcinoma, and malignant lymphoma. Analysis of DNA content in aspirated cells may also be helpful in delineating benign from malignant lesions.

III

Hyperthyroidism
H. Kim Lyerly, M.D.

Hyperthyroidism is caused by increased levels of thyroid hormone and loss of the normal feedback mechanism controlling the secretion of thyroid hormone. Common types of

See the corresponding chapter or part in the *Textbook of Surgery*, 14th edition, pp. 568–576, for a more detailed discussion of this topic, including a comprehensive list of references.

hyperthyroidism include diffuse toxic goiter (Graves' disease), toxic adenoma, and toxic multinodular goiter. Graves' disease is a systemic autoimmune syndrome with variable expression that includes goiter with hyperthyroidism, exophthalmos, pretibial myxedema, and acropachy. A thyroid adenoma is a benign neoplasia associated with excess secretion of thyroid hormone and is thus a localized disease. Uncommon causes of hyperthyroidism include thyrotoxicosis factitia, functioning metastatic thyroid carcinoma, trophoblastic tumors that secrete human chorionic gonadotropin having thyroid-stimulating properties, inappropriate secretion of thyrotropin by pituitary tumors, struma ovarii, iodide-induced hyperfunction, and thyroiditis.

GRAVES' DISEASE

The incidence of Graves' disease is 36 females and 8 males per 100,000 of the general population. The relative incidence of Graves' disease compared with adenomatous hyperthyroidism varies geographically, but Graves' disease is usually 3 to 10 times more common.

A hereditary component of Graves' disease is suggested by the increased incidence of clinical thyroid disorders and thyroid antibodies in families with Graves' disease and other autoimmune conditions that may be found in the same individual and within families. Susceptibility to the development of thyrotoxicosis in response to emotional upheaval appears to vary widely but has been reported. Consumption of iodide in excess of that normally available and use of thyroid hormone have also been implicated as activators of hyperthyroidism in various reports.

Although the origin of Graves' disease remains obscure, current evidence suggests it is an autoimmune disorder caused by thyroid-stimulating immunoglobulins that have been produced against an antigen in the thyroid. These polyclonal immunoglobulins appear to be directed to thyroid-stimulating hormone receptors and can be detected by radioreceptor assays. Substantial levels of thyroid-stimulating immunoglobulins are present in over 90 per cent of patients with active Graves' disease; these levels are sensitive and specific and correlate with the activity of hyperthyroidism. Thyroid-stimulating immunoglobulin levels have been reported to decrease to normal in approximately 50 per cent of patients treated with antithyroid medications or radioactive iodine and in 83 per cent after successful subtotal thyroidectomy.

The pathogenesis of ophthalmopathy is not understood as well as that of hyperthyroidism. Possibilities include pituitary exophthalmos-producing substances, circulating antibodies that bind specifically to eye muscle antigens, circulating lymphocytes sensitized to an antigen in the extraocular tissue, and a complex of thyroglobulin and antithyroglobulin antibody formed in the blood that is bound by the external orbital muscles.

CLINICAL FEATURES

The symptoms and signs of hyperthyroidism are well known and include heat intolerance, increased sweating, weight loss, hyperkinetic movements, insomnia, proximal muscle weakness, tremor, scant menses, tachycardia, and atrial fibrillation. The eye features of Graves' disease include a continuum from mere stare and lid lag to complete visual loss from corneal or optic nerve involvement. Hyperthyroidism is usually confirmed by measuring circulating thyroxin (T_4); however, other tests may be useful. Elevated radioactive iodine uptake is also diagnostic for hyperthyroidism. Thyroid suppression tests can diagnose hyperthyroidism because autonomously functioning thyroid should not be suppressible. Patients with Graves' disease also have a flat response to the thyroid-releasing hormone stimulation test.

TREATMENT

Thyroid hypersecretion can be controlled by reducing the functional mass of thyroid tissue with surgical removal of a large part of the gland or by destruction of most of the gland with radioiodine. Thyrotoxicosis can also be controlled with antithyroid drugs for reduction of the secretion of thyroid hormone, and by drugs that block beta-adrenergic receptors.

ANTITHYROID DRUGS. Thyrotoxicosis is effectively controlled by antithyroid drugs. Unfortunately, these agents may succeed in inducing a permanent remission in only a small minority of adults and in approximately 20 per cent of children. Prolonged use of these agents is limited because of toxic side effects such as rash, liver dysfunction, neuritis, arthralgia, myalgia, lymphadenopathy, psychosis, and the occasional development of irreversible agranulocytosis. Beta-receptor blockade, although effectively controlling some of the major effects of thyrotoxicosis, has not been effective as a sole means of therapy.

RADIOIODINE. Radioiodine therapy may be considered for thyrotoxicosis except in newborns, in pregnant females, or when it is precluded by a low iodine uptake. Treatment is highly effective, although progressive hypothyroidism requiring thyroid replacement is common.

SUBTOTAL THYROIDECTOMY. Indications for subtotal thyroidectomy for Graves' disease include (1) intolerance or noncompliance with antithyroid drug therapy and (2) contraindications to radioiodine therapy. Subtotal thyroidectomy is indicated for Graves' disease in children and adolescents, for women who are potential mothers, for patients under the age of 20 years who are unlikely to undergo remission because of a large goiter, and in those who do not experience a remission as indicated by persistent thyromegaly or the need to continue antithyroid medication beyond 1 or 2 years.

Surgical management of hyperthyroidism is directed to removal of sufficient thyroid tissue for rendering the patient euthyroid. Surgical risks are minimal but include recurrent laryngeal nerve injury, hypoparathyroidism, and permanent hypothyroidism.

PREOPERATIVE PREPARATION. Subtotal thyroidectomy should be performed after thyrotoxicosis is controlled medically. Propylthiouracil is used to inhibit thyroid hormone synthesis and limit peripheral conversion of T_4 and T_3. Thyroidectomy performed immediately after control of thyrotoxicosis is associated with a risk of thyroid crisis, and it is preferable to wait approximately 2 months after a patient is euthyroid.

Thyrotoxic patients are usually treated with iodide and iodine 10 days before operation to decrease the vascularity of the gland. Thyroid hormone, rather than iodine, can also be used to reduce the vascularity of the gland treated with propylthiouracil, because adequate doses of thyroid hormone suppress the thyroid-stimulating hormone increase associated with propylthiouracil and decrease the thyroid vascularity stimulated by that mechanism.

Beta-adrenergic blockade alone has been prescribed for preoperative preparation but is more commonly used as an adjunct to thionamides. Propranolol may be used alone or in conjunction with Lugol's solution in the preparation of the patient who is intolerant of antithyroid drugs or is noncompliant.

RESULTS. Subtotal thyroidectomy effectively and immediately controls thyrotoxicosis. The incidence of recurrent disease is inversely related to the incidence of hypothyroidism and is 1 to 5 per cent. Within 1 to 2 years, hypothyroidism may develop in 5 to 50 per cent of patients with a slight additional increase in subsequent years. The associated morbidity, related primarily to damage to the recurrent laryngeal nerves and parathyroid glands, is estimated to be 0.5 to 3 per cent.

THYROID STORM

The manifestations of thyroid storm include hyperthermia, tachycardia, intense irritability, profuse sweating, hypertension, extreme anxiety, eventual prostration, hypotension, and death. Sympatholytic treatment has been the most effective. Reserpine and guanethidine have been used to dissipate the thyroid crisis gently and effectively. Beta-adrenergic blockade is used to control the tachycardia, tremor, and anxiety. Oxygen is delivered, as well as liberal amounts of intravenous glucose. Intravenous sodium or potassium iodide (1 to 2.5 gm.) is also recommended. Large doses of adrenal steroids have been advised because cortisol breakdown is accentuated by excess thyroid hormone.

OPHTHALMOPATHY

Although exophthalmos frequently occurs in hyperthyroidism, the majority of patients require no heroic measures for a condition that is self-limiting and that to a variable degree regresses. Treatment is directed to reducing periorbital swelling and safeguarding against infection.

TOXIC ADENOMA

Hyperfunctioning adenomas are often first recognized on a thyroid scan, on which they appear as hot nodules. Often the patient is still euthyroid because even though the adenoma is hypersecreting independently of the pituitary feedback system, suppression of thyroid secretion from the normal gland maintains a physiologic net secretion rate of thyroid hormone. Only when the normal gland can no longer be suppressed does hyperthyroidism ensue.

CLINICAL FEATURES. In adenomatous disease, the recognition of symptoms is slower because an older age group is affected, especially in multinodular disease, since there is more commonly a predominance of cardiac symptoms. However, the only clinical aspect that clearly differentiates one from the other is the presence of ophthalmopathy, pretibial myxedema, or acropachy in patients with Graves' disease. The correct diagnosis may rest with the character of the goiter. When there is a toxic adenoma, paranodular tissue and the contralateral lobe are functionally suppressed and are usually minimally, if at all, palpable. The diagnosis is suggested by thyroid scanning after administration of radioiodine; when the diagnosis is in doubt, a suppression test can be useful. The autonomous nodule has persistently elevated radioactive iodine uptake, whereas normal thyroid tissue is suppressed.

TREATMENT. Surgical removal of the neoplasm can be offered to these patients. Thyroid nodules of various forms require a clear understanding for treatment, and these features are discussed in detail elsewhere. For purposes of control of hyperthyroidism, surgical excision of the thyroid lobe containing the hyperfunctioning adenoma is simple, safe, and effective. Radioactive iodine therapy for hot nodules is also effective, although there is a high risk of permanent hypothyroidism.

HYPERTHYROIDISM IN PREGNANCY

The management of such patients with hyperthyroidism is controversial. Radioactive iodine is absolutely contraindicated because destruction of the fetal thyroid would follow its use. Antithyroid drugs in conventional doses have a risk of development of fetal goiter that may obstruct the fetal airway at birth. Minimal-dose antithyroid drug therapy reduces this risk. In the middle trimester of pregnancy, subtotal thyroidectomy after a short course of antithyroid drugs and propranolol has been effective. So far as can be determined, the risks to the mother and to the fetus from the operation are comparable to those of nonoperative treatment.

IV

Thyroiditis
H. Kim Lyerly, M.D.

The term *thyroiditis* refers to the infiltration of the thyroid gland by inflammatory cells caused by a diverse group of infectious and inflammatory disorders. Inflammation of the thyroid may be organ-specific or part of a multisystem process and may be acute and self-limiting or chronic and progressive.

AUTOIMMUNE THYROIDITIS

The term *autoimmune thyroid disease* defines a group of conditions characterized by the presence of circulating thyroid antibodies and immunologically competent cells capable of reacting with certain thyroid constituents. These autoimmune thyroid diseases include Hashimoto's disease (lymphocytic thyroiditis), primary myxedema, and juvenile, fibrous, focal, and painless varieties of thyroiditis.

Hashimoto's Disease (Lymphocytic Thyroiditis)

Hashimoto's disease is the most common cause of goitrous hypothyroidism in adults and sporadic goiter in children. The incidence is 0.3 to 1.5 cases per 1000 population per year and is 10 to 15 times more common in women than in men; the highest incidence is in the age group of 30 to 50 years. In Hashimoto's disease, thyroid tissue damaged by immunologic factors is replaced by lymphocytes, plasma cells, and fibrosis. Antithyroid antibodies in the serum of patients with Hashimoto's disease were first discovered in 1957 by Doniach and Roitt. These antibodies have subsequently been demonstrated to be directed against elements in the thyroid cell or colloid. No antibodies to the thyroid-stimulating hormone receptor on the cell surface (as seen in Graves' disease) have been associated with Hashimoto's disease. Patients with Hashimoto's disease usually have detectable antithyroid antibodies at some time in the course of their disease. The mechanism causing antithyroid antibody formation and cell-mediated immune reactivity has not been fully established.

PATHOLOGY. The enlarged thyroid is pale and firm, with a finely nodular surface and a pale yellow color. On histologic examination, there is diffuse infiltration of the gland by lymphocytes and plasma cells, with formation of lymphoid follicles and germinal centers.

CLINICAL FEATURES. Symptoms of hypothyroidism in association with a painless, firm goiter are frequent present-

---

See the corresponding chapter or part in the *Textbook of Surgery*, 14th edition, pp. 576–579, for a more detailed discussion of this topic, including a comprehensive list of references.

ing complaints; however, patients may be euthyroid. The diagnosis of Hashimoto's disease begins by documenting hypothyroidism with thyroid function tests. Transient (2 to 8 weeks) hyperthyroidism may be present when inflammatory changes cause disruption of follicles with leakage of thyroid hormone into the circulation. Routine tests for thyroglobulin and microsomal antibodies should be performed because the presence and the titer of these antibodies correlate with the severity and extent of the autoimmune process. Hypothyroidism associated with a goiter but negative thyroid antibodies suggests use of goitrogen, a dyshormonogenetic goiter, or an endemic goiter.

If thyroid neoplasia is suspected clinically owing to asymmetry of the goiter, cervical lymphadenopathy, pressure symptoms, hoarseness, or enlargement of the goiter despite adequate thyroid replacement, fine-needle aspiration or open biopsy of the suspicious area should be performed. There is a strong relationship between thyroiditis and malignant thyroid lymphoma.

TREATMENT. Patients are usually followed medically, and replacement therapy with thyroxin (T_4) is begun in patients with hypothyroidism that is symptomatic or associated with a goiter that is causing pressure symptoms. Surgical reduction of goiter should be performed if severe pressure symptoms that have not responded to corticosteroid therapy are present; the operation usually consists of subtotal thyroidectomy. Biopsy for exclusion of malignancy in nodules suspicious for thyroid carcinoma (usually papillary) or lymphoma is performed as indicated.

DE QUERVAIN'S (SUBACUTE OR GIANT CELL) THYROIDITIS

Subacute thyroiditis represents approximately 1 per cent of all cases of thyroid disease, is much less common than is Hashimoto's thyroiditis, and has only one eighth the incidence of Graves' disease. It often follows upper respiratory tract infections, which suggests that it is due to a viral infection.

PATHOLOGY. There is generally moderate thyroid enlargement, which may be asymmetric. The inflammatory reaction involving the thyroid may cause adherence of the gland to the capsule and immediate extrathyroid tissues. Histologic features include desquamation of the follicular cells and disturbance and loss of colloid material.

CLINICAL FEATURES. Pain in the thyroid gland often develops relatively suddenly, often with radiation to the jaw and ears, and may be associated with marked tenderness and dysphagia. The gland is generally moderately enlarged. General laboratory findings include an increased erythrocyte sedimentation rate, a generalized increase in immunoglobulins, and a neutrophil leukocytosis or lymphocytosis in some patients. The changes in thyroid function are quite characteristic, with an early thyrotoxic stage followed by hypothyroidism and usually euthyroidism.

TREATMENT. This condition remits spontaneously after a variable period from a few days to a few months and relapses occasionally before the disease remits permanently. The treatment consists of analgesics such as aspirin or ibuprofen in mild cases. Steroids are effective in controlling symptoms in the more severe cases. However, spontaneous recovery is observed in over 90 per cent of patients, and therefore subtotal thyroidectomy is not indicated.

ACUTE SUPPURATIVE THYROIDITIS

This is a rare condition of the thyroid gland that is usually due to bacterial infection. Common pathogens include *Streptococcus, Staphylococcus, Pneumococcus,* and rarely *Salmonella* or *Bacteroides.* Normal thyroid glands are susceptible to infection, as are those with underlying disorders.

PATHOLOGY. Histologic examination of the gland reveals a marked polymorphonuclear leukocytic and lymphocytic infiltrate in the acute phase, which may be associated with frank thyroid necrosis and abscess formation. Fibrosis occurs with healing.

CLINICAL FEATURES. Symptoms occur with an acute onset and characteristically include tenderness, enlargement, warmth, erythema, and neck pain exacerbated by neck extension and swallowing. Septicemia or direct extension to the neck or chest may occur. Although the clinical characteristics of acute suppurative thyroiditis are usually straightforward, differentiation from de Quervain's thyroiditis is important.

TREATMENT. Primary treatment of suppurative thyroiditis consists of appropriate antibiotics against the causative organism. Thyroid abscesses should be drained, and cysts communicating with the piriform sinus or trachea require excision.

RIEDEL'S THYROIDITIS

Riedel's thyroiditis is a very rare inflammatory condition; it has been reported in only 20 of 42,000 surgical specimens of the thyroid at the Mayo Clinic. The etiology of invasive fibrous thyroiditis remains uncertain. It appears likely that the invasive fibrous thyroiditis represents one aspect of a generalized process that is not specifically related to the thyroid gland.

PATHOLOGY. The gland is involved wholly or in part by dense, invasive fibrosis that extends to include the surrounding tissues so that the capsule and anatomic margins of the gland cannot be precisely defined. There is no lymphocytic infiltrate in the tissue, but a lymphocytic perivasculitis is observed in most cases.

CLINICAL FEATURES. The patient generally presents with a history of rapid increase in thyroid size, which is frequently associated with symptoms of tracheal or esophageal compression. The gland is often described as "woody" in texture and is generally uniformly enlarged, nontender, and strikingly hard on palpation. It is often mistaken for thyroid carcinoma. There are no characteristic laboratory findings except absent to low titers of antithyroid antibodies. In late stages of disease, hypothyroidism may be present. The diagnosis can be confirmed only by biopsy.

TREATMENT. Medical therapy includes thyroid replacement if hypothyroidism is present. Surgical treatment is indicated if pressure symptoms in the neck require relief, and partial thyroidectomy is required in the majority of these patients. The operation requires meticulous dissection because fibrosis may involve surrounding structures such as the trachea, the carotid sheath, and the recurrent laryngeal nerve.

V

Nodular Goiter and Benign and Malignant Neoplasms of the Thyroid

George S. Leight, Jr., M.D.

MULTINODULAR GOITER

Goiter is a compensatory mechanism for inadequate thyroid hormone production. This may be caused by a deficiency of dietary iodine, dietary substances or medications that impair hormone synthesis, absence of an enzyme essential for hormone synthesis, or thyroiditis, which damages follicular cells and impairs hormone production. The final common pathway to goiter formation depends on the central role of thyroid-stimulating hormone (TSH) and its ability to promote thyroid growth.

Whereas large multinodular goiters rarely cause symptoms, the enlarging goiter can cause compression of neck structures, with resultant dysphagia, cough, respiratory compromise, or a feeling of fullness in the neck. Radiographs may show deviation or compression of the trachea. Presence of airway obstruction should be viewed with concern, since further airway compromise (foreign body, tracheitis with edema) could produce a respiratory emergency.

The treatment of goiter is based on suppression of TSH by administration of exogenous thyroid hormone. Although most multinodular goiters regress very little, these patients may be comfortable for many years on thyroid hormone replacement if the goiter remains stable. Indications for sur-

---

See the corresponding chapter or part in the *Textbook of Surgery*, 14th edition, pp. 579–590, for a more detailed discussion of this topic, including a comprehensive list of references.

gical therapy include the presence of obstructive symptoms or cosmetic problems related to the size of the goiter. Once obstructive symptoms occur, thyroid hormone replacement is unlikely to produce improvement. The goal of surgical therapy is to remove all the abnormal, nodular thyroid tissue, and this should correct the current problem and prevent recurrence of the goiter.

Substernal goiter is caused by the downward growth of the enlarged thyroid gland through the thoracic inlet into the mediastinum. Because the goiter is growing in a confined space with many critical structures, the potential for complications is significant. Substernal goiter rarely regresses with thyroid hormone suppression and is usually managed by surgical removal. The majority of substernal goiters can be removed through a standard cervical incision.

MANAGEMENT OF THYROID NODULES

Although thyroid nodules are common in the adult population (4 per cent), clinically evident thyroid carcinoma is quite rare. Thus, it is a challenge to select those patients who require surgical therapy from this large group with thyroid nodules. Physical examination findings suggestive of malignancy include firm texture, irregularity, fixation to surrounding structures, and enlarged ipsilateral cervical lymph nodes. Studies of thyroid function are of little value in establishing the benign or malignant nature of a thyroid nodule. Ultrasonography provides a noninvasive, radiation-free procedure that permits classification of a nodule as solid, cystic, or mixed; however, there are no specific ultrasonographic criteria for malignancy. Thyroid scintiscans using radioiodine or technetium have been widely used in evaluation of thyroid nodules. Malignant thyroid nodules usually do not organify iodine, and hypofunctional nodules are thus more likely to be malignant than are functioning nodules. Hyperfunctioning nodules are rarely malignant. Radionuclide scanning, however, does not clearly differentiate benign from malignant lesions.

Needle biopsy is now accepted as the most precise diagnostic screening procedure for differentiating benign from malignant thyroid nodules. Because it is safe, inexpensive, and accurate, needle aspiration biopsy is used routinely as the initial diagnostic technique in management of thyroid nodules. The important factors for a satisfactory test include a representative specimen from the nodule and an experienced cytologist to interpret the findings. Sampling errors may occur with lesions larger than 4 cm., and lesions smaller than 1 cm. may be difficult to aspirate. A correct diagnosis is achieved in over 90 per cent of papillary, medullary, and undifferentiated carcinomas. Accuracy in follicular carcinoma is approximately 40 per cent because of the difficulty in distinguishing benign from malignant follicular tumors. When a hypercellular aspirate is obtained, these lesions are classified as follicular tumors or suspicious for malignancy and should be removed surgically unless they are hyperfunctioning on radionuclide scanning. Those hypofunctioning by scan require surgical resection, since approximately 20 per cent are thyroid carcinomas. Nodules that are benign by needle aspiration biopsy must be followed with repeat aspirations periodically, since there is a 10 per cent false-negative diagnosis rate. Despite these limitations, needle biopsy has reduced the number of patients requiring surgery while increasing the incidence of malignancy in resected nodules.

THYROID CARCINOMA

Thyroid carcinoma occurs with an incidence of approximately 36 to 60 cases per million population per year. The annual mortality from thyroid carcinoma in the United States is only six persons per million. This discrepancy between the incidence and the mortality presumably reflects the favorable prognosis for most thyroid carcinomas. The importance of irradiation as an etiologic factor in the development of thyroid carcinoma in humans is well documented. Exposure of the thyroid gland to external radiation is directly related to the subsequent development of benign and malignant thyroid nodules. The malignancies that develop begin to appear within 3 to 5 years after radiation exposure and reach a peak incidence at 15 to 25 years after exposure. The types of thyroid cancer seen in this group are similar to those that develop in nonirradiated individuals of comparable age, with papillary or mixed papillary-follicular tumors predominating. A characteristic difference of the radiation-associated tumors is the presence of tumor multicentricity, which is found in up to 55 per cent of the irradiated patients. The natural history of radiation-associated thyroid carcinoma is basically the same as in nonirradiated patients in the same age group.

Age at the time of diagnosis has consistently been shown to have a profound influence on prognosis in patients with well-differentiated thyroid carcinomas. Children and young adults have an excellent prognosis despite the fact that a high percentage have nodal metastases at the time of diagnosis. Patients under 40 years of age have a better prognosis than do older patients in whom the disease is more aggressive. The prognosis in follicular carcinoma is slightly less favorable than with papillary carcinoma; the prognosis is generally poorer in patients with medullary carcinoma and is least favorable in those with undifferentiated cancer. The influence of nodal metastases on prognosis is controversial, but generally this represents a more extensive thyroid tumor and is associated with an increased recurrence rate and a poorer prognosis. Patients whose cancers have invaded into the adjacent neck structures have a poorer prognosis, and the presence of distant metastases is associated with the poorest prognosis.

Most experienced surgeons agree that thyroid lobectomy and isthmusectomy is the appropriate initial procedure for a thyroid nodule that might be cancer. Small anterior nodules or nodules at the isthmus may be locally resected with the anterior third of each lobe. If the nodule is found to be papillary carcinoma by frozen section, surgical options include lobectomy, near-total thyroidectomy, and total thyroidectomy. As the extent of thyroidectomy increases, the risk of complications such as recurrent nerve injury and hypoparathyroidism also increases. The extent of thyroidectomy is best determined by the extent to which the thyroid gland is involved with the tumor. Total thyroidectomy would be appropriate in patients with gross evidence of extensive bilateral carcinoma. Many surgeons feel that this procedure should be used in all patients whose tumors are larger than 1.5 cm. Others advocate thyroid lobectomy or near-total thyroidectomy for papillary carcinoma confined clinically to one lobe. They report that the more extensive total thyroidectomy does not improve survival but substantially increases the complication rate. Until more conclusive studies establishing the optimal surgical procedures for papillary carcinoma are available, and since papillary carcinoma usually has an excellent prognosis, the more extensive operations should be performed only if they can be done with very low morbidity.

Patients with papillary thyroid carcinoma frequently have metastatic involvement of regional lymph nodes, but routine prophylactic neck dissection in these patients is not indicated. When total thyroidectomy is performed for papillary carcinoma, the central neck nodes including nodes in the ipsilateral tracheoesophageal groove, in the pretracheal area, along the recurrent laryngeal nerve and inferior thyroid veins, and in the anterior mediastinum are removed with the operative specimen. In patients with palpably enlarged lateral cervical nodes, most surgeons feel that their removal by modified neck dissection is indicated.

Follicular carcinoma constitutes 15 to 20 per cent of thyroid cancers, and these tumors typically occur in older patients with a peak incidence in the fifth decade of life. This lesion has a marked propensity for vascular invasion but does not invade lymphatic channels, and lymph node metastases are much less common than in papillary carcinoma. Follicular carcinoma frequently disseminates hematogenously with bone, lung, brain, and liver as the most frequent sites of metastases. The minimally invasive follicular carcinoma is rarely multicentric, rarely metastasizes, and is generally associated with an excellent prognosis. These well-differentiated follicular carcinomas can be safely managed by total lobectomy as long as they are confined to one lobe. The widely invasive follicular carcinoma is the most aggressive of the well-differentiated thyroid cancers, frequently showing extension through the thyroid capsule into surrounding structures. The prognosis in these patients is poor, and those who present with locally aggressive tumors or proven metastatic disease are best treated with near-total or total thyroidectomy, which optimizes the effectiveness of ^{131}I treatment for residual or distant disease.

Undifferentiated or anaplastic carcinomas are predominantly seen in patients over age 50 years with a peak incidence of approximately 65 years of age. This tumor is the most aggressive of all thyroid malignancies and constitutes

5 to 10 per cent of thyroid cancers. By the time of diagnosis, the majority of undifferentiated carcinomas have spread locally to vital structures in the neck, precluding surgical resection. In patients with diffuse infiltrative lesions, surgical resection or debulking is rarely indicated. Instead, therapy with external radiotherapy and chemotherapy may provide limited palliation.

Primary malignant lymphoma of the thyroid is a rare malignancy that typically presents as a rapidly enlarging, firm, painless mass in older women. Following diagnosis, appropriate staging should be performed to determine the extent of disease. Patients with local disease are treated with radiation therapy, since the lesion is quite radiosensitive. In patients in whom lymphoma is discovered at the time of operation, survival is unaffected by the extent of operation even if only biopsy is obtained. The surgical procedure should be limited to securing a diagnostic specimen, since more aggressive procedures may increase morbidity without improving survival. Patients with more extensive disease or those who relapse are treated with chemotherapy.

The role of radioiodine in the postoperative management of patients with well-differentiated thyroid carcinoma remains controversial, but it must be remembered that numerous convincing studies have demonstrated that the lowest recurrence and death rates are found in patients who have received both radioiodine and thyroid hormone suppression. This survival advantage is seen primarily in patients with follicular and mixed papillary-follicular tumors. In order for the radioiodine to be most effective, the normal thyroid tissue must first be removed, since it accumulates the isotope more avidly than do thyroid cancers. Postoperative ^{131}I scans are usually performed 2 to 3 months following operation for well-differentiated thyroid carcinoma. Patients with significant residual functioning tissue and evidence of metastatic disease are candidates for radioiodine ablation. Ablation of residual thyroid tissue can usually be accomplished with one dose of 30 mc. of ^{131}I; patients with metastatic deposits in the neck are given 75 to 100 mc., and those with distant metastases are given 150 to 200 mc. Radioiodine scan and treatment are then repeated at 6- to 9-month intervals until tumor uptake of the isotope is abolished or adverse effects of radioiodine are encountered.

Nearly all patients who undergo operation for well-differentiated thyroid carcinoma should receive thyroid hormone. This may be necessary for preventing hypothyroidism, but in addition there is clear evidence that TSH can stimulate growth of differentiated thyroid carcinoma and that thyroid hormone given in adequate doses is beneficial because of its TSH suppressive effect. Serum thyroglobulin measurements are helpful in determining the presence of recurrent disease in patients who have undergone ablative therapy of all thyroid tissue. Increasing levels of thyroglobulin in these patients are suggestive of disease recurrence.

VI

The Multiple Endocrine Neoplasias

Terry C. Lairmore, M.D. and Samuel A. Wells, Jr., M.D.

Tumors of the endocrine system most often develop within a single gland. There are inherited disorders, however, that are characterized by the development of neoplasms in multiple endocrine glands. The multiple endocrine neoplasia (MEN) syndromes are classified according to the pattern of involvement. In its full expression, MEN I is characterized by the concurrence of parathyroid hyperplasia, pancreatic islet cell neoplasms, and adenomas of the anterior pituitary. Multiple endocrine neoplasia IIa (MEN IIa) is characterized by the concurrence of medullary thyroid carcinoma (MTC), pheochromocytoma, and parathyroid hyperplasia; MEN IIb consists of MTC, pheochromocytoma, mucosal neuromas, a distinctive "marfanoid" habitus, and the absence of parathyroid disease. These syndromes are all transmitted as Mendelian autosomal dominant traits.

MULTIPLE ENDOCRINE NEOPLASIA TYPE I

The clinical expression of MEN I most often develops in the third or fourth decade, and the onset of symptoms is rare before the age of 10 years. Males and females are affected equally. The gene for MEN I is transmitted with nearly 100 per cent penetrance, but with variable expressivity, such that each affected individual exhibits some but not necessarily all of the components of the syndrome. The most common abnormality in MEN I is parathyroid hyperplasia, which occurs in approximately 90 to 97 per cent of patients, followed by pancreatic islet cell neoplasms (30 to 80 per cent) and pituitary adenomas (15 to 50 per cent). The clinical manifestations of patients with MEN I are caused by either overproduction of hormones by the endocrine tumor or the effects of the tumor mass itself.

PARATHYROIDS. The most common endocrine abnormality in MEN I is hyperparathyroidism, which occurs in greater than 90 per cent of patients. The characteristic pathologic lesion is generalized parathyroid hyperplasia with involvement of all four glands. In contrast, fewer than 20 per cent of patients with sporadic primary hyperparathyroidism have multiglandular involvement.

Hyperparathyroidism is usually the first biochemical abnormality detected in patients with MEN I and may precede

---

See the corresponding chapter or part in the *Textbook of Surgery*, 14th edition, pp. 590–597, for a more detailed discussion of this topic, including a comprehensive list of references.

the clinical onset of an islet cell or pituitary neoplasm by several years. In many patients, asymptomatic hypercalcemia is present over a long period of observation. Symptomatic patients may develop renal or ureteral lithiasis or nephrocalcinosis. Skeletal manifestations of hyperparathyroidism occur but are uncommon. Diagnosis is made by measurement of serum calcium, phosphate, and parathormone levels.

Patients with parathyroid disease in MEN I have been treated with subtotal (3½ gland) parathyroidectomy in an attempt to resect almost all abnormal tissue. However, in contrast to patients with primary hyperparathyroidism, persistent or recurrent disease has been as high as 30 to 40 per cent. Alternatively, patients with multiglandular hyperplasia can be treated by total parathyroidectomy with autotransplantation of parathyroid tissue into the forearm. The advantage of this procedure includes easier management of recurrent disease by excision of grafted parathyroid tissue under local anesthesia.

PANCREAS. The most common pancreatic islet cell lesion in patients with MEN I is gastrinoma. Clinically, patients present with a severe peptic ulcer diathesis caused by autonomous gastrin hypersecretion. Gastrinomas associated with MEN I represent 20 to 50 per cent of all cases of the Zollinger-Ellison syndrome. The diagnosis of gastrinoma is made by documentation of hyperacidity with abnormally elevated levels of serum gastrin. Approximately 15 per cent of gastrinomas associated with MEN I are malignant. Owing to the characteristic diffuse nature of these neoplasms, preoperative and intraoperative localization may be difficult. A small percentage may be localized preoperatively by computed tomographic scanning or angiography.

Previously, the accepted surgical therapy for intractable peptic ulcer disease in patients with unresectable gastrinoma was total gastrectomy, since a total pancreatectomy would have been required to resect the multicentric tumor. The use of H_2-receptor antagonists has been effective in controlling the acid hypersecretion and its complications. Patients treated in this manner may have an indolent course and tolerate their metastases well for a long time.

The second most common islet cell neoplasm of the pancreas in patients with MEN I is insulinoma. Approximately 10 per cent are malignant. Insulinomas in association with MEN I are usually small (less than 1 cm.) and multiple. In contrast, approximately 80 per cent of sporadic insulinomas are solitary. Patients commonly present with recurrent symptoms of neuroglycopenia: sweating, dizziness, confusion, or syncope. The diagnosis of insulinoma is made by the measurement of plasma insulin during a prolonged fast. The documentation of hypoglycemia with inappropriately elevated plasma insulin levels strongly suggests the diagnosis of insulinoma. Surgical extirpation of macroscopic tumor is the treatment of choice when feasible. Patients with diffuse disease may respond to chemotherapy with streptozotocin, and some control of glucose levels may be achieved by the administration of diazoxide, an inhibitor of insulin secretion.

Other pancreatic islet cell neoplasms, such as glucagonoma, somatostatinoma, and tumors secreting vasoactive intestinal peptide or pancreatic polypeptide, occur less commonly in association with MEN I.

PITUITARY. Pituitary neoplasms occur in 15 to 50 per cent of patients. Most of these tumors were formerly thought to be nonfunctioning chromophobe adenomas, but prolactin-secreting microadenomas may be the most common abnormality. Pituitary tumors cause symptoms by either hypersecretion of hormones or compression of adjacent structures. Pituitary tumors, either functioning or nonfunctioning, may require ablation by surgical therapy or irradiation.

OTHER TUMORS. Patients with MEN I may also develop adrenocortical tumors (40 per cent) or nonmedullary thyroid carcinomas (15 per cent). Lipomas and carcinoid tumors rarely occur in association with the MEN I syndrome.

MULTIPLE ENDOCRINE NEOPLASIA TYPES IIa AND IIb

The traits for MEN IIa and MEN IIb are transmitted in an autosomal dominant pattern with nearly 100 per cent penetrance and variable expressivity. Males and females are affected equally.

MEDULLARY THYROID CARCINOMA. Bilateral MTC occurs in nearly every affected individual with MEN IIa and MEN IIb. In addition, patients with MEN IIa may have associated pheochromocytoma (less than 50 per cent) or parathyroid hyperplasia (less than 50 per cent). Medullary thyroid carcinoma is usually the first abnormality expressed in both MEN IIa and MEN IIb, and in the majority of patients MTC is diagnosed either before or concurrently with pheochromocytoma. The peak incidence of MTC in the setting of MEN IIa is in the second or third decade, compared with a peak incidence in the fifth or sixth decade for sporadic MTC. Whereas sporadic MTC is almost always unilateral, in patients with MEN IIa or MEN IIb, MTC is nearly always bilateral. A diffuse premalignant proliferation of C-cells in the thyroid of patients with familial MTC has been described and termed C-cell hyperplasia. The presence of bilateral MTC or microscopic evidence of C-cell hyperplasia in areas of the thyroid adjacent to foci of MTC should strongly suggest familial disease.

Medullary thyroid carcinoma cells are capable of great biosynthetic activity and have been reported to secrete adrenocorticotropic hormone, prostaglandins, melanin, and serotonin. However, the most important product of MTC cells is calcitonin, which serves as a sensitive plasma tumor marker for diagnosing and following patients with this neoplasm. Asymptomatic members of kindreds with MEN IIa or MEN IIb may be diagnosed by demonstrating increased plasma calcitonin levels after provocative testing with secretagogues. The best provocative test is the sequential intravenous administration of calcium gluconate followed by pentagastrin. Patients at risk should undergo annual calcium pentagastrin stimulation testing beginning as early as age 5 years and continuing until the age of 40 to 45 years.

Patients whose MTC is diagnosed by provocative testing have smaller primary tumors and a lower incidence of regional lymph node and distant metastases when compared with patients whose MTC is diagnosed by physical examination. Also, the incidence of curative thyroidectomy is significantly higher in the former group (a parameter easily determined by measuring stimulated plasma calcitonin levels postoperatively). It is imperative that patients with hereditary MTC be identified by an aggressive screening program, since with early diagnosis and early thyroidectomy, MTC is curable in a large percentage of patients.

Medullary thyroid carcinoma, whether sporadic or familial, should be treated by total thyroidectomy with a prophylactic dissection of the central zone lymph nodes between the jugular veins and from the hyoid bone to the sternal notch. Meticulous removal of all thyroid tissue should be undertaken at initial operation to prevent recurrence in a thyroid remnant.

PHEOCHROMOCYTOMA. The pheochromocytomas in patients with MEN IIa and MEN IIb usually appear in the second or third decade of life. Approximately 60 to 80 per cent are bilateral, compared with 10 per cent of sporadic pheochromocytomas. The pheochromocytomas are generally limited to the adrenal medulla and are almost always benign. A diffuse involvement of the adrenal medulla termed adrenal medullary hyperplasia may precede the development of pheochromocytoma in MEN IIa and MEN IIb. The pheochromocytomas in MEN IIa and MEN IIb may either be clinically silent or produce dramatic clinical symptoms. When symptomatic, the adrenal lesions can produce severe pounding frontal headaches, episodic diaphoresis, palpitations, vague feelings of anxiety, and paroxysmal hypertension.

The diagnosis of pheochromocytoma in patients with MEN IIa and MEN IIb is made biochemically by measurement of the urinary excretion of catecholamines and catecholamine metabolites (metanephrines and vanillylmandelic acid). Patients with elevated levels of one or more components of the 24-hour urine catecholamine determinations should be evaluated further by computed tomography of the adrenal glands bilaterally. If pheochromocytoma is detected, the patient should have a bilateral subcostal incision and exploration of both adrenal glands and the sympathetic chain. Bilateral involvement requires bilateral adrenalectomy. Although a matter of some controversy, in patients with unilateral pheochromocytoma and a palpably normal contralateral gland at operation, it is acceptable policy to perform a unilateral adrenalectomy.

PARATHYROIDS. Hyperfunction of the parathyroid glands in patients with MEN IIa is the most variable component of the syndrome. Many patients are asymptomatic, and recognition of the parathyroid lesions stems from the finding of hypercalcemia during routine laboratory studies. As in patients with MEN I, advanced signs of hyperparathyroidism, such as osteitis fibrosa cystica or nephrocalcinosis, are unusual.

The characteristic parathyroid lesion in patients with MEN IIa is hyperplasia with involvement of all four glands. In patients with documented hypercalcemia, one can expect to find enlarged parathyroid glands at operation. However, grossly enlarged parathyroid glands may be found during thyroidectomy for MTC in a patient in whom hyperparathyroidism has never been documented. Although some surgeons would perform a subtotal (3½ gland) parathyroidectomy in patients with parathyroid hyperplasia and MEN IIa, the authors prefer total parathyroidectomy with autografting of parathyroid tissue into the forearm musculature. In patients without hypercalcemia undergoing thyroidectomy for MTC, grossly normal parathyroid glands should be left in place with a carefully preserved blood supply.

NONENDOCRINE MANIFESTATIONS OF MEN IIb. The rarer MEN IIb syndrome occurs sporadically or is transmitted in an autosomal dominant pattern. Significantly, the MTC in MEN IIb occurs earlier and is a much more aggressive neoplasm biologically when compared with that in MEN IIa.

In addition to MTC and pheochromocytoma, patients with MEN IIb develop several nonendocrine derangements, principally involving the peripheral nerves and the musculoskeletal system. Unlike patients with MEN I or MEN IIa, these patients have a characteristic phenotype, including a tall, thin "marfanoid" body habitus. Multiple neuromas develop on the lips, tongue, and oral mucosa, producing thick, "bumpy" lips. Slit lamp examination of the eyes often reveals hypertrophied corneal nerves. Patients may develop diffuse ganglioneuromatosis of the gastrointestinal tract, characterized microscopically by hypertrophy and nerve fiber disarray of the myenteric and submucosal plexuses. A history of chronic constipation or recurrent crampy abdominal pain may be present owing to the disordered motility of the gut. Contrast studies may reveal evidence of colonic dilatation or megacolon. There is also a high incidence of skeletal anomalies, including congenital dislocation of the hip, pes planus or cavus, pectus excavatum, and kyphosis. Clinical hyperfunction of the parathyroid glands is not a component of the MEN IIb syndrome.

24

THE PARATHYROID GLANDS

Stanley W. Ashley, M.D., and Samuel A. Wells, Jr., M.D.

The physiologic role of the parathyroid glands is the endocrine control of calcium homeostasis. This function is mediated through the production of parathyroid hormone (PTH). The major clinical disorders affecting the parathyroids involve either over- or undersecretion of PTH—hyper- or hypoparathyroidism. *Primary hyperparathyroidism* occurs when the normal feedback control of serum calcium is disturbed and there is overproduction of PTH. *Secondary hyperparathyroidism* develops most commonly in patients with renal disease; there is a defect in mineral homeostasis causing a compensatory increase in gland function. Occasionally a hyperplastic compensatory gland develops autonomous function, a condition referred to as *tertiary hyperparathyroidism*. *Hypoparathyroidism* is most frequently seen as a surgical complication of either the thyroid or parathyroid glands.

EMBRYOLOGY AND ANATOMY

The superior parathyroids arise from the fourth branchial pouch along with the lateral thyroid. The origin of the inferior parathyroids is the third branchial pouch in conjunction with the thymus. Although the four glands are most commonly identified on the posterior aspect of the upper and lower lateral thyroid lobes, they may be found anywhere from the musculature of the pharynx to the deep mediastinum, spanning the origin and the end of migration of their respective *branchial pouch* structures. Ectopic superior glands tend to migrate posteriorly along the esophagus and into the mediastinum. Inferior glands are most commonly found in association with the thymus. There are nearly always at least four parathyroids. Five glands are found approximately 4 per cent of the time.

The parathyroid glands tend to be flat and ovoid in shape and are yellow-brown in color. Normally they measure 2 × 3 × 7 mm. with a combined weight of 90 to 200 mg. The arterial supply is most commonly from a branch of the inferior thyroid artery; the venous drainage is highly variable. On histologic examination, they are composed of a parenchyma of hormonally active cells and a stroma composed primarily of adipocytes. The functional significance of the various cell types remains unclear, although the chief cell appears to be the predominant type.

See the corresponding chapter or part in the *Textbook of Surgery,* 14th edition, pp. 598–615, for a more detailed discussion of this topic, including a comprehensive list of references.

PHYSIOLOGY

The parathyroid glands are critical in the normal control of calcium homeostasis. PTH and vitamin D are the major regulators of calcium and phosphate metabolism. *Calcium* is a critical constituent of all body fluids and is intimately involved in a number of physiologic processes ranging from blood coagulation to bone formation. It represents a major cellular messenger and is critical in muscle contraction and membrane repolarization. Calcium in the inorganic form is absorbed from the upper small intestine. On a regular diet, approximately 1 gm. is ingested daily. The calcium in the extracellular fluid is constantly being exchanged with that in the exchangeable bone pool, the intracellular fluid, and the glomerular filtrate. Normal plasma calcium measures 9 to 10.6 mg. per 100 ml. (4.5 to 5.2 mEq. per liter) and is about equally divided between an ionized, or metabolically active, and a protein-bound phase. Total serum calcium is affected by the concentration both of albumin, the major calcium-binding protein, and of hydrogen ion, which displaces calcium from albumin.

Plasma phosphate measures 2.6 to 4.3 mg. per 100 ml. and varies inversely with the calcium such that the product of their concentrations is constant and measures between 30 and 40.

The primary agents responsible for *regulation of calcium metabolism* are PTH, vitamin D, and calcitonin. Their major actions are summarized in Table 1. Briefly, a reduction in serum ionized calcium increases secretion of PTH, which secondarily stimulates hydroxylation of 25(OH) vitamin D to metabolically active 1,25(OH)$_2$ vitamin D$_3$ in the kidney. Through their actions on bone, renal reabsorption, and intes-

TABLE 1. Actions of Major Calcium-Regulating Hormones

	Bone	Kidney	Intestine
Parathyroid hormone	Stimulates reabsorption of calcium and phosphate	Stimulates reabsorption of calcium and conversion of 25(OH)D$_3$ to 1,25(OH)$_2$D$_3$ Inhibits reabsorption of phosphate and bicarbonate	No direct effects
Vitamin D	Stimulates transport of calcium	Inhibits reabsorption of calcium	Stimulates absorption of calcium and phosphate
Calcitonin	Inhibits reabsorption of calcium and phosphate	Inhibits reabsorption of calcium and phosphate	No direct effects

tinal absorption, these hormones act to increase serum calcium. Calcitonin's action actually tends to reduce serum calcium although it has never been demonstrated to be important in the control of serum calcium in man.

PARATHYROID DISORDERS

Primary Hyperparathyroidism

The *incidence* of hyperparathyroidism is approximately 25 per 100,000, and 50,000 new cases occur annually. The incidence increases markedly with age, and it is especially common in postmenopausal women.

ETIOLOGY. The etiology of hyperparathyroidism is unknown. A sustained stimulus to PTH production, such as the renal calcium leak that occurs with age, has been postulated but never proved. There appears to be an association with small-dose ionizing radiation to the neck, usually in childhood. Recent studies have suggested the presence of chromosomal deletions in some parathyroid adenomas, although the implications of this finding remain to be determined.

PRESENTATION. Whereas in the past most patients presented with severe bone or renal disease, as a result of increased routine screening for calcium and phosphate, approximately half of patients today are *asymptomatic*. When carefully questioned, however, many of these patients describe symptoms or associated conditions that can be related to hyperparathyroidism. The most frequent symptoms in 100 sequential patients evaluated in the authors' clinic are shown in Table 2. The earliest complaints are nonspecific and include muscle weakness, anorexia, nausea, constipation, and polyuria. *Renal complications* are generally the most serious. Of patients presenting with nephrolithiasis, approximately 5 to 10 per cent have hyperparathyroidism. Although renal stones may be removed, calcification of the renal parenchyma (nephrocalcinosis) seldom improves even after parathyroidectomy. Some abnormality in renal function is detectable in 80 to 90 per cent of patients with hyperparathyroidism. *Hypertension*

TABLE 2. Presenting Symptoms in 100 Patients with Primary Hyperparathyroidism

Symptoms	Percentage of Population
Nephrolithiasis	30
Bone disease	2
Peptic ulcer disease	12
Psychiatric disorders	15
Muscle weakness	70
Constipation	32
Polyuria	28
Pancreatitis	1
Myalgia	54
Arthralgia	54

with its complications (heart failure, arterial hemorrhage, and renal insufficiency) has been associated with hyperparathyroidism. The relationship is unknown although it appears related to the degree of renal impairment. The hypertension may or may not improve in patients after parathyroidectomy.

Symptomatic *bone disease* develops in 5 to 15 per cent of patients. In its most severe form, it is referred to as osteitis fibrosa cystica, a disease entity that is characterized by bone pain and secondary fractures. Radiologic findings include subperiosteal resorption most evident on the radial aspect of the middle phalanx of the second and third fingers and a mottled cystic appearance to the skull. Osteoclastomas or "brown tumors" may be present. In general, bone and renal disease tend not to occur in the same patients, and patients with bone disease often have a higher serum calcium and larger, more rapidly growing tumors.

Gastrointestinal manifestations including associations with peptic ulcer, pancreatitis, and cholelithiasis have been reported but not confirmed by all investigators. Their relationship with hyperparathyroidism remains controversial. The hypercalcemia is also associated with neurologic and *psychiatric disturbances* ranging from depression and anxiety to psychosis and coma. These abnormalities may resolve following parathyroidectomy.

Abnormal calcium deposition in hyperparathyroidism is associated with the development of chondrocalcinosis and pseudogout. Vascular calcification, skin necrosis, and band keratopathy of the cornea all occur. Muscle weakness and fatigue may also develop.

Diagnosis

The laboratory diagnosis of hyperparathyroidism depends on the documentation of an elevated *serum calcium* in conjunction with an elevated PTH. Normal values for calcium range from 8.5 to 10.5 mg. per 100 ml. Because of variations in serum protein and pH, the measurement of ionized calcium is the more accurate determination. This technique is still somewhat cumbersome but is becoming more readily available clinically.

On release from the parathyroid, *PTH* is cleaved into a biologically active amino-terminal fragment and an inactive carboxy-terminal fragment. The carboxy-terminal fragment has a longer half-life and has been more useful for radioimmunoassay determinations. An elevated PTH is diagnostic of hyperparathyroidism only in the presence of an elevated serum calcium.

Half of patients with hyperparathyroidism have hypophosphatemia, the normal range being 2.5 to 4.5 mg. per ml. They also often have a *hyperchloremic metabolic acidosis* as a result of increased bicarbonate excretion. The chloride:phosphate ratio, when elevated (greater than 33), is highly suggestive of hyperparathyroidism. In patients with bone disease, the *alkaline phosphatase* is frequently elevated.

Less Common Manifestations

Hyperparathyroidism can occur in a *familial* form both as an isolated disease and in association with multiple endocrine neoplasia (MEN) Types I and II. MEN I is characterized by parathyroid hyperplasia, pituitary adenomas, and pancreatic islet cell neoplasms. Type II consists of medullary thyroid carcinoma, pheochromocytoma, and parathyroid hyperplasia. Familial hypocalciuric hypercalcemia is a recently described entity characterized by generalized parathyroid enlargement that is associated with minimal morbidity and is very difficult to cure surgically.

Parathyroid Carcinoma

Parathyroid carcinoma is rare, representing less than 1 per cent of patients with hyperparathyroidism. The diagnosis is made on the basis of histologic evidence of local invasion or metastases. Characteristically, the serum concentrations of calcium, PTH, and alkaline phosphatase are markedly elevated when compared with levels in patients with benign parathyroid tumors. In half of patients, the parathyroid carcinoma is palpable. The majority of patients are symptomatic, and both the kidneys and the skeleton are commonly affected. Treatment involves radical resection of the involved gland, the ipsilateral thyroid, and the adjacent soft tissues and regional lymph nodes. Neither chemotherapy nor radiotherapy offers any benefit, and the 10-year survival is less than 20 per cent.

Hyperparathyroid Crisis

Occasionally hyperparathyroid patients may become acutely ill with urgent symptoms that can prove fatal. Serum calcium is almost always markedly elevated in the range of 16 to 20 mg. per 100 ml., and the symptoms are similar to those seen in *severe hypercalcemia* accompanying other diseases. They include rapidly developing muscle weakness, nausea and vomiting, weight loss, fatigue, and confusion. The evolution of this syndrome appears to involve uncontrolled PTH secretion followed by hypercalciuria, polyuria, dehydration, and subsequent worsening hypercalcemia. Initial *management* is similar to that for other causes of acute hypercalcemia. Diuresis is initiated, first with normal saline infusion, and then, when adequate hydration is assured, by the addition of furosemide. A variety of other agents are available if the free calcium in the serum remains elevated (Table 3). Definitive therapy in the case of hyperparathyroidism involves neck exploration and resection of the hyperfunctioning tissue.

Secondary Hyperparathyroidism (Renal Osteodystrophy)

Secondary hyperparathyroidism develops as a result of the metabolic alterations in chronic renal failure patients on

TABLE 3. Agents Used in the Treatment of Hypercalcemia

Agent	Dosage	Administration	Comment
Calcitonin	2–6 MRC units/kg. 10–20 MRC units	Subcutaneous, every 6–8 hr. Intravenously, hourly	Nausea and vomiting are side effects: allergy is the only contraindication; onset of calcium-lowering effect is rapid
Mithramycin	25 µg./kg.	Intravenously over 1 hr. in 100 ml. 0.9% saline or 5% dextrose	Contraindications are renal or hepatic dysfunction; calcium-lowering effect occurs within 24 hr.; drug is useful when diuretic and intravenous saline are contraindicated; nausea and vomiting are side effects
Glucocorticoids	Prednisone 40–50 mg./day Prednisolone phosphate 40 mg.	Oral Intramuscularly or intravenously every 8 hr.	Lag period may be 7–10 days; glucocorticoids are safe for short-term use; alternate-day oral program may be used for long-term use
Orthophosphate	1–2 gm./24 hr.	Oral	Dosage must be adjusted for renal impairment; soft tissue calcification may occur; intravenous phosphate is not recommended
Prostaglandin synthetase inhibitors	Indomethacin, 25–50 mg. 3 times a day	Oral	Unless increased prostaglandin secretion is measured, this drug should not be used alone

From Purnell, D. C., and van Heerden, J. A.: Management of symptomatic hypercalcemia and hypocalcemia. World J. Surg., 6:702, 1982.

dialysis. Phosphate retention and hyperphosphatemia in conjunction with a decrease in the renal production of $1,25(OH)_2$ vitamin D_3 reduce serum calcium and cause secondary hyperparathyroidism. In addition, aluminum from the dialysate and phosphate binder medications accumulates in the bone and contributes to the osteomalacia. Conservative therapy involves dietary calcium and vitamin D supplementation and phosphate restriction.

Differential Diagnosis

The *differential diagnosis* of hypercalcemia is listed in Table 4. No single test, short of neck exploration, establishes the diagnosis of hyperparathyroidism. In hospitalized patients, *malignancy* is the most common cause. Generally, these patients can be divided into three groups: (1) those with lytic bone metastases (50 per cent), (2) those with hematologic malignancies (myeloma, lymphoma) that appear to secrete an osteoclast-activating factor, and (3) those with solid tumors that secrete a substance that causes hypercalcemia.

Of the other more common causes, *artifactual elevations* due to laboratory error occur and can usually be eliminated by

TABLE 4. Causes of Hypercalcemia

Condition	Approximate Frequency (%)
Malignancy	35
Breast cancer	
Metastatic tumor	
PTH-secreting tumor (lung, kidney, others)	
Multiple myeloma	
Acute and chronic leukemia	
Hyperparathyroidism	28
Artifact (e.g., laboratory error, dirty glassware, cork stopper contamination, tight tourniquet)	10
Vitamin D overdose	7
Thiazide diuretics	3
Hyperthyroidism	3
Milk-alkali syndrome	3
Sarcoidosis	3
Benign familial hypocalciuric hypercalcemia	2
Other causes	6
Immobilization	
Paget's disease	
Addison's disease	
Idiopathic hypercalcemia of infancy	
Dysproteinemias	
Vitamin A overdose	
Myxedema	
Pancreatic cholera (WDHA) syndrome (VIPoma)	
Aluminum intoxication	
Rhabdomyolysis	

From Clark, O. H.: Thyroid and parathyroid. *In* Way, L. W. (Ed.): Current Surgical Diagnosis and Treatment, 8th ed. Norwalk, Appleton & Lange Co., 1988.

repeating the test. Hyperthyroidism, the milk-alkali syndrome, hypervitaminosis D and A, and immobilization can be excluded by a careful history and physical examination. In patients with sarcoidosis or multiple myeloma immunoglobulin levels are usually elevated, and there are characteristic radiologic findings.

Localization

Approximately 95 per cent of patients with primary hyperparathyroidism are cured at the initial neck exploration by an experienced surgeon. No study has yet demonstrated that preoperative *localization* reduces either the length of operation or the incidence of complications. Many surgeons believe that these techniques should be reserved for the patient undergoing re-exploration after a failed initial procedure, and they will be discussed in that context.

Treatment

The increasing percentage of patients with primary hyperparathyroidism who present with asymptomatic disease has raised the question of conservative, nonoperative management. The only prospective study addressing this question was reported in 1981 by Scholz and Purnell. They followed 142 patients with mild disease over a 10-year period. Twenty-three patients required surgical therapy for an increase in mean serum calcium to more than 11 mg. per 100 ml., roentgenographic evidence of bone disease, decreased renal function, nephrolithiasis, and gastrointestinal complications, or if observation became impractical. Twenty-three per cent died of apparently unrelated causes, 13 per cent were lost to follow-up, and 29 per cent had persistent disease. The investigators were unable to define criteria that would predict which patients would require surgical therapy and therefore concluded that operative treatment was indicated in most patients. More complete resolution of this question requires a randomized, controlled trial, and until that time the only curative treatment is surgical therapy. The complication rate is less than 3 per cent and includes injury to the superior and recurrent laryngeal nerves and the development of hypocalcemia.

Parathyroid exploration is performed under general anesthesia through a transverse cervical incision. The thyroid lobes are elevated, the recurrent laryngeal nerve and inferior thyroid artery are visualized, and all four (or more) parathyroids are identified. The upper glands are usually located dorsally on the upper surface of the thyroid lobe. The inferior glands are usually more anterior and may be found anywhere from the neck to the mediastinum along the course of migration of the thymus.

An assiduous primary operation is essential. A second exploration because of failure to find the gland initially is more difficult and damage to the recurrent nerve is more likely. If no parathyroid is found after meticulous exploration of the neck and removal of the thymic pedicle, which can usually be done through the cervical incision, the thyroid lobe on that side should be carefully palpated and even removed as a last resort. To ensure that the parathyroids have been identified, small biopsies should be taken of each gland. If, after diligent exploration of the neck, no abnormal parathyroid can be found, a decision must be made regarding *mediastinotomy*. This is required in only 1 to 2 per cent of patients. Most surgeons would delay at least 2 to 4 weeks after the initial procedure if the serum calcium remains elevated. The mediastinum is usually explored through a median sternotomy. Glands are most often located in association with the thymic remnant, but they may even be found in the posterior mediastinum.

Operative management depends on the number of enlarged glands. The most reliable index of abnormality is determination of gland size. If only one gland is enlarged, its resection is curative in nearly all patients. If two or three glands are enlarged, they are resected although this is associated with recurrent hypercalcemia in approximately 10 per cent of patients over prolonged periods of follow-up. The management of patients with *parathyroid hyperplasia* or generalized enlargement of four glands is more difficult. Standard therapy of subtotal (3½ gland) parathyroidectomy has been associated with recurrent hyperparathyroidism in 10 to 55 per cent of patients and hypoparathyroidism in 15 to 25 per cent. Because of these less than satisfactory results, the authors have elected to manage these patients by total parathyroidectomy and heterotopic autotransplantation.

RECURRENT HYPERPARATHYROIDISM. If *recurrent hypercalcemia* develops after neck exploration and the initial diagnosis was correct, most patients have a missed adenoma although inadequately excised hyperplastic tissue can also occur. It is in this setting that *localization procedures* are indicated. High-resolution, real-time ultrasonography, computed tomography, magnetic resonance imaging, and thallium-technetium subtraction scanning may all prove useful. If one or more of these studies prove negative, selective angiography and venous sampling for PTH may also help to localize the lesion. Arteriography has been associated with serious neurologic complications, and both techniques require special expertise. The precise role for both the noninvasive and the invasive localizing procedures remains to be defined.

Reoperation by an experienced surgeon is associated with resolution of the hypercalcemia in approximately 90 per cent of patients, although 10 to 15 per cent become permanently hypocalcemic.

MANAGEMENT OF SECONDARY HYPERPARATHYROIDISM. Although medical management of *secondary hyperparathyroidism* is generally effective, occasionally patients develop refractory hypercalcemia or bone pain and fractures. Patients can be managed by subtotal parathyroidectomy or total parathyroidectomy with autotransplantation.

PARATHYROID TRANSPLANTATION. Reoperation for recurrent hyperparathyroidism is accompanied by a significant increase in the risks of both recurrent laryngeal nerve injury and permanent hypoparathyroidism. This situation most frequently arises after subtotal parathyroidectomy for parathyroid hyperplasia, either primary or secondary. The technique of *total parathyroidectomy with heterotopic autotransplantation* was developed to circumvent this dilemma. Approximately 20 to 25 pieces of finely sliced parathyroid are autografted into the forearm musculature or viably frozen in cases in which there is uncertainty about the amount of remaining parathyroid. If the patient becomes hypercalcemic after the transplant, a few pieces can be removed from the arm under local anesthesia. If the patient becomes hypocalcemic, pieces of frozen tissue may similarly be reimplanted.

Hypoparathyroidism

The most common cause of *hypoparathyroidism* is injury to the glands during thyroid surgery, but it also occurs as a complication of neck exploration for hyperparathyroidism. Idiopathic lack of function has been reported, primarily in children, but it is extremely rare. In newborns it may be due to prenatal suppression as a consequence of maternal hyperparathyroidism. The major signs and symptoms are a direct consequence of the hypocalcemia that causes neuromuscular excitability. Patients first develop numbness and paresthesias followed by anxiety, depression, and confusion. This may progress to frank tetany with carpopedal spasm, tonic-clonic convulsions, and laryngeal stridor, which may prove fatal. Physical examination reveals contraction of the facial muscles on tapping of the facial nerve anterior to the ear (Chvostek's sign). Trousseau's sign is carpal spasm produced by occluding blood flow to the forearm for 3 minutes. The treatment of acute hypocalcemia is intravenous administration of calcium gluconate or calcium chloride. Vitamin D and oral calcium are used for long-term management.

25

THE PITUITARY AND ADRENAL GLANDS

David Soybel, M.D., and Samuel A. Wells, Jr., M.D.

ANATOMIC RELATIONSHIPS

Pituitary

The pituitary lies within a fossa, the sella turcica. The floor of the sella is the roof of the sphenoid sinus. The cavernous sinus lies lateral to the sella and transmits the carotid siphon and cranial nerves III, IV, and VI. The diaphragma sellae, a thick reflection of dura mater, forms the roof of the sella. In about 50 per cent of patients, the diaphragma does not provide a barrier to upward spread of tumor or hemorrhage arising in the pituitary. Above the diaphragma lies the suprasellar cistern, optic chiasm, and median eminence. Above these structures lies the hypothalamus.

The pituitary consists of two lobes: anterior (adenohypophysis) and posterior (neurohypophysis). Releasing and inhibitory factors synthesized by cells of the hypothalamus influence the endocrine secretions of the anterior pituitary. The posterior pituitary hormones, oxytocin and antidiuretic hormone (ADH), are synthesized in the hypothalamus and transmitted by neuronal axons for cleavage and release within the posterior pituitary. Six cell types, each secreting one hormone product, have been identified in the adenohypophysis. Secretory products include growth hormone (GH), adrenocorticotropic hormone (ACTH), thyroid-stimulating hormone (TSH), prolactin (PRL), follicle-stimulating hormone (FSH), luteinizing hormone (LH), and somatostatin (SRIF). Gonadotrope cells secrete both LH and FSH, but otherwise each pituicyte appears to secrete only one hormone product. No direct arterial supply to the anterior pituitary has been identified. Arterial flow to the median eminence ramifies into portal capillaries and vessels that carry blood to the anterior pituitary. These vessels rejoin and exit via the cavernous sinus.

Physiology

POSTERIOR PITUITARY. The two hormones secreted by the neurohypophysis include vasopressin (also called antidiuretic hormone or ADH) and oxytocin. ADH enhances the permeability of the cortical collecting system to water, leading to conservation of body water, concentration of the urine (i.e., higher osmolality), and prevention of inappropriate

---

See the corresponding chapter or part in the *Textbook of Surgery*, 14th edition, pp. 616–654, for a more detailed discussion of this topic, including a comprehensive list of references.

concentration of the plasma. ADH is released when serum osmolality rises above 285 mOsm. or when plasma volume contracts by 5 per cent or more. Trauma, sepsis, or administration of opiates stimulates release of ADH by the neurohypophysis. Oxytocin is released in response to suckling of the breasts and stimulates myoepithelial cells of the breast to produce milk ejection.

ANTERIOR PITUITARY. Hormones secreted by the adenohypophysis include FSH, LH, PRL, ACTH, GH, and TSH. In women, FSH stimulates maturation of the graafian follicle and its production of estradiol. At midcycle of the menstrual period, a surge of LH causes rupture of the follicle, ovulation, and development of the corpus luteum. In the male, LH stimulates Leydig cells to produce testosterone, and FSH binds to Sertoli cells to influence the rate of germ cell maturation and spermatogenesis. In women, PRL influences maturation of the breasts and their preparation for lactation; it influences progesterone synthesis by the ovary and testosterone synthesis by the testes. TSH stimulates thyroxine synthesis and release by the thyroid follicles. ACTH stimulates cortisol production and secretion by adrenal cortex; it also has a permissive role in aldosterone secretion by the adrenal cortex. The ACTH molecule is synthesized as part of a larger precursor molecule (proopiomelanocortin), which contains sequences of other peptides such as beta-endorphin and met-enkephalin. The role of pituitary hormones in the response of the organism to stress is not yet defined. Finally, GH exerts major stimulatory effects on longitudinal growth of bones and growth of muscle, cartilage, and other tissues. GH induces a generally catabolic state and insulin-resistant glucose intolerance.

Stimuli that release GH, TSH, ACTH and LH/FSH are synthesized in the hypothalamic nuclei and known as releasing hormones or factors (e.g., GHRH, TRH, CRH, LHRH). Releasing hormones for PRL are not well characterized. Inhibitory factors have also been described for some pituitary hormones. In most cases, a rise in the circulating level of a hormone or of the products of the target tissue activities (e.g., thyroxine, cortisol, estrogen, or testosterone) provides negative feedback and inhibition of the production of the releasing factors and pituitary hormones.

Evaluation of Hypothalamic/Pituitary Disturbance

SIGNS AND SYMPTONS. Ordinarily the pituitary occupies about 75 per cent of the sellar space. Lesions that expand beyond this space infringe on local structures, most notably the optic chiasm, suprasellar cistern, and cranial nerves III, IV, and VI. Characteristic symptoms thus include bitemporal hemianopsia and extraocular muscle palsies. Nonspecific signs or symptoms include headache and optic atrophy. Sudden hemorrhage, or apoplexy, is accompanied by visual loss, meningismus, and altered mental status. Specific syndromes of endocrine hypersecretion or deficit are described later.

DIAGNOSTIC IMAGING. *Plain films* of the skull provide dimensions of the sella and may provide clues to the presence of a pituitary mass lesion. These include asymmetric enlargement of the sella, focal bony erosion, or a double floor.

Computed tomography (CT) and *magnetic resonance imaging (MRI)* provide tomograms in coronal, sagittal, and transverse planes. CT scans, using intravenous contrast, and MRI provide dimensions of the sella and images of the pituitary lesions. Pituitary adenomas characteristically are well-circumscribed, focal, non-midline lesions. MRI provides additional details about the relationship of pituitary lesions to adjacent vascular structures and cranial nerves.

EVALUATION OF PITUITARY FUNCTION. Radioimmunoassays of plasma hormone levels provide rapid assessment of pituitary secretory reserve. Assessment of anterior pituitary function includes measurement of basal plasma hormone levels under standard conditions and reserve function after stimulation. A convenient protocol for testing reserve function utilizes insulin-induced hypoglycemia and infusions of L-dopa, TRH, and LHRH for testing reserves of GH, PRL, TSH, LH, FSH, and ACTH. Posterior pituitary function is evaluated indirectly by measurements of plasma and urine osmolality: high osmolality of plasma and low osmolality of the urine indicate diabetes insipidus; low plasma osmolality and concentrated urine indicate a syndrome of inappropriate ADH secretion.

Principles of Management of Pituitary Disorders

PITUITARY ADENOMA. Staging of pituitary adenomas is useful in directing therapy. A widely used system of classification is shown in Table 1. Lesions confined to the sella (Grades I, II, III) frequently are best managed by trans-

TABLE 1. Pituitary Tumor Classification

I. Enclosed microadenoma—sella of normal size with focal asymmetry of the floor or normal sella
II. Enclosed adenoma—sella enlarged with an intact floor
III. Localized invasive adenoma—sella enlarged with localized erosion of the floor
IV. Diffuse invasive adenoma—entire floor of sella destroyed by tumor
   A. Small suprasellar extension filling only the suprachiasmatic cistern
   B. Large suprasellar extension deforming the anterior recesses of the third ventricle

Data according to Hardy, J., and Vezina, J. L.: Transsphenoidal neurosurgery of intracranial neoplasm. Adv. Neurol., *15*:261, 1976; and Hardy, J., Somma, M., and Vezina, J. L.: Treatment of acromegaly: Radiation or Surgery? *In* Morley, T. P. (Ed.): Current Controversies in Neurosurgery. Philadelphia, W. B. Saunders Company, 1976, pp. 377–391.

sphenoidal hypophysectomy. This approach permits selective removal of the tumor with preservation of normal pituitary tissue. Many Grade III lesions (localized invasive) and Grade IV lesions (diffusely invasive) are best approached transfrontally. Radiation therapy is used as an adjunct to surgical therapy if the risk of recurrence is high or if the tumor is not amenable to resection. Complications of surgical therapy include cerebrospinal fluid infection or leak, cranial nerve deficits, or visual loss. Permanent panhypopituitarism occurs in less than 0.1 per cent of operations for microadenoma (lesions less than 1 cm. in diameter) and in 15 per cent of operations undertaken for larger lesions. The disadvantages of radiation therapy include permanent panhypopituitarism in as many as 25 to 40 per cent. In addition, the full benefits of radiation may require several months or even years to be realized. Some medical therapies can inhibit secretion of pituitary hormones (e.g., bromocriptine for prolactin- or growth hormone–secreting tumors) and reduce tumor size. These are used as adjuncts to surgical therapy and radiation. In some cases, medical therapy may be the primary mode of management, as discussed later.

PANHYPOPITUITARISM. Loss of pituitary function may occur suddenly owing to intrasellar hemorrhage (apoplexy), following pituitary surgery or irradiation, or secondary to enlargement of nonsecreting, space-occupying lesions. Enlarging functional lesions may also cause symptoms of panhypopituitarism in conjunction with the symptoms of a single hormone's excess. Replacement of adrenocortical and thyroid hormones is essential when the syndrome is recognized and when depletion of pituitary functional reserve is documented. Diabetes insipidus is treated by use of a parenteral preparation of vasopressin. Estrogens may be used to treat symptoms of FSH and LH loss.

Management of Specific Disorders of the Pituitary

Prolactinomas comprise about half of pituitary adenomas. In women, signs and symptoms of prolactin excess include amenorrhea for longer than 6 months, galactorrhea, infertility, and sometimes polycystic ovaries. In men, these lesions present as space-occupying lesions of the sella, with visual disturbance and headache. Basal levels of prolactin of 200 ng. per ml. or greater indicate a strong likelihood of pituitary prolactinoma. In women with Grade I or Grade II lesions, transsphenoidal hypophysectomy is the preferred management, since 80 per cent of patients will resume their menses and 40 per cent of childbearing age may actually be able to bear children. Relapse occurs in 15 per cent of patients so treated, and recurrences are managed with bromocriptine. Under selected circumstances, radiation and bromocriptine individually or together may be used for treatment, if restoration of menstrual function is not a primary goal of therapy. Larger lesions are approached transfrontally, if surgical resection is feasible. If resection is not possible, radiation and bromocriptine can palliate symptoms for prolonged periods.

Excess growth hormone levels produce the syndrome of acromegaly. Clinical features include a protracted history of coarsening of facial features; enlargement of hands, feet, and tongue; musculoskeletal degeneration; enlargement of viscera; and glucose intolerance. Menstrual disturbances are common in women with acromegaly. Elevated growth hormone levels (greater than 10 ng. per ml.) and elevated somatomedin C levels confirm the diagnosis. Ectopic sources of GH in carcinoids and islet cell tumors are rare. If CT and MRI do not reveal a pituitary lesion, ectopic sources should be sought before exploration of the sella is recommended. Transsphenoidal excision cures 80 per cent of Grade I or Grade II lesions. Surgical debulking plus radiation provides excellent palliation for diffusely invasive or locally recurrent lesions. In 20 per cent of cases, bromocriptine may palliate symptoms and elicit some regression of tumor.

ACTH-secreting tumors are discussed in the following section.

TSH-secreting tumors are rare and managed according to principles outlined previously.

Nonfunctioning adenomas present as space-occupying lesions of the sella, often with symptoms of amenorrhea and panhypopituitarism. Surgical therapy is the preferred management, with radiation reserved for lesions that are recurrent or unresectable. Replacement therapy with thyroid hormone, corticosteroids, and ADH may be required.

Craniopharyngiomas, gliomas, and metastatic tumors may arise in the region of the sella. They are treated as space-occupying lesions, preferably by surgical removal.

ADRENAL CORTEX

Anatomic Relationships

Each adrenal gland weighs approximately 4 gm. and is perched on the superior medial aspect of the kidney. Arterial supply to each gland derives from the inferior phrenic artery, aorta, and renal artery. The right adrenal gland is wide and short. It empties into the cava directly. The left adrenal vein drains via the left renal artery.

The adrenal cortex is composed of three zones that can be distinguished by routine histologic examination. The outer zona glomerulosa synthesizes aldosterone, whereas the middle zona fasciculata and inner zona reticularis synthesize cortisol and androgens. The adrenal medulla comprises the innermost region of the gland; it secretes catecholamines. Grossly, the cortex appears bright yellow, whereas the medulla is darker.

Physiology

As discussed in the preceding, ACTH is secreted by the corticotropin cells of the pituitary, under stimulation by corticotropin-releasing factor secreted by the hypothalamus. Cortisol, the major glucocorticoid secreted by the adrenal gland, can suppress the synthesis and release of ACTH. Adrenocortical hormones—aldosterone, cortisol, and androgens—are synthesized by a series of enzymatic conversions of the cholesterol molecule. A normal adult secretes 10 to 30 mg. of cortisol each day, 100 to 150 mg. of aldosterone, and minute amounts of androgen. Synthesis of aldosterone and androgen is only partly controlled by ACTH. Synthesis and secretion of aldosterone are regulated mainly by levels of renin and angiotensin, which are related to volume status and levels of sodium (Na^+) ions in the plasma. Serum potassium (K^+) levels also directly influence aldosterone secretion, and hypokalemia can markedly diminish the rise in aldosterone that normally occurs with hyponatremia and hypovolemia.

Physiologic effects of the corticosteroid hormones are well described: glucocorticoids (cortisol, corticosterone) enhance catabolism, promote insulin resistance, and have anti-inflammatory and immunosuppressive effects. They also retard wound healing and increase bone resorption. The major mineralocorticoid, aldosterone, acts on gastrointestinal and distal collecting segments of the nephron to conserve Na^+ at the expense of K^+ and H^+, thereby preserving volume. Adrenal sex steroids normally are produced in such small amounts that they do not influence development of fetal tissues or the later development of gonads and secondary sexual attributes. In excess, all the corticosteroid hormones have mineralocorticoid effects on Na^+ and volume homeostasis.

Diseases of the Adrenal Cortex

HYPERCORTISOLISM (CUSHING'S SYNDROME). In 1932, Harvey Cushing described eight patients with central obesity, glucose intolerance, hypertension, plethora, hirsutism, osteoporosis, nephrolithiasis, menstrual irregularity, muscle weakness, and emotional and psychological instability. Basophilic adenomas were found in six of the eight patients. The syndrome has become known as Cushing's syndrome and is attributable to high levels of plasma cortisol. Cushing's disease refers specifically to hypercortisolism associated with a pituitary lesion secreting excessive amounts of ACTH.

When the diagnosis of hypercortisolism is suspected, it must be confirmed through laboratory testing. Elevations in plasma cortisol, loss of the normal diurnal variation of plasma cortisol levels, and increased amounts of urinary excretion of free cortisol are required in the diagnosis of hypercortisolism. Obese patients often may have elevated free urinary cortisol levels without Cushing's syndrome. It may be necessary to control for difference in body size by measuring the urinary free cortisol excretion as a ratio of the urinary creatinine content. The diagnosis of Cushing's disease requires a demonstration of elevated ACTH levels and exclusion of ectopic sources of ACTH (e.g., small cell carcinomas of the lung, pancreas, or thymus). A diagnosis of hypercortisolism due to adrenal adenoma, nodular hyperplasia, or carcinoma requires measurement of suppressed ACTH levels and imaging of the adrenal lesion.

Two tests useful in helping to differentiate adrenal, pituitary, and ectopic lesions are the dexamethasone suppression test and the metyrapone stimulation test. Dexamethasone is a synthetic and highly potent glucocorticoid that suppresses ACTH release by the pituitary. Less than 2 per cent of individuals with hypercortisolism demonstrate normal suppression of 0800 plasma cortisol levels to less than 5 μg. per 100 ml. following an overnight dose of 1 mg. of dexamethasone. In a prolonged 6-day test, small doses (0.5 mg. every 6 hours for 2 days) and larger doses (2 mg. every 6 hours for 2 days) of dexamethasone are given, and urinary free cortisol and 17-hydroxycorticosteroid levels are measured. Following small doses of dexamethasone, patients with Cushing's syndrome do not exhibit suppression; following large doses, patients with pituitary adenoma demonstrate suppression, but those with autonomous adrenal lesions or ectopic sources of ACTH do not show suppression. Metyrapone inhibits conversion of 11-deoxycortisol to cortisol, thus lowering circulating cortisol levels and stimulating ACTH production. The result is accumulation of cortisol precursors and 17-hydroxycorticosteroid, which are measurable in the urine. Again, patients with pituitary lesions tend to show stimulation, whereas those with adrenal lesions or ectopic sources of ACTH do not.

Management of Cushing's syndrome depends on localization and removal of the source of ACTH or cortisol excess. With present imaging technologies (contrast-enhanced CT or MRI), 60 to 75 per cent of patients with Cushing's syndrome are found to have pituitary adenomas. Transsphenoidal surgical excision is usually feasible, since the majority of these lesions are Grade I, II, or III. Ten to 20 per cent of patients are found to have adrenal nodules. Of these cases, 90 per cent have a solitary lesion associated with atrophy of adjacent and contralateral cortical tissue. Ten per cent have bilateral nodular hyperplasia. A small subset of patients with nodular hyperplasia have pituitary lesions and elevated levels of ACTH, but most have lesions that suppress pituitary ACTH production. Adrenocortical carcinoma causing Cushing's syndrome is rare and often associated with virilizing signs and symptoms. Management of adrenal lesions requires removal of the involved adrenal (if a solitary adenoma or carcinoma) or of both adrenals (if nodular hyperplasia). When carcinoma recurs or when the patient is unfit for surgical therapy, medical approaches for reducing cortisol secretion (mitotane, metyrapone, aminoglutethimide, or ketaconazole, alone or in combination) are used. These medications are associated with severe side effects and are not recommended as primary therapy for lesions curable by surgical therapy. Bilateral adrenalectomy is now rarely recommended for patients with pituitary or ectopic lesions producing an excess of ACTH.

HYPERALDOSTERONISM (CONN'S SYNDROME). In

1955, Conn described a 34-year-old woman with diastolic hypertension, general weakness, polyuria, hypokalemia, hypernatremia, and alkalosis. Removal of an adenoma of the right adrenal gland cured her symptoms. Subsequent assays of stored urine samples from this patient revealed elevated levels of aldosterone. Primary hyperaldosteronism, known as Conn's syndrome, is associated with low renin levels in the plasma and is found in approximately 1 per cent of patients with diastolic hypertension (greater than 100 mm. Hg). The hypertension is generally mild. Only 20 per cent of patients have diastolic pressures greater than 120 mm. Hg. Perhaps 40 per cent of patients with diastolic hypertension and unexplained hypokalemia will have low-renin aldosteronism.

The diagnosis is usually established by measurement of high plasma and urinary aldosterone levels and low plasma renin levels. Before these measurements are performed, it is necessary to discontinue all diuretic medications, estrogens, and spironolactone and to replete serum K^+ levels. A high-sodium diet or intravenous saline infusions may be used to demonstrate lack of suppression of plasma aldosterone levels and urinary aldosterone excretion. Approximately 80 per cent of cases are attributable to a solitary, unilateral adrenocortical adenoma (APA), which is curable by surgical removal. Adrenocortical carcinomas causing aldosteronism are rare and managed by surgical removal or debulking followed by chemotherapy. Ovarian tumors ectopically producing aldosterone are managed in a similar manner. Another rare form of hyperaldosteronism, which is suppressible by administration of dexamethasone, is often familial and managed by administration of corticosteroid.

Fifteen per cent of cases with low-renin aldosteronism are associated with bilateral adrenocortical hyperplasia (IHA). This lesion is cured only in approximately one fifth of cases, even after bilateral adrenalectomy. Accordingly, surgical therapy should be avoided in this subset of patients. This subset can be distinguished from those with surgically curable adrenal adenomas by imaging studies. In addition, patients with IHA can be distinguished from those with APA by sensitivity of plasma aldosterone levels to movement from supine to standing position and by much lower levels (less than 100 ng. per 100 ml.) of plasma 18-hydroxycorticosterone levels. Patients with IHA are managed medically by use of spironolactone or other K^+-sparing diuretics such as amiloride. Angiotensin-converting enzyme inhibitors and calcium channel blocker medications are also useful in managing this subset of patients.

ADRENOGENITAL SYNDROMES. These conditions arise from a deficiency of one or several enzymes necessary for synthesis of cortisol. With loss of circulating cortisol, ACTH levels rise, stimulating hyperplasia of the cortex, which can produce only cortisol precursors. Shunting of these precursors into pathways that synthesize androstenedione and testosterone produces the characteristic virilization. In males, clinical signs and symptoms of these disorders may not appear until age 2 or 3 years, when there may be hypertrophy of the phallus and muscle mass and premature increase in body hair. In females, signs are apparent at birth, with clitoral hypertrophy and fusion of labioscrotal folds. Internal female organ development (ovaries, uterus, salpinx) is not affected. Enzyme deficiencies that can cause these syndromes include those of 21-hydroxylase, 11β-hydroxylase, 3β-hydroxydehydrogenase, 17-hydroxylase, and desmolase. Principles of therapy include early operative correction of external genital malformations and repletion of cortisol insufficiency in order to reduce circulatory ACTH levels.

ADRENOCORTICAL INSUFFICIENCY (ADDISON'S DISEASE). Thomas Addison described clinical features of adrenal insufficiency in 1855. Until recently, tuberculosis was the most common cause of this syndrome; at present, the idiopathic form of autoimmune destruction of the gland represents the majority of cases. Bilateral metastatic lesions, especially those from carcinoma of the lung, are encountered not infrequently as a cause of Addison's disease. Adrenocortical insufficiency also is encountered in patients on chronic corticosteroid therapy who are subjected to a systemic stress such as major surgical therapy, trauma, or sepsis. Characteristic symptoms and signs include fatigue, weight loss, nausea and vomiting, abdominal pain, temperature disturbance, hyponatremia, hyperkalemia, and eosinophilia. Infusion of ACTH and lack of cortisol secretion by the adrenal confirms a primary adrenocortical insufficiency. In acute situations, adult patients should receive large-dose glucocorticoid therapy (hydrocortisone phosphate 100 mg. intravenously every 6 to 8 hours) and mineralocorticoid therapy (fluorohydrocortisone, 0.10 mg. per day). Replacement therapy for chronic insufficiency in the absence of stress includes oral prednisone and fluorohydrocortisone.

ADRENAL MEDULLA

Physiology

The cells of the adrenal medulla secrete biologically active amines, including norepinephrine, epinephrine, and dopamine. Synthesis and secretion of catecholamines are regulated by the autonomic nervous system. The division between alpha and beta receptors has arisen from identification of specific activities and of characteristic inhibitors for each: alpha receptors are most receptive to norepinephrine and are antagonized by phentolamine and phenoxybenzamine; beta receptors are most sensitive to epinephrine and are antagonized by propranolol. Metabolism of catecholamines is mediated by two enzymes: monoamine oxidase and catechol-O-methyl transferase. Antagonists of these enzymes are prescribed occasionally for other disorders and can interfere with diagnosis and management of disorders affecting catecholamine production.

Pheochromocytoma

Approximately 0.1 per cent of patients with diastolic hypertension harbor a pheochromocytoma, that is, a tumor in an adrenal medullary or extramedullary site that secretes an excess of catecholamines. Hypertension is commonly paroxysmal, and paroxysms can be evoked by many factors. Sweating, palpitations, myocarditis, and obstipation are frequently observed in these patients. Although most tumors are sporadic, some are found in association with specific familial syndromes, including MEN IIa (medullary carcinoma of the thyroid, pheochromocytoma, parathyroid hyperplasia), MEN IIb (medullary carcinoma, pheochromocytoma, mucosal neuromas, ganglioneuromatosis), and the neuroectodermal dysplasias. Ten per cent of these lesions occur in children (under age 20), 10 per cent are found outside the adrenal gland, 10 per cent are multiple or bilateral, and 10 per cent are malignant. In familial cases, pheochromocytomas are almost always found bilaterally.

Diagnosis of a pheochromocytoma is suspected by clinical signs and symptoms or because the patient is part of a kindred with a hereditary disposition for the lesion. Measurement of 24-hour excretion of catecholamines, metanephrines, and vanillylmandelic acid is highly sensitive in detecting these lesions. Glucagon can be used to stimulate catecholamine release for screening in members of an affected kindred.

Pheochromocytomas are removed surgically whenever possible, since medical therapies do not reliably control symptoms of catecholamine excess. Preoperatively, patients receive alpha blockade with oral phenoxybenzamine or, less commonly, phentolamine. Adequate hydration is crucial. Intraoperative management includes intravenous nitroprusside and adrenergic blockade before the tumor is removed. With removal of the tumor and loss of excess catecholamine, volume replacement is the treatment of choice. In extreme cases, intravenous norepinephrine in small doses may be used to stabilize blood pressure while the re-expanded intravascular volume is repleted.

THE INCIDENTALLY DISCOVERED ADRENAL MASS

The application of CT scanning for evaluation of abdominal complaints has led to the incidental discovery of apparently nonfunctioning adrenal masses. Approximately 0.5 to 1 per cent of such scans reveal an adrenal mass in patients with no symptoms of adrenal cortical or medullary dysfunction. Most commonly these lesions prove to be benign adenomas. In unselected series, about one fifth of these lesions prove to harbor metastatic malignancy, primary adrenocortical carcinoma, or a functional adenoma. Lesions greater than 6 cm. in diameter should be removed because of the significant likelihood of malignancy. Adrenal masses greater than 3 cm. in diameter should be followed closely and removed if they increase in size.

26

THE ESOPHAGUS

I

Historical Aspects and Anatomy
Mark B. Orringer, M.D.

HISTORICAL ASPECTS

The modern surgical treatment of esophageal disease is the result of refinements in both anesthetic and operative techniques as well as methods of assessing normal and abnormal anatomy and physiology. In the early 1900s, Chevalier Jackson pioneered the use of the rigid esophagoscope and established guidelines for proper rigid endoscopic technique. LoPresti and Hilmi (1964) developed the flexible fiberoptic esophagoscope, which has revolutionized the evaluation of esophageal mucosal detail and the treatment of strictures, achalasia, and varices.

While techniques of resection of the thoracic esophagus awaited the development of anesthetic methods that would permit the chest to be opened safely, resection of the cervical esophagus for carcinoma by Billroth (1871) and Czerny (1877) followed by reconstruction of the cervical esophagus with a skin tube by von Mikulicz (1886) were surgical milestones. Turner (1933) performed the first successful transmediastinal blunt esophagectomy for carcinoma and established alimentary continuity with an antethoracic skin tube. This technique did not gain widespread use because the advent of endotracheal anesthesia made possible transthoracic esophageal resection. Transthoracic esophagectomy and an esophagogastric anastomosis were first successfully performed by Ohsawa (1933) and by Marshall (1937) and Adams and Phemister (1938). Sweet (1945) and Garlock (1946) established many principles of esophageal resection that are still used, and Ivor Lewis (1946) popularized the right-sided transthoracic esophagectomy for carcinoma. Techniques of esophageal replacement with stomach, jejunum, and colon were then refined. Orringer and Sloan (1978) repopularized the technique of transhiatal esophagectomy without thoracotomy.

Surgical milestones in the treatment of benign esophageal disease have included the addition of esophagomyotomy to resection of pulsion diverticula for eliminating the elevated intraesophageal pressure responsible for the pouch (Allen and Clagget, 1965; Belsey, 1966); treatment of achalasia with cardioesophagomyotomy (Heller, 1913; Zaaijer, 1923; Ellis, 1969); antireflux operations for restoration of a functioning distal esophageal sphincter mechanism (Nissen, 1961; Belsey,

---

See the corresponding chapter or part in the *Textbook of Surgery*, 14th edition, pp. 655–659, for a more detailed discussion of this topic, including a comprehensive list of references.

1967; Hill, 1967); and combined esophageal-lengthening Collis gastroplasty and fundoplication procedures for better control of reflux in patients with esophageal shortening (Pearson, 1971; Orringer and Sloan, 1976, 1978; Henderson, 1977). No less important in the treatment of benign esophageal disease has been the development and refinement of diagnostic studies for objective assessment of esophageal function: techniques of esophageal manometry (Code, 1958; Vantrappen, 1958); the intraesophageal pH electrode (Tuttle and Grossman, 1958); provocative pH reflux testing (Kantrowitz, 1969; Skinner and Booth, 1970); and 24-hour distal esophageal pH monitoring (Johnson and DeMeester, 1974).

ANATOMY

The esophagus is a hollow muscular tube that is 25 cm. (10 inches) long and extends from the pharynx to the stomach. The *pharyngoesophageal* segment includes the pharyngeal musculature and ends beneath the cricopharyngeal or upper esophageal sphincter, the most inferior portion of the inferior pharyngeal constrictor. The upper esophageal sphincter is unique in that it is the narrowest point of the gastrointestinal tract (14 mm.) and consists of a bow of muscle connecting the lateral borders of the cricoid cartilage. The *cervical* esophagus is 5 to 6 cm. long and extends to the top of the first thoracic vertebra. It lies anterior to the prevertebral fascia and courses behind and more to the left of the trachea; it is therefore more readily approached surgically through a left cervical incision. The *thoracic* esophagus enters the posterior mediastinum behind the aortic arch and great vessels, curves slightly to the left of the trachea and passes behind the left main stem bronchus and behind the pericardium, and enters the diaphragmatic hiatus at the level of the eleventh thoracic vertebra. The thoracic esophagus is bounded on either side by the right and left parietal pleurae, which are easily injured during esophageal operations. The *abdominal* esophagus is 1 to 2 cm. in length and extends from the esophageal hiatus to the point at which it joins the stomach, the *cardia*, or the esophagogastric junction. The esophagus is normally lined by squamous epithelium except for the distal 1 to 2 cm., which are junctional columnar epithelium. The squamocolumnar epithelial junction (or Z-line) typically occurs at the gastroesophageal junction.

The esophagus lacks a serosal covering and is surrounded by adventitia, loose fibroareolar mediastinal tissue. It has an outer longitudinal and an inner circular layer of muscle. Both muscle layers are striated in the upper third of the esophagus and are nonstriated (smooth) in the distal two thirds. The esophagus receives its *arterial blood supply* from the superior and inferior thyroid arteries and from four to six aortic esophageal arteries, supplemented by collaterals with the intercostal, bronchial, inferior phrenic, and left gastric arteries. The aortic esophageal arteries terminate in fine capillary networks before actually entering the muscle layer. *Sympathetic innervation* consists of fibers from the superior and inferior cervical sympathetic ganglia, the upper thoracic and splanchnic nerves, and the celiac ganglion. Intrinsic autonomic innervation is from Meissner's plexus in the submucosa and Auerbach's plexus between the circular and longitudinal muscle layers. *Parasympathetic* innervation is from the vagus nerves, which in the neck give rise to the external and internal laryngeal nerves. The external laryngeal nerve innervates the cricothyroid muscle and part of the inferior pharyngeal constrictor. The internal laryngeal nerves provide sensory innervation of the pharyngeal surface of the larynx and base of the tongue. The recurrent laryngeal nerves of the vagi provide parasympathetic innervation to the cervical esophagus and upper esophageal sphincter. Thus, injury to the laryngeal nerve may cause not only hoarseness, but also dysfunction of the upper esophageal sphincter with secondary aspiration on swallowing as well. The vagus nerves send fibers to the muscles of the thoracic esophagus. At the diaphragmatic hiatus, the left vagus nerve comes to lie anterior to the esophagus, and the right vagus lies posterior. There is an extensive esophageal lymphatic mediastinal drainage. Esophageal carcinomas metastasize along submucosal lymphatics and to the internal jugular nodes in the neck; paratracheal nodes in the superior mediastinum; subcarinal nodes in the midchest; paraesophageal and inferior pulmonary ligament nodes in the lower mediastinum; and perigastric and left gastric artery lymph nodes.

II

Physiology
Mark B. Orringer, M.D.

The basic function of the esophagus is transportation of swallowed material from the pharynx into the stomach. Secondarily, retrograde flow of gastric contents is prevented by the lower esophageal sphincter (LES); and air entry into the esophagus with each inspiration is prevented by the upper esophageal sphincter, which normally remains closed as a result of tonic contraction. Most current knowledge of esophageal physiology has been derived from esophageal manometry that permits recordings of intraesophageal pressure phenomena: the amplitude and length of the upper and lower sphincters, the extent and duration of relaxation of the sphincters with swallowing, and the characteristics of peristaltic activity in the body of the esophagus. The most

---

See the corresponding chapter or part in the *Textbook of Surgery*, 14th edition, pp. 660–663, for a more detailed discussion of this topic, including a comprehensive list of references.

common method of measuring intraluminal esophageal pressures currently in use involves the transmission of pressure changes through swallowed hollow tubes connected externally to transducers and a recording system. The standard motility catheter is a triple-lumen, constantly perfused system of polyethylene or polyvinyl tubing with either an open end or a lateral orifice. The addition of the intraesophageal pH electrode to this system permits objective documentation of the degree of abnormal gastroesophageal reflux present as determined with the standard acid reflux test. The standard acid reflux test measures the number of episodes of reflux (fall in intraesophageal pH below 4) detected by a pH electrode positioned 5 cm. proximal to the distal esophageal sphincter. A standard 250- to 300-ml. bolus of 0.1N HCl is placed in the stomach, and reflux is determined with the patient in a variety of standardized positions (supine, right side, left side, and Trendelenburg). Twenty-four hour distal esophageal pH monitoring further characterizes patterns of gastroesophageal reflux.

The action of *swallowing* begins with voluntary movement of the tongue, which initiates an involuntary peristaltic wave that rapidly traverses the pharynx and reaches the upper esophageal sphincter, producing a brisk, coordinated relaxation that is followed by a post-deglutitive contraction. The upper esophageal sphincter is approximately 3 cm. in length and has a mean resting pressure of 20 to 60 mm. Hg. Its duration of relaxation with swallowing is 0.5 to 1 second. Contraction of the upper esophageal sphincter after the relaxation phase produces an intraluminal pressure of 70 to 100 mm. Hg that lasts 2 to 4 seconds. As the swallowed bolus enters the esophagus, a *primary* peristaltic wave is activated and propels the swallowed material from the pharynx into the stomach in 4 to 8 seconds in an orderly, progressive manner. Normally, a progressive peristaltic contraction (primary wave) follows 97 per cent of all swallows. Pressures within the esophageal body parallel negative intrathoracic pressure, being maximally negative (-5 to -10 mm. Hg) during deep inspiration and highest (0 to 5 mm. Hg) during exploration. Esophageal peristaltic pressure ranges from 20 to 100 mm. Hg, with a duration of contraction between 2 and 4 seconds. If the entire swallowed bolus of food does not empty from the esophagus into the stomach, *secondary* peristaltic waves are initiated. These contractions, like the primary waves, are progressive and sequential but begin in the smooth muscle segment of the esophagus (near the level of the aortic arch) and continue until retained intraesophageal contents are emptied into the stomach. Unlike the primary wave, the secondary contraction is not initiated by a voluntary swallow but rather by local distention of the esophagus. *Tertiary* contractions are simultaneous, nonprogressive, nonperistaltic, mono- or multiphasic waves that occur throughout the esophagus and represent incoordinated contractions of the smooth muscle that are responsible for the classic "corkscrew" appearance of esophageal spasm on barium swallow examination. Increased resting pressures within the body of the esophagus and abnormal

TABLE 1. Factors Affecting Distal High-Pressure Zone (HPZ) Tone

Factors	Increased HPZ Tone	Decreased HPZ Tone
Hormonal	Gastrin Motilin Prostaglandin $F_{2\alpha}$ Bombesin	Secretin Cholecystokinin Glucagon Progesterone Estrogen Prostaglandins E_1, E_2, A_2

Drugs	Caffeine
	Alpha-adrenergic agents
	  Norepinephrine
	  Phenylephrine
	Anticholinesterase
	  Edrophonium
	Cholinergic agents
	  Bethanecol (Urecholine)
	  Methacholine
	  (Mecholyl)
	Betazole
	Metoclopramide
		Alpha-adrenergic blockers
		  Phentolamine
		Anticholinergics
		  Atropine
		  Theophylline
		Beta-adrenergic blockers
		  Isoproterenol
		Ethanol
		Epinephrine
		Nicotine
		Nitroglycerin

Foods	Protein meal	Fatty meal Chocolate
Myogenic	Normal resting muscle tone	? Aging ? Diabetes mellitus
Mechanical	Antireflux operation	Hiatal hernia Abnormal phrenoesophageal ligament insertion Short or absent intra-abdominal distal esophageal segment Nasogastric tube
Miscellaneous	Gastric alkalinization Gastric distention	Gastric acidification Gastrectomy Hypoglycemia Hypothyroidism Amyloidosis Pernicious anemia Epidermolysis bullosa

Modified from Hurwitz, A. L., Duranceau, A., and Haddad, J. K.: Disorders of Esophageal Motility. Philadelphia, W. B. Saunders Company, 1979, p. 120.

motor function are seen with obstruction, either mechanical or functional.

Manometric studies have demonstrated a well-defined *functional* lower esophageal sphincter that has a measurable elevated distal esophageal resting pressure, is 3 to 5 cm. in length, and serves as a barrier against abnormal regurgitation of gastric contents into the esophagus. Since there is no demonstrable *anatomic* lower esophageal sphincter, this valve mechanism is more accurately referred to as the lower esophageal sphincter *mechanism* or the distal esophageal high-pressure zone (HPZ). "Normal" resting pressure within the

HPZ ranges from 10 to 20 mm. Hg, but *no absolute HPZ value per se indicates either competence or incompetence of the lower esophageal sphincter mechanism.* HPZ pressures of 0 to 5 mm. Hg and HPZ lengths of 2 cm. or less are more likely to be associated with a mechanically incompetent LES and secondary gastroesophageal reflux. Much more meaningful in the demonstration of abnormal reflux, however, is the intra-esophageal pH electrode, the use of which has been expanded from the standard pH reflux test to 24-hour monitoring of distal esophageal pH. Esophagoscopy, the barium swallow examination, and the acid perfusion (Bernstein) test are poor and inconsistent indicators of gastroesophageal reflux. Within 1.5 to 2.5 seconds after a swallow is initiated, distal HPZ relaxation occurs, lasting 4 to 6 seconds. A post-deglutitive contraction then occurs, generating pressures of 25 to 35 mm. Hg for 7 to 10 seconds, after which HPZ tone returns to resting levels. Distal HPZ pressure varies continually and is influenced by a host of neural, hormonal, myogenic, mechanical, and environmental factors (Table 1).

III

Disorders of Esophageal Motility

Mark B. Orringer, M.D.

Functional disorders of the esophagus are those conditions that interfere with the normal act of swallowing or that produce dysphagia without any associated intraluminal organic obstruction or extrinsic compression of the esophagus. Among these disorders are the abnormalities of esophageal motility, most of which have now been precisely defined by esophageal manometry, a vital part of the evaluation of these patients. Generally, a barium swallow, esophagoscopy, and esophageal function tests, including manometry and intra-esophageal pH reflux testing, constitute the minimal evaluation of the patient with a suspected disorder of esophageal motility.

UPPER ESOPHAGEAL SPHINCTER DYSFUNCTION (Oropharyngeal Dysphagia or Cricopharyngeal Dysfunction)

A number of abnormalities of the central and peripheral nervous systems, metabolic and inflammatory myopathy, gastroesophageal reflux, and unknown factors cause diffi-

See the corresponding chapter or part in the *Textbook of Surgery*, 14th edition, pp. 663–678, for a more detailed discussion of this topic, including a comprehensive list of references.

culty in propelling liquid or solid food from the oropharynx into the upper esophagus. It has been difficult to characterize these abnormalities by use of standard esophageal manometric techniques owing to the limitations of this equipment in recording the rapid sequence of events that occurs with normal deglutition in a unique asymmetric sphincter that changes position with laryngeal excursions during swallowing. Other nonmotor causes of upper esophageal dysphagia such as carcinoma, caustic stricture, cervical vertebral bone spurs, thyromegaly, and trauma must be excluded. The term *globus hystericus*, indicating a purely psychological basis for a patient's complaint of cervical dysphagia, is a diagnosis of exclusion, made only after significant esophageal disease has been ruled out.

Upper esophageal sphincter dysfunction has a typical clinical presentation: cervical dysphagia, expectoration of saliva, intermittent hoarseness, and weight loss. Barium esophagogram findings may be normal in patients with intermittent symptoms. Alternatively, hypertonicity of the upper esophageal sphincter, a typical posterior cricopharyngeal "bar" at the level of the C7 or T1 vertebrae, or a pharyngoesophageal (Zenker's) diverticulum may be seen. Esophageal manometry should be performed, although standard recordings may fail to demonstrate any upper esophageal sphincter abnormality. Abnormalities of thoracic esophageal peristalsis or an incompetent lower esophageal sphincter may also be detected. Treatment varies with the cause of oropharyngeal dysphagia and must be individualized. In the presence of incapacitating cervical dysphagia and aspiration, for example, after a midbrain bulbar stroke, and a radiographically or manometrically documented abnormal upper esophageal sphincter, a cervical esophagomyotomy through the abnormal musculature may produce gratifying results.

DISORDERS OF THE BODY OF THE ESOPHAGUS

Achalasia

The term *achalasia* is of Greek derivation and literally means "failure of relaxation." It refers to the failure of the lower esophageal sphincter in patients with this disease to relax normally with swallowing. The term fails to recognize that achalasia is a disease that involves the entire body of the esophagus. In South America, the cause of achalasia is often Chagas' disease, a parasitic infestation by the leishmanial forms of *Trypanosoma cruzi*, which destroys the ganglion cells of Auerbach's plexus, causing motor dysfunction and progressive dilation of the esophagus, colon, ureters, and other viscera. In Europe and North America, however, the etiologic agent is obscure, the condition frequently following a number of physically or emotionally stressful situations. Regardless of the etiologic factor, degeneration of the ganglion cells of Auerbach's plexus is invariably found. The *classic triad* of presenting systems includes dysphagia, regurgitation, and weight loss. Retrosternal pain on ingestion of food is more characteristic of esophageal spasm, not achalasia. Hematemesis is rare but can occur as a result of retention esophagitis. Achalasia is a premalignant lesion of the esophagus; carcinoma develops as a late complication in approximately 10 per cent of patients after 15 to 25 years. The carcinomas are typically squamous cell and are located in the middle third of the esophagus.

The radiographic appearance varies with the stage of the disease: mild dilation early in the disease to a massively dilated sigmoid-shaped megaesophagus in advanced disease. Retained intraesophageal debris is common. The radiographic hallmark of achalasia on barium esophagogram is the distal "bird-beak" taper of the esophagogastric junction. The standard posteroanterior chest film shows a characteristic "double mediastinal stripe" (the dilated esophagus), and a posterior mediastinal air-fluid level is seen on a lateral view. Manometric criteria of achalasia are (1) failure of the distal esophageal high-pressure zone to relax reflexly with swallowing and (2) lack of progressive peristalsis throughout the length of the esophagus. Mean intraesophageal pressure is elevated relative to mean intragastric pressure, a reversal of the normal situation. Esophagoscopy is indicated to exclude carcinoma, to evaluate for retention esophagitis, and to determine if there is a distal stricture from reflux esophagitis that may have followed prior forceful dilations or esophagomyotomy. The treatment of achalasia is *palliative*, since the condition is incurable although compatible with normal longevity. In the early stages of the disease, sublingual nitroglycerin before meals, long-acting nitrates, and calcium channel blockers improve swallowing. Forceful pneumatic balloon dilation is the appropriate first line of defense, providing good to excellent relief of dysphagia in 65 to 77 per cent of patients so treated with a perforation rate of 1 to 5 per cent. If pneumatic dilation fails to provide lasting relief of dysphagia, it may be repeated a second time, but then a distal esophagomyotomy through the lower esophageal sphincter is recommended. The myotomy is 7 to 10 cm. in length, extending from the level of the inferior pulmonary vein through the lower esophageal sphincter. Controversy exists as to the distal extent of the esophagomyotomy. Some recommend complete division of the distal esophageal sphincter followed by a Belsey repair to prevent the subsequent development of gastroesophageal reflux. Others advocate extending the esophagomyotomy onto the stomach only far enough to relieve the obstruction but not to induce reflux through an incompetent lower esophageal sphincter. Esophagomyotomy provides good to excellent relief of dysphagia in 85 per cent of patients with a perforation rate of 1 per cent. For advanced disease (megaesophagus), esophageal resection provides excellent relief of dysphagia and regurgitation and eliminates the risk of late development of carcinoma.

DIFFUSE ESOPHAGEAL SPASM

This is a poorly understood and equally poorly treated hypermotility disorder in which patients complain of chest pain and/or dysphagia as a result of repetitive, simultaneous, high-amplitude esophageal contractions. Patients are characteristically anxious, and the chest pain mimics that of angina pectoris due to coronary artery disease. A history of irritable bowel syndrome, pylorospasm, spastic colon, or other functional gastrointestinal complaints is common, and gastroesophageal reflux, gallstones, peptic ulcer disease, and pancreatitis can all initiate diffuse esophageal spasm. Underlying psychiatric disease is common. A cardiac evaluation is indicated to exclude an etiologic cardiac factor for the chest pain. Barium esophagogram findings are highly variable, since symptoms and episodes of spasm tend to be intermittent. The classic radiographic appearance of diffuse esophageal spasm is "curling" or a "corkscrew" esophagus caused by segmental contractions of the circular muscle. A "long esophagomyotomy" extending from the level of the aortic arch to the lower esophageal sphincter that has been advocated by some for the treatment of diffuse esophageal spasm provides lasting relief of chest pain and dysphagia in less than 50 per cent of these patients. *Surgical procedures should be avoided* if at all possible and should be reserved only for patients incapacitated by chest pain or dysphagia. Better treatment options include avoidance of stress during meals and "trigger" foods or drinks; psychiatric and family counseling; treatment of associated gastroesophageal reflux; antispasmodics; H_2-blockers; nitrates; calcium channel blockers; and periodic esophageal dilations with mercury-weighted bougies (e.g., Maloney tapered dilators).

SCLERODERMA (Systemic Sclerosis)

This collagen vascular disease is characterized by induration of the skin, fibrous replacement of the smooth muscle of internal organs, and progressive loss of visceral and cutaneous function. Disruption of normal esophageal peristalsis is common and is a major diagnostic sign of the disease, particularly in patients with Raynaud's phenomenon. As fibrous replacement of esophageal smooth muscle progresses, the distal esophageal high-pressure zone loses its tone and normal response to swallowing, and gastroesophageal reflux occurs. In the distal two thirds of the esophagus, normal progressive peristalsis gives way to weak, simultaneous nonpropulsive contractions. These patients complain of slow emptying of the esophagus that requires them to wash food down with water, as well as severe heartburn and gastroesophageal reflux. The prolonged duration of contact between refluxed gastric acid and the esophageal mucosa that occurs because of the impaired ability of the atonic lower esophagus to clear refluxed gastric contents back into the stomach may dramatically accelerate reflux esophagitis. Treatment consists of an aggressive antireflux medical regimen and periodic esophageal dilations as indicated. Gratifying relief of reflux symptoms may be achieved with a combination of the esophageal-lengthening Collis gastroplasty-fundoplication procedures. In patients with severe reflux esophagitis and stricture formation, a transhiatal esophagectomy without thoracotomy and a cervical esophagogastric anastomosis appear to be a better option.

MOTOR DISORDERS OF THE LOWER ESOPHAGEAL SPHINCTER

A *hypertensive lower esophageal sphincter* may cause low retrosternal chest pain, which generally responds to intermittent bougienage but occasionally requires esophagomyotomy for relief of symptoms. A *hypotensive lower esophageal sphincter* in the absence of a hiatal hernia may be responsible for massive gastroesophageal reflux. Postvagotomy *dysphagia* associated with intraoperative injury to the vagus nerve is generally transient and responds to periodic esophageal dilation as needed.

IV

Diverticula and Miscellaneous Conditions of the Esophagus
Mark B. Orringer, M.D.

Esophageal diverticula are epithelium-lined mucosal protrusions from the esophageal lumen that are classified according to their location, the extent of the esophageal wall thickness that accompanies them, and their mechanism of formation. Almost all are acquired and occur in adults. A "true" diverticulum contains all layers of the normal esophageal wall (mucosa, submucosa, and muscle). A "false" diverticulum consists primarily of mucosa and submucosa protruding through the muscle layer. *Pharyngoesophageal* (Zenker's) diverticula occur at the junction of the pharynx and esophagus. *Parabronchial* (midesophageal) diverticula are located near the tracheal bifurcation, and *epiphrenic* (supradiaphragmatic) diverticula arise from the distal 10 cm. of esophagus. Pulsion diverticula arise as a result of elevated intraluminal pressure that forces the mucosa and submucosa to herniate through the esophageal musculature; they are therefore "false" diverticula (e.g., Zenker's and epiphrenic diverticula). Traction diverticula arise as a result of external inflammatory reaction in adjacent mediastinal lymph nodes that adhere to the esophagus and pull the entire wall toward them as they heal and contract. They are "true" diverticula (e.g., parabronchial diverticula).

See the corresponding chapter or part in the *Textbook of Surgery*, 14th edition, pp. 678–684, for a more detailed discussion of this topic, including a comprehensive list of references.

PHARYNGOESOPHAGEAL (ZENKER'S) DIVERTICULUM

This is the most common esophageal diverticulum, generally occurring in patients between 30 and 50 years of age as an acquired *pulsion* diverticulum. Zenker's diverticula characteristically arise within the inferior pharyngeal constrictor at a point of potential weakness (Killian's triangle) between the oblique fibers of the thyropharyngeus muscle and the horizontal cricopharyngeus muscle—the upper esophageal sphincter. Because of the unique characteristics of the upper esophageal sphincter and the speed with which neuromotor events in this area occur during deglutition, precise documentation of the exact abnormality in pharyngoesophageal motor function in these patients is difficult to obtain. However, these pulsion diverticula occur because *some* distal abnormality causes unusually elevated pharyngeal pressures during swallowing. The swallowed bolus exerts pressure within the pharynx, and mucosa and submucosa herniate through the anatomically weak area above the cricopharyngeus muscle. With time, the diverticulum enlarges and gradually dissects inferiorly in the prevertebral space behind the esophagus.

Typical symptoms of a Zenker's diverticulum include cervical dysphagia, effortless regurgitation of undigested food or pills consumed hours earlier, a gurgling sensation in the neck on swallowing, choking, and recurrent aspiration. The diagnosis is established with a barium esophagogram. In most symptomatic patients, surgical treatment is indicated, it is hoped before complications of malnutrition or pulmonary sepsis occur.

It is not the size of the pouch, but rather the degree of upper esophageal sphincter motor dysfunction that determines the severity of symptoms in the patient with a Zenker's diverticulum. Therefore, proper surgical therapy must be directed toward the underlying motor abnormality responsible for formation of the pouch and not toward the diverticulum *per se*. The most popular operation currently performed for a Zenker's diverticulum is a cricopharyngeal myotomy that divides the upper esophageal sphincter, thereby relieving the obstruction distal to the pouch. Most pouches 2.5 cm. or less in diameter require no additional treatment. Larger pouches may be either resected or suspended from the prevertebral fascia (diverticulopexy). Operative complications include salivary fistula from the resected diverticulum site and recurrent laryngeal nerve injury, both of which are rare. Endoscopic division of the common wall between the diverticulum and esophagus (i.e., the upper esophageal sphincter)—the Dohlman procedure—has been popularized in Europe but is not in widespread use. Regardless of the operation used, so long as the obstruction distal to the pouch is relieved, recurrence is rare and results are excellent.

MIDESOPHAGEAL (TRACTION) DIVERTICULA

These are invariably associated with mediastinal granulomatous disease (e.g., tuberculosis, histoplasmosis). They are characteristically very small (1 cm. or less) in size, asymptomatic, found incidentally on a barium esophagogram, and rarely require treatment. They have a blunt tapered tip that points upward to the adjacent subcarinal or parabronchial lymph node to which they are adherent and are quite different in appearance from the large, round, relatively narrow-mouthed pulsion diverticula. Midesophageal *pulsion* diverticula *can* occur in association with neuromotor dysfunction, but the most common pulsion diverticula of the esophageal body are epiphrenic diverticula.

EPIPHRENIC DIVERTICULA

These occur within the distal 10 cm. of the thoracic esophagus, are pulsion diverticula, and occur because of either esophageal motor dysfunction that produces distal obstruction or a mechanical distal obstruction (e.g., stricture). Associated esophageal disease—hiatal hernia with gastroesophageal reflux, diffuse esophageal spasm, achalasia, reflux esophagitis, and carcinoma—is common. Symptoms include dysphagia, regurgitation, and retrosternal pain from diffuse esophageal spasm. Mildly symptomatic patients with pouches less than 3 cm. in diameter often require no treatment, whereas those with progressive dysphagia and chest pain or anatomically dependent or enlarging pouches are surgical candidates. The surgical approach is a left thoracotomy, resection of the pouch, and a long extramucosal esophagomyotomy from beneath the aortic arch to the esophagogastric junction. The distal extent of the esophagomyotomy is controversial, but most favor extending the incision through the lower esophageal sphincter and onto the stomach for 1.0 to 1.5 cm. A partial fundoplication (e.g., modified Belsey repair) is then done to prevent gastroesophageal reflux. A 360-degree fundoplication is more likely to produce functional obstruction after a long esophagomyotomy and is not advocated.

MISCELLANEOUS CONDITIONS

Sideropenic Dysphagia (Plummer-Vinson or Patterson-Kelly Syndrome)

Sideropenic dysphagia refers to the development of cervical dysphagia in patients with iron deficiency anemia. Patients are typically elderly, malnourished women who are edentulous and have glossitis and spoon-shaped fingernails (koilonychia). They frequently have a cervical esophageal web. Treatment consists of esophageal dilation and correction of nutritional deficiency. This is a premalignant lesion with

10 per cent of patients developing squamous cell carcinoma of the hypopharynx, oral cavity, or esophagus.

Schatzki's Ring (Distal Esophageal Web)

A Schatzki's ring is a short annular constriction occurring at the esophagogastric junction in a patient with a sliding hiatal hernia. It is identified with a barium esophagogram. When the ring diameter is 13 mm. or less, dysphagia is likely. The rings are *not* true fibrotic strictures, but rather represent a prominent lower esophageal sphincter area in a patient with a hiatal hernia. They occur precisely at the squamocolumnar epithelial junction. The presence of a Schatzki's ring indicates *only* that there is a hiatal hernia, but *not* that there is either gastroesophageal reflux or esophagitis. Many patients with symptomatic rings have no reflux symptoms and respond well to intermittent esophageal bougienage. Those with dysphagia as well as reflux symptoms require dilation and an antireflux medical regimen. Those with refractory dysphagia or very symptomatic reflux despite adequate medical therapy respond well to intraoperative dilation combined with an antireflux operation. Resection of the ring alone, without repair of the associated hiatal hernia, should not be done.

Mallory-Weiss Syndrome (Emetogenic Mucosal Laceration)

Forceful emesis may cause a distal esophageal mucosal tear that presents as either melena or hematemesis. This may occur in a number of clinical settings: alcoholism, pregnancy, peptic ulcer disease, cirrhosis, bowel obstruction, drug withdrawal, or food poisoning. Esophagoscopy *may* establish the site of bleeding. In more than 90 per cent of cases, the bleeding stops in response to nasogastric decompression, iced saline gastric lavage, and blood replacement. With massive bleeding, however, the upper abdomen should be explored and a long proximal gastrotomy performed. After evacuation of clots from the stomach, the mucosal tear at the cardia is identified and oversewn. Results are excellent, and recurrent bleeding is rare.

MONILIAL ESOPHAGITIS

Candida albicans is a fungus that is normally a commensal inhabitant of the mouth, oropharynx, and gastrointestinal tract. The fungus may become pathogenic in severely debilitated or immunocompromised patients. Acute monilial esophagitis is therefore seen in transplant patients, oncology patients receiving chemotherapy, and surgical patients on potent broad-spectrum antibiotics. Submucosal inflammation produces the "cobblestone" pattern of luminal nodularity seen on barium esophagogram. Esophagoscopy demonstrates a whitish cheesy exudate or pseudomembrane overlying the mucosa. Treatment of acute monilial esophagitis is oral nystatin, 500,000 to 1,000,000 units of the suspension every 6 hours. Persistent or severe infection warrants intravenous amphotericin B, 1 to 10 mg. per day for 7 to 10 days, or oral flucytosine, 50 to 150 mg. per kg. per day. Late stricture formation from healing of the inflamed esophagus may occur and should be sought on barium esophagogram obtained within several weeks of the acute infection so that early dilation therapy can be instituted.

RARE ESOPHAGEAL PATHOLOGY

Cervical dysphagia may be caused by *extrinsic* esophageal disease: vertebral body osteophytic spurs, thyroid tissue, or parathyroid tissue. Infectious esophagitis may be due to syphilis, tuberculosis, and herpes. Stricture may occur in association with dermatologic conditions such as pemphigus vulgaris and epidermolysis bullosa.

V

Esophagoscopy
Mark B. Orringer, M.D.

Esophagoscopy is among the most vital diagnostic means of assessing the patient with esophageal symptoms from any cause. It should be borne in mind, however, that this procedure, particularly in association with dilation of a stricture, is one of the most dangerous operations performed, the complications of a perforation being associated with major morbidity and mortality.

INDICATIONS AND CONTRAINDICATIONS

Diagnostic esophagoscopy is warranted for symptoms of dysphagia, heartburn, odynophagia, hematemesis, or atypical chest pain and for assessing established disease: esophagitis, neuromotor disease, caustic injury, tumors, strictures, hiatal hernia, diverticula, varices, and extrinsic compression. It is used to assess postoperative problems: anastomotic stricture, tumor recurrence, bleeding, dysphagia, or recurrent gastroesophageal reflux. Therapeutically, esophagoscopy is used for dilation and biopsy of strictures, removal of foreign bodies, placement of endoluminal prostheses, sclerotherapy

---

See the corresponding chapter or part in the *Textbook of Surgery*, 14th edition, pp. 685–689, for a more detailed discussion of this topic, including a comprehensive list of references.

and laser photocoagulation, or tumor debulking. Esophagoscopy should not be performed in a struggling, uncooperative, agitated patient. Relative contraindications include recent myocardial infarction, severe cervical spine deformities, and large thoracic aortic aneurysm.

GENERAL PRINCIPLES

Elective esophagoscopy should not be performed without a prior barium esophagogram displayed in view of the endoscopist. The esophagogram defines the level and extent of the pathologic process being evaluated and identifies unsuspected disease, for example, a Zenker's diverticulum, which may complicate the procedure, before the instrument is passed.

Esophageal pathology seen on a barium esophagogram should be related to anatomic landmarks that can be used to approximate the level at which the abnormality will be seen endoscopically:

1. The cricopharyngeus sphincter is located on barium esophagogram at the level of C7 or T1 vertebral bodies, or approximately 15 cm. from the upper incisor teeth at esophagoscopy.

2. The angle of Louis (sternomanubrial junction) aligns with the tracheal bifurcation and the fourth thoracic vertebral body, approximately 25 cm. from the incisors on esophagoscopy.

3. The esophagogastric junction is located 40 cm. from the upper incisors endoscopically, at the level of the eleventh or twelfth thoracic vertebrae.

Most esophagoscopies can be performed with the *flexible* fiberoptic esophagoscope with use of topical anesthesia of the posterior tongue and mild intravenous sedation. General anesthesia should be used in anxious, combative, or uncooperative patients, and also in the *initial* evaluation of high-grade obstructing lesions. The rigid esophagoscope is best for evaluating lesions at or just below the cricopharyngeus sphincter, removing foreign bodies, dilating high-grade stenosis, and obtaining larger and more adequate biopsies. Mucosal detail is better seen with the flexible fiberoptic esophagoscope, which is therefore best for evaluating reflux esophagitis and following Barrett's mucosa for evidence of malignant degeneration.

ENDOSCOPIC EVALUATION OF REFLUX ESOPHAGITIS

The consistent use of a standardized grading system for endoscopic reflux esophagitis provides a more objective description of the gross pathologic changes seen and permits more meaningful evaluation of patients at different times by different endoscopists. Two commonly used classifications of reflux esophagitis are the following.

Skinner and Belsey Classification

Grade I   Distal mucosal erythema
Grade II   Mucosal erythema with superficial linear ulcerations
Grade III Mucosal erythema, ulceration, and submucosal fibrosis—a dilatable "early" stricture
Grade IV   Extensive ulceration and fibrous panmural stenosis

Savary and Miller Classification

Stage I   One or more nonconfluent longitudinal mucosal erosions
Stage II   Confluent ulcerations—noncircumferential
Stage III Erosive esophagitis with circumferential ulceration
Stage IV   Chronic changes of reflux (stricture, ulcer, Barrett's mucosa)

ENDOSCOPIC EVALUATION OF ESOPHAGEAL STRICTURE

Two questions must be answered about every esophageal stricture: Is the stricture benign or malignant? If benign, can the stricture be dilated? Both questions are answered by esophagoscopy, which is a mandatory part of the evaluation of *every* stricture. Comfortable swallowing requires that esophageal dilation be achieved to the range of a 46-French or larger bougie. Methods of esophageal dilation include passage of mercury-weighted tapered Maloney dilators, or dilators passed over a previously swallowed thread (Plummer dilator) or metal wire (Eder-Puestow or Savary-Gilliard bougies) or retrograde through a gastrostomy (Tucker dilators). The newer Savary-Gilliard dilators appear to be safer and more effective than the older instruments. A number of balloon dilators are now also available. Strictures should not only be biopsied, but also brushed for cytologic evaluation. The combination of biopsy and brushings establishes the diagnosis of carcinoma in 95 per cent of cases.

COMPLICATIONS OF ESOPHAGOSCOPY

Perforation is the leading and most serious complication of esophagoscopy and occurs in 1 to 2 per cent of patients. The most common sites of perforation in order of decreasing frequency are (1) just proximal to the upper esophageal sphincter in the neck, (2) just above the esophagogastric junction, and (3) at the level of aortic arch. *Pain or fever after esophageal instrumentation represents an esophageal perforation until proven otherwise* and is an indication for an immediate esophagogram. A contrast study with *both* a water-soluble agent (Gastrografin) and dilute barium, if no perforation is seen, should be obtained, because a perforation may not be seen when only Gastrografin is used. Cervical or high thoracic esophageal perforations are drained through a cervical incision; the upper two thirds of the thoracic esophagus are approached through a right thoracotomy; distal third perforations and those at the esophagogastric junction are approached through a left thoracotomy. Additional complications of esophagoscopy include laceration of lips or tongue, fracture or dislodgment of teeth, pharyngeal lacerations, and massive tracheobronchial aspiration.

VI

Tumors of the Esophagus
Mark B. Orringer, M.D.

BENIGN ESOPHAGEAL TUMORS AND CYSTS

Leiomyomas

Esophageal leiomyomas, the most common benign esophageal neoplasms, are smooth muscle tumors that occur in patients between 20 and 50 years of age and are multiple in 3 to 10 per cent of patients. More than 80 per cent occur in the middle and lower thirds of the esophagus. Calcification may occur within a leiomyoma, which must therefore be considered in the differential diagnosis of a calcified mediastinal mass. Most leiomyomas are asymptomatic, but tumors larger than 5 cm. may produce dysphagia, vague retrosternal pressure, and pain. Esophageal leiomyomas characteristically appear on barium esophagogram as a smooth concave defect with intact mucosa and sharp borders and abrupt sharp angles where the tumor meets the normal esophageal wall. Esophagoscopy is indicated to exclude carcinoma, but if a leiomyoma is suspected, a biopsy of the mass should *not* be performed so that subsequent extramucosal resection will not be complicated by scarring at the biopsy site. Symptomatic leiomyomas or those larger than 5 cm. should be excised. Asymptomatic or small leiomyomas discovered incidentally may be followed with periodic barium esophagograms, since these tumors grow slowly and the likelihood of malignant degeneration is low. Esophageal ultrasonography has recently provided a noninvasive means of diagnosing leiomyomas. When a leiomyoma is resected, the overlying longitudinal esophageal muscle is split in the direction of its fibers,

---

See the corresponding chapter or part in the *Textbook of Surgery*, 14th edition, pp. 689–700, for a more detailed discussion of this topic, including a comprehensive list of references.

the tumor is gently dissected away from contiguous tissues and underlying submucosa and is enucleated, and the longitudinal muscle is reapproximated. Multiple enucleations may be required for multiple leiomyomas. Results of resection of leiomyomas are excellent, and recurrence has not been reported.

Pedunculated Intraluminal Polyps

Benign esophageal polyps are rare but dramatic in their presentation. They arise in the cervical esophagus, develop progressively larger pedicles, and may intermittently extrude into and even out of the mouth. They may cause intermittent dysphagia, asphyxiation, hematemesis, or melena. On histologic examination, they consist of vascular fibroblastic tissue with varying amounts of fat. Despite their size, these tumors are easily overlooked at esophagoscopy. Resection through a lateral cervical esophagotomy is curative.

Esophageal Cysts

Esophageal cysts arise as diverticula of the embryonic foregut and similarly contain both stratified squamous and simple columnar ciliated epithelium, as well as fat and smooth muscle. A variation of the foregut cyst, the esophageal duplication cyst extends along the length of the thoracic esophagus, is lined by squamous epithelium, and has submucosal and muscle layers, the latter of which may interdigitate with the outer longitudinal muscle layer of the normal esophagus. Three quarters of duplication cysts present in childhood, over 60 per cent occur along the right side of the esophagus, and they are frequently associated with vertebral anomalies (e.g., Klippel-Feil deformity or spina bifida) and abnormalities of the spinal cord. More than 60 per cent of congenital esophageal cysts present in the first year of life with either respiratory or esophageal symptoms. Adults remain asymptomatic until bleeding or infection in the cyst causes enlargement with secondary dysphagia, choking, or retrosternal pain. The barium esophagogram shows a smooth extramucosal esophageal mass with occasional communication between the esophageal lumen and the cyst. Because of the potential for bleeding, ulceration, perforation, or infection, excision of the cyst is recommended. This is generally achieved by means of an extramucosal enucleation with excellent long-term results and no recurrence if the initial excision is complete.

MALIGNANT TUMORS OF THE ESOPHAGUS AND CARDIA

Esophageal squamous carcinoma is relatively uncommon in the United States, where the incidence is approximately 4 cases per 100,000 white men per year and 12 cases per 100,000 black men per year. Alcohol and tobacco are strong etiologic factors. The tumor is of epidemic proportion in northeast Iran (180 new cases per 100,000 population per year), the Transkei of South Africa, the Linxian County in Henan Province in northern China, and parts of southern Russia, India, and the Middle East. Epidemiologic studies have implicated carcinogenic nitrosamines in the soil, contamination of foods by fungi and yeast that produce mutagens, chronic irritation of esophageal mucosa by ingestion of hot beverages, the betel leaf, slaked lime, or resin from the acacia. A number of esophageal lesions are believed to be premalignant: achalasia, reflux esophagitis, Barrett's esophagus, radiation esophagitis, caustic burns, Plummer-Vinson syndrome, leukoplakia, esophageal diverticula, and familial keratosis palmaris et plantaris (tylosis).

PATHOLOGY. Approximately 95 per cent of esophageal carcinomas are squamous cell carcinomas, the vast majority being seen in men in the sixth and seventh decades of life and in an advanced stage (III or IV) (Table 1). Squamous cell esophageal carcinoma is most frequent in the upper and middle thoracic segments. It occurs in three common growth

TABLE 1. Tumor-Node-Metastasis (TNM) Staging System for Esophageal Carcinoma

Definition of TNM

Primary Tumor (T)

T_x	Primary tumor cannot be assessed
T_0	No evidence of primary tumor
T_{is}	Carcinoma in situ
T_1	Tumor invades lamina propria or submucosa
T_2	Tumor invades muscularis propria
T_3	Tumor invades adventitia
T_4	Tumor invades adjacent structures

Regional Lymph Nodes (N)

N_x	Regional nodes cannot be assessed
N_0	No regional node metastasis
N_1	Regional node metastasis

Distant Metastasis (M)

M_x	Presence of distant metastasis cannot be assessed
M_0	No distant metastasis
M_1	Distant metastasis

Stage Grouping

Stage	T	N	M
Stage 0	T_{is}	N_0	M_0
Stage I	T_1	N_0	M_0
Stage IIA	T_2	N_0	M_0
	T_3	N_0	M_0
Stage IIB	T_1	N_1	M_0
	T_2	N_1	M_0
Stage III	T_3	N_1	M_0
	T_4	Any N	M_0
Stage IV	Any T	Any N	M_1

From Beahrs, O. H., Henson, D. E., Hutter, R. V. P., and Myers, M. H.: Manual for Staging of Cancer, 3rd ed. American Joint Committee on Cancer. Philadelphia, J. B. Lippincott Company, 1988, pp. 63–67.

patterns: fungating (60 per cent), ulcerative (25 per cent), and infiltrative (15 per cent). Esophageal cancer is notoriously aggressive, infiltrating locally, invading adjacent intramural lymphatics and lymph nodes, and metastasizing widely by hematogenous spread. Extra-esophageal tumor extension is present in 70 per cent of cases at the time of diagnosis. Overall 5-year survival for treated tumors is 5 to 12 per cent. The 5-year survival is only 3 per cent when lymph node metastases are present compared with 42 per cent when there is no lymph node spread.

Adenocarcinomas constitute 2.5 to 8 per cent of primary esophageal cancers, although this frequency is increasing in the United States. They occur most commonly in the distal third of the esophagus, in the sixth decade of life, and with a male to female ratio of 3:1. Esophageal adenocarcinoma has one of three origins: malignant degeneration of metaplastic columnar (Barrett's) epithelium, heterotopic islands of columnar epithelium, or the esophageal submucosal glands. Patients with columnar-lined lower esophagus (Barrett's metaplasia) have been estimated to be 40 times more likely to develop adenocarcinoma than is the general population. It is estimated that adenocarcinoma arises in 8 to 15 per cent of patients with a columnar-lined esophagus. The finding of dysplasia in Barrett's mucosa is an ominous prognostic sign of impending malignant degeneration, *severe dysplasia* being nearly synonymous with carcinoma *in situ* and being an indication for resectional therapy. As with squamous cell carcinoma, esophageal adenocarcinoma is an aggressive tumor with frequent transmural invasion and lymphatic spread. Since many of these tumors arise in the distal esophagus, spread to paraesophageal, celiac axis, and splenic hilum lymph nodes is common. Metastases to lung and liver are frequent. Five-year survival is only 0 to 7 per cent. Other rare types of esophageal malignant tumors include anaplastic small cell (oat cell carcinoma), adenoid cystic carcinoma, malignant melanoma, and carcinosarcoma.

CLINICAL PRESENTATION AND DIAGNOSIS. Progressive dysphagia is the predominant symptom followed by weight loss, odynophagia, chest pain, and occasional hematemesis. A complaint of progressive dysphagia warrants *both* a barium esophagogram and esophagoscopy for excluding carcinoma. A stricture seen on barium esophagogram should be both biopsied and brushed for cytologic assessment, since the combination of these two studies establishes the diagnosis of carcinoma in 95 per cent of cases.

TREATMENT. Therapy is influenced by the knowledge that *in the majority of patients, local tumor invasion or distant metastases preclude cure*. Neither chemotherapy, radiation therapy, nor surgical resection for esophageal carcinoma has achieved significant and consistent long-term survival. The 5-year survival rate from esophageal carcinoma treated by either radiation or surgical therapy is less than 10 per cent, more than 80 per cent of patients dying within 1 year of diagnosis. Until very recently, the aim of therapy for esophageal cancer has been *palliation*, that is, restoring a patient's ability to swallow comfortably in the most simple and expeditious manner possible. Palliative transoral intubation of esophageal tumors by use of any number of available prosthetic tubes re-establishes a passage for saliva. This method, however, carries a 14 per cent mortality and a 25 per cent complication rate. Comfortable swallowing of food is often not achieved. The average survival after palliative intubation of esophageal cancer is less than 6 months. Operations that bypass the unresected esophagus (e.g., substernal colon interposition, reversed gastric tube) are associated with a high mortality (25 to 40 per cent) and a survival that averages only 6 months.

For most patients with localized esophageal carcinoma, resection, if possible, provides the best palliation. A transthoracic esophagectomy and intrathoracic esophagogastric anastomosis have been the standard operative approach for nearly 50 years. Although providing excellent palliation, this operation is associated with major morbidity—primarily respiratory insufficiency from combined thoracic and abdominal incisions in a debilitated patient and disruption of the intrathoracic anastomosis, which has a 50 per cent mortality from the resultant mediastinitis. Operative mortality figures of 15 to 40 per cent are common. In an effort to minimize the aforementioned complications of esophageal resection, the technique of transhiatal esophagectomy without thoracotomy has been popularized. In this operation, the entire thoracic esophagus is resected through upper midline abdominal and cervical incisions, the stomach is pulled into the posterior mediastinum in the original esophageal bed, and a cervical esophagogastric anastomosis is performed. This procedure avoids the morbidity of a thoracotomy, and should a cervical anastomotic leak occur, it is relatively easily managed by opening the neck wound for drainage. Operative mortality is approximately 5 per cent. Survival is equal to that achieved with standard transthoracic esophageal resection. Advocates of "radical" esophagectomy (extensive *en bloc* resection of the esophagus and contiguous tissues and lymph nodes) have not demonstrated consistently superior survival with this approach. Recently conducted uncontrolled Phase II trials of combined preoperative chemotherapy and radiation therapy before esophagectomy have yielded encouraging results that have justified prospective trials that are now under way.

VII

Perforation of the Esophagus
David B. Skinner, M.D.

Rupture of the esophagus, an uncommon condition, can be an unexpected cause of death in otherwise healthy individuals, is often difficult to diagnose, and continues to be a challenging surgical problem. The esophagus differs from the remainder of the alimentary tract in that it has no serosal layer, which makes it more likely to rupture. Perforations of the lower esophagus usually rupture into the left thoracic cavity, and ruptures of the mid-esophagus perforate into the right thorax, since there is no surrounding soft tissue to buttress the esophagus from negative intrathoracic pressure in these locations. During vomiting, the lower esophagus must momentarily increase in diameter by five times or more. This combination of factors—the absence of serosa, a pressure gradient across the esophageal wall, and rapid dilation— provides the setting in which rupture of the esophagus occurs. Perforations of the esophagus are classified according to etiology as well as location (Table 1).

SYMPTOMS AND PHYSICAL FINDINGS. Symptoms of esophageal rupture are usually dramatic, and death may occur within 24 hours in untreated cases. Pain is a nearly universal complaint. Abdominal pain may mimic a perforated gastroduodenal ulcer or severe pancreatitis, and chest pain may mimic an aortic dissection or myocardial infarction. Nausea is common, but vomiting may not occur. If the perforation occurs into the pleural cavity, respiratory symptoms predominate (dyspnea, cyanosis, air hunger), and tension pneumothorax may occur.

Early changes in vital signs following esophageal perfora-

TABLE 1. Causes of Esophageal Perforation

Spontaneous or stain-induced
Instrumental
  Esophagoscopy
  Dilation
  Intubation
Traumatic
  Penetrating missile
  Foreign body swallowed
  Blunt chest or abdominal
    injury
  Surgical dissection
  Ingested caustic agents
Intrinsic esophageal disease
  Carcinoma
  Acid-peptic ulceration
Anastomotic

See the corresponding chapter or part in the *Textbook of Surgery*, 14th edition, pp. 701–704, for a more detailed discussion of this topic, including a comprehensive list of references.

tion include fever, tachycardia, tachypnea, hypotension, and clinical evidence of shock are common. Extensive mediastinal emphysema may be palpable as crepitus at the base of the neck. Patients with thoracic perforations may have spasm, guarding, and tenderness of the upper abdomen, which may be misleading. Perforations limited to the neck cause less severe abnormalities often limited to fever, local tenderness, and crepitus.

When the diagnosis of ruptured esophagus is suspected, confirmation is generally easy. Chest radiographs alone may be diagnostic when a hydropneumothorax is seen combined with air in the mediastinum. Esophageal radiographic contrast studies are performed promptly with use of a water-soluble medium initially. If negative, the examination should be repeated with barium. Even if the perforation is obvious, the contrast study should be performed to document the level and extent of perforation. Only rarely is esophagoscopy necessary to confirm or establish the level of perforation, but it is useful if underlying esophageal disease is suspected.

TREATMENT. Surgical treatment is usually required for the recovery of patients suffering a ruptured esophagus. The operative approach depends on the cause and site of the perforation and the time elapsed before surgical therapy. In special circumstances, patients treated by nonoperative methods may survive.

For perforation of the cervical esophagus with limited extravasation and no thoracic involvement, nonoperative treatment including intensive antibiotic therapy, elimination of all feeding, and provision of intravenous alimentation is occasionally sufficient. When there is crepitus in the neck and dissection of extravasated material in fascial planes, operative drainage with intensive antibiotic therapy is the minimal treatment necessary. If it is technically possible, closure of the perforation site is advantageous. Alternatively, a cervical esophagostomy tube can be inserted through the perforation and drawn out through a stab wound for establishing a controlled fistula. Perforation of the cervical esophagus should be managed with low mortality.

Survival after perforation of the thoracic esophagus varies directly with the time elapsed between perforation and operation. In those treated within 24 hours, mortality in the range of 10 to 15 per cent can be achieved, whereas the mortality increases to 50 per cent or more for patients with delayed surgical treatment. When spontaneous or instrumental perforation is treated promptly, suture closure combined with chest drainage is often successful. Adjacent tissue such as a pleural flap or gastric fundus may be used as an onlay patch. If the perforation is related to intrinsic esophageal disease and early surgical treatment is performed, definitive therapy for the disease is desirable. Closure of a perforation above an obstructing esophageal lesion or in the presence of free gastroesophageal reflux cannot be expected to succeed.

When surgical treatment is delayed, the operative choices are often limited by the poor quality of infected and edematous tissue. Extensive drainage of infected secretion is essential in all cases and is coupled with intensive nutritional

support and antibiotics. Simple suture repair is unlikely to
be successful but should be supplemented by a patch overlay
if it is undertaken. When the poor quality of the tissue
precludes primary closure, a better alternative is diversion
including ligation or division of the cardia and a cervical
esophagostomy. If there is extensive destruction of the esophagus or intrinsic disease such as neoplasm, tight stricture, or
perforating Barrett's ulcer, an esophagectomy may be necessary with an end cervical esophagostomy, division of the
cardia, and gastrostomy. Reconstruction is performed at a
later time. Results from these several techniques for treating
late perforations vary and depend more on the time delay
and the underlying disease than on the specific surgical
procedure used.

The major complication following treatment of perforation
is continuing infection including mediastinitis; empyema;
lung, mediastinal, or subphrenic abscess; or breakdown of
the anastomosis. These infectious complications are the main
reason that perforation continues to cause a high mortality
and morbidity. Vigilance in the detection and treatment of
these complications and maintenance of adequate nutrition
are important in order to achieve better results, particularly
in patients with a delay in surgical treatment.

VIII

Hiatal Hernia and Gastroesophageal Reflux

David B. Skinner, M.D.

Hiatal hernia cannot be discussed separately from gastroesophageal reflux and its complications. Each has its own
history, method of evaluation, indications for treatment, and
therapy, but both conditions involve abnormalities of the
gastroesophageal junction and may coexist.

HIATAL HERNIA

Hiatal hernia is the herniation of an abdominal organ,
usually the stomach, through the esophageal hiatus in the
diaphragm. The Type I hiatal hernia, also called sliding or
axial, is a frequent radiographic diagnosis. It is not a true
hernia because the endoabdominal fascia remains intact but
protrudes upward through the hiatus. The intra-abdominal

See the corresponding chapter or part in the *Textbook of Surgery*,
14th edition, pp. 704–715, for a more detailed discussion of this topic,
including a comprehensive list of references.

segment of esophagus caudal to the insertion of the phreno-esophageal membrane is often of normal length. Because the fascia is intact, such a hernia does not necessarily enlarge and usually has no clinical significance. It is only when gastroesophageal reflux accompanies the hernia that symptoms or complications may develop.

The Type II hiatal hernia, also called paraesophageal or rolling hernia, is rare and represents a true herniation of a peritoneal sac through a defect in the phrenoesophageal membrane. Because intrathoracic pressure is less than atmospheric and abdominal pressure is positive throughout the respiratory cycle, the natural history of this type of hernia is progressive enlargement. The distal esophagus may remain fixed by the remaining phrenoesophageal membrane. The free intraperitoneal portion of the stomach may herniate completely upward into the intrathoracic peritoneal sac so that the pylorus comes to lie near the cardia. This causes a giant Type IIA hernia or an upside-down intrathoracic stomach that is prone to gastric volvulus. The Type II hernia may be completely asymptomatic and reach a large size without the patient's being aware of disabling symptoms. When symptoms do occur, they may include fullness after meals, gurgling noises in the chest, dysphagia, early satiety, and postprandial vomiting. Gastric obstruction may cause pain, and bleeding may occur from a chronic gastric ulcer in the pouch. Such a hernia is prone to sudden gastric volvulus with obstruction or strangulation, which may cause rapid death.

Because of the potential for catastrophic complications, surgical therapy is recommended provided that the patient's general condition is satisfactory. Even in an asymptomatic patient, a Type IIA hiatal hernia is itself an indication for surgical treatment. Approximately two thirds of patients with this type hernia have abnormal reflux when studied by pH monitoring. For this reason, an antireflux repair as well as a hiatal hernia repair is the preferred surgical treatment.

GASTROESOPHAGEAL REFLUX

Abnormal gastroesophageal reflux may occur from an incompetent cardia without a hiatal hernia. Approximately 80 per cent of patients with pathologic reflux do have a Type I hiatal hernia. Regurgitation of gastric contents occurs normally in human beings, particularly after a large meal. Gastric distention effaces the abdominal segment of esophagus and shortens its length. The gradual conversion of this segment to an inverted funnel shape permits postprandial reflux and belching to occur normally. It is only when reflux occurs with increased frequency that it is abnormal.

The symptoms of reflux are heartburn and regurgitation aggravated by postural change such as stooping or lying flat. The regurgitation is sour or bitter, reflecting stomach origin. These typical symptoms or abnormal reflux may be accompanied by symptomatic complications such as dysphagia, bleeding, substernal chest pain, a sensation of spasm in the throat, or respiratory symptoms. For upper digestive symptoms, it is important to observe the whole esophagus and stomach as a unit. If a radiologist sees spontaneous free reflux, it is clear evidence of pathologic reflux because it is somewhat difficult to induce reflux during a standard barium swallow examination.

If the symptoms and radiographic findings are not clear, esophageal function tests are indicated. These are always performed in patients being considered for antireflux surgery to be certain of the diagnosis. The techniques used for esophageal function tests include manometry for recording pressures in the stomach and esophagus and pH recordings in the distal esophagus for measuring reflux directly. As the manometric pressure transducers are withdrawn across the esophageal junction, a high-pressure zone of 10 to 20 mm. Hg is noted in the distal esophagus. Approximately 2 to 3 cm. of this is located caudal to the respiratory pressure inversion point representing the intra-abdominal esophagus. In the body of the esophagus, peristaltic or spastic contractions are noted. Manometry is essential in ruling out achalasia, scleroderma, or esophageal spasm, which may mimic symptoms caused by reflux.

For detecting reflux directly, a standard acid reflux test may be performed in which 300 ml. of 0.1 normal hydrochloric acid is placed into the stomach and the pH is recorded 5 cm. above the high-pressure zone while the patient performs a series of respiratory and postural maneuvers. The efficiency of the esophageal peristalsis and salivary production in clearing acid is measured by installing 15 mg. of 0.1 normal hydrochloric acid in the mid-esophagus and instructing the patient to swallow at intervals. The correlation of symptoms with acid in the esophagus is studied by the esophageal acid perfusion test, which alternates hydrochloric acid and normal saline for determination of whether the acid provokes symptoms not initiated by the saline infusion. A battery of esophageal function tests including manometry, standard acid reflux test, acid clearing test, and acid perfusion tests may be done on an outpatient basis and requires approximately 1 hour of technician time. These generally enable an accurate diagnosis to be made of esophageal functional disorders including pathologic reflux.

In more complicated cases or in patients who have had failed previous treatment, prolonged monitoring of pH in the distal esophagus over a 24-hour period offers the most precise and quantitative method for diagnosing reflux. In atypical syndromes such as angina-like chest pain, globus hystericus, or respiratory symptoms suspected of being caused by aspiration, prolonged intraesophageal pH monitoring is essential for demonstrating a cause and effect relationship between reflux and the symptoms.

When abnormal reflux is diagnosed, esophagoscopy is indicated to assess the degree of esophagitis and other abnormalities that may accompany reflux. Esophagitis is graded on a scale of 0 to 4 depending on the severity of inflammation and stricture. A careful observation must be performed to determine the exact location of the squamocolumnar mucosal junction. If this is 3 cm. or more above the junction of the peristaltic tubular esophagus with a gastric pouch, the diagnosis of Barrett's esophagus is made. Multiple biopsies are obtained to rule out dysplasia and to determine the cell type. Based on the analysis of symptoms, radiographs, esophageal function tests, and esophagoscopy, full information is available to decide on treatment.

TREATMENT. The indications for surgical treatment of reflux are primarily its complications including persistent Grade II ulcerative esophagitis, stricture, bleeding esophagitis, and aspiration shown to be caused by reflux. Patients without complications are treated medically to relieve symptoms. Surgical therapy is considered for symptoms alone only if medical therapy proves unsatisfactory for at least a 6-month trial and abnormal reflux is clearly documented. The patients with large paraesophageal or composite hernias are treated surgically with an antireflux repair as well as correction of the hiatal hernia.

Medical treatment of reflux starts with postural adjustment including sleeping with the bed elevated, avoiding stooping, and avoiding eating before bedtime. Antacids are prescribed initially after meals and at bedtime. The next stage of medical therapy includes cimetidine or ranitidine. If these fail, omeprazole should be given. Other medications such as metoclopramide or bethanechol are less effective. Weight loss is generally recommended but difficult to achieve.

When surgical treatment is indicated, the operation is an antireflux repair designed to restore the intra-abdominal segment of esophagus and to maintain this segment as a small-diameter tube as it enters the stomach. All repairs involve mobilization of the lower esophagus and cardia with some type of plication of the stomach around or onto the intra-abdominal segment of esophagus and narrowing of the esophageal hiatus. Three types of repairs include these principles and are used widely.

The Belsey Mark IV operation is performed through a thoracic approach. The esophagus is mobilized up to the aortic arch, and the cardia is freed completely. The fundus of the stomach is folded against the lower 4 cm. of esophagus with two rows of mattress sutures extending approximately 240 degrees around the circumference of the esophagus anterior to the vagus nerves. After the imbrication is reduced into the abdomen, sutures placed in the hiatus are tied to narrow the hiatal opening posteriorly.

The fundoplication described by Nissen can be performed through either a thoracic or abdominal approach. It involves full mobilization of the lower esophagus and gastric fundus including division of several short gastric arteries. The fundus of the stomach is brought posteriorly to encircle approximately 3 cm. of esophagus. This repair has the potential to cause obstruction, so the fundus must be well mobilized and the repair done over a large-diameter bougie. Again, the hiatus is narrowed posteriorly.

The Hill gastropexy and calibration of the cardia is performed through an abdominal incision. After mobilization, the posterior cardia is anchored to the arcuate ligament overlying the aorta. Sutures are placed from the anterior and posterior aspects of the lesser curvature as it blends with the cardia, and anchored to the arcuate ligament. This repair also has the potential to create obstruction. It is performed with the use of intraoperative manometry for adjustment of the pressure of the cardia with the plicating sutures so that an adequate barrier is achieved without its being too tight.

Each of these repairs gives excellent early results in approximately 90 per cent of patients. Side effects of the repairs include inability to belch and vomit, gaseous distention, and the risk of dysphagia from too tight a repair particularly with the total fundoplication. Another risk is injury to the esophagus or stomach from the placement of sutures. No one of these repairs has proved to be better than the others in long-range follow-up to date.

ESOPHAGUS LINED WITH COLUMNAR EPITHELIUM (BARRETT'S ESOPHAGUS)

In this condition, 3 cm. or more of the distal esophagus is lined with heterotopic glandular epithelium. Three cell types are seen: a specific metaplastic type of epithelium characterized by goblet cells; simple columnar epithelium; and gastric fundus epithelium lining what is clearly peristaltic esophagus. The squamocolumnar junction is frequently the site of a stricture. Penetrating ulcers may occur within the heterotopic gastric epithelium. The metaplastic epithelium has a potential for malignant degeneration. The risk of the development of carcinoma in this epithelium is approximately 1 in 75 patient years of follow-up.

Indications for antireflux surgery are similar to those for other types of reflux, that is, ulcerative esophagitis, stricture, bleeding ulcerations, and aspiration. If high-grade dysplasia is identified on one or more multiple biopsies, the case should be treated as early carcinoma and the patient should undergo an esophagectomy. Patients known to have this epithelium should be examined periodically with brush cytology or endoscopy for detection of dysplastic changes before the development of invasive carcinoma.

REFLUX-INDUCED STRICTURES

At an advanced stage, reflux may cause sufficient inflammation, ulceration, destruction, and scarring to cause a frank stricture just proximal to the squamocolumnar junction. For the initial treatment of a reflux-induced stricture, the inflammation, edema, and spasm should be reversed by intensive medical therapy and bougienage. When dilation to a No. 40 French bougie can be achieved easily before surgery, an antireflux repair alone has a high chance of success similar to a primary antireflux repair. For reoperative cases or if the stricture cannot be easily dilated, alternative procedures include a gastroplasty with antireflux repair, an intrathoracic total fundoplication, or a fundic patch operation. For patients who have had failures of previous surgery and extensive scarring in the mediastinum, a resection and intestinal inter-position is indicated. This is preferred to an esophagogas-trostomy for eliminating the risk of recurrent gastroesopha-geal reflux above the esophagogastric anastomosis.

IX

Corrosive Strictures of the Esophagus
James L. Talbert, M.D.

Despite an enhanced public and legislative awareness, caustic ingestions remain a significant health problem in the United States, affecting between 5000 and 15,000 citizens annually. The incidence is bimodal in age distribution, with over 75 per cent of injuries involving children less than 5 years of age and a much lower, secondary peak occurring in late adolescence and early adult life. The ingestion is almost always accidental in the young child, who all too frequently has been enticed by chemical solutions that have been care-lessly placed in familiar soft drink containers, or by crystalline caustics that resemble sugar or candy exposed in jars or cans. In the older patient, the event is usually linked to a suicide attempt. Immediate surgical attention is essential in such cases because of the high potential for inflicting serious damage to the airway and upper gastrointestinal tract. The agents most frequently involved are alkaline caustics (lye), acid or acid-like corrosives, and household bleaches. How-ever, severe localized esophageal burns can also follow inges-tion of Clinitest tablets, which are used for testing sugar in the urine and contain significant amounts of anhydrous sodium hydroxide, or swallowing of small, disc-shaped (but-ton) alkaline batteries, which may become entrapped in the esophagus of a young child.

DIAGNOSIS

Caustic injury is manifest by oral pain, drooling, excessive salivation, and inability or refusal to swallow or drink in association with visible erythema, blistering, or ulceration of the lips, oral mucosa, tongue, and pharynx. The presence of hoarseness, stridor, and dyspnea suggests laryngeal injury, whereas substernal, back, or abdominal pain and rigidity may signify mediastinal or peritoneal perforation. However,

See the corresponding chapter or part in the *Textbook of Surgery*, 14th edition, pp. 715–721, for a more detailed discussion of this topic, including a comprehensive list of references.

reported series have repeatedly emphasized that the absence of symptoms or identifiable oropharyngeal burns does not exclude the possibility of esophageal injury.

The most important element in the successful management of a corrosive burn of esophagus is immediate verification of the etiologic agent and accurate assessment of the depth and extent of injury. Induced vomiting or gastric lavage is usually contraindicated because of the dangers of compounding the original injury and of potentially incurring laryngeal damage. As soon as an appropriate period of time has elapsed to allow gastric emptying and stabilization of the patient, esophagoscopy should be performed expeditiously, preferably within the first 12 to 24 hours to confirm the extent and severity of the burn. In children, this procedure is best accomplished under general anesthesia. The only exceptions to this approach are those patients in whom esophageal or gastric perforation or impending airway obstruction is evident. The primary goal of the endoscopist is to confirm the presence or absence of a caustic burn, and past reports have cautioned against passing a rigid esophagoscope beyond the proximal point of injury because of the potential danger of perforation. In this circumstance, the status of the distal intestinal tract can be assessed only indirectly by radiographic techniques. Today's endoscopist must continue to maintain a high degree of caution, but the advent of the flexible gastroscope has increased the relative safety of such procedures, and when liquid caustics or acids have been ingested, it is especially important to visualize the stomach wall directly because of the potential of these agents to produce gastric injury, even when there is no identifiable esophageal burn.

INITIAL TREATMENT

As a consequence of the continually changing spectrum of ingested caustics over the past 30 years involving a variety of substances with differing potentials for injury, and the absence of any large, well-controlled reference series of patients comparable to that utilized nationally for randomized, coordinated trials of childhood cancer treatment, the management of this condition has remained controversial, with advocates espousing both pharmacologic and mechanical modification of wound healing, either separately or in combination. Regardless of the mode of treatment, clinical reports have increasingly emphasized that in the presence of a full-thickness esophageal injury, there is an inherent high potential for stricture formation. In those patients who sustain only superficial injuries, as manifest by erythema, edema, or blistering, the prognosis appears excellent, even in the absence of any specific treatment. However, the identification of ulcerations, especially when circumferential, warrants special concern, and in this group some form of treatment intervention for preventing stricture formation appears clearly justified.

Pharmacologic management of esophageal burns has been predicated on the use of steroids for modification of the inflammatory response to injury, and antibiotics for control of secondary bacterial infection. Experimental studies by Spain and colleagues in 1950 first suggested that early administration of cortisone produced an anti-inflammatory effect that inhibited fibroplasia in wound healing. Subsequent studies in both animals and humans utilizing steroids in concert with antibiotic coverage for control of secondary suppurative complications indicated a significant decrease in stricture formation when treatment was instituted within 48 hours following injury. This regimen may prove especially beneficial in alleviating the symptoms of impending airway obstruction induced by laryngeal edema and may also facilitate the early institution of oral feedings by minimizing pain and swelling. Indeed, the simplest approach to achieving esophageal dilation, especially in small children, is to encourage self-bougienage through the ingestion and swallowing of food.

Steroid treatment is contraindicated in cases of severe caustic injuries that are associated with clinical or roentgenographic evidence of perforation of the esophagus or stomach and has questionable efficacy in the treatment of acid ingestion, because it may not only mask evidence of peritonitis but also increase the potential for gastric ulceration and bleeding. In contrast, patients with signs of dyspnea, hoarseness, or stridor should be treated immediately with steroids and antibiotics, since they may prove effective not only in alleviating the underlying cause of the airway obstruction but also in managing the highly probable, associated esophageal injury. The steroid and antibiotic regimen that has been employed most frequently for treatment of esophageal burns consists of prednisone, administered in divided doses of 2 to 3 mg. per kg. of body weight every 24 hours, and ampicillin, administered in divided doses of 50 to 100 mg. per kg. of body weight every 24 hours, over a total of 3 weeks. If the patient is initially unable to take oral alimentation, these medications should be administered intravenously with hydrocortisone or methylprednisolone sodium succinate substituted in equivalent doses. Because the act of swallowing food probably contributes to the success of steroid therapy, oral feedings should be instituted as soon as they can be tolerated by the patient, beginning with a clear liquid diet and progressing to soft foods. When the initial edema of injury has resolved, usually within 2 to 3 days, the patient's ability to swallow should gradually improve. If dysphasia recurs and stricture formation is confirmed radiographically, the treatment regimen requires appropriate modification. In the absence of obstructive symptoms, the steroid dosage should be tapered and finally discontinued after completion of 3 full weeks of treatment. A complete radiographic evaluation of the esophagus is obtained at the termination of the steroid therapy and is reviewed again at 3 months, 6 months, and 1 year after injury. Because the reflux of acidic gastric secretions may potentiate the injury to the esophageal mucosa and further increase the likelihood of stricture formation, the concomitant administration of H_2-blockers or therapeutic doses of antacids for 6 to 8 weeks has been recommended.

Because there is a high incidence of stricture formation subsequent to severe esophageal caustic injuries, despite prompt treatment with steroids and antibiotics, an alternative method of management that has been increasingly advocated in such cases involves mechanical modification of wound healing through the placement of intraluminal Silastic stents either by mouth under fluoroscopic guidance or in concert with a gastrostomy. Several reports have indicated success with this technique, used with or without systemic antibiotics and steroids, in decreasing the incidence of residual significant scarring and stricture formation, even in the presence of severe, circumferential esophageal mucosal injury. Depending on the type and configuration of the stent, however, this form of treatment may require more intense monitoring and necessitate a longer period of hospitalization than the alternative approach of steroid and antibiotic management.

MANAGEMENT OF COMPLICATIONS

Early complications may include perforation of the esophagus or stomach demanding immediate celiotomy or thoracotomy, development of airway obstruction requiring a tracheostomy, and development of a tracheoesophageal fistula necessitating bipolar exclusion of the esophagus by proximal and distal division and closure in the neck and abdomen in conjunction with a cervical esophagostomy, gastrostomy, and tracheostomy. With identification of full-thickness necrosis of the esophagus and stomach, as may be incurred by the ingestion of concentrated solutions of alkalies or acids, emergency esophagectomy and/or gastrectomy may be required to prevent lethal complications such as overwhelming sepsis or aortoenteric fistula.

Stricture formation is usually manifest within the first few months but may be delayed until considerably later. When stenosis ensues, dilation should be attempted through the passage of bougies, either antegrade by mouth or retrograde through a previously constructed gastrostomy. An alternative method of dilation that has proved especially helpful in the management of complicated or persistent strictures involves the inflation of an intraluminal, Grüntzig-type balloon optimally positioned under fluoroscopic monitoring by means of an endoscopically directed guidewire. When a stricture proves refractory to all forms of dilation, esophageal reconstruction must be undertaken, most frequently with interposition of either a segment of colon or a reversed antiperistaltic gastric tube, based proximally on the greater curvature of the stomach and receiving its blood supply from the left gastroepiploic artery. Either of these techniques has been demonstrated in children to provide excellent long-term function and allow normal growth and development, but in adults, the alternative procedure of gastric transposition has gained increasing favor.

Late complications of corrosive burns of the esophagus include the development of achalasia or hiatal hernia as a consequence of progressive intramural scarring and contraction, as well as a thousand-fold increase in the frequency of esophageal cancer as a consequence of malignant degeneration in the previously injured tissues.

27

ABDOMINAL WALL, UMBILICUS, PERITONEUM, MESENTERIES, OMENTUM, AND RETROPERITONEUM

Kevin M. Sittig, M.D., Michael S. Rohr, M.D., Ph.D., and John C. McDonald, M.D.

ABDOMINAL WALL

The abdominal wall is a complex musculoaponeurotic structure that is attached to the vertebral column posteriorly, the ribs superiorly, and the bones of the pelvis inferiorly. It is derived embryonically in a segmental metameric manner, and this is reflected in its blood supply and innervation. The abdominal wall protects and restrains the abdominal viscera, and its musculature acts indirectly to flex the vertebral column. The integrity of the abdominal wall is essential to the prevention of hernias, whether they are congenital, acquired, or iatrogenic.

Anatomy, Innervation, Lymphatic Drainage

The abdominal wall is composed of nine layers. From superficial to deep they are (1) skin, (2) tela subcutanea (subcutaneous tissue), (3) superficial fascia (Scarpa's fascia), (4) external abdominal oblique muscle, (5) internal abdominal oblique muscle, (6) transversus abdominis muscle, (7) endoabdominal (transversalis) fascia, (8) extraperitoneal adipose and areolar tissue, and (9) peritoneum. The plane between the internal oblique and transversus abdominis muscles can properly be considered a neurovascular plane because it contains the segmental arteries, veins, and nerves that supply the abdominal wall. The anterior primary rami of thoracic spinal nerves T7 to T12 and lumbar nerve L1 supply the abdominal wall in a segmental, sequential manner from superiorly to inferiorly. The main trunks of the nerves are found in the neurovascular plane. The anterior cutaneus rami pierce the rectus sheath anteriorly to supply the anterior skin. The anterior cutaneus rami of T10 innervate a dermatome that includes the umbilicus. The lateral cutaneus rami of T7 to T9 supply skin of the thorax and lateral abdominal wall, and the lateral cutaneus rami of T12 and L1 supply the skin of the gluteal region.

The transversalis fascia is poorly named and often misunderstood. It more properly should be called the endoabdom-

---

See the corresponding chapter or part in the *Textbook of Surgery*, 14th edition, pp. 722–735, for a more detailed discussion of this topic, including a comprehensive list of references.

inal fascia, for it is a continuous lining of the abdominal cavity. Where this fascia lies in direct relation to certain muscles, it is given a special name. Over the psoas muscle, it is called the psoas fascia. Where it lies deep to the transversus abdominis muscle, it is properly called the transversalis fascia. The integrity of the endoabdominal fascia is absolutely essential for the integrity of the abdominal wall. If this layer is intact, no hernia exists. A hernia may, in fact, be defined as a hole in the endoabdominal fascia or transversalis fascia. This definition applies to esophageal hiatus hernia, umbilical hernia, inguinal hernia, femoral hernia, and incisional hernia. The peritoneum provides little strength in wound closure, but it affords remarkable protection from infection if it remains unviolated.

The lymphatic supply of the abdominal wall follows a simple pattern. Above the umbilicus, the lymphatic pathways drain into the ipsilateral axillary lymph nodes. Below the umbilicus, they drain into the ipsilateral superficial inguinal lymph nodes. Basically, the superficial lymphatics parallel the superficial veins, which above the umbilicus drain into the axillary vein and below it into the femoral vein.

The most common variant of normal anatomy seen in the abdominal wall is diastasis recti. This consists of an upper midline protrusion of the abdominal wall between the right and left rectus abdominis muscles. This abnormality represents a weakness of the linea alba and does not require treatment unless an epigastric hernia occurs in association with the diastasis recti.

Omphalocele may be seen in the newborn and represents a defect in the closure of the umbilical ring. The herniated viscera are usually covered with a sac composed of amnion. Gastroschisis is a defect of the abdominal wall that is located lateral to the umbilicus. It is due to failure of closure of the body wall in which abdominal viscera protrude through the defect. No sac is present to cover the herniated intestine.

Omphalomesenteric Duct Remnants

Remnants of the omphalomesenteric (vitelline) duct may present as abnormalities related to the abdominal wall. An umbilical polyp is a small excrescence of omphalomesenteric duct mucosa that is retained in the umbilicus. Such polyps resemble umbilical granulomas except that they do not disappear after silver nitrate cauterization. Appropriate treatment is excision of the mucosal remnant.

Umbilical sinuses are due to the continued presence of the umbilical end of the omphalomesenteric duct. The morphologic features of the sinus tract can be readily delineated with a sinogram. Treatment is excision of the sinus.

Persistence of the entire omphalomesenteric duct is heralded by the passage of enteric contents from the umbilicus. This is seen in the early neonatal period and should be treated promptly with laparotomy and excision of the duct to avoid intussusception or volvulus.

Meckel's diverticulum results when the intestinal end of

the omphalomesenteric duct persists. This is a true diverticulum of the intestine with all layers of the intestinal wall represented.

Urachal Anomalies

The urachus is a fetal structure that connects the developing bladder to the umbilicus. The urachus normally is obliterated by the time of birth. It may persist *in toto*, causing a vesicoumbilical fistula manifested by the drainage of urine from the umbilicus. Proper treatment is excision of the fistula after distal urinary obstruction has been excluded.

A persistent urachal sinus results when the umbilical end of the urachus does not obliterate normally. It may become infected and should be totally excised. Cystic remnants of the urachus may persist between the bladder and umbilicus when urachal obliteration is incomplete. These cysts may become symptomatic at any time and present as lower abdominal masses, or occasionally abscesses. They should be excised completely.

Omphalitis

Infection of the umbilicus may occur in infants and adults. It is generally an innocuous disease due to poor hygiene and is treated with appropriate cleansing and local care to the umbilicus. However, in the neonatal period, omphalitis may be the result of bacterial infection and may potentially be associated with serious sequelae such as portal vein thrombosis. In neonates, treatment should include systemic antibiotics.

Rectus Sheath Hematoma

Extravasation of blood into the rectus sheath that causes a hematoma is rarely a life-threatening illness. However, it may mimic other abdominal diseases and must be considered in the differential diagnosis to avoid unnecessary laparotomy. Patients with rectus sheath hematomas most often give a history of receiving anticoagulant drugs for various conditions. When the hematoma develops, it ordinarily occurs at the level of the semicircular line of Douglas where the inferior epigastric artery enters the rectus sheath.

Abdominal Wall Tumors

Benign tumors of the abdominal wall may arise from any of the elements contained within the abdominal wall. Desmoid tumors of the abdominal wall are benign fibrous tumors arising from the musculoaponeurotic abdominal wall. They should be widely excised to prevent local recurrence.

Primary malignancies of the abdominal wall are uncommon. Any of the cutaneous neoplasms may affect the abdominal wall and are treated in the same manner as skin cancers elsewhere. The abdominal wall is occasionally the site of metastasis from primary malignancies located elsewhere.

PERITONEUM

The peritoneal cavity is a potential space containing the abdominal viscera. It develops from the primitive coelom, which is formed by a splitting of the lateral mesoderm into somatic and splanchnic layers.

The peritoneum provides a frictionless surface over which the abdominal viscera can freely move, and the mesothelial lining secretes fluid that serves to lubricate the peritoneal surfaces. Normally, there is about 100 ml. of clear, straw-colored fluid present in the peritoneal cavity of the adult. The quality and quantity of this fluid may change with various pathologic conditions.

Peritoneal dialysis is possible because of bidirectional transport across the peritoneal membrane. By adjusting the composition of the dialysate, excess water, sodium, potassium, and products of metabolism can be removed from the bloodstream. In addition, a variety of drugs can be removed with peritoneal dialysis.

Normally, there is a balance between fluid secretion and absorption in the peritoneal cavity. Ascites occurs when either the secretion rate increases or the absorption rate decreases disproportionate to the other. This fluid may be a transudate or exudate, and its composition is determined by the etiology of the ascites.

Accumulation of lymph within the peritoneal cavity is usually the result of trauma or tumor involving lymphatic structures. It differs from other fluid accumulations in the peritoneal cavity in that it has bacteriostatic properties, making infection less likely.

Uninfected bile is a mild irritant to the peritoneal cavity. It causes an increased production of peritoneal fluid, resulting in bile ascites or choleperitoneum. Patients with this condition may be relatively well as long as the fluid remains sterile, exhibiting only a mild jaundice from absorption of bile pigments. Infected bile, however, causes a severe peritonitis and necessitates urgent surgical therapy.

Blood is not an irritating substance in the peritoneal cavity. The most common cause of hemoperitoneum is trauma to the liver or spleen. Approximately two thirds of the red blood cells in the peritoneal cavity are absorbed intact into the bloodstream.

Urine collections within the peritoneal cavity are generally due to trauma to the urinary tract.

Pneumoperitoneum is usually secondary to perforation of the gastrointestinal tract or to recent operation. It may follow alveolar rupture in patients on mechanical ventilators. Treatment is directed to the underlying cause of the pneumoperitoneum.

Peritonitis

Peritonitis is inflammation of the peritoneum. It can be septic or aseptic, bacterial or viral, primary or secondary, acute or chronic.

Primary peritonitis refers to inflammation of the peritoneal cavity without a documented source of contamination. It occurs more commonly in children than in adults, and in females more than in males. Children with nephrotic syndrome and, less commonly, systemic lupus erythematosus are particularly susceptible to primary peritonitis. In recent years, the bacterial flora has changed from gram-positive to gram-negative organisms. Thus, the distinction between primary and secondary peritonitis is more difficult to make by peritoneal aspirate alone.

Aseptic peritonitis is generally due to chemical or foreign body irritants. It may be followed by secondary bacterial peritonitis. Most chemical peritonitis is due to various irritative body fluids (bile, meconium, gastric contents).

MESENTERY AND OMENTUM

The intestine begins to elongate during the fifth week of development and forms a loop that extends out into the umbilical cord with the superior mesenteric artery extending to the apex of the loop. This is Stage I of midgut development. Stage II involves return of the duodenum to the abdominal cavity with its 270-degree counterclockwise rotation around the superior mesenteric artery. In Stage III, the right half of the colon returns to the abdomen and rotates 270 degrees in a counterclockwise direction to lie on the right side anterior to the superior mesenteric artery. This stage is completed with fixation of the intestine and its mesenteries. By the twelfth week of development, rotation is finished, but fixation may not be completed until birth.

The greater and lesser omenta and the intestinal mesentery are rich in lymphatics and blood vessels. In response to intraperitoneal inflammation, the omentum provides the major source of peritoneal macrophages and aids in removal of foreign material and bacteria. Torsion or infarction of the omentum, like mesenteric cysts or omental cysts, is best treated by excision.

RETROPERITONEUM

The retroperitoneum is an actual space located between the peritoneal cavity and the posterior body wall. Anteriorly this space is bounded by the posterior parietal peritoneum and the spaces between the leaves of the small and large bowel mesenteries. Posteriorly it is bounded by the vertebral column and the psoas and quadratus lumborum and tendinous portions of the transversus abdominis muscles. Embryologically, ectoderm, mesoderm, and embryonal remnants constitute the contents of the retroperitoneum. It is, therefore, only natural that the majority of abnormalities in the

TABLE 1. Structures that Can Be Approached Surgically via the Retroperitoneum

Adrenal glands
Kidneys
Ureters
Bladder
Lumbar sympathetic chain
Splenic artery and vein
Renal artery and vein
Distal abdominal aorta
Inferior vena cava
Common iliac artery and vein
Internal iliac artery and vein
External iliac artery and vein
Distal pancreas
Groin hernias

retroperitoneum arise from these cell lines. (See Table 1 for a list of the contents of the retroperitoneum.)

Several disorders that lend themselves to surgical treatment can be approached by an extraperitoneal or retroperitoneal exposure. This approach has many advantages over the more commonly used transabdominal approach. It is sound judgment to choose retroperitoneal or extraperitoneal exposure over transabdominal exposure when technically feasible.

Many intra-abdominal abscesses are localized in such a way that a part of the limiting wall is the parietal peritoneum. Such abscesses, when recognized, are best evacuated through the retroperitoneal portion of the abscess, thereby avoiding contamination of the general peritoneal cavity.

Retroperitoneal Fibrosis

This unusual disease, which has some similarities to hypersensitivity or autoimmune disease, is relatively rare. The etiology is unknown.

The important clinical aspect of retroperitoneal fibrosis is that the fibrotic process frequently entraps and constricts the ureters, thereby causing obstructive uropathy.

Surgical treatment of retroperitoneal fibrosis consists of freeing the encased ureters from their fibrous encapsulation. When freed, the ureters must be protected from recurrent fibrotic encasement. This has been successfully prevented by converting the ureters into intra-abdominal organs or wrapping them with omentum. Renal autotransplantation also has been used as a means to surgically treat retroperitoneal fibrosis.

Retroperitoneal Tumors

At the time of presentation, the majority of retroperitoneal tumors have invaded adjacent organs and have reached considerable size. The majority of these tumors (60 to 85 per cent) are malignant and are of mesodermal origin (75 per cent) and of nervous origin (24 per cent). Successful treatment of these tumors remains primarily surgical. An *en bloc* resection of these malignancies provides the most favorable 5-year survival of 67 per cent.

Retroperitoneal Vascular Procedures

Elective surgical procedures on the aorta and its branches are more commonly being approached from an extraperitoneal route today. The extraperitoneally exposed visceral aorta and its branches can be easily controlled for bypass, endarterectomy, splenorenal shunting, renal autotransplantation, and correction of aneurysmal disease.

28

THE ACUTE ABDOMEN

Arnold G. Diethelm, M.D., and Robert J. Stanley, M.D.

Acute abdominal pain continues to be a common diagnostic challenge to the surgeon, internist, family practitioner, obstetrician-gynecologist, and pediatrician. The complexity of the entity known as the acute abdomen is such that a careful, methodical diagnostic approach is necessary in order to arrive at a correct diagnosis. Rapid or quick decisions are usually not required and are often incorrect or misleading. A thorough knowledge of the etiology of abdominal pain and its natural history is essential in the proper management of these patients.

HISTORY

PRESENT ILLNESS. A careful and detailed history usually defines the time of onset of pain, its location, and change in character and position. The exact situation in which the onset of pain occurs may be important in establishing the diagnosis. Pain that is sharp, severe, and sudden in onset—awakening the patient from sleep or incapacitating the patient at work—suggests a perforated viscus. The character of the pain initially and later is important in the differentiation of small bowel obstruction from strangulation of the intestine. The former is a cramping intermittent type of pain, whereas the latter causes a dull constant pain. The original location of the pain and its shifting or changing of position may provide a clue to the diagnosis, as is commonly seen with acute appendicitis. Radiation of the pain may be helpful in the diagnosis. Pain of acute cholecystitis frequently radiates around the right costal margin to the right scapula and to the shoulder. Pain in acute pancreatitis is usually epigastric in origin, with subsequent radiation along both costal margins to the back. Ureteral calculi produce pain radiating to the testicle when the stone is in the cephalad portion of the ureter and perineal pain when the stone is near the ureterovesical junction. Vomiting may result from the severity of the pain, but in many instances the cause is related to the gastrointestinal tract. The temporal relationship of abdominal pain to vomiting is important and may provide valuable diagnostic clues to the underlying etiologic factor. The character of the emesis, including the color and content, is pertinent in regard to the site of obstruction. Clear vomitus suggests an obstructed pylorus, whereas bile-stained emesis indicates that the obstruction is distal to the entrance of the common bile duct into the duodenum. Anorexia is usually associated with acute abdominal pain, and in patients with acute appendicitis, it

---

See the corresponding chapter or part in the *Textbook of Surgery*, 14th edition, pp. 736–755, for a more detailed discussion of this topic, including a comprehensive list of references.

may precede the onset of pain. Constipation, diarrhea, and a recent change in bowel habits are important factors in the diagnosis of patients with abdominal pain. The failure to pass flatus associated with cramping pain and vomiting strongly supports mechanical obstruction of the gastrointestinal tract. An accurate menstrual history is especially valuable in the assessment of abdominal pain in the female, including the frequency of the cycle and the duration of the menstrual period. The type of contraception and its duration of use must be considered because there are specific complications for each method.

PAST ILLNESSES. The patient's history before the present illness is of special value, particularly in regard to previous surgery (e.g., appendectomy, cholecystectomy, gastric or intestinal surgery) or the previous diagnosis of an abdominal or inguinal hernia.

FAMILY HISTORY. The probability of acute abdominal pain relating to a familial disease is unlikely but may occur in some circumstances. Familial Mediterranean fever (familial recurring polyserositis) occurs in persons of Armenian or Sephardic Jewish background as an inherited autosomal recessive trait with spontaneous attacks of abdominal pain. Sickle cell anemia in black patients is another example of hereditary influence on the cause of abdominal pain.

PHYSICAL EXAMINATION

The physical examination begins with the patient's appearance, ability to answer questions, position in bed, and degree of obvious pain or discomfort. The position in bed is important regarding whether the patient lies in a supine position or on the side with knees and hips flexed.

Examination of the abdomen always begins with a visual inspection of the chest and abdomen for previous scars, hernia or obvious masses, or abdominal wall defects. The inspection should focus on the size, shape, and contour of the abdomen, with specific consideration given to the respiration of the patient including the rate and depth of breathing. Auscultation of the abdomen should include all four quadrants, with special attention given to the frequency and pitch of bowel sounds and rushes of gas audible to the examiner that correlate to the facial expression of pain by the patient. Percussion of the abdomen should begin in the quadrant free of pain and should be performed lightly so that elicitation of pain is avoided at the onset of the examination.

The presence of peritoneal irritation can be assessed either by palpation with a quick release of the examining hand (rebound tenderness) or by gently rolling the patient from side to side, with the examiner's hands placed on the patient's pelvis. The pelvic examination will note the presence of cervical discharge or vaginal bleeding, and bimanual examination will either confirm or exclude tenderness on uterine or adnexal palpation. A rectal examination should note the existence of pelvic tenderness or a mass and the presence of a perirectal abscess.

RADIOGRAPHIC STUDIES

The plain supine and erect radiographs of the abdomen remain the first step in the diagnostic imaging evaluation of patients with abdominal pain, although more sensitive and specific imaging methods, such as computed tomography and ultrasonography, play an increasing role in the evaluation of this complex, emergent clinical problem. Free intraperitoneal air can result from perforation of a gastric or duodenal peptic ulcer, perforation of the cecum due to obstruction and/or ischemia, and perforation associated with colonic diverticulitis. Plain radiographs of the abdomen are most valuable in the evaluation of mechanical obstruction of the gastrointestinal tract. Supine and erect radiographs of the abdomen should allow the distinction between obstruction of the gastric outlet and small and large bowel obstruction.

The indications for the use of computed tomography and ultrasonography in the evaluation of the acute abdomen have increased greatly in the past 5 years. Ultrasonography can provide rapid evaluation of liver, spleen, pancreas, and renal morphologic features. Aortic and visceral artery aneurysms, thrombi within veins, arteriovenous fistulas, and vascular anomalies all are amenable to evaluation with modern ultrasound equipment. Diagnostic arteriography serves a tertiary role in the evaluation of patients with an acute abdomen and should be considered only when the clinical presentation, supported by suggestive findings on computed tomography or ultrasonography, indicates a vascular lesion amenable to diagnostic as well as potentially therapeutic angiographic techniques.

CLINICAL PATHOLOGIC DIAGNOSTIC STUDIES

A complete blood count and urinalysis are essential in all patients evaluated for acute abdominal pain. The results need to be reviewed before a final decision is made regarding surgical intervention unless the urgency is such that immediate operation is required; additional laboratory tests that are especially helpful include a serum amylase for patients with acute pancreatitis, liver function studies for confirming the presence of acute hepatitis, and the human chorionic gonadotropin for excluding an ectopic pregnancy.

ORGAN SUBSYSTEM ANALYSIS

The etiology of acute abdominal pain can be separated according to the organ subsystem involved. The most common cause of acute abdominal pain in the gastrointestinal subsystem relates to an inflammatory or mechanical process of the stomach, small and large intestine, gallbladder, common bile duct, liver, or pancreas.

PERFORATED PEPTIC ULCER. Free perforation of peptic ulcer disease, more often resulting from duodenal ulcer than from gastric ulcer, is more common in male patients between the third and fourth decades. The pain is sudden in onset, severe, and located first in the epigastrium, later spreading over the entire abdomen. Shoulder pain is common and reflects referred pain from diaphragmatic irritation. The patient with generalized peritonitis from a perforated ulcer usually lies in the supine position, avoiding any undue motion that might increase the abdominal pain. The patient often appears acutely ill with tachypnea and tachycardia. Percussion reveals generalized abdominal tenderness, especially in the epigastric region. Palpation suggests a firm "boardlike" abdomen, with rigidity of the rectus muscles. Rebound tenderness that is present in all four quadrants and worse in the epigastric region is the most important diagnostic finding. Auscultation of the abdomen soon after perforation reveals hypoactive bowel sounds that progress to absent bowel sounds. Laboratory data usually include an elevated white blood cell count between 12,000 and 20,000 per cu. mm. with immature forms. The serum amylases may be slightly elevated but less than that seen in acute pancreatitis. Air underneath the diaphragm in erect films is present in about 75 per cent of patients.

ACUTE CHOLECYSTITIS. This disease most commonly occurs in women between the ages of 30 and 60 years who have had a previous history of pregnancy. The younger patients often have a family history of biliary tract disease. The attack is characterized by the onset of a constant dull pain in the right upper quadrant. Some patients move about, attempting to relieve the pain, whereas others lie restlessly in bed. Nausea and vomiting are common, with temporary improvement in the severity of pain after an episode of emesis. The pain may subside after several hours; if so, the episode is considered to be biliary colic. The disease process may progress to acute cholecystitis. Examination of the abdomen reveals mild to moderate distention, and on inspection from the patient's feet, the abdomen may show asymmetry in the right upper quadrant with a mass that distends on deep inspiration. Bowel sounds are hypoactive to auscultation. Tenderness is maximal in the right upper quadrant. In the absence of perforation and generalized peritonitis, tenderness to palpation confirms the right upper quadrant tenderness to be worse with deep inspiration. Frequently a mass can be palpated along the right costal margin, which represents a distended tense gallbladder that descends with deep inspiration. Laboratory data often reveal the white blood cell count to be elevated (10,000 to 13,000 per cu. mm.); however, a normal white blood cell count may occur in the presence of severe acute cholecystitis. An elevated serum bilirubin to 2.0 or 2.5 mg. per 100 ml. may exist with uncomplicated acute cholecystitis. If, however, the bilirubin exceeds 3.0 mg. per 100 ml., common duct calculi should be considered. Ultrasonography, currently the most common imaging method used, can rapidly assess the diameter of the biliary tree, the presence or absence of biliary calculi, and the appearance of the gallbladder wall and contents as well as the surrounding structures.

ACUTE PANCREATITIS. Pancreatitis may present with

sudden onset of severe epigastric pain radiating directly through to the back and around both costal margins with or without shoulder pain. Acute pancreatitis usually presents in patients between the ages of 25 and 50 years and has frequently been preceded by a similar episode with a previous diagnosis. The onset may be rapid, with the pain becoming intolerable in 3 to 4 hours. Anorexia, nausea, and vomiting are common, and emesis rarely provides relief. Abdominal tenderness, most evident in the epigastric region, is present with both percussion and palpation. Bowel sounds are usually hypoactive and may be absent. Routine laboratory tests show a leukocytosis ranging from 12,000 to 22,000 per cu. mm. The key diagnostic test is the serum amylase, which is elevated within a few hours in most patients who have the acute form of the disease. Plain radiographs of the abdomen are often nondiagnostic in patients with acute pancreatitis. Computed tomography and ultrasonography are the next studies performed for confirmation of the clinical diagnosis or assessment of suspected complications.

ACUTE RELAPSING PANCREATITIS. Acute relapsing pancreatitis differs from acute pancreatitis in that the pain is recurrent with each exacerbation of pancreatitis and is associated with an increase in serum amylase. The patient's previous history of pancreatitis will usually confirm the diagnosis. The physical findings are identical to those noted with acute pancreatitis. The diagnosis can be established by ultrasonography or a computed tomographic scan of the pancreas.

CHRONIC PANCREATITIS. Patients with chronic pancreatitis differ from those with recurrent episodes of acute pancreatitis (acute relapsing pancreatitis) in that the pain becomes constant. The history usually suggests the diagnosis from the patient's previous attacks, and radiographs of the abdomen often reveal pancreatic calcification.

ACUTE APPENDICITIS. Acute appendicitis, a common cause of abdominal pain, is especially difficult to diagnose in patients younger than age 3 and older than 70 years. A careful history is essential in making an accurate early diagnosis. Abdominal pain first begins in the epigastrium, then gradually migrates to the periumbilical region and finally to the right lower quadrant. Anorexia, nausea, and vomiting are common. The prodromal symptoms of indigestion, irregularity of the bowels, nausea, and vomiting are all common findings. There is localization of the pain to the right lower quadrant after 6 to 8 hours of onset, with tenderness to palpation and rebound tenderness. Guarding to palpation occurs when the process has progressed to localized peritonitis. Abdominal distention is rarely seen in the early stages of the disease. Regardless of all the presenting illnesses, the most common complaint is right lower quadrant pain, and the most frequent physical finding is right lower quadrant tenderness to palpation. Laboratory data are nondiagnostic and may be normal. The plain abdominal film findings are usually not helpful, although a visible fecalith may be diagnostic. Recent experience with ultrasonography and computed tomography has shown both imaging methods to be helpful in defining the pathologic changes characteristic of appendicitis as well as its associated complications.

PELVIC INFLAMMATORY DISEASE. Pelvic inflammatory disease with acute salpingitis is encountered in patients before menopause; it causes acute pelvic pain originating in the right lower and left lower quadrants. Acute pelvic inflammatory disease often becomes symptomatic at the completion of or just following a menstrual period. The pain is rarely associated with anorexia, nausea, or vomiting. The pain and tenderness are usually bilateral and associated with a temperature of 38 to 39° C. (100 to 102° F.). Tenderness to palpation usually exists in both lower quadrants; tenderness is associated with palpation of the cervix. Adnexal masses are present bilaterally with vaginal discharge.

RENAL CALCULI. Renal or ureteral calculi may cause severe abdominal pain; however, once the calculus begins to descend in the ureter, the pain pattern varies, with radiation to the groin, testicle, and perineum. The pain is sudden, is excruciating in severity, and may subside in a few minutes only to recur when the calculus descends in the ureter. Radiographs of the abdomen should be performed in patients in a supine position with an intravenous pyelogram, and urinalysis can usually differentiate renal pain from that of nonrenal origin.

MECKEL'S DIVERTICULITIS. This condition, which involves the persistence of a portion of the vitelline duct on the antimesenteric border of the distal ileum, may produce bleeding, intestinal obstruction, and, less often, acute abdominal pain from diverticulitis. The signs and symptoms of Meckel's diverticulitis are difficult to separate from those of acute appendicitis.

ACUTE DIVERTICULITIS. Acute diverticulitis may result from congenital or acquired diverticula. In most instances, the disease is a result of the acquired form of the disease; the incidence increases with age. The process may involve the entire colon but more commonly involves the left colon, particularly in the sigmoid. The disease presents with left lower quadrant pain, chills, and fever. Vomiting and anorexia are uncommon. Abdominal examination reveals the abdomen to be slightly distended with tenderness in the left lower quadrant. A mass is often palpable just medial to the anterior superior iliac spine.

ACUTE OBSTRUCTION OF THE SMALL INTESTINE. The first symptom of acute obstruction of the small intestine is sudden, sharp, colicky abdominal pain, often periumbilical and cramping in nature. Between episodes of colic, the patient is free of pain and may feel quite well. Nausea and vomiting occur soon after the onset of symptoms, and emesis may temporarily relieve the pain. The color of the vomitus is at first green, containing bile, and later changes to a yellow-brown color with a feculent odor. Auscultation of the abdomen reveals hyperactive bowel sounds of increased pitch and intensity with audible rushes as peristalsis increases in frequency. Laboratory data show an increase in hematocrit resulting from dehydration with the white blood cell count increased from 12,000 to 20,000 per cu. mm. Supine and erect radiographs of the abdomen are almost always diagnostic in the evaluation of patients with acute small bowel obstruction. If the level of obstruction is in the mid or distal small bowel, dilated loops of fluid- and gas-filled small bowel will be apparent, whereas the nonobstructed colon will appear devoid of gas or feces.

ACUTE OBSTRUCTION OF THE LARGE INTESTINE. Obstruction of the large intestine occurs more often in patients over the age of 40 years, is gradual in onset, and presents with constipation and abdominal distention. The most common causes of large bowel obstruction include carcinoma of the colon, acute diverticulitis, and volvulus. The abdomen appears distended and tympanitic to percussion. Unless peritonitis or peritoneal irritation exists, there is minimal abdominal tenderness to percussion and palpation. The distention may prevent the palpation of abdominal masses, and results of a pelvic and rectal examination are negative unless the obstructing lesion is within reach of the examining finger. The diagnosis can be suggested in most instances by a supine and an upright radiograph of the abdomen. The descending and sigmoid colon are dilated to the point of the obstruction, and the small intestine may be dilated if the ileocecal valve is competent. Acute diverticulitis with large bowel obstruction occurs most frequently in patients older than 45 years and has often been preceded by other attacks.

Volvulus of the large intestine causing acute intestinal obstruction can occur in the cecum or sigmoid portion of the colon. Sigmoid volvulus is more common than is cecal volvulus and occurs more frequently in patients over the age of 65 years. The diagnosis is established by the supine and upright radiographs of the abdomen; a contrast enema reveals the characteristic point of torsion and nonfilling of the obstructed loop of sigmoid colon. It should be noted that when a sigmoid or cecal volvulus is strongly suspected, a water-soluble contrast enema is preferable to barium. Cecal volvulus usually occurs in patients of the middle and older age group, with sudden onset of cramping right lower quadrant and epigastric pain associated with nausea and vomiting. The diagnosis is best established by supine and upright radiographs of the abdomen demonstrating a dilated cecum and ascending colon, often with the gas-distended cecum in the left upper quadrant. Nonobstructive colonic dilation, also described as pseudo-obstruction of the colon (Ogilvie's syndrome), refers to a clinical entity in which there are signs and symptoms of colonic obstruction but without mechanical obstruction.

Acute Gynecologic Disease

Acute abdominal pain resulting from disorders of the gynecologic subsystem is one of the most common and serious diagnostic problems encountered by the surgeon in which surgical therapy is often contraindicated.

ACUTE SALPINGITIS. This disease, most commonly due

to gonococcal infection, has an index of highest frequency in sexually active patients between the ages of 15 and 35 years and is rarely seen after menopause. The pain begins caudal to the umbilicus in the midline and radiates to the right and left lower quadrants. Examination of the abdomen reveals right and left lower quadrant tenderness to percussion and palpation. Bowel sounds are hypoactive. Cervical tenderness is marked to palpation on pelvic examination. A vaginal discharge is frequent, and a positive diagnosis can be established with a cervical smear and culture.

OVARIAN CYSTS. Ovarian cysts may present in an acute manner when torsion occurs. Pain is sudden, located in the lower abdomen, and most severe in either the right or left lower quadrant, depending on the ovary involved. Pelvic examination is the key diagnostic maneuver, and a palpable mass may confirm the suspicion.

ECTOPIC PREGNANCY. Tubal pregnancy may present as an acute intra-abdominal condition with sudden lower abdominal pain that is sharp in character and persistent, with or without nausea and vomiting. These symptoms indicate rupture of the fallopian tube and occur in the first trimester of pregnancy. A missed menstrual period or an abnormally short scanty period will have preceded the abdominal pain. The preoperative diagnosis may be established by a positive human chorionic gonadotropin test.

SUMMARY

Acute abdominal pain is a serious surgical emergency requiring the surgeon to combine the results of the history and physical examination with properly selected laboratory and radiographic studies. The indications for surgical therapy can be established in most situations, and a correct preoperative diagnosis will usually lead to a successful operation.

29

THE STOMACH AND DUODENUM

James C. Thompson, M.D., M.A.

The stomach and duodenum may be considered logically as a unit because many physiologic mechanisms and certain diseases are either shared by or interact with these two segments of the gut.

ANATOMY

The stomach arises as a spindle-shaped dilation of the foregut during the fourth week of embryonic life. With later growth, it undergoes a rotation so that the previous left side of the stomach becomes the anterior wall, and the previous right side comes to lie posteriorly (mnemonic—LARP). The duodenum, which was initially suspended between dorsal and ventral mesenteries, also rotates so that the second portion of the duodenum becomes retroperitoneal and encompasses the head of the pancreas in its C loop.

The fully developed stomach is the largest dilation of the gut and lies between the esophagus and the duodenum. The topographic anatomy of the stomach is quite simple, although it has been confused by the application of overlapping terms by anatomists, surgeons, endoscopists, and radiologists. For gross description, the stomach can be divided into fundus, body, and antrum. The fundus is the dome of the stomach, to the left of and superior to the esophagogastric junction. An angulation approximately 5 to 6 cm. proximal to the pylorus on the lesser curvature, at about the midline of the body, is termed the *incisura angularis*. The area between the fundus and a line drawn from the incisura angularis to the greater curvature of the stomach is the body of the stomach; the area distal to that line and proximal to the pylorus is the gastric antrum. The pylorus may be palpated as a thick ring of muscle and is marked externally by the prominent veins of Mayo.

PEPTIC ULCER AND OTHER SYNDROMES OF MUCOSAL INJURY

Peptic ulcer of the stomach and the duodenum afflicts more than 10 million citizens of the United States according to the best statistics, and probably only one half of the cases are recognized. The condition is most common in men between the ages of 20 and 60 years, and the cost to society

---

See the corresponding chapter or part in the *Textbook of Surgery,* 14th edition, pp. 756–787, for a more detailed discussion of this topic, including a comprehensive list of references.

is in excess of 1 billion dollars per year. Evidence indicates that the incidence of duodenal ulcer is decreasing.

Duodenal Ulcer

The association of duodenal ulcer with acid hypersecretion is firmly established. In most collected series, the mean basal and maximal acid output of patients with duodenal ulcer is one and one half to two times as great as that of control patients, and Cox has shown that the stomachs of patients with duodenal ulcer have almost twice the number of parietal cells as do normal stomachs (normal is about 1 billion). There is as yet no evidence that duodenal defense mechanisms are faulty in patients who develop duodenal ulcer.

Strong public opinion holds that emotional factors have an important role in the development of peptic ulcer. Feldman and associates have provided evidence that patients with ulcers handle ordinary life-stresses poorly. Diet and alcohol appear to have no role, but smoking does appear to predispose to ulcer.

Gastric Ulcer

Whereas duodenal ulcers appear to be caused by increased potency of the acid peptic forces attacking the mucosa, gastric ulcers may be related primarily to injury of the gastric mucosa, which renders it more susceptible to acid peptic damage. Most studies report that patients with gastric ulcer secrete either low-normal or below-normal amounts of acid, and only 5 per cent of patients with gastric ulcer demonstrate acid hypersecretion. The evidence is now abundant that reflux of bile and pancreatic juice is involved in the pathogenesis of gastric ulcer. Gastric reflux of bile after meals is increased in patients with gastric ulcer, which may be caused, at least in part, by dysfunction of the pyloric sphincter. Bile salts apparently damage the mucosa, which is then attacked by acid peptic digestion. Gastric ulcers invariably occur in areas of gastritis. Because the gastritis progresses proximally from the pylorus, patients with gastric ulcers have a larger distal area of alkaline mucosa, and gastric ulcers lie in achlorhydric zones of mucosa. The great majority of gastric ulcers (up to 95 per cent) occur on the lesser curvature near the incisura angularis.

Acute Mucosal Erosions (Stress Ulcers)

Acute superficial ulcerative lesions of the gastroduodenal area have been variously termed *acute mucosal erosions, stress ulcers, acute peptic ulcers, erosive gastritis, hemorrhagic gastritis,* and *Curling's* or *Cushing's ulcers.* The last two eponymic lesions have specific causes, burns and head injury, respectively; the other terms are approximately synonymous and are often used interchangeably. None of the terms is satisfactory.

Sepsis may well be the most important etiologic factor. Undrained pus is responsible for a high proportion of stress ulcers. Upper gastrointestinal bleeding occurring in a critically ill patient signals investigation for pus.

DUODENAL ULCER

Duodenal ulcer is a chronic disease that was formerly considered to be four times more common in men than in women; Kurata and associates suggest that there may currently be little difference in the sex distribution. Duodenal ulcer may appear at any age but occurs most frequently between the ages of 20 and 60 years and has previously been considered to have a peak incidence in the fourth decade of life; recent studies suggest an increasing incidence with increasing age. The clinical course is characterized by long periods of remission and periods of exacerbation that may last from days to months. The chief symptom is pain, which classically is perceived in the epigastrium in the midline. Pain is frequently absent in postbulbar ulcers. When pain is present, however, it often has bizarre characteristics and is often unresponsive to antacid therapy.

Diagnosis

A presumption of the presence of a duodenal ulcer may be made from a patient's history, but definitive diagnosis depends on either endoscopy or radiology. Formerly, radiologic diagnosis was given precedence, but fiberoptic endoscopy has now become the standard by which all diagnostic procedures are graded. Even so, if a duodenal ulcer is clearly shown on upper gastrointestinal radiography, there is usually no indication to confirm the finding by endoscopy unless the patient is bleeding. Radiography is less expensive than endoscopy, and this must be considered.

HISTORY. Most important in the history is the character of the pain. It may take various forms and be interpreted in various ways. Care should be taken to avoid misunderstanding because of different connotations given to the word *pain.* It is often necessary to use several synonyms, *discomfort, ache, pressure,* or even *hunger pain,* in order to be sure that disavowal of pain is valid.

RADIOLOGY. The radiologic diagnosis of duodenal ulcer is 75 to 80 per cent accurate. The patient may show an actual crater deformity indicative of active disease or may merely demonstrate scarring of the duodenal bulb caused by previous ulceration. About 95 per cent of duodenal ulcers occur in the duodenal bulb, and 5 per cent are postbulbar. An indeterminate number occur in the pyloric canal and are often termed *channel ulcers.*

The most important sign in the diagnosis of duodenal ulcer is the demonstration of the ulcer crater. Because ulcer craters are much more commonly located on the anterior or posterior wall of the duodenal bulb, the crater is more likely to be seen *en face.*

FIBEROPTIC ENDOSCOPY. The development of the flexible fiberoptic panendoscope has greatly facilitated diagnosis of peptic ulcer disease. A diagnostic accuracy of 95 per cent or even greater may be achieved, and the evidence is clear that endoscopy is superior to radiography in defining the presence of lesions of the esophagus, stomach, and duodenum.

Treatment

A large percentage of patients, perhaps most with duodenal ulcer, never have any formal treatment. Of patients whose ulcer diathesis is sufficiently severe to require medical attention, probably 85 per cent may be managed successfully by medical therapy.

MEDICAL TREATMENT. A legitimate aim of all ulcer therapy is to maintain the intraluminal pH above about 5.5 so that pepsinogen is not activated. The mainstay of this effort formerly was antacid therapy, but H_2-receptor blockade has proved so effective and acceptable that it is now the most common and most effective treatment. The choice among different drugs (cimetidine, ranitidine, famotidine, and others) is governed primarily by the cost and duration of action of the drugs. Omeprazole is a relatively new and highly potent suppressor of acid secretion that achieves its effect by blocking the proton-pump in the parietal cell that actually secretes H^+.

H_2-receptor blockade treatment was initially designed for a brief intensive period to heal the ulcer. When it became apparent that drug therapy did not alter the basic ulcer diathesis and that recurrence after the brief intensive period was approximately 70 to 80 per cent, the concept of maintenance therapy (usually one pill at night) was popularized. The true cost of lifelong maintenance therapy has never been accurately estimated. Costs are a vital consideration today, and governmental agencies are deeply involved in projecting long-term costs. Will surgical therapy, which offers a much higher cure rate and, with selective proximal vagotomy, a low rate of complications, ultimately prove to be more economical than lifelong medical therapy?

INDICATIONS FOR SURGICAL TREATMENT. Less than 1 in 5 patients with long-standing duodenal ulcer require operation. Surgical techniques in operations on the stomach are discussed in a subsequent section. The complications of duodenal ulcer that require surgical management are hemorrhage, perforation, obstruction, and intractability.

Hemorrhage. Bleeding is the most serious complication of peptic ulcer and represents about 40 per cent of deaths due to the disease. Bleeding may be chronic and insidious or brisk and life-threatening. Even when large vessels are eroded by enzymatic digestion, bleeding is usually self-limited, and it is rare for a patient to bleed and continuously bleed to death. Spontaneous remission of the hemorrhage occurs when the blood pressure falls because of hypovolemic shock and a clot then forms on the ulcer crater. Bleeding may be heralded by several days of exacerbation of pain or may arise *de novo* in a patient who has never had ulcer symptoms. Bleeding from duodenal ulcer is usually manifested by passage of black tarry stools (melena), but with rapid bleeding, bright red blood may appear per rectum, and blood may also regurgitate into the stomach and be vomited.

Mortality for operations on patients during acute bleeding episodes are several times greater than for elective operations. Everything possible must be done to control the bleeding so that the patient may be resuscitated and evaluated for elective operation. Obviously, however, if the patient begins to bleed and continues to bleed, as less than 10 per cent of patients do, emergency surgical therapy as a lifesaving measure is required.

The availability of fiberoptic endoscopy has revolutionized the emergency management of patients with massive upper gastrointestinal bleeding. The procedure is safe and accurate and provides critical information quickly.

What are the criteria for deciding which bleeding patients should be operated upon? Any patient who has suffered a massive blood loss, by any of the following criteria, should be considered a *candidate* for operation: (1) loss of 1500 to 2000 ml. of blood; (2) blood loss that causes an acute fall in the hematocrit to 25 or below; (3) acute blood loss causing syncope; (4) blood loss that, after the patient's vital signs have been stabilized, requires more than 1000 ml. of blood per 24 hours for maintaining a stable hematocrit and stable blood pressure.

If a patient is admitted to the hospital bleeding massively, ceases bleeding spontaneously and is completely resuscitated, and then has another massive hemorrhage while in the hospital, surgical therapy is indicated.

Perforation. Perforation of a duodenal ulcer initiates a remarkable series of dramatic changes. Immediately before perforation, the patient may feel entirely well, within a few minutes be in great pain, and within an hour be desperately ill. As already noted, hemorrhage is associated with *posterior* erosion of an ulcer; perforation occurs when an anteriorly or laterally placed ulcer erodes through the full thickness of the wall of the duodenum into the free peritoneal cavity, spilling acid peptic juice, bile, and pancreatic juice into the peritoneal cavity. Within a short time, massive amounts of extracellular fluid may be sequestered in the area of peritoneal injury, and hypovolemic shock may ensue from this loss of fluid. Perforated ulcers are usually not associated with significant loss of blood. Diagnosis in most cases is not difficult, but in atypical instances, it may be extraordinarily so.

Examination of the abdomen usually reveals considerable guarding and often boardlike rigidity of the abdominal musculature. With free air in the peritoneal cavity, there is often a loss of the normal dullness on percussion over the liver. If gastric contents have flowed into the right lower quadrant guided by the attachment of the small bowel mesentery, the patient may have signs and symptoms of peritonitis in the right lower quadrant, which may confuse the diagnosis and suggest appendicitis.

Approximately 75 per cent of patients show free air under the diaphragm on an upright chest film or on a lateral decubitus film if the patient is unable to sit. Conversely, this means that about one in four patients with perforated duodenal ulcer do not show free air, and that it is perfectly proper, if other evidence warrants, to make the diagnosis of perforation *without* the demonstration of free intraperitoneal air on upright chest film or on lateral abdominal decubitus films.

At operation, the site of perforation should be located and either closed with an omental patch (Graham closure) or incorporated into a pyloroplasty, which, when coupled with a vagotomy, not only repairs the perforation by reducing acid secretion but also serves as definitive treatment for the duodenal ulcer. Pyloroplasty of the scarred duodenum is often difficult. A parietal cell vagotomy may also be used.

Obstruction. Patients with chronic duodenal ulcer may develop gastric outlet obstruction caused by chronic cicatrization in which scar contracture gradually narrows the lumen. In this instance, patients with a massively dilated stomach may seek help after months of intermittent obstruction, or they may suddenly undergo complete obstruction of the pylorus and vomit perniciously for several days. Because of the massive loss of H^+ and Cl^{-} the patient may have a severe hypochloremic alkalosis along with hypokalemia. The potassium deficiency is due to a moderate loss from vomiting (gastric juice has about 10 mEq. K^+ per liter) and to an important renal loss caused by substitution of K^+ for H^+.

The operative procedure usually recommended is truncal vagotomy either with antrectomy or with gastroenterostomy. The author believes that gastroenterostomy is preferable because it avoids placing an anastomosis or closure in the scarred duodenum.

Intractability. An ulcer may be intractable because of the extraordinary virulence of the ulcer diathesis or, far more commonly, because the patient is unable to comply with a program of drug treatment. Intractability was formerly the most common indication for operation. Most such patients are now treated with H_2-blockade. Time will allow the opportunity to determine what percentage of patients can avoid operation. Some will fail on H_2-blockade, usually because of poor compliance. In patients with severe ulcer disease, some believe that long-term H_2-blockade may delay, rather than avoid, operative therapy. Only surgical therapy can effectively alter the natural history of the majority of patients with duodenal ulcer. Sufficient experience with omeprazole has not been obtained to predict its effectiveness, but the main difficulty is with compliance, not the efficacy of drug treatment. Omeprazole not taken is no better than cimetidine not taken.

On the basis of review of the results of various procedures, the author believes that selective proximal vagotomy is the procedure of choice for elective operations performed for intractability.

GASTRIC ULCER

Gastric ulcers generally appear later in life than duodenal ulcers and have a peak incidence in the fifth decade. They affect about twice as many men as women, and although variously estimated as only one third to one fifth as common as duodenal ulcers in this country, they are responsible for almost half the deaths due to peptic ulcer disease. The relative incidence of gastric to duodenal ulcer is increasing in the United States.

Diagnosis

HISTORY. Although the clinical findings in a patient with gastric ulcer may be quite similar to those in a patient with duodenal ulcer, there are often important differences. The pain pattern is not nearly as clear-cut; pain usually appears just at or slightly to the left of the midline.

RADIOLOGY. Although radiographic studies have long been the mainstay of diagnosis of gastric ulcer, gastroscopy is more accurate and affords the additional opportunity for biopsy. An important consideration in the diagnosis of gastric ulcer is the possibility of malignancy.

About 95 per cent of benign gastric ulcers are located on or near the lesser curvature, and a majority have been reported in the region of the incisura.

GASTROSCOPY. Fiberoptic gastroscopy examination allows the endoscopist to directly view the gastric ulcer, to obtain a radiograph of it, and to obtain with a biopsy forceps small fragments of the edges of the ulcer for histologic examination. Experienced endoscopists can often recognize malignant ulcers, but multiple (8 to 12) biopsies provide the most accurate answer to the question of possible malignancy. With multiple samples, endoscopic biopsy is remarkably accurate.

Treatment

Most patients with duodenal and gastric ulcers do well on medical (H_2-blockade or antacids) therapy, but there is a higher rate of recurrence in those with gastric ulcers. Because of this and because of the frequency (as high as 63 per cent) and the serious consequences of complications, operation should be considered strongly in patients with recurrent gastric ulcer. Although selective proximal vagotomy has been advocated in patients with gastric ulcer, resection of the distal 50 per cent of the stomach appears to provide the best result. Selective proximal vagotomy is not effective for channel (pyloric) ulcers; they should be resected.

The indications for operation in patients with gastric ulcer are hemorrhage, perforation, obstruction, intractability, and the need to exclude the possibility of carcinoma of the stomach. Since endoscopic biopsy, properly performed, is highly accurate, the last indication is rare. Because malignancy is a possibility in all gastric ulcers, at operation it is important either to remove the entire ulcer and obtain pathologic examination by frozen-section technique or to obtain biopsy specimens from four quadrants of the ulcer and examine them by frozen section.

ZOLLINGER-ELLISON SYNDROME

Zollinger and Ellison in 1955 described a clinical syndrome that is now recognized to consist of massive gastric hypersecretion, peptic ulceration (often multiple, often jejunal, and frequently fatal), and a non–beta cell islet tumor of the pancreas that produces gastrin. The gastrinoma metastasizes to the liver and regional lymph nodes in more than 50 per cent of cases. Diarrhea and malabsorption are frequently associated and may precede the development of peptic ulcers.

Zollinger and Ellison initially recommended total gastrectomy for patients with gastrinoma. This treatment proved effective and was adopted as standard therapy. Current experience with H_2 blockade or omeprazole treatment appears effective, however, and many patients are now managed without operation. Because of problems in compliance (not deficits in drug potency), the author and others have seen patients who have failed medical treatment and have required later operation. Because most gastrinomas are malignant, every patient with Zollinger-Ellison syndrome who meets standard criteria for operability should have a laparotomy for possible removal of tumor tissue.

PEPTIC ULCER IN CHILDREN

Although uncommon, peptic ulcer in patients under the age of 15 years often has a complicated and serious clinical course. Ulcers may be primary (true peptic) or secondary to overwhelming disease. True primary ulcers are rare; only 30 patients were seen with primary ulcers over a 30-year period at the Hospital for Sick Children in London. Whenever children develop peptic ulcer, gastrin levels should be measured and patients should be evaluated for the Zollinger-Ellison syndrome.

ACUTE MUCOSAL EROSIONS

For reasons that are not clear, the incidence of major bleeding from acute mucosal erosions (stress ulcers or hemorrhagic gastritis) has decreased drastically in the last decade, perhaps because of improvements in the nutrition of severely ill patients.

Diagnosis

Acute mucosal lesions should be considered whenever acute upper gastrointestinal bleeding or perforation occurs after a major injury or during the course of an important metabolic insult.

Gastroscopy is the most important diagnostic technique available. It is usually possible to demonstrate acute, superficial, bleeding gastric lesions when patients are examined during gastric hemorrhage. Upper gastrointestinal series obtained during bleeding episodes are rarely helpful because the erosions are quite superficial.

Treatment

Regardless of the initial mechanisms of mucosal damage, acid is required for mucosal destruction and bleeding, and *antacid therapy* is therefore a logical prophylaxis for all patients who are at risk of stress ulceration. Intravenous H_2-receptor blockade therapy has been widely used in prophylaxis. Neither antacids nor H_2-blockers can control established bleeding, and in the presence of sepsis, neither is effective in control of acid output. At the first sign of bleeding, antacid therapy may be combined or alternated with iced saline lavage. This regimen is often successful in halting further hemorrhage.

SURGICAL PROCEDURES ON THE STOMACH

The initial development of surgical procedures for peptic ulcer was empiric. The subsequent evolution has been guided by demonstration of physiologic mechanisms controlling gastric secretion.

Operations Currently in Use

The three operations in general use for peptic ulcer are gastric resection without vagotomy, truncal vagotomy and drainage (either gastroenterostomy or pyloroplasty), and truncal vagotomy plus antrectomy. Selective denervation of the acid-secreting portion of the fundus with preservation of innervation to the antrum and to the rest of the abdominal viscera is widely used in Europe and has achieved acceptance in North America.

Postoperative Complications

EARLY COMPLICATIONS

Hemorrhage in the immediate postoperative period may be due to failure to control bleeding from an ulcer or may be due to bleeding at the suture line. The use of gastrostomy tubes for postoperative gastric decompression is attended by a small but definite incidence of complications, including bleeding, leaking of gastric juice into the peritoneal cavity, and, rarely, persistent gastrocutaneous fistulas.

The most serious common complication following resection is leakage from the duodenal stump (Billroth II) or leakage at the gastroduodenostomy (Billroth I). Both result in peritoneal soilage with gastroduodenal contents and are associated with peritonitis, ileus, sepsis, and significant (10 to 15 per cent) mortality. Resection is associated with a higher incidence of breakdown of the suture line than are drainage procedures, because dissection is performed in areas of ulcer scarring and the blood supply to the remaining structures is often compromised.

LATE COMPLICATIONS

DUMPING SYNDROME. Any operative procedure that destroys or bypasses the pylorus may cause sudden emptying of hyperosmolar material into the jejunum, and this may result in a large inflow of extracellular fluid into the jejunum. This rapid fluid shift may clinically cause abdominal colic, nausea, vomiting, diarrhea, faintness, sweating, and pallor.

The dumping syndrome is often relieved by eating small dry meals and restricting all intake of fluid during meals. There is no standard operative treatment for the dumping syndrome; good results have been reported following conversion of Billroth I to Billroth II anastomoses (and vice versa) and with the use of a small segment of reversed jejunum to impede gastric emptying. The author believes it wise to delay reoperating on patients with the dumping syndrome and to treat them with alterations of diet together with mild sedation and small doses of anticholinergic drugs in order to avoid operation.

The foregoing complications are all more common after resection than after vagotomy and drainage procedures. Vagotomy appears to be associated with two complications. One, a suggested increased incidence of gallstones, is difficult to prove statistically and is therefore of questionable importance.

ALKALINE REFLUX GASTRITIS. A few postoperative patients are troubled with severe continuous burning epigastric pain, usually aggravated by meals. The pain is usually not relieved by vomiting. The condition is diagnosed by gastroscopy, which reveals bile reflux in the stomach and a beefy red, generally inflamed gastric mucosa, often with multiple superficial gastric erosions.

Although there is great interest in this condition and although the diagnosis achieved considerable popularity in a short period, the author believes that great restraint should be exercised in planning reoperation. These unfortunate patients have been around for a long time; many were miserable for years, but the majority survived and improved without operation.

MARGINAL ULCER. Ulcers recur in a small fraction of postoperative patients; 1 to 5 per cent of patients who undergo gastric resection for peptic ulcer may be expected to develop recurrent peptic ulceration. Recurrent ulcers after gastric resection and Billroth II anastomosis occur classically on the jejunal side of the margin of the anastomosis. The ulcer may produce periodic episodes of midabdominal pain, it may make its first appearance with massive hemorrhage, or it may erode into the free peritoneal cavity or into the colon, creating a gastrojejunocolic fistula.

I

Benign Tumors of the Stomach
Onye E. Akwari, M.D.

INCIDENCE. Benign tumors comprise 7 per cent of premortem gastric tumors but less than 2 per cent of true gastric neoplasms. A classification of benign tumors of the stomach is presented in Table 1. Approximately 40 per cent of the tumors are mucosal epithelial polyps, and another 40 per cent are leiomyomas. All other tumors are rare.

CLINICAL PRESENTATION. Benign gastric tumors occur predominantly in the middle decades of life and most commonly are located in the gastric antrum or corpus. Occult loss of blood causing iron deficiency anemia is common because these tumors ulcerate their overlying mucosal epithelium. Deep ulcerations overlying intramural tumors are notorious for their association with overt hemorrhage. Ulceration may cause a pain syndrome indistinguishable from that of peptic ulcer disease. Tumors of the cardia and pylorus may cause obstruction; if pedunculated, the tumor, usually pyloric, may create intermittent obstruction due to a ball valve effect. Frank gastroduodenal intussusception secondary to a prolapsing gastric tumor may occur.

DIAGNOSIS. Barium studies (with or without air contrast) and gastroscopy with biopsy through the fiberoptic gastroscope are the mainstay for diagnosis. However, even with biopsy, diagnosis of a specific type of polyp or hyperplastic gastropathy cannot be made with certainty. Biopsy of intramural tumors is an especially vexing problem, since the leiomyomas and other mesenchymal tumors are firm with rubbery consistencies that prevent deep enough penetration by the biopsy forceps for an adequate sampling of the tumor for histologic examination.

The indications for extirpation of the tumor are elimination of any significant clinical effects and the necessity to exclude a diagnosis of malignancy. Ultimately, the tumor must be *completely* excised either by endoscopic techniques or surgical excision before a final disposition can be made.

POLYPS

Almost all polyps (Greek *polypus*, "many footed") arise from the mucosal epithelium. That the nomenclature of

See the corresponding chapter or part in the *Textbook of Surgery*, 14th edition, pp. 787–794, for a more detailed discussion of this topic, including a comprehensive list of references.

TABLE 1. Benign Tumors of the Stomach

Polyps
  Hyperplastic (Type I and Type II polyps of Japanese authors)
  Neoplastic or adenomatous (Type III and Type IV polyps of
    Japanese authors)
  Mixed (hyperplastic and neoplastic)
  Fundic gland polyp
  Familial polyposis and other polyposis syndromes
  Peutz-Jeghers (hamartomatous) polyp
  Inflammatory fibroid polyp
  Retention (juvenile) polyp

Benign Hyperplastic Gastropathy
  Ménétrier's disease (polyadenomes en nappe)
  Associated with Zollinger-Ellison syndrome
  Glandular type, without hypergastrinemia
  Pseudolymphoma

Intramural Tumors
  Leiomyoma
  Other mesenchymal tumors (lipoma, neurogenic tumors, fibroma,
    vascular tumors)
  Osteoma and osteochondroma
  Heterotopic pancreas
  Brunner's gland adenoma
  Adenomyoma
  Xanthoma (xanthelasma)

Inflammatory
  Eosinophilic gastritis
    Diffuse
    Localized (inflammatory fibroid polyp—see above)
  Benign histiocytosis X
  Granulomatous (sarcoid, Crohn's disease)
  Syphilis
  Tuberculosis

Cysts
  Intramucosal (mucocele)
  Submucosal (gastritis cystica profunda)
  Duplication cyst

Miscellaneous Conditions
  Gastric varices
  Aneurysm of gastric vessels (Dieulafoy's disease)
  Antral vascular ectasia (watermelon stomach)

gastric polyps is confusing is in large measure due to early attempts at presenting them as being analogous to colorectal polyps in microscopic appearance and natural history. In fact, most gastric polyps have no exact counterparts in the large bowel. Unlike colonic polyps, gastric epithelial polyps are very uncommon tumors with an incidence of 0.4 to 0.7 per cent. No distinction exists between the histologic types of epithelial polyps (hyperplastic, neoplastic or adenomatous, fundic gland polyp) by age, sex, location, symptoms, or endoscopic appearance. The median age for gastric polyps is about 65 years, with an equal gender distribution, or at most a slight female predilection. The histologic appearance of a polyp cannot be predicted on the basis of location within the stomach. However, in the same patient, polyps are almost always of the same histologic type, should they be multiple. The nomenclature and characteristics of gastric polyps are summarized in Table 2.

TREATMENT. Polyps causing pain, bleeding, or gastric outlet obstruction should be removed. Total endoscopic excision is advocated so that the nature of the polyp can be firmly established. Open surgical excision is indicated when the benignity of a pedunculated polyp greater than 2 cm. in diameter has not been firmly established and/or safe total excision by endoscopic snare and cautery is judged not to be feasible; when examination of the tissue removed endoscopically is consistent with invasive malignancy; and when a sessile polyp is present that exceeds 2 cm. in diameter. Multiple polyps involving the distal stomach or a group of closely aligned polyps in the gastric corpus can be removed by resection of the segment or by wide local excision. In diffuse polyposis, a large portion of the gastric mucosal surface is involved with innumerable tumors. The decision in this situation must also include the fact that although benign, these polyps may be associated with coexisting adenocarcinoma elsewhere in the stomach. A total gastrectomy may be indicated in these cases, especially when the fundus is involved, since a coexisting fundal adenocarcinoma may be masked and difficult to identify. Local wedge excision is adequate treatment for polyps showing focal atypia or carcinoma *in situ*. Asymptomatic polyps should be biopsied by endoscopic snare-cautery excision. Hyperplastic polyps may be safely observed and repeat endoscopy advised on an annual basis for examination not only of the polyps but also of the entire intervening gastric mucosa.

Gastric Polyps in Polyposis Syndromes

Gastric involvement occurs in 50 per cent of patients with familial polyposis coli and the related Gardner's syndrome, in which patients may also harbor polyps in the duodenum. The gastric polyps can be adenomatous, hyperplastic, or the fundic gland hyperplasia type.

All patients confirmed as having familial polyposis coli should have gastroduodenoscopy. Any adenomas found should be eradicated by endoscopic destruction. Repeat examination should then be undertaken at 6- to 12-week intervals until no polyps remain. Thereafter 6-monthly examinations should be made.

In *Peutz-Jeghers syndrome,* hamartomatous gastric polyps occur in about 20 per cent of the cases, with an occasional coexisting adenocarcinoma. These patients require regular endoscopic surveillance.

Generalized juvenile polyposis and the related *Cronkhite-Canada syndrome* are associated with a high incidence of gastric retention (juvenile) polyps.

Cowden's syndrome (family name of index patient) may be associated with small sessile gastric polyps, most of which are of the hyperplastic type. The feature of disseminated polyposis (oral mucosa to anus) has recently been empha-

TABLE 2. Gastric Polyps

Type	Other Names	Comment	Cancer Risk
Hyperplastic	Regenerative, inflammatory, hyperplasiogenic, hamartomatous, Type I and Type II polyps of Japanese authors	Correspond to Ménétrier's polyadenomes polypeux. Peutz-Jeghers syndrome Cowden's syndrome	Cancer risk associated with atrophic gastritis that frequently accompanies hyperplastic polyps rather than the polyps themselves
Neoplastic or adenomas	Type III and Type IV polyps of Japanese authors	May be adenomatous or villoglandular Positive cells for peptide hormones and CEA reactivity may be present Incidence of cancer *in situ* and invasive adenocarcinoma increase with polyp size	Adenomatous polyp; cancer risk up to 24% in polyps 2 cm. or greater
Fundic gland polyp	Fundic gland hyperplasia, hamartomatous cystic polyps, polyps with fundic glandular cysts	Associated with familial polyposis syndrome but not specific for this disorder Presence of O-acylated sialic acid may indicate high probability of colorectal polyposis	
Inflammatory fibroid polyp	Eosinophilic granuloma, granuloblastoma, neurofibroma, hemangiopericytoma	Often associated with hypochlorhydria Usually antral Not true neoplasm Allergic cause and peripheral eosinophilia absent	

sized in this autosomal dominant disease. An increased, evidently genetically determined prevalence of malignant tumors of various organs (e.g., thyroid, breast) in patients with Cowden's disease and their family members mandates careful follow-up not exclusively focused on the stomach.

SMOOTH MUSCLE TUMORS

INCIDENCE. Leiomyomas are the most common benign tumor of the stomach reported at autopsy. It is rare for gastric leiomyomas less than 3 cm. in diameter to be symptomatic; therefore, considerably less than 2 per cent of gastric neoplasms resected surgically are smooth muscle tumors.

PATHOLOGY. The smooth muscle tumor may arise from the muscularis propria, the muscularis mucosae, or the smooth muscle present in the blood vessels. The mural tumor may protrude into the gastric lumen (endogastric), develop as an exogastric (exophytic) mass, or have both a submucosal and a subserosal component (dumbbell).

On microscopic examination, although they appear well circumscribed, leiomyomas are not encapsulated, and tumor cells at the margin may intermingle with cells of the surrounding gastric wall. Along with the marked cellularity and occasional large cells with bizarre hyperchromatic nuclei, this feature often causes confusion in distinguishing benign from malignant leiomyoma. A variant of gastric smooth muscle tumors, which has been termed leiomyoblastoma by Stout, is distinguished by a central nucleus in rounded rather than elongated smooth cells and a clear zone that surrounds the nucleus, which is thought by some to be an artifact of fixation. Carney has described a syndrome characterized by the triad of multiple malignant leiomyoblastoma, pulmonary chondroma, and functioning extra-adrenal paraganglioma.

TREATMENT. The principle of surgical treatment of smooth muscle tumors is local excision with a 2- to 3-cm. margin of surrounding gastric wall. Because of the difficulty of distinguishing benign and malignant variants, enucleation is an inappropriate method of treatment. When the tumor encroaches upon the esophagogastric junction, a conservative approach is indicated, although a standard gastric resection may be the most expeditious form of removal of a very large distal gastric tumor or a prepyloric tumor. Even when there is doubt about benignity, regional lymphadenectomy need not be added, since this is unlikely to be of value for a tumor that rarely involves lymph nodes and spreads preferentially by the hematogenous route.

HYPERPLASTIC GASTROPATHY

The general term *hyperplastic gastropathy* refers to a rare condition in which there is enlargement of the rugal folds in the stomach. The etiology of the hyperplastic process varies. *Ménétrier's disease (polyadenomes en nappe)* is a process in which gastric mucosal hypertrophy may be so great that the rugae assume the appearance of convolutions of the brain.

Although this gross appearance is common to all cases of Ménétrier's disease, in an individual case, either the gastric glandular elements or the superficial epithelial elements of the gastric mucosa may predominate. Thus, acid secretion may be high, normal, or low; hypoproteinemia, formerly considered an essential component of the disease, may not be present.

On microscopic examination, there is a striking *foveolar hyperplasia*, accompanied by tortuosity and some degree of cystic dilation with extension into the base of the gastric glands. The stomach is edematous and inflamed. Hyperrugosity may regress, atrophic gastritis may develop, and carcinoma of the stomach may ensue.

Ménétrier's disease may be diagnosed at any age. The etiology is unknown. Since spontaneous resolution of the acute signs and symptoms (abdominal pain, 80 per cent; blood loss, 34 per cent; hypoproteinemia, 40 per cent; weight loss; edema; malnutrition) may occur, nutritional support and a period of observation are justified when the precise diagnosis has been established. Anticholinergics and also H$_2$-blockers may be attempted for diminishing acid secretion and tightening gastric cell junctions, but a combination of these approaches is the norm. If pharmacologic therapy fails, *total* gastrectomy and reconstruction with a long Roux-en-Y jejunal limb is the best therapy. Any remaining gastric mucosa is the focus of a significant incidence of subsequent development of adenocarcinoma. An interesting aspect of the management of patients with Ménétrier's disease is their propensity to have a hypercoagulable state, sometimes associated with gastric carcinoma, which occurs in 1 to 15 per cent of all cases of Ménétrier's disease.

OTHER HYPERTROPHIC CONDITIONS

Other conditions associated with hyperrugosity are gastric cancer and malignant lymphoma. In "chronic hypertrophic gastritis," there is non-neoplastic proliferation of all epithelial elements—mucus-secreting cells as well as parietal cells and chief cells. The lesion is noninflammatory, and thus the term *gastropathy* is preferred to gastritis. *Zollinger-Ellison syndrome* may be associated with gastric changes, showing glandular (rather than foveolar) hyperplasia of the fundic gland, grossly similar to those of Ménétrier's disease.

CYSTIC LESIONS

The most important cystic lesion is a reduplication cyst. Usually encountered in the distal stomach, it may but does not usually communicate with the gastric lumen. When distention of the cyst with fluid causes obstruction and/or a palpable mass, surgical removal is indicated.

PSEUDOLYMPHOMA

Extensive lymphocytic infiltration of a portion of the stomach may be associated with benign gastric ulcer. Submucosal nodules, diffuse thickening, or enlarged rugal folds should be biopsied. The infiltrate often has a follicular pattern that may be confused with "follicular lymphoma." However, the presence of clearly reactive germinal centers throughout the lesion, including a mixed population of inflammatory cells, establishes the diagnosis of pseudolymphoma. Immunohistochemical stains for immunoglobulins show a polyclonal pattern, but the distinction from lymphoma can be extraordinarily difficult.

HETEROTOPIC PANCREAS

An aberrant rest of pancreatic tissue may project into the gastric lumen and occasionally cause pain from becoming inflamed, or cause pyloric obstruction or hemorrhage. Usually it is found incidentally at autopsy or laparotomy. The most characteristic gross feature is a central ductal orifice that tends to umbilicate the tumor, which is submucosal in 85 per cent of cases. Technically a hamartoma, the antral (61 per cent) or prepyloric (24 per cent) mass is composed of glands and intervening connective tissue. Islets of Langerhans are seen in only 30 per cent of the cases; if present, their number is generally less than in normal pancreas. From a practical point of view, most of these lesions are surgically excised because patients and physicians alike prefer surgical excision to the diagnostic uncertainty they create.

II

Lymphoma of the Stomach
Theodore N. Pappas, M.D.

Primary intra-abdominal lymphomas represent 10 to 20 per cent of all lymphocytic lymphomas, and gastric lymphomas comprise the majority of primary gastrointestinal lymphomas. In contrast, primary gastric lymphomas make up less than 5 per cent of all primary gastric tumors. Because of their common clinical presentation, gastric lymphoma and adenocarcinoma of the stomach exist in the same differential diagnosis and need to be distinguished by preoperative and intraoperative evaluation.

CLINICAL PRESENTATION AND DIAGNOSTIC TESTS. Clinical presentation of gastric lymphoma is similar to the presentation of adenocarcinoma of the stomach. Patients with primary gastric lymphoma present in their mid-50s; there is

See the corresponding chapter or part in the *Textbook of Surgery*, 14th edition, pp. 794–797, for a more detailed discussion of this topic, including a comprehensive list of references.

a male to female predominance of 1.7:1. Eighty per cent of patients present with abdominal pain, which can be associated with anorexia, early satiety, weight loss, nausea, and vomiting. Less than 10 per cent of patients present asymptomatically. Over 40 per cent of patients may present with an emergent complication of their gastrointestinal lymphoma, including bleeding, perforation, and obstruction.

On physical examination, patients may have an abdominal mass. Splenomegaly occurs because of direct extension of the tumor, but massive splenomegaly and diffuse adenopathy are more consistent with diffuse lymphoma. Barium studies have been classically used for diagnosis of gastric masses but usually do not distinguish between adenocarcinoma and lymphoma. Whereas lesions as small as 3 to 4 cm. in the stomach can be detected by upper gastrointestinal series, 10 to 20 per cent of patients have a completely normal upper gastrointestinal series when a primary gastric lymphoma is present. Abdominal ultrasound and endoscopic ultrasound have a relatively limited utility in the evaluation of gastric masses. Endoscopic ultrasound has been used in staging of these tumors and defining wall penetration. Computed tomography characterizes gastric masses but cannot distinguish between lymphoma and adenocarcinoma of the stomach.

Gastrointestinal endoscopy is essential in attempting to make the diagnosis of gastric lymphoma. Visual diagnosis of gastric lymphoma is correct in only half the patients examined. These lesions appear as superficial stellate ulcers involving large areas of the stomach where the margin between normal mucosa and the lesion is very sharp. Biopsies and cytologic examination of these gastric lesions in patients with lymphoma accurately make the diagnosis in 30 to 90 per cent of patients. Owing to insufficient tissue, many patients require exploratory laparotomy for definitive pathologic determination.

PATHOLOGY. There are five major classifications of the gross morphologic features of primary gastric lymphoma. These include (1) infiltrative, (2) ulcerative, (3) nodular, (4) polypoid, and (5) combined morphology (any combination of the other four). The histologic type of primary gastric lymphoma is characterized by mucosal or submucosally based lymphoid tissue with infiltration of the gastric glands by follicular cells forming characteristic lymphoid epithelial lesions.

Pseudolymphoma represents 10 per cent of all gastric lymphomas diagnosed. The patients present with ulceration and extensive fibrosis, commonly in the presence of chronic peptic ulcer disease. It is a benign gastric lymphomatosis that is characterized by lymphoid infiltration of the gastric wall predominantly in the mucosa without evidence of nodal disease. The *sine qua non* for the histologic diagnosis is the finding of germinal centers within the gastric lesions. Pseudolymphoma may represent a premalignant lesion that can convert to malignant lymphoma; therefore, current recommended management is conservative surgical resection, and nonoperative observation is reserved for patients at high risk for surgical therapy.

TREATMENT. The current recommendation for treatment of primary gastric lymphoma is attempted cure with surgical resection, including total gastrectomy in the appropriate patient. Approximately 75 per cent of patients are able to have resection on exploration; curative resection should yield a 5-year survival of 35 to 50 per cent for all stages. The stage of the tumor correlates well with 5-year survival (90 to 95 per cent for Stage I; 20 to 25 per cent for Stage IV). Surgical resection is also recommended for decreasing the complications of bleeding and perforation during adjuvant therapy.

Adjuvant therapy has been recommended for all stages of primary gastric lymphoma. This may include whole abdominal radiation with a boost to the stomach bed or combination chemotherapy, such as CMOPP or CHOP. Adjuvant therapy clearly improves survival, particularly in patients with nodal disease.

In summary, all Stage I and Stage II patients (disease confined to stomach and regional nodes) should undergo attempted curative resection followed by adjuvant chemotherapy and/or radiation therapy. Stage III and Stage IV patients who present with complications of bleeding, obstruction, and perforation should also undergo attempted primary resection followed by adjuvant therapy. Patients without complications who present with preoperative documentation of Stage III or Stage IV disease should be treated with radiation therapy and chemotherapy initially, with surgical resection reserved for persistent local disease in the stomach or for complications.

III

The Pathogenesis, Prophylaxis, and Treatment of Stress Gastritis

Laurence Y. Cheung, M.D.

Stress gastritis occurs primarily in patients following severe burn, trauma, hemorrhagic shock, respiratory failure, or sepsis. The lesions are multiple and superficial erosions. It has been shown by gastroscopy that the incidence of such gastric erosions was 100 per cent in 40 severely injured patients. In a similar study, gastric erosions were found by sequential endoscopic examinations in 27 of 29 patients with major burns. Fortunately, only a small number of these patients had significant gastrointestinal hemorrhage.

See the corresponding chapter or part in the *Textbook of Surgery*, 14th edition, pp. 797–801, for a more detailed discussion of this topic, including a comprehensive list of references.

PATHOGENESIS. Although the precise mechanisms involved in the development of stress gastritis remain unknown, current evidence supports a multifactorial etiology. Most of the factors contribute to the development of stress gastritis by reducing the ability of the stomach to protect itself against acid injury rather than by increasing the amount of acid secretion.

The Presence of Acid. There is no evidence that an increased quantity of acid secretion is the cause of stress gastritis. Although hypersecretion is an unlikely cause, it can be stated with certainty that some hydrogen ions are necessary for the development of stress gastritis.

Ischemia. Clinically, most patients who develop stress gastritis have experienced an episode of shock from hemorrhage, sepsis, or cardiac dysfunction. Diminished gastric mucosal blood flow is a common denominator in animal experiments that employ restraint, hemorrhage, or endotoxemia for the production of acute ulceration. There is near-agreement among all investigators that one basic pathogenetic feature of stress gastritis is mucosal ischemia. The cause-effect relationship between ischemia and stress erosions has been explained by the hypothesis of energy deficit of the gastric mucosa. Ischemia may adversely affect gastric energy metabolism, an important factor in mucosal defense against injury. The other leading hypothesis is that gastric mucosal blood flow has an important role in the disposal, or buffering, of the H^+ entering the tissue. Ischemia reduces the capacity of the gastric mucosa to neutralize acid that enters the tissue. This then causes accumulation of H^+ within the tissue, mucosal acidification, and ulceration.

Systemic Acid-Base Balance. Recent studies have suggested that the ability of the gastric mucosa to maintain its neutral pH is dependent not only on the rate of mucosal blood flow but also on the pH of the arterial blood perfusing the stomach. Therefore, systemic acidosis renders the gastric mucosa more susceptible to acid injury.

Secretory State of the Gastric Mucosa. It is well known that bicarbonate is released intrinsically within the mucosa during active secretion of acid. However, the importance of this intramural release of bicarbonate in mucosal protection against luminal acid has only recently been recognized. An actively secreting stomach is much more resistant to ulceration than is a metiamide-inhibited rabbit stomach, which supports the concept that the intrinsic release of bicarbonate protects the tissue against ulceration.

PREVENTION. On the basis of the various factors identified experimentally in the pathogenesis of stress gastritis, a number of prophylactic measures can be instituted in patients at high risk for its development. Vigorous efforts should be made to correct any shocklike state following blood loss and/or sepsis. In addition, efforts should be made to improve ventilatory support, to correct any systemic acid-base abnormality, and to maintain adequate nutrition in these critically ill patients.

From the "no acid, no ulcer" dictum, the concept that maintaining neutral pH of the gastric contents may prevent development of stress gastritis in critically ill patients evolved. In fact, titration of gastric pH with antacid has been shown to be effective in preventing gastrointestinal bleeding in intensive care unit patients in several controlled prospective trials. Other studies have reported that H_2-receptor antagonists are also useful in the prophylaxis of stress ulceration.

Most recently, several reports indicate that neutralization of gastric acid or inhibition of acid secretion may increase the risk of nosocomial pneumonia by favoring gastric colonization with gram-negative bacilli. In a prospective study (Driks), the rate of pneumonia was twice as high in the antacid/H_2-blocker group of patients as in the sucralfate group. Gram-negative bacilli were isolated more frequently from tracheal aspirates of patients with pneumonia who were receiving antacid or H_2-blockers. Although these results are still preliminary and not yet conclusive, they do suggest that in patients receiving mechanical ventilation for a prolonged period of time, the use of a prophylactic agent such as sucralfate, which preserves the natural gastric acid barrier against bacteria overgrowth, may be preferable to antacid or H_2-blockers.

TREATMENT. Initial management for control of gastrointestinal hemorrhage should consist of gastric lavage with chilled solutions through a large-bore nasogastric tube. Lavage of the stomach aids in the fragmentation of clots and avoids gastric distention. Fortunately, in most patients, bleeding appears to cease following gastric lavage. In occasional patients, specific nonoperative or operative treatment is required.

Endoscopic Therapy. Techniques for the treatment of stress gastritis via endoscopy include either electrocoagulation or laser photocoagulation. Initial clinical experience with endoscopic therapy reports over 90 per cent permanent hemostasis. However, only a small percentage of the total patients in these studies had bleeding from stress gastritis. At present, this technique provides an opportunity for direct control of bleeding from stress gastritis at institutions where this technique is available.

Angiographic Pharmacotherapy. Several earlier papers have reported a high success rate with this technique in the treatment of bleeding from stress gastritis. Conn and colleagues observed in a prospective trial that control of massive bleeding by the use of selective intra-arterial infusion of vasopressin was not associated with improved survival. They concluded from their study that vasopressin decreased the amount of blood transfusion required during episodes of hemorrhage and provided the interval of time required for a planned surgical approach to the problem. On the basis of these studies, it is recommended that this technique be attempted if facilities and trained personnel are available before surgical therapy is considered.

Surgical Therapy. Persistent or recurring bleeding that is refractory to all nonsurgical measures is an indication for operative intervention. The operative procedures used for the control of bleeding stress ulcers have ranged from total gastrectomy to procedures of much lesser magnitude, such as pyloroplasty and vagotomy. It can be generally stated that lesser procedures are associated with lower mortality but with higher incidences of rebleeding. There are no prospective clinical trials to substantiate the superiority of one form of therapy over another. Some surgeons have had fairly satisfactory results with vagotomy and pyloroplasty combined with oversewing the bleeding erosions as an initial operation for bleeding stress ulcers. Total gastric resection is reserved for those in whom bleeding continues after the initial operation or for those patients with diffuse bleeding lesions.

IV

Tumors of the Duodenum and Small Intestine
G. Robert Mason, M.D.

Approximately half the tumors of the small bowel are benign and half are malignant. The benign tumors are relatively evenly distributed throughout the length of the small bowel, whereas the malignant tumors are much more common in the duodenum. The influence of carcinogenic constituents of the bile versus the immunologic defenses of the intestine deserves further investigation. Of the benign tumors, leiomyomas and adenomas are the most common, whereas among the malignancies, adenocarcinomas and lymphomas are most frequently found.

INCIDENCE. Tumors of the small bowel are estimated to comprise approximately 1 to 6 per cent of gastrointestinal tract tumors. An incidence of 1 in 10,000 hospital admissions and 1 in 2000 general surgical procedures has been estimated. This indicates that a typical practicing general surgeon would see one case every decade.

SYMPTOMS. Because the numbers of small bowel tumors found at postmortem examination greatly exceed those coming to medical attention during life, the assumption is that many such tumors are asymptomatic. As tumors enlarge to compromise the passage of intestinal contents, the patient may notice postprandial cramping epigastric and periumbilical pain. Nausea and vomiting are indications of near or total obstruction of the lumen in that the content of the small bowel is generally liquid. Benign tumors most commonly present with obstruction, commonly as an intussusception, except for leiomyomas, which not only are the most common

---

See the corresponding chapter or part in the *Textbook of Surgery*, 14th edition, pp. 802–807, for a more detailed discussion of this topic, including a comprehensive list of references.

small bowel tumor but most frequently present with often vigorous bleeding.

Malignant tumors may also be associated with anorexia and weight loss or produce more persistent pain. Bleeding, when present, is more likely to be occult, presenting as an anemia. Periampullary tumors may interfere with normal drainage of bile or pancreatic juice, and the patient may present with painless jaundice. When a palpable gallbladder is also present, suspicion may be higher that a neoplasm is the cause (Courvoisier).

DIAGNOSIS. The presence of obvious hereditary genetic defects such as are observed in Gardner's syndrome and the Peutz-Jeghers syndrome should alert the surgeon to underlying intestinal associated anomalies. Duodenal lesions are most easily visualized and biopsied by fiberoptic endoscopy. Approximately half of the currently reported villous adenomas of the duodenum are malignant regardless of size, and as such the diagnosis of benign tumor on endoscopic biopsy must be considered carefully. Radiologic studies utilizing barium are the standard diagnostic method used to diagnose tumors of the mesenteric small intestine. The technique of passing a nasointestinal tube to a point just above a suspected lesion and instilling contrast at that point (enteroclysis) may add further information beyond the standard small bowel series. Lesions bleeding at a rate of 1 to 2 ml. per minute may be more readily identified by angiography. Nuclear scanning with labelled red blood cells may be useful for slower rates of bleeding. A long mercury-weighted polyethylene tube may also be useful in the preoperative localization of a minimally bleeding lesion. In addition, at operation, the use of rigid or fiberoptic endoscopes through the opened intestine may be diagnostic. The advantages of computed tomography, nuclear magnetic resonance, and sonography are probably less than the techniques listed above.

MANAGEMENT. Surgical excision of the tumor mass and its draining lymph nodes in the mesentery is the preferred treatment of lesions of the mesenteric small bowel. The techniques of resection and anastomosis are those introduced some decades ago and are not different in these circumstances. Malignancies of the duodenum in general are treated as are cancers of the pancreas and distal bile ducts with pancreatoduodenectomy, as is covered in the chapter on diseases of the pancreas. Resection of benign tumors of the duodenum may require some ingenuity on the part of the surgeon to avoid constriction of the pancreatic or bile ducts or the duodenum, or devascularization of the duodenum. The use of onlay serosal patches, Roux-en-Y loops, and ductal reimplantation is covered elsewhere. Villous adenomas of the duodenum have been successfully managed by local resection in some patients, and the surgeon may choose this alternative in selected patients, bearing in mind the incidence of malignancy in these lesions. Symptomatic management of APUD tumors such as carcinoids, gastrinomas, glucagonomas, and others may relate specifically to the end organ affected, such as the use of H_2-blockers for the Zollinger-Ellison syndrome or methysergide and antihistamines for carcinoid tumors. The use of somatostatin may supplant these agents. Lymphomas that are resectable appear to be best treated in this manner; however, the addition of radiation therapy appears to augment the 5-year survival of these patients. Chemotherapy for advanced metastatic cancers of the gastrointestinal tract is an evolving field that appears to indicate the benefits of multiple drug therapy.

OUTCOME. Patients with carcinomas of the duodenum, when treated by pancreatoduodenectomy, are reported to have 5-year survival rates in the range of 25 per cent. Patients with adenocarcinoma of the mesenteric small intestine are reported to have 5-year survival rates of 14 to 37 per cent. Patients with lymphomas treated by excision and adjunctive radiotherapy have 5-year survivals as high as 85 per cent, and those with carcinoid tumors without apparent metastases at the time of resection may have 5-year survivals of greater than 70 per cent; those with metastases may expect rates of 35 per cent. Since the growth of this tumor is very slow, it may be more appropriate to view the 10-year survival rates, which are reported as 60 per cent and 15 per cent, without and with known metastases at the time of original resections.

V

Vascular Compression of the Duodenum
Bruce D. Schirmer, M.D.

The syndrome of vascular compression of the duodenum was first described by von Rokitansky in 1842. Stavely performed the first successful operative bypass for this condition in 1908. The syndrome has received various names, including the superior mesenteric artery syndrome. They all represent the condition of duodenal obstruction from the overlying mesenteric vasculature.

The superior mesenteric artery arises from the aorta at an acute angle through which passes the duodenum as well as the left renal vein and the uncinate process of the pancreas. The third portion of the duodenum crosses from right to left and simultaneously from posterior to anterior, crossing upward and in front of the abdominal aorta and lumbar spine. It is at this location that the duodenum is most susceptible to obstruction from external compression. Patients with vascular compression of the duodenum have been shown to

See the corresponding chapter or part in the *Textbook of Surgery*, 14th edition, pp. 807–813, for a more detailed discussion of this topic, including a comprehensive list of references.

have both a narrower angle of takeoff of the superior mesenteric artery and a shorter distance between the beginning of the artery and the duodenum.

Conditions that are known to predispose to vascular compression of the duodenum include weight loss, excessive lumbar lordosis, the supine position, and congenital high fixation of the duodenum to the ligament of Treitz.

The clinical pattern of this syndrome involves symptoms of profound nausea and vomiting, abdominal distention, postprandial epigastric pain, and weight loss. Acute symptoms are classically relieved when the patient adopts the knee-chest, the left lateral, or occasionally the prone positions. Symptoms vary from intermittent to constant, depending on the severity of obstruction. If nausea and vomiting become protracted, dehydration can follow. Dehydration, cachexia, and aspiration pneumonia are known fatal complications of this problem.

The syndrome usually presents in thin patients with acute weight loss and is slightly more common among females and younger patients. It has been reported in association with other clinical conditions, including body casts, extensively burned patients and bedridden combat casualties, and anorexia nervosa. The syndrome has also been well described in the pediatric population. The true incidence is unknown, but it is uncommon, with one review showing an incidence of only 0.0024 to 0.0965 per cent of hospital cases.

The diagnosis is confirmed radiographically in the presence of the appropriate clinical symptoms. Hypotonic duodenography has been shown to be the best radiographic test. A pathognomonic "to and fro" peristalsis of contrast is seen in the duodenum on fluoroscopy along with an abrupt cutoff of distal flow of contrast. Changing the patient's position to one such as the knee-chest position that causes simultaneous relief of symptoms and passage of contrast distally is confirmatory.

The differential diagnosis for this syndrome includes peptic ulcer disease, biliary lithiasis, pancreatitis, metastatic or primary tumors of the periaortic lymph nodes, primary gastrointestinal tumors, scleroderma, primary neuromuscular disorders of the bowel, surgical adhesions, and postvagotomy symptoms. There is a known associated incidence of peptic ulcer disease and vascular compression of the duodenum, but the etiologic basis of this association is unclear.

The treatment of vascular compression of the duodenum should be conservative initially, since success has been achieved with nasogastric suction, patient repositioning for relief of the obstruction, and use of parenteral or enteral nutrition as tolerated for promoting weight gain. Surgical intervention should be undertaken if conservative measures fail. Simple division of the ligament of Treitz with mobilization of the duodenum has been successful in about 87 per cent of reported cases. Some authors advocate repositioning of the small and large bowel along with division of the ligament. Duodenojejunostomy has been the most commonly reported surgical treatment for this syndrome, and also the most successful (92 per cent). Where simple division of the

ligament of Treitz has failed, it has been then used successfully as a second procedure. Gastroenterostomy is less successful in general, for the operation relies on biliary reflux
into the stomach for decompression should the duodenal
obstruction persist.

30

CARCINOMA OF THE STOMACH

Aaron S. Fink, M.D., and William P. Longmire, Jr., M.D.

Gastric carcinoma remains a prominent cause of mortality worldwide. Fortunately, the death rate from gastric carcinoma is declining, primarily owing to its decreasing incidence.

PATHOGENESIS. Gastric carcinogenesis appears to be linked to several etiologic factors, especially environmental agents. Dietary factors have received the most attention, since the stomach is the first point of prolonged contact with food. In general, gastric cancer appears to be positively correlated with the ingestion of starch, pickled vegetables, and salted fish and meat, and negatively correlated with whole milk, fresh vegetables, vitamin C, and refrigeration. Dietary nitrates have also been implicated in the development of gastric cancer. These agents can be reduced to nitrites by various enteric bacteria. Nitrites, then, can combine with amines and amides to form nitroso compounds, which are gastric carcinogens in experimental animals. There may also be a genetic predisposition to gastric carcinoma.

Gastric cancer occurs more frequently in males than in females, and the incidence and mortality increase as age increases. Specific precursors of gastric cancer include pernicious anemia, adenomatous gastric polyposis, chronic atrophic gastritis with intestinal metaplasia, previous gastric operative procedures for peptic ulcer disease, and hypertrophic gastropathy (Ménétrier's disease). The degree of risk and latency associated with each of these precursors is variable. Thus, previous peptic ulcer surgery imposes a twofold increased risk of gastric carcinoma, but only after a 15- to 20-year latency period. As many as 10 per cent of patients with pernicious anemia and Ménétrier's disease may ultimately develop gastric adenocarcinoma. Gastric adenomatous polyps, like colonic polyps, have a variable risk of gastric cancer depending primarily on polyp size.

PATHOLOGY. Gastric adenocarcinoma develops from mucous cells, most commonly along the lesser curvature aspect of the pyloric and antral regions. These tumors are usually classified into *papillary, tubular, mucinous,* and *signet cell* varieties (World Health Organization) or *intestinal* and *diffuse* types (Lauren classification). These tumors tend to extend within the gastric wall and into regional lymphatics, as well as directly invading adjacent organs (liver, pancreas, transverse colon, or mesocolon). Hematogenous spread to the liver, lungs, bones, and elsewhere produces systemic metas-

---

See the corresponding chapter or part in the *Textbook of Surgery*, 14th edition, pp. 814–827, for a more detailed discussion of this topic, including a comprehensive list of references.

tases. In addition, peritoneal seeding from the involved gastric serosa to the omentum, parietal peritoneum, ovary (Krukenberg's tumor), and other sites also occurs.

The two major factors influencing survival are the extent of spread through the gastric wall and the presence or absence of regional lymph node involvement. These factors, along with the R description indicating postsurgical tumor status, are combined within the new TNM staging system (Table 1). The extent of penetration of the primary tumor through the stomach wall is expressed by the letter T; T_1 indicates mucosal and submucosal involvement, T_2 muscularis invasion, T_3 serosal infiltration, and T_4 invasion of contiguous organs. N denotes regional lymph node involvement from none (N_0) to involvement of unremovable intraabdominal nodes (N_3). Metastases are indicated as M_1 if present, or M_0 if absent. The anatomic and pathologic findings, together with the R descriptor indicating postoperative

TABLE 1. TNM Classification

Primary Tumor (T)

T_1	Tumor limited to mucosa and submucosa regardless of its extent or location
T_2	Tumor involves the mucosa and the submucosa (including the muscularis propria), and extends to or into the serosa, but does not penetrate through the serosa
T_3	Tumor penetrates through the serosa without invading contiguous structures
T_4	Tumor penetrates through the serosa and invades the contiguous structures

Nodal Involvement (N)

N_0	No metastases to regional lymph nodes
N_1	Involvement of perigastric lymph nodes within 3 cm. of the primary tumor along the lesser or greater curvature
N_2	Involvement of the regional lymph nodes, more than 3 cm. from the primary tumor, that are removable at operation, including those located along the left gastric, splenic, celiac, and common hepatic arteries
N_3	Involvement of other intra-abdominal lymph nodes that are not removable at operation, such as the para-aortic, hepatoduodenal, retropancreatic, and mesenteric nodes

Distant Metastasis (M)

M_0	No (known) distant metastasis
M_1	Distant metastasis present

Surgical Results (R)

R_0	No residual tumor
R_1	Microscopic residual tumor
R_2	Macroscopic residual tumor

From Davis, G. R.: Neoplasms of the stomach. *In* Sleisenger, M. H., and Fordtran, J. S. (Eds.): Gastrointestinal Disease. 3rd ed. Philadelphia, W. B. Saunders Company, 1983.

tumor status, are then used to stage the tumor. Five-year survival closely correlates with stage: 90 per cent for Stage 1, 50 per cent for Stage 2, 10 per cent for Stage 3, and 0 per cent for Stage 4.

The term *early gastric cancer* refers to gastric carcinoma involving only the mucosa or submucosa with positive lymph nodes in 5 to 20 per cent. Unfortunately, in contrast to the Japanese experience, this highly favorable lesion represents only 10 per cent of European and North American cases. *Advanced gastric cancer* suggests invasion of the muscularis or beyond. This situation is frequently associated with distant or contiguous spread. These tumors have a much graver prognosis and are often not amenable to curative resection.

DIAGNOSIS. Symptoms are rarely associated with early gastric cancer and, when present, are vague and nondescript. Symptoms generally do not occur until the tumor is of sufficient size to interfere with either the motor activity of a significant segment of the gastric wall or the normal gastric lumen. This causes symptoms of indigestion, postprandial fullness, eructation, loss of appetite, and heartburn. Vomiting occurs late in the disease. Pain, a common first symptom, may be similar to that of benign peptic ulcer disease and may be relieved by antacid. The disease may occasionally present with symptoms referable to distant spread including ascites, anemia, or pleural effusion. Physical findings, which are frequently nonrevealing until the disease is well advanced, may include an epigastric mass, hepatomegaly from metastatic disease, or ascites. Signs of distant metastases include Virchow's node (supraclavicular, especially on the left), Blumer's shelf (a firm metastatic mass palpable in the posterior pelvic cul-de-sac), Sister Mary Joseph node (infiltration of the umbilicus), and Krukenberg's tumor.

Radiologic examination of the stomach during barium meal is often obtained in patients with upper gastrointestinal symptoms. Advanced gastric cancer presents as a polypoid mass protruding into the lumen of the stomach, an ulcer crater, or a nondistensible stomach due to diffuse, infiltrating carcinoma (linitis plastica). Malignant ulcer craters lie within a mass and do not extend outside the boundary of the gastric wall. The mucosal folds maintain their usual contour up to and beyond the ulcer. These lesions are usually larger than 1 cm. and are frequently surrounded by a rigid gastric wall on fluoroscopic examination. Computed tomography is also an important radiologic modality; findings on computed tomographic scan have been shown to correlate closely with surgical findings.

Upper gastrointestinal endoscopy is an essential procedure in the evaluation and management of gastric cancer. It is much more effective in detecting early or minute gastric cancers; many now consider it to be the procedure of choice. Endoscopy with biopsy is well over 90 per cent accurate in the diagnosis of advanced gastric cancer. It is often combined with cytologic techniques including brushing, lavaging, or direct irrigation and aspiration. Endoscopic ultrasound has recently been introduced and may be as sensitive as computed tomography in evaluation of extent of the primary tumor and regional lymph node status. In addition, palliative or definitive endoscopic therapy may be a valuable option in carefully selected situations.

Any suspicious lesions (e.g., lymph nodes or skin nodules) detected on the physical examination should be biopsied before laparotomy. Liver biopsy, either percutaneous or laparoscopically directed, should also be considered for patients with suspicious computed tomographic or liver scans.

TREATMENT. Surgical resection of the involved portion of the stomach remains the only method capable of curing gastric malignancy. In early gastric cancer, operation is usually curative. A five-year survival rate of 95 per cent or higher has been reported following surgical resection of gastric cancer *confined to the mucosa*. Unfortunately, the majority of patients seen in the West have advanced gastric cancer when first seen. In over 50 per cent of such patients, the tumor is no longer localized when first identified, and gastric resection is only moderately beneficial in most.

Patients with gastric carcinoma should first be evaluated for serious cardiovascular, pulmonary, or renal disorders that may require special preoperative preparation or, rarely, contraindicate surgical therapy. The latter situation most frequently occurs following histologic confirmation of distant spread. However, even in the presence of local extension or distant spread, exploration should still be recommended if there is an opportunity for palliation. Total gastrectomy should not be performed as a palliative procedure.

At laparotomy, the initial exploration should be thorough, with careful examination and biopsy of any suspicious areas in the pelvis, lower abdomen, retroperitoneum, and right upper quadrant in addition to evaluation of fixation and local extension of the primary tumor. Tumors extend 6 cm. proximally within the gastric wall on average; duodenal extension is usually no greater than 3 cm. beyond the pylorus. Thus, "standard" resection for the usual distal gastric cancer should include the greater and lesser omenta, division of the duodenum 2 to 3 cm. distal to the pylorus (but with an adequate cuff for a secure closure), ligation of the left gastric artery at the celiac axis, division of the lesser curvature adjacent to the esophagogastric junction, and division of the greater curvature at the level of the vasa brevia just distal to the spleen. More extensive subtotal resection may require a splenectomy. Alimentary continuity is usually restored via antecolic gastrojejunostomy. Total gastrectomy is indicated only for distal gastric tumors if it allows complete extirpation of a large, fungating, or diffusely spreading tumor not removable by subtotal resection. Total gastrectomy is the procedure of choice for more proximal tumors (e.g., gastric corpus, cardia, or esophagogastric junction) as well as carcinomas in a gastric remnant following a previous subtotal resection, cancer in a patient with a diffuse mucosal lesion with malignant potential (e.g., chronic atrophic gastritis, Ménétrier's disease), and cancer developing within diffuse gastric polyposis. Proximal tumors in the last locations have the poorest prognosis and will often require a radical operation, most frequently via a thoracoabdominal approach.

Although elective total gastrectomy has been recommended for all patients with gastric carcinoma, especially in European centers, this approach has been based primarily on data from retrospective studies. A recent randomized prospective study indicated that although total gastrectomy could be performed without an increase in morbidity and mortality, routine adoption of this approach for the "routine distal tumor" offered no benefit in long-term survival. Extended lymph node resection has also been adopted by several Japanese and European surgeons. Benefits of this approach also remain unproven.

Chemotherapy has frequently been utilized in treating advanced gastric cancer. Combination chemotherapy rarely produces a high clinical response and has not been shown to be superior to single-agent chemotherapy in randomized studies. Adjuvant chemotherapy has not been demonstrated to provide any consistent benefit in early gastric cancers. Debulking of these tumors appears to improve chemotherapy results.

PROGNOSIS. The overall survival in most gastric cancer series in the United States is dismal. Average long-term survival is approximately 10 per cent at 5 years. Lymph node involvement and distant metastases are still the most consistent indicators of ultimate prognosis. The absence of lymphatic spread improves the 5-year survival three to four times. Lymph node involvement is correlated with the depth of invasion of the primary tumor, undoubtedly contributing to the poor prognosis for tumors with serosal penetration. Recent studies demonstrate appreciable improvement in operative mortality following operation for gastric carcinoma, as well as possibly improved 5-year survival.

The most promising aspect of this disease is its decreasing incidence worldwide. Given the excellent results obtainable following treatment of *early* gastric cancer, a practical mass screening technique facilitating early diagnosis might be of great benefit. Unfortunately, the low incidence of this disease in the United States argues against adoption of available mass screening procedures.

31

THE SMALL INTESTINE

I

Anatomy
R. Scott Jones, M.D.

The small intestine extends from the pylorus to the cecum and provides the environment for digestion and absorption. The essential anatomic characteristic of the small intestine remains its large surface area produced by (1) intestinal length, (2) mucosal folds, (3) villi, and (4) microvilli.

GROSS ANATOMY

The 21-cm. duodenum combined with the jejunum measures 261 cm. and composes about three fifths of the entire alimentary canal. The proximal two fifths of small intestine are arbitrarily termed the *jejunum* and the distal three fifths the *ileum*.

The *mesentery* suspends the small intestine from the posterior abdominal wall. The mesentery contains blood vessels, nerves, lymphatics, and lymph nodes as well as stored fat. The broad-based attachment of the mesenteric root stabilizes the small bowel to prevent it from twisting upon its blood supply.

The superior mesenteric artery supplies blood to the small intestine. This artery arises from the abdominal aorta; it courses dorsal to the neck of the pancreas and anterior to the uncinate process to enter the small bowel mesentery. The intestinal arteries branch within the mesentery and unite with adjacent arteries to form a series of arterial arcades before sending small straight arteries to the small intestine. The veins of the small intestine drain into the superior mesentery vein, a major tributary to the portal vein.

The submucosa of the small intestine, especially in the ileum, contains aggregated lymphatic nodules termed Peyer's patches. The lymphatic drainage from the small intestine passes first into lymph nodes close to the wall of the small intestine, then into a second set of nodes adjacent to the mesenteric arcades, and then into a third set of nodes along the superior mesenteric artery. Lymph drains into the intestinal trunk, then into the cisterna chyli.

The mucosal surface of the small intestine contains numerous circular folds, the *plicae circulares* (valvulae conniventes or valves of Kerckring). The intestinal villi, barely visible to the naked eye, are tiny, fingerlike processes projecting into the intestinal lumen.

See the corresponding chapter or part in the *Textbook of Surgery*, 14th edition, pp. 828–831, for a more detailed discussion of this topic, including a comprehensive list of references.

The small intestine receives its parasympathetic innervation from preganglionic fibers passing through the vagus nerves to synapse with neurons of the intrinsic plexuses of the intestine. Its sympathetic innervation is derived from preganglionic fibers arising from the ninth and tenth thoracic segments of the spinal cord passing to synapse in the superior mesenteric ganglion. Postganglionic fibers then pass along branches of the superior mesenteric artery. Thoracic visceral efferents mediate pain from the intestine.

MICROSCOPIC ANATOMY

Mucosa

The epithelium, the lamina propria, and the muscularis mucosa compose the mucosa of the small intestine. Two important structural features characterize the mucosal surface: the villi and the crypts of Lieberkühn. The villi of the jejunum, 0.5 mm. to 1 mm. in length, occur in a density of 10 to 40 per sq. mm. of mucosa. Each villus contains a central lymphatic vessel termed a lacteal, a small artery, a vein, and a capillary network. The crypts of Lieberkühn reside adjacent to the bases of the villi and extend down to but not through the muscularis mucosa.

CELLS OF THE EPITHELIUM

CELLS OF THE VILLI. The cells responsible for absorption, the columnar epithelial cells, are characterized by a luminal brush border and a basal placed nucleus. The microvilli provide the appearance to the brush border and are 1 μ tall and 0.1 μ wide. Each microvillus contains a glycocalyx containing high concentrations of digestive enzymes, particularly disaccharidases. The lateral plasma membrane contains tight junctions, intermediate junctions, and desmosomes. Goblet cells are present in both the villi and the crypts, and they contain a cytoplasm filled with mucous granules.

CELLS OF THE CRYPTS. Enterochromaffin cells reside in the crypts of the small intestine but also occur in other parts of the gastrointestinal system. These cells usually do not contact the intestinal lumen, and their secretory granules reside below the nuclei away from the lumen. This structure suggests an endocrine function.

Paneth cells occur in the base of the crypts, and their function is unknown.

Undifferentiated cells occur only in the crypts, particularly at their bases. These cells exhibit mitosis, multiply, and differentiate to replace lost absorptive cells.

Epithelial Renewal. Undifferentiated cells may (1) differentiate into an absorptive cell and migrate to the villus, (2) remain in the crypt and continue mitotic activity, or (3) remain in the crypt in a resting stage. The cells entering the villi migrate to the villus tips, which shed them into the lumen. This replaces the population of the intestinal epithelial cells every 3 to 7 days.

Muscular Layer and Intramural Neural Structures

Two distinct layers of smooth muscle, the outer longitudinal coat and an inner circular coat, form the muscular portion of the small intestine. Intestinal smooth muscle fibers are discrete spindle-shaped structures about 250 μ long. Nexuses approximate the plasma membranes of adjacent muscle cells to allow electrical continuity between smooth muscle cells and permit conduction through the muscle layer. There are four identifiable neural plexuses in the small intestine: (1) the subserous plexus, (2) the myenteric plexus between the longitudinal and circular muscle layers, (3) the submucosal plexus, and (4) the mucous plexus.

II

Physiology
R. Scott Jones, M.D.

DIGESTION AND ABSORPTION

CARBOHYDRATE. Dietary starch contains two glucose polymers, amylopectin and amylose. Amylase hydrolyzes amylose to maltose and maltotriose. Amylase splits amylopectin to maltose, maltotriose, and the residual branched saccharides, the dextrins. Brush border enzymes break down maltose, maltotriose, dextrins, and the dietary disaccharides lactose and sucrose to constituent monosaccharides. Glucose and galactose then are actively transported into the intestinal cells against a concentration gradient. This active transport of sugars requires metabolic energy, oxygen, and small concentrations of sodium ion. Fructose enters the intestinal cell by facilitated diffusion.

PROTEIN. The stomach initiates protein digestion by (1) the acidic environment, which denatures protein, and (2) the presence of pepsin, which hydrolyzes protein to polypeptides. Protein digestion is incomplete when gastric chyme enters the duodenum, where the higher pH inactivates pepsin. The pancreas secretes proteolytic enzyme precursors into the duodenum, where the intestinal enzyme enterokinase converts trypsinogen to trypsin. Trypsin also activates trypsinogen and other pancreatic proteolytic enzyme precursors. The pancreatic endopeptidases trypsin, chymotrypsin, and elastase split peptide bonds in the central portion of protein

---

See the corresponding chapter or part in the *Textbook of Surgery*, 14th edition, pp. 831–834, for a more detailed discussion of this topic, including a comprehensive list of references.

molecules; exopeptidases, such as carboxypeptidase, remove amino acids from the C-terminal position of protein molecules. Amino peptidases split amino acids from the end-terminal position of protein molecules. Amino acids, the final product of protein digestion, then undergo absorption. Some dipeptides are absorbed. Absorptive cell carrier-mediated active transport requiring oxygen and sodium removes luminal amino acids against a concentration gradient.

FAT. In the duodenum, the dietary triglycerides mix with biliary and pancreatic secretions, which contain bile salts, pancreatic lipase, and bicarbonate ion. Bile salts produce polymolecular aggregates termed micelles. Micelles permit solubilization of lipid in an aqueous environment to produce micellar solutions. Pancreatic lipase aided by colipase catalyzes the hydrolysis of dietary triglyceride into 2-monoglyceride and fatty acids. The bile salt, monoglyceride, fatty acid micelle also solubilizes other lipids such as cholesterol, phospholipid, and fat-soluble vitamins. An alkaline pH favors ionization of fatty acids and bile salts, which increases their solubility in micelles. When the micelles encounter the microvilli of the intestinal epithelial cells, the fatty acids and 2-monoglycerides pass into the epithelial cells by a process not requiring energy, probably diffusion. In the epithelial cells, the endoplasmic reticulum synthesizes 2-monoglycerides and fatty acids into triglyceride. Synthesized triglyceride, phospholipid, cholesterol, cholesterol esters, and lipoprotein then form chylomicrons. Chylomicrons pass from the epithelial cells into the lacteals, into the lymphatics, and then into the venous system. Medium-chain triglycerides can be absorbed without hydrolysis and pass into the portal blood rather than into the lymph. Most bile acids that form micelles are absorbed in the ileum by an active transport process.

WATER AND ELECTROLYTES. Approximately 5 to 10 liters of water enter the small bowel daily, whereas only approximately 500 ml. or less leave the ileum and enter the colon. Simultaneously, large quantities of water move from intestinal lumen to blood as well as from blood to intestinal lumen. Water absorption follows osmotic gradients established by the active transport of solutes such as sodium ion, glucose, or amino acids to the cells. In the jejunum, active transport is responsible for a portion of sodium absorption, whereas most jejunal sodium absorption occurs along osmotic gradients. The human ileum absorbs sodium against steep electrochemical gradients. This observation suggests a very efficient sodium transport in the ileum. The ileum also absorbs chloride against steep electrochemical gradients. Potassium is passively absorbed in the intestine according to its electrochemical gradient. The proximal small intestine absorbs calcium by active transport. Vitamin D and parathyroid hormone enhance calcium absorption. The small intestine regulates the body pool of iron. Normal iron stores permit only a slight transfer of iron from intestinal absorptive cell to plasma. In iron deficiency, the absorptive cells effectively transfer iron into the plasma.

MOTILITY

There are several types of visible small intestine muscular activity. *Segmenting contractions* occurring regularly and rhythmically in adjacent portions of the small intestine divide and subdivide the intestinal content, mixing it and exposing it to larger areas of mucosa, which facilitates digestion and absorption. *Pendular movements* are probably the same as or a minor modification of rhythmic segmentation. *Peristalsis* consists of intestinal contraction passing aborally at a rate of 1 to 2 cm. per second throughout several centimeters of intestine. The major function of peristalsis is distal movement of intestinal chyme. During the interdigestive period, cyclically occurring contractions termed the migrating myoelectrical complex move aborally along the intestine to sweep or cleanse the intestine during the interdigestive period.

Two types of electrical activity occur in the small intestine. Slow-wave electrical activity, the basal electrical rhythm (BER), begins in the longitudinal muscle layer of the duodenum and propagates distally. The BER can occur unrelated to motor activity. Intestinal spike potentials produce motor activity. The BER coordinates spike potentials.

The intrinsic nerve supply regulates rather than initiates motor action. Sympathetic activity inhibits whereas parasympathetic activity stimulates motor function.

Gastrin stimulates gastric and intestinal motility and relaxes the ileocecal sphincter. Cholecystokinin stimulates intestinal motility and decreases intestinal transit time. Secretin and glucagon inhibit intestinal motility.

ENDOCRINE FUNCTION OF THE SMALL INTESTINE

The duodenum and jejunum secrete secretin, cholecystokinin, vasoactive intestinal polypeptide, gastric inhibitory polypeptide, motilin, and somatostatin.

IMMUNOLOGIC FUNCTION OF THE INTESTINE

The intestine produces IgA. This immunoglobulin arises from plasma cells and, after linkage with a protein synthesized by epithelial cells, is secreted in the lumen.

III

Intestinal Obstruction

R. Scott Jones, M.D.

Any impediment to the aboral progression of gastrointestinal luminal content defines intestinal obstruction. Mechanical occlusion of the bowel lumen or paralysis of the intestinal muscle can produce intestinal obstruction.

Three types of abnormalities produce *mechanical obstruction:* (1) obturation of the intestinal lumen; (2) intrinsic bowel lesions, such as atresia, stenosis, or stricture; and (3) lesions extrinsic to the bowel, such as hernia or volvulus.

Paralytic ileus, a common disorder, occurs to some extent in most patients undergoing abdominal surgery. Neural reflexes, peritonitis, and electrolyte imbalance, particularly hypokalemia, produce ileus. Ischemia of the intestine rapidly inhibits motility.

Idiopathic intestinal pseudo-obstruction is a chronic illness characterized by symptoms of recurrent intestinal obstruction without demonstrable mechanical occlusion of the bowel. Patients with this disease have impaired motor responses to intestinal distention. Some patients have aperistalsis of the esophagus with failure of the lower esophageal sphincter to relax. Heredity may have a role. Controversy exists whether neural abnormalities, muscle abnormalities, or both produce the disease. The symptoms include cramping abdominal pain, vomiting, distention, diarrhea, and sometimes steatorrhea. Physical examination reveals abdominal distention. Intestinal pseudo-obstruction is difficult to distinguish from mechanical intestinal obstruction.

PATHOGENESIS. *Simple mechanical obstruction* of the small intestine is caused by accumulation of fluid and gas proximal to the obstruction, which produces distention of the intestine. One of the most important events during simple mechanical small bowel obstruction is the loss of water and electrolytes from the body. Vomiting and accumulation of water in the intestine contribute to water loss. Progressive dehydration may produce oliguria, azotemia, and hemoconcentration. If dehydration persists, circulatory changes such as tachycardia, low central venous pressure, and reduced cardiac output may cause hypotension and hypovolemic shock. Also during intestinal obstruction, bacteria proliferate rapidly in the intestinal lumen. Small intestinal contents thus become feculent during long-standing obstruction because of the large quantities of bacteria.

Impaired circulation of the obstructed intestine causes *strangulation obstruction.* Occlusion at two points along its length produces closed loop obstruction. This type of obstruction may proceed more rapidly to strangulation than does simple obstruction. Strangulation can cause loss of blood and

---

See the corresponding chapter or part in the *Textbook of Surgery*, 14th edition, pp. 835–842, for a more detailed discussion of this topic, including a comprehensive list of references.

plasma from the strangulated segment, which may be particularly severe if venous occlusion predominates. If the strangulation produces gangrene, peritonitis with its sequelae occurs. Another important factor in strangulation obstruction is the toxic material from the strangulated loop. Luminal fluid from a strangulated intestinal loop and the bloody, malodorous peritoneal fluid are lethal when administered to normal animals.

Generally, *colonic obstruction* produces less fluid and electrolyte disturbance than does mechanical small bowel obstruction. If the patient has a competent ileocecal valve, there may be little or no small bowel distention, and the colon will behave as a closed loop. In patients with an incompetent ileocecal valve, the signs of small bowel distention may accompany colon obstruction.

DIAGNOSIS. Abdominal pain, vomiting, obstipation, abdominal distention, and failure to pass flatus characterize the syndrome of intestinal obstruction. Intestinal obstruction typically produces crampy abdominal pain. After a longer period of mechanical obstruction, the crampy pain may subside because motility may be inhibited by bowel distention. Proximal intestinal obstruction may cause profuse vomiting and no abdominal distention.

Physical Examination. Tachycardia and hypotension may indicate severe dehydration or peritonitis. The abdomen is usually distended. Surgical scars should be noted because of the etiologic implication of previous operative procedures. Incarcerated hernias may be obscure, particularly in the obese patient. Abdominal masses should be sought. Abdominal tenderness is a characteristic finding in patients with intestinal obstruction; however, localized tenderness, rebound tenderness, and guarding suggest peritonitis and the likelihood of strangulation. The bowel sounds in intestinal obstruction are usually high-pitched. Rectal examination should be done.

Radiologic Examination. Films in patients with mechanical small bowel obstruction usually show multiple gas-fluid levels with distended bowel. Occasionally, ordinary films fail to distinguish a colonic from a small intestinal obstruction. A barium enema identifies an obstructed colon.

Laboratory Tests. Any patient suspected of having intestinal obstruction should have laboratory measurements of serum sodium, chloride, potassium bicarbonate, and creatinine. The hematocrit and white blood cell count should be measured also.

TREATMENT. In many cases, the appropriate treatment for intestinal obstruction includes surgical relief of the obstruction. The mortality from intestinal obstruction with intestinal gangrene exceeds the mortality in simple mechanical obstruction. Patients with severe fluid and electrolyte imbalance and concomitant illnesses profit from supportive treatment. Intravenous therapy should begin with an infusion of isotonic sodium chloride solution. Potassium chloride infusion should begin after adequate urine formation occurs. After pulse, blood pressure, central venous pressure, and urinary output are normal, surgical therapy may be considered. Antibiotics should be given during the period of resuscitation, particularly if strangulation is suspected. Nasogastric suction empties the stomach, reducing the hazard of pulmonary aspiration of vomitus as well as minimizing further intestinal distention from swallowed air during the preoperative period. In some cases, a long intestinal tube can be passed into the intestine for deflating the bowel. There is controversy concerning the urgency for early operation on patients thought to have partial small bowel obstruction due to adhesions. Partial adhesive small bowel obstruction resolves with nasogastric suction usually within 24 hours in the majority of patients. Operations may be delayed under the following circumstances: (1) in patients with pyloric obstruction; (2) in patients with postoperative intestinal obstruction; (3) in infants with ileocecal intussusception; adults with intussusception should be operated upon because of the high frequency of underlying causes for the intussusception; (4) in patients with sigmoid volvulus decompressed with a sigmoidoscope or a colonoscope; (5) in patients with intestinal obstruction due to an exacerbation of Crohn's disease; and (6) in patients with chronic partial obstruction.

Operative Treatment. Four approaches are available for providing operative relief of intestinal obstruction. (1) In simple obstruction, the obstructed segment of bowel can be freed surgically. (2) A second approach to obstructing lesions is an intestinal bypass. (3) The placement of a cutaneous fistula such as a colostomy proximal to the obstruction is a standard form of therapy. (4) Excision of a lesion with restoration of intestinal continuity by anastomosis may be used frequently, also. With few exceptions, operations for intestinal obstruction should be performed under general anesthesia with endotracheal intubation for minimizing the risk of vomiting and tracheobronchial aspiration of the vomitus. The criteria generally used to assess viability of the obstructed bowel are (1) color, (2) motility, and (3) arterial pulsation. The approach to colon obstruction differs from that to small bowel obstruction. The method of treating obstruction of the left colon entails two or three separate operative steps, including (1) relief of gaseous distention by colostomy proximal to the obstruction, (2) removal of the diseased segment of colon and anastomosis, leaving the colostomy intact, and (3) closure of the colostomy when healing of the anastomosis is complete. In many cases, for example, in obstructing left colon cancer, it may be possible to resect the cancer, perform a colostomy, and then reunite the ends of the colon at a later date after the patient has recovered from the ill effects of intestinal obstruction. In treating cecal or right colon obstruction due to cancer, one usually would perform a right colectomy and ileotransverse colostomy.

Treatment of Paralytic Ileus. Paralytic ileus is treated by nasogastric suction and intravenous fluid administration. Correction of electrolyte imbalance, particularly hypokalemia, is especially important in managing this disorder.

IV

Crohn's Disease (Regional Enteritis)

Keith A. Kelly, M.D., and Bruce G. Wolff, M.D.

Crohn's disease is a chronic, nonspecific inflammatory disease of the gastrointestinal tract of unknown cause. It involves mainly the ileum, colon, and rectum, most often producing symptoms of obstruction or localized perforation with fistula. Both medical and surgical treatment are palliative. Nonetheless, operative excision provides effective symptomatic relief and reasonable long-term benefit.

INCIDENCE AND ETIOLOGY

The incidence of Crohn's disease in the general population is approximately 6 or 7 per 100,000 subjects at risk. The incidence in recent years has been described by some as increasing, whereas others have found it stable. The disease is as common in men as in women and can occur in individuals of any age, although the peak age of onset is between the second and fourth decades of life. No specific cause of the disease has been identified. Some data, however, suggest that environmental factors have an etiologic role. The disease is more common among individuals living in temperate climates than among those living in tropical climates. Also, spouses of those with Crohn's disease have a higher incidence of the disease than does the general population.

PATHOLOGY

Crohn's disease is a generalized inflammatory disorder of the gastrointestinal tract, but it is discontinuous and segmental. One of the earliest macroscopic signs of Crohn's disease is the appearance of aphthous ulcers in the mucosa of the gastrointestinal tract. These small, flat, soft ulcers have a whitish center and a red border. They are scattered in the mucosa with normal areas of intervening mucosa. As the disease progresses, the aphthous ulcers deepen and coalesce, penetrating through the entire mucosa and forming longer ulcers that may reach 1 cm. in size or larger. They often appear first on the mesenteric border of the bowel and have a linear pattern along the wall of the intestine. Islands of normal mucosa can remain between the ulcers to give the surface of the bowel a cobblestone appearance. Noncaseating granulomas are associated with the inflammation in about 50 per cent of patients and are a hallmark of the disease.

As the ulcers grow and the inflammation spreads, the

See the corresponding chapter or part in the *Textbook of Surgery*, 14th edition, pp. 843–851, for a more detailed discussion of this topic, including a comprehensive list of references.

lesions extend transmurally deep into the wall of the bowel. The inflammatory response on the serosa and adjacent mesentery thickens these structures, and the fat of the mesentery creeps around the side of the bowel to add to the thickening. The intestinal lymphatic vessels are engorged, and the lymph nodes in the adjacent mesentery are enlarged. Two main intestinal complications develop from these lesions: obstruction and perforation with abscess or fistula to other organs. Bleeding and toxic megacolon can also develop. Long-standing lesions of the small and large intestine are premalignant. Carcinomas can develop in both the small bowel and the large bowel in patients with Crohn's disease. Extraintestinal manifestations of the disease are also common and include erythema nodosum and pyoderma gangrenosum, iritis, uveitis, arthritis, and pericholangitis/hepatitis (Table 1).

SYMPTOMS

The most common symptoms of Crohn's disease are those from the intestinal lesions, with abdominal pain, especially of a cramping nature, being the primary complaint. Diarrhea is frequent. The stools may contain blood, although often they do not. Patients experience abdominal distention or flatulence and sometimes nausea and vomiting. Eating becomes difficult because it induces symptoms. The patients, therefore, decrease their food intake and lose weight.

The course of the disease is one of exacerbations and remission, but as the lesions mature and complications develop, the symptoms continue unabated and the disease becomes relentlessly progressive. About 70 per cent of patients eventually are operated upon despite medical or dietary therapy.

TABLE 1. Extraintestinal Manifestations of Crohn's Disease

Skin	Liver
Erythema multiforme	Nonspecific triaditis
Erythema nodosum	Sclerosing cholangitis
Pyoderma gangrenosum	
	Kidney
Eyes	Nephrotic syndrome
Iritis	Amyloidosis
Uveitis	
Conjunctivitis	Pancreas
	Pancreatitis
Joints	
Peripheral arthritis	General
Ankylosing spondylitis	Amyloidosis
Blood	
Anemia	
Thrombocytosis	
Phlebothrombosis	
Arterial thrombosis	

DIAGNOSIS

The diagnosis is based on the history, physical findings, and appropriate laboratory tests, including endoscopy and radiography. On physical examination, thickened bowel wall or an adjacent inflammatory response or abscess may be palpable in the abdomen. When fistulas are present, probes and catheters can be passed through the cutaneous openings and into the lumen of the bowel through the tracts. Proctoscopy often reveals the characteristic rectal aphthous ulcer with surrounding normal-appearing mucosa. Anoscopy can demonstrate perianal abscesses, perianal fistulas, and even rectal-vaginal fistulas. Colonoscopy delineates the extent of the ulcerating lesions in the large intestine. At times, the colonoscope can be passed through the colon and into the ileum for identification of the ileal lesions of the disease. Roentgenographic examination of the gastrointestinal tract with use of barium sulfate reveals the ulcerating lesions scattered in a segmental, irregular pattern along the wall of the involved intestine, producing areas of ulceration, narrowing, and thickened bowel wall. The differential diagnosis includes both specific microbiologic causes of intestinal inflammation and nonspecific causes, such as chronic ulcerative colitis (Table 2).

THERAPY

Medical and Dietary Therapy

Medical therapy consists of sulfasalazine, 5-aminosalicylic acid, corticosteroids, antibiotics such as metronidazole and ampicillin, and immunosuppressive agents such as azathioprine and cyclosporin A. Because no specific etiologic agent has been identified for Crohn's disease, treatments are also not specific. They suppress inflammation and improve symptoms, but are not curative. Manipulations of the diet ordinarily have little effect on the progress of Crohn's disease.

Surgical Therapy

INDICATIONS FOR OPERATION. Patients with small intestinal Crohn's disease are usually operated upon because an intestinal complication of the disease, such as obstruction, perforation, or bleeding, mandates the operation. In contrast, patients with large intestinal Crohn's undergo operation because of intractability to medical therapy and chronic debility.

GENERAL PRINCIPLES OF OPERATION. Because Crohn's disease involves nearly the entire gastrointestinal tract in most patients, the possibility of totally excising the disease is not reasonable. Thus, surgical treatment is directed to the most severe areas of involvement, including those that represent complications of obstruction, bleeding, or perforation. The two main operative approaches are to excise the lesions or to bypass them. Currently, most surgeons advise

TABLE 2. Diagnosis of Crohn's Colitis Versus Ulcerative Colitis

Observations	Crohn's Colitis	Ulcerative Colitis
Symptoms and Signs		
Diarrhea	70%–90%	80%–90%
Rectal bleeding	Less common	Prominent
Abdominal pain (cramps)	Moderate to severe	Mild
Palpable mass	At times	No (unless large cancer)
Anal complaints	Frequent (<50%)	Infrequent (<20%)
Radiologic Findings		
Ileal disease	Common	Rare (backwash ileitis)
Nodularity, fuzziness	No	Yes
Distribution	Skip areas	Rectum extending upward and continuously
Ulcer	Linear, cobblestone, fissures	Collar-button
Toxic dilation	Yes	Yes
Proctoscopic Findings		
Anal fissure, fistula, abscess	Common	Rare
Rectal sparing	Common (50%)	Rare (5%)
Granular	No	Yes
Ulceration	Linear, deep	Superficial erosion

391

excision rather than bypass. Bypass allows the diseased intestine to remain in place where it can cause continuing symptoms, require treatment, and perhaps even develop malignancy. The risk of cancer in bypassed small and large intestine with Crohn's disease is greater than the risk in healthy bowel. Excision is done with 5-cm. "disease-free" margins on both sides of the area of involvement. The disease-free margins are established by gross inspection. Most surgeons do not use microscopic confirmation of healthy borders. After excision, bowel continuity is restored by an enteroenterostomy.

After resection of the index segment (or segments) of intestine requiring operation, fistulas from the index segment to adjacent organs, such as the stomach, colon, duodenum, bladder, or vagina, can usually be closed by suture of the entrance of the fistula into the adjacent segment. Resection of the adjacent segment is seldom required unless it, too, is primarily involved with gross Crohn's disease.

SURGICAL TREATMENT AT SPECIFIC SITES. The three most common sites requiring operation for Crohn's disease are the ileum, the colorectum, and the anorectum, with other sites needing surgical treatment less often. With ileal involvement, obtaining 5-cm. grossly disease-free margins on the proximal and distal end usually means resecting the adjacent ileocolic valve, the cecum, and a small portion of ascending colon. No attempt should be made to resect the entire thickened adjacent mesentery. Only that amount of mesentery should be resected as needed to facilitate the removal of the diseased bowel and the anastomosis. Intestinal continuity is then restored with an end-to-end ileal-ascending colostomy. For extensive Crohn's disease of the jejunoileum, either bypass of the involved segments with a side-to-side anastomosis between the uninvolved proximal small intestine and the adjacent large intestine or the performance of multiple "stricturoplasties" on the narrowed, diseased segments of bowel can be done. The stricturoplasties are performed by making a longitudinal incision through the narrowed areas and closing these incisions in a transverse direction. This relieves obstruction but avoids excision.

Crohn's disease involving the ileum, cecum, and ascending colon should be removed again with 5-cm. gross disease-free margins. An anastomosis is made between the ileum and the transverse colon in end-to-end manner.

The operative approach to Crohn's disease of the colorectum varies depending on the exact sites of colorectal involvement and their severity and can include colectomy with ileorectostomy, colectomy with ileostomy and closure of the rectal stump, or proctocolectomy with permanent ileostomy. Sphincter-saving operations such as the continent ileostomy (Kock pouch) or the ileal pouch–anal anastomosis, both of which are commonly used in ulcerative colitis, are not often used for Crohn's disease because of the likely recurrence of Crohn's in the ileal pouch.

Conservative operations directed to relieving symptoms from anorectal Crohn's disease have been done with increasing frequency in recent years. Abscesses have been drained, fissures excised, and anal fistulas opened and débrided, sometimes aided by use of a "seton" when the fistula goes through the anal sphincter. Rectal-vaginal fistulas have been closed by débridement and direct suture of the opening of the fistula, followed by advancement of a rectal mucosal flap from the upper rectum over the opening of the fistula and down to the dentate line.

COMPLICATIONS OF OPERATION

The main early complications of operation are intestinal obstruction from adhesions, intra-abdominal abscess, wound infection, anastomotic leaks, bleeding from areas of operation, phlebothrombosis and pulmonary embolism, atelectasis and pulmonary infections, urinary retention, and enterocutaneous fistulas. Most of these complications can be managed nonoperatively and reoperation should be required in less than 10 per cent of patients. Operative mortality is unusual and should be less than 2 per cent of patients at risk. Late complications include steatorrhea, diarrhea, gallstones, urinary stones, and the short bowel syndrome.

RESULTS

Operations directed to Crohn's disease are palliative. They provide the patients with symptomatic relief, but not cure. Overall, rates of recurrence are about 6 per cent of patients at risk per year or 30 per cent at 5 years and 60 per cent at 10 years. Recurrences usually occur at or just proximal to an anastomosis or stoma. The mortality from Crohn's disease increases slowly with time and is about twofold that of a matched control group of healthy subjects drawn from the general population over the long term.

V

The Surgical Approach to Morbid Obesity
Walter J. Pories, M.D.

Morbid obesity is a serious disease associated with a high incidence of medical complications and a significantly shortened life span. Obesity is "morbid" when the patient is 100

See the corresponding chapter or part in the *Textbook of Surgery*, 14th edition, pp. 851–866, for a more detailed discussion of this topic, including a comprehensive list of references.

pounds or more over ideal body weight. The problem, unfortunately, is common. People in the United States tend toward obesity, with an estimated 12 million individuals being seriously overweight. Of these, at least 3 million are morbidly obese but some have estimated the number to be closer to 7 million.

THE COMPLICATIONS OF MORBID OBESITY

There is a direct relationship between the amount of excess weight and the incidence of arthritis, coronary heart disease, cerebrovascular disease, congestive heart failure, hypertension, diabetes mellitus, cancer of the stomach, and cholecystitis. *Mortality* accelerates steeply when an individual becomes 50 per cent overweight; morbidly obese young males have a 12-fold increase in mortality. In females of this age group, the situation is equally bleak. Sudden, unexplained deaths are common.

Hypertension is the most common complication associated with morbid obesity; it occurs in over 60 per cent of patients. As might be expected, the principal cause of death in the morbidly obese is directly related to cardiovascular disease in the form of stroke, acute coronary thrombosis, or arrhythmias. The role of the obesity is underscored by the observation that weight reduction alone lowers blood pressure in over half of hypertensive obese patients.

Adult onset diabetes (non-insulin-dependent diabetes mellitus, NIDDM) or impaired glucose tolerance occurs in one third of the morbidly obese, with the frequency and severity of glucose intolerance being directly related to the degree of excess weight. The NIDDM is not due to a lack of insulin; in fact, these patients generally exhibit significant hyperinsulinemia. When diabetes complicates morbid obesity, mortality increases 40 per cent. *Pulmonary insufficiency* develops in almost all of the morbidly obese to some degree as the expiratory reserve volume falls with the continuing gain in weight. In those who develop the fully developed pickwickian hypoventilation syndrome, the mortality exceeds 30 per cent. *Cholelithiasis* is increased threefold. Infertility and amenorrhea are common. Pregnancy, when it does occur, is frequently associated with a high risk of complications. Other complications of obesity include *degenerative arthritis, gout, skin diseases, proteinuria, increased hemoglobin concentration, and immunologic impairment.* In fact, morbid obesity probably affects every organ system.

Of greater immediate concern to the patients, however, and the major reason for seeking surgical therapy, are the *psychological and socioeconomic consequences* of morbid obesity. Fat people are frequently objects of public scorn and malicious ridicule. Obese patients are often unable to fit into armchairs, find suitable clothing, obtain access to public toilets, and enter public conveyances. If they can enter an automobile, they may be unable to get out. Employers usually consider the morbidly obese poor candidates because of their unfavorable appearance, their inability to fit into office furniture or into factory environments, and their high absenteeism due to illness. The environment of the morbidly obese is neither happy nor filled with opportunities. The morbidly obese are severely handicapped by every measure: physically, emotionally, economically, and socially. Morbid obesity is indeed a serious disease.

THE ETIOLOGY OF HUMAN OBESITY

Although there is wide acceptance of the observation that "obesity runs in families," the cause of that obesity, whether genetic or environmental, continues to be disputed. Both etiologic factors probably have a role. The genetic argument rests on several findings: (1) the demonstration that most of the offspring of thin parents are thin, and most of the children of fat parents are fat; (2) that the strong inverse relationship between the current socioeconomic status and obesity in women holds just as strongly when analyzed for socioeconomic status of origin; (3) analysis of the Twin Register of the National Academy of Sciences/National Research Council shows that the concordance rates for obesity in monozygotic twins were approximately twice that at lesser degrees of overweight and even higher at greater degrees of overweight; and (4) body mass index of adoptees is strongly related to the body mass index of the biologic parents and not to that of the adoptive parents.

Similarly, there is evidence that environmental factors are also strong: (1) adoptees who are raised in a rural environment are more overweight than those who have been raised in an urban setting; (2) studies of Danish draftees showed no change in the average weight of these men from 1943 to 1960, but in the following 12 years there was an eightfold increase in the number with severe obesity, certainly too short a time for a change in the gene pool; and (3) the higher attendance at "smorgasbord restaurants" by the obese on the nights that buffets were featured. Currently, most authorities concur that both genetic and environmental factors have a role and that the genetic influences appear to be stronger.

THE DEFINITION OF OBESITY

The term *morbid obesity* reflects the life-threatening consequences of being more than 100 pounds (45 kg.) over ideal body weight. For patients of short stature, that is, less than 5 feet, morbid obesity cannot be defined as easily and is generally described as 100 per cent or more over ideal body weight. Recently, some authors have adopted the term *malignant obesity* to identify those who exceed their ideal weight by 200 per cent or 200 pounds.

A number of indices have been developed for the quantification of obesity. The most useful is the list of 1983 Height and Weight Standards of the Metropolitan Life Insurance Company. The midpoint of the medium weights listed on that table has been arbitrarily accepted, for bariatric studies, to be the ideal body weight for an individual of given sex and size. Also useful is the body mass index (weight [kg.]/ height [m.]), which can be related to health risks. The most accurate and clinically useful measure of obesity, however, is probably provided by hydrodensitometry, that is, by assessing the proportion of fat with the measurement of buoyancy when the subject is immersed in water. By this measure, morbid obesity begins at 45 per cent fat.

Other indices of relative adiposity include skinfold thickness, total body potassium, total body water, uptake of fat-soluble inert gases, energy balance, nitrogen balance, and various combinations of height versus weight calculations. Except for special research protocols, no clinical advantage is evident for any of these approaches.

Fat distribution appears to be a more important risk factor for morbidity and mortality than is overweight or obesity *per se*. The risk of death and/or an increased risk of diabetes, hypertension, or stroke appear to be far higher in those individuals with large bellies and narrow hips versus those with a more gynecoid distribution. Unfortunately, accurate measures of fat distribution are not yet available.

NONOPERATIVE TREATMENT OF MORBID OBESITY

THE FAILURE OF DIETING. Although dieting remains the most useful method of weight control for most patients, it is generally ineffective for the morbidly obese. Weight loss is usually disappointingly low. In most cases, even when massively obese patients are aided by groups such as Weight Watchers, by psychotherapy, by diuretics, by thyroid preparations, or by anorectic agents such as amphetamines, the lost pounds are usually regained together with a few extra ones as soon as the intense weight-reducing regimen has ceased. The long-term success rate by any of the conservative (that is, nonoperative) methods (diets, medications, behavior modification) is generally conceded to be less than 10 per cent in the morbidly obese. Similarly, wiring the teeth, a method of limiting the diet to liquids, has fallen into disuse for three reasons: (1) many morbidly obese patients are edentulous and therefore are not suitable candidates; (2) they tolerate the wiring poorly because of their personality patterns and generally demand removal of the wires within a few days; and (3) most important, as soon as the wires are removed, even if a major change in appearance is apparent, they resume previous eating habits and quickly return to their original weight. There may still be limited indications for wiring teeth in poor-risk obese patients who are in cardiac or pulmonary failure and who are being prepared for surgical therapy. However, if this is done, it must be remembered that many morbidly obese patients are severely malnourished despite their size and that their liquid diets may require considerable nutritional enrichment in order to minimize postoperative complications.

SURGICAL THERAPY FOR
MORBID OBESITY

Because diets are ineffective in the management of morbid and malignant obesity, most authorities now agree with the recommendation in Conn's *Current Therapy:* "During the past ten or so years, surgery has become the treatment of choice of that small percentage of persons who suffer from severe obesity."

The first operations for morbid obesity were a variety of intestinal bypasses that interfered with absorption and digestion by shortening the small intestine. The most successful of the bypasses was a procedure that excluded all but 14 inches of jejunum and 4 inches of ileum by joining these segments end-to-end and by connecting the inactivated segment to the sigmoid colon for drainage. Good results, in terms of weight loss, were reported in about 80 per cent of patients, with an average weight loss of 45 kg. or 100 pounds. Massively obese individuals lost more than those less obese and younger patients lost more than those in middle age. Most weight loss occurred during the first year after operation, with the jejunocolic bypass averaging total weight loss of 41 per cent and the jejunoileal bypass averaging weight loss of 35 per cent. By the second or third year almost all patients reached a plateau, and many regained their weight as adaptations for better absorption occurred in their intestines.

The intestinal bypasses were finally discarded because of an unacceptably high complication rate. The operative mortality varied from 1 to 8 per cent, and the major early complications included wound problems (10 to 20 per cent), pulmonary emboli (1 to 4 per cent), and hepatic failure (1 to 2 per cent). Of even greater concern were the long-term metabolic problems. Some followed the severe loss of minerals associated with diarrhea, including hypocalcemia, hypokalemia, hypomagnesemia, and iron and zinc deficiency. Hypoproteinemia and anemia were common. The diarrhea usually began about the fifth postoperative day and soon reached 12 to 20 liquid movements per day, gradually subsiding to 6 to 10 semiformed movements per day. Serum electrolyte, mineral, and vitamin levels had to be carefully monitored and corrected in order to avoid serious and occasionally uncontrollable symptoms. Vitamin B_{12} and folic acid deficiencies were common.

Gastrointestinal complications included intractable diarrhea with associated rectal problems, hemorrhage, and "bypass enteritis." The last is a syndrome that is probably due to pathologic bacterial colonization of the bypassed bowel from the colon and is characterized by diarrhea, abdominal pain, fever of up to 39° C., and occasionally even pneumatosis cystoides.

Biliary or urinary calculi developed in 8 per cent of patients following intestinal bypass, possibly as a result of increased bile salt and glycine synthesis and hyperoxaluria.

Liver disease was the most feared complication of intestinal bypass, and a number of fatalities were reported. Many morbidly obese patients were particularly vulnerable because fatty metamorphosis is common among the morbidly obese even before operation, that is, their fatty livers resemble those of force-fed geese. Abnormalities in liver function occurred in about 40 per cent of patients with an intestinal bypass. These changes were unpredictable and dangerous, appearing as early as 3 weeks or as late as 2 years after operation. Nausea, vomiting, jaundice, and enlargement of the liver were reported frequently; however ascites and anasarca were rare. Hepatic coma and death occurred in 1 per cent of all bypass patients. Although many patients showed improvement 6 to 12 months after operation, in 3 to 5 per cent the changes were progressive and associated with marked fibrosis. In severe cases, the terminal changes were histologically indistinguishable from alcoholic cirrhosis. Hepatic deterioration progressed in some patients despite restoration of good nutrition by hyperalimentation.

In addition to hepatic dysfunction and urinary and biliary calculi, a large number of case reports cited a variety of problems, including unmanageable diarrhea, polyarthrosis, fatigue, lethargy, muscle cramps, uncontrollable nausea and bloating, tuberculosis, and nontuberculous granulomas. Besides the various metabolic problems, patients developed mechanical complications, including obstruction of the bypassed small intestine and intussusception of the blind loop into the colon. These two problems can be particularly puzzling and dangerous because roentgenographic findings may not be helpful, since the characteristic small bowel loops with air-fluid levels may not be present.

Moreover, 20 per cent of the patients failed to lose weight satisfactorily, and some lost no weight at all. A significant number regained some of the lost weight during the second and third year after operation, and some of these required another procedure in which an additional segment of the now adapted small bowel was removed.

In summary, following intestinal bypass, most patients lost one third of their total body weight with some improvement of insulin resistance, hypertension, cardiac failure, pulmonary function, and hyperlipidemia. Unfortunately, the long-term complications were serious with persistent diarrhea, hypokalemia, profound hypomagnesemia and hypocalcemia, arthralgias, neurologic signs, enteropathies, intussusceptions, avitaminoses, trace element deficits, cholelithiasis, renal disease, and liver failure.

Conversion from Intestinal to Gastric Bypass

Because the intestinal bypass is associated with so many long-term complications and because these complications are unpredictable, most bariatric surgeons agree that patients with these intestinal configurations should be converted to either a gastric bypass or a vertical banded gastroplasty. Simple reversal is, of course, another option, but in almost all cases the patients quickly revert to morbid obesity, merely trading one complication for another. Since many of these patients are severely malnourished, 2 to 3 weeks of parenteral nutrition may be required for preparing them for surgical therapy.

Gastric Operations for Morbid Obesity

In 1966, Mason, concerned by the frequency and seriousness of the complications from intestinal bypass, devised the gastric bypass, which was designed to interfere with food intake rather than with digestion and absorption. Since then there have been a number of modifications based on similar principles: (1) reduction of gastric capacity to a small pouch of 20 to 30 ml.; (2) delayed emptying of that pouch with the creation of a small outlet of about 8 mm.; and (3) in the gastric bypass versions, the bypass of the antrum and duodenum with a Roux-en-Y loop of intestine. The two most commonly done operations, Mason's vertical banded gastroplasty and the Greenville gastric bypass, have now become widely accepted as the procedures of choice because of their safety and efficacy.

Results of the Vertical Banded Gastroplasty

Mason recently reported a combined series of 1000 patients from the University of Iowa Hospitals and clinics in Iowa City and the St. Francis Memorial Hospital in San Francisco. The operative mortality was 0.33 per cent. Three-year results show sustained weight control with a loss of 35 kg. (54 per cent excess weight loss) in 45 patients whose initial weight was greater than 225 per cent of ideal. The vertical banded gastroplasty is an effective procedure that can be performed with an acceptable morbidity and mortality.

The Greenville Gastric Bypass

Of the Roux-en-Y gastric exclusion procedures, the Greenville gastric bypass (GGB) appears to be the most effective operation. The operation produced significant *weight loss* and, during the 9 years of observation, maintained that loss well. If morbid obesity is defined as 100 pounds over ideal weight, 94 per cent of the 462 patients were no longer morbidly obese within 2 years. There was, however, some weight gain between 24 and 96 months (178 to 194 pounds) reflecting (1) the individuals who learn to "outeat" their pouch with high-calorie liquids and who continue snacking as well as (2) those 26 individuals who had a staple line breakdown.

The GGB effectively reduced the proportion of *body fat:* the females fell from a preoperative mean of 50.92 to 38.46 per cent fat and males from 46.70 to 31.93 per cent fat.

The GGB produced remarkable improvement in the abnormal glucose metabolism of those morbidly obese individuals who either were glucose-impaired or had frank adult onset *diabetes mellitus.* NIDDM was present in 100 (21.6 per cent) and impaired glucose tolerance was present in another 62

(13.4 per cent) of 462 patients. All but three of these (97 per cent) became euglycemic after operation. Of these, 42 patients were studied intensively; 12 had been maintained on insulin, nine were on sulfonylureas, and two were on both medications before the gastric bypass. None now receive any antidiabetic medication or special diets. Fasting plasma glucose, fasting insulin, and glycosylated hemoglobin were restored to normal levels in all patients while insulin release, insulin resistance, and utilization of glucose were sharply improved.

The GGB also favorably affected *hypertension.* Of the 462 patients, 267 (58 per cent) were hypertensive before operation, and of these, 151 (33 per cent) were on antihypertensive medication. After the GGB, 91 (20 per cent) remained hypertensive and 74 (16 per cent) were maintained on medication by their physicians.

Although the GGB produced long-term improvement in the health and physical functioning of the morbidly obese, the emotional and social changes for the better proved to be temporary. The RAND measures of mental health improved significantly after operation, but after 12 months there was a gradual return to the preoperative personality pattern as reflected by such indices as anxiety, depression, self-control, and vitality. Improvement in health was not necessarily associated with a better personality.

The perioperative mortality of 0.4 per cent (2 of 462) is low for this group of high-risk patients with such complicating preoperative factors as pickwickian syndrome, inadequately managed diabetes, cardiopulmonary failure, asthma, chronic skin infections, and disabling arthritis. The average length of stay was 8.6 days (range 5 to 34 days). Of the 462 patients, 11 per cent had a complication serious enough to prolong hospital stay. The most common perioperative complications included wound problems (minor infections 10.2 per cent, seromas and liquefied fat 10.1 per cent, major infections 3.9 per cent, dehiscence 1.1 per cent) and anastomotic leak or subphrenic abscess in 2.4 per cent. Infectious complications were most common in patients with NIDDM or glucose impairment. Reoperation was required in 1.7 per cent; 7.8 per cent were readmitted during the first 30 days after GGB.

There were 16 late deaths among the 462 operated patients (3.5 per cent) during the 9 years of follow-up. The high rate of depression seen among the morbidly obese may be responsible for the three deaths from suicide, the death from malnutrition bulemia, and the two deaths due to progressive cirrhosis from extensive alcohol abuse.

Patients with bariatric surgery require rigorous follow-up because late complications are common. The most common was dumping (75.7 per cent), an initially bothersome but desirable outcome because it alters behavior and probably is responsible for the long-term effectiveness of the procedure. The other complications are generally temporary, induced by the nutritional deficits associated with the period of major weight loss: hair loss 46.8 per cent, constipation 46.4 per cent, anemia 39.2 per cent, vitamin B_{12} deficiency 38.9 per cent, psychiatric problems 28.2 per cent, nausea and vomiting usually due to initial overeating 27.1 per cent, incisional hernias 17.9 per cent, neuropathies usually due to vitamin B complex deficits 14.9 per cent, cholelithiasis 9.8 per cent, bile reflux and esophagitis 5.9 per cent, small bowel obstruction due to adhesions 5.3 per cent (usually self-limited), marginal ulcer (all healed, but one healed with H_2-blockers) 3.9 per cent, pouch dilation 3.1 per cent, staple line failures 2.6 per cent, anastomotic dilation 1.8 per cent, and anastomic stenosis requiring dilation 1.5 per cent. During the 9-year follow-up, 31.3 per cent of the patients with gastric bypasses reentered the hospital, primarily for cholecystectomies, incisional hernia repairs, abdominal pain, psychiatric problems, and nutritional deficits.

The most serious complications are the neuropathies that may occur when these patients fail to take their vitamin B complex or vitamin B_{12} supplements. These syndromes, which are manifested by weakness, peripheral tingling, dizziness, anorexia, and confusion, should be treated promptly because they can progress rapidly. Hospitalization with total parenteral nutrition may be required.

Despite these problems, only one patient has requested and undergone reversal of the gastric bypass; and in those patients in whom the operation failed owing to pouch dilation, anastomotic widening, and staple failure, all but one requested that the defect be corrected as quickly as possible before they regained their previous weight. There are few operations that have that high a level of patient satisfaction.

A Comparison of the Gastric Bypass, the Gastroplasties, and Gastric Banding

Only one well-controlled series comparing the gastric bypass with the true Mason's vertical banded gastroplasty has been published. Sugerman stopped the randomization at 9 months after 20 patients had undergone each procedure because greater weight loss ($p < 0.05$) was noted after the gastric bypass. The difference increased ($p < 0.01$) with each 3-month interval through 3 years. In a later study, the same authors obtained their best results by assigning sweet-eaters to the gastric bypass and recommended that vertical banded gastroplasty should not be performed in patients who are addicted to sweets.

In summary, both procedures, the Greenville gastric bypass and Mason's vertical banded gastroplasty, have been shown to be effective therapies for morbid obesity. Each has been reported to produce effective weight loss, to reverse hyperglycemia and hypertension, and to provide significant rehabilitation. All can be done with surprisingly low operative mortalities (<1 per cent) and acceptable morbidity.

At present, the vertical banded gastroplasty is still the most commonly performed bariatric operation. Even though the data remain incomplete, it would appear that the gastric bypass produces the greatest weight loss but is also associated with the highest rate of complications and nutritional deficiencies. The vertical banded gastroplasty is less effective in terms of weight reduction but is technically easier and has fewer long-term nutritional problems.

Details concerning the criteria for patient selection, preoperative preparation, operative technique, postoperative care, long-term follow-up, and revision of failed procedures are included in the main text chapter.

CONCLUSION

Morbid obesity is a serious and increasingly common disorder that represents a severe handicap and that is associated with major health problems including diabetes, hypertension, biliary disease, arthritis, and a number of other disorders. Because diets rarely produce sustained weight loss in these patients, surgical therapy has become the treatment of choice. Two operations, the Greenville gastric bypass and Mason's vertical banded gastroplasty, have produced the best results to date; both are no longer experimental and can be considered effective procedures that can sharply ameliorate or reverse not only the excessive weight but also the complications of the disorder. The operations are difficult, and the management of these patients is challenging but rewarding. Long-term follow-up is essential for the proper management of such late complications as nutritional deficiencies and psychological problems. Failures due to pouch distention, anastomotic dilation, and staple line breakdown are unusual, but revisions, although technically challenging, can be done with acceptable results.

VI

Meckel's Diverticulum
Ward O. Griffen, Jr., M.D., Ph.D.

Meckel's diverticulum, the most frequently encountered diverticulum of the small intestine, was described by Johann Meckel in 1808. It is a true diverticulum consisting of all elements of the bowel wall. It is a congenital abnormality representing a persistence of the omphalomesenteric or vitelline duct, a tubular structure that connects the two portions of the primitive yolk sac in the embryo. This tube is contained within the umbilical cord and ordinarily is obliterated by the seventh week.

Persistence of the vitelline duct produces the various forms of Meckel's diverticulum encountered in children and adults.

See the corresponding chapter or part in the *Textbook of Surgery*, 14th edition, pp. 866–868, for a more detailed discussion of this topic, including a comprehensive list of references.

The anatomic entities seen are are (1) a fistula between the umbilicus and the ileum when the entire duct remains patent; (2) the usual Meckel's diverticulum due to failure of closure of the intestinal end of the duct; the diverticulum is located 45 to 90 cm. proximal to the ileocecal valve on the antimesenteric border of the ileum; (3) an umbilical sinus when the umbilical end of the duct does not obliterate; (4) a fibrous cord between the umbilicus and the ileum representing the obliterated duct and its vessels; or (5) any combination of these four. An additional abnormality is the presence of heterotopic tissue in the mucosal lining, for example, gastric and pancreatic tissue.

This pathologic anatomy is responsible for the symptoms seen in patients with Meckel's diverticulum, although it should be emphasized that the majority of patients with Meckel's diverticulum are asymptomatic. The most common symptom associated with this congenital lesion is gastrointestinal bleeding, usually melena or bright red blood per rectum. The ileal mucosa is particularly sensitive to acid-peptic digestion so that a small amount of gastric mucosa in the diverticulum produces an ileal ulcer with bleeding after erosion into bowel wall blood vessels ensues. Because gastric mucosa takes up ^{99m}Tc-pertechnetate, scintiscanning with this agent has been used to make the diagnosis preoperatively. Occasionally a small bowel enema demonstrates the diverticulum. The treatment is either diverticulectomy if the bleeding has subsided or ileal resection to include the diverticulum with primary anastomosis if bleeding is active.

The second most common symptom associated with Meckel's diverticulum is intestinal obstruction. The mechanism of obstruction may be due to

1. intussusception when the diverticulum is the leading point. Crampy abdominal pain and "currant jelly" stools occur and the intussusception can be reduced by low-pressure barium enema. If the diverticulum is identified during this procedure or if the intussusception cannot be reduced, a celiotomy is indicated either to remove the diverticulum or to reduce the intussusception and remove the diverticulum.

2. volvulus of the bowel around either a patent persistent duct or an obliterated fibrous cord, provided it is tethered to both the ileum and the anterior abdominal wall. Therapy consists of reduction of the volvulus and complete resection of the diverticulum or fibrous cord.

3. incarceration of the diverticulum in an inguinal hernia, first described by Littre. Treatment should include both hernia repair and diverticulectomy.

The third complication associated with Meckel's diverticulum is diverticulitis. This entity mimics appendicitis and should be treated with the same alacrity. To delay in operating on the patient because the diagnosis is not firm is to invite the serious life-threatening events of perforation and resultant peritonitis. A more recent finding associated with this uncommon entity is the rare development of malignancies in the diverticulum. Leiomyosarcoma and carcinoid are the most common although other neoplasms have been reported.

Controversy still surrounds the question of what should be done about a diverticulum found incidentally. Although diverticulectomy under these circumstances is safe, the probability of developing symptoms from the diverticulum is small, particularly if the patient is over 40 years old. Therefore, the current recommendations are (1) do not remove the diverticulum if there is no evidence of ectopic tissue, and if the orifice is wide, and (2) perform a diverticulectomy if there is evidence of ectopic tissue, such as localized thickening, if the orifice is narrow, or if there is any concern that the symptoms that necessitated the operation may be secondary to the diverticulum.

VII

Carcinoid Tumors and the Carcinoid Syndrome

Haile T. Debas, M.D., and Susan L. Orloff, M.D.

Carcinoid tumors arise from cells with APUD characteristics and represent 55 per cent of all gut eudocrine tumors. The incidence is 1 to 5 cases per 100,000 of the general population.

CARCINOID TUMORS

SITE OF ORIGIN. These derive from the three portions of the embryonic gut. Foregut carcinoids develop primarily in the stomach, pancreas, and lungs and frequently produce atypical carcinoid syndrome. Midgut carcinoid tumors are most common and arise primarily in the appendix and terminal ileum. They produce multiple secretory products and are often associated with the typical carcinoid syndrome. Hindgut carcinoid tumors arise almost exclusively in the rectum. They do not produce secretory products and, therefore, do not cause carcinoid syndromes.

CLINICAL MANIFESTATIONS

Foregut Tumors. Gastric carcinoid tumors may be silent but may cause upper abdominal pain or bleeding. Bronchial carcinoid tumors have initial clinical manifestations of hemoptysis, recurrent pneumonitis, or localized wheezing or present as a "coin-lesion" on chest film. Both gastric and bronchial carcinoid tumors may be associated with the carcinoid syndrome.

See the corresponding chapter or part in the *Textbook of Surgery*, 14th edition, pp. 869–873, for a more detailed discussion of this topic, including a comprehensive list of references.

Midgut Carcinoid Tumors. Appendiceal and small intestinal tumors may be silent. Appendiceal carcinoid tumors may cause acute obstructive appendicitis. Small intestinal tumors may cause bowel obstruction due to fibrotic kinking or intussusception. They may also have initial clinical manifestations of diarrhea, bleeding, and weight loss and rarely may present as an abdominal mass.

Hindgut Tumors. These present as rectal lesions on endoscopy or may cause bleeding.

DIAGNOSIS. The most useful diagnostic finding is an elevated level of 5-hydroxyindoleacetic acid (5-HIAA). In foregut carcinoid tumors, the urine contains little (but above normal) 5-HIAA but large amounts of 5-hydroxytryptophan (5-HTP) and serotonin (5-HT) since these tumors are deficient in dopa-decarboxyls and cannot convert 5-HTP into 5-HT. Plasma levels of neurotensin, substance P, motilin, somatostatin, and vasoactive intestinal polypeptide are sometimes elevated.

Treatment. Early resection, while the tumor is small, offers the patient the best likelihood for cure. Resection is often necessary regardless of the presence or absence of metastases. Appendiceal tumors less than 1.5 cm. in diameter may be treated by routine appendectomy. When they are greater than 1.5 cm. or are associated with invasion of the ileum or lymphatic spread, a right hemicolectomy is required. Rectal carcinoid tumors less than 1 cm. may be removed endoscopically. Tumors measuring 1 to 2 cm. should be excised operatively with margins. Those larger than 2 cm. require anterior resection.

CARCINOID SYNDROME

CAUSES. The carcinoid syndrome occurs in fewer than 10 per cent of patients with carcinoid tumors. The syndrome occurs when venous drainage from the tumor gains access to the systemic circulation so that vasoactive secretory substances escape hepatic degradation. Three conditions under which this occurs are (1) when hepatic metastases are present, (2) when venous blood from retroperitoneal metastases drains into paravertebral veins, and (3) when the primary carcinoid tumor is outside the gastrointestinal tract, for example, bronchial, ovarian, or testicular.

CLINICAL MANIFESTATIONS. The syndrome consists of (1) flushing, (2) diarrhea, (3) wheezing, and (4) tricuspid and/or pulmonic valve insufficiency. Other symptoms include sweating, abdominal pain and borborigimi, and pellagra dermatosis.

BIOCHEMICAL MEDIATORS. Serotonin is thought to be responsible for the diarrhea and fibrosis including that in cardiac valves. The vasomotor changes are thought to be mediated by kinins and such vasoactive peptides as substance P, neuropeptide-K, neurokinin-A, and neurotensin.

DIAGNOSIS. Elevated urinary 5-HIAA and elevated 5-HT in whole blood or platelet-poor plasma provide the best confirmation of the diagnosis. Occasionally, pentagastrin-

provocative test may be used to induce symptoms and to
elevate circulating levels of 5-HT and peptides secreted by
the tumor.

TREATMENT. Primary tumors should be resected. Debulking procedures of either the primary or secondary tumors
in the liver may provide significant palliation. Liver transplantation, when the primary has been eradicated and the
tumor is confined to the liver, has been recently suggested.
This form of treatment is as yet unproved. Pharmacologic
treatment with antisecretion agents or interferon is relatively
ineffective. The best symptomatic treatment has been produced with the use of long-acting somatostatin analog. The
best cancer chemotherapeutic regimen is a combination of
streptozotocin and 5-fluorouracil.

VIII

Malabsorption Syndromes
John P. Grant, M.D.

Malabsorption is any disorder with impaired absorption of
fats, carbohydrates, proteins, vitamins, electrolytes, minerals,
and/or water. This abnormal physiologic state is seen following several surgical procedures.

ESOPHAGECTOMY. The amount of nitrogen excreted in
the stool is usually normal. Both D-xylose and vitamin B_{12}
absorption and small bowel biopsies are normal. Seventy-
two–hour stool collections demonstrate mild steatorrhea. This
is most likely related to the vagotomy performed as a part of
the esophageal resection.

TOTAL GASTRECTOMY. Malabsorption of fat and protein occurs owing to performance of a truncal vagotomy and
to inefficient mixing of food with digestive enzymes. Xylose
and lactose absorption are normal. Pernicious anemia occurs
infrequently because of large hepatic reserves of intrinsic
factor and the relatively poor survival of those patients with
gastric cancer.

Reduced dietary intake follows loss of gastric storage capacity and dysphagia with reflux alkaline esophagitis. Although creation of a jejunal pouch improves storage capacity
and Roux-en-Y esophagojejunostomy decreases reflux alkaline esophagitis, anorexia often persists and poor dietary
intake remains a major cause of nutritional depletion.

PARTIAL GASTRECTOMY. Partial gastrectomy reduces
the gastric reservoir as the percentage of gastric resection

See the corresponding chapter or part in the *Textbook of Surgery*,
14th edition, pp. 873–880, for a more detailed discussion of this topic,
including a comprehensive list of references.

increases. Increasing meal frequency may compensate, but patients often do not comply. In addition, malabsorption is often present. There are decreased gastric digestion, more rapid and less regulated gastric emptying, and decreased intestinal transit time. Small bowel biopsies are usually normal.

A Billroth II procedure may cause more malabsorption than does a Billroth I because of (1) defective stimulation of biliary and pancreatic secretions with bypass of the duodenum, (2) possible inadequate mixing of pancreatic enzymes and bile salts with gastric contents, (3) possible stasis in the afferent loop causing bacterial overgrowth and abnormalities of bile salt metabolism, and (4) loss of the duodenum as the principal surface for iron, calcium, fat, and carotene absorption. Approximately 50 per cent of patients develop steatorrhea following a Billroth II procedure, with fecal fat levels greater than 8 gm. per 24 hours. Fewer than 20 per cent develop clinically significant malabsorption. Only 25 per cent of patients following a Billroth I procedure demonstrate steatorrhea, and fewer than 10 per cent show clinically significant malabsorption.

Anemia occurs in up to 30 per cent of patients within 15 years following subtotal gastrectomy. Malabsorption of iron, folate, and occasionally vitamin B_{12} occurs. A metabolic bone disease similar to osteomalacia occurs in up to 33 per cent of patients after 10 to 20 years owing to malabsorption of vitamin D and calcium.

FOLLOWING VAGOTOMY. Malabsorption following truncal vagotomy may be due to diarrhea, poor mixing of pancreatic secretions and bile salts with food, and diminished release of secretin and cholecystokinin. The reported incidence varies from 28 to 68 per cent, but significant diarrhea occurs in only about 5 per cent. The incidence following selective vagotomy is less than 10 per cent. The diarrhea may be due to rapid small bowel transit resulting from vagal denervation or stasis of food in the stomach and small bowel with periodic bacterial overgrowth and dumping. In addition, truncal vagotomy alters competence of the ileocecal valve, reducing dwell time of the sulcus entericus in the terminal ileum. This causes malabsorption and depletion of bile salts with steatorrhea. Steatorrhea may also be due to abnormalities of gastric grinding and sieving of food particles, with larger fat particles being malabsorbed. There is little difference between fecal fat levels after truncal vagotomy and selective vagotomy.

Vagotomy with drainage reduces glucose absorption approximately 30 per cent. Rapid gastric emptying and small bowel transit time overload the limited glucose-absorbing capacity of the gut. Plasma glucose and insulin peaks, however, are two to four times higher than normal, reflecting rapid gastric emptying and initial glucose absorption. The relatively short absorption period with normal glucose clearance causes "reactive" hypoglycemia.

ENTEROCUTANEOUS FISTULAS. Enterocutaneous fistulas located distally in the gastrointestinal tract cause little malabsorption. If the fistula is proximal, however, significant loss of ingested food may occur. Low-output (less than 200 ml. per day) fistulas seldom cause significant malnutrition. High-output (especially greater than 800 ml. per day) fistulas cause significant nutrient losses. Biliary and pancreatic fistulas may cause malabsorption of fat, protein, and starch depending on the amount of daily loss.

PANCREATIC INSUFFICIENCY. Subtotal pancreatectomy is well tolerated if the remaining gland is normal. Resection of a major portion or all of the pancreas or ligation or obstruction of its duct can, however, cause both diabetes and malabsorption. Although insulin requirements are not as high as might be expected, control of the diabetes may be difficult. Intestinal function is normal with no evidence for bacterial overgrowth or rapid transit. Lack of lipase and protease is responsible for all the malabsorption.

BILIARY TRACT DISEASE. Reduction or absence of bile salts in the duodenum, due to biliary obstruction or biliary-cutaneous fistulas, causes steatorrhea. Loss of vitamin D and calcium can cause bone changes of both osteoporosis and osteomalacia. Loss of vitamin K can cause prolonged prothrombin times and bleeding.

SMALL BOWEL RESECTION. Malabsorption increases as more small bowel is removed. With greater than 50 per cent reduction, malabsorption is a significant clinical problem. (1) Malabsorption is due to loss of the ileocecal valve with rapid transit. (2) Resection of the absorption site for vitamin B_{12} and bile salts causes vitamin B_{12} and bile salt diarrhea. Bile salt depletion causes steatorrhea, incrased stool calcium, and increased absorption of soluble oxalate salts. Oxaluria may cause renal stone formation. (3) Resection of the proximal small bowel removes sites of calcium and iron absorption. (4) Intestinal resection causes gastric hypersecretion and hyperacidity in direct proportion to the amount of small bowel removed. The high solute load may exceed the absorptive capacity of the remaining small bowel. Acid injury to the mucosa may impair absorption, increase secretions, and inactivate lipase and trypsin. (5) Finally, reduction in lactase may increase intolerance to lactose.

BLIND LOOP SYNDROME. "Blind loop syndrome" can occur whenever there is stasis of the intestinal contents. It is most commonly seen when a blind loop is created, as with a Billroth II or intestinal bypass. The syndrome is characterized by diarrhea, steatorrhea, anemia, loss of weight, abdominal pain, and multiple vitamin deficiencies. The diagnosis can be confirmed by a Schilling test, which should demonstrate reduced absorption. When the test is repeated with the addition of intrinsic factor, however, there is no increase in uptake as would occur in true pernicious anemia.

Vitamin B_{12} deficiency occurs either from utilization of vitamin B_{12} by bacteria in the stagnant intestine or from bacterial production of a toxin-inhibiting enzymatic transfer of vitamin B_{12} across the small bowel mucosa. Steatorrhea also occurs, probably because of structural alterations of bile salts brought about by bacteria.

MISCELLANEOUS SMALL BOWEL LESIONS OF SURGICAL INTEREST. Radiation enteritis may cause malabsorption as a result of injury to the bowel mucosa or lymphatics, or stasis due to partial obstruction. Resection of involved segments may be required. Occlusion of the superior mesenteric artery and either the celiac or inferior mesenteric artery with intestinal angina commonly causes altered intestinal motility and malabsorption with slow but progressive malnutrition. If done before permanent scarring, percutaneous dilation of the involved vessels or surgical revascularization can be curative. Intestinal lymphangiectasis and intestinal lymphatic obstruction due to tumor or infection are rare causes of malabsorption.

IX

Radiation Injury to the Intestine
Jerome J. DeCosse, M.D., Ph.D.

The goal of radiation therapy is local control of tumor with minimal damage to normal tissue. The danger of such damage to the intestine is a major constraint on radiation therapy of the abdomen and pelvis.

Intensive radiation therapy administered to the pelvis for carcinoma of the cervix, endometrium, ovary, bladder, or prostate places the patient at risk for acute radiation-induced or factitial proctitis or for injury to the small intestine. Usually, such injuries are transient, self-limited, and localized. Patients with mucosal lesions and steatorrhea may have few or no gastrointestinal symptoms. Patients with proctitis usually present with diarrhea, tenesmus, and rectal bleeding. Nausea is common, and crampy abdominal pain may be present. Usually, these symptoms subside shortly after completion of radiation therapy, and patients require only supportive therapy with antidiarrheal, anticholinergic, and antispasmodic medication. An elemental diet, cholestyramine, and glutamine may be beneficial.

Some patients with acute injury progress to chronic injury with a continuous display of intestinal symptoms; others experience a long symptom-free period before their chronic radiation injury becomes evident. Subclinical injury may become overt when low-flow states, such as congestive heart failure or vascular narrowing from hypertension and arteriosclerosis, further diminish tissue perfusion already limited by radiation-induced vasculitis until, finally, cellular oxygenation and nutrition are reduced below critical levels.

Prior operation or intra-abdominal infection may increase

See the corresponding chapter or part in the *Textbook of Surgery*, 14th edition, pp. 880–884, for a more detailed discussion of this topic, including a comprehensive list of references.

the risk of injury by causing loops of small or large intestine to be fixed in the radiation field. Surgeons may reduce such risks by outlining the intended portal with radiopaque markers; by reperitonealization; by excluding small bowel from the pelvis through, for example, omental transposition; and by scrupulously cleansing the peritoneal cavity before closure.

Chemotherapeutic drugs, even if administered at another time, also may increase the risk of intestinal injury to irradiated patients.

DIAGNOSIS AND TREATMENT. Chronic radiation injury of the intestine is frequently associated with injury to cutaneous, bony, and other visceral structures encompassed by the radiation portals. Patients should be examined for cystitis, urethral injury, and radiation nephritis.

Radiation injury of the small or large intestine may cause malabsorption, acute or chronic obstruction, ulceration, perforation, abscess formation, or fistulization. Other than biopsy, there are no specific tests for distinguishing radiation damage from recurrent tumor. However, computed axial tomography and magnetic resonance imaging may provide useful information. A patient who appears well and maintains body weight but continues to have crampy abdominal pain often has a radiation injury. Malabsorption with steatorrhea and hypocalcemia also suggests radiation injury to the small intestine.

Patients with limited nausea, no vomiting, only slight crampy pain, and modest distention may have a partial obstruction. A small intestinal barium examination is necessary but not always sufficient for confirmation. Constricted, narrow loops of intestine or puddling of barium is indicative of partial obstruction. Vascular compromise heralds an emergency. Symptoms include continuous abdominal pain between cramps, involuntary guarding, localized and persistent tenderness to percussion or palpation, reduced or absent peristaltic sounds, a rectal temperature above 38° C., and a white blood count in excess of 12,000 cells per cu. mm. Back pain suggests mesenteric torsion.

Both vascular compromise and complete obstruction require exploration: in the former case, exploration is urgent; in the latter, it should be preceded by nasogastric intubation and drainage as well as volume repletion. Wide resection of the diseased bowel is preferable, but occasionally a bypass is necessary. Normal, unirradiated intestine should be used for the enteroenterostomy.

Partial obstruction from radiation-induced stenosis of the small intestine may not require surgical therapy and should be managed initially by conservative intestinal decompression and fluid replacement. Oral steroids, sulfasalazine, and a low-residue diet may control symptoms adequately.

Obstruction and vascular occlusion can cause hypoxia, necrosis, and perforation of the intestine. Perforation can cause a diffuse peritonitis; a localized abscess; or fistulization into the bladder, ureter, vagina, intestine, or an operative wound agglutinated to the injured intestine. Operative management requires exteriorization of the perforated bowel, drainage, and proximal defunctionalization. It is important to determine the injury site by endoscopy, oral and rectal contrast studies, computed tomographic scan, and fistulograms (by instillation of iodinated water-soluble dyes) and to exclude recurrent cancer.

Intestinal fistulas generally require excision. However, most patients with fistulas are severely ill; a preliminary program of gastrointestinal decompression, resolution of pelvic sepsis, and nutritional repletion by total parenteral nutrition reduces operative risk and promotes healing.

Patients who have persistent proctitis with severe pelvic pain, pain on defecation, and rectal bleeding also require endoscopic assessment and barium enema examination. Generally, radiation-induced proctitis can be managed successfully with a low-residue diet, stool softeners, sedation, antispasmodics, and general supportive measures. Oral steroids, sulfasalazine, and steroid enemas are beneficial in more severe injuries. Some patients with severe rectal bleeding or intractable pain may require a proximal defunctionalizing colostomy, but this procedure does not always relieve pain. Rectal stenosis usually can be managed by conservative measures including instrumental or digital dilations but sometimes requires a sigmoid or descending colon colostomy for defunctionalization of the rectum.

Proctitis may progress to ulceration and ulceration to rectovaginal fistula. Rectovaginal fistulas are associated with recurrent carcinoma and therefore must be biopsied. Rectovaginal fistulas from radiation injury usually require defunctionalization of the rectum by colostomy. In recent years, some patients have had gut continuity restored successfully by coloanal "sleeve" anastomosis or by interposition of a rotated flap of sigmoid colon.

X

Appendicitis
Gordon L. Telford, M.D.,
and Robert E. Condon, M.D., M.S.

Acute appendicitis must be considered in any patient with abdominal pain or symptoms of peritoneal irritation. It is rare in infants, reaches maximal incidence in the teens and twenties, and thereafter declines. The mortality of acute but not gangrenous appendicitis is less than 0.1 per cent; mortality rises in gangrenous appendicitis to about 0.6 per cent and

See the corresponding chapter or part in the *Textbook of Surgery*, 14th edition, pp. 884–898, for a more detailed discussion of this topic, including a comprehensive list of references.

with perforated appendicitis is approximately 5 per cent. Although the mortality has declined progressively, morbidity continues to be high and involves 10 per cent of patients with appendicitis. The presence of gangrene or perforation increases the morbidity risk four- or fivefold, with wound infection occurring in 15 to 20 per cent of patients. Delay in diagnosis and treatment causes mortality and serious morbidity; exploration for discovering the cause of minimal but unexplained symptoms, even in poor-risk patients, is safer than waiting.

CLINICAL MANIFESTATIONS

The sequence of symptoms in acute appendicitis usually begins with diffuse abdominal pain, most prominently in the epigastrium or around the umbilicus, followed by anorexia; nausea and vomiting, if they are to occur, appear next. If vomiting precedes pain, the diagnosis should be questioned. After a variable time, pain shifts toward the right side and then into the right lower quadrant. Atypical abdominal pain that fails to follow the classic sequence is common, occurring in 45 per cent of patients. A patient with an abnormally located appendix is also likely to have an atypical history, particularly of pain.

The physical signs of appendicitis are local and rebound tenderness and muscle guarding. Moderate fever (up to 38° C.) is found, but higher fever is unusual with uncomplicated appendicitis and the temperature is often normal. Tenderness to palpation corresponds to the position of the appendix and typically is in the right lower quadrant. Muscle guarding, or resistance to palpation, eventually is replaced by reflex involuntary rigidity. On occasion, especially in patients who seek care late, a periappendiceal mass may be palpated in the right lower quadrant due to an abscess or to omentum and coils of bowel adherent about the inflamed appendix. Although seldom diagnostic, rectal examination is essential in every patient suspected of appendicitis. In addition, a pelvic examination in women is necessary for exclusion of lesions such as ovarian cyst or tubal abscess.

Following rupture, physical signs usually become much more definite. Tenderness encompasses the whole right lower quadrant. Rebound tenderness and muscular rigidity are more marked. The temperature and pulse may rise. If the rupture fails to localize, signs of spreading peritonitis ensue.

LABORATORY EXAMINATIONS. Far too much stress has been placed on the alleged value of laboratory values in the diagnosis of acute appendicitis. Up to one third of patients, particularly older adults, have a normal leukocyte count. Most patients have a left shift in the differential even when the total count is normal. Whenever the clinical findings are at variance with the white cell count, clinical findings should take precedence.

RADIOLOGIC EXAMINATION. The presence of an appendiceal fecalith is the only pathognomonic radiographic sign of early acute appendicitis. When plain films demonstrate other signs suggestive of appendicitis, such as a mass extrinsic to the cecum, the appendix generally is gangrenous and often perforated.

Barium enema examination is safe in patients with appendicitis. This procedure is unnecessary in most cases but can be of diagnostic aid in two clinical situations in which avoidance of a negative laparotomy is desirable: patients with a pre-existing debilitating systemic disease, such as leukemia, which increases operative risk; and young women in whom the diagnosis continues to be obscure after 6 to 12 hours of observation.

DISTINCTIVE CLINICAL SETTINGS OF APPENDICITIS

APPENDICITIS IN INFANTS AND YOUNG CHILDREN. Because an accurate diagnosis is difficult in this age group, treatment often is delayed and complications develop. Every child with appendicitis has abdominal pain, but the pattern can mimic nonspecific gastroenteritis. Vomiting, fever, irritability, flexing of the thighs, and diarrhea are early complaints with appendicitis. The most consistent physical finding is abdominal distention. Because of the high incidence of perforation, the mortality of acute appendicitis in this age group remains at about 5 per cent.

APPENDICITIS IN YOUNG WOMEN. The diagnosis of acute appendicitis in women 20 to 30 years of age has a higher rate of error than at other ages. Pain or discomfort associated with ovulation (mittelschmerz), diseases involving the ovary, tube, or uterus, and infections or other disorders of the urinary system represent some, but not all, of the misdiagnoses. Observation is in order if pain is atypical, there is no muscular spasm in the right lower quadrant, and fever and leukocytosis are absent. If symptoms and signs do not progress over several hours, a barium enema examination that visualizes the appendix may help exclude appendicitis.

APPENDICITIS DURING PREGNANCY. The incidence of appendicitis during pregnancy parallels that in nonpregnant women of the same age. Appendectomy should be performed upon suspicion of the diagnosis, just as if the pregnancy were not present. During the third trimester, the clinical situation is slightly altered; displacement and lateral rotation of the cecum and appendix by the enlarged uterus causes localization of pain higher in the abdomen or in the right flank. Premature labor occurs in about half of women who develop appendicitis during the third trimester; the prognosis for the infant in cases of uncomplicated appendicitis is directly related to the infant's birth weight.

APPENDICITIS IN THE ELDERLY. Acute appendicitis among older patients has a higher mortality owing both to delay by the patient in seeking medical care and to delay by physicians in removing the appendix. The classic symptoms of pain, anorexia, and nausea are present but are less pronounced. Physical examination differs mainly by the paucity of findings in the presence of severe disease, although tenderness in the right lower quadrant is elicited eventually in most patients. Distention of the abdomen is prominent, even in the absence of perforation. Symptoms and signs mimicking mechanical small bowel obstruction are not uncommon. More than 30 per cent of elderly patients have a ruptured appendix at the time of operation. Delay in operation is responsible for the high incidence of perforation.

DIFFERENTIAL DIAGNOSIS

In young children, the diseases most frequently mistaken for appendicitis are acute gastroenteritis, mesenteric lymphadenitis, pyelitis, Meckel's diverticulitis, intussusception, enteric duplication, Henoch-Schönlein purpura, and primary peritonitis. In this age group, basilar pneumonia (even on the left side) may mimic appendicitis.

In teenagers and young adults, the differential diagnosis is directed by the patient's sex. In young women, obstipation, diseases of the ovary and tube, ruptured ectopic pregnancy, mittelschmerz, endometriosis, and salpingitis (pelvic inflammatory disease) must be differentiated. In a young man, the list of alternative diagnoses is smaller: acute regional enteritis, right renal or ureteral calculus, torsion of a testis, and acute epididymitis.

In older adults, diseases to be considered are diverticulitis, perforated duodenal or gastric ulcer, acute cholecystitis, pancreatitis, intestinal obstruction, perforating cecal carcinoma, torsion of an ovarian cyst, perforated ileal diverticulum, mesenteric vascular occlusion, rupturing aortic aneurysm, and idiopathic infarction of an epiploic appendage or the omentum.

TREATMENT

PREOPERATIVE PREPARATION. Aggressive fluid resuscitation is initiated to establish a good urinary output. This rarely requires more than 2 hours. Patients with a palpable periappendiceal mass may, in selected cases, be managed initially without operation. Nasogastric suction is helpful. Hyperpyrexia is treated with salicylates in addition to hydration and antibiotics. Preoperative antibiotics are administered to all patients; administration is continued postoperatively only in patients with complicated appendicitis. The authors' current choice of antibiotic is a second-generation cephalosporin such as cefoxitin or cefotetan.

EXAMINATION UNDER ANESTHESIA. After the patient has been anesthetized, the abdomen should be carefully and systematically palpated for other possible causes of the illness and for an appendiceal mass.

MANAGEMENT OF THE PATIENT WITHOUT A PALPABLE MASS (PRESUMED UNCOMPLICATED APPENDICITIS). A transverse incision is made on the right side, 1 to 3 cm. below the umbilicus and centered on the midclavicular-midinguinal line. The aponeurosis and muscles of the abdominal wall are split in the direction of the skin wound. The appendix is identified by following the anterior cecal taenia and is coaxed into the wound. If the appendix is retrocecal or retroperitoneal, or if local inflammation and edema are intense, exposure is improved by dividing the lateral peritoneal reflection of the cecum.

The mesoappendix is transected between clamps beginning at its free border. After transection of the mesoappendix, a suture should be passed through the mesoappendix and into the wall of the cecum close to the base of the appendix in order to secure the intramural accessory branch of the posterior cecal artery. If exposure of a long appendix is difficult, the mesoappendix can be transected in a retrograde manner beginning at the cecum.

In most cases, inversion of the unligated stump by use of a Z stitch, rather than the more conventional pursestring suture, is preferred. If the appendix is edematous, turgid, or otherwise unsuitable for inversion, it should be doubly ligated at its base, the distal ligature being placed as a suture ligature.

ERRONEOUS DIAGNOSIS (APPENDIX NORMAL). If exploration reveals a normal appendix, orderly investigation for the cause of the symptoms must be accomplished. Obtain a specimen of peritoneal fluid or exudate for Gram's stain and culture for aerobes and anaerobes. The cecum is inspected for evidence of a perforated diverticulum. The small intestine is examined for regional enteritis or a Meckel's diverticulum. The pelvic organs are palpated and inspected. The intra-abdominal colon, the gallbladder, the duodenum, and the stomach should be palpated. If enlarged lymph nodes are present in the mesentery, a node should be excised and sent for culture. Exploration should not cease until the cause of the acute abdominal symptoms has been identified or the surgeon is certain that no remediable lesion is present within the abdominal cavity.

WOUND CLOSURE. Closure of the peritoneum is not necessary. Each fascial layer is closed separately with nonabsorbable sutures. If there has been contamination of the subcutaneous tissue, that portion of the wound is loosely packed open and the skin reapproximated about the fifth postoperative day.

HOSPITAL DISCHARGE. The patient with uncomplicated appendicitis may be discharged as early as the third postoperative day provided there is no undue wound tenderness or fever and antibiotics have not been administered for 48 hours before discharge.

MANAGEMENT OF THE PATIENT WITH A MOBILE PERIAPPENDICEAL MASS (PRESUMED GANGRENOUS OR LOCALLY PERFORATED APPENDICITIS) DETECTED AFTER INDUCTION OF ANESTHESIA. A transverse incision should be made over the most prominent portion of the mass and the muscles and aponeuroses split. Fluid and pus, if present, are aspirated after a specimen has been obtained for culture and sensitivity tests. The tissues are dissected sufficiently for exposure of the appendix, which should be removed unless the base of the cecum is very inflamed. If a periappendiceal abscess is present or the tissues are so turgid as to create a dead space, the cavity should be drained with a soft suction drain brought out through a separate stab incision.

Systemic antibiotics should be continued for 4 to 5 days after operation. A rectal examination is conducted daily for detecting development of pelvic abscess. Discharge from the hospital is delayed until the patient has been afebrile for 2 days, has not had antibiotics for 72 hours, and has no evidence of wound infection or intraperitoneal or pelvic abscess.

MANAGEMENT OF THE PATIENT WITH A FIXED PERIAPPENDICEAL MASS ON INITIAL PHYSICAL EXAMINATION. If a patient is first seen when symptoms are subsiding and a well-localized periappendiceal mass is found on physical examination, it is reasonable in most adults to initiate systemic antibiotics and to continue expectant treatment. In two of three adults in whom expectant treatment of the appendiceal mass is indicated, symptoms continue to subside and a subsequent interval appendectomy can be accomplished. Children, pregnant women, and most elderly patients should not be managed by expectant treatment of an appendiceal mass.

If an operation is deemed appropriate, the incision for drainage is made just medial to the crest of the ileum at the level of the most prominent portion of the periappendiceal mass. The muscles are split and the peritoneum exposed and pushed medially so that the mass surrounding the appendix is approached from its lateral retroperitoneal aspect. A finger should be slowly introduced into the abscess and its loculations broken down by blunt dissection. In infants, appendectomy should be accomplished in addition to drainage of the abscess. In adults, if the appendix is not removed, interval appendectomy should be done 6 to 8 weeks after drainage from the abscess has ceased and the wound has healed.

A sump drainage tube is inserted into the abscess cavity and extracted through a stab wound in the flank. The wound is irrigated with dilute antibiotic solution, the muscular layers are closed, and the subcutaneous tissues are packed open. The sump tube should be left undisturbed until it is draining less than 50 ml. each day. Systemic antibiotics should be continued for at least 5 days postoperatively. A daily rectal examination is made to detect a developing pelvic abscess. Criteria for discharge are the same as those noted for patients with a mobile periappendiceal mass.

RECURRENT, SUBACUTE, AND CHRONIC APPENDICITIS. In patients in whom an initial attack of acute appendicitis subsides spontaneously, the risk of a recurrent episode is high. Elective appendectomy within 6 to 8 weeks should therefore be advised. If abdominal films demonstrate the presence of a fecalith, if a barium enema shows nonfilling of the obstructed appendix, or if observation of repeated attacks provides evidence that the patient is suffering from recurrent subacute appendicitis, elective appendectomy should be undertaken.

COMPLICATIONS OF APPENDECTOMY

Postoperative complications occur in only 5 per cent of patients if an unperforated appendix is removed intact but in more than 30 per cent of patients with gangrenous or perforated appendicitis. The incidence of perforation is less than 20 per cent in the first 24 hours of symptoms but rapidly increases to over 70 per cent after 48 hours. The more frequent complications of appendectomy include wound infection; pelvic, subphrenic, and intraperitoneal abscesses; fecal fistula; pylephlebitis; and intestinal obstruction. Wound infections in cases of appendicitis are caused by fecal organisms. The early signs of a fecal wound infection are undue pain and modest edema around the wound. If such signs are present, the skin and subcutaneous tissues should be opened. Pelvic, subphrenic, or intra-abdominal abscesses occur in up to 20 per cent of patients with gangrenous or perforated appendicitis. An abscess causes recurrent fever, malaise, and anorexia, usually beginning about a week after appendectomy. Abscesses must be drained, percutaneously or surgically. Fecal fistula usually is not a dangerous complication of appendectomy because most close spontaneously. Pylephlebitis, or portal pyemia, a serious illness characterized by jaundice, chills, and high fever, is due to septicemia of the portal venous system, causing development of multiple liver abscesses. Pylephlebitis is associated with gangrenous or perforated appendicitis and may appear either preoperatively or postoperatively.

32

THE COLON AND RECTUM

I

Surgical Anatomy and Operative Procedures

Joel J. Roslyn, M.D., and Michael J. Zinner, M.D.

SURGICAL ANATOMY

Although the colon is generally considered to be an intra-peritoneal organ, the ascending and descending segments are frequently fixed by retroperitoneal attachments, which render a portion of the circumference of the lumen to a retroperitoneal location. In addition to anatomic variations secondary to developmental anomalies that frequently affect the ascending or sigmoid colon, the transverse colon is usually supported by a mesentery and is found in a horizontal position or in a more dependent position traversing freely into the lower abdomen.

Blood Supply of the Colon

The cecum, ascending colon, hepatic flexure, and proximal portion of the transverse colon derive their arterial blood supply from the ileocolic, right colic, and middle colic branches of the superior mesenteric artery. The inferior mesenteric artery supplies blood to the distal transverse colon, splenic flexure, descending colon, and sigmoid via the left colic artery and branches of the sigmoid and superior hemorrhoidal vessels. The rectum is supplied by a rich network of vessels from the middle hemorrhoidal and inferior hemorrhoidal arteries. As the main vessels course through the mesentery toward the bowel wall itself, they frequently bifurcate, and arcades are formed 1 to 2 cm. from the mesenteric border of the bowel. In this manner, a continuous chain of communicating vessels is formed, and this has been referred to as the marginal artery of Drummond. The anastomosis or linking of arcades between the superior and inferior mesenteric vessels has been referred to as the long anastomosis of Riolan.

OPERATIVE PROCEDURES

When a colon resection is being planned, certain specific factors should be carefully considered by the surgeon. It is

---

See the corresponding chapter or part in the *Textbook of Surgery*, 14th edition, pp. 899–903, for a more detailed discussion of this topic, including a comprehensive list of references.

essential to ensure adequate vascularity to all colonic anastomoses. Ideally, the surgeon should be able to palpate pulsating vessels in the colonic mesentery, and at the very least, active bleeding from the cut edges of the colon should be documented. Adequate mobilization of the colon should be accomplished for minimizing tension on an anastomosis. The bacterial flora of the colon is significantly different both qualitatively and quantitatively from that of the small bowel, and efforts should be exercised to achieve adequate bowel preparation before colonic anastomoses.

The basic principles of surgical oncology apply to tumors involving the colon. Ideally, curative operations on the colon should be performed whenever possible. An attempt should be made to remove all of the malignant tissue from both the primary organ and any other structures that are locally involved. In addition, early control of the venous drainage from the primary tumor is recommended for decreasing the likelihood of tumor embolization during manipulation. Similarly, the surgeon should attempt to remove the lymphatic channels and tissue through which the primary tumor is likely to spread. In the context of tumors involving the large intestine, adherence to these principles would require ligation of the appropriate vessels at their origin. The exact distance of proximal and distal bowel that should be removed with a tumor has been the subject of considerable debate in recent years. Nonetheless, certain standard principles remain. These include (1) obtaining tumor-free margins and (2) removal of all lymphatic drainage. The goals and concepts that govern treatment of benign lesions of the colon are different from those for neoplastic disease. As such, the nature of the recommended operations also differs. In general, with benign conditions of the colon, it is not necessary to remove the mesentery, and one can stay closer to the bowel wall.

Colostomy

The term *colostomy* refers to the creation of a stoma, which in effect is an opening of the bowel onto the surface of the abdomen. Colostomies, whether temporary or permanent, are performed for a number of indications in patients with colonic and gastrointestinal disorders.

General indications for colostomy include (1) to function as the site of elimination of feces when the distal colon or rectum has been removed, (2) to divert the fecal stream to protect a distal anastomosis, (3) to decompress a more distal colonic obstruction and to serve as a "vent," and (4) to divert the fecal stream from a more distal pathologic process that will be definitively managed at a later date. Depending on the specific indication and individual setting, the surgeon may choose to construct either a temporary colostomy or a permanent stoma. The ideal temporary colostomy should provide adequate fecal diversion as necessary, be safe to construct, and be easy to reconstruct when gastrointestinal continuity is restored. A loop or double-barreled colostomy is typically performed when diversion is temporary. This is generally achieved by exteriorizing a segment of the colon and then making an opening in the loop of bowel through the taeniae. This procedure is relatively straightforward and can be performed expeditiously without significant manipulation or dissection.

When distal resection of the colon is indicated, but primary anastomosis is ill-advised because of associated inflammation and/or intra-abdominal sepsis, a simpler procedure is often performed. The Hartmann procedure involves sigmoid resection with oversewing or closure of the distal rectal pouch and creation of an end descending colostomy. This type of stoma, although generally temporary, should be constructed with use of the same principles and techniques for a more permanent stoma. A permanent colostomy is generally created following abdominoperineal resection in patients with rectal tumors. The ideal stoma should be situated in the left iliac fossa and pierce the abdominal wall through the rectus muscles. Positioning of the stoma in this location reduces the likelihood of peristomal herniation. Internal hernias around the colostomy can be avoided by securing the mesentery to the left paracolic gutter and closing this defect with a series of interrupted sutures.

Colostomy takedown with restoration of gastrointestinal continuity is not an innocuous procedure and has been associated with significant morbidity. Before colostomy closure, the patient should undergo radiographic or endoscopic evaluation and bowel preparation as is the custom of the individual surgeon. These procedures should be approached and managed with the same concern and principles that govern primary colon resections.

II

Physiology

Joel J. Roslyn, M.D., and Michael J. Zinner, M.D.

The four primary functions of the human colon are to (1) absorb sodium and water and thereby concentrate fecal contents, (2) secrete potassium and bicarbonate, (3) serve as a storage reservoir for fecal contents, and (4) facilitate elimination of intestinal waste. The mechanism governing this last function and maintenance of continence is quite elaborate and is focused in the rectum.

See the corresponding chapter or part in the *Textbook of Surgery*, 14th edition, pp. 903–904, for a more detailed discussion of this topic, including a comprehensive list of references.

ABSORPTION

Whereas the small intestine is largely responsible for the absorption of essentially all nutrients that enter the gastrointestinal tract, the large intestine or colon is incapable of absorbing carbohydrates, protein, and so on. Nonetheless, the colon is responsible for absorption of large amounts of water from the feces, thus in essence drying the fecal mass. Although the entire length of the colon (approximately 135 cm.) has the capacity to absorb water and specific electrolytes, the majority of this absorptive activity actually goes on in the ascending colon. The total absorptive area of the large bowel has been estimated to be approximately 900 sq. cm. The capacity of the colon to absorb water and electrolytes is reflected by the 10-fold reduction in water volume that occurs on a regular basis. Numerous studies have suggested that approximately 1000 to 1500 ml. of water are delivered from the ileum into the cecum during any 24-hour period. This effluent has a sodium concentration of approximately 200 mEq. per liter. Nonetheless, the total volume of stool water is estimated to be only 100 to 150 ml. per day with a sodium concentration of 25 to 50 mEq. per liter. Therefore, despite the significant concentration effect and absorption of water, which is ongoing, the sodium concentration is paradoxically quite low in the stool effluent. Numerous *in vivo* and *in vitro* electrophysiologic studies have demonstrated that the mechanism by which this occurs is an active transport process directed against a combined transepithelial chemical concentration and electropotential difference. Many factors have been identified that influence water and electrolyte movement by the colon. These include mucosal cyclic adenosine monophosphate level, pH, osmolarity, and ions such as fatty bile acids. More recent information would suggest that water and electrolyte movement is also controlled to some extent by the hormonal milieu. The net effect of the active sodium transport is that this process influences the return of water from the lumen, and therefore absorption of water is a passive process.

In addition to being the site of sodium and water absorption, the colon also has an important role in the enterohepatic circulation of bile acids insofar as these solutes are absorbed from the colon by nonionic or passive fusion. This activity assumes even greater significance in patients in whom the terminal ileum is either diseased or surgically absent. In addition, the colon is the site of bile acid dehydroxylation, the process by which primary bile acids are converted to secondary bile acids. Bile acids affect colon transport of water and electrolytes.

SECRETION

Studies in both animals and humans suggest that potassium is actively secreted by colonic epithelium. This activity is stimulated by exogenous or endogenous mineralocorticoids. There is also evidence that bicarbonate is secreted by the human colon as an active process that is directed against both a chemical concentration difference and an electrical potential difference. Alterations in net fluid and electrolyte movement in the colon have been documented following administration of a number of laxatives as well as in disease states, such as ulcerative colitis, granulomatous colitis, congenital chloridorrhea, and watery diarrhea syndrome.

During the past 15 years, considerable attention and investigative efforts have focused on the hormonal regulation of ion transport in the small and large intestine during both health and disease. Although there is considerable evidence that several peptides and bioactive amines modulate small intestinal ion transport, several studies suggest that cyclic adenosine monophosphate, prostaglandins, and gut peptides, including vasoactive intestinal polypeptide, influence colonic ion transport. The true physiologic role of these substances on colonic absorptive and secretory function remains to be defined.

COLONIC MOTILITY

The storage and excretory functions of the colon are closely correlated and are dependent on a series of neurally mediated reflexes and smooth muscle contractions that are probably regulated to some extent by the autonomic nervous system. Current thinking suggests that ingestion of food stimulates the production of mass movements that are strong, propulsive contractions moving in a caudal direction, which serves to move fecal material down into the descending and distal segments of the colon. These propulsive contractions may be altered in patients with irritable bowel syndrome and may actually be modified by laxatives or antidiarrheal drugs. The importance of understanding colonic motor activity is underscored by the recent description of "dysmotility" syndromes, which can mimic mechanical bowel obstruction.

III

Diagnostic Studies

Joel J. Roslyn, M.D., and Michael J. Zinner, M.D.

The astute physician recognizes the colon as the site of a pathologic process based on the patient's complaints and history. Given the critical nature that the colon has in storage and evacuation of feces, diseases of the colon, whether inflammatory or neoplastic, frequently cause some alteration

---

See the corresponding chapter or part in the *Textbook of Surgery*, 14th edition, pp. 905–906, for a more detailed discussion of this topic, including a comprehensive list of references.

of gastrointestinal function. This is generally reflected by change in the caliber of the stool, diarrhea (as opposed to steatorrhea), constipation or obstipation, hematochezia, melena, or rectal tenesmus or urgency. All patients in whom a diagnosis of colonic disease is being considered should undergo a thorough and complete physical examination including a pelvic (in women) and rectal examination. Considerable information can often be gleaned from visualization and palpation, with specific attention being paid to consideration of systemic disease processes that may affect the colon and the presence of stigmata of portal hypertension, malnutrition, or the palpation of masses that may be either inflammatory of neoplastic in origin. Examination of the stool for blood either directly or by guaiac testing is an essential part of all physical examinations, especially in the setting in which carcinoma of the colon is being considered. The efficacy of mass screening, however, remains to be defined.

Other diagnostic studies should be considered based on the individual clinical setting. Baseline biochemical tests assessing the patient's nutritional status can provide important information about the patient's current situation and may help the clinician plan the timing of definitive therapy. Liver function tests are particularly helpful in the clinical evaluation of patients in whom some systemic process is suspected or in whom liver metastases may be a consideration. The utility of carcinoembryonic antigen continues to be a source of considerable controversy.

The recognition of motor disturbances involving the anorectal mechanism has been facilitated by the development of several new diagnostic modalities that attempt to quantify motor activity in this region. The ultimate clinical role of these tests remains to be defined.

RADIOGRAPHIC EVALUATION

Plain abdominal radiographs and contrast studies of the large intestine continue to be invaluable diagnostic methods in the evaluation of patients with suspected colonic diseases. These tests are rapid, easy to perform, noninvasive, and associated with essentially zero morbidity. They are frequently quite helpful in directing the endoscopist and/or surgeon to the site of pathologic change and in general provide important information. Contrast studies of the colon and colonoscopy should be viewed as complementary procedures. Although barium enema can fail to reveal small polyps and/or carcinomas, this study continues to be an important screening test in patients with colon disease. It is essential when a barium enema is ordered that the clinician communicate to the radiologist what the presumptive diagnosis is and in addition provide as much clinical information as possible. This dialogue facilitates the interpretation of the radiograph by the radiologist and enhances the ability to make an accurate diagnosis. The communication between clinician and radiologist is particularly important when the concern is colonic obstruction and/or perforation. In these settings, consideration should be given to the use of a water-soluble agent such as Gastrografin.

ENDOSCOPY

With an ever-expanding technology, the ability to inspect the colon visually from the rectum to the cecum is such that this can now be performed safely in outpatient endoscopic units on a routine basis. With improving optics in a higher quality instrument, diagnostic and therapeutic colonoscopies have become routine and have in effect revolutionized diagnostic capabilities in the management of patients with colonic disorders. Whereas full colonoscopy should be performed only by trained surgical and gastrointestinal endoscopists, the recent introduction of a 60-cm. "flexible sigmoidoscope" has allowed the nonspecialist to participate in the diagnostic evaluation of patients. Nonetheless, a certain amount of expertise is required for manipulation of the flexible sigmoidoscope, and all individuals practicing this technique should have basic training. Currently, endoscopic evaluation of the colon remains the cornerstone for the accurate diagnosis of colonic disease, especially carcinoma.

Colonoscopy is the most accurate method of assessing colonic disease. A skilled endoscopist can maneuver the scope so as to visualize the entire colon from the anus to the cecum. There are seven general indications for flexible sigmoidoscopy or for colonoscopy: (1) diagnosis, (2) biopsy to confirm or establish the nature of a disease process or malignant lesion, (3) therapeutic removal of polyps, (4) management of bleeding lesions, (5) surveillance and follow-up of lesions that have previously been removed endoscopically or surgically, (6) detection and removal of foreign bodies, and (7) as part of an early cancer detection or other screening process. Whereas vast experience throughout the world has suggested that colonoscopy is a safe procedure that can be performed with minimal morbidity and essentially no mortality, a number of potential contraindications should be considered. These include (1) suspected colonic perforation, (2) acute fulminating inflammatory bowel disease, (3) peritonitis with secondary paralytic ileus, and (4) acute inflammatory disease of the anus. Unlike rigid or flexible sigmoidoscopy, satisfactory performance of colonoscopy generally requires varying degrees of intravenous sedation. Therefore, the general medical condition of the patient and specifically the cardiopulmonary status should be carefully considered before it is elected to proceed with a colonoscopic procedure.

The efficacy and safety of diagnostic and/or therapeutic colonoscopy is dependent on the presence of a well-cleansed bowel. Satisfactory bowel preparation can be achieved by use of a number of techniques including a mechanical preparation with enemas or simple irrigation of the gastrointestinal tract with either saline, with or without mannitol, or commercially available physiologic preparations. The commercially available preparations, including Golytely, are easy and safe and can be completed in a matter of hours. In the authors' experience, these preparations have largely replaced the more traditional regimens that required the patient's being maintained on clear liquids for 24 to 48 hours before the procedure as well as the administration of citrate of magnesia, castor oil, and tap water enemas.

IV

Intestinal Antisepsis
Joel J. Roslyn, M.D., and Michael J. Zinner, M.D.

MICROBIOLOGY OF THE COLON

The human colon contains more than 400 bacterial species. Unlike the stomach and proximal small bowel, both of which have a bacterial count generally considered to be no greater than 10^5 organisms, the colon has a bacterial concentration that approaches 10^{12} CFU ml. The organisms found in the colon vary widely depending on the clinical situation but in general include large numbers of both aerobic and anaerobic bacteria. Nearly one third of the fecal dry weight consists of bacteria. The predominant bacteria are anaerobic and include *Bacteroides*, *Bifidobacterium*, and *Eubacterium*. Perhaps the most important clinical manifestation of colonic microflora has to do with the risk of infection following colonic surgery. Analysis of the available literature suggests that the rate of wound infection in patients undergoing colonic surgery who have not received prophylactic antibiotics may be as high as 75 per cent. This concept has been largely responsible for the development of differing approaches for intestinal antisepsis.

MECHANICAL PREPARATION

As previously stated, much of the dry weight of feces is in fact bacteria. For reducing the bulk of feces and bacteria within the colon, mechanical cleansing of the colon has long been an integral feature of intestinal antisepsis and colon preparation. Nonetheless, it appears that mechanical cleansing does not in fact produce a significant reduction in the colony count of bacteria within the colon. For many years, mechanical preparation of the bowel consisted of a 3-day period during which the patient was maintained on clear liquids and received a variety of purgatives and laxatives. Although the details of the specific regimens may have varied from institution to institution, they all shared certain potential

---

See the corresponding chapter or part in the *Textbook of Surgery*, 14th edition, pp. 907–909, for a more detailed discussion of this topic, including a comprehensive list of references.

problems. They were time-consuming, frequently requiring several days of hospitalization preoperatively, and were associated with varying degrees of physical exhaustion, patient compliance, and dissatisfaction. During the past 10 years, colonic lavage with a variety of solutions has been introduced as a viable alternative to the 3-day mechanical preparation component of the intestinal antisepsis program. The earliest attempts at colonic lavage with saline were associated with some problems and potential risks specifically in elderly patients because of sodium and water retention. This system was modified to include the use of oral mannitol. During the last several years, a commercially available electrolyte–polyethylene glycol solution has been introduced and widely tested. Clinical trials have examined the efficacy of this solution as compared with more conventional mechanical preparations for colonoscopy and have clearly determined the newer solution to be safe, well-tolerated, and cost-effective. This type of solution is administered orally, and consumption of 4 liters the day before operation generally provides excellent mechanical preparation of the bowel. Use of this solution has become the standard regimen for mechanical bowel preparation for elective colon surgery.

ORAL VERSUS PARENTERAL ANTIBIOTICS FOR COLON SURGERY

The rationale for the use of antibiotics preoperatively for patients undergoing colon surgery is to reduce the number of bacteria within the colon. This concept is well accepted and there is no basis for challenging it. However, controversy continues about the most efficacious way of achieving this goal. The role of oral antibiotics compared with parenteral agents, as well as the selection of specific agents, continues to be debated and studied. In 1973, Nichols and associates demonstrated the benefit of orally administered, nonabsorbable antibiotics in combination with mechanical cleansing compared with mechanical cleansing alone. The findings of this rather limited study were confirmed several years later in a prospective randomized multi-institutional trial. The subsequent study of over 1000 patients undergoing colon surgery suggested that there was no significant benefit from the addition of parenteral antibiotic prophylaxis to an appropriate mechanical preparation with oral nonabsorbed antimicrobial agents. A large number of studies have subsequently tried to identify the ideal agents for either oral antimicrobial therapy or parenteral administration. There are certain characteristics that any ideal prophylactic antibiotic regimen, whether oral or parenterally administered, should include. The regimen selected should provide broad suppression of fecal flora with high activity against aerobic and anaerobic organisms. Toxic effects from this regimen should be minimal, and there should be no emergence of resistant organisms. Additionally, a single agent is preferable to multiple drugs, there should be a short term of administration, and the drugs should be cost-effective. Orally administered neomycin and erythromycin base or metronidazole have become the most common agents used for oral antibiotic preparation. These drugs are generally administered at 1:00 P.M., 2:00 P.M., and 11:00 P.M. the day before operation. It was initially thought that absorption of these drugs was not desirable. This has been somewhat changed over the last several years, and it is now thought that increased tissue levels of the drug at sites distant from the colon aid the normal host resistance mechanisms should contamination of a wound occur.

Appropriate regimens for parenteral antibiotics should include agents that have considerable activity against aerobes and anaerobes. There are a number of studies that have assessed multiple-drug regimens including aminoglycosides and either metronidazole or clindamycin in contrast to single agents. In recent years, the second-generation cephalosporins have gained considerable popularity as useful agents for antimicrobial prophylaxis. More recent studies have compared the third-generation cephalosporins used as a single dose with multiple-dose administration of the second-generation cephalosporins. These types of studies may ultimately help to define the nuances of antibiotic utilization in patients undergoing colon surgery. Undoubtedly, in the future, techniques in management of patients undergoing elective and emergent colon surgery will evolve. New antibiotics will be described, and perhaps understanding of the host factors that dictate the response to clinical infection will be such that whole new techniques will be described for colon and intestinal antisepsis.

V

Diverticular Disease of the Colon
Anthony L. Imbembo, M.D., and Robert W. Bailey, M.D.

Diverticula are saclike protrusions of the colonic wall that vary in size from a few millimeters to several centimeters. *True diverticula* are congenital and contain all layers of the bowel wall present in normal colon. They are quite uncommon. *False or pseudodiverticula* represent acquired herniations of the mucosa and submucosa through the muscular layer of the bowel wall. These constitute the predominant lesion and are the focus of the remainder of this discussion. The *prevalence* is estimated to be less than 5 per cent at age 40, increasing to 30 per cent by age 60, and being as high as

---

See the corresponding chapter or part in the *Textbook of Surgery*, 14th edition, pp. 910–920, for a more detailed discussion of this topic, including a comprehensive list of references.

65 per cent by age 85. Males and females appear to be affected equally. Geographically, diverticular disease is much more common in the United States and Western Europe than in less industrialized regions such as Africa, South America, and Asia. Although dietary factors are thought to contribute significantly to the development of diverticular disease, the complete etiologic basis is likely to involve other as yet unrecognized influences.

Clinical and experimental studies have implicated *low-fiber diets* as a prominent etiologic factor. Diets lacking vegetable fiber are presumed to predispose to the development of diverticula by *altering colonic motility*. There is evidence that patients with diverticular disease manifest exaggerated contractile responses to feeding and hormonal stimuli. These abnormal muscular contractions are believed to cause *increases in intraluminal pressures* with resultant smooth muscle hypertrophy and the formation of diverticula.

Anatomically, diverticula form at *"weak" points* where the nutrient blood vessels (vasa recta) penetrate the circular muscle layer en route to the mucosa. These "perforating" vessels tend to penetrate the colonic wall along the mesenteric border of the two antimesenteric taeniae. It is estimated that *90 to 95 per cent* of patients with diverticulosis have involvement of the sigmoid colon, and *65 per cent* of patients have disease limited to the sigmoid colon alone. Conversely, only 2 to 10 per cent of patients have disease confined to the ascending or transverse colon.

DIVERTICULOSIS

Only 10 to 25 per cent of patients with diverticula develop *symptoms of diverticulitis*. An overall mortality of less than 5 per cent follows an initial attack of diverticulitis. Almost one third of patients experience *recurrence of diverticulitis* within 3 to 5 years. Another 30 to 40 per cent suffer from intermittent abdominal pain, whereas the remainder can be expected to remain symptom-free. The *morbidity* from recurrent attacks (60 per cent) is higher than that associated with an initial episode (20 per cent). Only 30 per cent of patients demonstrate *radiologic evidence of progression* of their disease, in the form of either an increased number of diverticula or involvement of other segments of the colon. *Progression of disease following resection* also is unusual and occurs in less than 10 to 15 per cent of patients.

COMPLICATIONS. *Bleeding* can be expected to develop in *15 per cent of patients with diverticulosis*, and diverticular disease is responsible for 30 to 50 per cent of massive colonic bleeding. Angiodysplasia is the second most common source of massive colonic bleeding. Diverticular hemorrhage arises from the *right colon in 70 to 90 per cent* of patients, and 70 per cent of patients with diverticular hemorrhage cease bleeding *spontaneously*. The risk of rebleeding is only 30 per cent but increases to 50 per cent in patients who have suffered a second episode of hemorrhage. Diverticular hemorrhage is thought to follow injury and subsequent rupture of blood vessels lying adjacent to a diverticulum.

Most individuals with diverticular hemorrhage present with only minor or occult bleeding. One third of patients with diverticular hemorrhage (5 per cent of all patients with diverticulosis) present with *massive, exsanguinating hemorrhage.* Abdominal pain secondary to active diverticulitis is extremely uncommon during a bleeding episode. A 10 to 20 per cent morbidity and mortality is associated with massive diverticular hemorrhage. All patients should undergo *proctoscopy* for excluding the rectum as the bleeding source. Patients who cease bleeding spontaneously should undergo elective evaluation, whereas continued massive bleeding is an indication for emergent surgical therapy. In *actively bleeding patients who maintain relative hemodynamic stability*, attempts at *localization*, by selective mesenteric arteriography, radioisotope scanning, or colonoscopy, should be made. Emergent selective mesenteric arteriography successfully identifies the site of hemorrhage in 40 to 60 per cent of patients. In order for arteriography to be diagnostic, bleeding must be occurring at a *minimal rate of 0.5 ml. per minute.*

Alternatives include *combined upper and lower endoscopy* (with an 86 per cent diagnostic accuracy in localizing the site of bleeding) and *radioisotope scanning*, either labeled red blood cells or sulphur colloid. Although accurate in the detection of active bleeding, radioisotope scans have only a 40 to 50 per cent localization accuracy. Segmental colon resection based solely on the results of a positive bleeding scan should be undertaken with *extreme caution*. Nuclear scanning can be used as a *screening test* for determination of the need for subsequent arteriography. Patients with positive bleeding scans proceed to selective arteriography, whereas those with no evidence of active bleeding are observed for signs of further hemorrhage. The diagnostic accuracy of arteriography can be *substantially improved* (up to 70 to 100 per cent) by limiting its use to patients with *documented ongoing hemorrhage.*

TREATMENT. About 15 per cent of all patients presenting with massive diverticular hemorrhage require *emergency surgical therapy* before further diagnostic information can be obtained. Their mortality approaches 30 to 50 per cent. In patients with an identifiable site of bleeding, *selective intraarterial infusion of vasopressin* controls hemorrhage in over 90 per cent of cases. Vasopressin treatment is associated with a 50 per cent rate of rebleeding. *Complications* include myocardial, mesenteric, and cerebral ischemia, arrhythmias, hypertension, and fluid overload. Embolic, thrombotic, and septic problems due to the indwelling arterial catheter contribute to an *overall complication rate* of 4 to 6 per cent. However, selective arterial infusions may convert an emergent situation to an elective or semielective one, thereby decreasing the operative mortality in this elderly, high-risk patient population. Diverticular hemorrhage is usually *not* amenable to endoscopic therapy.

Indications for emergent surgical intervention include *persistent hemodynamic instability*, a large *transfusion requirement*, and *recurrent hemorrhage*. If the bleeding site has been identified, a *segmental resection* can be performed with control in 90 per cent of patients. Segmental resection should not be

performed when the site of hemorrhage has not been identified, since the rebleed rate is 35 to 50 per cent and the
resultant mortality about 30 per cent. *Subtotal* colectomy is
the preferred treatment when preoperative localization has
been unsuccessful.

DIVERTICULITIS

The term *diverticulitis* refers to *inflammation* of one or more
diverticula and represents, at an anatomic level, *perforation of
a diverticulum* into the pericolic space. Unfortunately, a clear
distinction between diverticulitis and painful colonic spasm
is often difficult. *Simple diverticulitis* can be expected to resolve
in most cases with standard medical therapy. Patients with
complicated diverticulitis develop problems such as colonic
obstruction, abscess formation, free perforation, or fistulization. Such patients generally require surgical intervention.
Diverticulitis ultimately develops in 15 to 20 per cent of
patients with diverticulosis. Inflammation is *limited to the
sigmoid colon* in over 90 per cent of cases. Isolated right-sided
diverticular inflammation occurs in only 5 per cent of patients
with diverticulitis. The inflammatory process is usually
walled-off by pericolic fat and mesentery. Involvement of
other abdominal organs in this walling-off process may cause
intestinal obstruction or fistulization. A contained perforation
causes intra-abdominal abscess formation; generalized peritonitis may occur if a perforation is not well contained.

Clinically, patients with diverticulitis usually manifest signs
and symptoms of ongoing inflammation, such as *progressive
left lower quadrant pain* (70 per cent of patients), *anorexia,
nausea, and vomiting* (20 per cent), diarrhea (30 per cent), low-
grade fever, and urinary tract symptoms (15 per cent). The
pain is usually present for several days before presentation,
unlike other acute surgical conditions such as appendicitis or
perforated peptic ulcer that typically are more rapidly progressive. A *tender abdominal mass* is found in 20 per cent of
cases, and its presence portends a poorer prognosis.

Most patients can be *diagnosed* on the basis of their *clinical
presentation.* However, *confirmation* of the diagnosis by radiographic or endoscopic means is of importance. Routine abdominal films are helpful in *excluding* other acute surgical
problems such as intestinal obstruction or a perforated viscus.
Contrast radiography or colonoscopy may cause free rupture
of a previously well-localized peridiverticular abscess and,
therefore, should be undertaken with *extreme caution* in patients with suspected *acute* diverticulitis. *Computed tomography*
has been shown to be as accurate as barium enema in
diagnosing diverticulitis and therefore has substantially reduced the use of contrast studies. Computed tomography
demonstrates pericolic inflammation, bowel wall edema, abscess formation, and even fistulization in 63 to 95 per cent of
patients. *Elective evaluation* of a patient following *resolution* of
diverticulitis should include colonoscopy, barium enema, or
both.

TREATMENT. Most patients require *hospitalization.* Standard therapy consists of *bowel rest, intravenous antibiotics,* and *fluid resuscitation.* Antispasmodics and analgesia often are added in order to improve patient comfort. The antibiotic regimen should provide *coverage of normal colonic flora.* Therefore, an aminoglycoside in combination with either clindamycin or metronidazole often is prescribed. With resolution, patients should be placed on a high-fiber diet. Barium enema or colonoscopy should be scheduled within several weeks of the acute episode for confirmation and definition of the extent of disease.

Patients who *fail to respond or deteriorate* within the first 24 to 48 hours usually require urgent surgical treatment. Occasionally, patients who are known to have a diverticular abscess can be *stabilized temporarily* by percutaneous, computed tomography–guided drainage. This may permit adequate resuscitation of a critically ill patient. Such drainage should *never* be construed as definitive treatment.

Approximately 20 per cent of patients who develop *acute diverticulitis* eventually require surgical therapy. Following a second attack, the *incidence of complications* approaches 50 to 60 per cent, with mortality *twice* that associated with an initial attack. *Recurrence* of acute diverticulitis warrants surgical resection when active inflammation has subsided. Septic complications such as abscess formation and free perforation constitute the most common reasons.

SURGICAL OPTIONS. Patients undergoing elective surgical procedures are best served by *resection of the involved segment and primary anastomosis.* Bowel preparation usually has been possible, and antibiotics (both systemic and oral) can be administered safely and easily. The mortality for elective colon resection after the resolution of inflammatory diverticular disease should be less than 2 per cent.

In patients with fulminant disease, bowel preparation is not usually possible. Therefore, a two-stage procedure usually is required. Numerous studies have documented that primary resection is associated with a significantly lower mortality (up to 10 per cent) and morbidity (25 to 30 per cent) compared with simple drainage of the abscess with proximal colostomy (mortality and morbidity of 30 per cent and 50 per cent, respectively).

The distribution of the various *complications* of diverticulitis in patients requiring surgical therapy is *abscess formation* (40 to 50 per cent), *intestinal obstruction* (10 to 30 per cent), *free perforation* (10 to 15 per cent), and *fistulization* (4 to 10 per cent). Each of these conditions may coexist in any patient. Complications develop in up to 25 per cent of patients with active diverticulitis, and surgical intervention is necessary in almost all such instances.

Diverticulitis may cause progressive large bowel *obstruction,* which is usually partial. Primary resection of the involved segment with either anastomosis or temporary colostomy is the treatment of choice. Occasionally, a loop of *small intestine* may become densely adherent to the colonic inflammatory process, causing partial or complete small bowel obstruction.

Although most episodes of perforated diverticulitis are confined to the peridiverticular region, an occasional patient presents with signs of *generalized peritonitis* due to *perforation*. These patients require emergent surgical intervention. The overall mortality is high (20 to 40 per cent), largely owing to septic shock and multiple organ failure. *Resection* of the perforated segment with *diversion* of the fecal stream, coupled with copious irrigation of the peritoneal cavity, is the appropriate treatment.

Diverticular *abscesses* are quite common and are characterized according to their location as peridiverticular, retroperitoneal, mesenteric, or pelvic. *Primary resection* of the involved segment with *colostomy* and *adequate local drainage* is the most appropriate treatment. *Percutaneous drainage* may help to *stabilize* critically ill patients and, thereby, enable them to undergo elective, one-stage resection at a later date.

Over 90 per cent of cases of acute diverticulitis are localized to the sigmoid colon; therefore, *fistulization* most commonly involves this segment. The most common type is the *colovesical fistula*, which represents up to two thirds of all internal diverticular fistulas. *Colocutaneous fistulas* are the second most common type followed by colovaginal and coloenteric fistulas in decreasing order of frequency. Colovesical fistula is three to five times *more common* in men. This has been attributed to the presence of an intervening uterus in females, which serves as a protective anatomic barrier between the inflamed colon and the bladder. Patients with colovesical fistula present with *dysuria* (94 per cent), *fecaluria* (75 per cent), and *pneumaturia* (75 per cent) as the most frequent complaints. Only 25 to 30 per cent of patients present with abdominal pain or evidence of systemic infection. The diagnosis of a colovesical fistula can be made by a history of *pneumaturia* and the finding of *fecaluria* on urinalysis. These findings do not, however, identify the underlying cause of the fistulization. Therefore, further evaluation is necessary. *Cystoscopy* (80 to 95 per cent diagnostic accuracy), *computed tomographic scanning* (50 to 90 per cent accuracy), and *barium enema* (30 per cent accuracy) are the studies most likely to confirm the presence of a colovesical fistula and to define its cause. The *low diagnostic yield* (20 per cent) of cystography and colonoscopy has limited their use. Segmental colon resection, primary bladder repair, and primary colon anastomosis is the preferred treatment. The mortality associated with a colovesical fistula is 4 to 5 per cent.

VI

Benign Neoplasms of the Colon Including Vascular Malformations

Anthony L. Imbembo, M.D.,
and J. Lawrence Fitzpatrick, M.D.

A variety of *submucosal lesions* occur throughout the colon and rectum and include lipomas, fibromas, leiomyomas, and carcinoids. Many remain asymptomatic. Clinical problems, when they occur, are due to a mass effect or blood loss secondary to ulceration of the overlying mucosa.

Hyperplastic polyps are not premalignant but appear to be because of impaired sloughing of apical cells. *Juvenile or retention polyps* occur mainly in children. They are considered to be hamartomatous and consist of large, dilated, mucus-filled glands. They are not considered to be premalignant. In the multiple juvenile polyposis syndrome, there is an increased incidence of adenocarcinoma of the colon arising from coexistent adenomatous polyps. *Inflammatory polyps* or pseudopolyps are foci of regenerating mucosa against a background of denuded mucosa seen with inflammatory processes such as idiopathic ulcerative colitis.

Neoplastic polyps or adenomas are very common, with a 10 per cent incidence in the general population. Their incidence increases with age. Adenomas may be broad-based (sessile) or may have a stalk produced by the traction of peristalsis (pedunculated). These polyps may be classified as *tubular* or *villous,* depending on their glandular pattern. There are intermediate polyps having characteristics of both.

Neoplastic polyps are thought to be premalignant with the polyp-cancer sequence well established and a generally accepted latency period of about 15 years. Several features increase malignant potential and include *villous characteristics, size over 1 cm., dysplasia,* and *ulceration.* All pedunculated polyps should be endoscopically removed. Such excision usually constitutes adequate treatment if carcinoma *in situ* is present. However, involvement of the muscularis mucosa and stalk defines invasion mandating segmental resection. Whereas tubular adenomas occur throughout the colon with a modest left-sided predilection, villous adenomas occur predominantly in the sigmoid colon and rectum. Villous adenomas have a *marked predilection for malignant degeneration,* and complete excision is required.

There are a number of *familial syndromes* characterized by *multiple neoplastic colonic polyps.* Whereas 100 polyps must be present for diagnosis, the mean number present is about 1000. Familial polyposis coli, Gardner's syndrome, and Turcot's syndrome are each examples of familial syndromes and are probably related entities characterized by multiple ade-

See the corresponding chapter or part in the *Textbook of Surgery,* 14th edition, pp. 921–927, for a more detailed discussion of this topic, including a comprehensive list of references.

nomatous colonic polyps and a number of extracolonic features that may include osteomas of the mandible or skull, exostotic lesions in long bones, soft tissue tumors such as lipomas, fibromas, or desmoid tumors, or adenomatous lesions elsewhere in the gastrointestinal tract. Malignant degeneration is considered to be essentially inevitable, and prophylactic resection of the colon is warranted.

Total colectomy with ileostomy eliminates the risk of malignancy. The consequent creation of a permanent abdominal stoma and loss of continence make this procedure unacceptable to many patients. *Total abdominal colectomy with ileoproctostomy* mandates continued endoscopic surveillance of the retained rectum. Unfortunately, even though residual rectal polyps may regress transiently, the risk of malignancy is not eliminated. An increasingly attractive alternative is *total abdominal colectomy, rectal mucosectomy, and ileoanal pullthrough*. Although this procedure is not without significant problems, satisfactory continence is achieved in many patients, and the risk of colonic malignancy is eliminated.

Cronkhite-Canada syndrome is a nonfamilial condition characterized by diffuse hamartomatous polyps throughout the gastrointestinal tract, accompanied by skin and nail changes, weight loss, diarrhea, and malnutrition. It is not premalignant. Therapy is supportive and directed to nutritional repletion.

Peutz-Jeghers syndrome has an autosomal dominant inheritance. It is characterized by *diffuse hamartomatous polyps* throughout the gastrointestinal tract with associated melanin pigmentation about the face, mouth, and buccal mucosa. The most frequent complications are bleeding, obstruction, and intussusception. There is an *increased risk* of carcinoma of the small bowel due to the presence of associated adenomatous polyps.

Angiodysplasia or arteriovenous malformations may occur anywhere in the gastrointestinal tract. The most frequently encountered subset is an acquired lesion that tends to localize in the right colon. These malformations are thought to develop secondary to altered vascular dynamics in the bowel wall. They occur primarily in older patients, and there may be an increased incidence in patients with aortic valvular disease and chronic renal failure. Angiodysplasias may cause chronic blood loss with anemia or acute gross hemorrhage. Indeed, angiodysplasia constitutes the second leading cause of lower gastrointestinal hemorrhage in adults. Diagnosis of these lesions may be difficult, with angiography or endoscopy being most useful. When they have been identified, endoscopic electrocoagulation or laser photoablation may be effective. Segmental resection is reserved for failure of endoscopic therapy, particularly in the presence of ongoing hemorrhage, when definitive localization has been accomplished.

Gastrointestinal hemangiomas are less frequent than angiodysplasias and are most frequently of the cavernous type. They may be associated with similar lesions in the central nervous system or other organs. Because of their vascularity, endoscopic coagulation should not be attempted. Segmental resection is the definitive treatment.

Kaposi's sarcoma is a neoplastic vascular malformation seen frequently with acquired immunodeficiency syndrome (AIDS). One half of these lesions occur in the gastrointestinal tract with the majority in the duodenum. Treatment is relief of symptomatic lesions.

VII

Ulcerative Colitis
James M. Becker, M.D., and Frank G. Moody, M.D.

Chronic ulcerative colitis is a diffuse inflammatory disease of the mucosal lining of the colon and rectum. The disease is characterized by bloody diarrhea that exacerbates and abates without apparent cause and without a clearly identified etiologic agent or specific medical therapy. Total removal of the colon and rectum provides a complete cure. New surgical alternatives have eliminated the need for a permanent ileostomy following definitive resection of the involved colon and rectum.

The cause of ulcerative colitis remains unknown despite intensive work by many investigators. The examination of bacterial and viral agents continues to be an area of considerable activity, although there is uncertainty as to the fundamental role that infectious agents have in the primary pathogenesis of ulcerative colitis. Genetic factors appear to have an important role, since most studies have demonstrated that ulcerative colitis is two to four times more common in Jewish than in non-Jewish white populations and is approximately 50 per cent less frequent in nonwhite than in white populations. In addition, there is a 10 to 15 per cent greater frequency of ulcerative colitis in family members of patients with confirmed ulcerative colitis. Psychological factors may have a role in exacerbations of the disease but are not of primary importance in the pathogenesis of the disorder. There has been considerable speculation that ulcerative colitis is an autoimmune disease. A number of immunologic studies have supported this concept, and there is currently much interest in the role of cytokines and immunoregulatory molecules in control of the immune response in patients with inflammatory bowel disease. Other studies have suggested that ulcerative colitis represents an energy-deficient disease of the colonic epithelium. It has also been suggested that there might be alterations in colonic mucosal glycoprotein composition in patients with ulcerative colitis.

See the corresponding chapter or part in the *Textbook of Surgery*, 14th edition, pp. 927–940, for a more detailed discussion of this topic, including a comprehensive list of references.

Ulcerative colitis, for the most part, is a disease confined to the mucosal and submucosal layers of the colonic wall. It is a continuous colonic disease with the rectum essentially always involved. This is in contradistinction to the transmural inflammatory changes found in Crohn's disease of the colon in which all layers of the colonic wall may be involved in a granulomatous inflammatory process.

CLINICAL MANIFESTATIONS. Ulcerative colitis usually presents with bloody diarrhea, abdominal pain, and fever. Occasionally arthritis, iritis, hepatic dysfunction, skin lesions, or other systemic manifestations may be paramount. The disease presents as a chronic, relatively low-grade illness in most patients. In a small number of patients (15 per cent), it has an acute and catastrophic fulminating course. Such patients present with frequent bloody bowel movements, high fever, and abdominal pain. Onset of the disease occurs in patients less than 15 years of age in approximately 15 per cent of cases, and presentations over 40 years of age are not uncommon. The incidence of ulcerative colitis is 3.5 to 6.5 per 10^5 population, and the prevalence is 60 per 10^5.

Physical findings are directly related to the duration and presentation of the disease. Weight loss and pallor are usually present. In the active phase, the abdomen, in the region of the colon, is usually tender to palpation. During acute episodes or in the fulminant form of the disease, there may be signs of an acute abdomen accompanied by fever and decreased bowel sounds. It is also in these patients with toxic megacolon that abdominal distention may be identified.

Sigmoidoscopy is the first step in diagnosis, since ulcerative colitis involves the distal colon and rectum in 90 to 95 per cent of patients. The mucosa of the rectum and sigmoid colon is erythematous and friable. Normal colonic vascular markings may be lost or the mucosa may be hyperemic, and the intracolonic haustra are thick and blunted. Superficial mucosal ulcerations are seen. In advanced disease, the areas of ulceration may surround areas of accumulated granulation tissue and edematous mucosa, which are termed pseudopolyps. The use of flexible sigmoidoscopy has improved diagnostic accuracy and patient acceptability. Colonoscopy may be useful in determining the extent and activity of the disease, particularly in patients in whom the diagnosis is unclear or if cancer is suspected.

A plain abdominal film shows colonic dilation, which has been termed *toxic megacolon*, in approximately 3 to 5 per cent of patients. Most frequently seen is dilation of the transverse colon, although there may be free air within the peritoneal cavity from perforation of the diseased colon. Barium enema examination of the colon is useful in most patients although potentially dangerous in those with toxic megacolon. Radiographic signs suggesting ulcerative colitis on barium enema include loss of haustral markings and irregularities of the colon wall, which represent small ulcerations. Later in the course of the disease, pseudopolyps may be identified. In long-standing chronic ulcerative colitis, the colon assumes the appearance of a rigid contracted tube, the "lead pipe" appearance.

In all patients presenting for the first time, it is necessary to exclude infectious causes of the enterocolitis. Therefore, stool specimens must be obtained for smears and cultures to exclude colitis due to viruses, *Chlamydia*, bacterial pathogens, and parasites. It has become increasingly important to differentiate ulcerative colitis from Crohn's colitis. Crohn's disease of the colon, compared with ulcerative colitis, would be suggested by the findings of small bowel involvement, rectal sparing, absence or infrequency of gross bleeding, perianal disease, focal lesions, segmental distribution (skip lesions), asymmetric involvement, fistulization, granulomas or transmural involvement on biopsy, and the distinct endoscopic appearance.

MEDICAL MANAGEMENT. Patients who present with advanced signs of acute illness require hospitalization and supportive as well as specific therapy for associated metabolic and hematologic derangements. Because of the massive fluid and electrolyte loss per rectum, such patients usually present with metabolic acidosis, contracted extravascular volume, and prerenal azotemia. Intravenous potassium and blood transfusion are often needed. Symptoms of toxicity are treated by nasogastric suction, intravenous corticosteroids, antibiotics, and total parenteral nutrition.

Corticosteroids and immunosuppressive agents have both been demonstrated to be effective in the management of ulcerative colitis. These agents, however, are capable of producing significant side effects. Corticosteroids remain the mainstay of therapy during acute episodes. Forty to 60 mg. of prednisolone in a single daily dose is effective in most cases in inducing remission. Patients with more active disease or toxicity may require parenteral steroids in the form of hydrocortisone or methylprednisolone. Although maintenance steroids may be useful in controlling symptoms of patients with continuing activity, maintenance therapy with small-dose corticosteroids for patients with inactive disease has not been demonstrated to prevent relapse. Sulfasalazine has not been of significant value in treating patients with severe ulcerative colitis but may have a role in controlling acute exacerbations in patients with chronic disease. In an effort to eliminate the side effects associated with the sulfa carrier, newer forms of the drug, such as 5-ASA, have been developed and are available for clinical use. A number of immunosuppressive agents have been utilized for the management of ulcerative colitis, including azathioprine, 6-mercaptopurine, and cyclosporine. Before these immunosuppressive agents are prescribed, familiarity with the dosing, monitoring, toxicity, and possible induction of lymphoma or other malignancies associated with these drugs is mandatory. Although widely prescribed for both ulcerative colitis and Crohn's disease, metronidazole and other antibiotics are of no proven value in the treatment of inflammatory bowel disease.

INDICATIONS FOR SURGICAL TREATMENT. Common indications for surgical intervention include (1) massive unrelenting hemorrhage, (2) toxic megacolon with impending or frank perforation, (3) fulminating acute ulcerative colitis that is unresponsive to steroid therapy, (4) obstruction from strictures, and (5) suspicion or demonstration of colonic cancer. Surgical therapy is also recommended in children who fail to mature at an acceptable rate. For most patients with ulcerative colitis, a colectomy is performed when the disease enters an intractable, chronic phase and becomes a physical and social burden to the patient.

Acute perforation occurs infrequently, with the incidence directly related to both the severity of the initial episode and extent of the disease of the bowel. Specifically, although the overall incidence of perforation during the first attack is less than 4 per cent, if the attack is severe, the incidence rises to approximately 10 per cent. If there is pancolitis, the perforation rate is approximately 15 per cent, and if the attack is both severe and involves the entire colon, it increases to almost 20 per cent. The site of perforation is most often in the sigmoid colon or splenic flexure. Perforation occurs usually in patients with toxic megacolon. This complication causes more deaths than does any other complication of ulcerative colitis.

Obstruction due to benign stricture formation occurs in approximately 10 per cent of patients with ulcerative colitis, with one third of these occurring in the rectum. It is important that the obstructive lesions be differentiated from carcinoma by biopsy or excision and particular attention given to excluding Crohn's disease.

Massive hemorrhage is a rare complication of acute ulcerative colitis that occurs in fewer than 1 per cent of patients. Prompt surgical intervention is indicated if transfusion of more than 3000 ml. of blood is required within 24 hours. It must be remembered that 50 per cent of patients with acute colonic bleeding have toxic megacolon. Uncontrollable hemorrhage from the entire colorectal mucosa may be the one clear indication for an emergency total proctocolectomy. In selected cases, the rectum can be spared for a later sphincter-saving operation, with the realization that this may be a continued source of bleeding.

Toxic megacolon occurs in approximately 10 per cent of patients with ulcerative colitis. If toxic colitis, with or without megacolon, does not improve within 48 hours, an emergency operation is indicated. The operation of choice in this setting is abdominal colectomy with Brooke ileostomy and Hartmann closure of the rectum. Emergency operation for acute toxic megacolon has a high operative morbidity and a mortality of 3 to 30 per cent. The mortality appears to be higher following a total proctocolectomy than following abdominal (subtotal) colectomy. Subtotal colectomy also preserves the rectum, thus allowing subsequent mucosal proctectomy and ileoanal anastomosis.

Although recent studies have suggested that previous reports may have overestimated the risk of cancer in the adult population with ulcerative colitis, patients with this disease remain at a 10 to 20 per cent risk of developing carcinoma within 20 years of the diagnosis of ulcerative colitis. Adenocarcinoma, in association with ulcerative colitis, is multicentric in 50 per cent of cases. In addition, the cancers tend to be more infiltrated and more difficult to identify colonoscopically. These tumors are evenly distributed throughout the colon, with approximately 50 per cent found proximal to the splenic flexure. The likelihood of carcinoma in patients with ulcerative colitis appears to relate to both the extent of colonic involvement and the duration of disease. Although it was held for some time that the carcinoma associated with ulcerative colitis was more aggressive than that of the general population, recent studies have demonstrated that the natural evolution of the cancer is probably the same in both groups. The question of timing of surgical therapy for cancer prophylaxis remains controversial. After 10 years of follow-up, prophylactic colectomy needs to be considered because of the accelerating risk of cancer. The role of colon or rectal biopsy in directing the timing of colectomy remains controversial. Patients followed more than 5 to 7 years should undergo an annual colonoscopy and multiple biopsies for detection of epithelial dysplasia. Severe dysplasia on several biopsies is associated with cancer of the colon in up to half the patients. A number of studies have demonstrated that surveillance programs are associated with a high false-negative and false-positive rate. In addition, to date no study has demonstrated that surveillance lowers the mortality from colorectal cancer associated with ulcerative colitis.

The relationship between systemic extracolonic manifestations of ulcerative colitis and colectomy is not entirely clear. Although arthritis and skin lesions respond to colectomy, ankylosing spondylitis and liver dysfunction or failure may not respond.

The most common indication for operation remains intractability. Elective operations for medically intractable ulcerative colitis include total proctocolectomy and Brooke ileostomy or continent ileostomy (Kock pouch), subtotal colectomy with ileostomy or ileorectal anastomosis, and colectomy with mucosal proctectomy and ileal pouch–anal anastomosis. Because of the availability of the sphincter-sparing operations, patients and their physicians are now electing surgical therapy for intractability earlier in the course of their disease. Criteria regarding timing of operation and indications for operation are therefore undergoing considerable revision.

SURGICAL MANAGEMENT. Since chronic ulcerative colitis is cured when the colon and rectum are removed, single-stage total proctocolectomy has until recently been the operation of choice for elective surgical treatment. Despite the fact that proctocolectomy eliminates the diseased mucosa and the risk of malignant transformation, it has remained controversial and poorly accepted by patients and their physicians. This is primarily due to the fact that a permanent abdominal ileostomy is required after standard proctocolectomy. Although most patients adjust to their ileostomy, a significant percentage have chronic appliance-related problems, and there are significant psychological and social implications of an ileostomy for young and active patients. Fortunately, a number of other surgical alternatives to total proctocolectomy and ileostomy are currently available.

Subtotal colectomy with ileorectal anastomosis has been employed as a compromise operation for ulcerative colitis for decades. The operation eliminates an abdominal stoma, and since the pelvic autonomic nerves are not disturbed, impotence and bladder dysfunction are not risks. The operation, however, does not eliminate the proctitis, and thus patients may have persistent, severe rectal disease and a poor functional result. In addition, there is a 15 to 20 per cent risk of developing cancer in the rectal stump after many decades.

Kock first proposed the concept of a continent ileostomy in 1969. In constructing the continent ileostomy, the colon and rectum are removed just as in proctocolectomy with a standard ileostomy. However, the creation of the ileostomy incorporates the concepts of an intestinal pouch or reservoir and a one-way valve at the abdominal wall. Patients can then empty the pouch by passing a tube through the valve into the pouch via the stoma. The pouch has the advantage that a definitive or curative procedure may be performed and the majority of patients are continent. Nevertheless, at least 15 per cent of patients are incontinent owing to failure of the nipple valve, and ultimately 40 to 50 per cent of patients may require reoperation for technical or anatomic complications. With the success of ileoanal anastomosis as described in the following, the Kock pouch is being performed much less frequently. Continent ileostomy is currently most useful in patients who have already undergone total proctocolectomy and ileostomy and who strongly desire a continence-restoring operation.

In 1947, Ravitch and Sabiston proposed an anal sphincter-sparing operation that consisted of abdominal colectomy, mucosal proctectomy, and endorectal ileoanal pull-through and anastomosis. As initially proposed, the operation was performed by first resecting the abdominal colon in a standard manner. Rather than removing the entire rectum and anus, the disease-bearing mucosa of the rectum was dissected free and resected, preserving an intact rectal muscular cuff and anal sphincter mechanism. Continuity of the intestinal tract was re-established by extending the terminal ileum into the pelvis within the muscular tube and circumferentially suturing it to the anus. Potential advantages of this approach are elimination of all diseased mucosa, preservation of parasympathetic innervation to the bladder and genitalia, thus avoiding impotence, avoiding a permanent abdominal ileostomy, and preservation of the anorectal sphincter apparatus that is responsible for fecal continence. Despite these theoretic advantages, the operation was associated initially with a high complication rate and an unpredictable functional result and was performed on very few patients until the early 1980s. Improved success with the operation was noted, in part, because of a generalized advancement in perioperative and intraoperative surgical care, but more specifically because of a number of technical improvements in the operation. Perhaps the most important modification of the operation was the creation of an ileal pouch or reservoir proximal to the ileoanal anastomosis. Several pouch configurations exist: J, S, and W. Studies comparing the functional results following ileoanal anastomosis, with and without an ileal reservoir, have found that 24-hour stool frequency was significantly reduced in patients with ileal pouches, particularly in the early postoperative period.

The selection of patients for this operation is key to a good result. Crohn's disease contraindicates the operation, although patients with indeterminant colitis do well after this operation. The patient must have a good anal sphincter for control of the semisolid stool, and this can be tested using anorectal manometric techniques. Anorectal sepsis precludes this operation. Obesity is a relative contraindication. Chronologic age may be a relative contraindication, but more important is the physiologic age and pre-existing continence. The functional results in most large series of patients undergoing ileoanal anastomosis have been encouraging. By providing an adequate intestinal reservoir and preserving nearly normal anal sphincter function, the operation provides anal continence and acceptable stool frequency. The number of bowel movements is four to nine daily, with an average of six. Nocturnal bowel movements occur one to two times nightly, with a mean of slightly more than one. Of greater importance are control and urgency of bowel movements, which are variable, depending on the time after operation. Daytime incontinence is extremely uncommon, although nocturnal incontinence occurs in 10 to 50 per cent of patients. Improvement in these factors continues for more than 2 years after operation. In an effort to control stool output, patients have been placed on loperamide hydrochloride, a synthetic opioid antidiarrheal agent, and supplementary fiber in the form of psyllium hydrophilic mucilloid. In addition, patients are placed on a high-fiber diet.

Mortality for elective surgical therapy for ulcerative colitis is 0 to 2 per cent; for emergency operation, it is about 4 to 5 per cent; and for toxic megacolon, it rises to 17 per cent. A major complication in all reported series is sepsis, either in the wound or in the intra-abdominal cavity. The most common late complication of proctocolectomy with a Brooke or continent ileostomy or an ileoanal anastomosis is intestinal obstruction, which occurs in about 10 per cent of patients. Other complications following proctocolectomy include delay in perineal closure, sexual dysfunction, and renal stones. The most frequent late complication in patients undergoing ileoanal anastomosis is ileal pouch dysfunction or pouchitis, which has been reported to occur in 10 to 20 per cent of patients undergoing this procedure for ulcerative colitis. Pouchitis is an incompletely defined and poorly understood clinical syndrome consisting of increased stool frequency, watery stools, cramping, urgency, malaise, and fever. Fortunately, treatment with a short course of metronidazole is successful in most patients. All patients undergoing surgical therapy for ulcerative colitis benefit from support through ileostomy clubs, enterostomal therapists, and patient-oriented support groups.

Thus, ulcerative colitis is a chronic inflammatory disease of the mucosa of the colon and rectum. It can be effectively controlled in most patients with diet, sulfasalazine, and steroids. Eventually, a significant proportion of patients require operation, particularly if the inflammatory process involves the entire colon and rectum. Ulcerative colitis is cured if the colon and rectum are removed. In the past, definitive treatment required total proctocolectomy and permanent ileostomy. In recent years, surgical alternatives that provide continence but are associated with distinct morbidity have become available.

VIII

Volvulus of the Colon
Anthony L. Imbembo, M.D., and Karl A. Zucker, M.D.

Volvulus is the abnormal twisting or rotation of a portion of the bowel about the mesentery. This may cause occlusion of the lumen at each end of the segment with resultant obstruction and/or vascular compromise. The sigmoid colon, cecum or right colon, transverse colon, or splenic flexure may be involved. Colonic volvulus generally occurs in the setting of a large redundant colonic segment with a narrow mesenteric base. The redundant segment is freely mobile whereas the points of fixation are quite close, serving as foci for development of volvulus or twisting of that segment of bowel. These features may be acquired, as in sigmoid volvulus, or congenital in origin, as is likely with cecal volvulus. Left untreated, volvulus generally progresses rapidly from colonic obstruction to strangulation and gangrene. Volvulus is an uncommon cause of obstruction in English-speaking countries, representing only 1 to 3 per cent of all admissions for bowel obstruction. It remains, however, a major health problem in parts of Russia, Iran, and Africa, where volvulus may constitute the most common cause of intestinal obstruction.

SIGMOID VOLVULUS

Approximately three quarters of all cases of large bowel volvulus involve the sigmoid colon. An incidence of 1.47 episodes of sigmoid volvulus per 100,000 population per year has been reported in Minnesota. Advancing age appears to be an important factor, since sigmoid volvulus was found to be 20 times more common in individuals over the age of 60 years.

The age and sex distribution of patients with sigmoid

See the corresponding chapter or part in the *Textbook of Surgery*, 14th edition, pp. 940–944, for a more detailed discussion of this topic, including a comprehensive list of references.

volvulus appear to have two distinct patterns. Patients in Iran, Africa, and Eastern Europe are predominantly middle-aged males (mean age 40 to 50 years); the pathogenesis has been ascribed to an acquired redundancy of sigmoid colon secondary to high-residue diets. In the United States, Australia, the United Kingdom, and Canada, sigmoid volvulus occurs in elderly individuals (mean age 60 to 70 years) of either sex with almost all patients reporting a long history of disordered bowel habits. Many patients are referred from chronic care facilities with disorders such as Parkinson's disease, Alzheimer's disease, multiple sclerosis, paralysis, chronic schizophrenia, pseudobulbar palsy, and senility. The usual bedridden state of these patients and the use of various neuropsychotropic drugs are both known to alter bowel motility. Adhesions from prior abdominal surgical procedures have also been implicated as a causative factor, with the scar tissue serving as a pivot point around which bowel can twist.

Acute sigmoid volvulus generally presents with the sudden onset of severe, colicky abdominal pain, obstipation, and abdominal distention. Generalized abdominal pain, tenderness, fever, and hypovolemia suggests that strangulation has already occurred. Occasionally, patients present with a history of intermittent pain and distention consistent with chronic recurrent volvulus.

Plain abdominal radiographs often reveal a dilated colon forming the "bent inner tube" or "omega loop" sign. The convexity of the loop points toward the right upper quadrant, or away from the point of obstruction. The narrowed segment of colon, the "bird's beak," generally points toward the site of obstruction. Barium enema is usually not required for diagnosis and is contraindicated whenever strangulation is suspected.

Initial treatment of sigmoid volvulus consists of attempted nonoperative reduction, which is successful in 70 to 80 per cent of patients. Successful detorsion permits deferral of surgical therapy in acutely ill patients with unprepared bowel. The most widely used nonoperative procedure for reduction of sigmoid volvulus is the combination of proctoscopy and rectal tube placement. Following successful nonoperative reduction of a sigmoid volvulus, delayed sigmoid colonic resection with appropriate bowel preparation is recommended for most patients. In such a setting, primary anastomosis may be safely performed. In patients who fail nonoperative reduction, the appropriate surgical approach is less clear. Colostomy alone is contraindicated because this procedure does not prevent strangulation of the segment or recurrent volvulus. Operative detorsion alone is associated with up to a 40 per cent recurrence. Other procedures that have been used include tube sigmoidostomy, extraperitonealization of the sigmoid colon, sigmoidopexy, and resection with end-colostomy (with or without mucous fistula). Unfortunately, there is insufficient experience reported for evaluating the efficacy of these procedures. If gangrene is present at the time of laparotomy, immediate resection is indicated, usually with an end-colostomy and a mucous fistula or Hartmann's procedure.

The main determinant of patient mortality from sigmoid volvulus is viability of the colon. Successful nonoperative reduction followed by elective resection has an expected mortality of 6 to 10 per cent, whereas patients operated upon for gangrenous colons have a mortality of 50 to 70 per cent.

CECAL VOLVULUS

Cecal volvulus represents 20 to 40 per cent of all cases of colonic volvulus. Approximately 90 per cent of patients with cecal volvulus have an axial twist of a segment of the proximal colon or even the entire right colon; in the remainder, there is a cephalad fold of the cecum across the ascending colon (cecal bascule). A mobile cecum is a prerequisite for the development of a cecal volvulus. As many as one half to two thirds of these patients have undergone previous abdominal surgical procedures. Colonic distention following distal obstruction has also been implicated in the development of cecal volvulus and should be excluded.

Cecal volvulus presents with the acute onset of severe, colicky pain, nausea, vomiting, and obstipation along with a compressible mass extending from the right lower quadrant to the midabdominal region. Abdominal films reveal marked distention of the cecum; barium enema may show the narrowing of bowel lumen accompanying the twisting of the colon ("bird's neck deformity). Nonoperative techniques for the reduction of cecal volvulus have been much less successful than for sigmoid volvulus. Approximately 25 per cent of patients are found to have gangrenous changes at the time of laparotomy, and the mortality in this setting approaches 40 per cent. Therefore, when the diagnosis of cecal volvulus has been made, prompt surgical intervention is advised. When the cecum is gangrenous, resection is mandatory, usually with ileotransverse colostomy. However, in the setting of viable bowel, the procedure of choice is again less clear. Right hemicolectomy is recommended in many institutions. Other options include detorsion alone, cecopexy, or cecostomy.

VOLVULUS OF THE TRANSVERSE COLON

Less than 100 cases of transverse colon volvulus have been reported. Patients present with the typical signs and symptoms of colonic obstruction. Diagnosis of transverse colon volvulus is difficult on plain abdominal films and is often not suspected preoperatively. Reported attempts at nonoperative reduction have been few and generally unsuccessful. Urgent surgical intervention is advised, and if gangrenous bowel is encountered, resection is mandatory. In patients with viable colon, detorsion alone is associated with a high rate of recurrence and mortality. Transverse colectomy, colopexy, and transverse tube colostomy have been used successfully.

VOLVULUS OF THE SPLENIC FLEXURE

Less than 50 cases have been described in the literature. Congenital absence or iatrogenic division of the gastrocolic, splenocolic, or phrenocolic ligaments may predispose to splenic flexure volvulus. Approximately two thirds of reported patients have undergone prior abdominal surgical procedures. Urgent surgical intervention is recommended. Resection is mandated in cases of ischemic bowel. The majority of patients with nongangrenous bowel have also been treated by resection.

IX

Carcinoma of the Colon, Rectum, and Anus

Anthony L. Imbembo, M.D., and Alan T. Lefor, M.D.

Carcinoma of the colon and rectum is the second most common malignancy and cause of cancer deaths in the United States. It is estimated that there will be 157,500 new cases in 1991, and 60,500 deaths. Aggressive approaches for identifying patients with early lesions are needed to improve overall survival. It is generally a disease of older individuals, with equal incidence in men and women.

The *pathogenesis* of colorectal cancer is unclear, but there is almost certainly a strong *environmental influence*. This is suggested by studies of individuals who emigrate from an area of low incidence, such as Japan, to an area of higher incidence, such as the United States. Such individuals have a likelihood of developing colorectal cancer similar to that of their new country, suggesting environmental and dietary influences. Western diets, high in animal fat and relatively low in fiber, are associated with a higher incidence. In addition, groups with familial polyposis have a very high incidence of colorectal cancer, suggesting genetic influences as well.

Current recommendations of the American Gastroenterologic Association include *digital rectal examination and fecal occult blood testing annually beginning at age 40 years* and *flexible sigmoidoscopy to begin at age 50 years* for the average-risk individual. A negative endoscopy in 2 consecutive years is followed by endoscopy every 3 years thereafter. Patients in *high-risk groups*, including those with long-standing ulcerative

---

See the corresponding chapter or part in the *Textbook of Surgery*, 14th edition, pp. 945–958, for a more detailed discussion of this topic, including a comprehensive list of references.

colitis, Crohn's disease, previous colorectal carcinoma, familial colon cancer, Gardner's syndrome, and familial polyposis, require earlier and more frequent endoscopic studies.

The *signs and symptoms* of colorectal cancer generally are nonspecific. The optimal time for diagnosis is when the patient is still asymptomatic, since it has been shown that the existence of symptoms significantly worsens the prognosis. Right-sided lesions are classically associated with *dull abdominal pain and occult bleeding*, whereas left-sided lesions are associated with a *change in stool caliber, red blood, and a change in bowel habits*. Rectal lesions can be associated with bright red blood–coated stool, tenesmus, or a *sense of incomplete evacuation*.

Digital rectal examination with fecal occult blood testing should be a part of every *diagnosis*. A Valsalva maneuver often pushes a high rectal lesion within reach of the examining finger. Proctosigmoidoscopy can identify as many as one half of colonic malignancies. Flexible sigmoidoscopy allows examination of the distal 40 to 60 cm. of colon and is somewhat better tolerated by the patient than is rigid sigmoidoscopy. Colonoscopy allows examination of the entire colon. Barium enema allows imaging of mucosal detail through the entire colon. Good preparation is essential. *The entire colon must be evaluated for synchronous lesions when a tumor has been found.* Chest films, liver function studies, carcinoembryonic antigen titer, and abdominal computed tomography scan are also obtained preoperatively. *Carcinoembryonic antigen* can be used to follow the patient postoperatively, frequently serving as an indication of recurrence.

STAGING OF DISEASE

The true extent of disease can be determined only after resection of the specimen and staging. Carcinoma of the colon and rectum extends by six routes: *intramural extension, direct invasion of adjacent structures, lymphatic spread, hematogenous spread, intraperitoneal spread, and anastomotic implantation.* There are a number of staging systems in use today. The original system was developed by Dukes and was further modified by Astler and Coller in 1954. Most recently, the *TNM system* has been recommended by the American Joint Committee on Cancer. A number of new technologies are being applied to these tumors in the hope of obtaining better prognostic information.

TREATMENT

The objective of therapy is excision of the primary lesion with *adequate margins* of normal tissue. The exact procedure is dependent on the location of the tumor in the colon. Preoperatively, the patient undergoes bowel preparation, including whole-gut lavage with polyethylene glycol–electrolyte solution and oral erythromycin base and oral neomycin. Intravenous antibiotics are administered just before operation and continued for two doses postoperatively. Patients should be psychologically prepared if either a temporary or permanent colostomy is anticipated. Males should be counseled about postoperative sexual dysfunction if extensive pelvic dissection is anticipated.

Lesions in the right colon are treated with a *right hemicolectomy*. This encompasses about 10 cm. of terminal ileum and the right colon distal to the hepatic flexure, including the right branch of the middle colic artery. Continuity is reestablished with an ileotransverse colostomy. Lesions in the transverse colon are treated with *transverse colectomy* or by *extended right hemicolectomy*. The entire middle colic artery is included in the specimen. Carcinomas arising in the splenic flexure or proximal descending colon are treated with resection of the entire left colon, down to the first branch of the inferior mesenteric artery. Sigmoid carcinomas are treated with *left hemicolectomy*, including the inferior mesenteric artery. The sigmoid colon is resected down to the peritoneal reflection in the pelvis. Adjuvant therapy with 5-fluorouracil and levamisole is indicated for patients with Duke's class C lesions of the colon.

Therapy of *rectal carcinomas* depends on their location in the rectum. Those lesions near the anal verge require *abdominoperineal resection* for adequate treatment. Those lesions that are high up, generally more than 12 cm. from the anal verge, may be resected by *low anterior resection*. Those lesions in between pose a dilemma resolved only by judgment at the time of the procedure. Those lesions that can be safely reconstructed are treated with low anterior resection; otherwise, abdominoperineal resection is performed. The use of *stapling devices* has made possible the construction of low anastomoses, which have been shown to compare well with handsewn anastomoses. *Local excision* can be considered in patients with small, well-differentiated lesions limited to the mucosa; in patients with normal preoperative computed tomography scans; and particularly in older patients with compromised cardiovascular status. Whereas there have been a number of techniques described for improving the results of surgical therapy in these patients, data are sparse as to their true efficacy.

Despite complete preoperative evaluation, the identification of metastatic disease at the time of laparotomy is not uncommon. *Excision of the primary lesion* is desirable, if only for prevention of obstruction in the future, even in the presence of widespread metastatic disease. If resection is not possible, then proximal diverting colostomy is indicated. In patients with rectal lesions and accompanying tenesmus or bleeding, even abdominoperineal resection is indicated as a palliative procedure. A single small hepatic metastatic lesion can be considered for resection at the time of treatment of the primary, if this can be accomplished with a wedge resection and minimal morbidity. The performance of a hepatic lobectomy concurrently with a colon resection is not indicated. Identification of a single large hepatic metastasis should prompt curative colon surgery to be followed by a complete imaging work-up and possible hepatic resection at another time.

Patients with *right-sided* obstructing lesions should undergo resection and anastomosis, whereas those with *left-sided obstructing carcinomas* should have resection with proximal colostomy and distal mucous fistula. The latter approach is mandatory for perforated lesions in order to control sepsis. Direct extension to adjacent organs necessitates *en bloc resection* of these organs, since the adhesions are filled with tumor cells. Patients with an abdominal aortic aneurysm and a colon carcinoma should have resection of the symptomatic lesion first. If both are asymptomatic, the aneurysm should be resected first, regardless of size. *Concurrent oophorectomy* is recommended in all postmenopausal women with carcinoma of the colon for decreasing morbidity. It should be considered in all premenopausal women with ovarian abnormalities at operation or in the presence of peritoneal implants.

A benefit from *adjuvant radiation therapy* in patients with *rectal lesions* has been demonstrated in several studies as evidenced by improved local control but *not* by improved overall survival. Some workers have shown improved survival in patients treated with combined radiation therapy and chemotherapy. Adjuvant therapy is recommended for those *patients at highest risk for recurrence*, namely, for those with transmural spread of disease, with or without regional nodal involvement (Astler-Coller Dukes B_2, C_1, and C_2).

Colonoscopy or barium enema, for imaging the entire colon, is recommended in the postoperative period, usually within 2 to 3 months. Colonoscopy should be repeated annually for at least the first 4 years following resection. Routine physical examination with complete blood count and liver function tests should be obtained every 3 months for 2 years, then every 6 months for 2 years, then annually. A chest film should be obtained every 6 months for 3 years, then annually. *Carcinoembryonic antigen* level should be assessed every 2 months for 2 years, then every 4 months for 2 years, then annually.

The majority of *recurrences* are either hepatic metastases or local recurrences. Most patients with recurrent disease have *combined recurrences* at more than one of these sites. Approximately 35 per cent of all patients with colorectal carcinoma *develop hepatic metastases* during the course of their disease. It is estimated that 10 to 20 per cent of these patients may benefit from hepatic resection. Hepatic resection may be undertaken in the absence of demonstrable extrahepatic disease after complete evaluation. At laparotomy, extrahepatic disease may be identified in some of these patients despite negative work-up. In one study of 607 patients who underwent liver resection, 25 per cent remained disease-free at 5 years. *Negative resection margins and unilobar disease* correlate with the best survival. Patients with unresectable hepatic metastases have been treated with a number of modalities, including hepatic *intra-arterial chemotherapy*. However, because of toxicity of the therapy and the inability to demonstrate a clear survival advantage from intra-arterial therapy using 5-fluorouracil, this approach remains investigational. Anastomotic recurrences represent a major form of treatment failure and occur in 2 to 15 per cent of all curative resections.

Re-exploration is necessary to determine resectability. Patients who develop local recurrence after low anterior resection usually must undergo abdominoperineal resection for achievement of local control.

MALIGNANCIES OF THE ANUS

Anal cancers are relatively *uncommon tumors*, with squamous cell comprising about 70 per cent of all cases. The most common treatment for these lesions has been surgical excision by abdominoperineal resection. Combination therapy strategies have been developed with use of radiation therapy and chemotherapy. In one program, after a radiation dose of 3000 cGy. to the primary tumor, systemic chemotherapy is given. The area of the primary lesion is excised, and if tumor remains, abdominoperineal resection is performed. The results with this approach are *similar to those with radical surgery alone*. Local excision may be appropriate for small lesions of the anal margin.

X

The Anus
Onye E. Akwari, M.D.

ANATOMY AND PHYSIOLOGY

The anal canal is the terminal 4.4 to 4.5 cm. of the gastrointestinal tract, extending from just below the level of the puborectalis muscle to the anal opening. Embryologically the upper part of the canal is formed from the cloacal expansion of the hindgut in which a longitudinal septum eventually separates the alimentary tract posteriorly from the genitourinary tract anteriorly. The lower part of the canal is derived from the proctodeal dimple of the ectoderm. The structure of the anal canal and its junction with the distal rectum may be conceptualized as two tubular parts that ensheathe each other over the length of the anal canal. The inner component is the termination of the gut tube, the inner circular layer of smooth muscle expanding to form the internal sphincter. The outer component is composed of striated muscle of the pelvic floor, which consists of the levator ani muscle, the puborectalis muscle, and the external sphincter. The internal sphincter tone is normally maximal with relax-

---

See the corresponding chapter or part in the *Textbook of Surgery*, 14th edition, pp. 958–972, for a more detailed discussion of this topic, including a comprehensive list of references.

ation being triggered in response to rectal distention (recto-sphincteric reflex).

The columnar epithelium of the rectum is replaced by a mixture of columnar and squamous epithelium in the upper anal canal. This mucocutaneous junction at the level of the anal valves is termed the *dentate* or *pectinate line*. Distal to this line, the anal canal is lined by stratified squamous epithelium (the pecten), which is tightly bound onto the internal sphincter. At the anal orifice, this changes to normal skin with hair follicles and a number of apocrine sweat glands. The *pecten*, which extends into the canal about 2 cm., is devoid of hair, sweat glands, and sebaceous glands. In the zone that extends cephalad from the anal valves for a distance of about 3 to 11 mm., the epithelial type has been described as transitional.

COMPLETE RECTAL PROLAPSE (PROCIDENTIA)

The most important pathophysiologic abnormality of the pelvic floor encountered by the surgeon, procidentia, must be distinguished from simple mucosal prolapse. Procidentia occurs most commonly at the extremes of life (in children below the age of 5 years and in elderly women), causing frank incontinence and social embarrassment of these patients. In children it usually resolves spontaneously by the age of 5 years, and operative treatment is seldom required in this age group. In adults, the condition is more common in women who have not borne children and therefore cannot be ascribed to birth trauma. Treatment of chronic prolapse has followed a trend in recent years of performing major surgical therapy at an earlier stage. The operation performed is one of several types of abdominal rectopexy, a procedure that causes the rectum to become adherent to the sacrum, which prevents it from prolapsing. The success rate from the point of view of correction of the prolapse is high, but one third of the patients are still incontinent to some degree. Rectal prolapse may rarely be complicated by incarceration, strangulation, and gangrene. Complicated prolapse may require emergency rectosigmoidectomy and creation of a colostomy.

HEMORRHOIDS

Hemorrhoids may be complicated early by bleeding that is characteristically arterial in type. In time, with increasing mucosal prolapse, the prolapse may require manual replacement after defecation. The presence of the hemorrhoidal mass through the anal sphincter mechanism may cause such irritation that the sphincter undergoes paroxysms of severe spasm. The severe pain of sphincter spasm may be further compounded by the pain from the relative ischemia of the hemorrhoidal mass trapped by the sphincter in spasm. Successful manual replacement of the acutely prolapsing hemorrhoidal mass provides immediate and often dramatic relief. Some patients have an associated laxness of the external

sphincter, and their large internal hemorrhoids tend to prolapse with any transitory rise in intra-abdominal pressure
such as may occur with walking or during a coughing
episode. When this stage, which is sometimes termed third-
degree hemorrhoidal change, has been reached, the patient
may develop acute discomfort at any time. The prolapsed
hemorrhoid causes perineal itching and soilage from persistent mucus discharge. Third-degree hemorrhoids and those
prone to recurrent episodes of thrombosis should be considered for surgical therapy.

An *uncommon* complication of hemorrhoidal bleeding is
anemia. However, so uncommon is anemia as a result of
hemorrhoidal disease that other causes of this condition
should be sought, such as carcinoma of the stomach or colon,
before a firm diagnosis is made. The most significant change
in the operative treatment of hemorrhoids is that it is now
often performed in an ambulatory setting.

ANORECTAL SUPPURATION

The most common cause of anorectal suppuration is an
abscess or a fistula, or both. The pathogenesis of these two
apparently separate conditions is often the same: the abscess
is the acute phase and the fistula the chronic phase.

ABSCESS. Infection starts in the intersphincter space and
is thought to begin in one of the anal glands. A small abscess
may form in this space (intersphincteric abscess), and the
infection may spread vertically, horizontally, or circumferentially. All abscesses in this area should be drained as soon
as diagnosed, since dramatic necrotizing infection of the
entire perineum may complicate the situation. Diabetic patients are especially at risk for the rapid spread of infection
sometimes involving clostridial and mixed anaerobic infections. A preliminary computed tomographic scan of the
perineum and pelvis may identify unsuspected collections of
pus.

FISTULA IN ANO. The incidence of *fistula in ano* complicating anorectal suppuration either in the acute phase or
during follow-up within 6 months is about 26 per cent. In a
recent study, half of the fistulas were unrecognized by the
patient, and no fistulas developed in patients when the
original pararectal abscess pus culture revealed only skin-
derived bacteria. Fistulas occurred when intestinal microorganisms were cultured from the anorectal abscess. Whereas
the management of fistulas may be complex and protracted,
the key principles to be observed in planning surgical management are (1) abscess drainage and (2) careful postoperative
care of the wound. Suprasphincteric and extrasphincteric
fistulas are very unusual, and their difficult management
requires specialists in the field.

ANAL FISSURE

The squamous mucosa of the lower half of the anal canal
is prone to superficial linear ulceration, usually situated in

the posterior commissure. There may be a skin tag protruding from the anal margin, the sentinel pile. The fissure situated just within the anus is easily overlooked. Because it involves the highly sensitive squamous epithelium, it is often a very painful condition. Bleeding, especially upon wiping, is characteristically anal in type. Anorectal sphincter *spasm* compounds the problem of pain in these patients who then avoid defecation, and the formation of hard, constipated stools results. The condition tends to be cyclic. Early conservative treatment with use of local anesthetic for diminishing the pain and abolishing the exaggerated anal reflex, avoidance of constipation by the use of bland laxatives, and sitz baths for keeping the ulcer clean during the acute phase usually produce a satisfactory outcome. Surgical *division* of the lower half of the internal sphincter is nearly always curative. The operation, which is usually performed laterally in the anal canal, enlarges the lower anal canal and eliminates defecation trauma.

CROHN'S DISEASE OF THE ANORECTUM

Distinct from granular proctitis, Crohn's disease of the anorectum occurs in as many as 75 per cent of patients with Crohn's disease. Simultaneous occurrence of Crohn's disease in the ileum and colon is common. The initial treatment is conservative, including a trial of immunosuppressive drugs such as prednisone. Anorectal sepsis may respond to antibiotic therapy along with conservative incisional drainage of local abscesses. Metronidazole (Flagyl) has become the drug of choice. Occasionally the disease is so destructive that excision of the anorectum is the only possible course. An abdominoperineal resection is performed with emphasis on dissection close to the rectal muscle to avoid damage to the other pelvic structures, particularly the *nervi erigentes*. Failure to observe this precaution in young individuals may cause severe bladder and/or sexual dysfunction.

TUMORS OF THE ANUS

Condyloma acuminatum (perianal warts) is the perineal homologue of common papovavirus warts. The warts may be extensive, involving the vulva, vagina, cervix, anal canal, and even the lower rectum. Although dysplasia is *not* usually a feature, transformation to invasive squamous carcinoma is recognized. The giant variety of condyloma acuminatum (Buschke-Lowenstein tumor) may also occur in the anorectum but less commonly than in the genital area. Its clinical and histologic resemblance to *verrucous carcinoma* is such that most observers regard them as essentially identical. Giant condylomata can also evolve into conventional invasive squamous carcinoma. Perianal warts, when few and isolated, may be treated by the local application of podophyllin. When the warts are extensive, excisional treatment under general anesthesia is required followed by a program of frequent examination and podophyllin ablation of persistent or new lesions.

Malignant Tumors

Tumors of the *proximal* anus are adenocarcinomas derived from the colorectal type of glandular epithelium. The lymphatic drainage of these tumors is largely via the superior hemorrhoidals and to the pelvic organs. Tumors arising in the transitional zone may be histologically squamous, pseudoadenoid, pseudosarcomatous, cloacogenic, mucoepidermoid, melanoma, carcinoid, perianal mucinous carcinoma, lymphoma, small cell carcinoma, or neuroendocrine. The lymphatic drainage from this zone is directly from the inferior and middle hemorrhoidals to the hypogastric and obturator nodes or indirectly via the submucosal plexus of nodes to the rectal nodes and pelvic organs.

The most distal anus is a zone of nonkeratinized squamous epithelium, devoid of hair, sweat glands, and sebaceous glands. This zone then merges into the keratinized perianal skin with glands and follicles. Well-differentiated keratinizing squamous carcinoma arising in this distal zone may spread to the superficial inguinal nodes.

Patients with malignant neoplasms of this region have for years been treated by abdominoperineal resection, with 5-year survival ranging from 24 to 70 per cent with an average of about 55 per cent in larger series. External irradiation combined with 5-fluorouracil and mitomycin provides a 5-year survival of 78 per cent. This is superior to abdominoperineal resection combined with chemotherapy, or abdominoperineal resection combined with radiation. Combined chemotherapy and radiation therapy may also negate a permanent colostomy.

Malignant Melanoma and Other Nonepithelial Tumors

These tumors constitute 0.4 to 0.8 per cent of colorectal malignancies and less than 2 per cent of all melanomas. Commonly presenting with intermittent rectal bleeding and pain, these lesions may be ignored as hemorrhoids. The tumor may be positively identified on electron microscopy and S-100 protein analysis. Malignant melanoma spreads rapidly, causing death from widespread blood-borne deposits, predominantly in the liver and lungs. Leiomyosarcoma arising from the internal sphincter and perianal rhabdomyosarcomas and myoblastomas arising from the external sphincter have been reported. Endocrine tumors (carcinoids) have been classified as arising in the rectum but originate from the endocrine cell population of the anal canal. Abdominoperineal resection is advocated for those carcinoids exceeding 2 cm. in diameter although lymph nodal spread may be associated with smaller lesions.

ANAL EROTICISM, FOREIGN BODIES, AND TRAUMA

Insertion of foreign bodies (some specially designed for the purpose) into the anorectum may lead to tears, avulsion of the sphincter, bleeding, perforation of the rectum or intra-abdominal colon, and retention of the foreign body. Perirectal or deep abscesses may be associated with the very unimpressive finding of an intact perineum in these patients. Extraction of a foreign body should be performed under excellent anesthesia so that the injury can be fully assessed. Extensive anorectal damage may require diversion of the fecal stream by the creation of an end colostomy. If intraperitoneal involvement is suspected, laparotomy should be undertaken. Today, any patient with cramping abdominal pain presenting with unexplained diarrhea, especially if there is evidence of perineal trauma, should alert the surgeon to the possibility of "gay bowel syndrome." The term refers to proctocolitis due to trauma or a wide variety of enteric organisms including herpes simplex, cytomegalovirus, *Salmonella, Shigella, Entamoeba histolytica*, and others. The diagnosis may be made by tissue biopsies and careful microbiologic cultures.

I

Anatomy and Physiology
William C. Meyers, M.D.

ANATOMY

The liver is the largest gland in the body, weighing approximately 1500 gm. in the adult and representing about one fiftieth of the body weight. The liver conforms to the undersurface of the diaphragm, and its inferior surface is in contact with the duodenum, colon, kidney, adrenal gland, esophagus, and stomach. It is under the protection of the ribs.

Lobar Anatomy

The topographic lobes do not correspond to the true lobar anatomy. Distribution of the major branches of the veins, arteries, and bile ducts divides the liver into two relatively equal masses by a plane (the portal fissure) passing from the left side of the gallbladder fossa to the left side of the inferior vena cava, creating the *right* and *left* lobes. The left lobe consists of a *medial segment* lying to the right of the falciform ligament and a *lateral segment* to the left of the falciform ligament. The right lobe consists of an anterior and posterior segment for which there is no visible superficial demarcation.

French "Segmental" System

Another nomenclature takes into greater consideration the hepatic venous drainage but also applies to the portal biliary and arterial anatomy. Instead of four, there are eight segments: four on the right, three on the left, and one corresponding to the caudate lobe. The three hepatic veins divide the liver into four *sectors*. The planes contain the right, middle, and left hepatic veins and are termed *portal scissurae*; the planes containing portal pedicles are termed *hepatic scissurae*. Segments, according to the French system, correspond generally to the *subsegments* described in the lobar anatomic classification.

Biliary System

The biliary ductal pattern becomes more variable distally. Basically, one duct drains each segment and joins into two

---

See the corresponding chapter or part in the *Textbook of Surgery*, 14th edition, pp. 976–992, for a more detailed discussion of this topic, including a comprehensive list of references.

main trunks. However, it is not uncommon to have three or even four relatively equally converging ducts into one confluence. The left hepatic duct joins the right at a much more anterior and acute angle, an anatomic consistency that becomes important during common duct exploration or cholangiography. The upper limit of the normal diameter of the common duct is controversial, although most references list 6 to 8 mm. except after cholecystectomy, when it may dilate. The gallbladder is a pear-shaped distensible appendage of the extrahepatic biliary system containing 30 to 50 ml. of bile. The valves of the cystic duct are extremely tortuous, sometimes making cholangiography difficult. The sphincter of Oddi has three principal parts: the sphincter of the choledochus, the pancreatic sphincter, and the ampullary sphincter. Knowledge concerning possible biliary variations is extremely important in avoidance of injury even in seemingly simple procedures such as cholecystectomy.

The liver "acinar unit" is a concept of microscopic masses of liver cells functionally situated around terminal portal venules. Blood flow is from the venules into the sinusoids coming into contact with hepatocytes until it drains into the terminal hepatic venules. Zones of hepatocytes have been arbitrarily divided into three sections, Zone 1 being the area immediately adjacent to the portal venule and Zones 2 and 3 being farther away. Certain functions are readily explained by this concept, such as Zone 1 cells being the first to receive blood and oxygen and therefore the last to undergo necrosis.

PHYSIOLOGY

The liver is an amazingly dynamic organ, active in the uptake, storage, distribution, and disposition of various nutrients from the intestine or blood, and responsible for the synthesis, transformation, and metabolism of many endogenous and exogenous substrates.

The liver expends approximately 20 per cent of the body's energy and consumes 20 to 25 per cent of the total oxygen utilized despite constituting only 4 to 5 per cent of the body weight. About 70 to 75 per cent of the total hepatic blood flow is derived from the portal vein and the remaining 25 to 30 per cent from the hepatic artery. There is a reciprocal increase in hepatic arterial flow in response to reduction in portal venous flow, but the converse does not occur. Approximately 1000 ml. of blood can be made available to the body by the liver in periods of stress. The portal and arterial systems converge in the sinusoidal bed where the pressure remains remarkably constant and low. Deprivation of portal flow causes deterioration in hepatic structure and function, marked pathologically by Zone 3 "centrilobular" hepatocyte atrophy and fatty infiltration.

Bile Formation

Bile formation is an active process relatively independent of total hepatic blood flow except during conditions simulating shock. Bile is formed at two sites: (1) the canalicular membrane of the hepatocyte and (2) the bile ductules or ducts. The bile canaliculus is a long, narrow channel that begins as a space of approximately 1μ in diameter bounded by two or three hepatocyte canalicular membranes. The best method of estimating canalicular flow is by the clearance of metabolically inert, freely permeable neutral solutes such as erythritol and mannitol, although there is some question whether the bile duct epithelial cells are also slightly permeable to these sugars. There appears to be both a transcellular and a paracellular route for canalicular and probably ductular bile formation. The paracellular route is of lesser importance under physiologic conditions.

The principal organic compounds in bile are the conjugated bile acids, cholesterol, phospholipid, bile pigments, and protein. Because of the excellent correlation between bile acid output and bile flow, the term bile acid–dependent flow describes this fraction of bile formation. In addition, canalicular flow may be generated in near absence of bile acids or during stabilized bile acid–dependent flow, and this fraction is termed the bile acid–independent canalicular fraction. Abundant evidence now exists that this bile salt–independent fraction may not be as "independent" as was previously thought. Both canalicular and ductular bile salt–independent flow appear to be under the regulation of gastrointestinal hormones, which include glucagon, secretin, and probably cholecystokinin. Total unstimulated bile flow in a 70-kg. man has been estimated to be between 0.41 and 0.43 ml. per minute. Of this, 0.15 to 0.16 ml. per minute is bile acid–dependent flow, another 0.16 to 0.17 ml. per minute is bile acid–independent canalicular flow, and approximately 0.11 ml. per minute is from ductular secretion. Under physiologic conditions, total bile flow in 1 day is estimated to be 600 to 1000 ml. The total flow varies considerably depending on the presence or absence of various physiologic stimulants or inhibitors. The two most important factors in this variability in the surgical setting are the presence or absence of a fistula and fasting versus feeding.

Lymph Formation

Hepatic lymph collection transports large and small molecules, plasma protein, debris, bacteria, other foreign substances, and fluid. Lymph is 3 to 5 per cent protein, mainly albumin, and its electrolyte composition estimates that of plasma. Greatly increased numbers of lymph channels are present in cirrhosis.

Enterohepatic Circulation

Bile salts are secreted into the biliary system and empty into the intestine where they are efficiently reabsorbed into the portal circulation. The liver extracts the bile acids and transports them to the canalicular membrane where they are resecreted into the biliary system. This process is referred to as the *enterohepatic circulation*. Total bile salt pool size in humans is 2 to 5 gm. and undergoes this circulation two to three times per meal and six to ten times daily, depending on dietary habits. In addition, 0.2 to 0.6 gm. is lost per day in the stool, and this quantity is replaced by newly synthesized bile acids.

Bilirubin Metabolism

The primary breakdown product of heme, bilirubin, is excreted almost entirely in the bile. With hepatocellular disease or extrahepatic biliary obstruction, free bilirubin may accumulate in blood and tissues and cause toxic effects. A number of disorders of bilirubin metabolism have been described that vary from kernicterus, which is an extreme example of bilirubin toxicity occurring in children, to Gilbert's syndrome, which is benign.

Other Hepatocyte Functions

Hepatic protein synthesis and catabolism are vitally important, and measurement of these functions often provides a useful indication of the degree of liver impairment. Albumin is the most studied of the various proteins synthesized in the liver. Synthesis of the protein is influenced by nutrition, various hormones, and oncotic pressure. Much information is presently being accumulated on the genes expressed by the liver. A large number appear to be expressed primarily in the liver compared with other organs, such as albumin and tyrosine aminotransferase.

II

Pyogenic and Amebic Liver Abscess

Gene D. Branum, M.D., and William C. Meyers, M.D.

Abscess of the liver remains a challenging diagnostic and therapeutic problem for the clinician despite modern imaging techniques for the diagnosis of the disorder, effective antibiotics, and a range of effective methods for drainage. Pyogenic (bacterial) and amebic organisms are the most common pathogens encountered, with bacteria the cause in 80 to 90

See the corresponding chapter or part in the *Textbook of Surgery*, 14th edition, pp. 992–999, for a more detailed discussion of this topic, including a comprehensive list of references.

per cent of the cases in the United States. Early diagnosis and treatment are critical in successful management of liver abscess.

PYOGENIC LIVER ABSCESS

INCIDENCE AND PATHOGENESIS. The incidence of pyogenic liver abscess is probably increasing owing to the aggressive treatment of malignant disorders. The current estimate of prevalence is 13 to 22 patients per 10,000 hospital admissions. The pathophysiologic mechanism of liver abscess in general, or pyogenic abscess in particular, involves two basic elements: (1) the presence of the organism and (2) vulnerability of the liver. The spread of bacterial or other organisms to the hepatic parenchyma may occur via (1) the portal system, (2) ascension from the biliary tree, (3) the hepatic artery during generalized septicemia, (4) direct extension from subhepatic or subdiaphragmatic infection, or (5) a direct route as a result of trauma. Most organisms arise in the liver via the portal route, and hepatic clearance of portal bacteria is probably a common event in healthy individuals. Bacterial organisms superimposed on necrotic tissue, hepatic injury, malignant tumors, or acquired biliary or vascular obstruction, however, may cause multiplication, tissue invasion, and abscess formation.

Appendicitis was formerly the most common source of bacterial organisms, but it has been replaced in recent series by benign and malignant biliary obstruction as the most common source. Other significant sources include diverticulitis, regional enteritis, trauma, generalized sepsis, and pelvic inflammatory disease. Patients receiving chemotherapy for hematologic or solid malignancies are at increased risk. Despite great advances in diagnostic techniques and aggressive searches for a source, no probable cause of hepatic abscess was identified in 13 to 35 per cent of cases since 1984.

PATHOLOGY AND MICROBIOLOGY. Pyogenic hepatic abscesses have some characteristic gross and microscopic pathologic features. Right lobe involvement predominates by a 3:1 ratio. Bilobar metastases occur in approximately 10 per cent of patients. Most series indicate a nearly equal distribution between solitary and multiple liver abscesses. Hepatic abscesses appear yellow, compared with the normal deep maroon hepatic parenchyma that surrounds them. The organ is usually enlarged, and palpation may reveal a fluctuant area corresponding to the pus-filled cavity. On microscopic examination, acute inflammatory reaction is seen with necrosis and hepatocyte cords in the portal triad regions. Cholestasis may be evident in adjacent tissue.

Organisms recovered from liver abscesses vary greatly in reported series but generally reflect biliary or enteric flora. Solitary abscesses are more likely than multiple ones to grow multiple organisms. Presently, the most common aerobic organisms cultured are *Escherichia coli*, *Klebsiella*, and enterococcus. The most common anaerobes are *Bacteroides*, anaerobic streptococci, and *Fusobacterium* species. Streptococcal species (aerobic, anaerobic, or microaerophilic) are found in 25 to 30 per cent of cultured abscesses and are believed to be of increasing importance in the pathogenesis of pyogenic abscess.

AMEBIC ABSCESS

INCIDENCE. Recent epidemiologic data in the United States are lacking concerning the incidence of amebic infestation. In general, the prevalence is higher in (1) countries in tropical or subtropical zones, (2) locations with poor sanitation, (3) mental institutions, and (4) cities in the United States with large immigrant populations. American tourists to tropical areas are more likely to develop invasive amebiasis than are permanent residents, presumably owing to a partial immunity of local inhabitants. Amebic abscess affects males more than females in a 9 to 10:1 ratio. In general, the patients are younger than their counterparts with pyogenic abscess, with the peak incidence in the fourth decade. There does not appear to be any particular racial susceptibility except for that related to living conditions.

PATHOLOGY. Amebic liver abscess follows intestinal infestation by *Entamoeba histolytica*. *Entamoeba* infestation occurs via contaminated drinking water, food, or person-to-person contact. *Entamoeba* cysts are ingested and resist digestion in the gastrointestinal tract. Trophozoites then colonize the colon and are transported via the portal circulation to the liver where they either degenerate in the portal venous radicles or migrate to an adjacent area, causing necrosis and liquefaction. Areas of destruction then coalesce to form, most commonly, a single large cavity in the right lobe. The contents are a mixture of necrotic hepatic parenchyma and blood, which yields the classic "anchovy paste" appearance. Bacterial superinfection occurs in approximately 10 per cent of cases, which may change the color and odor of the contents. Greater than 90 per cent of the abscesses are in the right lobe, and older abscesses have a well-formed fibrous capsule. The lesions may grow to an extremely large size and rupture intraperitoneally, intrathoracically, or into the pericardial space.

DIAGNOSIS

The diagnosis of hepatic abscess is challenging because clinical signs are usually not specific. Early differentiation between pyogenic and amebic liver abscess may be difficult but is important because the treatments are radically different. Hepatic abscess is apparent at the time of admission in a minority of patients but if suspected is readily diagnosed by ultrasonography or computed tomography in over 95 per cent of patients.

The majority of patients with hepatic abscess have an illness of less than 2 weeks' duration, although a third have been ill for a month or longer. The primary symptoms are fever, malaise, chills, anorexia, weight loss, abdominal pain, or nausea. With amebic abscess, a recent diarrheal syndrome is present only in a minority of patients. Physical findings include right upper quadrant tenderness, pleural dullness to percussion, fever, hepatomegaly, and jaundice. Most patients have leukocytosis and some liver enzyme abnormality. The most common findings on plain abdominal or chest radiographs are right-sided atelectasis, an elevated hemidiaphragm, pleural effusion, or pneumonia. Occasionally, a subdiaphragmatic air-fluid collection is seen with pyogenic abscess or superinfected amebic abscess.

Ultrasonography has become the most useful screening test when the suspicion of hepatic abscess arises. The test is highly sensitive, is more accurate than computed tomography in imaging the biliary tree, and allows diagnostic or therapeutic drainage or biopsy at the time of performance. Computed tomographic scanning is the most sensitive of the imaging procedures (95 to 100 per cent) and allows diagnostic or therapeutic intervention to be performed. ^{99m}Technetium sulfur colloid scanning has been useful in diagnosis of abscesses for 4 decades. Although very sensitive, the test has significant limitations of (1) being unable to detect lesions smaller than 2 cm. and (2) not allowing diagnostic or therapeutic procedures at the time of performance.

DIFFERENTIAL DIAGNOSIS. When an abscess has been demonstrated, a distinction must be made between pyogenic and more unusual types. Serum antibody titer for *Entamoeba histolytica* or counterimmunoelectrophoresis is highly specific and of great benefit when positive. Percutaneous aspiration may help in the identification of a bacterial organism; however, such aspiration is not usually helpful in the diagnosis of amebae. If amebic serologic study is not available or the results are delayed, the best method of early distinction between pyogenic and amebic abscess is a trial of an amebicidal agent. If the patient has not clinically responded in a 24- to 36-hour trial, pyogenic abscess should be the primary diagnosis. Clinical response is determined by relief of pain, fever, and leukocytosis.

MANAGEMENT

Untreated pyogenic abscesses are 95 to 100 per cent fatal, with death following rupture, sepsis, or both. Prognostic factors include the patient's age, multiplicity of abscesses, multiplicity of organisms, and the presence of associated malignant or other immunosuppressive disease. Survival has improved in recent years, and mortality should be less than 20 per cent with current therapy.

Effective management involves elimination of the abscess and the underlying source. Treatment of the abscess usually requires both intravenous antibiotics and effective drainage. Drainage may be accomplished by either *percutaneous* or *open* surgical methods. Recent series have documented the ease, effectiveness, and safety of *percutaneous drainage* of most hepatic abscesses. Solitary abscesses in the peripheral posterior of the right lobe are particularly amenable to percutaneous treatment. However, a combination of appendiceal or diverticular abscess and hepatic abscess is usually best treated by open drainage. Multiple abscesses remain difficult management problems by percutaneous, open, or even a combination of the two approaches.

Adjunctive antibiotic therapy is critical to effective treatment of hepatic abscesses. Directed therapy is based on the results of Gram stain and culture of diagnostic abscess aspirates. The most common isolates are gram-negative aerobes, colonic anaerobes, and microaerophilic streptococcal species. An appropriate regimen might include an aminoglycoside, an antibiotic directed primarily against anaerobes such as clindamycin or metronidazole, and a penicillin. This regimen is adjusted appropriately after definitive culture results become known.

Surgical approaches available for use include the transpleural, extraperitoneal, and transperitoneal approaches. Most surgeons presently prefer the transperitoneal route because it allows inspection of the entire abdominal cavity for an underlying source as well as the best mobilization for appropriate drainage. The transpleural route is occasionally useful for high posterior lesions.

AMEBIC ABSCESS. Except where there is rupture or secondary infection, amebicidal agents are the treatment of choice for hepatic amebiasis. The drug of choice is metronidazole, and the usual dosage is 750 mg. orally 3 times daily for 7 to 14 days. If the patient is too ill to receive oral agents, intravenous administration is effective.

If clinical symptoms do not resolve within 48 hours of treatment, an incorrect diagnosis or secondary bacterial infection should be suspected. At that time, percutaneous aspiration or surgical drainage may be considered. Surgical therapy also has a role in suspected rupture, erosion, or perforation of an adjacent viscus or extrahepatic problems such as colonic obstruction. Mortality from amebic liver abscess should be less than 5 per cent in the absence of secondary bacterial infection.

III

Neoplasms of the Liver
William C. Meyers, M.D.

PRIMARY MALIGNANT TUMORS
Hepatocellular Carcinoma

The most prevalent malignant disease worldwide today is *hepatocellular carcinoma*. The tumor is much more common in

---

See the corresponding chapter or part in the *Textbook of Surgery*, 14th edition, pp. 999–1012, for a more detailed discussion of this topic, including a comprehensive list of references.

Africa and Asia than in the United States, where it may be increasing in incidence. Epidemiologic and laboratory studies have now firmly established a strong and specific association between hepatitis B virus and hepatocellular carcinoma. Other etiologic factors include cirrhosis from other causes, aflatoxin, oral contraceptives, and Thorotrast. Symptoms of hepatocellular carcinoma are extremely variable, but over half of the patients have metastatic disease at the time of initial presentation. A large number of paraneoplastic manifestations are associated with hepatocellular carcinoma including protein abnormalities, the most important of which is elevation of the alpha-fetoprotein level.

Alpha-fetoprotein is of particular diagnostic significance—over half of the patients with tumor exhibit the antigen. During the past several years in the Orient, the combination of alpha-fetoprotein level and real-time ultrasonography has been used as a screening method for hepatocellular carcinoma. Other radiologic investigations of importance in the diagnosis of hepatocellular and other tumors of the liver include computed tomography, magnetic resonance imaging, endoscopic or percutaneous cholangiography, and radionuclide scanning. Recently, the technique combining computed tomography and angiography has been developed that appears to be more sensitive in the identification of primary liver and metastatic liver lesions. This technique takes advantage of differential blood flow between the hepatic artery and portal vein to the hepatic tumor. In most cases, neoplasms of the liver are fed more by the artery than by the portal vein. Primary treatment of hepatocellular carcinoma is resection whenever possible. Liver transplantation sometimes achieves resectability, but the long-term survival is relatively poor. Five-year survival for patients with hepatocellular carcinoma is generally considered to be about 20 per cent.

Bile Duct Cancer (Cholangiocarcinoma)

Bile duct cancers represent 5 to 30 per cent of all hepatobiliary neoplasms and may occur anywhere within the biliary system. Both intra- and extraheptic bile duct cancers have been associated with ulcerative colitis and may be confused with sclerosing cholangitis. The tumor is often a markedly sclerotic adenocarcinoma. Approximately 20 to 25 per cent of the tumors are resectable, which is usually advised if possible. Biliary intubation without resection may provide excellent palliation. With more aggressive invasive treatment, survival has often been extended from several weeks to many months or even years. Although patients with bile duct cancer might be expected to be a favorable group for hepatic transplantation, this has not been substantiated.

Other Primary Malignant Tumors

These tumors represent approximately 5 per cent of cases and include *combined hepatocellular-cholangiocarcinoma, bile duct cystadenocarcinoma, squamous cell carcinoma,* and the incurable *angiosarcoma.* Sarcomas, carcinoid, and other mixed malignant tumors more rarely occur. *Epithelioid hemangioendothelioma* is considered a malignant neoplasm because of the diffuse involvement within the liver and the metastatic characteristics.

Metastatic Tumors

Metastatic cancer comprises the largest group of malignant tumors in the liver. Most occur in the liver probably as a result of primary tumor cells shedding into the vascular system. According to one autopsy study, bronchogenic carcinoma was the most common primary lesion causing hepatic metastases. Next in frequency were colonic, pancreatic, breast, and stomach tumors.

The liver is the most common site of metastatic colorectal cancer. Approximately one fourth of metastatic colorectal cancers to the liver are resectable. Several studies have documented the unfavorable prognosis of untreated hepatic metastases from colorectal cancer. Three-year survival in recent reports of resection for metastatic colorectal cancer is approximately 35 to 40 per cent. Five-year survival appears to be 20 to 30 per cent. Although there is little question that aggressive surgical therapy benefits selected patients, the precise numbers of and methods for selecting those patients preoperatively are still lacking. The probable significant prognostic factors include size and number of metastatic lesions. Undoubtedly, the most important predictor is the presence or absence of extrahepatic or residual local disease. Recently, improved response rates with the combination of 5-fluorouracil and calcium leucovorin or levamisole as well as with intra-arterial chemotherapy have produced a number of ongoing chemotherapeutic protocols.

BENIGN HEPATIC NEOPLASMS

A number of primary benign lesions may occur in the liver. Some require resection whereas others do not. Therefore, it is important to be familiar with the types of lesions that affect the liver and the methods of diagnosis. Liver cell *adenoma* and *focal nodular hyperplasia* are frequently difficult to differentiate although each has distinct pathologic and clinical features. Both affect women and are associated with the use of oral contraceptives. Hepatic adenomas are usually solitary but vary in size up to 38 cm. in diameter. Occasionally, they are multiple and cluster in families. The lesions are prone to rupture, and malignant change is possible. In contrast, focal nodular hyperplasia typically does not produce symptoms, and bleeding, rupture, and malignant changes do not occur.

Nodular regenerative hyperplasia is by definition a noncirrhotic diffuse hepatocellular process characterized by multiple nodules in intervening areas of hepatic atrophy. Like cirrhosis, this lesion is frequently associated with portal hypertension, but it is distinguished by the absence of severe fibrosis. Probably the most common benign tumor to come to the attention of surgeons is *cavernous hemangioma*, which is found in approximately 2 per cent of livers at autopsy. Spontaneous rupture is unusual but can be dramatic. Complications include congestive heart failure, arteriovenous shunting, and consumptive coagulopathy. Resection is usually determined by the presence of symptoms, danger of rupture, and the amount of liver tissue involved. *Hemangioendotheliomas* are rare vasoformative cellular tumors usually occurring in the first 2 years of life. Resection may be indicated when there is no response to prednisone. A number of other benign solid tumors that may occur in the liver include *lipoma, leiomyoma, myxoma, teratoma, carcinoid tumor,* and *mesenchymal hamartoma.*

CYSTS

Cysts of the liver can be divided into those that are parasitic and nonparasitic. Large solitary *parenchymal (developmental) cysts* are rare; they most commonly occur in the right lobe of the liver, probably representing an arrest of development. By definition, a cyst contains epithelium, often resembling biliary epithelium. Most small cysts require no treatment although they may be difficult to differentiate from cystadenoma or cystadenocarcinoma. Preferred treatment of large cysts that are causing symptoms is resection although other surgical treatments may be attempted. One consideration in the surgical treatment of large hepatic cysts is whether there is communication with the biliary system. *Polycystic liver disease* often accompanies polycystic kidneys. A surgical procedure of choice for a symptomatic dominant cyst in polycystic disease is the fenestration operation, in which the symptomatic cyst is made to communicate with the peritoneal cavity. A cyst *(pseudocyst)* may also form as a consequence of trauma or inflammation; however, these are not true cysts, since they have a fibrous rather than an epithelial lining.

Choledochal cysts are more common in the Orient than elsewhere and may be associated with supraduodenal entry of the pancreatic duct. There is a premalignant potential of choledochal cysts. The extreme form of choledochal cysts consists of multiple cystic dilations in the intrahepatic ducts termed *Caroli's disease.*

Echinococcus is the most frequent cause of parasitic liver cysts. The problem is endemic in Greece and other parts of Eastern Europe, South America, Australia, and South Africa. It is rare in the United States. The most common form is due to *Echinococcus granulosus.* The other primary form is *Echinococcus multilocularis* and is endemic to Alaska. The eggs of *E. granulosus* are passed in the stool and ingested by cows, sheep, moose, caribou, or humans. The primary treatment of echinococcus (hydatid) cysts is surgical resection without peritoneal contamination.

MAJOR HEPATIC RESECTION

Because of reduction of operative mortality in hepatic resection to less than 5 per cent, and in many centers to less than 1 per cent, it has become the primary therapy for resectable primary or metastatic tumors as well as selected benign conditions. The four classic types of major hepatic resection are (1) right hepatic lobectomy, (2) left hepatic lobectomy, (3) right trisegmentectomy, and (4) left lateral segmentectomy. With improved techniques and recognition of the segmental vasculature, numerous other types are now performed. Segmental resection has become increasingly popular. In addition, techniques such as the use of the ultrasonic dissector have improved.

IV

Hemobilia
William C. Meyers, M.D.

Bleeding into the biliary tract is a common, usually inconsequential problem but may also be life-threatening. By far the most common cause of hemobilia is trauma. Some degree of hemobilia often accompanies hepatobiliary diagnostic and therapeutic techniques, such as liver biopsy, transhepatic or endoscopic cholangiography, and lithotripsy.

The bleeding can occur anywhere within the biliary system: liver parenchyma, intra- or extrahepatic bile ducts, gallbladder, pancreas, or ampullary region. In an early review (1972), trauma comprised 48 per cent of the cases, infection 28 per cent, and gallstones 10 per cent. The classic cause of dramatic hemobilia is blunt trauma causing injury deep within the liver without disruption of Glisson's capsule. As the resultant hematoma expands, rupture occurs into the biliary system, or a false aneurysm forms that creates the same problem in a more delayed manner. An important cause of hemobilia in the Far East is parasites, most notably *Clonorchis* or *Ascaris*, which may cause hemobilia associated with cholangitis or pericholangitic abscesses. Other relatively common causes of hemobilia include pancreatic disease, various types of aneurysms, hepatoma, other tumors, and sickle cell anemia.

The classic triad of hemobilia is gastrointestinal bleeding, right upper quadrant pain, and jaundice. These symptoms also suggest other diseases such as terminal cancer, but in the setting of trauma, general good health, or biliary tract manipulation, the triad should suggest the possibility of hemobilia. Other findings may include a palpable mass in the right upper quadrant or right upper quadrant bruit.

Arteriography remains the single most accurate and helpful

See the corresponding chapter or part in the *Textbook of Surgery*, 14th edition, pp. 1012–1015, for a more detailed discussion of this topic, including a comprehensive list of references.

diagnostic test in the evaluation of patients in whom bleeding into the biliary ducts is suspected. Cholangiography may also be helpful. However, these procedures may also confuse the diagnosis because manipulation may also create a new source of bleeding. Technetium-labeled red blood cell scans may occasionally be an efficient way of establishing the diagnosis. An external biliary drainage catheter may, of course, also demonstrate the bleeding.

Management of hemobilia can be divided into two phases. The first phase is general evaluation and resuscitation with blood transfusions as needed. The second phase is treatment, for which there are several options. The majority of cases of severe hemobilia are best treated by arteriographic embolization. Generally, operation should be considered a last resort.

V

Surgical Complications of Cirrhosis and Portal Hypertension

Layton F. Rikkers, M.D.

Cirrhosis is the result of a variety of mechanisms that cause the combination of hepatocellular injury, fibrosis, and regeneration. Although only 15 per cent of alcoholics are afflicted, alcoholic cirrhosis is the most common type of chronic liver disease in the United States, making cirrhosis the fifth leading cause of death between the ages of 35 and 54 years. Cirrhosis causes two major phenomena, hepatic failure and portal hypertension. Complications of portal hypertension include variceal hemorrhage, portal systemic encephalopathy, ascites, and hypersplenism. The most life-threatening complication is variceal hemorrhage, which ranks second to hepatic failure as a cause of death in patients with cirrhosis.

PATHOGENESIS OF PORTAL HYPERTENSION AND VARICEAL RUPTURE

Since increased portal venous resistance is usually the cause of portal hypertension, classifications of cirrhosis are generally based on the site of elevated resistance. However, increased portal venous inflow secondary to a hyperdynamic systemic circulation and splanchnic hyperemia is often a significant contributor to the maintenance of portal hyperten-

---

See the corresponding chapter or part in the *Textbook of Surgery*, 14th edition, pp. 1015–1029, for a more detailed discussion of this topic, including a comprehensive list of references.

sion. Prehepatic, presinusoidal portal hypertension is usually due to extrahepatic portal vein thrombosis and is most common in the pediatric age group. Hepatic function remains normal because portal flow is restored through collaterals. The most common cause of intrahepatic, presinusoidal portal hypertension is schistosomiasis. Again, liver function is generally well preserved. Depending on the etiologic agent of cirrhosis, the site(s) of increased resistance within the liver may vary. Alcoholic cirrhosis usually involves sinusoidal and postsinusoidal levels, whereas some types of nonalcoholic cirrhosis have a presinusoidal component as well. Elevated portal vein pressure stimulates portal systemic collateralization. The most important pathway clinically is through the esophagogastric venous network to the azygous system.

Esophagogastric varices do not develop until portal pressure exceeds 12 mm. Hg and bleed in only one third to one half of patients when present. The pathogenesis of variceal rupture is probably multifactorial with variceal size, magnitude of portal pressure, and thickness of the overlying epithelium all contributing (Laplace's law). In 90 per cent of patients, variceal rupture occurs within 2 to 3 cm. of the esophagogastric junction. The remaining 10 per cent of patients bleed from gastric varices. Gastritis secondary to portal hypertension (portal hypertensive gastropathy) usually involves the proximal stomach and may also be a cause of hemorrhage.

PATIENT EVALUATION

Key components of evaluating a patient with cirrhosis and portal hypertension include (1) diagnosis of the underlying liver disease, (2) estimation of hepatic functional reserve, (3) hepatic hemodynamic assessment and definition of portal venous anatomy if a shunt operation is anticipated, and (4) identification of the site of bleeding if present.

Patient evaluation begins with a detailed history and physical examination. Stigmata of chronic liver disease include spider angiomas, palmar erythema, gynecomastia, testicular atrophy, and altered mental status. Splenomegaly, ascites, and visible abdominal wall veins each indicate the presence of portal hypertension. A chemistry profile, hepatitis serology, and liver biopsy may be helpful in making a specific diagnosis.

Child's classification, composed of three clinical variables (ascites, encephalopathy, and nutritional status) and two biochemical tests (serum bilirubin and albumin), is an indirect but useful estimate of hepatic functional reserve. This classification scheme is particularly valuable in predicting outcome after surgical intervention. Operative mortality for Child's A, B, and C class patients is 0 to 5 per cent, 10 to 15 per cent, and greater than 25 per cent, respectively.

In patients with alcoholic cirrhosis and many types of nonalcoholic cirrhosis, portal pressure can be indirectly estimated by measurement of hepatic venous wedge pressure. This variable is normal in patients with presinusoidal portal hypertension. Selective visceral angiography has been the most frequently used method for definition of portal venous anatomy, qualitative estimation of hepatic portal perfusion, and determination of postoperative shunt patency. Duplex ultrasonography is a less accurate but noninvasive alternative to angiography for assessment of these same parameters.

Endoscopy is the procedure of choice for diagnosing the site of upper gastrointestinal hemorrhage in a patient with portal hypertension. In approximately 90 per cent, bleeding is secondary to portal hypertension (esophageal varices, gastric varices, or portal hypertensive gastropathy). The remaining 10 per cent of bleeding episodes in portal hypertensive patients are usually due to duodenal ulcer, gastric ulcer, or Mallory-Weiss tear.

MANAGEMENT OF ACUTE VARICEAL HEMORRHAGE

Since the greatest risk of death from variceal bleeding is within the first few days after the onset of hemorrhage, prompt and effective therapy is essential for maximal patient salvage. Many patients have decompensated hepatic function secondary to either recent alcoholism or hypotension and are high risks for surgical therapy. Therefore, emergency treatment should be nonoperative whenever possible. However, failure of nonoperative therapy should be promptly recognized so that the appropriate operation can be performed before the patient is moribund.

The highest priority of emergency treatment is restoration of circulating blood volume, which should be accomplished before endoscopy. At present, endoscopic sclerotherapy is the most commonly used treatment for management of the acute bleeding episode. This technique offers the opportunity for control of hemorrhage at the same time the diagnosis is made. Sclerotherapy is usually done through a flexible endoscope without accessories. Both intravariceal and paravariceal injections are effective, with acute hemorrhage ceasing in over 80 per cent of patients. Failure of acute sclerotherapy can be defined as persistent bleeding after two sclerotherapy sessions. Sclerotherapy is generally ineffective for bleeding gastric varices.

Since the reintroduction of endoscopic sclerotherapy, pharmacotherapy and balloon tamponade have been less frequently used. The mainstay of pharmacotherapy is intravenous infusion of vasopressin, a potent splanchnic vasoconstrictor. Simultaneous administration of nitroglycerin decreases the incidence of adverse side effects of vasopressin and may also enhance therapeutic effectiveness. Approximately 50 per cent of acute variceal hemorrhages are controlled by vasopressin, but no trial has shown an improvement in survival. Pharmacotherapy is an important component of treatment for patients awaiting endoscopy, for sclerotherapy failures, and for individuals bleeding from gastric varices or portal hypertensive gastropathy.

The advantage of variceal tamponade with the Sengstaken-

Blakemore tube is immediate control of hemorrhage in over
85 per cent of patients. For avoidance of complications, this
device is used according to a strict protocol. It may be
lifesaving for individuals with exsanguinating hemorrhage
and for patients who do not respond to sclerotherapy and
pharmacotherapy. Because rebleeding is common after balloon deflation, either surgical therapy or endoscopic sclerotherapy should be planned.

Although routine emergency surgical intervention has been
advocated by some, there is no evidence that this approach
is superior to acute sclerotherapy followed by elective operation or by chronic sclerotherapy. The major disadvantage of
emergency surgical therapy is that operative mortality exceeds 25 per cent in most series. The most frequently used
emergency operations are stapled esophageal transection and
portacaval shunt.

PREVENTION OF RECURRENT VARICEAL HEMORRHAGE

Although only one third to one half of patients with varices
bleed, when hemorrhage has occurred, it recurs in over 70
per cent of untreated individuals. Available definitive therapies include pharmacotherapy, chronic sclerotherapy, three
types of portal systemic shunts (nonselective, selective, and
partial), a number of nonshunt procedures, and hepatic
transplantation.

Long-term drug therapy for prevention of recurrent variceal
bleeding is presently an area of intensive clinical investigation. Most trials have evaluated propranolol and other beta-
blockers given in a titrated dose for reducing heart rate by 25
per cent. Results with respect to rebleeding, survival, and
hemodynamic effects of the administered drugs have varied
widely. Thus, although attractive because of its noninvasive-
ness and minimal associated morbidity, pharmacotherapy
remains experimental at the present time.

During the past decade, chronic endoscopic sclerotherapy
has become the most frequently used treatment for prevention of recurrent variceal hemorrhage. Varices can be completely eradicated in approximately two thirds of patients.
Although rebleeding after sclerotherapy approaches 50 per
cent in most trials, many episodes of recurrent hemorrhage
can be successfully treated by further sclerotherapy. However, this therapeutic approach eventually fails in approximately one third of patients, most of whom require surgical
therapy. Nevertheless, chronic sclerotherapy is a reasonable
initial approach for many patients so long as surgical rescue
is readily available.

Portal systemic shunts are the most effective means of
preventing recurrent variceal hemorrhage. In addition to
providing adequate variceal decompression, nonselective
shunts (end-to-side and side-to-side portacaval, interposition,
and conventional splenorenal shunts) divert the entire portal
venous flow away from the liver. Since portal blood contains
hepatotrophic hormones and cerebral toxins, adverse conse-

quences of these procedures are accelerated hepatic failure and frequent post-shunt encephalopathy (20 to 50 per cent of patients). Because of these side effects, controlled trials have failed to show a survival advantage of nonselective shunts over conventional medical management. All nonselective shunts, except the end-to-side portacaval shunt, decompress the hepatic sinusoidal network in addition to the portal venous system. Therefore, these procedures effectively relieve ascites in addition to preventing recurrent variceal bleeding.

The distal splenorenal shunt is a selective shunt that compartmentalizes the portal venous circulation into a decompressed gastrosplenic component and a high-pressure mesenteric component. Because hepatic portal perfusion is maintained into the late postoperative interval in approximately 40 to 50 per cent of patients undergoing this procedure (greater in nonalcoholic and less in alcoholic cirrhotics), the majority of series have reported less frequent encephalopathy (10 to 15 per cent of patients) following the distal splenorenal shunt than after nonselective shunts (20 to 50 per cent). No controlled trial has shown a survival advantage of selective over nonselective shunts. Contraindications to the distal splenorenal shunt are medically intractable ascites and incompatible anatomy (prior splenectomy or splenic vein diameter less than 7 mm.). Splenopancreatic disconnection is an extension of the distal splenorenal shunt that more effectively preserves hepatic portal perfusion in alcoholic cirrhotics. However, this addition makes the operation more technically demanding, and clinical benefits of splenopancreatic disconnection have not yet been proved.

The small-diameter (8 to 10 mm.) portacaval H-graft is a partial shunt that also preserves hepatic portal perfusion in some patients. Initial experience with this procedure suggests that the frequency of postoperative encephalopathy is low when portal flow is maintained. Controlled trials are presently in progress.

Nonshunt operations extend from simple stapled transection and reanastomosis of the distal esophagus to extensive esophagogastric devascularization (the Sugiura procedure). The advantage of these operations is minimal alteration of hepatic portal perfusion and liver function. A significant disadvantage is a high rebleeding rate (20 to 40 per cent) in Western series. Nonshunt procedures are the only applicable operations for patients with diffuse splanchnic venous thrombosis.

Hepatic transplantation is the only definitive therapy for variceal hemorrhage that addresses the underlying liver disease. Variceal bleeders who are transplant candidates include nonalcoholic cirrhotics and abstinent alcoholic cirrhotics with either limited functional hepatic reserve (Child's Class C) or a poor quality of life secondary to their disease. Future transplant candidates (Child's Class A and Class B) who receive other therapy initially (chronic sclerotherapy or shunt) should be carefully monitored so that transplantation is accomplished before they become high operative risks for this procedure. Patients are first grouped according to their transplant candidacy. Immediate transplant candidates should undergo this procedure as soon as a donor liver is available. Most future transplant and nontransplant candidates should receive initial sclerotherapy unless they bleed from gastric varices or have limited access to emergency surgical care. These individuals and those who fail sclerotherapy should receive the appropriate shunt or nonshunt operation depending on their clinical circumstances and portal venous anatomy.

VI

Peritoneovenous Shunts for Intractable Ascites

Paul D. Greig, M.D., F.R.C.S.(C), F.A.C.S., and Bernard Langer, M.D., F.R.C.S.(C), F.A.C.S.

PATHOGENESIS OF ASCITES IN CIRRHOSIS

Ascites in the cirrhotic patient follows the interaction of portal hypertension, hypoalbuminemia, and renal sodium and water retention. The increased hydrostatic pressure and reduced oncotic pressure cause an imbalance of Starling forces and the net movement of fluid from the capillary into the peritoneal cavity. Renal dysfunction with reduced glomerular filtration and increased renin and aldosterone cause sodium and water retention with resultant fluid overload, which aggravates the ascites. This may progress to uremia and oliguria ("hepatorenal syndrome"), an uncommon form of functional renal failure in which the kidneys are histologically normal.

CLINICAL MANIFESTATIONS OF ASCITES IN CHRONIC LIVER DISEASE

The development of ascites usually is chronic and progressive and indicates an advanced degree of liver dysfunction. Resistant ascites occurs in only 10 per cent of patients and carries with it a poor prognosis with less than 50 per cent 1-year survival. Transient ascites may develop in cirrhotic patients following laparotomy or from aggressive resuscitation following variceal bleeding. Severe ascites is associated with pleural effusions, atelectasis, leg edema, and the devel-

---

See the corresponding chapter or part in the *Textbook of Surgery*, 14th edition, pp. 1030–1035, for a more detailed discussion of this topic, including a comprehensive list of references.

opment of umbilical and inguinal hernias. Patients are at risk of developing spontaneous bacterial peritonitis.

TREATMENT OF ASCITES

Treatment includes dietary restriction of sodium (400 mg. per day) and fluid (1 liter per day). Diuretics are administered with an aldosterone antagonist (spironolactone or amiloride) with the addition of a diuretic such as thiazide or furosemide when necessary for mobilizing up to 1 liter per day. Complications include hypokalemia, metabolic alkalosis, and hyponatremia. Excessive diuresis can produce acute tubular necrosis or precipitate the hepatorenal syndrome.

Therapeutic paracentesis with albumin infusions may be necessary in patients with tense ascites. Physiologic side-to-side portal systemic shunts (side-to-side portacaval, mesocaval, or proximal splenorenal anastomoses) lower intrahepatic and portal pressure and decrease ascites formation. These operations have a high surgical risk and incidence of postoperative encephalopathy.

PERITONEOVENOUS SHUNTING

The peritoneovenous shunt involves the implantation of a prosthetic conduit with a one-way valve between the positive-pressure peritoneal cavity and the negative-pressure intrathoracic vascular compartment. The LeVeen shunt has received the widest use and consists of a pressure-activated valve with Silastic peritoneal and venous catheters. Other valves (e.g., the Denver shunt) have a pumpable valve.

Indications for a peritoneovenous shunt are (1) cirrhosis with chronic ascites that becomes refractory to medical management, (2) hepatorenal syndrome, and (3) ascites that develops following an abdominal operation in a cirrhotic patient, usually a portosystemic shunt.

The peritoneovenous shunt is contraindicated in infected ascites or other sepsis, acute viral or alcoholic hepatitis, or end-stage liver disease. Relative contraindications are gastrointestinal bleeding or peritonitis within the previous month, hepatic encephalopathy greater than Grade 1, other complications of alcoholism, an uncomplicated hernia, severe malnutrition, a serum bilirubin more than 3 times normal, a prothrombin time more than 4 seconds prolonged, or a serum creatinine more than 2.3 times normal. Patients with a previous variceal hemorrhage are better treated with a physiologic side-to-side portosystemic shunt.

Preoperative assessment includes a diagnostic paracentesis, a liver biopsy, liver biochemical tests, and coagulation studies. Broad-spectrum prophylactic antibiotics are administered.

The shunt may be inserted under local or general anesthetic. The LeVeen valve is placed in the abdominal wall deep to the rectus muscle. A pumpable valve is placed over the chest wall. The peritoneal end lies freely in the ascites. The venous limb is tunneled subcutaneously and inserted into the superior vena cava via either the internal jugular or the subclavian vein. The tip is directed under radiologic control to lie just within the right atrium. Postoperative coagulopathy may be reduced by replacing the ascitic fluid with Ringer's lactate.

Postoperatively, furosemide is used for maintaining the urinary output over 60 ml. per hour. Weight, girth, hematocrit, electrolytes, renal function, and coagulation are monitored. An initial diuresis follows increases in circulating volume, cardiac output, renal blood flow, and glomerular filtration and corresponding decreases in circulating levels of renin and aldosterone. Ultimately there is reduction of ascites.

Complications occur in up to 80 per cent of patients. All develop a coagulopathy, and up to 20 per cent develop disseminated intravascular coagulation that is treated by temporary ligation of the shunt and provision of fresh frozen plasma, cryoprecipitate, and platelets. Epsilon-aminocaproic acid may also be useful. Shunt infection is a serious complication requiring removal of the shunt and systemic antibiotics. Shunt blockage may be diagnosed by an intraperitoneal injection of [99m]technetium sulfur colloid and scanning the chest or by a direct injection of radiopaque contrast into the shunt. The operative mortality ranges up to 30 per cent.

The renal and hemodynamic changes persist in the late postoperative period. Even with a blocked shunt, most patients become ascites-free and have an improvement in nutrition. Late complications include shunt blockage, infection, superior vena caval thrombosis, and bowel obstruction. The patency rate of 5-year survivors has been only 40 per cent, and the incidence of superior vena caval thrombosis has been over 25 per cent. Most late deaths are due to bleeding esophageal varices and hepatic failure.

The peritoneovenous shunt should be considered only a palliative procedure that may temporarily control ascites but has not been shown to prolong life. It should be avoided in potential liver transplant patients.

PERITONEOVENOUS SHUNT FOR MALIGNANT ASCITES

Malignant ascites occurs most commonly with intraperitoneal spread of ovarian, colonic, or breast cancer. About half such patients obtain adequate palliation from diuretics, paracentesis, chemotherapy, and/or radiotherapy. In selected patients unresponsive to medical therapy, the peritoneovenous shunt may be indicated. Complications and operative mortality are similar to those in patients with cirrhosis. Median reported survival, however, is only 3 months.

VII

Viral Hepatitis and the Surgeon
John D. Hamilton, M.D.

DEFINITION AND ETIOLOGY. Viral hepatitis is an infection of the liver caused by one of five distinct groups of viruses: hepatitis A (HAV), formerly infectious hepatitis; hepatitis B (HBV), formerly serum hepatitis; hepatitis C (HCV), the recently recognized virus that is associated with parenterally transmitted non-A, non-B hepatitis (PT-NANB); hepatitis D (HDV), known also as delta-associated hepatitis; and hepatitis E (HEV), the virus responsible for enterically transmitted non-A, non-B hepatitis (ET-NANB).

To date, no antigens common to two or more viral agents have been identified. Within each class of virus, no differences in the virulence or the nature of the ultimate disease have been found between subtypes or strains. In 1988, 26,000 cases of hepatitis A, 22,000 cases of hepatitis B, and 2500 cases of non-A, non-B hepatitis were reported to the Centers for Disease Control. From these figures, it is projected that there are 300,000 cases of hepatitis B, and 5000 deaths due to viral-induced cirrhosis and hepatocellular carcinoma per year in the United States. Hepatitis A has been generally decreasing but represents about 50 per cent of all reported cases of hepatitis. Hepatitis B and PT-NANB hepatitis (HCV) have been increasing and are responsible for 40 and 10 per cent, respectively, of the reported cases. A fatality of 0.8 per cent has been associated with these cases.

HAV and HEV are transmitted by the fecal-oral route, as might occur with close personal contact or the ingestion of contaminated food or water. Both HAV and HEV are present in the feces of infected patients during the 1 to 2 weeks preceding and the 1 to 2 weeks following the onset of clinical disease, but there is no known chronic fecal or blood carrier. Hepatitis A and hepatitis E, therefore, do not appear to constitute any special risk for the surgeon.

HBV, HCV, and HDV are typically, but not exclusively, transmitted by parenteral routes. HBV is present in high concentrations in the blood and in essentially all other body fluids but may not be present in an infectious form in feces owing to enzymatic inactivation.

The classic route of transmission of HBV and HCV is by transfused blood. This mechanism is facilitated by the capability of HBV and HCV to exist as asymptomatic but infectious viruses in the serum of otherwise normal blood donors or patients with other conditions, making the period of infectivity potentially very long. HDV, a defective virus that requires HBV for replication, is not known to exist as a chronic, asymptomatic viremia. Moreover, since no tests are available for the exclusion of HCV and HDV viruses from blood or

---

See the corresponding chapter or part in the *Textbook of Surgery*, 14th edition, pp. 1036–1041, for a more detailed discussion of this topic, including a comprehensive list of references.

blood products, no measures are known to eliminate these viruses. As might be expected, posttransfusion hepatitis is most often due to HCV. Recently, however, donated blood is subjected to testing for elevation of alanine aminotransferase and hepatitis B core antigen (HBcAg) as surrogate markers for identification of blood more likely to be infected with HCV. Hepatitis due to HBV, HCV, or HDV may be acquired by other parenteral routes more commonly in the individual who uses intravenous drugs. The prevalence of hepatitis in this group approaches 100 per cent. Other predictable means of exposure include accidental needle stick or accidental injury such as might occur during a surgical procedure. It is this occupational risk that represents a continuous threat over the period of a surgical career and that constitutes the basis for individual protection through careful surgical procedures, appropriate surveillance when necessary, and HBV vaccine for all surgical personnel.

There is strong evidence that HAV and HEV certainly but also HBV and HCV viruses may be transmitted by close, personal contact including sexual transmission. Vertical transmission *in utero* and perinatal transmission occur with HBV, HCV, and HDV.

CLASSIFICATION AND CLINICAL DISEASE. All five hepatitis viruses cause a wide spectrum of clinical disease, and in the majority of instances the resultant syndromes are indistinguishable. Typically, there are three more frequent types of infection: (1) inapparent and asymptomatic, (2) anicteric but symptomatic, and (3) icteric and symptomatic. The precise incidence of these alternatives is unknown, but inapparent disease appears to occur several to many times more frequently than does symptomatic clinical disease, especially in children. The clinical illness typically found in about 90 per cent of symptomatic patients may include lassitude, anorexia, weakness, nausea, dark urine, fever, vomiting, headache, chills, and abdominal discomfort with other miscellaneous symptoms occurring somewhat less commonly. Laboratory abnormalities reflect liver cell necrosis including primarily an elevation of aminotransferase and, less commonly, elevations of alkaline phosphatase and bilirubin. Tests for viral antigens and antibodies are helpful in making specific diagnoses.

HBV and HCV, however, have variants of typical disease. Extrahepatic manifestations of HBV, HCV, and HDV most frequently occur in the form of arthralgias, predominantly involving the small joints. Other reported "immune phenomena" include arteritis, nephritis, and dermatitis.

Acute HBV infections produce long-term carriage of hepatitis B surface antigen (HBsAg) and sometimes other markers of HBV in approximately 5 per cent of clinically identified cases. Lack of a history before infection is not unusual, and the carrier may or may not be infectious. From a practical point of view, all carriers should be considered potentially infectious, particularly when an invasive procedure is contemplated.

Of some concern to the surgeon is the possibility that he or she may be or will become a carrier of HBV or HCV.

Although the risk to patients has not been conclusively defined, most agree that disease transmission from physician to patients is a very unusual event and that common hygienic measures, not to mention scrupulous surgical technique, reduce that risk perhaps to zero.

Of the serious sequelae, *acute fulminant viral hepatitis* occurs unpredictably with all types of viral hepatitis. *Chronic aggressive hepatitis* occurs after either HBV or HCV, and either may progress to *cirrhosis*. Finally, there is an association between *hepatoma* (hepatocellular carcinoma) and HBV.

PREVENTION. General measures are the basis of disease prevention for all hepatitis viruses. These include case identification and attention to standard principles of cleanliness and hygiene and specific measures directed toward the interdiction of recognized modes of transmission. Immune serum globulin for HAV and hyperimmune hepatitis B immune globulin for HBV are useful adjuncts. Active immunization is now commercially available for HBV with a highly immunogenic, effective, and safe vaccine manufactured with recombinant DNA technology.

TREATMENT. There are no currently accepted, effective modes of specific therapy for any of the types of viral hepatitis. Management is generally supportive. A variety of agents including interferon-alpha have been used for chronic hepatitis, but critical analysis of these trials does not reveal compelling evidence of efficacy.

34

THE BILIARY SYSTEM

David L. Nahrwold, M.D.

Detailed knowledge of the anatomy of the biliary duct system and its associated arteries and veins is essential for safe biliary surgery. Anomalies of the duct system that are surgically important include a very long or very short cystic duct, a cystic duct that courses behind the common bile duct to enter it on the left or posteriorly, and fusion of a long cystic duct to the common duct, with which it may share a common wall. Anomalies of the cystic artery are very frequent, but less dangerous.

CONGENITAL ANOMALIES OF THE GALLBLADDER

Agenesis of the gallbladder is very rare. Patients may be asymptomatic or have symptoms suggestive of biliary tract disease. One third of symptomatic patients have dilation of the common duct, and approximately one fourth have choledocholithiasis. When the gallbladder cannot be found in symptomatic patients, operative cholangiography should be done to exclude common duct stones.

Double and triple gallbladders are also rare. When multiple gallbladders do not share a common outlet, the cystic ducts open separately into the common duct or, less commonly, into the right hepatic duct.

Ectopic gallbladders may be located within the falciform ligament or within the substance of the right or left lobe. Retrodisplaced gallbladders may be located behind the duodenum or posterior and inferior to the liver. Torsion of the gallbladder may occur when the organ is completely covered with peritoneum and "floating" free of the liver, or when the attachment to the liver is by a long mesentery.

CHOLEDOCHAL CYSTS

Choledochal cysts are of several types. The most common is the fusiform-shaped extrahepatic cyst thought to be caused by a distal stricture and destruction of the proximal duct epithelium by pancreatic juice. Sometimes they are associated with fusiform cysts within the intrahepatic ducts. Another type is a diverticulum from the common duct. In addition, the entire distal duct may be a cyst, referred to as a choledochocele. The symptoms are abdominal pain, jaundice, and an abdominal mass. Episodes of cholangitis are frequent. Choledochal cysts can be imaged by ultrasonography, but

---

See the corresponding chapter or part in the *Textbook of Surgery*, 14th edition, pp. 1042–1049, for a more detailed discussion of this topic, including a comprehensive list of references.

the definitive diagnosis is made by cholangiography. The treatment is excision and biliary tract reconstruction by Roux-en-Y hepaticojejunostomy. A high incidence of carcinoma within the cyst and recurrent pancreatitis militate against leaving the cyst in place.

CHOLEDOCHOLITHIASIS

Bile duct stones may migrate from the gallbladder (secondary stones) or form within the duct (primary stones). Arbitrarily, a stone detected 2 years after cholecystectomy is designated a primary common duct stone. Secondary stones are predominantly cholesterol, and primary stones are predominantly calcium bilirubinate. The latter are associated with the presence of bacteria in bile and often are found in patients with a benign biliary stricture, sclerosing cholangitis, or Oriental cholangiohepatitis.

CLINICAL MANIFESTATIONS AND DIAGNOSIS. Jaundice, chills and fever, and upper abdominal pain (Charcot's triad) are the hallmarks of choledocholithiasis, but one or two of these symptoms may be absent. Charcot's triad plus shock and central nervous system symptoms (Reynold's pentad) are pathognomonic for acute toxic cholangitis caused by complete obstruction and the presence of infected bile under pressure in the duct. In most cases of choledocholithiasis, the physical examination is normal, but jaundice and mild abdominal tenderness may be present. The white blood cell count may be elevated when cholangitis is present, and elevation of serum bilirubin and alkaline phosphatase is characteristic. The definitive diagnosis is made by percutaneous transhepatic or endoscopic retrograde cholangiography.

TREATMENT. Cholangitis should be treated with antibiotics. Acute toxic cholangitis should be treated immediately by percutaneous transhepatic decompression of the duct, or by endoscopic sphincterotomy and extraction of the offending stone. If these are unsuccessful or unavailable, emergency operation and decompression of the duct by insertion of a T-tube should be done. Common duct stones in patients with symptomatic cholelithiasis or those discovered at operative cholangiography should be removed at the time of cholecystectomy. Endoscopic removal should be done in patients who have had previous cholecystectomy. The best method of treatment of patients who present with stones in both the gallbladder and the common duct is not clear. If the symptoms are clearly due to cholelithiasis, cholecystectomy and choledocholithotomy are indicated, but preliminary endoscopic removal of the common duct stones followed by cholecystectomy may be more economical. The elderly or high-risk patient with symptomatic common duct stones usually also has gallbladder stones; endoscopic removal of the common duct stones should be done. The experience is that only about 20 per cent of such patients require cholecystectomy later, although the follow-up period is short.

BILE DUCT STRICTURES

Most bile duct strictures are due to iatrogenic injury during biliary tract surgery. Other causes are chronic pancreatitis, abdominal trauma, impaction of a stone within the duct system, and chemical injury. Bile duct injuries heal with extensive scarring and fibrosis, probably because of damage to the blood supply of the bile ducts.

CLINICAL MANIFESTATIONS AND DIAGNOSIS. In the immediate postoperative period, strictures present with drainage of bile and, in some instances, sepsis. Late strictures are heralded by cholangitis or jaundice. Liver function tests show elevated bilirubin and alkaline phosphatase, and this is an indication for cholangiography by the percutaneous transhepatic or the endoscopic retrograde route. The author prefers the former with simultaneous insertion of a Ring catheter for facilitating duct identification at operation.

TREATMENT. End-to-side Roux-en-Y choledochojejunostomy or hepaticojejunostomy is indicated for high strictures, whereas choledochoduodenostomy may suffice for distal strictures, especially those caused by chronic pancreatitis. The mucosa-to-mucosa anastomosis should be stented for at least 3 months. Percutaneous balloon dilation successfully dilates benign strictures, but long-term studies are sparse. This technique, combined with stenting, may be useful in elderly or high-risk patients.

BILE DUCT CANCER

Bile duct cancer occurs sporadically but is also associated with chronic ulcerative colitis, sclerosing cholangitis, infestation with *Clonorchis sinensis*, the typhoid carrier state, choledochal cyst, and Caroli's disease. Most patients present with jaundice, frequently accompanied by weight loss and mild pain. Sometimes patients present with cholangitis. Liver function studies reveal an obstructive pattern. Cholangiography is essential, and computed tomography is used to assess the radial extent of the growth. Angiography should be done to assess hepatic arterial or portal venous invasion. Cytologic diagnosis is possible from brushings obtained at cholangiography. Preoperative stenting may be useful.

TREATMENT. When resection for cure is precluded by invasion of surrounding structures, the malignant stricture should be stented at operation or percutaneously. Radiation therapy appears to prolong life. Potentially curable lesions in the upper and middle thirds of the extrahepatic duct system should be managed by resection and a Roux-en-Y reconstruction. In high lesions, separate anastomoses of the right and left hepatic ducts stented by Silastic tubes brought out through the liver and skin are usually necessary. The tubes should be changed periodically under fluoroscopic guidance. Cancers in the lower third of the duct system require resection by the Whipple procedure. Only about 10 per cent of patients with bile duct cancer are cured. The value of adjuvant radiation therapy and chemotherapy has not been established.

SCLEROSING CHOLANGITIS

This inflammatory disease of the bile ducts causes fibrosis and thickening of their walls and short, concentric strictures. About 70 per cent of cases are associated with ulcerative colitis, and other rare associations have been noted. Most cases occur in individuals less than 45 years of age. The male to female ratio is 3:2. The signs and symptoms include fatigue, anorexia, weight loss, jaundice, pruritus, and vague abdominal pain. The diagnosis is made by the typical appearance on cholangiography and liver biopsy.

TREATMENT. The primary treatment is medical; steroids have been the mainstay until recently, with early results suggesting that ursodeoxycholic acid causes marked improvement. Surgical exploration may be necessary when cholangiocarcinoma cannot be excluded. When a dominant stricture is present at the bifurcation of the right and left hepatic ducts, some have advocated resection of the distal duct system and anastomosis of the hepatic ducts to a Roux-en-Y segment of jejunum, with individual stenting by Silastic tubes brought through the liver and the abdominal wall. In general, surgical treatment can occasionally be helpful in unique anatomic situations, but the definitive treatment of the disease is transplantation of the liver, for which 5-year survival rates are about 60 per cent.

I

Acute Cholecystitis
David L. Nahrwold, M.D.

Acute cholecystitis is a bacterial or chemical inflammation of the gallbladder. Stones are present in the gallbladder in 95 per cent (calculous cholecystitis) and absent in 5 per cent (acalculous cholecystitis).

ACUTE CALCULOUS CHOLECYSTITIS

The incidence is higher in females than in males and increases with age. Approximately 20 per cent of cholecystectomies are done for acute cholecystitis. The disease is probably caused by obstruction of the cystic duct or gallbladder outlet by a stone, producing edema, ischemia, and inflammation. Bacteria are found in 50 to 75 per cent of patients. Untreated, the process produces complications of

See the corresponding chapter or part in the *Textbook of Surgery*, 14th edition, pp. 1050–1057, for a more detailed discussion of this topic, including a comprehensive list of references.

acute cholecystitis, which are pericholecystic abscess, perforation, and cholecystoenteric fistula with or without gallstone ileus.

CLINICAL MANIFESTATIONS. Persistent pain in the right upper quadrant or the epigastrium is present in almost all patients. Often, the pain radiates around the right side toward the tip of the scapula. Nausea and vomiting are the only other frequent symptoms. The greater severity and longer duration of the pain distinguish acute cholecystitis from an attack of gallbladder colic.

Tenderness in the right upper quadrant or epigastrium is generally present. Voluntary or involuntary guarding is a common feature. Inspiratory arrest during palpation of the right upper quadrant, Murphy's sign, is an inconsistent albeit pathognomonic sign. Mild jaundice, probably due to bile pigment absorbed from the diseased organ, is frequent. Concomitant choledocholithiasis is found in 10 to 15 per cent of patients.

LABORATORY FINDINGS. The white blood cell count is usually elevated, and mild increases in serum amylase and serum bilirubin are frequent. Approximately 15 per cent of stones are seen on an abdominal roentgenogram owing to the presence of calcium. The specific test for acute cholecystitis is cholescintigraphy with a derivative of ^{99m}technetium, a test with an accuracy rate of over 90 per cent in patients with calculous cholecystitis. Ultrasonography detects stones but is not specific for the diagnosis of acute cholecystitis.

DIFFERENTIAL DIAGNOSIS. The differential diagnosis includes acute appendicitis, pancreatitis, penetrating or perforated duodenal ulcer, acute pyelonephritis, and right-sided pneumonia. Conditions that cause pain from acute hepatic enlargement, such as hepatitis, must also be considered.

TREATMENT. Antibiotic therapy should be administered as soon as the diagnosis is made. A second-generation cephalosporin suffices in most cases, but the combination of ampicillin, clindamycin, and an aminoglycoside may be necessary in patients who are seriously ill with sepsis. The antibiotic should be discontinued after 24 hours unless peritonitis is present, in which case it should be continued for 7 days.

The definitive therapy is cholecystectomy. The patient should be thoroughly evaluated for risk factors, especially cardiac and cerebrovascular disease. Early operation, usually within 6 to 24 hours of admission, is indicated in patients without significant risk factors. The alternative is to treat the patient medically until the acute inflammation is resolved and delay the operation for 4 to 6 weeks. Delayed operation is advisable in patients who have significant risk factors, including unstable angina, clinically significant carotid artery disease, congestive heart failure, cirrhosis, and other conditions known to significantly increase the risk of operation. At operation, decompression of the gallbladder with the use of a trochar facilitates the dissection. Although some disagree, the author believes that an operative cholangiogram should be obtained unless the inflammation and friability of the tissue makes it dangerous to do so. Cholecystostomy should be done when cholecystectomy is too dangerous, a circumstance that arises only rarely.

ACUTE ACALCULOUS CHOLECYSTITIS

Acute acalculous cholecystitis represents 4 to 8 per cent of all cases of acute cholecystitis and is more common in males than in females. The disease has a tendency to be associated with other diseases or conditions, including major trauma, burns, major surgical procedures, multiple transfusions, childbirth, bacterial sepsis, and debilitating diseases such as sarcoidosis, lupus erythematosus, and polyarteritis nodosa. No precipitating factor is apparent in about 50 per cent of cases. Patients who develop the disease after major operations or after trauma often have gallstones.

The etiology is not known. The theories include stasis of gallbladder bile that could produce a functional gallbladder outlet obstruction, ischemia of the gallbladder causing the development of gangrene, and sepsis causing bacterial infection directly or through the adverse effects of endotoxin or other bacterial products.

CLINICAL MANIFESTATIONS AND DIAGNOSIS. The diagnosis may be delayed because the patient cannot communicate well owing to a concomitant disease or the postoperative or posttraumatic state. Pain in the right upper quadrant or the epigastrium is present in 70 per cent, and vomiting occurs in about 35 per cent of patients. Right upper quadrant tenderness, fever, abdominal distention, and absent or hypoactive bowel sounds are the predominant physical findings. Cholescintigraphy should be done when the disease is suspected, but in acute acalculous cholecystitis, the test is only 85 to 90 per cent accurate because of a high rate of false-positive tests.

TREATMENT. Percutaneous aspiration of bile for microscopic examination and culture followed by immediate establishment of a percutaneous tube cholecystostomy has been used increasingly as a combined diagnostic and therapeutic maneuver. However, the standard treatment has been cholecystectomy. Mortality and morbidity are higher than for uncomplicated acute cholecystitis because of the associated diseases and the frequent delay in diagnosis.

II

Chronic Cholecystitis and Cholelithiasis

David L. Nahrwold, M.D.

Approximately 20 million Americans have gallstones, and approximately 475,000 cholecystectomies are done annually. The incidence is three times higher in women than in men, and the prevalence of stones increases with age. Approximately 80 per cent of gallstones are composed predominantly of cholesterol, and 20 per cent are pigment stones. Pigment stones are classified as black pigment stones, which are associated with hemolysis and cirrhosis, and calcium bilirubinate stones, which are associated with infection in the biliary tract.

Biliary lecithin and bile salts form micelles, which solubilize cholesterol. When the relative amounts of these three substances are such that not all the cholesterol present can be solubilized, the bile is said to be lithogenic. Stone formation involves saturation of cholesterol in bile, nucleating factors, and stasis of bile in the gallbladder.

PATHOLOGY. Chronic cholecystitis may occur primarily (primary chronic cholecystitis) or follow an attack of acute cholecystitis (secondary chronic cholecystitis). The secondary type is characterized by granulomas containing cholesterol clefts, fibrosis of the muscular layer, loss of the villous appearance of the mucosa, and thickening of the entire organ. The gallbladder retains its thin-walled appearance in the primary type, and the mucosa retains its villous appearance. The inflammatory cell infiltrate is predominantly lymphocytes. Stones are almost always present in both types.

CLINICAL MANIFESTATIONS AND DIAGNOSIS. Chronic cholecystitis and cholelithiasis are manifest by repeated attacks of right upper quadrant or epigastric pain that typically radiates around the right side toward the tip of the scapula. Nausea and vomiting are frequent. Attacks often follow large meals, and patients often have a sensation of fullness or bloating between episodes. The cardinal symptom is pain. Physical findings are present only during an attack and include right upper quadrant or epigastric tenderness to palpation and voluntary muscle guarding, but no signs of peritonitis.

The diagnosis should be confirmed by ultrasonography, which has an accuracy rate of over 95 per cent when carefully performed. Oral cholecystography, which is less accurate, should be done when the symptoms are typical and ultrasonography is normal or equivocal.

TREATMENT. Treatment of an attack of gallbladder colic is parenteral administration of a narcotic for relief of pain.

See the corresponding chapter or part in the *Textbook of Surgery*, 14th edition, pp. 1057–1063, for a more detailed discussion of this topic, including a comprehensive list of references.

Avoidance of dietary fat may be helpful in some patients. The definitive treatment of symptomatic gallstones is cholecystectomy. The mortality for elective cholecystectomy is approximately 0.5 per cent and is lower in patients under age 50 years. The higher risk in elderly patients emphasizes the need of detecting cerebrovascular and cardiovascular disease. Elective cholecystectomy should be delayed until after coronary artery bypass or carotid artery revascularization, when they are indicated.

Prophylactic antibiotic administration is indicated in patients over age 60 years, those recovering from acute cholecystitis, and patients known to have bile duct stones. The author always performs operative cholangiography for detection of anomalies of the duct system and unsuspected stones, but some disagree with this policy.

Gallstone Dissolution. Ursodeoxycholic acid reduces the amount of cholesterol in bile and effectively dissolves cholesterol gallstones in approximately 50 per cent of properly selected patients within 2 years. Patients should have radiolucent stones less than 2 cm. in diameter in a functioning gallbladder. Criteria that favor dissolution are ideal body weight, small stones, few stones, and stones that float on bile. The recurrence rate approximates 10 per cent per year for the first 5 years, following which it remains relatively stable.

Extracorporeal Shock Wave Lithotripsy. Lithotripters generate acoustic shock waves under water and focus them on gallstones within the gallbladder. Shock waves pass through soft tissue, which has a high water content, without causing injury but create forces within gallstones that cause them to fragment. The procedure can be done on an outpatient basis with intravenous analgesia. Typically, 1500 to 2000 shock waves are applied over approximately an hour, and the stones are fragmented into pieces less than 5 mm. in diameter. Retreatments may be necessary. Adjuvant (ursodeoxycholic acid) therapy is essential. Patients should have fewer than four radiolucent stones, each less than 3 cm., in a functioning gallbladder. In highly selected patients, the stone-free rates are approximately 35 per cent at 6 months, 65 per cent at 12 months, and over 90 per cent at 2 years. The best success is with small, single stones. Pain on passage of the fragments is common, but serious complications are infrequent. Stone recurrence is inevitable in some patients.

Stone Dissolution. Percutaneous catheterization of the gallbladder and instillation of methyl *tert*-butyl ether (MTBE) is highly effective in dissolving cholesterol gallstones. Small aliquots are infused and withdrawn by use of an automatic system designed for preventing overflow of MTBE into the duodenum, which may produce duodenitis and anesthesia. In carefully selected patients, 95 per cent of the stone mass was dissolved in almost all patients within an average of 12.5 hours. As in all techniques in which the gallbladder is not removed, recurrence of stones is likely.

Laparoscopic cholecystectomy, in which the gallbladder is removed with use of instruments and scopes passed through quite small incisions in the abdomen, has gained rapid popularity recently with several large series in the literature. It is currently the operative therapy of choice in most instances. The procedure is followed by less postoperative pain, smaller scars, more rapid mobilization, and faster return to full-time work. It is also somewhat less costly.

Other Techniques. Percutaneous cholecystolithotomy, in which the gallbladder is catheterized, the tract is dilated after several weeks, and the stones are extracted, is currently being evaluated. Before extraction, large stones can be fragmented by the rigid ultrasonic lithotripter, an electrohydraulic lithotripter, or a laser fiber.

III

Cholangitis
David L. Nahrwold, M.D.

Cholangitis is a bacterial or parasitic infection of the biliary duct system that is always associated with partial or complete bile duct obstruction. In practice, the term is used to denote the signs and symptoms of bacterial inflammation of the bile ducts without regard for the presence or absence of inflammatory changes in the walls of the ducts or surrounding structures.

PATHOGENESIS. Bacteria probably enter bile through the portal venous system. Normally, they are phagocytosed in the liver by the reticuloendothelial system, but colonization of bile apparently is facilitated when an obstructing lesion or foreign body is present in the biliary tract. The symptoms of cholangitis occur when bacteria or their products enter the circulation from the biliary tract, usually in association with an increase in pressure caused by partial or complete obstruction. Bile canaliculi communicate with the hepatic sinusoids at their terminal ends, and cholangiovenous reflux of particles approximating the size of bacteria has been demonstrated experimentally. The organisms most frequently found in the blood of patients with cholangitis are, in decreasing order, *Escherichia coli*, *Klebsiella pneumoniae*, and *Streptococcus faecalis*. Anaerobic organisms, most commonly *Bacteroides fragilis*, are found less frequently.

ASSOCIATED PATHOLOGY. Calculi are the most frequent cause of cholangitis. They may migrate from the gallbladder or form *de novo* in the bile ducts. The latter are usually predominantly calcium bilirubinate, the formation of which involves beta-glucuronidase produced by biliary bac-

---

See the corresponding chapter or part in the *Textbook of Surgery*, 14th edition, pp. 1064–1069, for a more detailed discussion of this topic, including a comprehensive list of references.

teria. Occasionally, cholangitis is caused by the malignant strictures of cholangiocarcinoma, pancreatic cancer, or ampullary carcinoma. Benign strictures, caused by operative trauma or sclerosing cholangitis, are frequently associated with cholangitis. Most patients with stricture have bacterbilia and are prone to develop calcium bilirubinate stones as well. An episode of cholangitis in the patient with a biliary-enteric anastomosis is evidence of stricture formation or the presence of a stone. The fibrosis of chronic pancreatitis is an increasingly frequent cause of stricture in the distal portion of the common duct. Procedures such as T-tube cholangiography, the removal and replacement of indwelling stents, and endoscopic retrograde cholangiography frequently precipitate an episode of cholangitis. The presence of a T-tube or stent in the biliary system causes bacterbilia within a week in over 90 per cent of cases. The parasites *Clonorchis sinensis*, *Trichuris trichiura*, and *Ascaris lumbricoides* cause obstruction and bacterbilia; they are frequent causes of cholangitis in the Orient.

CLINICAL MANIFESTATIONS. Charcot's original description of the symptoms, chills and fever, jaundice, and abdominal pain, remain the hallmarks of acute cholangitis and are known as Charcot's triad. These symptoms plus shock and central nervous system depression, Reynold's pentad, are manifestations of acute toxic cholangitis, in which complete obstruction of a duct converts the duct system to an abscess under pressure. The entire system may be filled with pus.

The complete triad of symptoms occurs in only 50 to 70 per cent of patients with cholangitis, and fever is the most common (90 per cent), followed by pain and jaundice (80 per cent). The most consistent physical finding is tenderness in the right upper quadrant or epigastrium. Abnormal laboratory findings include elevation of the white blood cell count, serum bilirubin, and alkaline phosphatase. Bacteremia, manifested by positive blood cultures, is present in slightly less than half of patients.

TREATMENT. The principles of therapy are control of the infection and correction of the underlying cause. Antibiotic therapy is indicated in all patients who have significant symptoms. A second- or third-generation cephalosporin is adequate for mild cases, but the author treats patients with severe acute cholangitis or acute toxic cholangitis with the combination of ampicillin, clindamycin, and an aminoglycoside.

Patients who have acute toxic cholangitis with central nervous system depression and circulatory instability should have immediate definitive therapy. Percutaneous transhepatic decompression of the duct system is preferred, but endoscopic sphincterotomy and extraction of the obstructing stone is also effective. If these therapies are not successful or available, immediate laparotomy and decompression of the duct system by insertion of a T-tube is mandatory.

After the infection has been controlled in routine cases, the cause of the obstruction must be located and corrected. Ultrasonography and computed tomography are useful in the detection of masses and calculi, but the definitive test is cholangiography done by either the percutaneous transhepatic or the endoscopic route. When the underlying cause of cholangitis is delineated, appropriate therapy should be instituted.

IV

Gallstone Ileus and Fistula
Francis E. Rosato, M.D.

BILIARY FISTULAS

A biliary fistula is an abnormal communication between any portion of the biliary tree and some other area. If the communication is to the outside, it is termed an external fistula, whereas connection with other body structures is termed internal fistula. External fistulas are most often due to trauma, especially operative trauma on the biliary tree, and present as bile leaks externally. Internal fistulas are most often the result of inflammatory or neoplastic disease, and presentation depends on the structure in connection with the biliary tree. Biliary-intestinal fistulas may allow gallstones to enter the intestinal tract with resultant distal small bowel obstruction (see later); biliary-bronchial connections can cause biloptysis (bile-stained sputum); biliary to urinary bladder connections could produce bile-stained urine. All such connections—external and internal—allow bacterial contamination of bile and resultant cholangitis, a prominent mode of presentation in any and all fistulas.

COMPLICATIONS. There are four important complications of fistula: (1) hyponatremia due to the external loss of the sodium content of bile either externally or into other structures; (2) weight loss—the loss of bile to the gastrointestinal tract in all but biliary–high intestinal fistulas can cause the malabsorption syndrome; (3) infection—all bile fistulas potentially allow bacterial contamination of bile (cholangitis); the classic presentation of such cholangitis is Charcot's triad of jaundice, fever, and shaking chills; (4) gallstone ileus (see following section on gallstone ileus).

TREATMENT. There are five major components to treatment.

1. Define the fistula. This is most easily done through an external fistulogram with the injection of contrast material into the external opening of the fistula. For internal fistulas, other studies including a gastrointestinal series, barium

---

See the corresponding chapter or part in the *Textbook of Surgery*, 14th edition, pp. 1070–1072, for a more detailed discussion of this topic, including a comprehensive list of references.

enema, cholangiography, bronchoscopy, or cystography may be necessary for delineation of the fistula.

2. Discover the cause of the fistula. The studies mentioned for delineating the extent of the fistula may also provide evidence as to the cause. Cytologic studies of aspirated material may also help to establish neoplasm when it is the cause of the fistula. Presently 85 per cent of all internal fistulas are due to gallstone disease, with inflammation establishing a cholecystoenteric fistula, whereas 8 per cent are due to peptic ulcer disease. Operative trauma is responsible for most external fistulas.

3. Control infection. Cholangitis is a prominent part of the problem. Bile cultures can be useful in choosing the most appropriate antibiotic, but those with a high enterohepatic recirculation and a spectrum against gram-negative aerobic and anaerobic organisms are ideal.

4. Correct electrolyte abnormalities, particularly regarding sodium depletion.

5. Surgical therapy. The initial approach is usually percutaneous drainage of any bile collections associated with internal or external biliary fistulas, usually aided by computed tomographic scan or ultrasound guidance. This measure alone suffices to allow the resolution of most external biliary fistulas. Where indicated, the relief of distal common ductal obstruction through papillotomy by endoscopic retrograde cholangiopancreatography may allow normal flow of bile with resolution of many external and internal fistulas. When continuing jaundice, sepsis, electrolyte abnormalities, or worsening nutrition continue despite such measures, surgical therapy is indicated. At operation, an attempt is made to establish the cause of the fistula. For external fistulas, relief of obstruction may suffice. At times, formal biliary-enteric anastomoses must be constructed and bile duct repairs done in conjunction with attempts at relieving obstruction. For internal fistulas, separation of the partner structures is done with surgical closure of each. When neoplasia is the underlying cause, separation is often not possible, but relief of obstruction to bile flow is the objective. For fistulas secondary to gallstone disease, a simple cholecystectomy with repair of the biliary partner structure is sufficient. When peptic ulcer disease is the underlying cause, separation of the communicating structures, repair of both, and definitive acid-reducing procedures are combined for definitive treatment.

GALLSTONE ILEUS

When an antecedent cholecystointestinal or choledochointestinal fistula occurs, the potential exists for the migration of gallstones into the intestine. They cause obstruction when they can no longer negotiate the more narrow reaches of the small intestine. These are most common (4:1) in women, and 80 per cent occur in those over the age of 70 years. Although a relatively rare occurrence, it is always to be borne in mind when small bowel obstruction presents in older individuals, particularly in the absence of previous surgical procedures.

The diagnosis is based on a recognition of the following diagnostic features: air in the biliary tree (from the antecedent biliary-enteric fistula); a typical presentation of dilated small bowel loops; the finding of an opaque stone in the intestinal tract by radiography; and, more recently, the finding of nonopaque stones in the distal small bowel with the use of ultrasound.

TREATMENT. The first priority in gallstone ileus is the removal of the obstructing stone, usually located in the distal small bowel. If the patient is at high risk or if there has been instability of vital signs in the course of the operation, this suffices. If definitive "take down" of the underlying biliary-enteric fistulas (usually cholecystoenteric) is not performed, there is a 10 per cent likelihood of recurrence of the phenomenon. Where possible, therefore, definitive correction of the underlying fistula should be performed either as a part of the initial procedure or as a planned second operation when the patient is judged well enough.

V

Carcinoma of the Gallbladder
David Fromm, M.D.

Carcinoma of the gallbladder is the most common malignant lesion of the biliary tract and is more frequent in those at least 50 years old and female. There is a well-established association between this type of cancer and gallstones, which are present in at least 70 per cent of cases. Cancer of the gallbladder associated with cholelithiasis occurs in approximately 0.5 per cent of autopsies, whereas this figure is approximately 1 to 2 per cent in patients undergoing cholecystectomy. There is no predilection for the development of carcinoma in a gallbladder containing single or multiple stones. However, there may be a relationship to larger stones. Other conditions presumably associated with the development of carcinoma are cholecystoenteric fistula, porcelain gallbladder, congenital biliary dilation, a long common biliary channel distal to the entry of the pancreatic duct, and ulcerative colitis. Adenomatous residue has been found in 19 per cent of cases of invasive carcinoma.

Adenocarcinoma comprises 82 per cent of cases; undifferentiated carcinoma occurs in 7 per cent, and squamous cell occurs in 3 per cent. Unusual tumors include adenoacanthoma, lymphosarcoma, rhabdomyosarcoma, reticulum cell

---

See the corresponding chapter or part in the *Textbook of Surgery*, 14th edition, pp. 1070–1072, for a more detailed discussion of this topic, including a comprehensive list of references.

sarcoma, fibrosarcoma, melanoma, carcinoid, and carcinosarcoma. The tumor spreads by several routes: lymphatic, vascular, intraperitoneal seeding, neural, intraductal, and direct extension. The various forms of liver involvement include spread along the bile ductules, veins, and lymphatics and by direct extension.

The symptoms of carcinoma of the gallbladder are not specific. Pain occurs in 66 per cent, weight loss in 59 per cent, jaundice in 51 per cent, anorexia in 40 per cent, and right upper quadrant mass in 40 per cent of patients. Malignancy in patients with pre-existing biliary symptoms generally produces a noticeable change in symptoms. A right upper quadrant mass may be apparent and is usually tender. Jaundice most often is due to invasion of the common duct or compression from involved pericholedochal lymph nodes and, less frequently, involvement of the liver; rarely, it is due to concurrent stones in the biliary tract. The diagnosis is infrequently made by radiographic studies or even preoperatively. Those with early, resectable lesions tend to have symptoms of benign biliary disease.

Malignancy of the gallbladder usually is associated with a dismal prognosis. Approximately 88 per cent die within a year of diagnosis, and only approximately 4 per cent are alive after 5 years. Most of the long-term survivors are those in whom the surgeon was unaware of the presence of the tumor at the time of cholecystectomy (approximately 12 per cent of cases of carcinoma), the diagnosis being made by the pathologist. Nearly all patients with invasion confined to the mucosa and muscularis and who survive operation are alive at 5 years, whereas only about 7 per cent with serosal (or adventitial) involvement are alive at 5 years. It is a rare patient who is symptomatic from the tumor and who enjoys prolonged survival following operative treatment.

There continues to be debate concerning the utility of radical resection of the tumor. Proponents of a radical approach optimistically maintain that up to 30 per cent of patients present with tumors that could be encompassed by radical cholecystectomy, which includes in-continuity resection of the hepatic bed or right hepatic lobectomy (or even trisegmentectomy) and regional lymph node dissection. Yet, only a few long-term survivors have been reported following radical surgical therapy. Radical excision may be followed by death from disseminated metastases as soon as 2 months later, despite what appeared to be adequate resection at operation.

Moderate palliation is occasionally achieved by operation, although benefits are usually of short duration. Palliation is primarily directed to relief of common duct obstruction or bypassing an obstructed portion of the gastrointestinal tract. Some palliation may also be achieved by removing the gallbladder, when feasible, in the hope of delaying obstruction of surrounding structures. There are few reports concerning chemotherapy and/or radiation therapy, which thus far have questionable benefit.

Obstructive jaundice occurring some time after cholecystectomy can be difficult to treat by operation because of tumor encroachment in the porta hepatis. Placement of a prosthesis endoscopically or percutaneously through a malignant stricture in the common duct or hepatic bifurcation can successfully reduce symptoms relating to biliary obstruction. However, long-term palliation appears more related to tumor extent than to resolution of jaundice.

35

THE PANCREAS

Charles J. Yeo, M.D., and John L. Cameron, M.D.

ANATOMY

The pancreas is a retroperitoneal organ that extends obliquely from the duodenal C loop to the hilum of the spleen. It is divided into four portions: head, neck, body, and tail. The head is intimately associated with the second portion of the duodenum, and these two structures are jointly supplied by the pancreaticoduodenal arteries. The blood supply to the body and tail of the pancreas is via a more variable complex of arteries. The venous drainage of the pancreas corresponds to the segmental arterial supply and terminates in the portal vein. Multiple lymph node groups drain the pancreas, largely corresponding to the venous drainage patterns. A dual sympathetic and parasympathetic innervation subserves the pancreas.

HISTOLOGY

The pancreas incorporates both an endocrine and exocrine organ system. The endocrine portion resides in nearly spherical collections of cells scattered throughout the pancreatic parenchyma, the islets of Langerhans. Each islet is composed of several distinctive cell types. Beta cells produce insulin and comprise the majority of the islet cell population. Alpha cells produce glucagon and constitute approximately one quarter of the total islet cell number. Other cells found within the islets include somatostatin-producing delta cells as well as cells that produce pancreatic polypeptide, gastrin, and vasoactive intestinal polypeptide. The acini and ductal systems constitute the exocrine portion of the pancreas. Each acinus is composed of a single layer of acinar cells, which contain zymogen granules in their narrow, centrally located apical portion. The pancreatic ductal system originates in the centroacinar cells of each individual acinus and includes intercalated duct cells and cells of the main excretory duct.

PHYSIOLOGY

EXOCRINE. The final product of the exocrine pancreas is a clear isotonic solution with a pH in the range of 8. The two distinct components of pancreatic exocrine secretion are enzyme secretion originating from acinar cells and water and electrolyte secretion originating from the centroacinar and intercalated duct cells. Cholecystokinin is the most potent

---

See the corresponding chapter or part in the *Textbook of Surgery*, 14th edition, pp. 1076–1107, for a more detailed discussion of this topic, including a comprehensive list of references.

endogenous hormone known to stimulate pancreatic enzyme secretion. Secretin is the most potent endogenous stimulant of pancreatic electrolyte secretion.

ENDOCRINE. The release of *insulin* into the portal blood is controlled by the concentration of blood glucose, vagal interactions, and local concentrations of somatostatin. The major stimulus for *glucagon* release is a fall in serum glucose. *Pancreatic polypeptide* appears to function physiologically for regulation of pancreatic exocrine secretion and biliary tract motility. *Somatostatin* has a broad inhibitory spectrum of gastrointestinal activity.

ACUTE PANCREATITIS

Acute pancreatitis can vary from mild parenchymal edema to severe hemorrhagic destruction associated with loss of pancreatic viability, gangrene, and subsequent necrosis. Nine of 10 patients experience mild to moderate symptoms and improve with supportive care alone, whereas 10 per cent of patients develop a severe life-threatening form of acute pancreatitis.

ETIOLOGY. There are many causes of acute pancreatitis (Table 1). In 90 per cent of the cases, the cause is related to excessive alcohol intake or biliary tract disease.

CLINICAL PRESENTATION. The predominant clinical feature of acute pancreatitis is midepigastric abdominal pain. Nausea and vomiting frequently accompany the abdominal pain. Typical findings on examination include fever, tachycardia, epigastric tenderness, and abdominal distention. Patients with severe pancreatitis may manifest hypotension, hypovolemia, hypoperfusion, and obtundation.

DIAGNOSIS. The diagnosis of acute pancreatitis is supported by appropriate laboratory determinations and radiographic findings. Measurement of the serum amylase is the most widely used laboratory test for diagnosing acute pancreatitis. Hyperamylasemia is commonly observed within 24 hours of the onset of symptoms but gradually returns to normal levels. Persistent hyperamylasemia beyond the initial week of the illness may indicate the development of pan-

TABLE 1. Etiologic Factors of Acute Pancreatitis

Alcohol	Pancreatic duct obstruction
Biliary tract disease (gallstones)	Tumor
Hyperlipidemia	Pancreas divisum
Hypercalcemia	Ampullary stenosis
Familial	*Ascaris* infestation
Trauma	Duodenal obstruction
External	Viral infection
Operative	Scorpion venom
Retrograde pancreatography	Drugs
Ischemia	Idiopathic
Hypotension	
Cardiopulmonary bypass	
Atheroembolism	
Vasculitis	

TABLE 2. Diagnosis of Acute Pancreatitis

Laboratory Tests	Radiographic Procedures
Serum amylase	Plain chest roentgenogram
Serum amylase isoenzymes	Plain abdominal roentgenogram
Urinary amylase	Upper gastrointestinal contrast
Amylase: creatinine clearance ratio	series
	Ultrasonography
Serum lipase	Computed tomography
Serum methemalbumin	Magnetic resonance imaging
Peritoneal fluid analysis	

creatic pseudocyst, phlegmon, abscess, or ongoing acute pancreatic inflammation. The measurement of serum amylase is not an ideal marker for the diagnosis of acute pancreatitis. In an effort to improve the accuracy of the laboratory diagnosis of acute pancreatitis, several other tests have been utilized (Table 2). Radiographic findings can support the clinical and laboratory evidence of acute pancreatitis. Results of chest and abdominal radiographs are nonspecific. Abdominal sonography can be useful in assessing for cholelithiasis and choledocholithiasis in patients with suspected gallstone-associated pancreatitis. Currently the most widely accepted and sensitive radiographic method used to confirm the diagnosis of acute pancreatitis is computed tomography (CT). A correlation exists between the degree of CT abnormality and the clinical course and severity of acute pancreatitis.

CLINICAL COURSE. The severity and prognosis of an attack of acute pancreatitis can be predicted by use of routinely available clinical and laboratory determinations (Table 3). Patients with two or fewer prognostic signs generally require simple supportive care and have no major morbidity or mortality. In contrast, patients with three or more prognostic signs have a stepwise increase in morbidity and mortality rates.

NONOPERATIVE MANAGEMENT. The initial management of patients with acute pancreatitis is nonoperative. Therapy includes intravenous fluid and electrolyte replacement with crystalloid solutions. Nasogastric decompression is used in patients with significant ileus in an effort to prevent

TABLE 3. Ranson's Early Prognostic Signs of Acute Pancreatitis

At Admission	During Initial 48 Hours
Age over 55 years	Hematocrit fall >10 percentage points
WBC >16,000 cells/cu. mm.	
Blood glucose >200 mg./100 ml.	BUN elevation >5 mg./100 ml.
	Serum calcium fall to <8 mg./100 ml.
Serum lactate dehydrogenase >350 IU/liter	Arterial P_{O_2} <60 mm. Hg
AST >250 units/100 ml.	Base deficit >4 mEq./liter
	Estimated fluid sequestration >6 liters

emesis and aspiration. Abdominal pain is treated with careful administration of meperidine. Oral intake is initially prohibited but is resumed when abdominal pain and tenderness subsides and ileus has resolved. Antibiotics are not indicated in the routine treatment of mild to moderate pancreatitis. However, it appears prudent to advise the use of prophylactic antibiotics in patients with three or more Ranson prognostic signs. Respiratory complications require appropriate supportive care.

OPERATIVE MANAGEMENT. Operative intervention is indicated in four specific circumstances.

Uncertainty of Clinical Diagnosis. In this uncommon situation, exploratory laparotomy may be indicated for exclusion of a surgically correctable disease that has a potentially fatal outcome without surgical therapy. The widespread availability of abdominal CT scanning has made these situations less frequent.

Treatment of Pancreatic Sepsis. The development of a pancreatic abscess occurs in up to 5 per cent of all patients with pancreatitis and represents a serious, life-threatening complication. Pancreatic abscess occurs with increasing frequency in direct proportion to the severity of acute pancreatitis. The diagnosis of pancreatic abscess is suspected by clinical and laboratory abnormalities and assisted by CT. The combination of abdominal CT scan with CT-guided percutaneous aspiration appears to be highly reliable in differentiating pancreatic abscess from sterile peripancreatic fluid collections. The treatment of pancreatic abscess combines antibiotic therapy with prompt surgical drainage. Operative débridement is necessary for removal of the thick, pastelike collections of infected necrotic material. Following débridement, the two accepted alternatives for achieving drainage are liberal use of sump drains and open packing of the abscess cavity.

Correction of Associated Biliary Tract Disease. Definitive biliary tract surgery during the index admission is now favored for the majority of patients with gallstone-associated pancreatitis. In the subset of patients with severe disease and a deteriorating clinical course, both the use of endoscopic retrograde cholangiopancreatography (ERCP) to document the presence of choledocholithiasis and subsequent endoscopic sphincterotomy to retrieve stones should be considered.

Deterioration of Clinical Status. The most controversial indication for surgical therapy involves patients with a deteriorating clinical condition. In such cases, proponents of early operative intervention recommend operative procedures ranging from local débridement of necrotic tissue to formal total pancreatectomy. Currently, no controlled randomized clinical trials allow realistic evaluation of the efficacy of such early resectional therapy.

CHRONIC PANCREATITIS

Chronic pancreatitis is an entity encompassing recurrent or persistent abdominal pain of pancreatic origin combined with evidence of exocrine and endocrine insufficiency and marked pathologically by irreversible parenchymal destruction.

ETIOLOGY. Chronic pancreatitis is associated with alcohol abuse, hyperparathyroidism, congenital anomalies of the pancreatic duct, and pancreatic trauma. It may also be idiopathic.

CLINICAL PRESENTATION. Patients typically present in the fourth or fifth decades of life with a history of alcohol abuse and with epigastric and back pain. Anorexia and weight loss may be present. Up to one third of patients have insulin-dependent diabetes, and up to one quarter have steatorrhea. Narcotic abuse is common.

DIAGNOSIS. Chronic pancreatitis is usually suspected on the basis of the clinical setting. Plain abdominal films may reveal pancreatic calcifications. A CT scan of the abdomen is used to evaluate the size and texture of the gland, to inspect for pancreatic parenchymal calcifications and nodularity, and to assess the pancreatic ductal system. Pancreatography can document ductal abnormalities not seen by CT.

NONOPERATIVE MANAGEMENT. Nonoperative management encompasses control of abdominal pain and treatment of endocrine and exocrine insufficiency. In some patients, pain relief may be obtained by abstinence from alcohol. Pain control begins with non-narcotic analgesics, followed later by narcotic analgesics. Diabetes may require cautious insulin therapy. Exocrine insufficiency is treated with exogenous pancreatic enzyme supplementation.

OPERATIVE MANAGEMENT. Surgical treatment is categorized as ampullary procedures, ductal drainage procedures, or ablative procedures. Before consideration of surgical intervention, mandatory evaluation involves pancreatic imaging by CT as well as assessment of pancreatic ductal anatomy by ERCP. *Ampullary procedures* currently have limited application. In patients with the rare finding of focal obstruction at the ampullary orifice, transduodenal sphincteroplasty of the major pancreatic duct may be helpful. The *ductal drainage procedure* most commonly utilized involves a side-to-side pancreaticojejunostomy. Determinants of success for the side-to-side pancreaticojejunostomy include a pancreatic duct greater than 1 cm. in diameter, the presence of pancreatic calcifications, and a pancreatic-jejunal anastomosis longer than 6 cm. Ductal drainage does not improve established pancreatic exocrine or endocrine dysfunction, although it may delay the rate of progressive impairment. *Ablative procedures* are generally reserved for patients who are not candidates for or who have failed ductal drainage procedures. In carefully selected patients with parenchymal disease localized to the body and tail of the pancreas, limited distal pancreatectomy (40 to 80 per cent pancreatectomy) has success. Subtotal distal pancreatectomy (95 per cent pancreatectomy) has been applied to patients with severe diffuse parenchymal disease. Pylorus-preserving pancreaticoduodenectomy is an option in cases without ductal dilation in which parenchymal disease primarily affects the head of the gland. Total pancreatectomy, combined with the necessary duodenal resection, is a last resort measure in carefully selected patients who have failed lesser procedures.

DISRUPTIONS OF THE PANCREATIC DUCT

Disruptions of the pancreatic duct usually occur in the setting of alcoholic pancreatitis, following pancreatic trauma, or as a result of an operative intervention. Disruptions of the pancreatic duct can cause internal or external pancreatic fistulas.

INTERNAL PANCREATIC FISTULA. *Pancreatic pseudocysts* are localized collections of pancreatic secretions that lack an epithelial lining; they are caused by the walling off of a pancreatic duct disruption by surrounding tissues. Pancreatic pseudocysts may develop in up to 10 per cent of patients after acute alcoholic pancreatitis. Patients with pseudocysts most often present with upper abdominal pain, nausea, and vomiting. The majority of patients have elevations of serum amylase. Definitive diagnosis is made by CT scan or ultrasonography. Recent evidence suggests that up to 50 per cent of pseudocysts can be managed nonoperatively without complication. Strict size criteria alone are not sufficient for determining the need for operative versus nonoperative management. For pseudocysts that require operative intervention, preoperative endoscopic retrograde pancreatography may be useful. Options for the management of pseudocysts include *internal drainage* via cystojejunostomy, cystogastrostomy, or cystoduodenostomy; *excision; external drainage;* and *percutaneous* or *endoscopic* drainage techniques. When possible, treatment includes biopsy of the pseudocyst wall for excluding the presence of a cystic neoplasm.

Pancreatic ascites occurs when exocrine secretions extravasate anteriorly from the pancreatic duct and drain freely into the peritoneal cavity. *Pancreatic pleural effusion* can result when exocrine secretions extravasate into the retroperitoneum and track cephalad through the diaphragm into the thorax. Both entities most commonly occur from alcohol abuse, often in the absence of a history of clinical pancreatitis. Patients with pancreatic ascites usually present with painless massive ascites. The diagnosis is best made by paracentesis. Analysis of the ascitic fluid reveals it to be high in amylase (greater than 1000 units per liter) and high in albumin (greater than 3 gm. per 100 ml.). Patients with pancreatic pleural effusion generally present with primary pulmonary symptoms such as dyspnea, chest pain, and cough. The diagnosis of pancreatic pleural effusion is made by thoracentesis. Nonoperative treatment is indicated initially and is recommended for a 2- to 3-week period, since it may resolve the clinical entity in 50 per cent of patients. In patients not cured by nonoperative management, operative intervention follows delineation of pancreatic duct anatomy by ERCP.

EXTERNAL PANCREATIC FISTULA. An external pancreatic fistula is defined as drainage of exocrine secretions through a drain site or a wound that persists for greater than 7 days. Complications of such fistulas include sepsis, fluid and electrolyte abnormalities, and skin excoriation. Sinography and CT are used to delineate the anatomy of the fistulous tract. Total parenteral nutrition is often utilized to avoid pancreatic stimulation by oral intake and to maximize tissue anabolism. Somatostatin analog may accelerate fistula closure. The majority of external pancreatic fistulas close with nonoperative management. Refractory fistulas require surgical management after delineation of the ductal anatomy by ERCP.

NEOPLASMS OF THE PANCREAS

Exocrine Tumors

Approximately 28,000 new cases of *cancer of the exocrine pancreas* are diagnosed each year in the United States. Cancer of the pancreas is more common in blacks, cigarette smokers, and males, and it appears to be linked to the presence of diabetes mellitus and the use of alcohol. Over 90 per cent of these tumors are duct cell adenocarcinomas, with two thirds arising in the pancreatic head.

PERIAMPULLARY CARCINOMA. Four malignant neoplasms are classified as periampullary neoplasms: cancer of the head of the pancreas (85 per cent), ampullary carcinomas (10 per cent), duodenal carcinomas (less than 5 per cent), and carcinomas of the distal common bile duct (less than 5 per cent). The most common clinical features are jaundice, weight loss, and abdominal pain. The majority of patients will have elevated serum bilirubin and alkaline phosphatase with mild elevations of hepatic transaminases. Currently available serologic tests (such as carcinoembryonic antigen, CA 19-9, and others) are not sufficiently accurate for diagnosis or screening. CT scan is used to determine the size of the primary neoplasm and to detect hepatic metastases. The site of the biliary obstruction is defined by cholangiography, with use of either the percutaneous transhepatic or the endoscopic retrograde route. In patients with potentially resectable tumors, selective celiac and mesenteric angiography is combined with portal venography for staging for resectability.

Nonoperative therapy is an option in patients with documented distant metastases, unresectable local disease, or acute or chronic debilitating illnesses. Efforts should be made to acquire a tissue diagnosis and to palliate abdominal pain and biliary obstruction. Palliation of biliary obstruction can be achieved percutaneously with a transhepatic drainage catheter or endoscopically with an endoprosthesis. Duodenal obstruction is poorly palliated nonoperatively.

The majority of patients with periampullary carcinoma are candidates for *operative therapy*. Hepatic metastases, serosal implants, and lymph node metastases outside of the resection area indicate unresectable disease. For all patients with a preoperative diagnosis of periampullary carcinoma explored with a curative intent, the resectability rate approaches 40 per cent and is lowest for adenocarcinoma of the head of the pancreas (less than 20 per cent) and highest for ampullary carcinoma (approximately 80 per cent). Standard resection for periampullary carcinoma involves a pancreaticoduodenectomy, or Whipple's resection. A modification of the standard Whipple resection, the pylorus-preserving pancreaticoduodenectomy, has gained popularity. Accumulated data indicate no compromise in survival in patients undergoing pylorus preservation. The overall 5-year survival rate for patients with resected periampullary carcinoma approaches 25 per cent. The major determinant of survival is the site of origin of the tumor, with resectable cancers of the duodenum, distal bile duct, and ampulla approaching a 60 per cent 5-year survival rate, whereas resectable carcinoma of the head of the pancreas is associated with a 5-year survival rate of up to 20 per cent.

Palliative surgery for periampullary carcinoma is performed in patients with unresectable disease discovered at the time of laparotomy or in patients with prohibitive risk for resectional therapy whose symptoms are poorly managed nonoperatively. Palliative surgery seeks to alleviate biliary obstruction, duodenal obstruction, and tumor-associated pain.

Chemotherapy alone has yielded no significant improvement in survival after curative resection or as palliative therapy. The combination of radiation and chemotherapy has been shown to prolong survival following curative Whipple's resection. Unresectable periampullary cancer treated adjuvantly by use of either external beam or intraoperative radiation therapy has shown some improvement in local tumor control but little improvement in long-term survival.

CARCINOMA OF THE BODY AND TAIL OF THE PANCREAS. This comprises up to 30 per cent of all cases of pancreatic cancer. Patients generally present with weight loss and abdominal pain. Abdominal CT is the best initial radiographic study. ERCP commonly documents a pancreatic duct cutoff. Prior to laparotomy, visceral arteriography may be helpful. Good-risk patients without evidence of metastatic disease and with favorable arteriographic findings are best served by abdominal exploration with curative intent. The resectability rate for carcinoma of the body and tail of the pancreas is less than 7 per cent, and the prognosis is generally poor (mean survival 5 to 6 months).

BENIGN NEOPLASMS OF THE EXOCRINE PANCREAS. *Cystadenomas* comprise less than 10 per cent of cystic pancreatic lesions. There is a female predilection. Symptoms are often vague and may include abdominal pain and gastrointestinal obstructive symptoms. Cystadenomas may be difficult to differentiate from malignant cystic neoplasms or pancreatic pseudocysts. These tumors have no malignant potential and may be cured by appropriate resection.

Endocrine Tumors

Pancreatic islet cell endocrine tumors are rare and are presumed to originate from neural crest cells. Functional endocrine tumors are conventionally named according to the major hormone produced by the tumor (Table 4). Malignancy

TABLE 4. Classification of Functional Pancreatic Endocrine Tumors

Tumor Name	Major Hormone(s)	Cell Type	Syndrome	Malignancy Rate	Extrapancreatic Location
Insulinoma	Insulin	beta	Hypoglycemia	<15%	Rare
Gastroinoma (Zollinger-Ellison syndrome)	Gastrin	non-beta	Peptic ulcer Diarrhea	50%	Frequent
VIPoma (Verner-Morrison syndrome)	Vasoactive intestinal polypeptide Prostaglandins	non-beta	Hypokalemia Achlorhydria	Majority	Occasional
Glucagonoma	Glucagon	alpha	Hyperglycemia Dermatitis	Majority	Rare
Somatostatinoma	Somatostatin	delta	Hyperglycemia Steatorrhea Gallstones	Majority	Rare

is determined by the presence of local invasion, the spread to regional lymph nodes, or the existence of hepatic or distant metastases. The general principles applicable to the management of patients with suspected functional pancreatic endocrine tumors involve, first, the recognition of the abnormal physiologic mechanism or characteristic syndrome; second, the detection of hormone elevations in serum by radioimmunoassay; and third, the localization and staging of the tumor in preparation for operative therapy. Standard radiographic techniques used for tumor localization include CT with intravenous and oral contrast, visceral angiography, transhepatic portal venous sampling, and intraoperative ultrasonography. The distribution of pancreatic endocrine tumors varies, with gastrinomas and somatostatinomas most commonly being found in the head of the pancreas, whereas insulinomas and glucagonomas tend to be evenly distributed throughout the gland. The goals of surgical therapy include control of symptoms due to hormone excess, excision of maximal neoplastic tissue, and prevention of tumor recurrence.

Insulinoma is the most common endocrine tumor of the pancreas. Symptoms can be categorized as either hypoglycemia-induced catecholamine-surge or neuroglycopenic symptoms. The most reliable method for diagnosing insulinomas involves a monitored 72-hour fast. Other supportive tests include documentation of elevations in serum C-peptide and proinsulin levels, absence of sulfonylureas on serum screening, and absence of anti-insulin antibodies. Following biochemical diagnosis and appropriate localization studies, the treatment of insulinoma is surgical. Up to 90 per cent of patients have benign solitary pancreatic adenomas amenable to surgical cure, often by simple enucleation techniques. Malignant insulinomas occur in 10 to 15 per cent of cases. Pharmacologic therapy with diazoxide may be useful in patients with residual tumor following resection when symptomatic hypoglycemia cannot be avoided by frequent feedings.

Gastrinoma is the second most common functional pancreatic endocrine tumor. Clinical manifestations are related to hypergastrinemia and include peptic ulcer disease, abdominal pain, and reflux esophagitis. The fasting serum gastrin is almost always elevated above normal (100 to 200 pg. per ml.) and may be over 1000 pg. per ml. Gastric acid analysis differentiates ulcerogenic from nonulcerogenic states. Basal acid output in excess of 15 mEq. per hour or a basal acid output/maximal acid output ratio in excess of 0.6 supports the diagnosis of gastrinoma. Provocative testing with the secretin stimulation test should be employed in patients with fasting serum gastrin levels in the range of 200 to 1000 pg. per ml. After confirmation of the diagnosis, patient management involves control of gastric acid hypersecretion and alteration of the natural history of the gastrinoma. All patients undergo radiographic study for localization of the primary tumor and for assessment of metastatic disease. In the absence of documented unresectable disease, all patients undergo exploration with curative intent. Improvements in preoperative localization and intraoperative assessment have yielded surgical cure rates approaching 35 per cent. Survival rates have not been significantly altered by the use of chemotherapy.

VIPoma (Verner-Morrison syndrome) is associated with watery diarrhea, hypokalemia, and either achlorhydria or hypochlorhydria. Preoperative preparation must include correction of fluid and electrolyte deficits. Definitive treatment is surgical excision of the tumor. Over one half of the reported cases have been malignant.

Mild diabetes and severe dermatitis are the hallmarks of the *glucagonoma* syndrome. The characteristic skin rash (necrolytic migratory erythema) usually exhibits cyclic migrations with spreading margins and a healing point of resolution within its center. Most tumors have been large, with metastatic disease present in up to 80 per cent of cases.

Somatostatinoma syndrome is marked by gallstones, diabetes, and steatorrhea. This rare pancreatic endocrine tumor is difficult to diagnose because the early findings are nonspecific. Management encompasses preoperative treatment of hyperglycemia and malnutrition combined with standard radiographic localization and staging studies.

Up to 25 per cent of pancreatic endocrine tumors are classified as *nonfunctional* based on the absence of a clinical syndrome and the lack of elevated serum hormone levels. Nonfunctioning tumors frequently have clinical manifestations similar to the more common exocrine malignancies, such as abdominal pain, jaundice, and gastric outlet obstruction. Nonfunctioning tumors are associated with a higher malignancy rate than are their functioning counterparts. Surgical exploration follows routine radiographic and staging efforts.

PANCREATIC TRAUMA

Less than 2 per cent of patients with abdominal trauma have pancreatic injuries. Pancreatic trauma is commonly associated with injuries to adjacent organs and major vascular structures. No laboratory test is sufficiently accurate for the specific diagnosis of pancreatic injury. CT has gained importance in the serial evaluation of pancreatic trauma. Stable patients with suspected pancreatic injury lacking a specific indication for exploration are usually managed nonoperatively with serial clinical and laboratory follow-up and interval CT scan. Patients who undergo laparotomy for abdominal trauma require complete assessment of the pancreas. Four classes of pancreatic injury are described: *Class I injury,* pancreatic contusion without capsular rupture; *Class II injury,* pancreatic capsular or parenchymal rupture without injury to the main pancreatic duct; *Class III injury,* parenchymal injury associated with rupture or destruction of the main pancreatic duct; and *Class IV injury,* combined severe injuries to the pancreas and duodenum. Class I and Class II injuries are treated by drainage alone. Class III injuries to the body and tail are treated by distal pancreatectomy encompassing the site of the injury. Class III injuries to the head may be débrided and externally drained or drained via Roux-en-Y pancreaticojejunostomy. Surgical options for treatment of Class IV injuries include the serosal patch technique, duodenal decompression with triple ostomy, duodenal diverticularization, or pancreaticoduodenectomy.

PANCREATIC TRANSPLANTATION

There are approximately one million Type I diabetics in the United States. Until recently, their primary therapy involved intermittent administration of subcutaneous insulin. Newer treatment methods include sophisticated insulin delivery systems, pancreatic islet cell transplantation, and vascularized segmental or whole pancreas transplantation. Contraindications for pancreas transplantation include the presence of malignancy, active infection, advanced cardiovascular disease, and major amputations or blindness. The transplantation of pancreatic islet cells alone is theoretically attractive because it avoids vascular and ductular anastomoses and because it has the potential to allow harvesting of islets for multiple recipients from a single donor. Unfortunately, to date there have been no successful human islet allotransplants. In the last two decades, enthusiasm for segmental or whole pancreas transplantation has increased. Whole organ grafts are generally performed, with provision of exocrine drainage via a duodenal segment to the urinary bladder. Bladder-drained grafts allow the serial measurement of urinary amylase excretion as a measure of graft function. Immunosuppressive regimens usually involve quadruple drug therapy with prednisone, azathioprine, cyclosporine, and polyclonal anti–T lymphocyte antibody. The current results of pancreatic allotransplantation indicate a 60 to 80 per cent 1-year graft survival for synchronous pancreas and kidney grafts. Posttransplant patients with functioning grafts demonstrate nearly normal glucose tolerance. Successful grafting appears to be protective against the development of diabetic nephropathy and is associated with subjective improvement in peripheral neuropathy and diabetic retinopathy.

36

THE SPLEEN

Robert D. Croom, III, M.D., George F. Sheldon, M.D.,
and Anthony A. Meyer, Ph.D., M.D.

INDICATIONS FOR SPLENECTOMY

An improved understanding of immune anemia, thrombocytopenia, and neutropenia has clarified the role of splenectomy in many hematologic diseases. Some diseases, such as immune thrombocytopenic purpura, appear to be increasing in incidence. Splenectomy as a means of staging Hodgkin's disease is no longer such an important diagnostic test in the overall approach to that disease, which now can be controlled in most patients by use of radiotherapy and chemotherapy. Splenectomy for splenomegaly associated with selected leukemias and non-Hodgkin's lymphomas is less commonly indicated, since chemotherapy and radiation therapy have become more effective. The most frequent indications for splenectomy are now traumatic injury, immune thrombocytopenic purpura, and hypersplenism.

Splenic Trauma

The spleen is the most common intra-abdominal organ injured in blunt trauma and is a frequently injured organ in penetrating abdominal injury. Injury to the spleen should be suspected in blunt upper abdominal injuries, which commonly occur in motor vehicle or bicycle accidents. Splenic injuries are commonly associated with fractured ribs of the left chest. The signs and symptoms of splenic trauma are those of hemoperitoneum. Generalized and nonspecific abdominal pain in the left upper quadrant occurs in approximately one third of patients with splenic injury. Pain referred to the left shoulder (Kehr's sign) is inconstant.

Diagnostic peritoneal lavage may reveal gross blood or an elevated red blood cell count indicating intraperitoneal hemorrhage. When intraperitoneal hemorrhage is diagnosed by peritoneal lavage, laparotomy is performed for diagnosis and treatment of all bleeding viscera including the spleen. A number of imaging techniques are useful in the diagnosis of splenic injury and include standard abdominal or contrast radiography, splenic arteriography, ultrasonography, isotope scan (^{99m}technetium sulfur colloid), and computed tomography. Computed tomography is probably the most accurate method available for diagnosing splenic injury.

In selected splenic injuries, segmental resection of the spleen is practical and safe. In addition to partial splenectomy, splenorrhaphy, ligation of segmental vessels, and

---

See the corresponding chapter or part in the *Textbook of Surgery*, 14th edition, pp. 1108–1133, for a more detailed discussion of this topic, including a comprehensive list of references.

capsular repair are useful techniques for splenic salvage. Although technically more difficult than splenectomy, splenic repair can be performed with comparable transfusion requirements, reoperation rates, and morbidity. Conservatism in the management of splenic injury has extended beyond repairing and preserving an injured spleen when possible. Because bleeding from splenic trauma appears to be more self-limited in children than in adults, nonoperative therapy has proved to be safe in selected pediatric patients. Nonoperative therapy requires a stable patient who is found by diagnostic tests to have an isolated splenic injury. One pitfall of nonoperative management of splenic trauma is the significant possibility of failing to diagnose and treat concomitant intra-abdominal injuries. An additional concern is that most reported series of nonoperative management of splenic injuries include patients with blood transfusion requirements sufficiently substantial for the expectation of an incidence of transfusion-related hepatitis greater than the statistical probability of postsplenectomy sepsis.

SPLENOSIS AND SPLENIC IMPLANTS. Splenosis is the autotransplantation of splenic tissue following splenic trauma. Appearing as sessile or pedunculated dark red nodules, splenic implants vary in size from a few millimeters to several centimeters in diameter. Splenosis seldom causes symptoms and usually is discovered as an incidental finding at reoperation years after splenic trauma. Isolated reports have described splenosis producing intestinal obstruction from adhesions.

Immune Thrombocytopenic Purpura

Immune thrombocytopenic purpura (ITP, previously idiopathic thrombocytopenic purpura) is a syndrome characterized by a persistently low platelet count. The thrombocytopenia is caused by a circulating antiplatelet factor that causes platelet destruction by the reticuloendothelial system. In most patients, the antiplatelet factor is an immunoglobulin antibody directed toward a platelet-associated antigen. The majority of patients with ITP are young women. ITP is increasing in frequency, and the disease is being diagnosed more often now in men. This increase in part is due to the association of immune thrombocytopenia with the acquired immunodeficiency syndrome (AIDS) and an increasing occurrence of ITP in homosexual men positive for the human immunodeficiency virus, parenteral drug abusers, and hemophiliacs receiving multiple transfusions. The propensity for hemorrhage is reflected by the level of thrombocytopenia.

Diagnosis of immune thrombocytopenia requires the exclusion of drug-dependent antibodies, isoantibodies, collagen vascular disease, lymphoproliferative disorders, thyroid disease, recent viral illness, and spurious thrombocytopenia. Patients with "classic" ITP rarely have a palpable spleen (less than 2 per cent), whereas a palpable spleen that reflects mild to moderate enlargement and an associated high incidence of generalized lymphadenopathy have been found in ITP associated with AIDS. Except for thrombocytopenia, patients with ITP usually have normal blood counts. A peripheral blood smear shows thrombocytopenia, occasionally with an increased number of large platelets. A bone marrow aspirate reveals normal granulocytic and erythrocytic elements with an increased megakaryocyte count.

Thrombocytopenia in patients with ITP usually occurs from a combination of intramedullary platelet removal by reticuloendothelial cells causing ineffective platelet production and decreased survival of circulating platelets due to peripheral sequestration and destruction in the spleen and liver. Successful therapy may produce an increase in the platelet count either by increasing the effective production of platelets or by decreasing peripheral platelet sequestration and destruction. Splenectomy appears to increase platelet survival by removing a major organ of peripheral destruction.

The goal of therapy in chronic ITP is to obtain a complete and sustained remission of the disease and to remove the patient from the risks of hemorrhage. This can be achieved in 80 to 90 per cent of patients. Corticosteroid therapy (prednisone 1 mg. per kg. per day or the therapeutic equivalent) is instituted at the time of diagnosis. Most patients with ITP are improved with steroids, an increase in the platelet count occurring within 3 to 7 days and reaching a maximum in several weeks. Complete and sustained remission with steroids is rare. Splenectomy should be performed in patients with ITP that is refractory to corticosteroid therapy. In the majority of patients, splenectomy is performed electively. Emergent splenectomy is necessary in patients with ITP who have evidence of central nervous system bleeding.

ITP DURING CHILDHOOD. In children, particularly those under the age of 6 years, ITP often appears following a viral upper respiratory infection. In contrast to the adult form of the disease, childhood ITP usually undergoes spontaneous remission without specific therapy. Intracranial hemorrhage is a life-threatening complication of childhood ITP and is an indication for emergency splenectomy. Spontaneous and complete remission occurs in approximately 85 per cent of children with ITP. Those in whom spontaneous remission does not occur within 1 year are considered to have chronic ITP and usually undergo elective splenectomy for avoidance of the risks of chronic thrombocytopenia.

During the immediate postoperative period, steroid therapy is continued intravenously and the platelet count is monitored. It usually is possible to begin tapering the steroid dose immediately, and in patients demonstrating a satisfactory thrombocytosis, steroids are gradually reduced over 4 to 6 weeks and discontinued.

Thrombotic Thrombocytopenic Purpura

Thrombotic thrombocytopenic purpura (TTP) is a syndrome characterized by thrombocytopenia, microangiopathic hemolytic anemia, fluctuating neurologic abnormalities, progressive renal failure, and fever. TTP is produced by widespread deposition of platelet microthrombi, and the pentad of clinical manifestations follows occlusion of arterioles and capillaries by subendothelial and intraluminal deposits of "hyaline" material composed of aggregated platelets and fibrin. The etiology of TTP is unknown. TTP has a peak incidence in the third decade of life and occurs more frequently in females than in males.

Prognosis for untreated patients with TTP is very poor with less than 10 per cent surviving beyond 1 year. A combined therapeutic approach using plasma therapy, antiplatelet agents (aspirin and dipyridamole), and large-dose corticosteroid therapy is instituted immediately after the diagnosis is established. Plasma infusion or plasma exchange using plasmapheresis and replacement with fresh frozen plasma achieves response rates between 70 and 90 per cent. If combined modality therapy fails, splenectomy should be performed. Splenectomy occasionally produces spectacular improvement, particularly when combined with large-dose corticosteroid therapy and antiplatelet drugs.

Hypersplenism

Hypersplenism occurs as a result of a number of ill effects from increased splenic function that may be improved by splenectomy. Hypersplenism is classified as *primary* when the responsible underlying disease cannot be identified for the exaggerated splenic function. Those cases in which a specific or more or less well defined disorder has been diagnosed are classified as *secondary hypersplenism*. Primary hypersplenism is a diagnosis of exclusion and should be accepted only after an exhaustive search for a specific cause of hypersplenism has been unrewarding. Secondary hypersplenism includes a number of diseases sharing the common feature of splenomegaly. Work hypertrophy from immune response and/or red blood cell destruction, venous congestion, myeloproliferation, infiltration, and neoplastic proliferation within the spleen produce variable degrees of splenomegaly. Diverse pathophysiologic mechanisms are involved in the resulting hypersplenism.

Hodgkin's Disease

Hodgkin's disease is a malignant lymphoma characterized by the presence of typical, multinucleate giant cells. The unique cell, described by Sternberg and later Reed, is essential for diagnosis. The disease is slightly more common in men than in women. Most patients with Hodgkin's disease have asymptomatic lymphadenopathy at the time of diagnosis. The site of initial nodal involvement is the cervical area in most patients (65 to 80 per cent) followed by the axillary (10 to 15 per cent) and inguinal (6 to 12 per cent) regions. Constitutional symptoms (B symptoms) such as fever, night sweats, weight loss, and pruritus usually are indicative of widespread involvement and are unfavorable prognostic signs. They may appear simultaneously with lymph node enlargement or may precede development of lymphadenopathy.

There are four histopathologic subtypes of Hodgkin's disease: lymphocyte predominance, nodular sclerosis, mixed cellularity, and lymphocyte depletion. Lymphocyte predominance and nodular sclerosis subtypes have a more favorable prognosis than do mixed cellularity and lymphocyte depletion subtypes. Hodgkin's disease metastasizes initially in a predictable, nonrandom pattern via lymphatic channels to contiguous lymph node groups and organs with a prominent lymphatic tissue component. The predictable mode of spread of Hodgkin's disease provides the basis for irradiation of adjacent lymph node areas in patients with apparently localized disease. Treatment and ultimately survival of patients with Hodgkin's disease depend on the anatomic distribution of the disease and the presence or absence of specific symptoms, the stage of the disease, and the histopathologic subtype.

Since the concept of staging was introduced approximately 25 years ago, the staging process has undergone continued modification with the intent of accurately defining the anatomic sites of involvement and thus improving patient selection for the most appropriate type of therapy. Stage I disease indicates nodal involvement in only one lymph node region. Stage II disease is limited to two or more lymph node regions on the same side of the diaphragm. Stage III involves disease in lymph node regions on both sides of the diaphragm (the spleen is considered a lymph node). Stage IV disease encompasses diffuse or disseminated involvement of one or more distant extranodal organs with or without associated lymph node involvement. The subscripts E and S are used to denote selected patients having localized extranodal disease (e.g., lung, bone, muscle, skin) contiguous to involved nodes and patients having splenic involvement, respectively. Stage is further classified as A (absence) or B (presence) with regard to fever, night sweats, weight loss, and pruritus. *Clinical stage* is dependent on history and physical examination, the initial diagnostic biopsy, laboratory tests, and the results of radiographic and imaging studies. Lymphangiography and abdominal computed tomographic scanning are reliable and complementary tests for evaluating retroperitoneal and abdominal nodal involvement. *Pathologic stage* is more accurate than is the clinical stage because histopathologic data from the bone marrow, liver, spleen, intra-abdominal lymph nodes, and other involved tissues (e.g., bone, skin, lung) provide precise knowledge of the extent of the disease.

Staging laparotomy, which in the past was frequently employed for pathologic staging of Hodgkin's disease, now is being used less frequently. The role of staging laparotomy continues to be re-evaluated as a routine staging procedure for Hodgkin's disease. Diagnostic advantages and contributions of staging laparotomy have helped to significantly change the understanding and therapeutic management of patients with Hodgkin's disease, and the current success and widespread use of combination chemotherapy has challenged the need to know the precise anatomic extent of the disease required for treatment by radiation therapy. Staging laparotomy is not applicable to all patients with Hodgkin's disease and should be performed only in patients in whom the results may change management decisions and plans for therapy. Current treatment of Hodgkin's disease integrates radiation therapy and combination chemotherapy for achievement of the maximal potential for cure.

Non-Hodgkin's Lymphomas

Non-Hodgkin's lymphomas (NHL) constitute a diverse group of primary malignancies of lymphoreticular tissue. The clinical course and natural history of NHL are more variable than those of Hodgkin's disease, the pattern of spread is irregular, and more patients have leukemic features. In contrast to Hodgkin's disease, only about two thirds of patients with NHL initially have asymptomatic lymphadenopathy. In 20 to 35 per cent of patients, the onset of NHL occurs in an extranodal site. In addition to peripheral and mediastinal lymphadenopathy, NHL commonly is found initially as an abdominal mass (retroperitoneal or mesenteric) or as hepatic and/or splenic enlargement. Constitutional symptoms such as fever, weight loss, and night sweats are frequently present. In NHL the mode of spread generally is unpredictable, and most patients have disseminated disease at the time of presentation. As with Hodgkin's disease, chemotherapy and/or radiation therapy are the primary forms of treatment.

NHL having primary presentation in the spleen may present as asymptomatic splenomegaly. If parenchymal expansion secondary to tumor infiltration and congestion becomes massive, splenic pooling and increased regional blood flow may cause hypersplenism. NHL with primary presentation in the spleen may be diagnosed as "idiopathic splenomegaly" until splenectomy permits accurate histopathologic diagnosis.

Splenectomy in NHL also is performed for hematologic depression secondary to hypersplenism or for relief of symptomatic splenomegaly or discomfort from recurrent splenic infarctions. Significant therapeutic benefit can be achieved by splenectomy in 80 to 90 per cent of patients with advanced lymphomas (including Hodgkin's disease).

Chronic Myeloid Leukemia

Chronic myeloid (granulocytic, myelocytic) leukemia is a myeloproliferative abnormality characterized by marked elevation of the leukocyte count from myeloid cells in all stages of maturation and by neoplastic overgrowth of granulocytes in the bone marrow.

Hairy Cell Leukemia

Hairy cell leukemia (leukemic reticuloendotheliosis) is an uncommon form of leukemia characterized by pancytopenia, splenomegaly without significant lymphadenopathy, and characteristic mononuclear cells (hairy cells) in the blood and bone marrow.

Approximately 10 to 15 per cent of patients with hairy cell leukemia have an indolent course with a nearly normal life expectancy and require no specific therapy. These are usually elderly men who have minimal splenomegaly, relatively few hairy cells in the blood, and asymptomatic neutropenia. The remaining 85 to 90 per cent require treatment because of one or more cytopenias that cause symptomatic anemia requiring transfusion, thrombocytopenic bleeding, and repeated infections attributable to neutropenia. For the majority of patients who require some form of therapy shortly after diagnosis, splenectomy continues to be an early consideration. Splenectomy is most appropriate for those patients with severe cytopenias, a large spleen, and patchy bone marrow infiltration. Splenectomy provides rapid palliation, and almost all patients have hematologic improvement.

Patients with hairy cell leukemia with diffuse infiltration of the bone marrow, minimal splenomegaly, and severe cytopenias gain only minor or short-term benefit from splenectomy and require additional therapy. In the past 5 years, interferon-alpha and pentostatin (deoxycoformycin) have been found to be highly effective systemic therapy for hairy cell leukemia.

SPLENECTOMY FOR ANEMIA

Hemolytic anemia is the result of an increase in the rate of red cell destruction. Diagnostic evaluation should include a detailed family history because many hemolytic anemias benefited by splenectomy have a hereditary basis. Congenital hemolytic anemias have a defect intrinsic to the red cell that may involve the cell membrane (hereditary spherocytosis), cellular metabolism (pyruvate kinase deficiency, G-6-PD deficiency), hemoglobin structure (sickle cell anemia), or hemoglobin chain synthesis rates (thalassemia). Acquired hemolytic anemias have an extracorpuscular factor that affects normal red cells.

Hereditary Spherocytosis

Hereditary spherocytosis is a relatively common, genetically determined red blood cell membrane disorder that causes hemolytic anemia. The erythrocyte membrane defect is due to a deficiency in spectrin, a major component of the membrane skeleton that is thought to be responsible for the shape, strength, and reversible deformability of the red blood cell. The membrane abnormality causes a gradual loss of red cell surface area, so that instead of remaining a flexible biconcave disc, the red cell becomes small and spherical. Lacking adequate deformability to traverse the splenic microcirculation, spherocytes are trapped in the splenic red pulp and are eventually destroyed by reticuloendothelial cells.

Hereditary spherocytosis occurs primarily by autosomal

dominant inheritance with variable expression. Twenty to 25 per cent of the cases appear sporadically. Aplastic crisis, which usually is precipitated by a viral illness such as human parvovirus, may produce a rapidly worsening anemia that may be life-threatening. Fluctuating jaundice due to hemolysis is common, and pigment gallstones are frequent, the incidence being directly related to the severity of the hemolysis and patient age. Cholelithiasis develops in 20 to 25 per cent of patients with hereditary spherocytosis but is uncommon before the age of 10 years. Moderate splenomegaly is a characteristic physical finding. Diagnosis is established by the presence of spherocytes in the peripheral blood, reticulocytosis (usually 5 to 20 per cent), an increased osmotic fragility, and a negative Coombs' test.

Splenectomy is indicated in nearly all patients. Following splenectomy, hemolysis is alleviated and clinical cure of the anemia is achieved in most patients. The intrinsic red cell membrane defect is unaltered by splenectomy, but red cell survival becomes normal. With resolution of hemolysis, jaundice disappears, and the increased risk of calculous biliary tract disease is removed.

Hereditary Pyropoikilocytosis

Hereditary pyropoikilocytosis (HPP) is a rare congenital hemolytic anemia that is catalogued along with hereditary elliptocytosis because of certain molecular and morphologic similarities. Distinguished from hereditary elliptocytosis (and hereditary spherocytosis) by marked alterations in red cell morphologic features and by the pattern of inheritance, this severe hemolytic disorder occurs most commonly in blacks. The decision for splenectomy in HPP is deferred until the natural course of the disease has been established. In some newborns, HPP gradually evolves into a morphologic pattern characteristic of hereditary elliptocytosis. "True" HPP persists as a severe hemolytic anemia that usually requires early splenectomy, which greatly reduces hemolysis.

Sickle Cell Anemia

Sickle cell anemia is a hereditary hemolytic anemia occurring in blacks who are homozygous for the sickle hemoglobin (HbS) gene. Sickle hemoglobin (HbS) differs from normal adult hemoglobin (HbA) only in the substitution of valine for glutamic acid in the sixth position of the beta chain. HbS, which results from this single amino acid substitution, imparts the sickle shape to deoxygenated red cells and is responsible for the wide spectrum of clinical features that characterize sickle cell anemia. A combination of two variant hemoglobin genes or a combination of a variant hemoglobin and an interacting thalassemia gene produces doubly heterozygous states designated by both aberrant gene products, for example, HbS/C, HbS/beta-thalassemia.

Patients with sickle cell crisis often have severe abdominal pain and signs of peritoneal irritation similar to those of acute surgical illnesses such as acute cholecystitis and appendicitis. Clinical features of abdominal crisis in patients with sickle cell anemia tend to be similar for a specific individual, and deviation from previous patterns may be an important differentiating feature of an acute surgical illness in patients with sickle cell anemia. The incidence of pigment gallstones in patients with sickle cell anemia increases with age. Calculi appear first in childhood (2 to 4 years of age) and are present in approximately 70 per cent of adult patients.

Thalassemia (Thalassemia Syndromes)

These hereditary anemias are the result of a defect in hemoglobin synthesis in which one of the hemoglobin polypeptide chains is synthesized at a markedly reduced rate. Thalassemia is classified by the deficient peptide chain. Beta-thalassemia, in which there is a quantitative reduction in the rate of beta chain synthesis, is the most common type of thalassemia. When the abnormal gene is inherited from both parents (homozygous), severe anemia termed *thalassemia major* results. Heterozygous patients have a mild anemia termed *thalassemia minor*.

Thalassemia major causes a severe anemia and clinical manifestations usually within the first year of life. Pallor, retarded growth, and enlargement of the head with "thalassemic facies" are present together with splenomegaly and hepatomegaly. The intense erythroid hyperplasia in the bone marrow causes expansion of the medullary cavities and attenuation of the cortex, producing bone abnormalities and a predisposition to fractures. Owing to defective iron utilization coupled with increased iron absorption and frequent blood transfusions, iron overload is a common complication. Treatment consists of transfusion therapy and iron chelation, and splenectomy is effective in selected patients. Although the basic hematologic disease is not influenced, splenectomy decreases blood transfusion requirements and relieves discomfort from splenomegaly.

Autoimmune Hemolytic Anemia

Autoimmune hemolytic anemia (AIHA) is an acquired hemolytic anemia caused by an antibody that is produced by the body against its own red cells. Patients with AIHA have the usual manifestations of hemolysis with anemia, reticulocytosis, a shortened erythrocyte survival time, fluctuating jaundice, and splenomegaly. The blood smear in AIHA shows spherocytes and microspherocytes in numbers exceeded only in hereditary spherocytosis. The distinguishing feature of AIHA is a positive direct Coombs' test, which identifies antibody on the red cell surface. Treatment is directed toward the hemolytic anemia and any underlying disease. Blood transfusion, corticosteroid therapy, and splenectomy are important aspects of treatment for the anemia. Splenectomy usually is performed in patients with AIHA in whom steroids are ineffective or an excessive steroid dose is required, or when complications preclude steroid use.

MISCELLANEOUS ANEMIAS SOMETIMES BENEFITED BY SPLENECTOMY

Splenectomy occasionally is performed for rare disorders such as hereditary hydrocytosis and xerocytosis, acquired idiopathic sideroblastic anemia, congenital dyserythropoietic anemia, and porphyria erythropoietica. In these disorders, splenectomy may offer significant benefits by improving the hemolytic anemia and reducing transfusion requirements.

Treatment of patients with myeloid metaplasia is directed toward the anemia, thrombocytosis, and splenomegaly. Splenectomy is effective in controlling anemia and thrombocytopenia and relieving symptoms due to painful or massive splenomegaly. Splenectomy should be performed early rather than late in the course of illness, since the risk of complications following splenectomy increases with progression of the disease. Indications for splenectomy are (1) an increasing transfusion requirement, (2) thrombocytopenic bleeding episodes, (3) symptomatic splenomegaly, (4) high output cardiac failure, and (5) portal hypertension with bleeding varices.

Gaucher's Disease

Gaucher's disease is a disorder of lipid metabolism that may cause massive splenomegaly and hypersplenism. Caused by a deficiency of beta-glucocerebrosidase, an enzyme responsible for breaking down certain lipid complexes, Gaucher's disease ultimately causes retention of glucocerebroside in macrophages, especially those of the spleen, liver, bone marrow, and lungs. Of the three clinical forms of the disease, the adult form is most common. Splenomegaly, which may be massive, is usually the presenting feature and may be discovered incidentally or as a result of symptoms of early satiety, abdominal fullness, or painful infarctions. Moderate to severe thrombocytopenia is present in most patients and is the most troublesome hematologic manifestation. Moderate normocytic anemia and leukopenia are common. Splenectomy is almost uniformly effective in correcting the cytopenias and relieves symptoms due to splenomegaly and recurring splenic infarction, although there is no evidence that splenectomy influences other aspects of the disease. In an effort to reduce the risk of postsplenectomy sepsis, subtotal splenectomy has been used successfully.

Cysts and Tumors of the Spleen

Splenic cysts and primary tumors are rare but must be considered in the differential diagnosis of a left upper quadrant mass. Cystic lesions of the spleen comprise parasitic and nonparasitic cysts. Parasitic cysts are due almost exclusively to echinococcal disease and represent 60 to 70 per cent of splenic cysts in countries where hydatid disease is endemic (South America, Australia, and Greece). Because echinococcal disease is rare in the United States, nonparasitic cysts are classified as primary or true cysts, which have an epithelial lining, and pseudocysts. Pseudocysts are much more common and probably are the result of liquefaction of old hematomas or areas of infarction and inflammation. True cysts of the spleen are very rare and include epidermoid and dermoid cysts, cystic hemangiomas, and cystic lymphangiomas. Symptoms of splenic cysts are vague and primarily the result of mass effect, compression of adjacent viscera, and diaphragmatic irritation. Although selected nonparasitic cysts may be effectively managed by aspiration, splenectomy should be performed for all large cysts and those with uncertain diagnosis. In some patients, a splenic cyst may be suitably located for excision by partial splenectomy.

Malignant and benign primary tumors of the spleen are rare. Most primary malignant tumors are angiosarcomas, although primary splenic lymphoma may occur. Benign splenic tumors include hamartomas, lymphangiomas, hemangiomas, and lipomas. Except for involvement with Hodgkin's disease and non-Hodgkin's lymphomas, metastatic disease to the spleen is diagnosed infrequently.

OVERWHELMING POSTSPLENECTOMY SEPSIS

Asplenic patients and those with deficient splenic function have an increased susceptibility to the development of overwhelming infection characterized by fulminant bacteremia, meningitis, or pneumonia. Singer's review of 2796 patients with splenectomy described a 4.2 per cent incidence of sepsis and a 2.5 per cent mortality. The risk of overwhelming sepsis is approximately 60 times greater than normal following splenectomy and may be as high as 0.5 to 1 per cent per year. Although a lifetime risk of fulminant sepsis is incurred with splenectomy, the risk is greatest in children under 4 years of age and within 2 years of splenectomy (80 per cent of cases). The risk for overwhelming postsplenectomy sepsis is highest in patients requiring splenectomy for thalassemia and reticuloendothelial system diseases such as Hodgkin's disease, histiocytosis X, or the Wiskott-Aldrich syndrome. It is lowest for patients with splenectomy for trauma, ITP, and hereditary spherocytosis.

The postsplenectomy sepsis syndrome typically occurs in a previously healthy individual following a mild upper respiratory infection associated with fever. Within hours, nausea, vomiting, headache, confusion, shock, and coma occur, and death follows within 24 hours. Blood cultures reveal *Streptococcus pneumoniae*, *Neisseria meningitidis*, *Escherichia coli*, or *Haemophilus influenzae* in 75 per cent of the cases, with *S. pneumoniae* representing 50 per cent. The fulminant nature of the syndrome makes it difficult to diagnose sufficiently early for therapy to be effective. Adrenal hemorrhage is a common autopsy finding.

Antibiotic prophylaxis or early antibiotic therapy may be effective in reducing the incidence of postsplenectomy sepsis. Because half of the patients develop sepsis from *S. pneumoniae*, penicillin can be administered prophylactically or immediately with the onset of a febrile upper respiratory illness. In patients who have had splenectomy for Hodgkin's disease staging, the incidence of overwhelming sepsis has been reduced by penicillin prophylaxis. Considerable hope exists for preventing postsplenectomy sepsis by immunization with specific vaccines. Ideally patients should be immunized well in advance of splenectomy (2 to 3 weeks preoperatively) to allow development of protective antibodies. Polyvalent vaccines against capsular polysaccharides from pneumococcal strains responsible for the majority of serious pneumococcal disease (Pnu-Imune 23 [23 strains] and Pneumovax 23 [23 strains]) are available. Polyvalent meningococcal vaccines also are available, and *Haemophilus influenzae* type *b* conjugate vaccines provide immunization against type *b* *Haemophilus*, a leading cause of serious systemic bacterial disease.

SPLENIC ABSCESS

Splenic abscess occurs rarely and usually is the result of bacteremia associated with a primary septic focus, such as bacterial endocarditis or lung abscess, or secondary infection in an area of the spleen damaged by infarction (sickle cell anemia or leukemia), trauma, or parasitic infestation. Clinical features of splenic abscess are those of left subphrenic suppuration and include fever, chills, left upper quadrant tenderness, and often splenomegaly. Computed tomographic scanning is probably the most direct approach in evaluating the spleen and establishing an early diagnosis. Splenectomy has been the preferred treatment for most patients in the past and remains a standard means of safe and rapid management. Image-guided percutaneous drainage may be appropriate in the management of some patients with splenic abscess.

37

HERNIAS
Lloyd M. Nyhus, M.D., and Michael S. Klein, M.D.

HISTORICAL ASPECTS

In 1884, Bassini described a technique for reconstructing the inguinal floor with transposition of the cord. Halsted developed an operation similar to that of Bassini but transposed the spermatic cord above the external oblique aponeurosis. The use of the iliopectineal ligament (Cooper's ligament) to anchor the repair is credited to Lotheissen. The use of this structure as an integral part of hernial repair was popularized later by McVay. Recognition of the role of the posterior inguinal wall in the causation and repair of hernias represents a significant advance in the understanding of groin anatomy.

GROIN HERNIA

ANATOMY OF INGUINAL AND FEMORAL CANALS. The abdominal wall in the groin is composed of multilaminar arrangements of muscle, their aponeuroses, fascia, fat, and either skin or peritoneum. This may be divided into outer and inner laminae, which are mirror images of each other.

Endoabdominal Fascia. The endoabdominal fascia is crucial for the prevention of groin and other abdominal wall hernias. This fascial layer forms a compartment that holds abdominal viscera separate from the muscular layers of the abdominal wall. Condensations within endoabdominal fascia, termed analogs, are found at critical inserting points of muscle groups or attachments of aponeurotic structures.

The *transversalis fascial sling* reinforces the medial margin of the internal inguinal ring. As cord structures exit the ring, they have a projection of the transversalis fascia, the internal spermatic fascia.

The *transversus abdominis aponeurotic arch* forms the upper margin of the area through which inguinal hernias of all types protrude. In 5 per cent of cases, transversus abdominis aponeurosis fuses with the arch of the internal oblique aponeurosis to form the "conjoined tendon."

The *iliopubic tract* arises from the iliopectineal arch, a fibrous condensation of endoabdominal fascia spanning the iliopsoas muscles as it exits the pelvis. Shortly beyond the origin, the iliopubic tract arches over the femoral vessels, forming the anterior portion of the femoral sheath. The medial fanlike curved portion ordinarily closes the femoral canal, and not the lacunar ligament, which is external to it. Periosteum of the pelvis along the iliopectineal line is intimately fused with

---

See the corresponding chapter or part in the *Textbook of Surgery*, 14th edition, pp. 1134–1148, for a more detailed discussion of this topic, including a comprehensive list of references.

another condensation of the transversalis fascia and iliopubic tract, forming *Cooper's ligament*.

PHYSIOLOGY OF INGUINAL CANAL STRUCTURES. Normally, two mechanisms prevent the extrusion of contents through the internal ring. First, the sphincter action of the transversus abdominis and internal oblique muscles operates at the internal ring. The second is a shutter mechanism comprising the convex transversus abdominis arch, which is flattened when muscles are tensed. This tensing action brings the arch in apposition to the inguinal ligament, thereby covering the cord and buttressing the floor of the inguinal canal.

DIAGNOSIS, INCIDENCE, AND PROGNOSIS. The diagnosis of hernia is usually made on the basis of physical examination rather than the history. In children, however, the mother's report of a lump in the groin should alert the surgeon to the presence of a groin hernia even if it is not apparent on the first examination. The ultimate diagnosis of direct or indirect type of hernia is based on the intraoperative determination. A femoral hernia must be distinguished from an inguinal hernia during examination because a different operative approach is necessary, and a femoral hernia will be overlooked if the exposure is incorrect.

Approximately 50 per cent of all hernias are indirect inguinal and 25 per cent are direct inguinal; 6 per cent are femoral. Approximately 90 per cent of all groin hernias occur in males. Although 85 per cent of all femoral hernias occur in females, the most common groin hernia in women is the indirect inguinal type.

The Danger of Hernia. Incarcerated hernias are sometimes difficult to distinguish from those that are strangulated and therefore are surgical emergencies. Femoral and indirect inguinal hernias are more likely to cause strangulation because the hernial sacs have small necks. All patients with intestinal obstruction should be carefully examined for exclusion of an occult groin hernia, which may be the cause.

Inguinal Hernias in Adults. The indirect inguinal hernia requires a patent processus vaginalis and is therefore a true congenital defect. Various anomalies of processus obliteration are related. An undescended testicle is always associated with an indirect inguinal hernia. Indirect inguinal hernias may be classified according to the extent of dilation of the internal inguinal ring. If enlargement impinges on the floor of the inguinal canal, a combined indirect-direct (pantaloon) hernia is formed. In the direct inguinal hernia, the weakness is in the floor of the inguinal canal medial to the internal inguinal ring and the inferior deep epigastric vessels. Most recurrent hernias following the repair of a primary indirect inguinal hernia are direct. A recurrent indirect inguinal hernia may be attributed to the surgeon's failure to ligate the patent processus vaginalis (hernial sac).

INGUINAL HERNIA REPAIR. A single operative technique is not appropriate in all patients. The approach must be designed at operation for management of the following variations:

Small Indirect Inguinal Hernia. The basic feature is a

patent processus vaginalis with minimal dilation of the internal ring. After high ligation of the hernial sac, tightening of the transversalis fascia around the spermatic cord at the internal ring suffices. This is the simplest of all hernial defects to correct and is also the most common.

Medium Indirect Inguinal Hernia and Attenuated Posterior Inguinal Floor. Occasionally, the internal ring has enlarged farther medially, and the posterior inguinal wall appears attenuated. In addition to the closure of the internal ring, the posterior inguinal floor should be strengthened. This is achieved by suturing the aponeurotic arch of the transversus abdominis to the iliopubic tract from the internal ring medially toward the pubis.

Standard Anterior Inguinal Wall Repairs. The classic Bassini operation is suited for the repair of small or medium indirect inguinal hernias. This repair sutures the transversus abdominis aponeurotic arch to the lacunar-inguinal ligaments with satisfactory results.

Large Indirect and Direct Inguinal Hernia. These are the most difficult to repair because the surgeon must reconstruct the entire posterior inguinal wall and form a new internal ring. McVay popularized the Cooper's ligament repair for this problem with a reported 3.6 per cent recurrence rate. The Canadian method uses an imbrication technique to repair the floor of the inguinal canal in several layers for greater strength. Excellent results have been reported after primary inguinal hernia repairs.

Femoral Hernia. Interest in the preperitoneal or posterior approach to femoral hernia has grown. This method facilitates operative exposure, and its technical advantages are numerous. The hernial sac is found protruding into the femoral canal medial to the external iliac vein, lateral to the curved fibers of the iliopubic tract, and anterior to Cooper's ligament. The femoral canal is closed by suturing the iliopubic tract to Cooper's ligament. The McVay Cooper's ligament repair is a good alternative for the repair of a femoral hernia.

SPECIAL PROBLEMS

Incarcerated and Strangulated Hernias. Efforts to reduce an incarcerated hernia should be tempered by the awareness of possible complications. *Reduction en masse* can occur if the hernia is reduced in the endoabdominal fascia with disappearance of the external hernial bulge but without relief for the hernia, which remains incarcerated within the sac. Therefore, after an attempt at reduction, the patient must be carefully observed for signs of evolving obstruction or peritonitis.

Lipoma of the Cord. Lobulated preperitoneal fat may project down the cord at the internal ring and be mistaken for an indirect inguinal hernia. It should be excised.

Obturator Hernia. This "hidden hernia" passes through the obturator foramen, and diagnosis is difficult. Strangulation frequently occurs because of the rigid walls of the orifice. Most patients who have this type are elderly or emaciated, and these hernias are five times more common in women. The defect, which may be repaired by various routes, usually requires a prosthetic patch.

Perineal Hernia. Defects occur in the muscle floor of the pelvis through which peritoneal sacs project. Fortunately, these hernias are usually reducible, and strangulation seldom occurs.

Sliding Inguinal Hernias. Occasionally, the cecum on the right or the sigmoid colon on the left composes a portion of the sac wall in an indirect inguinal hernia. In women and young females, the sliding hernia may also contain portions of the genital tract. Special care must be taken to avoid opening the bowel or devascularizing it when managing the hernial sac. As a precaution, the sac of an indirect hernia is always opened at its anterior medial aspect.

ABDOMINAL WALL HERNIA

This may be defined as any protrusion of the abdominal viscera through the endoabdominal fascia.

UMBILICAL HERNIA. This is a true congenital defect present in 10 per cent of Caucasian infants and 40 to 90 per cent of blacks. In a majority, the patent umbilical ring closes spontaneously by the age of 2 years. In contrast, an umbilical hernia in an adult should be repaired because of a tendency for incarceration or strangulation. The classic repair for umbilical hernia, the "pants over vest" method, was proposed by Mayo in 1907. Recurrence is rare.

EPIGASTRIC HERNIA. Midline-occurring, also termed *hernias of the linea alba*, these hernias are more common above the umbilicus. Most are small and asymptomatic. Pain may be caused by a tag of omentum herniating through the defect.

VENTRAL (INCISIONAL) HERNIA. This is a true iatrogenic hernia. The most common cause is wound infection. Because of the intricate nature of the defect and the absence of healthy contiguous tissue, a number of operative procedures using prosthetic mesh techniques are often necessary.

SPIGELIAN HERNIA. This spontaneous lateral ventral hernia is a protrusion through the spigelian fascia often at a point just below the umbilicus in the region of the semilunar line of Douglas. The diagnosis may be difficult because of the frequent absence of a palpable mass; however, ultrasound or a computed tomographic scan may be helpful. The operative repair is straightforward. The hernial sac is ligated in the usual manner, and the fascial defect can be closed with a few interrupted nonabsorbable sutures.

LUMBAR HERNIA (PETIT'S TRIANGLE HERNIA AND GRYNFELTT'S HERNIA). These are relatively rare hernias. Only 250 to 300 cases have been reported in the literature. The more common of the two is Grynfeltt's, or superior lumbar hernia. More likely to be encountered in the same anatomic region are incisional hernias after nephrectomy.

38

PEDIATRIC SURGERY
Jay L. Grosfeld, M.D.

GENERAL CONSIDERATIONS

The newborn infant is a unique surgical patient who is physically and physiologically different from the adult. The cardiorespiratory dynamics in the newborn relate to conversion of a fetal circulation that bypasses the lungs to a postnatal state, with an elevated pulmonary artery pressure, patent ductus arteriosus, and patent foramen ovale causing a 15 to 20 per cent shunt. Cardiac output is rate-dependent, and stroke volume is limited when bradycardia occurs. The lung is not fully mature at birth. The more immature the infant, the fewer pulmonary units available and less surfactant produced, causing alveolar collapse, atelectasis, and hyaline membrane formation. Persistent pulmonary hypertension may cause significant extrapulmonary shunting and severe hypoxemia. The airways are quite small (tracheal diameter 2.5 to 4 mm.), and the tidal volume is 6 to 10 ml. per kg. Infants are nasal and diaphragmatic breathers and have a relatively rapid respiratory rate (up to 60 per minute is normal). Respiratory distress is heralded by tachypnea, nasal flaring, retractions, and cyanosis. The normal Pao_2 is 70 to 80 mm. Hg., $Paco_2$ 30 to 35 mm. Hg., and pH 7.3 to 7.4. The neonate has reasonably good renal function and manages a water load quite well despite a reduced glomerular filtration rate and immature tubular function that interfere with normal concentrating ability. Urine osmolality greater than 400 mOsm. may reflect dehydration, and less than 150 mOsm. overhydration. Normal urinary output is 1 to 2 ml. per kg. per hour. The neonate is relatively immunodeficient with decreased levels of IgG, opsonins, IgM, and the C3B component of complement. The more immature the infant, the less the ability to phagocytize bacteria, leaving the infant at a greater risk for serious infection. The infant must be maintained in a thermoneutral environment, and the body temperature is best monitored by a skin probe (36 to 36.5 °C. being normal). The baby's relatively large body surface area, lack of hair and subcutaneous tissue, and increased insensible losses make the infant vulnerable to hypothermia. Continued exposure to cold produces metabolic acidosis despite non-shivering thermogenesis. This is due to an increased metabolic rate caused by metabolism of brown fat.

Liver function in the neonate is immature, and physiologic jaundice due to relative deficiencies of glucuronosyltransferase is a common observation. Because of limited glycogen stores, the infant is prone to hypoglycemia (particularly small

See the corresponding chapter or part in the *Textbook of Surgery*, 14th edition, pp. 1149–1186, for a more detailed discussion of this topic, including a comprehensive list of references.

for gestational age infants), which may be manifested by seizures. Hypocalcemia and hypomagnesemia are other causes of seizure activity.

The infant has a total body water space that represents 80 per cent of body weight at birth and is mainly due to an increased extracellular fluid volume. Insensible losses are high (30 to 35 ml. per kg. per day) and are increased by fever, radiant warmers, phototherapy for hyperbilirubinemia, and respiratory distress. Intravenous water requirements are 100 to 125 ml. per kg. per day in full-term infants and as high as 140 to 150 ml. per kg. per day in the premature. Ten per cent glucose in 0.25 per cent saline is used for maintenance fluids. The potassium and sodium requirements are 2 to 3 mEq. per kg. per day. Body weight, skin turgor, urine and serum osmolality, and urine specific gravity are good parameters for assessing fluid requirements. Fluid losses from gastric drainage or stomal losses are replaced with lactated Ringer's solution. The total blood volume can be estimated at 80 ml. per kg. Transfusion with packed red blood cells at 10 ml. per kg. is a safe volume. Platelet and fresh frozen plasma infusions for thrombocytopenia or coagulation problems can be administered at a rate of 10 ml. per kg. as well.

The neonate has a metabolic rate 2.5 times that of the adult and a caloric requirement to grow of 120 calories per kg. per day. Most formulas contain 20 calories per ounce, and 6 ounces per kg. therefore delivers an adequate caloric load. Caloric requirements are increased by fever, major illness, trauma, or sepsis. If the infant cannot tolerate an enteral diet, total parenteral nutrition is required. The calorie:nitrogen ratio is maintained at greater than 150:1. A solution containing 25 per cent glucose, 2.5 gm. amino acids per kg. per day, and 3 to 4 gm. fat per kg. per day delivers an adequate caloric intake. Adequate vitamins, minerals, iron, and folate are required additives. Total parenteral nutrition is administered through a Silastic catheter placed in the superior vena cava at the entrance of the right atrium.

ALIMENTARY TRACT OBSTRUCTION

The cardinal signs of alimentary tract obstruction in the neonate are maternal polyhydramnios, bilious vomiting, abdominal distention, and failure to pass normal amounts of meconium in the first day of life.

Esophageal Atresia and Tracheoesophageal Fistula

Infants with variants of esophageal atresia may present with excess salivation, coughing, choking, and cyanosis. Aspiration of saliva and reflux of gastric juice through a tracheoesophageal (TE) fistula cause these symptoms. A high rate of associated anomalies may coexist (especially cardiovascular defects). Infants with proximal esophageal atresia and distal TE fistula (Type C) show a blind pouch in the upper thorax and air in the stomach and intestine on chest films. Infants with atresia but without a fistula (Type A) have mothers with polyhydramnios and no air beneath the diaphragm on abdominal films. Extrapleural division of the TE fistula and one-layer esophageal anastomosis is the procedure of choice. If the atretic ends are too far apart, a proximal esophagomyotomy is a useful adjunct and allows primary esophageal repair. Type A atresia (without a fistula) requires dilation for stretching of the proximal pouch and a single myotomy or occasionally multiple myotomies, which usually permit a primary anastomosis and avoid the need for esophageal replacement procedures. "H-type" TE fistula (Type E) is best detected by bronchoscopy and can be divided with a cervical approach. Type B proximal atresia and fistula and Type D proximal atresia with proximal and distal TE fistulae are less common anomalies. Complications include anastomotic leak, stricture, pneumonia, tracheomalacia, and severe foregut motility disorders including gastroesophageal reflux. The overall survival is greater than 85 to 90 per cent, with most deaths occurring in infants with severe associated anomalies (usually cardiac) or chromosomal syndromes.

Pyloric atresia presents with nonbilious vomiting, maternal polyhydramnios (66 per cent), and a single gastric bubble on abdominal films. The treatment program includes resection of a prepyloric web and pyloroplasty or a pyloroduodenal anastomosis when a gap separates the tissues. Duodenal atresia can be diagnosed *in utero* by the appearance of a double bubble on ultrasonography. Polyhydramnios is observed in 40 to 50 per cent, one third of the infants have Down's syndrome, and one third are premature. Associated anomalies are observed in more than half, with cardiovascular defects being most common. The diagnosis is confirmed following birth when a double bubble is seen on abdominal films and bilious gastric aspirate is observed or bilious vomiting occurs. Annular pancreas, malrotation, and anterior portal vein occur more commonly in these cases. The operative procedure of choice is a duodenoduodenostomy. The distal segment should be inspected for a second web. Occasionally, a windsock web deformity is identified, and this can be managed by duodenotomy and web excision. Survival is currently 90 per cent. Mortality is often due to serious cardiac anomalies. Jejunoileal atresia is due to a late intrauterine mesenteric vascular accident from volvulus, intussusception, and internal hernia. Most present with a single atresia, but 10 to 15 per cent may be multiple. The Type IIIa atresia with a mesenteric gap defect is the most common variant noted. These infants present with abdominal distention and bilious vomiting, and often they fail to pass meconium. Abdominal films demonstrate dilated intestinal loops often with air-fluid levels. A barium enema shows a microcolon, indicating that the colon is unused and pinpointing the site of obstruction to the small intestine. At laparotomy, the dilated atretic bowel end is resected and bowel continuity restored with an end-to-oblique anastomosis. In babies with short bowel syndrome and a proximal jejunal atresia, bowel length can be preserved by the performance of a tapering jejunostomy. Most infants with jejunoileal atresia have no other abnormalities and are more frequently full-term or small for gestational age patients. Approximately 35 per cent require total parenteral nutrition, and 20 per cent have short bowel syndrome. Survival is currently 87 to 90 per cent. All babies with jejunoileal atresia require a sweat chloride determination before discharge for excluding cystic fibrosis.

Meconium ileus is a manifestation of cystic fibrosis and occurs in 10 to 15 per cent of infants born with this hereditary disorder. This intraluminal form of obstruction is characterized by bilious vomiting, abdominal distention, and failure to pass meconium. Abdominal radiographs show dilated loops of similar sized bowel without air-fluid levels. A ground glass (soap-bubble) appearance may be seen in the right lower quadrant due to admixture of inspissated meconium and air. Barium enema shows a microcolon, and in some cases the barium refluxes into the distal ileum and demonstrates the obstructing meconium pellets. Treatment of choice for uncomplicated meconium ileus is nonoperative therapy by use of a hypertonic Gastrografin enema. Unsuccessful Gastrografin enema attempts require surgical intervention. The author favors an enterotomy and irrigation for clearance of the intraluminal obstruction; however, an enterostomy may occasionally be necessary. Complicated cases of meconium ileus include those instances associated with atresia, perforation, volvulus, and giant cystic meconium peritonitis. Gastrografin enema is contraindicated in these cases. At operation, resection and enterostomy may be required. Atresia can be managed by resection and anastomosis as outlined earlier. The mortality has been significantly reduced in recent years, with more than 90 per cent surviving the neonatal period.

Other causes of neonatal small bowel obstruction include infants with internal hernia due to volvulus around a congenital band, mesenteric cyst, or Meckel's diverticulum; an incarcerated inguinal hernia; or duplication of the jejunum or ileum.

Colon atresia is less common than either duodenal or jejunoileal atresia. The atresia usually occurs in the transverse or left colon and is probably related to intrauterine volvulus of these more floppy segments of the colon. Colon atresia usually occurs in large infants with no other serious anomalies. Preliminary colostomy and subsequent closure at 3 to 6 months of age has been a very successful method of management (100 per cent survival). Hirschsprung's disease is caused by colonic obstruction related to a lack of ganglion cells in the submucosal and myenteric plexus. Aganglionic megacolon occurs more frequently in males (80 per cent); most of the infants are full term, and 3 to 5 per cent have Down's syndrome. Presenting symptoms include bilious vomiting and abdominal distention, and 96 per cent fail to pass meconium in the first 24 hours of life. Perforation and enterocolitis may also be presenting findings. The differential diagnosis includes meconium plug syndrome, small left colon syndrome, colonic neuronal dysplasia, maternal narcotic addiction, and hypothyroidism. Diagnosis is usually achieved with a barium enema, which may show a cutoff point in the rectosigmoid or, in the newborn, a normal-sized colon with significant delays (more than 24 hours) in emptying the contrast material. Confirmation requires a rectal biopsy which shows an absence of ganglion cells in the submucosa. Acetylcholinesterase staining of neurofibrils may be useful. Anal manometry may demonstrate an absent rectoanal reflex. The treatment of choice in the neonatal period is a preliminary sigmoid colostomy with verification of the presence of ganglion cells at the stomal site. Aganglionosis is limited to the rectosigmoid in 80 per cent of cases but can extend proximal to the splenic flexure in 10 per cent and involve the entire colon, extending into the small bowel in 10 per cent. In these last instances, the preliminary stoma requires multiple frozen section biopsies for determining the proper site of stomal formation. Definitive therapy is a pull-through operation at 6 to 12 months of age by use of the Soave endorectal pull-through, the Duhamel retrorectal pull-through, or the Swenson procedure (surgeon's choice). The modified Duhamel procedure is the most popular procedure for total colonic disease in which the ileum or even more proximal intestine is brought down to the anus at the time of the pull-through procedure. Survival is greater than 90 per cent. Mortality is highest in patients with Down's syndrome and those with extensive disease or in cases complicated by enterocolitis.

Anorectal anomalies are now classified as high, low, or intermediate lesions according to whether the rectal atresia is above, at, or below the level of the puborectalis sling. Eighty-five to 90 per cent of infants with variants of imperforate anus and rectal atresia have an associated fistula to the perineum, urethra, or vagina. Low lesions with imperforate anal membrane or rectoperineal fistula can be treated in the neonatal period with a perineal anoplasty with avoidance of the need for colostomy. Intermediate or high-level rectal atresia is treated initially with a high sigmoid colostomy and a formal posterior sagittal anorectoplasty with division of a rectourethral fistula (in males) or rectofourchette or vaginal fistula (in females) or complete cloacal repair at 6 months to 1 year of age. Many patients have significant associated anomalies including cardiac defects, other gastrointestinal atresias (esophagus, duodenum), musculoskeletal disorders, urinary tract disorders, dysraphic spinal syndromes, other central nervous system abnormalities, and sacral abnormalities (hemivertebrae, sacral dysgenesis, and rarely sacral agenesis) that may contribute to their ability to survive early and achieve continence at a later time. The lower the rectal atresia, the better the prognosis. In intermediate and high lesions, the colostomy is maintained in place until the new anoplasty site has been dilated adequately for avoidance of a stricture. Long-term success in achieving socially acceptable continence is possible in greater than 90 per cent with low lesions and 50 to 60 per cent of those infants with intermediate or high rectal atresia requiring posterior sagittal anorectoplasty.

ACUTE NEONATAL EMERGENCIES

Necrotizing Enterocolitis

Necrotizing enterocolitis is a life-threatening intra-abdominal condition affecting 1 to 2 per cent of all neonatal intensive care unit admissions. The majority of cases occur in premature or low-birth-weight infants. Predisposing factors include shock, hypoxia, respiratory distress syndrome, apneic episodes, sepsis, polycythemia-hyperviscosity syndrome, exchange transfusion, patent ductus arteriosus, cyanotic heart disease with failure, and hyperosmolar feedings. The pathophysiologic insult involves splanchnic vasoconstriction, hypoperfusion, and mucosal injury compounded by bacterial invasion. Symptoms and signs include increased gastric residuals, abdominal distention, lethargy, vomiting, occult or gross rectal bleeding, fever or hypothermia, an abdominal mass, abdominal wall erythema, oliguria, and instances of apnea/bradycardia. Radiologic findings include pneumatosis intestinalis, portal vein air, pneumoperitoneum, fixed dilated loops, and ascites. Laboratory data usually show a leukocytosis with a shift to the left on differential smear, anemia, hypoalbuminemia, acidosis, electrolyte disturbances, disseminated coagulopathy, and a progressively decreasing platelet count. Resuscitation includes cessation of feedings, insertion of an orogastric tube for gastric drainage, repletion of intravascular volume with crystalloid and colloid infusions, ventilator support (if not already in place), triple antibiotics, and administration of blood, platelets, and fresh frozen plasma as indicated.

Infants who show a prompt response to medical therapy can be treated conservatively (nonoperatively). Babies with free air, massive rectal bleeding, abdominal wall erythema, and abdominal mass and those who deteriorate on conservative therapy require operative intervention. Infants with portal vein air have advanced disease and are candidates for early surgical intervention as well. In most cases, resection of infarcted bowel and a temporary enterostomy is the procedure of choice. Rarely, the process is so limited that a primary anastomosis may be reasonable. In colonic involvement, a proximal stoma and distal Hartmann's pouch procedure can be performed. Survival is 60 to 75 per cent and varies with the severity of illness and the extent of bowel necrosis. Many infants have short bowel syndrome as a result of extensive enterectomy. There is a subsequent late mortality due to underlying disease factors that affected the premature infant before the development of necrotizing enterocolitis.

Malrotation and Midgut Volvulus

Anomalies of intestinal rotation and fixation cause the development of abnormal fixation bands across the duodenum and jejunum and make the infant vulnerable to a clockwise twist of the intestine and midgut volvulus. One third of the cases of midgut volvulus occur in the first month of life. Infants with midgut volvulus present with the sudden onset of bilious vomiting and rapidly become seriously ill. If it is not recognized promptly, midgut infarction may occur with massive enterectomy and short bowel syndrome or death ensuing. The abdomen may be tender and distended. Bilious gastric returns are observed following passage of an orogastric tube. Occasionally the infant passes blood and tissue (sloughed mucosa) per rectum. Abdominal radiographs may show distended bowel with air-fluid levels or a distended stomach and duodenum with a gasless abdomen beyond that point. Barium enema shows the cecum in an abnormal upper abdominal position, whereas barium swallow demonstrates a duodenal cutoff with a corkscrew appearance consistent with a twist. The infant is given triple antibiotics and fluid resuscitation; at operation, the bowel is reduced in a counterclockwise manner, and Ladd's bands (across the duodenum) or duodenojejunal bands are lysed. The cecum is placed in the left lower quadrant next to the sigmoid colon, and an appendectomy is performed because of the atypical location of this appendage at the conclusion of the procedure. The Doppler probe or fluorescein dye and a Wood's lamp can usually predict bowel viability. If the entire small bowel and right colon appear necrotic, the bowel is detorsed, the abdomen is closed, and the infant is treated supportively. If the infant survives more than 48 hours, a second-look laparotomy is performed for evaluation of bowel viability. The mortality for midgut volvulus remains high (18 to 25 per cent). Most patients with incomplete or intermittent volvulus respond to a Ladd procedure and appendectomy as outlined, and almost all survive.

Gastroschisis

Gastroschisis refers to an evisceration of the gastrointestinal tract *in utero*. The defect lies just to the right of an intact umbilical cord. The herniated bowel is exposed to the irritating effects of amniotic fluid, which cause an inflammatory reaction and foreshortening of the mesentery and intestine. The infant has malrotation and a small abdominal cavity and is prone to hypothermia and hypovolemia due to increased insensible losses and evaporative losses from the exposed viscera. Bowel atresia as a result of volvulus or restraining of the blood supply to the herniated bowel in a very tight small defect may be seen in 10 to 15 per cent of cases. Associated anomalies are otherwise uncommon. Aggressive fluid resuscitation is required beginning with a bolus of 20 ml. per kg. of lactated Ringer's solution or colloid. An orogastric tube is passed, and broad-spectrum antibiotic coverage is initiated. Extending the incision 2 cm. cephalad and caudad allows a mechanical advantage for attempting reduction of the exposed viscera. The abdominal wall is manually stretched and the colon emptied of meconium so that more room is made within the small abdominal cavity for the herniated viscera. Primary closure is possible in 70 per cent of cases. This is monitored by the ventilatory pressure and pulse oximeter. Excessive ventilatory pressure (greater than 35 cm. H_2O) and hypoxemia indicate the need for application of a Dacron-reinforced temporary Silastic housing and a staged closure. Postoperative care may require short ventilation and adequate fluid resuscitation. Due to a prolonged adynamic ileus, total parenteral nutrition is often necessary for a 2- to 3-week period. Most infants can tolerate full enteral feedings by 1 month of age. Infants with associated atresia require a temporary enterostomy and subsequent anastomosis. The length of hospitalization for complicated cases (e.g., atresias, perforations) is significantly longer than for uncomplicated cases. The current survival for infants with gastroschisis is 90 per cent.

Omphalocele

An omphalocele is a covered defect of the umbilical ring into which abdominal contents herniate. The sac is composed of an outer layer of amnion and an inner layer of peritoneum. The incidence is 1 per 5000 births. More than 50 per cent of patients have significant associated anomalies affecting the cardiovascular, gastrointestinal, musculoskeletal, urinary tract, and central nervous systems. Many of the infants are premature (25 per cent); others are affected by a number of chromosomal syndromes including the Beckwith-Wiedemann syndrome, trisomy 13–15 and 16–18, or exstrophy of the bladder or cloaca and the pentalogy of Cantrell (epigastric located omphalocele, anterior diaphragmatic defect, sternal cleft, ectopia cordis, and intracardiac defects, usually a ventricular septal defect and occasionally a diverticulum of the left ventricle). The size of the defect varies from a small herniation of the umbilical cord to a 10-cm. defect containing the liver and entire gastrointestinal tract. The abdominal cavity may be quite small, and most cases have malrotation. An orogastric tube is inserted to prevent gastric distention, and the patient is placed feet first into a sterile bowel bag that is gently tied across the upper abdomen and transferred to a tertiary neonatal care center in a thermally neutral environment. Wet dressings macerate the sac and may cause hypothermia. The patient's general condition should be carefully assessed for severe anomalies, chromosomal defects, prematurity, and so on; the covered sac provides a number of treatment options. Small defects can be managed by direct primary closure of the abdominal wall. Medium to large defects may require a staged closure with use of a Dacron-reinforced Silastic silo as a temporary housing for the herniated viscera. The prosthetic material is sutured to the edge of the defect with continuous 3–0 polypropylene suture. The silo can gradually be reduced over a 3- to 7-day period on the newborn unit, and the infant is then returned to the operating room for removal of the prosthesis and abdominal wall repair. Giant (greater than 10 cm.) defects, infants with chromosomal syndromes, premature infants with hyaline membrane disease, or infants with severe cardiac defects in failure or requiring ventilator support can be treated initially by topical therapy with 0.25 per cent Mercurochrome or 0.5

per cent silver nitrate solution as an escharotic agent. Higher concentrations of Mercurochrome can occasionally cause mercury poisoning and should be avoided. Continued nonoperative treatment with topical agents is advised for infants with chromosomal syndromes such as trisomy 13–15 or 16–18 when long-term survival is not expected. Other patients can be treated definitively when their underlying illness is controlled and their general condition stabilizes. The overall survival for infants with omphalocele depends on the size of the defect, sac rupture and sepsis, complications of prematurity, and the number and severity of associated anomalies. Infants with chromosomal syndromes and those with the pentalogy of Cantrell have a very high mortality. The overall mortality at the author's institution is 37 per cent.

ACUTE RESPIRATORY EMERGENCIES

Congenital Diaphragmatic Hernia

Congenital posterolateral diaphragmatic hernia of Bochdalek is a defect of the developing pleuroperitoneal fold. The fetal intestine usually ascends through the defect and enters the chest in the eighth to tenth week of gestation. The herniated bowel acts as a space-occupying lesion and prevents normal lung development, which causes pulmonary hypoplasia. The risk of occurrence is 1 in 2200 births and is more common in males. The infants are usually full-term and weigh more than 3 kg. The defect can be detected by prenatal ultrasound and is frequently associated with maternal polyhydramnios, which is a poor prognostic marker. At birth, these infants develop symptoms of respiratory distress in the delivery room or shortly thereafter. The infant appears dyspneic, tachypneic, and cyanotic and has severe retractions with an increased chest diameter and a relatively scaphoid abdomen. Bowel sounds may be heard on auscultation of the affected chest. Chest films demonstrate air-filled viscera in the thorax on the side of the hernia. The left side is affected in 88 per cent, the right side in 10 per cent; bilateral hernias are observed in 2 per cent. In 10 per cent of cases there is a peritoneal sac. The infant develops extrapulmonary shunting owing to pulmonary hypoplasia accompanied by hypercarbia, severe hypoxemia, and a combined respiratory and metabolic acidosis.

Treatment can be conveniently divided into three categories: (1) stabilization and preoperative preparation, (2) operative treatment, and (3) postoperative respiratory, circulatory, metabolic, and nutritional support. The infant with diaphragmatic hernia should have direct endotracheal intubation and ventilatory support with high oxygen concentration ($FiO_2 = 1.0$). The respiratory rate is set intentionally rapid for induction of a respiratory alkalosis, which causes pulmonary vascular dilation. Excessive ventilatory pressures are avoided for prevention of contralateral pneumothorax. An arterial catheter is inserted, preferably in the right radial artery, for monitoring preductal pH and blood gas tensions.

An umbilical artery catheter is an alternative but measures postductal blood gas tensions. An orogastric tube is inserted for decompression of the stomach and prevention of air from entering the gastrointestinal tract and further compressing the lung. If the infant becomes stabilized and demonstrates a PaO_2 greater than 100 mm. Hg and $PacO_2$ less than 60 mm. Hg and an arterial-alveolar gradient of less than 600, operative correction of the defect is attempted. This is best accomplished with a transabdominal approach with use of a subcostal incision on the affected side. The bowel is carefully reduced from the chest, with care being taken to avoid injury to the spleen on the left or the liver on the right, which may be displaced into the thorax. A chest tube is inserted under direct vision, and the defect is then repaired with 3–0 silk interrupted mattress sutures. If the defect is too large or the diaphragm is absent, a prosthetic Goretex patch is used to replace the diaphragm. The abdomen is closed in layers when possible; however, occasionally the abdominal cavity is too small to accommodate the viscera from the chest, and either a skin closure or temporary Dacron-reinforced Silastic housing may be necessary. Postoperatively, the infant is returned to the neonatal intensive care unit to be monitored. The endotracheal tube is left in place, and the infant is given ventilatory support with $FiO_2 = 1.0$ for maintaining the PaO_2 above 150 mm. Hg for 48 to 72 hours to avoid deterioration following this temporary period of stability. This may occur when the FiO_2 and PaO_2 are reduced too quickly. This type of deterioration is related to the sudden onset of pulmonary vascular vasoconstriction and persistent pulmonary hypertension. Pharmacologic agents such as tolazoline, prostaglandins, and acetylcholine are used to induce pulmonary vascular vasodilation; however, the response to these medications has been disappointing. Infants older than 24 hours at diagnosis survive; however, the survival for infants who are symptomatic shortly after birth has been less than 30 per cent and is even lower (16 per cent) if polyhydramnios was present. The mortality is directly related to the degree of pulmonary hypoplasia (especially if the contralateral lung is also hypoplastic) or if associated congenital anomalies including congenital heart disease or chromosomal defects were present.

Since the advent of extracorporeal membrane oxygenation (ECMO), a number of innovative clinical programs have developed. Infants who develop persistent pulmonary hypertension following repair of a diaphragmatic hernia can usually be salvaged by ECMO. However, infants with pulmonary hypoplasia have not had the same postoperative benefits from treatment with ECMO and continue to have a significant mortality. Recently, some centers have been placing infants on ECMO preoperatively. When the infant's general condition improves, the baby can be successfully weaned from the ECMO circuit and repair of the defect performed. In some centers, repair of the diaphragmatic hernia is performed while the infant is still on the ECMO circuit. There have been encouraging survivors in each setting; however, not enough data are available for definitive recommendations at this time. Whereas ECMO has a significant role in the management of certain patients with diaphragmatic hernia, it is not a panacea for all cases. Recent reports indicate survival rates of 70 to 90 per cent with use of ECMO for all diaphragmatic hernia candidates who fail conventional treatment and have no other contraindications for life support therapy. An oxygenation index (O.I.) greater than 40 has a mortality risk of greater than 80 per cent and is an indication for ECMO. Oxygenation index is determined by O.I. = MAP (mean airway pressure) $\times$ Fio_2 $\times$ $100/Pao_2$ based on three of five postductal Pao_2 determinations. Gestational age less than 34 weeks, intracranial hemorrhage, neurologic impairment, anomalies incompatible with a meaningful life expectancy, and irreversible lung disease are contraindications for ECMO.

Other Causes of Respiratory Distress

Other congenital abnormalities affecting the diaphragm include the anterior diaphragmatic hernia through the foramen of Morgagni (which is relatively uncommon in infants and children) and eventration of the diaphragm. Eventration of the diaphragm is most often related to birth injury following a breech delivery when the phrenic nerve is stretched and may also be associated with Erb's palsy and torticollis on the same side. The diaphragm is paralyzed and becomes attenuated, allowing the intra-abdominal contents to push up the thin muscle into the chest and compress the lung tissues, causing atelectasis and hypoxemia. Morgagni hernias can be repaired through the abdomen, the author favors a transthoracic diaphragmatic plication for correcting eventration.

Congenital cystic lung disease can cause respiratory distress in the neonate. These lesions are derived from the primitive foregut from which the lung bud originates and are categorized as congenital lobar emphysema, cystic adenomatoid malformation, solitary lung cyst, pulmonary sequestrations (intra- and extralobar), bronchogenic cyst, and enteric duplication. Each condition either traps air in the lung or compresses the tracheobronchial tree or pulmonary tissues, causing respiratory compromise due to obstruction or compression atelectasis. The treatment for each of these congenital cystic lesions is resection. Additional causes of respiratory distress in the newborn include pulmonary interstitial emphysema, pneumothorax, and pneumomediastinum, which are sequelae of the air-block syndrome in the neonate. Micrognathia associated with Pierre Robin's syndrome and Stickler's syndrome, choanal atresia or stenosis, hemangiomas, lymphangiomas, and teratomas of the pharynx or tongue can cause airway obstruction. The extent of the lesion can be defined by computed tomographic examination. Tracheomalacia, subglottic stenosis, laryngotracheal cleft, and congenital tracheal stenosis are also conditions that must be considered when the neonate presents with obstructive stridorous

breathing. The appropriate diagnosis can usually be made
with a careful physical examination, air tracheograms, laryngoscopy, and bronchoscopy. Emergency intubation may
be lifesaving, and in some infants a temporary tracheostomy
is required for securing the airway.

39

OTOLARYNGOLOGY

James B. Snow, Jr., M.D.

THE EARS

The external auditory canal makes a slightly S-shaped curve. The outer one third has a cartilaginous skeleton, and the inner two thirds has a bony skeleton. Cerumen glands and hair are borne in the outer third. The plane of the tympanic membrane makes an angle of 55 degrees with the long axis of the external auditory canal. The long process of the malleus is embedded in the fibrous layer of the tympanic membrane, and the head of the malleus articulates with the body of the incus. The lenticular process of the incus articulates with the head of the stapes. The footplate of the stapes articulates with the oval window.

The cochlea makes two and three-quarters turns in the human. A cross section through the modiolus, or central bony framework, shows in each turn the scala vestibuli, the scala media, and the scala tympani. The scala vestibuli is separated from the scala media by Reissner's membrane. The scala media is separated from the scala tympani by the basilar membrane. The organ of Corti with its hair cells rests on the basilar membrane. The hairs of the hair cells are in contact with the tectorial membrane. Dendrites of the neurons, the cell bodies of which are in the spiral canal of Rosenthal in the modiolus, arborize about the base of the hair cells.

The principal components of the vestibular labyrinth are the saccule, utricle, and semicircular canals. The saccule is spherical and is connected with the scala media through the canalis reuniens of Hensen. The saccular duct joins the utricular duct to form the endolymphatic duct. The utricle is larger than the saccule and is ovoid. The utricle has five openings for the three ampullated ends of the semicircular canals, the crus simplex of the horizontal semicircular canal, and the crus commune of the superior and posterior semicircular canals.

Sound waves impinging upon the tympanic membrane set the tympanic membrane in motion. Movement of the tympanic membrane then causes movement of the malleus, incus, and stapes. Movement of the stapes causes pressure changes in the fluid in the inner ear. These pressure changes produce a traveling wave in the basilar membrane, from the base to the apex of the cochlea. Along the length of the basilar membrane, a point of maximal displacement occurs with each traveling wave. The location of the point of maximal displacement depends on the frequency of the stimulating tone. High-frequency tones cause maximal displacement

---

See the corresponding chapter or part in the *Textbook of Surgery*, 14th edition, pp. 1187–1208, for a more detailed discussion of this topic, including a comprehensive list of references.

near the base of the cochlea. As the frequency of the stimulating tone is decreased, the point of maximal displacement moves from the base to the apex.

Displacement of the basilar membrane causes movement of the organ of Corti and deformation of the hairs of the hair cells. A chemical transmitter is released in the region of the end boutons of the afferent eighth nerve fibers that attach to the hair cells. This chemical transmitter initiates depolarization of the dendritic terminals of the afferent nerve fibers.

Trauma and Foreign Bodies

Foreign bodies in the external auditory canal are a common problem. Beads, erasers, beans, and other objects may be inserted by children and their siblings into their ears. An insect may find its way into the ear canal and is particularly annoying to the patient until it is killed or removed. Foreign bodies are removed by passing a blunt hook deep to the foreign body and raking it out. A forceps is likely to push smooth foreign bodies ahead of it. If the foreign body is far medial, it is difficult to remove without injuring the tympanic membrane and ossicular chain. If a child is uncooperative or the mechanical problem is difficult, a general anesthetic is used for the removal of a foreign body. Metal and glass beads may be removed by irrigation, but care is used to be certain that the foreign body is not hygroscopic like a bean, because swelling with the addition of water complicates its removal. An insect is killed to give the patient immediate relief and facilitate its removal by filling the ear canal with mineral oil. The dead insect is removed with a forceps.

The tympanic membrane may be perforated with twigs of a tree, cotton applicators, and other objects placed in the ear canal, missiles such as hot slag in welding, and a sudden overpressure in an explosion (acoustic trauma). Perforations of the tympanic membrane may be associated with dislocations of the ossicular chain. Vertigo or a sensorineural hearing loss suggests that a portion of an ossicle or a missile has been driven into the inner ear or that there is a fistula between the perilymphatic space of the vestibule and the middle ear. These conditions require prompt exploration of the middle ear with an operative microscope and repair of the labyrinthine fistula. Most perforations of the tympanic membrane heal spontaneously in 6 weeks. For avoidance of infection during the healing period, the patient must be careful to avoid getting water in the ear. Prophylactic antibiotic therapy in the form of oral penicillin for the first 7 days is recommended. If the perforation fails to heal or if there is a persisting conductive hearing loss suggesting discontinuity of the ossicular chain, the middle ear is explored and repaired.

FRACTURES OF THE TEMPORAL BONE. Basal skull fractures follow blunt trauma to the head, particularly to the occipital area. Basal skull fractures are in essence fractures of the temporal bone, and they are a frequent cause of profound sensorineural hearing loss. Bleeding from the ear following an injury to the skull is pathognomonic of a fracture of the temporal bone whether the bleeding is medial to an intact tympanic membrane, from the middle ear through a rupture of the tympanic membrane, or from a fracture line in the ear canal. Hemotympanum gives the tympanic membrane a blue-black color. Usually, there is a communication with the subarachnoid space through the fracture line. Often there is cerebrospinal fluid otorrhea. The immediate danger to the patient is the development of meningitis. Therefore, prophylactic antibiotic therapy is initiated and continued for 7 to 10 days. More fractures of the temporal bone are longitudinal (80 per cent) than transverse (20 per cent) to the long axis of the petrous pyramid. Longitudinal fractures extend through the middle ear into the ear canal and cause rupture of the tympanic membrane. Transverse fractures extend across the cochlea and fallopian canal to produce a profound, permanent sensorineural hearing loss and a facial paralysis. Approximately 35 per cent of longitudinal fractures produce a sensorineural hearing loss, and approximately 15 per cent produce facial paralysis. The fracture extending through the middle ear may cause dislocation of the ossicular chain that requires subsequent repair. Persistence of a facial paralysis requires decompression of the facial nerve under certain circumstances.

Infectious Diseases

ACUTE OTITIS MEDIA. Acute otitis media is an infectious inflammatory process in the middle ear, usually secondary to an upper respiratory tract infection. It is the most common localized infection in children. Most children between 1 and 5 years of age have two or three episodes of acute otitis media each winter. Acute otitis media may be viral or bacterial.

A myringotomy is indicated if bulging of the tympanic membrane persists despite antibiotic therapy or if the pain and systemic symptoms and signs such as fever, vomiting, and diarrhea are severe. A large curvilinear incision is made parallel to the annulus in the inferior quadrants midway between the umbo and the canal wall. The appearance and movement of the tympanic membrane, tympanometry, and the patient's hearing are followed until there is complete resolution.

The infectious complications of acute otitis media are acute mastoiditis, petrositis, labyrinthitis, facial paralysis, conductive and sensorineural hearing loss, epidural abscess, meningitis, brain abscess, lateral sinus thrombosis, subdural empyema, and otitic hydrocephalus. The most common intracranial complication of acute otitis media is meningitis.

SEROUS AND SECRETORY OTITIS MEDIA. Serous and secretory otitis media are manifested as effusions in the middle ear. Such effusions are the result of incomplete resolution of acute otitis media or from eustachian tube obstruction due to inflammatory processes in the nasopharynx, allergic manifestations, hypertrophic adenoids, or benign or malignant nasopharyngeal neoplasms. Normally the middle ear is ventilated three to four times per minute as the eustachian tube opens during swallowing. If the patency of the eustachian tube is compromised, a relative negative pressure develops. At first there is mild retraction of the tympanic membrane. Soon a transudate of fluid occurs from the blood in the vessels in the mucous membrane of the middle ear. The presence of fluid in the middle ear may be recognized by an amber or dark gray color of the tympanic membrane, immobility of the tympanic membrane, a tympanogram indicating negative pressure in the middle ear, and conductive hearing loss.

Myringotomy for aspiration of the fluid and insertion of a tympanostomy tube for ventilation of the middle ear ameliorate the problem of eustachian tube obstruction regardless of the cause. In children, thorough adenoidectomy is frequently a necessary part of the treatment.

In children with middle ear effusions, initial treatment consists of antibiotic therapy appropriate for acute otitis media. Antibiotic therapy may sterilize the middle ear as well as ameliorate the eustachian tube obstruction secondary to purulent rhinitis, sinusitis, or adenoiditis and resolves the middle ear effusion in one third to one half of the patients.

CHRONIC OTITIS MEDIA. Chronic otitis media means a permanent perforation of the tympanic membrane. Perforations follow acute otitis media, mechanical trauma, thermal and chemical burns, and blast injuries. Chronic otitis media can be divided into two major categories depending on the type of perforation present. There is a benign tubotympanic type, with a central perforation of the tympanic membrane, and a dangerous type, with a pars flaccida or marginal perforation.

A central perforation is one in which there is some substance of the tympanic membrane between the rim of the perforation and the bony sulcus tympanicus. These perforations most commonly follow acute otitis media produced by relatively virulent microorganisms. Exacerbations of the chronic otitis media produce painless, purulent otorrhea, which may be foul-smelling and occur secondary to upper respiratory infections and when water gains access to the middle ear in bathing and swimming.

The middle ear can generally be repaired in chronic otitis media with a central perforation. A tympanoplasty provides sound protection for the round window and restores sound-pressure transformation to the oval window. Tympanoplastic procedures can be categorized into five types. The Type I tympanoplasty is applicable to the patient with a perforation of the tympanic membrane in which the ossicular chain is intact and mobile. The Type I tympanoplasty, sometimes termed a myringoplasty, restores the tympanic membrane by the use of a graft of soft tissue such as temporalis muscle fascia. A Type II tympanoplasty is required if there has been greater damage to the middle ear. Disruption of the ossicular chain, which often occurs as a result of necrosis of the long process of the incus, must be repaired in addition to grafting of the tympanic membrane. Often the remnant of the incus or the head of the malleus can be remodeled and repositioned to re-establish the continuity of the ossicular chain. Preserved homograft ossicles or alloplastic materials are also used to restore the sound-conducting mechanism. A Type III tympanoplasty is required for a still more severely damaged middle ear in which the malleus and incus are not usable and only the stapes remains. Under these circumstances, the graft is placed in contact with the head of the stapes to produce a columellar effect similar to the single middle ear ossicle or columella found in birds. In more severe degrees of damage to the middle ear in which the superstructure of the stapes has been destroyed, only sound protection of the round window can be achieved by grafting from the promontory to the inferior remnant of the tympanic membrane. This Type IV tympanoplasty creates a small closed space that communicates with the eustachian tube and provides an air-filled cushion over the round window. A Type V tympanoplasty is utilized when the footplate of the stapes is fixed. It provides sound protection for the round window as in a Type IV tympanoplasty and fenestration of the horizontal semicircular canal for the admission of acoustic energy into the inner ear.

A cholesteatoma occurs when the middle ear is lined with stratified squamous epithelium. The stratified squamous epithelium desquamates in this closed space. The desquamated epithelial debris cannot be cleared and accumulates in ever-enlarging concentric layers. This debris serves as a culture medium for microorganisms. Cholesteatomas have the ability to destroy bone, including the tympanic ossicles. The presence of a cholesteatoma greatly increases the probability of the development of a serious complication such as a purulent labyrinthitis, facial paralysis, or intracranial suppurations.

Cholesteatomas are usually recognized by the small bits of white, amorphous debris in the middle ear and by the destruction of the external auditory canal bone superior to the perforation. Cholesteatomas are often associated with aural polyps, which may conceal the epithelial debris and bone destruction. Computed tomography of the temporal bone may demonstrate destruction of bone due to the cholesteatoma. Destruction of the scutum of Leidy (lateral wall of the epitympanum) and enlargement of the antrum greater than 1 cm. in diameter should be considered suspicious of cholesteatoma.

Cholesteatomas require surgical treatment. The objective of surgical therapy is to exteriorize the cholesteatoma and, if possible, remove it. In a radical mastoidectomy, the middle ear, including the attic and the antrum, and the mastoid air cell area are converted into one cavity that communicates with the exterior through the ear canal. If the cholesteatoma lies superficial to the remnants of the tympanic membrane and ossicles, a modified radical mastoidectomy can be performed. The modified radical mastoidectomy spares the tympanic membrane remnants and ossicles and preserves the remaining hearing. Under favorable circumstances, the cholesteatoma can be completely removed and the middle ear reconstructed. Exteriorization or removal of the cholesteatoma greatly reduces the likelihood of intracranial complications. The primary goal of surgical therapy for cholesteatoma is to make the ear safe, and the secondary goal is to maintain or improve the hearing.

Idiopathic Disease

OTOSCLEROSIS. Otosclerosis is the most common cause of a progressive conductive hearing loss in the adult with a normal ear drum. Otosclerosis is a disease of the bone of the inner ear with predilection for the anterior part of the oval window. On histologic examination, foci of otosclerosis show irregularly arranged, immature bone interspersed with numerous vascular channels. As the focus of the otosclerotic bone enlarges, it causes ankylosis of the footplate of the stapes and produces a conductive hearing loss. A second site of predilection is the posterior part to the oval window.

Otosclerosis tends to occur in families. It is more common in women than in men. Approximately 10 per cent of the adult white population have foci of otosclerosis. Only 1 in 10 of these, or approximately 1 per cent of the white population, has clinical otosclerosis as evidenced by conductive hearing loss. Otosclerosis is rare in blacks, Native Americans, and Japanese. It is common in Asiatic Indians. Otosclerosis also produces a sensorineural hearing loss if the focus is adjacent to the scala media. The conductive hearing loss becomes clinically evident in the late teenage and early adult years. The fixation of the stapes may progress rapidly during pregnancy. The conductive hearing loss can be corrected surgically in most instances. With microsurgical techniques, the superstructure (head, neck, and crura) of the stapes is removed and replaced with a prosthesis. A widely used prosthesis is one composed of a stainless steel wire and a Teflon piston. The wire, which is shaped like a shepherd's crook, is crimped around the long process of the incus, and the piston is placed through a hole created in the footplate of the stapes. The sound conduction characteristics of this arrangement are excellent. The complication of a profound sensorineural hearing loss occurs in 2 to 4 per cent of patients. If a good initial hearing result is obtained, ordinarily a good result is maintained.

Neoplasms

Chemodectomas arise in the middle ear. These nonchromaffin paragangliomas are termed glomus jugulare or glomus tympanicus tumors, depending on their site of origin. The glomus tympanicus tumor arises from the area of Jacobson's nerve in the tympanic plexus on the promontory of the middle ear. The glomus jugulare tumor arises from the glomus jugulare body in the jugular bulb. Both tumors consist of rich networks of vascular spaces surrounded by epithelioid cells. Usually the neoplasms grow slowly, and symptoms may not be evident until the neoplasm is quite large. Pulsatile tinnitus, facial nerve paralysis, otorrhea, hemorrhage, vertigo, and paralysis of cranial nerves IX, X, XI, and XII are often the presenting symptoms and signs. Characteristically, a red mass that pulsates and blanches with compression with a pneumatic otoscope can be seen in the ear canal or middle ear. The pulsation can also be demonstrated with tympanometry. There may be evidence of bone erosion in the mastoid process, middle ear, or petrous pyramid on computed tomography. Treatment consists of excision of the smaller neoplasms with or without a radical mastoidectomy. With large lesions, radiation therapy is the treatment of choice.

Acoustic neurinomas represent approximately 7 per cent of all intracranial neoplasms. They arise twice as often from the vestibular division of the eighth nerve as from the auditory division. These neoplasms are derived from Schwann cells. Initially, they produce tinnitus and a neural hearing loss. The patient complains of unsteadiness or imbalance. True vertigo is not a common complaint. The hearing loss is predominantly a high-tone loss with greater impairment of the speech discrimination than would be expected with a cochlear lesion producing the same amount of puretone hearing loss. The structure of the five waves in brain stem response audiometry is disrupted, the interwave latency is increased, and the interaural latency difference of the fifth peak is increased. Initially, the tumor is confined to the internal auditory meatus. As it increases in size, it projects into the cerebellopontine angle and begins to compress the cerebellum and brain stem. Early diagnosis is based on auditory findings suggesting a neural loss of hearing. Auditory brain stem responses have become the most effective means of differentiating sensory from neural hearing losses. Acoustic neurinomas as small as 5 mm. in diameter can be visualized with magnetic resonance imaging with enhancement with gadolinium. For the removal of small tumors, microsurgical approaches have been developed that utilize a translabyrinthine route if no useful hearing remains and a middle cranial fossa route for the preservation of the remaining hearing. Both routes allow preservation of the facial nerve. For very large neoplasms, the combined suboccipital and translabyrinthine approach offers the best likelihood of complete removal.

THE NOSE AND THE PARANASAL SINUSES

Trauma and Foreign Bodies

NASAL FRACTURE. Fractures of the nose are the most common fractures of the facial bones. Nasal fractures may involve the ascending processes of the maxillae and the nasal processes of the frontal bones as well as the nasal bones. A fracture of the nose is usually an open fracture. The skin of the dorsum of the nose may be lacerated, and the mucous membrane in the nasal cavity is usually torn. The most common deformity is a deviation of the nasal bones to the right with depression of the nasal bones on the left, characteristically occurring with a right hook. Fractures of the nose may be associated with septal fractures and hematomas.

Fractures of the nasal bones are generally associated with bleeding from the nose owing to the tear of the mucous membrane. A fracture should be suspected if blunt injury causes bleeding from the nose. Soft tissue swelling occurs fairly promptly and may tend to obscure the underlying bony deformity. The diagnosis can ordinarily be established by gentle palpation of the dorsum of the nose. Any deformity suggests a fracture. Radiographs of the nasal bones will tend to confirm the diagnosis.

Fractures of the nasal complex are often associated with fractures of other facial bones, and computed tomography of the paranasal sinuses is obtained. Trauma to the facial bones is often associated with a cerebrospinal fluid rhinorrhea.

Nasal fractures in adults may be reduced under local anesthesia. General anesthesia is necessary for the reduction of nasal fractures in children. The fracture is manipulated into a good position by internal traction on the fracture fragments with a blunt periosteal elevator in association with external traction with the fingers. The need for internal and external splinting depends on the postreduction stability of the fracture.

Septal hematomas lie between the quadrangular cartilage and the perichondrium. If the perichondrium has been elevated from both sides of the septal cartilage, the cartilage will undergo avascular necrosis. Septal hematomas frequently become infected, and abscess formation produces avascular and septic necrosis of the septal cartilage, which causes a saddle deformity of the nose. Septal hematomas are incised and drained as soon as the diagnosis is made. The perichondrium is placed in contact with the septal cartilage by packing the nasal cavity with petrolatum gauze.

Septal abscesses are located between the cartilage and the perichondrium. They may involve both sides of the cartilage. Septal abscesses are incised and drained under general anesthesia as soon as the diagnosis is established. Incisions are made bilaterally if there is pus on both sides of the septum. A small rubber drain is sutured to a lip of the wound until the drainage subsides. Vigorous systemic antibiotic therapy is employed.

FOREIGN BODIES. Children put all manner of objects in their noses. Erasers, beans, buttons, pebbles, wool nap, paper, and sponge rubber are common foreign bodies. A foreign body in the nasal cavity produces a severe inflammatory reaction and causes a foul-smelling, bloody, unilateral discharge. Removal of the foreign body is facilitated by producing vasoconstriction anterior to it with a topical sympathomimetic amine such as phenylephrine. The foreign body is removed by placing a blunt hook posterior to it and raking it anteriorly. Attempts at grasping smooth, firm foreign bodies with forceps tend to push them farther posteriorly. General anesthesia is used if good cooperation from a child cannot be obtained by gentle reassurance.

If a foreign body dwells long in the nose, mineral salts are deposited on it and produce a rhinolith. The rhinolith tends to conform to the contour of the nasal cavity, and its removal is usually difficult.

Sinusitis

Acute rhinitis is the usual manifestation of a common cold. Acute sinusitis is usually initiated by an acute respiratory tract infection of viral cause. Nearly all cases of acute sinusitis and most cases of chronic sinusitis respond well to antibiotic therapy. The complications of acute and chronic sinusitis often require surgical therapy, as does unresponsive chronic sinusitis. Complications of maxillary sinusitis are rare. Ethmoid sinusitis is frequently complicated in children by orbital cellulitis and abscess. Eighty per cent of all cases of orbital cellulitis are secondary to ethmoid sinusitis. In the patient who presents with erythema and swelling of the eyelids, proptosis, and displacement of the globe laterally and inferiorly, the source of the infection is sought by inspection of the nose for mucopus in the middle meatus and by computed tomography of the paranasal sinuses for ethmoid sinusitis. Computed tomography of the orbits may allow differentiation of orbital cellulitis from orbital abscess. Ethmoid sinusitis and orbital cellulitis respond well to systemic antibiotic therapy. If the proptosis fails to subside or progresses, incision and drainage of the abscess, which is between the lamina papyracea and the orbital periosteum, is performed through a Killian incision that extends from the lateral aspect of the nose to the eyebrow. The orbital periosteum is elevated from the medial wall of the orbit so that the abscess cavity can be reached. The optic nerve tolerates 11 to 14 mm. of proptosis. The point at which extraocular motion is lost is also the limit of stretch of the optic nerve. Therefore, incision with drainage of an orbital abscess is performed before complete loss of extraocular motion for prevention of blindness.

Frontal sinusitis may cause intracranial complications such as meningitis, epidural abscess, subdural empyema, and brain abscess. In severe acute frontal sinusitis that fails to respond promptly to systemic antibiotic therapy, the floor of the frontal sinus is trephined through an incision just inferior to the medial part of the eyebrow. An opening of approximately 7 to 8 mm. is made, and a catheter is placed in the sinus for maintaining drainage. Trephination is performed in an attempt to prevent the intracranial complications of frontal sinusitis.

Fractures of the frontal sinus cause development of mucoceles. Mucoceles are due to duplication of the mucous membrane. They gradually enlarge and destroy the floor of the frontal sinus, and as they expand into the orbital cavity, they produce proptosis and inferior and lateral displacement of the eye. Mucoceles and other forms of chronic frontal sinusitis that do not respond to medical management can be managed surgically by an osteoplastic flap approach for obliteration of the frontal sinus. The incision in the bone is made at the periphery of the frontal sinus, and the anterior wall is rotated inferiorly on the hinge of periosteum at the floor of the sinus. Infected mucous membrane is removed with a gas-driven burr under microscopic control, and the cavity of the frontal sinus is obliterated by the implantation of fat taken from the abdominal wall.

Approximately 25 per cent of cases of chronic maxillary sinusitis are secondary to a dental infection. In chronic maxillary sinusitis, radiographs of the apices of the teeth should be obtained for excluding the possibility of a periapical abscess.

Chronic maxillary sinusitis that does not respond to medical management may be controlled with the Caldwell-Luc operation, which is a maxillary sinusotomy performed through an incision in the canine fossa. The bone of the anterior wall of the maxillary sinus is resected to permit access to the interior of the sinus for removal of infected mucous membrane, cysts, and epithelial debris. Drainage of the maxillary sinus is improved by creating a nasoantral window in the inferior meatus.

Chronic ethmoid sinusitis is often associated with allergic rhinitis and the formation of nasal polyps. In those individuals in whom the formation of nasal polyps and the symptoms of ethmoid sinusitis cannot be controlled adequately by intranasal polypectomy and medical management including topical corticosteroid therapy and immunotherapy, an ethmoidectomy is indicated. Ethmoidectomy is performed intranasally with endoscopic guidance and through an external approach by utilization of a Killian incision. In the external ethmoidectomy, the orbital periosteum is elevated, and the lamina papyracea is removed to give access to the ethmoid air cells. Infected mucous membrane, polypoid tissue, and epithelial debris are removed. The anterior half of the middle turbinate is excised to create a large opening between the ethmoid air cells and the nasal cavity. In essence, an ethmoidectomy incorporates the ethmoid air cell area into the nasal cavity.

Chronic sphenoid sinusitis that does not respond to medical management may be controlled by an operation in which the sphenoid sinus is approached through an external ethmoidectomy. After an external ethmoidectomy has been accomplished, the anterior wall of the sphenoid sinus is resected to remove infected mucous membrane, polypoid tissue, and epithelial debris. The anterior and inferior walls of the sphenoid sinus are removed. In this way, the interior of the sphenoid sinus is incorporated in the posterior part of the nasal cavity and the nasopharynx, and in essence, the sphenoid sinus is eliminated as a separate entity.

Epistaxis

Bleeding from the nose is a common clinical problem. Ninety per cent of the time, epistaxis occurs from a plexus of vessels in the anteroinferior part of the septum. In the other 10 per cent of cases, nasal bleeding occurs from the posterior part of the nose, particularly from far posterior in the inferior meatus at the junction of the inferior meatus and the nasopharynx. It is from this area that individuals with arteriosclerosis and hypertension are likely to bleed. This type of bleeding may be difficult to control and is associated with a 4 to 5 per cent mortality. Mild epistaxis from the anterior part of the nasal septum is usually effectively controlled by steady pressure applied by squeezing the mobile portion of the nose between the index finger and thumb for 5 to 10 minutes. Treatment for epistaxis that is not controlled by this simple measure requires visualization of the bleeding point. The bleeding point can be controlled temporarily and anesthesia achieved with pressure applied over a cotton pledget impregnated with a vasoconstrictor and a topically active local anesthetic such as lidocaine. The bleeding point can be cauterized chemically or with electrocautery. Silver nitrate is preferred as the cauterizing agent, since it produces satisfactory intravascular coagulation without a severe burn of the mucous membrane. If the bleeding cannot be easily controlled with cautery or if the bleeding point cannot be visualized, strips of ½-inch petrolatum gauze are used to apply pressure to the bleeding point. Pressure is applied as atraumatically as possible. This method is preferred in a patient with a bleeding tendency because the periphery of a cauterized area may begin to bleed.

In order to pack the posterior part of the nasal cavity, the choana is obstructed with the balloon of a Foley catheter. If the bleeding point is in the inferior meatus, this area is packed tightly. The packing is left in place for 4 days. Prophylactic antibiotic therapy is indicated to prevent sinusitis and otitis media. Patients requiring postnasal packing generally have serious systemic vascular diseases. They have a low arterial Po_2 while the packing is in place and should be given supplemental humidified oxygen by mask.

An alternative method of treatment of patients with severe bleeding from the posterior part of the nose is ligation of the internal maxillary artery.

Severe epistaxis is often associated with pre-existing liver disease. Large amounts of blood may have been swallowed before the nasal packing. Blood is eliminated from the gastrointestinal tract as promptly as possible by the use of cathartics and enemas. Sterilization of the gastrointestinal tract for preventing the breakdown of blood by microorganisms and the absorption of ammonia is indicated by the presence of liver disease.

Replacement of blood that has been lost as a result of the epistaxis is accomplished as indicated by the hemoglobin and hematocrit determinations as well as by the patient's vital signs.

Neoplasms

BENIGN NEOPLASMS OF THE NOSE AND PARANASAL SINUSES. Squamous cell papillomas occur in the nasal cavity and are thought to be caused by papovaviruses. Exophytic papillomas occasionally recur after excision but have a benign course. Inverted papillomas are invasive and behave in a locally malignant manner. They arise from the lateral wall of the nasal cavity and invade bone. Inverted papillomas require removal of a margin of normal tissue through a lateral rhinotomy. Fibromas, hemangiomas, and neurofibromas occur occasionally in the nasal cavity. Fibromas, neurilemomas, and ossifying fibromas occur in the paranasal sinuses.

MALIGNANT NEOPLASMS OF THE NOSE AND PARANASAL SINUSES. The most common malignant neoplasm occurring in the nose and paranasal sinuses is squamous cell carcinoma. Adenoid cystic carcinomas, adenocarcinomas (particularly in the ethmoid sinuses), mucoepidermoid carcinomas, malignant mixed tumors, lymphomas, fibrosarcomas, osteosarcomas, chondrosarcomas, and melanomas also occur in the nose and paranasal sinuses. Metastatic tumors may involve the paranasal sinuses, and the most common neoplasm to metastasize to the paranasal sinuses is the hypernephroma.

A combination of radiation therapy and radical resection provides the best survival rates in carcinomas and sarcomas of the nasal cavities and paranasal sinuses.

THE PHARYNX

Nasopharynx

THE ADENOIDS. Adenoid hypertrophy in childhood often causes obstruction of the eustachian tubes and the choanae. Obstruction of the eustachian tubes produces serous or secretory otitis media, recurrent acute otitis media, and exacerbations of chronic otitis media. Obstruction of the choanae produces mouth breathing, a hyponasal voice, and rhinorrhea.

Recurrent serous or secretory otitis media is the most common indication for the removal of the adenoid tissue.

An adenoidectomy is performed under general anesthesia. The adenoid tissue is sheared from the posterior nasopharyngeal wall with a guillotine-type adenotome placed posterior to the soft palate.

BENIGN NEOPLASMS OF THE NASOPHARYNX. Juvenile angiofibromas are very vascular neoplasms that occur in pubescent males. Angiofibromas may extend into and obstruct the nasal cavity and encroach upon the paranasal sinuses, the orbit, and the intracranial cavity. These neoplasms are composed of fibrous tissue and numerous thin-walled vessels without contractile elements.

Epistaxis is the major problem with angiofibromas, and the magnitude of the bleeding can be very great. The extent of the neoplasm can be determined with computed tomography and angiography. The main blood supply is usually from the branches of the internal maxillary artery, although the branches of the internal carotid artery and the middle meningeal artery also may contribute. Usually, they are removed through a transpalatal approach. The blood loss during excision is often very great, and rapid blood replacement is required. Treatment with estrogens and embolization of the internal maxillary artery at angiography have been used to reduce the operative blood loss. These neoplasms are responsive to radiation therapy. This is often the treatment of choice for the neoplasm that has invaded the orbit or the intracranial cavity or receives a large blood supply from intracranial vessels.

MALIGNANT NEOPLASMS OF THE NASOPHARYNX. Malignant neoplasms of the nasopharynx include squamous cell carcinomas, adenocarcinomas, adenoid cystic carcinomas, mucoepidermoid carcinomas, malignant mixed tumors, melanomas, chordomas, sarcomas including fibrosarcoma, rhabdomyosarcoma, liposarcoma and myxosarcoma, plasmacytomas, and lymphomas. Among children, lymphomas are the most common malignant neoplasms arising from and secondarily involving the nasopharynx. Among the carcinomas, lymphoepithelioma or squamous cell carcinoma is the most common type.

Carcinoma of the nasopharynx occurs at relatively young ages, and there is an unusually high incidence among the Chinese. The majority of patients with carcinoma of the nasopharynx present with nasal or eustachian tube obstruction. Obstruction of the eustachian tube may produce a middle ear effusion. The nasal obstruction may be associated with purulent, bloody rhinorrhea and frank epistaxis. The more dramatic symptoms following cranial nerve paralysis and cervical lymph node metastasis are, unfortunately, common presenting complaints.

The diagnosis is made by biopsy of the primary tumor. Adequate access to the nasopharynx ordinarily requires general anesthesia. General anesthesia also allows the opportunity to judge the extent of the primary lesion by palpation. Biopsy of the metastasis in the neck should be avoided until the nasopharynx has been inspected and palpated and any suspicious lesion has been biopsied. Biopsy of the cervical metastasis violates the integrity of the block of tissue that is removed in a radical neck dissection. It may cause implantation of the neoplasm in the skin and subcutaneous tissue. The necessity for demonstrating the neoplasm in the nasopharynx before treatment remains, even if a histologic diagnosis is obtained from biopsy of the cervical metastasis.

The treatment of choice for carcinoma of the nasopharynx is irradiation with a supervoltage source. The radiation should be delivered to the primary tumor-bearing area of the nasopharynx and to both sides of the neck whether there is clinically demonstrated metastasis or not. Those cervical metastases that remain clinically palpable following radiation therapy or that subsequently become apparent should be eradicated by radical neck dissection. The overall 5-year survival for carcinoma of the nasopharynx is approximately 35 per cent.

Oropharynx

PERITONSILLAR ABSCESS. Peritonsillar cellulitis and abscess are complications of acute tonsillitis in which the infection has spread deep to the tonsillar capsule. Pus forms between the tonsillar capsule and the superior constrictor of the pharynx, and the tonsil is displaced medially. The uvula becomes tremendously edematous and is displaced to the opposite side. The soft palate is very red and displaced forward. There is marked trismus due to irritation of the pterygoid muscles, and the head is held tilted toward the side of the abscess. It is painful for the patient to talk and to swallow. Peritonsillar cellulitis or abscess is usually caused by a group A beta-hemolytic streptococcus or anaerobe. If a cellulitis without pus formation exists, it will respond in a matter of 24 to 48 hours to penicillin therapy. If pus is present, it may resolve or require incision and drainage. The incision need only split the mucous membrane, and the pus is obtained by spreading gently with a hemostat. No drain is required because the abscess cavity is emptied by each swallow.

These abscesses tend to recur and are an indication for tonsillectomy. Some advocate that the tonsillectomy be performed within a day or two after the antibiotic therapy is initiated.

PARAPHARYNGEAL ABSCESS. Parapharyngeal abscess may occur in infants and young children as well as in adults. The abscess is usually secondary to streptococcal pharyngitis or tonsillitis. Pus forms in the parapharyngeal space secondarily from the breakdown of lymphadenitis. The pus is located lateral to the superior constrictor of the pharynx and adjacent to the carotid sheath. There is marked swelling in the anterior cervical triangle. Penicillin is the antibiotic of choice. Pus formation can be demonstrated with computed tomography or magnetic resonance imaging before the abscess becomes fluctuant. When pus formation has been demonstrated, the abscess is incised and drained. The abscess is not drained through the lateral pharyngeal wall because of the proximity of the internal carotid artery and the internal jugular vein. An incision is made parallel to the skinfolds over the anterior border of the sternocleidomastoid muscle. The anterior border of the muscle is identified, and blunt dissection is carried toward the carotid sheath where the pus is encountered. A drain is sewn in place and removed when the drainage subsides.

RETROPHARYNGEAL ABSCESS. Retropharyngeal abscess occurs in infants and young children. These infections are located between the constrictors of the pharynx and the prevertebral fascia. They are secondary to pharyngitis and are due to the breakdown of retropharyngeal lymphadenitis. Infants with retropharyngeal abscesses usually present with stridor and hyperextension of the neck. A lumbar puncture is the appropriate diagnostic procedure in a febrile infant who presents in opisthotonos. If the cerebrospinal fluid is normal, the possibility of a retropharyngeal abscess must be excluded. The diagnosis is made by palpating the posterior pharyngeal wall. The infant is held in the prone position for the examination so that if the abscess is ruptured during the examination, the pus will flow out of the infant's mouth and not be aspirated. The abscess has a boggy fluctuant texture, and the bodies of the cervical vertebrae are not palpable. Inspection of the pharynx may not demonstrate the abscess because the whole posterior pharyngeal wall may be displaced forward and there may be no inflammatory reaction in the mucous membrane. The abscess can also be demonstrated by a radiograph of the lateral neck in which the posterior pharyngeal wall is displaced anteriorly, or by computed tomography of the neck. For maintaining the airway, the child should be allowed to hyperextend the neck. A tracheotomy is rarely necessary. In addition to penicillin therapy, the posterior pharyngeal wall should be incised under general endotracheal anesthesia with the patient in the Rose position. The mucous membrane at the posterior wall of the pharynx is incised vertically. The incision need only split the mucous membrane. The pus is obtained by gently spreading a hemostat in the wound toward the retropharyngeal space. No drain is necessary because the abscess cavity tends to be emptied on swallowing.

TONSILLECTOMY. Recurrent acute bacterial tonsillitis caused by a group A beta-hemolytic streptococcus occurring three to four times during the year in children from 2 to 7 years of age can be adequately managed with penicillin or other appropriate antibiotics given for 12 days. The rationale for this length of treatment is that a shorter period may not eliminate a streptococcal infection. In addition to inappropriate selection of antibiotics and inadequate duration of therapy, passage of the streptococcus among family members is a cause of failure in the medical management of tonsillitis. This situation requires simultaneous cultures of the whole family and simultaneous treatment of all carriers. Despite these precautions, in some patients tonsillitis repeatedly develops within a few days after the completion of adequate treatment. When this pattern cannot be altered by medical management, tonsillectomy is indicated.

Chronic tonsillitis with persistent sore throat, either briefly relieved or not at all relieved by antibiotic therapy, constitutes another indication for tonsillectomy. Peritonsillar abscess is another indication for tonsillectomy.

In adults, tonsillectomy is performed under local or general anesthesia. In children, general anesthesia is required. The technique involves an incision in the free edge of the tonsillar pillars. The dissection of the tonsil from the tonsillar fossa is performed in the plane between the tonsillar capsule and the superior constrictor muscle of the pharynx and is completed by closing a snare placed inferior to the lower pole of the tonsil. The objective is to remove the tonsil and its capsule intact and spare the musculature of the tonsillar fossa.

CARCINOMA OF THE TONSIL. Carcinoma of the tonsil represents 1.5 to 3 per cent of all cancers and is second in frequency only to carcinoma of the larynx among malignant neoplasms of the upper respiratory tract. It is predominantly a disease of males, and smoking of cigarettes and consumption of more than 100 ml. of ethanol per day are etiologic factors. Squamous cell carcinoma is the predominant histologic type. Carcinoma of the tonsil usually remains asymptomatic until it has reached considerable size. Sore throat is the most common presenting complaint, and pain often radiates to the ear on the same side. Not infrequently the patient presents with a metastatic mass in the neck as the first symptom. The diagnosis is established by biopsy of the primary lesion. Treatment requires combined radiation therapy and operation. Radiation therapy may be given preoperatively or postoperatively. If preoperative irradiation is utilized, 5000 rads are delivered to the primary lesion and both sides of the neck over a 5-week period. The patient is given a 6-week rest. The operation consists of radical resection of the tonsillar fossa, hemimandibulectomy, and radical neck dissection if there are palpable metastases. If postoperative irradiation is utilized, 6000 rads are delivered to the primary site and 5000 rads to both sides of the neck. The 2-year disease-free survival approximates 50 per cent.

LARYNX

Structural Changes in the True Vocal Cords Secondary to Misuse and Abuse of the Voice

Abuse and misuse of the voice can produce structural changes in the true vocal cords. Using the voice too loudly and too long produces acute and chronic changes in the true vocal cords. Prolonged use of intensity rather than frequency for emphasis, the employment of a monotone, the affectation of a frequency that is too low, and a very abrupt onset of high intensities (sharp glottal attack) produce structural changes in the true vocal cords.

POLYPS OF THE VOCAL CORDS. Polyps of the true vocal cords develop in response to use of the voice too loudly and too long. Chronic subepithelial edema develops in the lamina propria of the true vocal cords. Such polypoid swellings of the free edge of the true vocal cord interfere with the approximation of the true vocal cords and with the maintenance of periodicity and synchrony of the vibration of the vocal cords. They produce hoarseness and give a breathy quality to the voice. For restoration of the voice, polyps are removed by use of an operating microscope at direct laryngoscopy under general anesthesia.

VOCAL NODULES. Vocal nodules are caused by using a fundamental frequency that is unnaturally low and using the voice too loudly and too long. Vocal nodules occur in children as well as in adults and are likely to occur in robust, athletic boys 8 to 12 years of age who yell a great deal. Men affect an unnaturally low pitch to give an air of authority; women do it to give an impression of sexiness; and young boys probably do it to identify with older males in the family or community. Vocal nodules are condensations of hyaline connective tissue in the lamina propria at the junction of the anterior one third and the posterior two thirds of the true vocal cords. These nodules produce hoarseness and give the voice a breathy quality. In adults, these lesions are removed at direct laryngoscopy for restoration of the voice. However, it is necessary to begin voice therapy before the surgical therapy because if the underlying misuse of the voice is not corrected, the nodules will recur. In children, surgical removal is not usually necessary because the vocal nodules will regress with voice therapy.

Trauma

Trauma has replaced infectious diseases such as diphtheria, streptococcal croup, syphilis, tuberculosis, rhinoscleroma, and typhoid fever as the most common cause of laryngeal stenosis. Automobile accidents in which the patient is thrown forward and the larynx is crushed between the cervical vertebrae and the object against which it decelerates are the single most important cause of laryngeal stenosis. Children may fracture the larynx by falling against the handlebars of a bicycle or riding a horse or bicycle under a taut line. Another cause of laryngeal stenosis is the high tracheotomy in which a perichondritis of the cricoid cartilage follows pressure of the tube on the cartilage. Prolonged endotracheal intubation frequently produces subglottic stenosis, as do infectious processes.

Patients with crush injuries of the larynx complain of pain on swallowing. Hoarseness may progress to aphonia. Hemoptysis is usually present. Progressive dyspnea due to upper respiratory obstruction is to be anticipated. Subcutaneous emphysema is usually present in fractures of the larynx or trachea. The laryngeal cartilages cannot be distinctly palpated, nor can the trachea, owing to soft tissue swelling. On indirect laryngoscopy, the laryngeal lumen may appear disrupted or obliterated, and there may be exposed cartilage and lacerated mucous membrane. Vocal cord paralysis may be noted. Radiographs of the lateral neck and computed tomography of the neck may indicate the type and degree of injury. Lateral neck radiographs may demonstrate associated fractures or dislocations of the cervical vertebrae.

In the initial management of the patient with a laryngeal fracture, a tracheotomy is performed and followed by direct laryngoscopy and tracheoscopy.

The repair of the fracture is done through a transverse incision in the neck. For gaining access to the interior of the larynx, a laryngofissure is performed by dividing the thyroid cartilage at its isthmus, or the fracture in the thyroid and cricoid cartilage is utilized. Mucous membrane lacerations are repaired, and the cartilages are returned to their normal alignment. Internal splinting is maintained with a solid-core mold for as long as 6 weeks.

In addition to external trauma, tracheal stenosis occurs secondary to pressure necrosis of the tracheal walls caused by the inflated cuff in prolonged endotracheal intubation. Tracheal stenosis also occurs secondary to tracheotomy, particularly when the wound becomes infected and there is cicatricial healing of large eroded tracheostomas. Tracheal stenosis may be managed by dilations, excision of the stenotic area with internal splinting for 6 weeks or more, or excision of the stenotic area with end-to-end anastomosis of the trachea. As much as 50 per cent of the length of the trachea can be resected and end-to-end anastomosis performed.

Foreign Bodies of the Larynx, Tracheobronchial Tree, and Esophagus

Foreign bodies are retained in the larynx generally because they are sharp and stick into the mucous membrane or are irregular and soft and are caught between the two vocal cords in laryngospasm. A frequently fatal laryngeal foreign body is a bolus of meat. The resulting laryngospasm completely occludes the larynx and makes a choking individual mute. This "café coronary" may be distinguished from a myocardial infarct by the respiratory effort without exchange and the marked suprasternal, intercostal, and subxiphoid retraction. Death occurs rapidly unless an alternative airway is established or the foreign body is dislodged. As long as adequate respiratory exchange occurs, the individual should be allowed to employ protective reflexes to manage the problem. Maneuvers such as striking the choking individual on the back or turning a choking child upside down may make it more difficult for the individual to handle the problem successfully and may convert the situation into one that is less easily managed. If the individual is mute and makes no respiratory exchange, the Heimlich (abdominal thrust) maneuver should be attempted. In this maneuver, the operator places his arms around the choking individual from behind, grasps the fist of one hand in the other hand, and brings both hands up in the subxiphoid area briskly to apply pressure to the diaphragm. The pressure increases the intrathoracic pressure and may expel the foreign body. Should this maneuver fail, an alternative airway must be established by the prompt performance of a tracheotomy.

Smooth objects such as nuts, kernels of corn, watermelon seeds, beans, peas, and plastic toys pass through the larynx into the tracheobronchial tree. At the onset, there is severe spasmodic coughing that continues for approximately 30 minutes. During this period of time, the foreign body migrates from one portion of the tracheobronchial tree to another. It more frequently comes to rest in the right bronchus because the right bronchus is larger than the left and makes less of an angle with the long axis of the trachea, and the carina is to the left of the midline of the tracheal lumen. As it finally comes to rest, the coughing subsides, and a latent period begins during which the patient is free of symptoms. The mistaken inference is often made by the family and the physician in attendance that the foreign body has been expelled. However, careful auscultation of the chest may demonstrate an expiratory wheeze and the signs of obstructive emphysema. The most common mechanism of the bronchial obstruction due to a foreign body is a one-way valve through which air may enter the bronchus distal to the foreign body during inspiration, but which affords limited egress on expiration. This type of obstruction produces emphysema distal to the foreign body. The obstructive emphysema may become apparent radiographically only on expiration. The mediastinum shifts away from the obstructed lung, and the obstructed portion of the lung becomes radiolucent compared with the normal lung.

A foreign body that completely obstructs the bronchus causes the rapid development of a more serious pathophysiologic state. Complete atelectasis of the obstructed lung occurs as a result of absorption of the remaining air in the lung. The mediastinum shifts toward the atelectatic lung, and the remaining lung undergoes compensatory emphysema. The atelectatic lung is useless as far as ventilatory exchange is concerned, and the efficiency of the emphysematous lung is greatly reduced. Rapid cardiorespiratory failure occurs unless the foreign body is removed. This type of complete bronchial obstruction is likely to occur with smooth hygroscopic foreign bodies, such as beans, that swell in the bronchus.

Vegetable foreign bodies are very poorly tolerated. Metallic and plastic foreign bodies that cause partial obstruction of the bronchus may be tolerated for long periods. Nuts, particularly peanuts, produce a very severe tracheobronchitis. After a latent period of 24 hours, the patient develops a cough productive of purulent sputum, and a febrile course begins. A long-indwelling foreign body of the bronchus may produce bronchiectasis, recurrent pneumonitis, lung abscess, and empyema. Tracheobronchial foreign bodies are removed under general anesthesia through an open bronchoscope with forceps designed specifically for each type of foreign body.

Foreign bodies of the esophagus are likely to lodge just below the cricopharyngeus muscle. Ninety-five per cent of esophageal foreign bodies are found in this location. Other locations are the gastroesophageal junction and the indentations of the esophagus caused by the left bronchus and the arch of the aorta. The constrictors of the pharynx are very strong and can propel almost any irregular object through the cricopharyngeus muscle. When the foreign body has passed the cricopharyngeus, the muscular activity is very weak, and progress occurs mainly by gravity. Therefore, irregular objects are brought to a very abrupt stop just below the cricopharyngeus muscle.

The symptoms of a foreign body of the esophagus are dysphagia and pain in the suprasternal area on swallowing. Bulky foreign bodies in the cervical esophagus may produce upper airway obstruction by extrinsic pressure through the membranous posterior wall of the trachea. Foreign bodies can be identified on a lateral neck radiograph if they are radiopaque. If they are radiolucent, evidence of a foreign body may still be obtained, because the foreign body tends to hold the esophageal walls apart and air may be seen in the cervical esophagus. If the foreign body cannot be located on a lateral neck film, posteroanterior and lateral chest films are taken. If the foreign body cannot be located in this manner, an esophagogram may demonstrate it. A small pledget of cotton saturated with a solution of barium sulfate may hang on a sharp foreign body. A foreign body of the esophagus is removed under general anesthesia through an open esophagoscope. The foreign body is grasped, disengaged, and removed as a trailing foreign body or through the esophagoscope with a foreign body forceps appropriate to the object. The longer a foreign body remains in the esophagus, the greater the risk of perforation of the esophagus. Perforation of the esophagus produces air and soft tissue swelling in the paraesophageal tissue that may be demonstrated on physical examination and radiographically.

Infectious Diseases

CROUP. There are two forms of croup, epiglottitis and laryngotracheobronchitis. Croup occurs primarily in children over 1 year and under 5 years of age. It may be viral or bacterial. Parainfluenza type I is the most frequently isolated agent in viral croup. *Haemophilus influenzae* is the most frequently isolated agent in bacterial croup, but *Staphylococcus* and *Streptococcus* may also cause croup.

Haemophilus influenzae type b is the predominant microorganism in epiglottitis and frequently causes a bacteremia. Both epiglottitis and laryngotracheobronchitis may produce the rapid onset of upper respiratory obstruction with inspiratory stridor and suprasternal, supraclavicular, intercostal, and subxiphoid retractions. The voice may be hoarse, and the cough has a brassy quality with subglottic edema.

Epiglottitis is more likely to cause abrupt and complete airway obstruction. When the diagnosis of epiglottitis is made, nasotracheal intubation is performed and maintained for 48 hours until the supraglottic swelling subsides. In laryngotracheobronchitis, the airway obstruction results in part from edema, but there are also tenacious mucoid secretions. Humidification of the inspired atmosphere liquefies the material, and the patient may cough it out to reduce the degree of airway obstruction. Antibiotic therapy is initiated at the onset of both diseases; amoxicillin is the drug of choice because the infection is frequently caused by *Haemophilus influenzae*. Corticosteroid therapy is also initiated in an attempt to reduce the inflammatory swelling. If the degree of airway obstruction becomes severe in laryngotracheobronchitis, a tracheotomy is performed in preference to prolonged endotracheal intubation, because the rate of complications, such as laryngeal and subglottic stenosis, is quite high with prolonged endotracheal intubation. The decision regarding a tracheotomy depends on the evaluation of the amount of ventilatory exchange, the degree of fatigue of the patient, and the respiratory and pulse rates. Development of cyanosis is a late sign, and the decision to perform a tracheotomy should be made before the advent of this ominous sign. Blood gas determinations are helpful, but the clinical situation may change very rapidly. If it appears that the ventilatory exchange is inadequate, the necessary ventilatory effort cannot be maintained, or there is a progressive increase in the pulse rate above 140 per minute, a tracheotomy should be performed. The airway emergency is converted to an elective tracheotomy by inserting an endotracheal tube or a bronchoscope. General anesthesia is induced, and the tracheotomy is performed in a relaxed patient under unhurried and ideal circumstances. This approach reduces the incidence of complications such as pneumothorax.

Neoplasms

Benign neoplasms, including papillomas, fibromas, myxomas, chondromas, neurofibromas, hemangiomas, and so forth, may involve any part of the larynx including the true vocal cords. Such lesions can ordinarily be removed at direct laryngoscopy with restoration of the voice, the airway, and the functional integrity of the laryngeal sphincter.

MALIGNANT NEOPLASMS OF THE LARYNX. The majority of malignant neoplasms of the larynx are squamous cell carcinomas. Squamous cell carcinoma of the larynx represents approximately 2 per cent of all cancer deaths. It is a disease mainly of males, with a sex ratio of 8:1. The peak incidence of carcinoma of the larynx is in the fifth and sixth decades of life. Laryngeal carcinoma occurs more commonly in individuals with a large ethanolic intake. It rarely develops in those who do not smoke.

Carcinoma may arise from the mucous membrane of any part of the larynx; however, there is a predilection for the true vocal cords, particularly the anterior portions of the true vocal cords. The epiglottis and pyriform sinus are common sites of origin of carcinoma. The natural history of the carcinoma varies considerably from one location to another. The early symptom of carcinoma of the true vocal cords is hoarseness. In any patient with hoarseness lasting 2 weeks, indirect laryngoscopy should be performed. Any discrete lesions of the mucous membrane of the larynx should be biopsied. Carcinomas of the true vocal cord limited to the middle third of the true vocal cord and not impairing the mobility of the cord are treated with radiation therapy or cordectomy with an overall 5-year survival rate of 85 to 95 per cent. Because cordectomy causes permanent hoarseness and the use of irradiation usually returns the voice to normal, radiation therapy is the treatment of choice. Cordectomy is reserved for the 5 to 15 per cent who have persistent carcinoma following radiation therapy. The likelihood of metastasis in early carcinoma of the true vocal cord is very slight.

The mobility of the vocal cord becomes impaired in more advanced carcinomas as a result of invasion of the intrinsic musculature and cartilage. With invasion of the intrinsic musculature, the rate of metastasis increases. With invasion of the thyroid cartilage, the rate of 5-year survival with radiation therapy decreases precipitously. Operation becomes the treatment of choice for lesions that involve the anterior commissure where cartilage is very early invaded and for larger glottic lesions in which the mobility of the true vocal cord is impaired. Often a vertical hemilaryngectomy can be performed for preservation of the phonatory and sphincteric functions of the larynx. In more advanced cases, total laryngectomy is required, and the laryngectomy may be combined with a radical neck dissection if palpable metastases are present.

Supraglottic carcinomas tend to be asymptomatic until they reach considerable size. They may produce hoarseness by secondary involvement of the vocal cords, or they may produce pain on swallowing as the first symptom. Often the pain radiates to the ears. Not infrequently, a patient with a supraglottic carcinoma presents with the chief complaint of a swelling in the neck that represents a metastasis. The likelihood of nonpalpable metastasis being present is 35 per cent. Early supraglottic carcinoma is successfully treated with radiation therapy; but in advanced lesions, better survival rates are obtained with a combination of radiation and surgical therapy. Better local and regional control is obtained with postoperative radiation therapy than with preoperative radiation therapy. The 2-year disease-free survival approximates 70 per cent. In many patients with supraglottic carcinomas, the neoplasm can be completely removed by performing a supraglottic partial laryngectomy with preservation of the phonatory and sphincteric function of the larynx. If the glottis is involved, a total laryngectomy is usually required. These procedures are often combined with a radical neck dissection if there are palpable metastases.

Pyriform sinus carcinomas tend to remain asymptomatic for long periods of time. Often the patient presents with dysphagia and pain on swallowing that may radiate to the ear on the same side. Often the presenting complaint is a mass in the neck that represents a metastasis. A combination of preoperative or postoperative radiation therapy and operation yields better survival rates than does operation alone. Depending on the location of the lesion in the pyriform sinus, a partial laryngectomy can sometimes be accomplished with preservation of the phonatory and sphincteric functions of the larynx. More often, a total laryngectomy is required. Either of these procedures is combined with a radical neck dissection if there are palpable metastases. The 5-year survival rate for all stages is 30 per cent.

A total laryngectomy requires the formation of a permanent tracheostomy in which the trachea is transected and anastomosed to the skin of the lower part of the neck. Rehabilitation of the postlaryngectomy patient requires the development of alaryngeal or esophageal speech. In this technique, the patient draws air into the esophagus during inspiration and gradually eructs the air through the cricopharyngeus muscle. The opening of the esophagus vibrates and serves as the sounding source. The sound is articulated by the pharynx, palate, tongue, teeth, and lips into speech. For those individuals who, because of age or other physical or emotional reasons, cannot develop alaryngeal speech, an electrolarynx can serve as the sounding source for modification by the articulators. The oscillator of the electrolarynx is placed in the submandibular area, and the sound is articulated into speech. Most patients who require a laryngectomy may return to their former occupation. With proper guidance in their rehabilitation, laryngectomees may resume all activities except swimming.

40

THE MOUTH, TONGUE, JAWS, AND SALIVARY GLANDS

Milton T. Edgerton, M.D., Michael F. Angel, M.D., and Raymond F. Morgan, M.D., D.M.D.

LIPS

Clefts are caused by lack of fusion of a single central prolabium with one or both of the lateral mesodermal masses. Cleft lip is usually associated with a cleft palate and occurs three times as frequently as does cleft palate alone.

Clefts of the lip are usually closed surgically during the first 3 months of life. Many surgeons apply the rule of tens, delaying closure of the lip until the child weighs 10 pounds, has a hemogloblin of 10 gm. or greater, and is 10 weeks old.

The pathologic process involves a transverse gap in soft tissues and a loss of vertical length of the lip. In general, internal lip tissue is obtained by some modification of the Z-plasty principle for adding tissue to the cleft area.

Macrostomia is a rare condition characterized by lateral displacement of the oral commissure producing an enlarged mouth. *Microstomia*, which is a small mouth, usually occurs with a small retruded mandible (micrognathia). It may cause feeding difficulties requiring surgical intervention.

Lacerations of the lip frequently involve both the mucosa and skin with division of the intervening muscularity. Because of the circular and radial distribution of the perioral muscularity, full-thickness lacerations tend to open widely when the muscle is divided. This may cause the inexperienced clinician to suspect tissue loss when the problem is only tissue retraction.

In repair of a lip, it is most important to accurately align the vermilion-cutaneous junction because even a slight disparity in reconstituting this line produces an obvious cosmetic deformity.

Thermal burns of the lips generally involve the exposed skin and mucosal surfaces. They are treated according to the depth of the burn in much the same way as are cutaneous burns elsewhere on the body.

One of the most frequently seen chemical burns of the lips is due to the use of lye for suicide. Treatment consists of early, copious irrigation with cold water. Systemic steroids are also helpful in diminishing the inflammatory reaction.

Electrical burns of the lips are most frequently seen in small children who are prone to chew on electrical cords or place the ends of extension cords in their mouths. Saliva creates a short circuit across the terminal within the plug, causing an

---

See the corresponding chapter or part in the *Textbook of Surgery*, 14th edition, pp. 1209–1234, for a more detailed discussion of this topic, including a comprehensive list of references.

electrical burn. Tissue destruction is sudden, extensive, and progressive. Initial treatment of electrical burns of the lips should be conservative.

Herpetic stomatitis is a viral infection that presents as yellowish papulovesicular lesions that may be discrete or occur in groups. After approximately 10 days, the lesion clears spontaneously. Acyclovir has been beneficial in the treatment of severe herpetic lesions.

Tumors

Tumors may arise from any of the tissues forming the lips. Treatment of these lesions is usually surgical excision with microscopic examination of surgical margins.

Most *cancers* of the lip arise at the skin-vermilion junction and represent approximately 15 per cent of all malignancies of the head and neck. Sunlight, excessive use of tobacco and alcohol, prior gamma radiation, and syphilis are etiologic factors. Squamous cell carcinoma is responsible for 99 per cent of all lip cancers. Management is individualized. Factors involved in the treatment plan are age of the patient, reliability of the patient, size of the lesion, histologic grade of the tumor, staging of the lesion, and ability of the surgeon.

ORAL CAVITY

Congenital Malformations

Clefts of the secondary palate (incisive foramen, posterior to the uvula) develop during the seventh to twelfth weeks of embryonic life. The defect is due to failure of the lateral mesodermal shelves to develop and fuse in the midline. The severity may vary from total, complete bilateral cleft of the hard and soft palate with wide communication between the oral and nasal cavities to a cleft manifested by only a slight notching of the uvula.

Clefts of the palate are repaired surgically when the child is between 1 and 2 years old. It is desirable to have the palate repaired by the time the child begins attempts to speak. If the repair is delayed, the child develops faulty speech habits that are difficult, if not impossible, to correct later with speech therapy.

PIERRE ROBIN'S SYNDROME. This anomaly is characterized by a small mandible, retrodisplacement of the chin and posterior displacement, and ptosis of the tongue that produces airway obstruction. The cause is unknown, although some believe that retrognathia is secondary to intrauterine pressure on the chin caused by fetal positioning, delaying forward development of the mandible. The degree of airway obstruction varies. In the most severe cases, operative management is indicated. Tracheotomy may be avoided by fixing the tongue to the lip. The ultimate growth potential of the mandible is unpredictable.

Trauma

Bleeding from the mouth following trauma is often profuse because of the extreme vascularity of this area. Hemorrhage is initially best controlled by digital pressure. The application of multiple hemostats in the emergency room is unnecessary and may cause neural damage. Local anesthesia with epinephrine (1:100,000) is helpful. Chromic catgut sutures or silk sutures should be used. Monofilament nylon sutures, which are stiff and uncomfortable to the patient, should not be used.

CHRONIC TRAUMA. Chronic trauma to the intraoral mucosa may induce hyperkeratosis or leukoplakia; if prolonged, cancer may result. Snuff, smoke, chewing tobacco, alcohol, and oral trauma from various dental sources have all been implicated in the development of leukoplakia. Initial treatment should consist of identification and elimination of all irritating factors. Recently, vitamin A analogs have shown some efficacy. If the lesion does not resolve, surgical excision is required for prevention of invasive cancer.

Infections

The majority of intraoral infections are odontogenic in origin. Laceration of soft tissues and fractures of the maxilla and mandible represent only a small percentage of infections. The etiologic bacteria are usually mixed flora. Nearly all bacteria are penicillin sensitive.

If an infection is not controlled, it can extend through neighboring fascial planes. This may rarely threaten the airway and require a tracheotomy. Most infections readily respond to antibiotics and drainage procedures.

Benign Tumors of the Oral Cavity

Nonmalignant tumors within the oral cavity usually arise from the gingival tissues or mucoperiosteal membrane. These include pyogenic granulomas, hemangioma, and giant cell tumor. Second in frequency are hyperplastic reactions of the cheeks and lips to chronic trauma. Third are tumors found beneath the mucosa of the cheek, such as fibromas, hemangiomas, and benign tumors of the roof of the mouth. The least common site for benign tumors is the floor of the mouth.

Most benign tumors are readily diagnosed by observation, palpation, and radiographic studies. When diagnosis is not readily apparent, a biopsy is indicated. Treatment is total excision. Radiotherapy is never indicated for management of these benign lesions.

Malignant Soft Tissue Tumors of the Oral Cavity

Although sarcomas, adenocarcinomas, and other cancers occur, the majority of intraoral cancers are squamous cell cancers representing 97 per cent. Carcinoma of the oral cavity is best classified by anatomic location.

Fifteen per cent of oral cavity cancers occur in the floor of the mouth. Because of its dependent position, this area has increased contact time with saliva-laden carcinogens (alcohol, tobacco). Carcinoma of the floor of the mouth presents as an infiltrating lesion that often extends across the midline, into the tongue, and into the first-echelon lymph nodes (submandibular). Assessment of extent is obtained visually, by palpation, and by use of computed tomographic scanning. Treatment is dictated by size of tumor, extent of invasion of neighboring structures (tongue, mandible), and presence of lymph node metastases. Smaller lesions are currently treated by surgical therapy or radiotherapy alone, whereas larger lesions often require combined therapy.

Cancer of the buccal mucosa usually occurs in an older age group. It is often preceded by leukoplakia and tends to be well differentiated. Diagnosis is by direct inspection and bimanual palpation. Treatment often requires resection of the overlying cheek skin, which produces a through-and-through defect. Reconstruction is by pedicle flaps or free tissue transfer.

Cancer of the gingiva occurs frequently in the lower jaw, and like buccal cancer, it is well differentiated. Surgical therapy is the treatment of choice.

The oropharynx includes the soft palate, pharyngeal wall, tonsil, and posterior one third of the tongue. Cancer of the tonsil is the most common cancer of this area. It often presents with pain to the ear (otalgia) and an enlarged neck mass. Cancer in this area is often less differentiated, and the patient sometimes presents late in the course. Treatment is surgical therapy if possible with radiation therapy postoperatively. Survival remains distressingly low, so newer combinations with chemotherapy are now being tried.

Tongue cancer represents 15 per cent of all head and neck cancers. Premalignant changes frequently proceed to frank carcinoma. Patients often present with chronic nonhealing ulcers. Small lesions can be accurately assessed, but as the tumor grows and infiltrates muscle, judgment of the extent of tumor becomes more difficult and requires imaging techniques. Lymph node metastases are common.

The primary reason for surgical failure is too small a resection of tongue and failure to clear nodal drainage areas. Reconstruction is by use of pedicle and free tissue transfer with bone if needed.

JAWS

The bony upper and lower jaws in the human are sometimes referred to as the upper and lower maxillae. The maxilla is composed of several membranous bones fused together: two maxillary bones, two palatine bones, and laterally the two zygomas that form the bony prominence of each cheek. The lower jaw is more commonly known as the mandible. Surgical diseases of the jaw may be conveniently divided according to the etiologic basis.

Congenital Malformation

Micrognathia is probably most commonly seen with Pierre Robin's syndrome as previously described. Other hypoplasias occur. Lack of development of the mandibular condyles may produce ankylosis. Very rarely, total absence (agnathia) of the mandible may be encountered.

Mandibular overgrowth is most commonly symmetrical and causes prognathism. *Hyperplasia (prognathism)* usually does not become evident until late childhood. Failure to correct the condition may produce a severe deformity and premature loss of dentition.

Injuries

Most injuries to the jaw are due to falls, fights, or automobile accidents. Membranous bone of the upper jaw has a great capacity to absorb force with deceleration injuries. This property has saved many lives by protecting the brain from lethal injury.

The muscles of the upper jaw are small and lack the strength and leverage of those inserting on the mandible. Consequently, reduction of maxillary fractures does not require strong or prolonged fixation. The fractures usually occur in well-defined patterns located at a weak point in the bone. LeFort in 1900 first recognized this and classified maxillary fractures into three types.

Diagnostic features of the upper jaw fractures include malocclusion, open-bite deformity, and mobility of the midface. Standard radiographs provide information, but computed tomographic scanning in multiple planes (axial, coronal) and, most recently, the three-dimensional technique provide more information.

The treatment of these fractures requires direct surgical exposure. With use of craniofacial techniques, the entire facial skeleton can be exposed by combining full coronal, subciliary, and upper buccal sulcus incisions. Bone fragments can be accurately reduced and fixed, and primary bone grafting can be done if needed.

The malar bone (zygoma) is an extremely dense base that forms the prominence of the cheek; it is commonly fractured. Clinical features are flattening of the cheekbone with inferior displacement of the lateral canthus with a laterally based subconjunctival hemorrhage. The floor of the orbit may be disrupted, producing blood within the maxillary sinus and diplopia. The globe can sometimes be injured. Treatment includes accurate reduction, fixation, and exclusion of significant globe injury.

Location, number and direction of fractures, and presence of teeth dictate the severity of the injury. There are several means of treating mandibular fractures. Simple intermaxillary wiring is a common, effective means of treating many of these fractures. Sometimes open reduction and application of metal plates are required.

Tumors of the Jaw

Most benign tumors of the upper and lower jaw can be readily excised when the diagnosis is established. Radiolucent lesions are often dental or root cysts. Radiopaque benign tumors such as cementomas, osteomas, and fibromas are quite common.

Both osteogenic sarcoma and osteochondrosarcomas occur in the jaws, and the prognosis is grave. Current treatment is combination surgical therapy, radiation, and chemotherapy. Rarely, the jaws can be a site of metastatic disease. The most common sources are breast, thyroid, and prostate; biopsy confirms the diagnosis.

SALIVARY GLANDS

The salivary glands are tubuloacinar glands arising from ectodermal and entodermal invaginations. There are six major salivary glands consisting of three pairs (parotid, submandibular, and sublingual). There are also numerous minor salivary glands located submucosally throughout the oral cavity and pharynx.

Trauma

Trauma to the face may cause division of parotid glandular tissue or Stensen's duct. When the duct is divided, the two ends must be carefully identified and repaired over a small plastic catheter that emerges into the oral cavity. Closure of skin over injured glandular tissue usually heals without difficulty. Late complications of injury to the parotid may include development of salivary-cutaneous fistulas. Chronic fistulas may require operative reconstruction.

Parotitis

Acute suppurative parotitis occurs generally in the very young or old. Dehydration and poor oral hygiene are important etiologic factors. If treated early, the condition responds to conservative therapy. If left untreated, however, it may produce abscess formation and sepsis, at which time surgical excision of necrotic tissue is often lifesaving.

Metabolic Disorders

Calculi may form in the salivary glands. Damaged ducts and abnormal pH are important contributing factors. Infection often occurs secondarily. Diagnosis is made by palpation and radiography. When located, the stone can be removed intraorally, although total removal of the gland may be necessary.

Tumors

Neoplasms of the salivary glands constitute 5 per cent of all head and neck tumors. They are a major cause of salivary gland surgery. Approximately 70 per cent of tumors occur in the parotid gland; 70 per cent of these are benign. Approximately 60 per cent of submandibular gland tumors, however, are malignant.

Most parotid tumors are slow-growing, firm, nodular masses that are sometimes mistaken for lymph nodes or cysts. Physical examination sometimes assisted by fine-needle aspiration and radiographic studies allows the surgeon to plan the surgical procedure.

The facial nerve that innervates the mimetic muscles of the face traverses the parotid gland. Damage to the entire nerve causes total paralysis, whereas division of branches of the nerve is variable in the clinical outcome.

The technique of lateral lobectomy with facial nerve dissection is useful for tumors of the lateral lobe. For benign and low-grade malignancy, it is both diagnostic and therapeutic. Most surgeons prefer locating the facial nerve as it exits the stylomastoid foramen and tracing it distally. The operation is tedious and should be done by those very familiar with the anatomy of the region. Even with great gentleness, transient paralysis of the face is common. Any injury to a major branch of the facial nerve should be repaired immediately.

The mixed tumor (pleomorphic adenoma) constitutes 70 per cent of all neoplasms of the parotid gland. It is followed by Warthin's tumor, adenomas, and oncocytomas. Malignant tumors are classified as low-grade (acinic cell, mucoepidermoid, and adenocystic) and high-grade (adenocarcinoma, high-grade mucoepidermoid, and squamous cell). This classification aids in assessing speed of tumor growth and type of surgical therapy.

SUBMAXILLARY GLAND TUMORS. Because of the deep location of the submaxillary gland and high incidence of malignancy, lymph node dissection is performed more often than in parotid cancer. Often the mylohyoid muscle and portions of the mandible must be resected for achieving adequate margins. Sometimes, the lingual and hypoglossal nerves must be resected.

The most frequent tumor of the minor salivary gland occurs in the palate and is a mixed tumor, more than 75 per cent of which are malignant. Patients with such tumors often require full-thickness resection of portions of the hard and soft palate.

41

NEUROSURGERY

I

Neuroradiology
William J. Meisler, M.D.

The most important modalities for imaging central nervous system disease are computed tomographic (CT) scanning and magnetic resonance imaging (MRI). Both allow direct visualization of pathologic processes of the central nervous system in several planes and, except for the administration of contrast agents intravenously, are totally noninvasive. Specialized studies such as angiography and myelography remain as supplements to CT and MRI but are much less commonly used. Before the introduction of MRI, CT scanning was the most important diagnostic test in neuroradiology. At present, it has its greatest utility in the evaluation of acute neurologic problems and bone abnormalities.

In most acute situtations, a noncontrast CT scan should be obtained, because the noncontrast study most clearly defines acute hemorrhages, acute infarcts, or fractures. On a noncontrast study, acute hemorrhage appears hyperdense (white). This hyperdensity may be very difficult to distinguish from hyperdensity related to contrast enhancement on contrast-enhanced scans; therefore, all patients being evaluated for acute hemorrhage must at least initially be evaluated with a noncontrast study. The other common acute condition requiring evaluation by CT scanning is "stroke-like" symptoms. This frequently is the result of cerebral infarction. Infarction never shows contrast enhancement acutely and usually appears as a lucency that is easily seen on the noncontrast study. In addition, the noncontrast study easily excludes other conditions mimicking an infarct, such as an acute subdural hematoma or hypertensive hemorrhage. For these reasons, in almost all acute situations, a noncontrast CT scan is sufficient.

In chronic situations, such as exclusion of tumors, abscess, or vascular malformation, a contrast-enhanced CT scan is required for determining the presence and total extent of the disease. Only rarely is a noncontrast study helpful in these instances. Thus, a contrast examination alone is usually appropriate for evaluation of chronic disease.

Because MRI does not visualize the bones well, CT remains the best examination for evaluation of bone problems. This would include examination of fractures of the spine and skull as well as primary bone problems such as abnormalities of the temporal bone and dysplasias such as fibrous dysplasia.

See the corresponding chapter or part in the *Textbook of Surgery*, 14th edition, pp. 1236–1241, for a more detailed discussion of this topic, including a comprehensive list of references.

Whereas CT scanning demonstrates most tumors, abscesses, and other masses extremely well, these abnormalities are demonstrated even better and often with greater sensitivity with MRI. MRI not only displays greater anatomic detail but also is more sensitive for detection of many disease processes. An MRI study typically consists of several different types of images. The T1 sequence can be recognized by the fact that water-containing tissues are of low intensity (black) and fat-containing tissues are of high intensity (white). The T1 sequence shows excellent anatomic detail and is the appropriate sequence to use with contrast enhancement. On the T2 images, water-containing tissues are of high intensity and fat-containing tissues are of low intensity. Whereas the anatomic detail is not as great on T2 sequences as it is on T1 sequences, the T2 sequences have greater sensitivity for the disease; therefore, the two studies usually complement one another. MRI can provide certain unique information such as tumor encasement of vessels. It is also excellent in the evaluation of lesions at the base of the skull, such as pituitary tumors and cerebellopontine angle masses. MRI has superseded almost all modalities in evaluation of disease of the spine.

Indications for cerebral angiography have been sharply circumscribed since the introduction of CT and MRI. This is indeed fortunate inasmuch as cerebral angiography is an invasive procedure with the risk of precipitation of an infarct during the course of the procedure. It is most useful in evaluation of cerebral aneurysms, vasculitis, carotid artery disease particularly at the carotid bifurcation and carotid siphon, arteriovenous malformations, and occasionally vascular displacement related to tumor or in localization of superficial cortical veins before surgery. More recently a number of therapeutic procedures have been developed that require an endovascular approach. Two types of angiographic examination are possible. The "cut film" method provides superior resolution and is best for evaluation of intercerebral aneurysms or vasculitides where fine detail is needed. "Digital" imaging refers to studies performed with computer-enhanced images. The digital examination is performed more quickly than is the cut film method but has poorer resolution. Digital angiography is frequently used for evaluation of carotid artery disease. The choice of imaging is most often left to the discretion of the radiologist.

Myelography has been almost completely supplanted by MRI in evaluation of diseases of the intraspinal contents. MRI is superior not only because it is a noninvasive test but also because it provides much information about the surrounding soft tissues that myelography cannot demonstrate. MRI has proved to be a very effective test in evaluation of congenital abnormalities of the spinal contents and in evaluation of both primary and metastatic tumors of the spine. In most cases of lumbar disc disease, an MRI or noncontrast CT scan of the spine proves superior to a myelogram. In certain instances in which an MRI does not give sufficient information, particularly with cervical and thoracic disc disease, a

myelogram may be performed followed by CT scanning of
the spine, the "CT-myelogram."

II

Intracranial Tumors
Robert H. Wilkins, M.D.

Primary intracranial tumors arise from tissues of the brain
or pituitary gland or their coverings. Often, these lesions are
not clearly separable into benign and malignant forms. Secondary intracranial tumors represent local extensions from
regional tumors or metastases from a primary malignancy
elsewhere in the body. The most common location of brain
tumors in childhood is below the tentorium within the
posterior cranial fossa. In contrast, the most common location
of brain tumors in adult life is above the tentorium. Within
the various intracranial locations, certain types of tumors
occur more commonly than others, both in childhood and in
adulthood.

SYMPTOMS AND SIGNS. Intracranial tumors can present
in several different ways. By their growth, they can cause an
increase in intracranial pressure, either directly by the mass
of the tumor or indirectly by obstructing the circulation of
the cerebrospinal fluid and producing hydrocephalus. In
addition, bleeding may occur into the tumor, with a sudden
increase in its mass effect. The symptoms that may be
produced by a generalized increase in intracranial pressure
are headaches (especially prominent in the morning, with a
dependent head position, or during straining), nausea, vomiting, and a reduction in the level of consciousness. Such a
patient may exhibit papilledema and unilateral or bilateral
abducens paresis. A generalized increase in intracranial pressure may be tolerated for a period of time, but with further
tumor growth, brain herniation may occur with a rapid
decline in the patient's neurologic function.

A second way in which an intracranial tumor may present
is by the loss of function of the portion of the nervous system
that is involved by the tumor. In contrast to the symptoms
and signs caused by an increase in intracranial pressure, the
symptoms and signs caused by the loss of function of a
specific area of the nervous system often permit an accurate
presumptive diagnosis based on the neurologic history and
physical examination.

In addition, an intracranial tumor may be manifested by

See the corresponding chapter or part in the *Textbook of Surgery,*
14th edition, pp. 1241–1246, for a more detailed discussion of this
topic, including a comprehensive list of references.

hyperactive function. The tumor can be the cause of this hyperfunction, such as a pituitary adenoma that overproduces one or more hormones or a choroid plexus papilloma that overproduces cerebrospinal fluid, or the tumor may stimulate seizures that arise from the adjacent or infiltrated brain.

DIAGNOSIS. The most common radiographic screening examination is CT scanning. Most intracranial tumors are demonstrated by such scanning, especially if scans made after the intravenous injection of an iodinated contrast agent (contrast-enhanced scans) are compared with analogous unenhanced scans. The bony structures forming the base of the skull are especially well demonstrated by CT scanning. However, these same bony structures are often the source of artifacts that degrade the images of the adjacent portions of the brain. MRI does not demonstrate bony detail but provides excellent visualization of the brain at the cranial base and at the craniocervical junction. MRI also offers much clearer and more easily obtained coronal and sagittal views. Among other types of radiologic studies are those done for specific purposes rather than for screening. For example, cerebral angiography may be useful for determining the vascularity of the tumor and its effect on the major adjacent vessels.

TREATMENT. The mainstay of the treatment of intracranial tumors is surgical removal. The major advances that have been made in the past two decades in diagnostic and therapeutic technology have made this task easier and safer than previously. With CT–guided or MRI–guided stereotactic techniques, tumors within the nervous system can now be biopsied through a burr hole with low morbidity. The introduction of the operative microscope into neurosurgery and the development of neurosurgical microtechnique have permitted tumor exposure through a small cranial opening with the double aids of magnification and excellent illumination. The simultaneous evolution of bipolar electrical technology for tissue coagulation and cutting and the development of devices that employ laser energy, ultrasonic vibration, suction, or mechanical cutting for removal of tissue permit resection of intracranial tumors more easily and safely. These technological advances have improved the outlook for patients with certain types of intracranial tumors, such as meningiomas, pituitary adenomas, and neurinomas of the cranial nerves, but they have not had a large impact on the gliomas, which in most instances cannot be cured by surgical resection.

III

Spontaneous Intracranial and Intraspinal Hemorrhage
Allan H. Friedman, M.D.

SUBARACHNOID HEMORRHAGE

Subarachnoid hemorrhage is characterized by the sudden onset of a severe headache. The headache is recalcitrant to minor analgesic medications and usually persists for days. Concomitant with the headache, the patient suffers a change in level of consciousness ranging from momentary confusion to persistent coma. Over the ensuing hours, the blood induces a sterile meningitis that produces a stiff neck, minor fever, and photophobia. Physical examination may reveal retinal hemorrhages. Approximately one third of patients suffer a "warning leak" manifest as a severe headache before a life-threatening hemorrhage. Unfortunately, these warning events frequently go unrecognized. The clinical diagnosis of spontaneous subarachnoid hemorrhage is verified by brain computed tomographic scan or lumbar puncture. When the diagnosis of subarachnoid hemorrhage is made, a cerebral angiogram should be performed for localizing the source of the hemorrhage.

ETIOLOGY. The most common cause of a nontraumatic subarachnoid hemorrhage is a ruptured intracranial aneurysm. The second most common cause is a ruptured arteriovenous malformation. In a smaller number of patients, the hemorrhage is the result of hypertensive cerebrovascular disease, primary or metastatic tumor, mycotic aneurysm, blood dyscrasia, anticoagulation therapy, eclampsia, intracranial infection, or spinal angiomatous malformation. In approximately 10 per cent of cases, the etiologic factor is never discovered.

CEREBRAL ANEURYSMS

Intracranial berry aneurysms are thin-walled outpouchings that most often originate at the bifurcation of the large intracranial vessels that reside at the base of the brain. Berry aneurysms have been postulated to be due to congenital deficiencies or degenerative changes in the vessel's wall. As the aneurysm enlarges, its internal elastic lamina and muscularis fragment so that the dome of the aneurysm consists only of intima and flimsy adventitial connective tissue.

Aneurysms usually present with a subarachnoid hemorrhage, but they may on occasion present as an intracranial mass. When presenting as a mass, berry aneurysms most frequently manifest as an optic or oculomotor nerve dysfunc-

---

See the corresponding chapter or part in the *Textbook of Surgery*, 14th edition, pp. 1246–1252, for a more detailed discussion of this topic, including a comprehensive list of references.

tion. Although berry aneurysms are sometimes referred to as congenital aneurysms, they seldom rupture during childhood. The median age of patients presenting with a subarachnoid hemorrhage from a berry aneurysm is 50 years. Patients who survive the first hemorrhage from a berry aneurysm are at risk for recurrent bleeding and vasospasm. One in 5 patients who have a ruptured intracranial aneurysm experience a second bleeding episode in the 2 weeks following the initial hemorrhage. Approximately 50 per cent of patients experience a second hemorrhage within 6 months if the lesion remains untreated.

Cerebral vasospasm is an idiopathic narrowing of the intracranial vessels that occurs within 2 weeks after the subarachnoid hemorrhage. The phenomenon is encountered on the angiograms of approximately 60 per cent of patients. Vasospasm is associated with decreased cerebral blood flow and becomes clinically manifest as cerebral ischemia or stroke.

THERAPY. The definitive treatment of an intracranial aneurysm is surgical. Most frequently the base of the aneurysm is ligated with a metal clip, with preservation of the continuity of the parent vessel. In the few cases in which this is not possible, techniques have been devised for reducing the pressure within the aneurysm or for reinforcing its thin wall. The effects of vasospasm are prevented by treating the patient with nimodipine, a calcium channel blocking agent. Cerebral ischemia from vasospasm is treated by increasing the patient's intravascular volume and elevating the patient's systemic arterial blood pressure.

ARTERIOVENOUS MALFORMATIONS

Arteriovenous malformations are a collection of abnormal arteries and veins that shunt blood without an intervening capillary network. They may present as an intraparenchymal or sometimes subarachnoid hemorrhage. They can also come to clinical attention by precipitating seizures or headaches. Occasionally the shunt within the malformation sumps blood from a critical portion of the brain, causing a progressive neurologic deficit. Arteriovenous malformations may bleed at any time during a patient's life, with the peak incidence in individuals between 30 and 39 years of age. The incidence of rehemorrhage from an arteriovenous malformation is much lower than that from an intracranial aneurysm. Treatment consists of surgical resection of the malformation when the lesion lies outside functionally important regions of the brain. Radiation therapy has proved effective in treating smaller deeply placed lesions.

HYPERTENSIVE HEMORRHAGE

Hypertensive hemorrhage within the parenchyma of the brain presents as a rapid loss of neurologic function. General physical examination reveals findings consistent with long-standing hypertension. The hemorrhage emanates from small deep perforating arteries that have suffered degenerative changes secondary to long-standing hypertension. These hemorrhages most frequently begin in the putamen or external capsule. Patients with a hemorrhage in this location typically experience a rapidly progressive hemiparesis, hemisensory loss, and hemianopsia contralateral to the hemorrhage. Hypertensive hemorrhages within the cerebellum present with headache, nausea, and vomiting. As the brain stem is compressed by the cerebellar hemorrhage, the patient develops progressive difficulty with lateral gaze, sixth nerve dysfunction, and facial paralysis culminating in a loss of consciousness.

The best treatment for a hypertensive hemorrhage is prevention with medical control of blood pressure. Surgical evacuation of supratentorial hemorrhage is reserved for patients who manifest a deterioration in their level of consciousness. However, evacuation of a cerebellar hemorrhage may be lifesaving and is performed on an emergency basis.

IV

Craniocerebral Injuries
Allan H. Friedman, M.D.

Accidental injury is the fourth leading cause of death in the United States and the leading cause of death in individuals between the ages of 1 and 44 years. Head injuries are present in more than 50 per cent of trauma-related deaths.

The final neurologic status of the patient who has sustained brain trauma is the sum of the irreversible damage acquired at the time of the initial injury and the damage that follows secondary insults. At the time of the initial head injury, the brain may suffer damage secondary to contusion, laceration, and shearing injuries. A portion of the brain sustains irreversible damage. Other areas of the brain sustain a lesser injury that has the potential to recover. Although several forms of intervention have been proposed for enhancement of the brain's normal repair processes, at this time the physician can do nothing to replace those cells that have suffered a fatal injury or to accelerate the restoration of recovering tissue. The physician's role is the prevention, recognition, and treatment of secondary brain insults.

SECONDARY BRAIN INSULTS

Secondary insults that further injure the already traumatized brain include metabolic abnormalities, expanding intra-

---

See the corresponding chapter or part in the *Textbook of Surgery,* 14th edition, pp. 1252–1257, for a more detailed discussion of this topic, including a comprehensive list of references.

cranial masses, and sustained increased intracranial pressure. Systemic metabolic abnormalities are common after a head injury. The comatose patient is prone to oral airway obstruction and aspiration pneumonia. At the scene of the accident, an oral airway should be placed, and hypoventilation should be treated with positive-pressure ventilation. Concomitant injury to the chest or upper airway may produce hypoxia or hypercapnia, and abdominal or orthopedic injury may cause hypotension.

Secondary injury may be due to an expanding intracranial mass such as a subdural, an epidural, or, rarely, an intraparenchymal hematoma. Focal brain contusion with ensuing edema can also act as a focal mass. An expanding intracranial mass not only raises intracranial pressure, but it can cause herniation of the brain through the tentorial notch or the foramen magnum. Transtentorial herniation follows downward movement of the supratentorial contents through the tentorial notch and secondary distoration of the midbrain, ocular motor nerve, and posterior cerebral artery. Clinically this manifests as one of two syndromes outlined in Table 1. The treatment of a large epidural or subdural hematoma is early recognition and rapid surgical evacuation. Intracranial pressure can be monitored by measuring pressure in the epidural space, subarachnoid space, or intraventricular fluid. Mortality is reduced without a concomitant increase in morbidity by aggressively lowering an increased intracranial pressure.

PATIENT EVALUATION

Following stabilization of the respiratory and cardiovascular systems, attention is turned to the central nervous system. The initial examination is recorded in detail so that it can be compared with subsequent examinations in order to detect a deterioration in the patient's condition. The head is inspected for scalp lacerations, compound skull fractures, or signs of a basilar skull fracture. In the awake patient, a detailed neurologic examination is performed with special attention to abnormalities in the patient's mentation, asymmetries in pupillary size, unilateral weakness, and asymmetries in deep tendon reflexes. In the comatose patient, the neurologic examination is confined to an observation of neurologic reflexes. Special attention is given to the patient's respiratory pattern, pupillary size and response to light, oculocephalic reflexes, motor response to noxious stimuli, and deep tendon reflexes.

The patient's overall neurologic status is denoted by using the Glasgow Coma Scale (Table 2). This 15-point scale assesses the patient's neurologic responsiveness in three categories (eye opening, verbal response, and best motor response) and has a high concordance among different observers.

MANAGEMENT

Patients who have sustained a transient loss of consciousness but are alert and awake upon arrival in the emergency

TABLE 1. Signs of Transtentorial Herniation

	Level of Consciousness	Respiratory Pattern	Pupillary Size; Response to Light	Oculovestibular Reflex	Motor Response to Pain
Uncal Herniation					
Early oculomotor nerve compression	Normal to obtunded	Normal	Unilaterally dilated; fixed	Full, conjugate gaze	Appropriate
Late oculomotor nerve compression	Normal to obtunded	Normal	Unilaterally dilated; fixed	Unilateral third nerve palsy	Appropriate
Midbrain compression	Comatose	Hyperventilation	Bilaterally midposition; fixed	Dysconjugate gaze	Decerebrate posturing
Central Herniation					
Early diencephalon compression	Obtunded	Deep sighs, yawns	Small; reactive	Conjugate gaze	Appropriate
Late diencephalon compression	Barely arousable to comatose	Cheyne-Stokes	Small; reactive	Conjugate gaze without nystagmus	Cortical
Midbrain compression	Comatose	Hyperventilation	Midposition; fixed	Dysconjugate gaze	Decerebrate

TABLE 2. Glasgow Coma Scale

Eye opening	
Spontaneous	E4
To speech	3
To pain	2
Nil	1
Best motor response	
Obeys	M6
Localizes	5
Withdraws	4
Abnormal flexion	3
Extension response	2
Nil	1
Verbal response	
Oriented	V5
Confused conversation	4
Inappropriate words	3
Incomprehensible sounds	2
Nil	1
Coma score = E + M + V	

room have suffered a mild head injury. These patients are given a detailed neurologic examination for detection of early manifestations of an enlarging intracranial hematoma that could cause a delayed neurologic deterioration. Patients with a severe headache, lethargy, or restlessness should be admitted to the hospital for 24 hours of observation. Although these patients are expected to make an uneventful recovery, they frequently have post-injury disability in the form of persistent headaches, unsteadiness, memory deficits, and difficulties with activities of daily living that persist for weeks to months after the accident.

Patients who have sustained a moderate head injury are lethargic, stuporous, or combative when seen in the emergency room. Approximately 10 per cent of patients entering the hospital with a moderate head injury are found to be harboring a focal intracranial lesion. Following assessment and stabilization of their cardiopulmonary systems and neurologic evaluation, these patients should have a brain CT scan. If no secondary insults occur, these patients become oriented and alert in the weeks following head injury. A high percentage of patients who have sustained a moderate head injury manifest some permanent alterations in mental acuity.

Patients who have a sustained loss of consciousness and have a Glasgow Coma Scale of less than 8 have sustained a severe head injury. These patients should undergo tracheal intubation for protection of the airway. Because 40 per cent of patients who have sustained a severe head injury harbor an intracranial mass lesion, an immediate brain CT scan should be obtained. Patients should be treated in an intensive care setting with special attention given to changes in neurologic examination, respiratory care, and management of increased intracranial pressure. The potential for recovery is inversely proportional to the patient's age and proportional to the Glasgow Coma score. Poor prognostic factors include abnormal brain stem reflexes, focal intracranial lesions, concomitant abdominal or chest injury, systemic arterial hypotension, and elevated intracranial pressure.

V

Intracranial Infections
Robert H. Wilkins, M.D.

The number of patients with infections amenable to neurosurgical treatment is relatively small, but because of the wide variety of infectious agents and the different pathologic lesions they can incite, this area remains a challenge for the neurosurgeon.

CRANIAL OSTEOMYELITIS, EPIDURAL ABSCESS, SUBDURAL EMPYEMA

A cranial bone may be the site of hematogenous spread of a bacterial infection from another area of the body, but more often it becomes involved by adjacent spread from an infected paranasal sinus, by a penetrating wound, or by an operative infection involving a craniotomy flap. Pott's puffy tumor is such a frontal osteomyelitis with marked overlying soft tissue swelling that is secondary to frontal sinusitis.

Treatment consists of the surgical removal of the infected bone with simultaneous treatment of any coexisting sinusitis. Appropriate systemic antibiotics are administered, and an adequate margin of normal bone is removed with the specimen to minimize the risk of recurrent infection.

An epidural infection is usually a well-confined bacterial abscess associated with one or more of the previously mentioned infections, and it is drained at the same time the coexisting osteomyelitis or sinusitis is treated. A subdural infection, however, is usually a more widespread empyema rather than a localized abscess, since the developing infection easily dissects open the subdural space to cover the surface of an entire cerebral hemisphere. Subdural empyema may begin by the extension of infection through the dura mater from without or through the arachnoid from within, or it may follow the operative infection of a subdural hematoma. In any event, a subdural empyema is usually treated by immediate evacuation through multiple trephine openings or

See the corresponding chapter or part in the *Textbook of Surgery*, 14th edition, pp. 1258–1259, for a more detailed discussion of this topic, including a comprehensive list of references.

a craniotomy flap in order to avert death or serious neurologic morbidity. Drains are usually left in the subdural space to be removed days later after all drainage has ceased.

ENCEPHALITIS, CEREBRITIS, BRAIN ABSCESS

The neurosurgeon may be deceived into exploring and resecting an area of severe viral encephalitis, believing it is a malignant glioma. Herpes simplex, for example, may cause a necrotic and cystic mass in the temporal lobe that closely resembles a brain tumor. However, even if the correct diagnosis is suspected preoperatively, biopsy of the lesion may be of value for verification. In addition, resection of such a lesion, or some type of decompressive operation, may also be necessary if steroids and other medical measures are inadequate to control the severe elevations of intracranial pressure that frequently accompany encephalitis.

The term *cerebritis* is usually reserved for describing the focal area of cerebral inflammation that immediately precedes the development of a brain abscess. Such areas of cerebritis may arise from the following:

1. Extension of an infection through the meninges. In this way, mastoiditis may cause an abscess in the ipsilateral temporal lobe or cerebellar hemisphere, or frontal sinusitis may produce a frontal lobe abscess.

2. Hematogenous spread from some other site, especially from the lungs, pleura, or heart, or from other areas of the body via congenital heart defects that permit the paradoxical embolism of infected material. Brain abscesses that originate in this manner are distributed among the various areas of the brain in proportion to the vascular supply, so a large number occur in the distribution of the middle cerebral arteries.

3. Inoculation through the meninges, as by a compound depressed skull fracture.

Typically, the patient with a brain abscess uncomplicated by meningitis has no systemic signs of infection, such as fever, tachycardia, or leukocytosis. The abscess presents clinically and by electroencephalography, computed tomography, magnetic resonance imaging, and cerebral angiography as an intracranial mass that must be differentiated from a neoplasm, hematoma, or some other type of space-consuming lesion.

Formerly, the preferred treatment of a brain abscess was total surgical excision. Now that such abscesses can be followed closely by CT or MRI, stereotactic aspiration and drainage are frequently employed, at least initially, to reduce the mass effect, provide information about the causative organism(s), and lower the risk of intraventricular rupture while the abscess is treated by the systemic administration of antibiotics. A patient with a brain abscess may also require treatment with a steroid medication for reduction of reactive brain edema. No matter which operative technique is used, there is a high incidence of seizures among survivors of abscesses of the cerebral hemispheres, which justifies the prophylactic administration of anticonvulsants in most of these patients.

VI

Intraspinal Tumors
Robert H. Wilkins, M.D.

Intraspinal tumors can be divided into three groups according to location: extradural, intradural extramedullary, and intramedullary. The neoplasms that occur in each of these three locations have clinical and radiologic characteristics that are different from those of the neoplasms in the other locations.

EXTRADURAL NEOPLASMS

Extradural (epidural) tumors are usually malignant. The most common example is a metastasis to a vertebra from a primary carcinoma of the lung, breast, or prostate. Other examples of malignant extradural spinal tumors are lymphoma and myeloma. The most common location for an extradural neoplasm is in the thoracic area of the spine. The typical symptoms relate to the directions of tumor growth: the patient first develops back pain centered where the tumor involves the vertebral bone, then the patient experiences radicular pain and dysfunction (radiculopathy) extending around the trunk at the same level on one or both sides as the tumor involves the exiting spinal nerve roots, and eventually the patient develops a progressive interference with spinal cord function (myelopathy) with eventual paraplegia. If a patient presents with progressive back pain (and especially pain that is not improved by recumbency), radicular pain, and neurologic loss, the preliminary assessment should include plain roentgenograms and computed tomographic scanning or magnetic resonance imaging, or both. If such studies do not provide sufficient information, they can be supplemented by other studies such as radionuclide bone scanning and positive contrast myelography accompanied by postmyelographic computed tomographic scanning.

There are generally two treatment options, radiation therapy or surgical resection followed by radiation therapy. With either option, steroid administration is often advantageous;

See the corresponding chapter or part in the *Textbook of Surgery*, 14th edition, pp. 1259–1262, for a more detailed discussion of this topic, including a comprehensive list of references.

it can be given immediately and reduces the bulk of the tumor (and the degree of neural compression) temporarily while the primary treatment modality is being accomplished. Surgical resection before radiotherapy is usually preferred if the patient is not known to have a malignancy or if the loss of neurologic function is proceeding rapidly. The goals of surgical treatment are to establish the diagnosis, to decompress the spinal cord or cauda equina, and to stabilize that area of the spine if the tumor has produced instability. Ordinarily, the tumor cannot be removed entirely, and radiotherapy is required postoperatively. Depending on the nature of the tumor, hormonal therapy or chemotherapy may also be beneficial.

INTRADURAL EXTRAMEDULLARY NEOPLASMS

Tumors occurring in the spinal subarachnoid space are of two types. The first type are benign neoplasms that arise from the meninges (meningiomas) or the nerve roots (neurofibromas, schwannomas). The second type are malignant tumors that have spread through the spinal subarachnoid space from a primary intracranial location (e.g., medulloblastoma, ependymoma, certain pineal region tumors) or from a malignancy elsewhere in the body (meningeal carcinomatosis).

The treatment of intraspinal meningiomas, neurofibromas, and schwannomas is their surgical excision, which may include excision of the involved portion of the dura mater (meningioma) or the involved nerve rootlets or root (neurofibroma, schwannoma). If the gross total removal of a solitary intraspinal meningioma, neurofibroma, or schwannoma can be achieved, which is usually the case, the patient is usually cured.

Metastases within the subarachnoid space are not treated surgically. These are generally managed with radiotherapy and hormonal therapy or chemotherapy.

INTRAMEDULLARY NEOPLASMS

This type of tumor develops within the spinal cord, enlarging it in a fusiform manner. The patient experiences a progressive myelopathy, and the radiographic studies demonstrate evidence of spinal cord expansion. Intramedullary tumors are usually treated surgically through a laminectomy. If an ependymoma is encountered, it may be possible to excise it completely with maintenance of the surrounding spinal cord. If only a partial resection can be achieved, radiotherapy can be given postoperatively.

An intramedullary astrocytoma ordinarily cannot be completely removed surgically. The decision regarding postoperative radiotherapy is based on the exact histologic type of the tumor, the degree of surgical resection, and the age of the patient. In contrast, the intramedullary hemangioblastoma is a benign tumor that can be cured by surgical excision without the need for radiotherapy.

Intraspinal dermoid and epidermoid tumors and lipomas are benign lesions that can be found within the subarachnoid space or the spinal cord, or both. They are most common in the lumbosacral area and may be associated with spinal dysraphism. These various benign tumors can be resected surgically, with the risks and difficulties of such treatment being related to the degree of involvement of the tumor with critical areas of the spinal cord and to the extent of any associated dysraphic changes.

VII

Ruptured Lumbar Intervertebral Disc

Robert H. Wilkins, M.D.

CLINICOPATHOLOGIC FEATURES. Degenerative changes in an intervertebral disc consist of two main forms: (1) the nucleus pulposus can herniate from its normally confined space (soft disc protrusion), or (2) the entire disc can lose substance, with loss of disc height and the formation of osteophytes that project outward from the adjacent rims of the vertebral body above and the vertebral body below the involved disc (hard disc protrusion).

Soft Disc Protrusion (Herniated Nucleus Pulposus, Herniated Disc, Ruptured Disc). The disc herniation that is important clinically begins with the development of a posterolateral or posterior fissure through the concentric rings of the anulus fibrosus. The nucleus pulposus may then begin to extend into this fissure. The patient at this stage may experience low back pain and perhaps some referred pain into the buttock or hip on the affected side. Further protrusion of the nucleus pulposus may then occur, causing bulging of the outer layers of the anulus and of the posterior longitudinal ligament sufficient to pinch the adjacent nerve root between the protruding disc and the lamina or the intervertebral facet. In addition, a fragment of the disc may actually be extruded completely through the remaining layers of the anulus fibrosus and posterior longitudinal ligament and become wedged anterior to the nerve root; this is referred to as a *free fragment*. When the nerve root is compressed by a protruding or extruded disc, the patient develops radiating

---

See the corresponding chapter or part in the *Textbook of Surgery*, 14th edition, pp. 1262–1264, for a more detailed discussion of this topic, including a comprehensive list of references.

pain along the distribution of the sciatic nerve (sciatica) on the involved side in addition to low back pain. The patient may also have neurologic deficits (hypesthesia, weakness, or reduction of the deep tendon reflex) in the distribution of the involved nerve root. This clinical pattern of radiating pain, perhaps with neurologic deficits, is referred to as a *radiculopathy*.

Approximately 95 per cent of lumbar disc herniations occur at the L5–S1 or L4–L5 level, with a slight numerical preponderance at one or the other level being reported by various authors. About 4 per cent occur at the L3–L4 level, and less than 1 per cent at the L2–L3 or L1–L2 level.

Hard Disc Protrusion (Degenerative Disc Disease with Spinal Osteoarthritis, Lumbar Spondylosis). Degeneration in a lumbar intervertebral disc with narrowing of the disc space and generalized bulging of the anulus fibrosus is frequently associated with the formation of osteoarthritic bony ridges (osteophytes) along the rims of the vertebral bodies adjacent to the involved disc. The posterior elements (laminae, facet joints, ligamenta flava) may become thickened, and osteophytes may project anteriorly from the facets. All of these changes tend to narrow the spinal canal (especially its lateral recesses) and the intervertebral foramina. Such narrowing may cause compression of an individual nerve root or multiple nerve roots of the cauda equina. The resulting symptoms and signs are similar to those caused by disc herniation but tend to be more gradual in onset and more protracted in course. If significant narrowing of the spinal canal occurs (acquired spinal stenosis), the cauda equina may be compressed when the lumbar spine is placed into certain positions, such as extension; when the patient walks, disagreeable paresthesias, numbness, or weakness in the lower extremities (neurogenic intermittent claudication) may develop.

SYMPTOMS AND SIGNS. The typical patient with a posterolateral lumbar disc herniation has intermittent low back pain for several weeks to several years and then develops sciatica as well. The pain is usually aggravated by back movement, by sitting or standing for long periods, by lifting an object from the bent position, and by coughing or straining. It usually is relieved temporarily by bed rest; the most comfortable position is horizontal, usually on the side, with the hips and knees flexed. The patient may also notice tingling paresthesias or numbness in certain aspects of the involved leg and foot, weakness in some muscle groups in that limb (less frequent), or, rarely, urinary retention.

On physical examination, the patient may demonstrate one or more of the following mechanical signs: lumbar scoliosis, paravertebral muscle spasm, tenderness over one or more of the lower lumbar spines, limitation by pain of low back motion (especially forward flexion), limitation by pain of straight leg raising on one or both sides, or the initiation or intensification of sciatic and back pain by the popliteal compression test. Neurologic deficits, if present, have a typical pattern for each of the commonly involved lumbar discs: (1) L3–L4 disc lesions involve the L4 nerve root with reduced sensation along the anterior thigh and anteromedial calf and motor loss of the quadriceps femoris with a reduction or loss of the knee jerk; (2) lesions of the L4–L5 disc involve the L5 nerve root with reduced sensation over the anterior calf and medial dorsum of the foot and with motor loss of the foot dorsiflexors; and (3) L5–S1 lesions involve the S1 nerve root with sensory loss over the lateral calf, lateral dorsum of the foot, and small toe, motor loss of the plantar flexors of the foot, and a reduction or loss of the abnormal ankle jerk.

MANAGEMENT. Radiographs are made of the lumbosacral spine and pelvis for assessment of disc narrowing and osteophyte formation, but especially for identification of causes of back and leg pain other than disc disease. The initial treatment of the acute symptoms of lumbar disc disease consists of bed rest on a firm mattress with medication to combat pain and muscle spasm as needed. Locally applied heat, anti-inflammatory medication, pelvic traction, or the use of a lumbosacral corset may also be helpful at times. If these measures provide relief of the acute episode, recurrences may be minimized by a daily maintenance program of low back exercises and the avoidance of certain activities such as frequent bending at the waist, lifting heavy objects, and sitting in an automobile for prolonged periods. Anti-inflammatory medication may be beneficial over a prolonged period for reducing the discomfort of lumbar osteoarthritis.

If conservative measures fail to relieve the patient's pain or if the patient develops significant weakness or urinary retention, a more aggressive approach to treatment should be taken. The patient should have further diagnostic tests such as an electromyogram, a spinal computed tomographic scan or magnetic resonance imaging examination, or a lumbar myelogram (usually followed by a computed tomographic scan while the contrast agent is still within the spinal canal). If all available evidence indicates that a soft or hard lumbar disc protrusion is present, it should be treated surgically.

Although a disc herniation usually can be managed effectively, with resolution or improvement of the symptoms and signs, the underlying (and poorly understood) biochemical abnormality that caused the herniation continues. Therefore, some of these patients are destined to have problems from disc disease at the same or a different spinal level at a later time.

VIII

Cervical Disc Lesions
Robert H. Wilkins, M.D.

Lesions of the cervical intervertebral discs are analogous to those that affect the lumbar discs. However, in the cervical region, the anatomy is somewhat different, and those differences introduce variations in symptoms, signs, and treatment.

CLINICOPATHOLOGIC FEATURES. As with a lumbar disc, degenerative changes in a cervical intervertebral disc can assume two main forms: (1) the nucleus pulposus can herniate out of its normal confined space (soft disc protrusion), or (2) the entire disc can lose substance with loss of disc height and the formation of osteophytes that project outward from the adjacent rims of the vertebral body above and the vertebral body below the involved disc. The second process is often combined with osteoarthritis of the apophyseal joints and the joints of Luschka. The combination of degenerative disc disease and osteophyte formation is termed *spondylosis.*

Soft Disc Protrusion (Herniated Nucleus Pulposus, Herniated Disc, Ruptured Disc). The pathologic process and the development of a cervical disc herniation are similar to those of a lumbar disc herniation. Cervical disc herniations are most frequent at the C6–C7 level but also occur at C5–C6 and to a lesser extent at C4–C5 and other levels.

With the usual posterolateral disc rupture, the patient experiences pain in the neck, and then as the nerve root is compressed, the patient develops pain radiating into the ipsilateral upper extremity and may also develop paresthesias, numbness, or weakness in an appropriate distribution. The pain and paresthesias may be intensified by neck movement, especially by extension or by lateral flexion to the side of the herniation, and by coughing or straining. They may be improved by bed rest.

On examination, the patient frequently exhibits restriction of neck movement, especially extension. Downward head compression by the examiner increases the patient's radicular pain and paresthesias, especially if the neck is simultaneously flexed to the side of the involvement. Hypesthesia, weakness, or the reduction of a deep tendon reflex may be present and should provide a clue to the level of the disc rupture and nerve root compression. Patterns of radiculopathy caused by cervical disc herniation or osteophyte formation for specific disc levels include (1) for C4–C5, the nerve root involved is C5 with reduced sensation over the deltoid area and weakness of the deltoid muscle; (2) for C5–C6, the nerve root involved is C6 with reduced sensory function of the thumb and index finger, biceps weakness, and a reduction or loss

See the corresponding chapter or part in the *Textbook of Surgery,* 14th edition, pp. 1265–1267, for a more detailed discussion of this topic, including a comprehensive list of references.

of the biceps reflex; (3) for C6–C7, the nerve root is C7 with reduced sensation of the index and long fingers, triceps weakness, and a reduction or loss of the triceps reflex; and (4) for C7–T1, the nerve root involved is C8 with reduced sensation in the ring and small fingers and weakness of grip.

If the disc herniation occurs more toward the midline (i.e., is a more direct posterior herniation), it compresses the spinal cord in addition to, or instead of, a nerve root. This produces cervical myelopathy manifested by lower motor neuron dysfunction (muscle weakness and hypotonia, reduction or loss of appropriate deep tendon reflexes, dermatomal sensory impairment) at the level of the compression and upper motor neuron dysfunction (spasticity, clonus, increased deep tendon reflexes, Babinski's sign, reduction of sensation) below that level. Loss of voluntary control of bowel, bladder, and sexual function may also develop.

Hard Disc Protrusion (Degenerative Disc Disease with Spinal Osteoarthritis, Cervical Spondylosis). As in the lumbar area, these changes tend to narrow the spinal canal and the intervertebral foramina, which may cause compression of one or more cervical nerve roots or of the spinal cord at one or more levels. The resulting symptoms and signs are similar to those caused by disc herniation but tend to be more gradual in onset and more protracted in course.

MANAGEMENT. Radiographic films are made of the cervical spine for assessment of the presence and degree of spondylosis, but especially for identification of a cause of neck and arm pain other than disc disease, such as a neoplasm or infection. The initial treatment of the patient with acute radiculopathy consists of bed rest with medication for pain and muscle spasm. Locally applied heat may provide additional comfort. Intermittent cervical halter traction (e.g., 7 pounds starting at 30 minutes four times per day and increasing to 2 hours four times per day) is often beneficial as well, but the direction of traction must be comfortable. Traction with the neck extended may actually increase the pain. Anti-inflammatory medication may be of value over a prolonged period for reducing the discomfort of cervical spondylosis.

If these measures do not provide adequate pain relief, or if the patient shows evidence of spinal cord compression, a more aggressive approach should be taken. The patient should have further diagnostic tests. Although electromyography, plain computed tomographic scanning, and magnetic resonance imaging may be useful, the best current study for assessing the presence and extent of cervical disc herniation or cervical spondylosis is the cervical myelogram followed by computed tomographic scanning while the contrast material is still present in the cervical subarachnoid space.

Surgical treatment to provide nerve root decompression can be accomplished by a posterior approach through a hemilaminectomy or by an anterior approach through the intervertebral disc.

If a patient is being treated for the unusual circumstance of a single midline disc herniation with spinal cord compression, an anterior discectomy is the procedure of choice.

Provided the myelopathy is not too severe or too long-standing, improvement can be expected.

In contrast, the surgical treatment of spinal cord compression from spondylosis usually requires a larger operation, and the results are not as good. If the operation is done via a posterior approach, it necessitates a full laminectomy (removal of the spinous process and the lamina on each side) at multiple levels. If an anterior approach is chosen, it involves either a discectomy/osteophytectomy at one or more levels or the resection of the central aspects of one or more vertebral bodies, usually with the insertion of a bone graft to ensure the postoperative maintenance of vertebral alignment and stability. These procedures have additional risks, but more significantly, the results are less satisfactory.

IX

Peripheral Nerve Injuries
Robert H. Wilkins, M.D.

ANATOMY AND PATHOPHYSIOLOGY. For correctly diagnosing and treating peripheral nerve injuries, the surgeon must understand the anatomy and pathophysiology of peripheral nerves. The "wiring diagram" of the human body is complex, in part because peripheral nerves contain varying proportions of motor, sensory, and sympathetic axons from diverse sources, and in part because of the mixing that occurs in the cervical, brachial, lumbar, and sacral nerve plexuses. In addition, the fascicles within a peripheral nerve divide and recombine along their course (funicular plexuses), and intercommunications between peripheral nerves (such as the ulnar and median nerves) are not uncommon. There also may be shared innervation by adjacent nerves and variations in nerve distribution from one individual to the next. In assessing the patient with a peripheral nerve injury, the surgeon must keep these facts about normal anatomy in mind while evaluating the changes caused by the injury.

In the Sunderland classification, there are five degrees of nerve injury. Seddon used only three terms to classify nerve injuries: neurapraxia, axonotmesis, and neurotmesis.

Neurapraxia is equivalent to first-degree nerve injury. Anatomic continuity is preserved, but there is selective demyelination of large nerve fibers that typically causes complete motor paralysis with little muscle atrophy and considerable sparing of sensory and autonomic function. Electrical con-

See the corresponding chapter or part in the *Textbook of Surgery*, 14th edition, pp. 1267–1269, for a more detailed discussion of this topic, including a comprehensive list of references.

ductivity of the nerve distal to the lesion is preserved. Surgical repair is not necessary, and recovery is rapid (within days or weeks). Recovery does not depend on regeneration, and there is no orderly sequence in the recovery of innervation. The quality of recovery is excellent.

Axonotmesis is equivalent to Sunderland's second-degree nerve injury. Anatomic continuity of the nerve and the Schwann sheaths is preserved, but the axons are interrupted and must recover by axonal regeneration. There is complete motor, sensory, and autonomic paralysis and progressive muscle atrophy. Surgical repair is not necessary. Recovery occurs at the rate of approximately 1 mm. per day (1 inch per month); it occurs according to the order of innervation, and the quality of recovery is excellent.

Neurotmesis is a more severe injury. There is significant disorganization within the nerve or actual disruption of its continuity, which precludes recovery without surgical repair. Wallerian degeneration occurs. In association with this, there is gradual loss of electrical conductivity in the distal portion of the nerve over a period of 3 days. At 10 to 20 days, fibrillations in the denervated muscles may first be detected by electromyography. From the time of the injury there is complete motor, sensory, and autonomic paralysis and progressive muscle atrophy.

At 10 to 20 days, axonal sprouting begins. If scar tissue blocks entrance into the distal portion of the nerve, these sprouts coil into a disorganized, painful neuroma. In contrast, if the nerve has been repaired, axonal regrowth proceeds at approximately 1 mm. per day. After the initial lag of 10 to 20 days, there is usually a further delay in the forward progress of nerve restitution if the regenerating axons have to bridge a narrow gap (e.g., where a divided nerve has been reapproximated) and another delay at the end organ before function resumes. The march of recovery occurs according to the order of innervation, and recovery is always imperfect.

DIAGNOSIS. A standard neurologic examination reveals the extent of the neurologic deficits following peripheral nerve injury. The examiner must not be deceived, however, by trick movements such as a movement that occurs when an uninvolved muscle or gravity compensates for a paralyzed muscle, a movement permitted by an accessory tendon slip or an anomalous muscle insertion or nerve supply, or a movement caused by strong contraction and sudden relaxation of an antagonist. Because of the overlap of sensory nerve distributions and the tendency for fibers to grow from adjacent nerves into a denervated area after injury, the sensory deficits may involve smaller areas than the examiner expects.

The Hoffmann-Tinel sign refers to the radiating tingling paresthesia that is felt in the cutaneous distribution of an injured nerve when the nerve is percussed lightly. If the distal aspect of the nerve is percussed progressively proximally, the level at which the sign is first elicited marks the most distal point of small fiber regeneration. The progress of nerve regeneration may thus be followed over a period of days to months by periodic charting of the location of the most distal point.

There are a number of electrical examinations that may add significant diagnostic information to that gained from the history and physical examination. Electromyography shows changes of denervation (increased insertional activity, spontaneous fibrillation, positive waves, and absence of voluntary action potentials) and of early reinnervation (decreased insertional activity, decreased fibrillation, and nascent polyphasic potentials). Disappearance of fibrillations may antedate the reappearance of voluntary action potentials. Muscle contraction in response to electrical stimulation may precede voluntary recovery by weeks. Although electromyographic evidence of reinnervation may precede recovery, it does not guarantee recovery.

SURGICAL THERAPY. Since surgeons first began to repair injured nerves there has been controversy about the timing of such repair. For many years, delayed repair was favored; the rare exceptions involved clean lacerations made by sharp objects. With the recent development of microsurgery and replantation surgery, there has been increased interest in primary nerve repair at the time of injury.

If a clinically nonfunctioning nerve is in continuity when it is explored some weeks after the initial injury, the surgeon may find it helpful to electrically stimulate the nerve proximal to the injury and distally identify evidence of muscle contraction or transmission of nerve action potentials. If there is no evidence of transmission across the area of injury, the injured portion of the nerve should be excised and the cut ends of the nerve should be sutured together. If there is transmission across the area of injury, surgical treatment should be limited to an external neurolysis.

If the nerve was initially divided in the accident or is divided by the surgeon, it should be reapproximated carefully and without tension after each end has been trimmed back to healthy fascicles. For regaining length so that the nerve can be sutured without tension, the nerve ends can be mobilized and rerouted, the adjacent joints can be flexed, and even a portion of the adjacent bone (e.g., humerus) can be removed if necessary. If the ends cannot be brought together with these maneuvers, an interposed graft of an available cutaneous nerve, such as the sural nerve, can be used. Grafts of this type add another suture line that the regenerating axons must cross, and the results are not as favorable as with direct nerve anastomosis.

X

Congenital Malformations of the Central Nervous System

W. Jerry Oakes, M.D.

Congenital malformations of the central nervous system are relatively common problems that are usually apparent at birth. The tremendous emotional impact of a deformed newborn should be borne in mind when the physician first discusses the problem with the parents. A sensitive and understanding approach is mandatory for the development of the trust and confidence necessary in managing these difficult and emotionally charged problems.

MYELOMENINGOCELE

Neural tube closure defects occur most commonly at each end of the neural tube. Improper closure of the anterior neuropore causes anencephaly. This lesion is not compatible with survival. Improper closure of the posterior neuropore causes the development of a myelomeningocele. This is the most common central nervous system birth defect. The etiologic basis of this defect is complex, with laboratory and epidemiologic evidence implicating both genetic and environmental agents. Among the most pursued investigations currently is the relationship of diet and, in particular, folic acid to the development of these lesions. Since the neural tube closes during the third and fourth week of gestation, frequently before the woman's pregnancy is confirmed, dietary supplementation must begin during the time of attempted conception. Myelomeningoceles represent a complex anomaly associated with hydrocephalus and herniation of the brain stem and cerebellar vermis into the upper cervical spine (Chiari II malformation). The distal spinal cord malformation (neuroplacode) is usually associated with the development of a neurogenic bladder and with variable degrees of weakness of the lower extremities. The current usual method of care is for early closure of the spinal defect and the insertion of a valve-regulated ventriculoperitoneal shunt for compensation of the frequent association of hydrocephalus. With aggressive therapy, most patients have an ample opportunity to lead productive and meaningful lives.

CRANIOSYNOSTOSIS

Deformity of the skull secondary to premature closure of one or more cranial sutures presents as a cosmetic and sometimes a medical problem. Single suture closure produces

---

See the corresponding chapter or part in the *Textbook of Surgery*, 14th edition, pp. 1269–1275, for a more detailed discussion of this topic, including a comprehensive list of references.

accentuation of skull growth parallel to the closed suture and restriction perpendicular to this suture. Most commonly, the result is a long narrow skull with forehead prominence as a result of closure of the sagittal suture (scaphocephaly). Surgical manipulation of the skull usually produces a dramatic improvement in the appearance and a normal globular shape to the brain. The risks involved with most skull remodeling procedures are relatively low. Because of this relatively low risk and significant improvement that can be accomplished with surgical intervention, most families choose to proceed with skull remodeling early in life.

HYDROCEPHALUS

The successful treatment of hypertensive hydrocephalus was one of the most significant therapeutic advances in the field of neurosurgery since its inception. With the ease of current imaging techniques (computed tomography and magnetic resonance imaging), clinical evidence of increased intracranial pressure in the neonate can easily and accurately be investigated. The level of cerebrospinal fluid obstruction is assessed, and associated primary processes (intracranial tumor, subarachnoid hemorrhage, intraventricular hemorrhage) are evaluated. Currently, the outcome of patients with hydrocephalus is determined by the prognosis for their underlying condition more than by the hydrocephalus itself. Premature infants with intraventricular hemorrhage or term infants who present with hydrocephalus from meningitis, encephalitis, trauma, or some neoplastic process in large part will have their eventual outcome determined by this primary problem. The follow-up of patients with ventricular peritoneal shunts in place is demanding. Problems with shunt infection and malfunction persist throughout life and demand vigilance from both the family and the treating physician for maximizing continued adequate function of the shunt system.

OCCULT SPINAL DYSRAPHISM

The entities that are comprised in occult spinal dysraphism share a common etiologic basis and presentation. The seven pathologic entities involved in the group include diastematomyelia, syringomyelia, lipomyelomeningocele, dermal sinuses and intraspinal dermoid tumors, meningocele manqué, tethered spinal cord, and neuroenteric cysts. These lesions frequently coexist or may be seen in association with a myelomeningocele. When found outside the setting of myelomeningocele, they are rarely associated with a pathologic intracranial process. The presentation of these lesions is protean and can range from simply the presence of a cutaneous abnormality (focal hirsutism, capillary hemangioma, midline lipoma, or dermal sinus) over the lumbar spine at birth to the development of scoliosis later in life. Neurogenic bladder and motor weakness in the lower extremities are common presentations. With the advent of magnetic resonance imaging of the spine, the ease with which these lesions can be diagnosed has increased. With early operative intervention, the likelihood of retention of neurologic function is higher; delayed intervention is inappropriate. Documentation of progression of neurologic loss before acceptance of surgical therapy is unwise, since bladder function is not available for evaluation at the bedside in young infants. In addition, when a patient develops a neurogenic bladder, it is unlikely that surgical therapy will return this lost function. Early investigation and therapy are thus advised.

XI

Neurosurgical Relief of Pain
Eben Alexander, III, M.D.,
and Blaine S. Nashold, Jr., M.D.

The success of the spinal cordotomy in relieving pain is associated with the neuroanatomic organization of pain and thermal fibers in the lateral spinothalamic tract. Although the lateral spinothalamic tract is of considerable importance in the transmission of painful and thermal sensation, neuroanatomic evidence indicates that additional pathways are available for the transmission of pain. The lateral spinothalamic tract is a phylogenetically recent pathway in man with its input directly into the sensory thalamus. Pain perception over the spinothalamic route has a rapid transit time to the thalamus where higher levels of integration occur through the thalamocortical connection. A definite topographic scheme of the body's image exists within the cord and thalamus, the input from the facial region being medial to that of the body and from the leg areas lateral to that of the body. Pain following electrical stimulation of the spinothalamic pathways is usually experienced by the patient as a sharp, well-demarcated painful sensation referred to a localized region of the body.

In contrast to this, the diffuse pain pathways appear to have multiple routes through the spinal cord with distribution to the midbrain, thalamus, and hypothalamus; these spinoreticular pathways are phylogenetically older than the lateral spinothalamic tract and have been designated as the paleothalamic system. They may be crossed or uncrossed tracts that are composed of short chains of the neurons that make synaptic connections at successive rostral levels in the central nervous system. Pain transmitted via these routes appears to be slowed in transit to higher levels, and the sensation

See the corresponding chapter or part in the *Textbook of Surgery,* 14th edition, pp. 1275–1281, for a more detailed discussion of this topic, including a comprehensive list of references.

experienced by alert patients during stimulation is ill-defined and unpleasant, being diffusely localized to regions in the central parts of the body including the head, chest, and abdomen.

Pain can be considered as either a primary or secondary symptom. In most patients, it is a secondary symptom usually originating from some underlying pathologic cause, the correction of which relieves the pain. However, when the pathologic state cannot be eradicated, as may be the case in metastatic malignancy, the pain may be relieved by a specific neurosurgical operation.

Pain is the primary symptom that follows neurophysiologic and neuropathologic involvement of the pain pathways within the central nervous system. A painful dysesthesia occurring after a surgical cordotomy, tractotomy, or thalamotomy is an example of a primary central pain syndrome. Other examples include the pain of the thalamic syndromes that often occur after trauma, vascular occlusion, tumor, degenerative disease of the central nervous system (multiple sclerosis), or infections (herpes zoster). The patient describes this type of pain as intense burning, crushing, or tearing and aggravated by the slightest sensory stimulation. An emotional upset intensifies the patient's pain, as can psychological disturbance. These patients often become drug addicts and undergo permanent personality changes. Numerous theories have been proposed to explain central pain as the presence of highly irritable neurons at the site of the central nervous system injury involving the diffuse pain tracts, the diversion of noxious impulses from the spinothalamic tract into the paleothalamic system, or the possible release of the thalamus from higher cortical inhibition.

Neurosurgical treatment of central pain has not been completely successful, although midbrain tractotomy and thalamotomy have been used in a limited number of patients.

THE NEUROSURGICAL OPERATIONS FOR PAIN

The neurosurgeon must consider certain facts before recommending an operation for relief of pain. The neurosurgical operation must not be done as a last resort or in desperation. Most failures to relieve pain are due to delay in surgical treatment. The neurosurgeon should be consulted early and before the occurrence of drug addiction or prolonged suffering. Long-established pain produces a state of suffering that should be avoided; ideally, benefit from operation should extend throughout the lifetime of the patient. Neurosurgical operations for the relief of pain can be divided into four types: (1) anatomic interruption of pathways serving pain or the destruction of sensory integration regions in the central nervous system (rhizotomy, cordotomy, tractotomy, thalamotomy, and cingulotomy); (2) sympathectomy for relief of causalgia and sympathetic dystrophy; (3) pituitary ablation for relief of generalized bone pain from metastatic tumors (breast, prostate) under hormonal influence; and (4) electroanalgesia for relief of pain by stimulation of peripheral nerves, dorsal columns, or central brain structures.

The simplest operation for pain relief is the section, avulsion, or alcohol injection of a peripheral nerve. It has the advantage of relieving pain originating in a small localized area. In trigeminal neuralgia, injection or avulsion of one of the peripheral branches of the fifth cranial nerve may provide several years of relief. The disadvantage of sectioning of the peripheral nerve is the return of the pain with neural regeneration. The sensory loss from a dorsal rhizotomy involves a large area, but at least three or four nerve roots must be sectioned to produce an analgesic zone equal to the dermatome. The dorsal rhizotomy may be useful in relieving pain originating from the neck, shoulder, thorax, or abdominal wall, but it is usually unsuitable for pain that involves an entire arm or leg, since the sensory loss in these regions may often reduce the functional usefulness of the limb.

Tic douloureux or trigeminal neuralgia is a common symptom in facial pain. The discomfort is frequently described as a sudden lancinating pain that spreads into one or more of the representative divisions of the trigeminal nerve, more commonly in the lower face, often causing the patient to wince because of the severity—thus the term *tic*. These paroxysms usually continue for seconds to less than a minute, and although there is often an aching background sensation, onset is either spontaneous or due to stimulation of a "trigger zone" in the form of touching skin areas. Speaking, chewing, and talking may also activate the pain. Medical treatment is the first priority in these patients with use of carbamazepine, phenytoin, or baclofen, but when medical treatment becomes ineffective, neurosurgical operation should be considered.

Percutaneous Radiofrequency Rhizotomy

One of the earliest surgical methods for management of trigeminal neuralgia is percutaneous radiofrequency lesions. Patients with multiple sclerosis as well as those infirm or over 70 years of age with pain in multiple divisions are especially suited to this procedure. Radiofrequency (RF) rhizotomy involves destruction of part of the trigeminal ganglion by use of heat from an electrode connected to an RF generator. The procedure is performed under local anesthesia and guided by electrical stimulation. Motor and sensory effects produced by stimulation may be helpful in precise placement of the lesion electrode in the trigeminal ganglion. Preliminary electrode placement is accomplished with use of roentgenograms or cinefluoroscopy.

The major advantages of the percutaneous technique include low morbidity and mortality with a high success rate. Patients who experience recurrence of pain are often improved by repeated lesions. One disadvantage of this method is reduction of corneal sensation with the possible development of keratitis, of which the patient must be forewarned. A cervical sympathectomy may have a protective effect on the cornea against the development of keratitis.

Glycerol Injection of the Gasserian Ganglion

Indication for percutaneous retroganglionic glycerol rhizotomy is similar to that for radiofrequency rhizotomy. Possible advantages are (1) significant reduction in facial deafferentation compared with the RF rhizotomy; (2) elimination of intraoperative sensory testing of RF lesion equipment provides a simpler technique; and (3) intraoperative trigeminal water-soluble contrast cisternography allows precise anatomic location.

MICROVASCULAR DECOMPRESSION FOR RELIEF OF TRIGEMINAL NEURALGIA

Microneurosurgical decompression for trigeminal neuralgia is appealing in that it addresses the possible cause of the disorder and does not rely on substantial ablation of part of the nervous system. However, it is a major cranial operation and is best performed on younger patients. Microvascular decompression is of no benefit in the pain of anesthesia dolorosa or multiple sclerosis and should not be used in painful conditions of the trigeminal nerve due to peripheral involvement. A partial section of the trigeminal nerve as it exits from the pons and posterior fossa is an alternative, or even an adjunct, to microvascular decompression. The most serious complications following microvascular decompression are intracerebral hematoma with acute hydrocephalus, cerebellar swelling, supratentorial subdural hematoma, status epilepticus, and infarction of the brain stem.

TRIGEMINAL NUCLEUS CAUDALIS DREZ LESIONS

Pain associated with post-trigeminal dysesthesia and anesthesia dolorosa has always been very difficult to control medically and surgically. Recently the DREZ (dorsal root entry zone) lesion technique has been applied to the trigeminal nucleus caudalis for pain relief. The trigeminal nucleus caudalis receives the majority of pain afferents from the face via the trigeminal nerve and can be lesioned at the cervicomedullary junction by use of a microsurgical technique and a special RF electrode. Best results are noted in patients with post-trigeminal dysesthesia and anesthesia dolorosa and postherpetic neuralgia. One of the major operative risks is the development of ipsilateral dysmetria in the arm or leg, which usually is transient and disappears within a short period of time.

MISCELLANEOUS THERAPIES

Use of electrical stimulation of the gasserian ganglion was proposed by Meyerson in 1980 and consists of chronic implantation of an electrode in the gasserian ganglion. Of five patients with trigeminal pain and partial sensory loss, three had relief of pain for a period of 2 years.

Generalized Somatic and Visceral Pain

Spinal cordotomy remains the most useful operation for relief of widespread somatic and visceral pain. It is especially helpful when pain originates from thoracic and abdominal regions. The surgical section is performed opposite the site of the pain in the anterolateral quadrant of the spinal cord at least six cord segments above the origin of the pain to allow some degree of postoperative regression of the sensory level. The analgesia following the cordotomy covers the opposite half of the body with the level beginning several segments below the cord section. An open surgical cordotomy has a mortality of 10 per cent. The cord section can be done at two different spinal levels, usually cervical (C1 to C3) and thoracic (T1 to T2). In the cervical operation, the analgesic level reaches the clavicle involving the arm to varying degrees, but the densest analgesia occurs over regions of the thorax, abdomen, and leg. A thoracic cordotomy produces contralateral analgesia beginning in the lower thorax. A well-executed unilateral lumbar cordotomy should provide good pain relief in 85 per cent of patients, whereas with a high cervical cordotomy, relief occurs in 50 per cent. After unilateral cordotomy, generally there are few complications with normal bladder, bowel, and sexual functions. Postoperative complications such as ipsilateral hemiparesis or monoparesis can occur if the surgical incision involves a nearby corticospinal tract. Bilateral cervical cordotomy at either level seriously interferes with bladder, bowel, and sexual functions.

Percutaneous spinothalamic cordotomy is a good technique for interrupting the pain pathways for somatic and visceral pain anywhere below the level of the mandible. This technique is best used in patients with unilateral pain who have malignant disease and are not expected to survive for more than 1 to 2 years. The reason for this stipulation is that there is a significant complication with anesthesia dolorosa in long-term survivors after cordotomy.

The percutaneous cordotomy is done with local anesthesia under roentgenographic control guiding an RF needle into the anterolateral quadrant of the spinal cord between the first and second cervical vertebrae. Electrical stimulation can be used to test the localization of the needle tip within the spinal cord tissue. The lateral spinothalamic tract can be coagulated unilaterally by means of a high-frequency electrical current. A percutaneous cordotomy is best suited for poor-risk patients with a short life expectancy.

Pain involving overlapping areas of the head and neck or arm can be difficult to control by a single surgical operation owing to overlapping of the cranial and cervical nerves in the head and neck region. Stereotactic operations in the midbrain or thalamus have relieved these widespread cervical cranial pains. A stereotactic medullary tractotomy can be performed to selectively interrupt pain involving the individual divisions of the trigeminal nerve, although a caudalis DREZ procedure is probably preferable at this time. One serious problem with the medullary tractotomy is the risk of postoperative dysesthesia. The mortality has been reduced to 1 per cent with good relief of pain, and although postoperative dysesthesia has occurred, this is less frequent. Postoperatively, there is usually loss of upward gaze and occasionally diplopia that may complicate the lesion. With improvements in the stereotactic technique, it is now possible to place lesions below the posterior commissure, which reduces the risk of ocular dysfunction and successfully relieves pain of the thalamic syndrome.

Stereotactic lesions in the thalamus or the cingulum have been successfully employed to relieve widespread pain causing suffering. A unilateral thalamic lesion (center median or parafascicular nucleus or both) is often sufficient for relief of the pain of extensive carcinoma. The relief is thought to be due to interruption of the sensory integration at high levels in the central nervous system. A thalamic lesion does not alter the threshold for pain, and no analgesia occurs despite the relief of the patient's pain. An added risk of the thalamic operation may be an interference with memory or speech mechanisms. In some patients, the relief of pain is short-lived.

When suffering is the most prominent clinical feature in a patient with intractable pain associated with maximal intake of narcotic drugs, it can best be relieved by a medial dorsal thalamic or cingulum gyrus lesion interrupting the cingulum bilaterally. The beneficial effect of the thalamic lesion is thought to be due to interruption of thalamofrontal connections, whereas the cingulate lesion exerts its effects by interfering with some circuits in the limbic system. Frontal leukotomy can no longer be recommended as an operation for the relief of pain.

PAIN OF BRACHIAL AND LUMBAR PLEXUS AVULSION, PARAPLEGIA, AND HERPES

Intractable pain associated with avulsion injury to the brachial plexus has been refractory to treatment until the use of a new surgical procedure in which small thermal lesions are made in the injured dorsal root entry zone (DREZ). Pain can be significantly relieved in over 70 per cent of these patients. Ten per cent of paraplegics develop intractable pain described as burning, crushing, or electrical in nature and involving the paralyzed limb. The onset of pain may be immediately after the injury or delayed for several years. The DREZ procedure has been successful in relieving this pain.

Herpes zoster is followed by chronic pain syndrome in 10 per cent of patients and has been intractable to treatment. The patients are often elderly and rapidly become debilitated because of the pain. Therapeutic lesions involving the dorsal roots can relieve pain in approximately 50 per cent of these patients. One objection to this operation is a 5 per cent risk of ipsilateral leg weakness.

PAINFUL PHANTOM LIMB

The loss of an arm, leg, or breast can cause phantom sensation. After an amputation, the phantom image appears to be fixed in the patient's awareness of the traumatic episode surrounding the loss of the limb, and it appears to influence whether the individual may experience a phantom sensation. Normally the phantom sensation fades by retracting into the end of the stump, but the patient is often aware of the phantom limb and may be able to "move" the missing fingers or toes.

When the phantom sensation is accompanied by pain, surgical treatment may be necessary, since the presence of the pain intensifies and prolongs the phantom sensation. When the pain is relieved, the phantom sensation fades. A painful phantom limb often follows a traumatic avulsion of the brachial plexus where the dorsal roots are disconnected from their attachment to the spinal cord. The arm becomes insensitive and flaccid. The pain is described as burning, tearing, or crushing, and the intensity appears to heighten the patient's awareness of the phantom limb. Injury to the substantia gelatinosa in the spinal cord at the point where the dorsal roots exit may be the site of the origin for the phantom pain. Recently, successful relief of pain has followed the use of the DREZ lesion involving the dorsal roots of the phantom.

SURGICAL SYMPATHECTOMY FOR RELIEF OF CAUSALGIA AND SYMPATHETIC DYSTROPHY

Causalgia is a syndrome characterized by intense "burning pain" and autonomic dysfunction caused by partial injury to a large nerve trunk. The etiology of this disorder is unknown, but the symptoms occur most often after injury to large peripheral nerves such as the brachial plexus or the median or sciatic nerves. Usually the nerve lesion is incomplete with partial sensory loss in the involved painful limb. The physiologic basis for the pain and its association with autonomic dysfunction are not understood. It has been postulated that the burning dysesthesia may be due to short-circuiting of C fiber impulses or the cross-circuiting of efferent sympathetic impulses via the peripheral nerves, which activate the pain fibers. The burning pain of causalgia usually involves the hand or foot. The skin may appear smooth with loss of hair, and vasomotor disturbance appears such as sweating involving the limb. Symptoms can be relieved temporarily by block of the sympathetic ganglion of the involved limb. Cure often results following sympathectomy.

RELIEF OF PAIN BY PITUITARY ABLATION

Intractable pain caused by metastasis from cancer of the breast or prostate dramatically subsides after ablation of the pituitary gland. Pain relief is immediate after the ablation procedure; and as the pain subsides, the tumor nodules also diminish in size, and lesions in the bone observed on the roentgenogram often resolve with recalcification. Pituitary ablation should be considered after oophorectomy in women or following the removal of the gonads in men. Complete surgical removal of the pituitary can be accomplished through a frontal craniotomy, but more recently stereotactic ablations have been performed by introducing lesion probes into the sella turcica. The gland can be destroyed by freezing, heat coagulation, implanting radioactive yttrium, or injecting absolute alcohol. Postoperatively these patients must be maintained on hormone replacement often combined with vasopressin (Pitressin) if diabetes insipidus appears.

RELIEF OF PAIN BY ELECTROANALGESIA

Sweet originally employed the electrical stimulation technique for successful relief of pain originating from an injured peripheral nerve. A pair of platinum electrodes is placed in contact with the nerve trunk above the level of the injury, and a miniature RF receiver attached to the stimulating platinum electrode is buried beneath the skin. The patient self-activates the painful nerve by electrical signal transmitted through the skin of the RF receiver by a small portable RF generator. The patient can vary the frequency or strength of the stimulating current in order to find a level of stimulation that relieves the pain. Later, in 1970, Shealy and Mortimer reported the implantation of stimulating electrodes for activating the dorsal columns of the spinal cord in patients with pain from widespread carcinoma. The device can be inserted percutaneously or through a laminectomy in the cervical, thoracic, or lumbar areas, but always above the segmental level of the body from which the pain originates. Self-activation of the dorsal columns by the patient causes paresthesia in the painful region with an associated reduction of pain. The technique has been used in a wide number of chronic pain problems with success.

XII

Neurosurgical Treatment of Epilepsy
Blaine S. Nashold, Jr., M.D.

Epilepsy is a disease in which repeated seizures occur. A seizure is a synchronous electrical discharge from the brain with or without alteration of consciousness or motor manifestations. Only patients with epilepsy that cannot be controlled by medical therapy should be considered candidates for surgical treatment. The medical treatment of epilepsy is

See the corresponding chapter or part in the *Textbook of Surgery*, 14th edition, pp. 1281–1286, for a more detailed discussion of this topic, including a comprehensive list of references.

the domain of neurologists, and a team approach to the analysis of patients who are candidates for surgical treatment involves participation of a neurologist throughout the patient's care. Most neurologists and neurosurgeons who manage patients with medically intractable epilepsy require documentation of persistent seizure activity with therapeutic levels of one or more anticonvulsant medicines. Moreover, the seizure frequency and character must interfere with the daily life of the patient, that is, a partial seizure every 6 months would not qualify the patient for surgical therapy. After it has been established that a patient's seizures are medically intractable, two other criteria must be met for a patient to qualify for surgical treatment: the seizure focus must be localized, and the location of the seizure focus can be removed surgically and with a low risk of a new neurologic impairment.

In addition to the clinical criteria for identifying patients, there are a battery of tests available for the pre- and perioperative evaluation of patients who fulfill these criteria. Most patients have had electroencephalograms, computed tomographic scans, and magnetic resonance imaging scanning. Positron emission tomography and Amytal angiography with physiologic testing are also used in the preoperative evaluation of patients. Many groups use simultaneous electroencephalography and videotaping to capture the behavioral manifestations of seizures and their relationship to the electrical activity in the brain. Each center has its own protocol established for the analysis of operative candidates. These protocols vary according to the availability of tests and the opinions of the team regarding the importance of the different criteria for identifying surgical candidates.

Most patients who qualify for surgical treatment of epilepsy have a type of epilepsy known as *complex partial seizures*. In older nomenclature, these seizures were termed *temporal lobe seizures*, since they often originate from a unilateral temporal lobe focus. Patients with this type of seizure activity are treated by temporal lobectomy. This operation is the most frequently performed procedure for the control of epilepsy and represents 80 per cent of the operations performed. Other operations performed for patients with medically intractable seizures include frontal lobectomy for seizures originating in one frontal lobe; corpus callosotomy for patients with bilateral foci and drop attacks as part of their seizures; and hemispherectomy, a rarely performed operation, for very young patients with infantile hemiplegia or Sturge-Weber disease and intractable epilepsy.

A successful outcome for patients with medically intractable epilepsy is measured by a reduction or elimination of seizure activity. Each operation discussed has a specific success rate reported in the literature. Most would agree that temporal lobectomy for partial complex seizures is the most successfully performed operation, with many groups reporting a 70 to 90 per cent rate of improvement in seizure frequency.

The pathologic processes that cause medically intractable epilepsy are quite variable. The most common pathologic finding in temporal lobes removed from patients with medically intractable seizures is sclerosis of the amygdala and hippocampus. However, every series of patients reported also contains cases of low-grade tumors of the brain, vascular malformations, and chronic inflammatory lesions.

XIII

Stereotactic Neurosurgery
Robert P. Iacono, M.D., and Blaine S. Nashold, Jr., M.D.

Rapid evolution of stereotactic methods has followed the development of computerized brain-imaging systems, allowing new application of therapeutic modalities to neurosurgery. These advances originated in 1906 when Horsley and Clarke reported the use of a stereotactic instrument for neurophysiologic exploration of deep brain centers. By 1950, Spiegel and Wycis and others had applied stereotactic techniques to man for the purpose of treating psychiatric disturbances and, in the 1960s, for the tremor and rigidity of Parkinson's disease. The advent of computed tomographic scanning and the availability of quality imaging techniques by 1980 were responsible for a rapid resurgence of interest in stereotactics.

CONVENTIONAL STEREOTACTIC TECHNIQUE FOR FUNCTIONAL NEUROSURGERY

In conventional stereotactic surgery, the main intent is the highly accurate placement of lesions and sometimes electrodes for neurophysiologic purposes; the use of a precision instrument that can direct a probe into deep brain targets with submillimeter accuracy is required. The intracerebral target is determined from the coordinates of a special stereotactic atlas of the human brain with sections in three planes. Localization of the target is made from an outline of landmarks of the third ventricle (anterior and posterior commissures) seen on intraoperative films. Following localization and probe insertion, anatomic variability errors are minimized by the use of electrophysiologic methods, either stimulation or recording of the target area, for monitoring the neurologic reactions of the patient under local anesthesia. The most ideal technique for producing a therapeutic lesion in the

---

See the corresponding chapter or part in the *Textbook of Surgery*, 14th edition, pp. 1287–1290, for a more detailed discussion of this topic, including a comprehensive list of references.

central nervous system of man has been radiofrequency thermocouple-monitored thermal coagulation.

FUNCTIONAL STEREOTACTIC SURGICAL INDICATIONS

Current indications for functional stereotactic intervention remain those patients with Parkinson's disease with hemiparkinsonism, severe tremor or tremor without rigidity, levodopa-induced dyskinesia, asymmetrical symptoms, or unsatisfactory treatment with medication. Patients with persistent hemiballismus, although rare, and essential tremor may benefit from lesions designed to interrupt pallidothalamic pathways or tremor generators from the ventrobasal thalamus. Tremor or unilateral rigidity as the major disabling symptom can be permanently and reliably arrested by such a therapeutic lesion in the ventrobasal complex of the thalamus.

Stereotactic procedures have also been used for the treatment of psychiatric disorders recalcitrant to conventional therapy. The use of stereotactic methods for the control of intractable pain has grown with understanding of neurophysiology and neuropharmacology. Placement of stimulating electrodes into the hypothalamus or into the periaqueductal-gray area of the upper midbrain can be effective treatment for pain of somatic origin. The pain relief, which lasts hours after a brief period of stimulation, is thought by some to be based on release of endorphin into the surrounding reticular areas of the brain. This general method is referred to as stimulation-induced analgesia or deep brain stimulation. The use of chronically implanted depth electrodes for diagnostic awake recording in complex-partial seizures often identifies deep epileptogenic foci, which may be followed by temporal lobectomy with marked improvement.

IMAGE-GUIDED STEREOTACTIC METHODS AND INDICATIONS

Numerous indications for stereotactic neurosurgery guided by computed tomography and magnetic resonance imaging have developed in the decade since its introduction. These include biopsy of primary and metastatic tumors, drainage of abscesses and cysts, evacuation of intracerebral hematomas, tissue transplantation, endoscopy, implantation of multiple afterloading catheters for interstitial radiation (brachytherapy), or hyperthermia. In addition, localization for laser resection or for craniotomy and localization for linear accelerator or proton beam radiotherapy and focused gamma emission radiosurgery have been applied with use of stereotactic instruments and principles.

These procedures can be performed under local anesthesia and are especially appropriate for minimizing morbidity, postoperative convalescence in the hospital, and treatment delays for several groups of patients including those with primary malignant brain tumors. For benign lesions such as colloid cysts of the third ventricle, cyst aspiration may be curative, whereas aspiration of pus from an abscess followed by appropriate antibiotics often proves adequate therapy, as does evacuation of intracerebral hematomas.

Radiobrachytherapy via stereotactically implanted arrays of afterloading cannulas combined with geometric dosimetry simulation for catheter placement and treatment planning is becoming increasingly important in the management of malignant gliomas. From a radiobiologic standpoint, large doses of radiation in the range of 60 Gy. can be administered by use of [192]iridium to a target volume delivering a protracted dose over 24 to 96 hours through cell cycle–sensitive phases (M, G_2). Hyperthermia may be used in conjunction with brachytherapy by ferromagnetic induction-heating of metallic seeds implanted through the same array of catheters as the [192]iridium.

Complications of these methods include intraparenchymal bleeding, infection, and increased neurologic deficits due to local damage or to exacerbation of mass effect. There is an overall morbidity of about 5 per cent, but this can be expected to vary with the extent of the procedure and preoperative condition of the patient. In patients with significant mass effect or shift, care should be taken with regard to fluids and steroid doses.

FUTURE DIRECTIONS

The field of stereotactic technique is being widely incorporated into general neurosurgery and radiation therapy. Stereotactic radiosurgery delivers externally directed gamma radiation, particles such as protons, or x-rays produced by a linear accelerator to restricted volumes of intracranial lesions in such a way as to produce focal tissue destruction, the result of which is analogous to surgical resection. Pioneering work has been accomplished for extracting tumor boundaries from computed tomography and magnetic resonance imaging data to allow the reconstructed target volume (tumor) to be resected by stereotactically directed CO_2 laser, mechanically directed and computer monitored in three-dimensional space. In summary, future possibilities for stereotactic surgery based on computer technology are essentially unlimited.

42

DISORDERS OF THE MUSCULOSKELETAL SYSTEM

I

Fractures and Dislocations: General Principles

John M. Harrelson, M.D., and John A. Feagin, M.D.

Fractures are as old as mankind; the method of treatment, however, has changed with better understanding of the pathophysiologic mechanism, the ingenuity of the surgeon, and the economic pressures for return to function. Because of high-speed vehicular trauma, improved life support, and improved care through specialization afforded by trauma centers, orthopaedic surgery for fractures and dislocations with the attendant acute and late complications has become vital.

MECHANISM AND CLASSIFICATION OF FRACTURES

Fractures may be classified as *simple* (a single fracture line) or *comminuted* (multiple fracture lines and fragments). Fractures may also be classified as *closed* (skin intact) or *open* (skin penetrated). The distinction between simple and comminuted and open and closed is important because these states reflect the forces at work and the risk of contamination and infection. The extent of soft tissue injury associated with a fracture is usually greater in comminuted and open fractures. The appreciation and care of the soft tissue injury associated with the fracture is frequently the key to the successful treatment, and the prognosis of open fractures is significantly different from that of closed fractures.

Fractures in children deserve special consideration. The periosteum is extremely strong in children; children's bones are more resilient, and they sometimes bend (greenstick) rather than break. Also, fractures may occur through the physeal plates and cause growth disturbance.

Pathologic fractures occur with osteoporosis, osteomalacia, diseased bone, infection, and tumors. The practitioner must be alert for these fractures, particularly in the elderly, and in the spine and hips. One clinical characteristic of the pathologic fracture is persistent pain interfering with sleep.

Healthy bone may fracture with repetitive application of

See the corresponding chapter or part in the *Textbook of Surgery*, 14th edition, pp. 1291–1294, for a more detailed discussion of this topic, including a comprehensive list of references.

minor trauma. Such fractures are termed *fatigue* or *stress fractures* and are seen most frequently in the metatarsals, tibia and fibula, and femur. Individuals actively involved in regular athletic activities are at risk.

ACUTE COMPLICATIONS

Initial evaluation of the patient with a fracture requires a careful neurologic and vascular examination. Adjacent organ injury should be suspected with fracture of the ribs, spine, and pelvis. Hypovolemia, fat embolization, and the adult respiratory distress syndrome are systemic complications of fracture. The earliest clinical signs of a developing syndrome are rising pulse and respiratory rate, which may occur within the first 12 to 72 hours following injury. A falling arterial PO_2 is a sensitive indicator of impending problems. Patients with long bone fracture and severely traumatized patients should have continuous PO_2 monitoring.

FRACTURE REDUCTION

Fractures displace as a result of either the etiologic trauma, the muscle pull, or both. *Manipulative reduction* can be accomplished when it is possible to overcome the pull of the muscles bridging the fracture site and there is no intervening soft tissue between the bone ends. *Traction reduction* is sometimes used by inserting a transverse pin distal to the fracture site and placing continuous pull on the pin. Some fractures cannot be reduced by either manipulation or traction and may require surgical therapy and *open reduction*. When open reduction is required, it is usually accompanied by some form of internal fixation of the fracture. The decision regarding *open reduction and internal fixation* is a critical one to be undertaken only where appropriate skills and facilities are available. *Prosthetic replacement* may be required in fractures such as the neck of the femur in elderly patients. Rehabilitation may be significantly reduced by appropriate operative intervention, particularly in the elderly.

FRACTURE IMMOBILIZATION

Fractures may be immobilized by splinting, casting, traction, and internal or external fixation. All forms of treatment must take into consideration the swelling that occurs after fracture. Increasing pain, progressive numbness, and decreased circulation in the extremity are ominous. All patients are cautioned to watch for these signs, and they should be examined immediately and repeatedly should they occur.

Immobilization is accomplished by *internal fixation* with intermedullary rods, percutaneous pins, and plates and screws, or by *external fixation*. The trend in recent years in multiple trauma has been toward the operative fixation of fractures, allowing the benefits of early mobilization. Appropriate techniques for internal fixation are discussed in the sections that follow.

OPEN FRACTURES

An *open fracture* should be treated as an emergency. Surgical débridement of the wound is required.

Repair of nerves and tendons in an open fracture is rarely indicated. Vessels require repair if the circulation to the extremity is in jeopardy. When débridement is completed, a decision must be made about stabilization of the fracture. The characteristics of the wound, the nature of the fracture, and the surgical environment determine treatment. A decision also must be made regarding wound closure. If there are any questions regarding viability of muscle tissue or degree of contamination, the wound should be dressed open. *When in doubt, dress the wound open.*

FRACTURE HEALING

Following fracture, a hematoma rapidly develops about the bone ends. Primitive mesenchymal cells within the periosteum and the medullary canal differentiate into primitive osteoblasts and proliferate. This proliferation of osteogenic cells and the early primitive bone produced constitute the "fracture callus." If there is motion at the fracture site, the primitive mesenchymal cells may differentiate into chondroblasts. If motion or distraction at the fracture site is allowed to persist, a dense, fibrous scar develops between the bone ends, producing a *fibrous nonunion.* Compression of a fracture enhances healing. This principle is used in treatment. Fractures of the tibial shaft may be treated in a walking cast, allowing the patient to bear weight across the fracture site. The compression principle may also be used with internal fixation devices for enhancement of healing.

LATE COMPLICATIONS

Late complications consist of soft tissue contracture, limitation of joint motion, delayed union or nonunion, malunion, avascular necrosis, and traumatic arthritis. Active and passive exercises are usually necessary for restoration of motion and strength. Delayed union or nonunion of a fracture may develop when motion is present; operative intervention may be indicated. When a fracture heals with unacceptable angulation or rotation, a *malunion* has occurred. The disability from malunion may be cosmetic, functional, or both. Malunion may require surgical intervention with correction through osteotomy. In some fractures, there is a loss of circulation of the involved bone with subsequent avascular necrosis. *Avascular necrosis* usually causes collapse of the articular surface of the involved bone and the development of subsequent degenerative arthritis. Fractures that involve articular surfaces may cause traumatic arthritis.

II

Fractures of the Spine
William T. Hardaker, Jr., M.D.,
and William J. Richardson, M.D.

Trauma may subject the vertebral column to one or a combination of violent forces including flexion, extension, axial compression, rotation, and shearing. If these forces produce motion greater than the physiologic range of the spine, a fracture or dislocation occurs.

The anatomic relationship for the vertebral supporting structures, the neural elements, and the types of forces producing the injury determines the amount of displacement, stability, and neurologic involvement within a given spinal injury. Spine fractures are considered stable if the fragments are unlikely to move when the spine is physiologically loaded. Conversely, if movement and neural damage are likely, the injured spine is labeled unstable. The instability may be acute or chronic, depending on whether the displacement is immediately threatening or if progressive deformity is likely to occur during the extended healing process.

A complete neurologic evaluation is essential in all individuals with suspected spine injuries. The intercostal and abdominal muscles should be examined along with motor, sensory, and reflex testing of the extremities. The anal sphincter tone and bulbocavernosus reflexes must be included in the evaluation. Complete loss of motor and sensory function, including perianal sensation, during the first 24 hours after injury indicates complete cord injury. The bulbocavernosus reflex usually recovers within the first 24 hours. Recovery of this reflex and the presence of complete anesthesia and paralysis is compelling evidence that the patient will not recover functional motor power of the lower extremity muscle groups innervated below the level of fracture.

Anteroposterior and lateral roentgenographic views demonstrate most fractures involving the vertebral bodies. Computed axial tomography and water-soluble contrast agents greatly improve the ability to thoroughly evaluate fractures and dislocations in the spinal canal. In addition, the computed tomographic scan provides valuable data for suspected fractures of the posterior elements.

THE CERVICAL SPINE

Fracture of the Atlas (Jefferson's Fracture)

This injury occurs from an axial load on the top of the head. The resultant forces are exerted laterally on the ring of C1, and the arches fracture at their thinnest and weakest points. Usually the spinal cord is not damaged because the

---

See the corresponding chapter or part in the *Textbook of Surgery,* 14th edition, pp. 1294–1300, for a more detailed discussion of this topic, including a comprehensive list of references.

canal of the atlas is normally large, and with fracture, the fragments spread outward to further increase the dimensions of the neural canal. Computed tomography represents the best available roentgenographic study for evaluation of the injury. When considerable instability is present, the halo-vest is the preferred method of treatment.

Fractures of the Odontoid

Odontoid fractures occur as a result of falls, blows to the head, and automobile accidents. If the injured patient complains of neck or occipital pain, experiences headaches, or has torticollis, the odontoid area should be examined thoroughly. Lateral views centered on the C2 vertebra and open-mouth views of the odontoid usually allow adequate visualization of the dens. However, tomograms may be necessary for demonstrating the fracture.

Three basic types of fractures are described based on the anatomic level of the injury. Type I fractures are oblique and occur at the extreme upper level of the odontoid process. A hard cervical orthosis provides satisfactory stability of this fracture. Type II fractures occur through the junction of the odontoid process and the C2 vertebral body. Union occurs in most cases of Type II injuries with prompt diagnosis, satisfactory reduction, and rigid external fixation with use of the halo-vest. Operative arthrodesis by use of autogenous iliac bone graft and wiring of C1–2 through a posterior approach is indicated if union is not achieved. Type III fractures extend through the cancellous bone of the C2 vertebral body. These injuries are rarely unstable and unite following 3 months of immobilization in a four-poster brace or a halo-vest.

Fractures of the Pedicles of the Atlas (Hangman's Fracture)

A fracture through the pedicles of C2 usually occurs from a severe extension injury such as an automobile accident or fall. Nonunion is uncommon in this fracture. If the injury is stable with little or no displacement, the four-poster brace is usually satisfactory treatment. In unstable circumstances, more rigid stabilization by use of the halo-vest may be required.

Fractures and Dislocations of the C3 to C7 Vertebrae

Fractures and dislocations of the lower cervical spine are common. Dislocations of the cervical spine occur most commonly at the interspaces between C3 and C7. The injury is caused by a flexion-distraction force. These forces combine to dislocate the facet joints with concomitant fracture of the disc bond and varying degrees of failure of the longitudinal cervical ligaments. Dislocations of the cervical spine are managed by prompt realignment by means of serial traction under direct radiologic control and with concomitant serial neurologic examinations. If closed reduction cannot be achieved, operative reduction under direct vision followed by wire fixation and fusion with use of autogenous bone graft should be performed.

THE THORACOLUMBAR SPINE

Fractures or dislocations of the lumbar area require considerably more displacement for injury of the neural elements than do fractures in the cervical and thoracic spine. A bursting fracture in the cervical or thoracic region may cause devastating neurologic loss, whereas a similar fracture in the lumbar area may produce no permanent neurologic deficit.

Flexion Injuries

Pure flexion injuries are the most common thoracolumbar fracture. These injuries usually involve only the anterior column and therefore are acutely stable. Neurologic loss is uncommon. If the compression is mild, a three-point brace will be satisfactory. When wedging is greater than 50 per cent of the anterior body height, a modified polypropylene jacket may be necessary for prevention of progressive angulation.

Axial Compression Injuries

Burst fractures follow axial compression of the spine frequently associated with varying degrees of flexion. These injuries, which most commonly occur at the thoracolumbar junction, are characterized by circumferential expansion of the entire involved vertebra with failure of the anterior, the middle, and, in some cases, the posterior spinal columns. Middle-column failure in burst fractures is produced by retropulsion of the posterosuperior portion of the vertebral body into the spinal canal, compressing the dural tube, often with associated neurologic deficit.

Mild burst fractures with minimal anterior body deformation, minimal retropulsion of fragments into the spinal canal, no posterior element involvement, and minimal kyphotic angulation can be treated satisfactorily with a molded polypropylene body jacket. If there is incomplete neurologic involvement with bone fragments impinging on the neural elements, surgical management may be indicated. The goal of surgical therapy is to provide an optimal environment for potential spinal cord recovery. Fundamental to this goal are (1) decompression of the spinal canal for removal of impinging bone and disc fragments, (2) restoration of the normal alignment of the spine at the thoracolumbar junction, (3) immediate stabilization of the fracture site with restoration of the normal vertebral body height, and (4) long-term stabilization by means of a posterior spine fusion with use of autogenous iliac bone graft.

Anterior exposure of the vertebral body for decompression is gained by a transthoracic, by a transabdominal, or through a transpedicular approach. The Harrington or Cotrel-Dubousset instrumentation allows acute realignment and stabilization. Realignment of the spinal canal and restoration of the height will not, in many cases, effectively decompress the spinal canal. The procedure should, therefore, be combined with definitive removal of bone fragments under direct observation.

Fracture-Dislocations

Fracture-dislocations usually involve translation of one spinal motion segment, or a portion of one spinal segment, in relationship to the remaining spine. A number of failure modes including shear, compression, tension, and rotation can occur within the individual columns and produce characteristic radiographic fracture patterns. In the lumbar region, these injuries are usually grossly unstable, and great care must be exercised in managing patients with such injuries. Operative reduction and internal fixation are the most reliable means of creating a stable environment for potential maximal neurologic return.

Flexion-Distraction Injuries

Flexion-distraction forces classically occur in seatbelt injuries in which the individual is subjected to sudden deceleration and the torso is flexed forward over the restraining belt. Tension failure occurs in the posterior and middle columns. The failure mode of the anterior column depends on the location of the fulcrum of rotation. These injuries may be associated with marked displacement and are usually very unstable. Open reduction with realignment and internal fixation is usually required in order to regain stability.

III

Fractures and Dislocations of the Shoulder, Arm, and Forearm

Robert D. Fitch, M.D.

TRAUMATIC ANTERIOR DISLOCATION OF THE SHOULDER

The shoulder demonstrates remarkable range of motion owing to the anatomic peculiarities of this unconstrained joint. However, these features also render it susceptible to dislocation. There is little contact between the shallow glenoid and the humeral head, and the capsular and ligament stability must be augmented by the surrounding rotator cuff musculature.

Following traumatic dislocation of the shoulder, the arm is held at the side. The acromion process is prominent, and the normal fullness of the shoulder is replaced by a concave contour just below the acromion. Evaluation must include complete neurologic and vascular examination because of the proximity of the brachial plexus and axillary artery to the site of injury. Anteroposterior and lateral views confirm the presence of dislocation and any associated fractures.

Treatment consists of prompt reduction of the dislocation. The longer the shoulder remains unreduced, the more muscle spasm there is to overcome. Reduction is accomplished by longitudinal traction on the arm, with countertraction applied in the axilla. An alternative method is the Stimson technique. The patient is placed prone with the arm allowed to drop off the table. Progressive weight is added to the extremity until a gradual gentle reduction is obtained. Following reduction, neurovascular status to the extremity is again reassessed. The arm is then immobilized in a sling held in internal rotation for approximately 3 weeks. Protected range-of-motion exercises are then begun, but excessive abduction and external rotation should be avoided for 3 months. Recurrence is a common complication in patients under 40 years of age.

FRACTURES OF THE PROXIMAL HUMERUS

Fractures of the proximal humerus occur more frequently with advancing age, and loss of normal trabecular bone with aging makes this area susceptible to injury. Minor trauma can cause fractures in the elderly; otherwise, fractures require considerable force. The major segments that can be involved include the anatomic neck, greater tuberosity, lesser tuberosity, and surgical neck. The fractures are described as

---

See the corresponding chapter or part in the *Textbook of Surgery*, 14th edition, pp. 1300–1308, for a more detailed discussion of this topic, including a comprehensive list of references.

nondisplaced or two-, three-, or four-part fractures depending on how many segments are involved and displaced. Most fractures occur as a result of a fall on the outstretched arm, which causes forced abduction, extension, and external rotation.

Clinically, some degree of ecchymosis and swelling about the shoulder should be present. The vascular supply to the limb must be assessed and a thorough neurologic examination performed for excluding associated arterial or nerve injury. Anteroposterior and lateral radiographs identify the extent of the injury and guide treatment.

Most proximal humeral fractures are minimally displaced, and treatment consists of temporary immobilization in a sling and swathe or commercially available shoulder immobilizer for 2 to 3 weeks followed by range-of-motion exercises. The prognosis for these fractures is quite good. Two-part fractures can generally be treated by closed reduction and immobilization. If significant displacement of the shaft or greater tuberosity persists following closed reduction, open reduction may be required. Three-part fractures generally require open reduction and internal fixation. In four-part fractures, prosthetic replacement of the humeral head has provided postoperative results superior to open reduction and internal fixation of all fracture fragments.

FRACTURES OF THE SHAFT OF THE HUMERUS

Humeral shaft fractures are caused by either direct trauma or a fall on the outstretched arm. Direct blow or bending movements usually cause a transverse fracture, whereas indirect torsional forces cause spiral fractures. The radial nerve is susceptible to injury because of its proximity to the bone at the junction of the middle and distal thirds of the shaft of the humerus. Clinical examination should include evaluation of the radial nerve function. Pain and swelling at the fracture site and crepitance are usually easily detectable. Radiographs identify the fracture location, pattern, and amount of comminution.

Nondisplaced fractures can usually be treated by simple immobilization of the arm to the chest with a sling and swathe followed by early active range-of-motion exercises in 2 to 3 weeks. Displaced fractures are managed by a coaptation splint or a hanging-arm cast. Occasionally, open reduction and internal fixation are indicated if there is an associated vascular injury or if the radial nerve function is lost during manipulation of the fracture fragments. A radial nerve injury that occurs before any manipulation does not require surgical exploration, since most of these injuries are a result of stretching or contusion; function will return within several weeks. In the occasional case of nonunion, open reduction with internal fixation and bone grafting is indicated.

FRACTURES OF THE DISTAL HUMERUS AND ELBOW

Supracondylar and Intercondylar Fractures

Supracondylar fractures of the humerus represent 50 to 60 per cent of all fractures about the elbow. There are two types: *flexion* and *extension*. The most common extension injury occurs as a result of a fall on the outstretched arm, which produces a compression and hyperextension force applied indirectly to the distal humerus. Clinically, pain and swelling are present. Neurovascular status must be carefully assessed because arterial or neurologic injury can occur by laceration and direct or indirect compression. Evaluation of the radiographs reveals the degree of displacement and amount of comminution. Subtle changes such as rotary malalignment and varus impaction must be identified.

In children, undisplaced fractures are treated by immobilization of the arm with the elbow flexed to 90 degrees. The period of immobilization is approximately 3 weeks. A varus impacted fracture may at first appear as a nondisplaced fracture, but if it is not recognized, a cubitus varus deformity will occur. Baumann's angle is a useful measurement for determining if varus position is present. If the fracture is significantly displaced, a reduction under anesthesia is warranted. If the fracture is unstable with the elbow flexed to 90 degrees, percutaneous pinning is recommended.

In the severely swollen, displaced supracondylar fracture without neurovascular compromise, preliminary sidearm traction or overhead traction may be useful. This can be provided by Dunlop skin traction or by olecranon pin traction. Attempts at obtaining and maintaining reduction while in traction are worthwhile. If the fracture cannot be aligned with traction after the swelling has subsided, a closed reduction with or without percutaneous pinning under general anesthesia is indicated.

Occasionally fractures cannot be reduced by traction or closed reduction because of soft tissue interposition. These fractures require open reduction and pinning. Similarly, in the case of neurologic deficit or vascular insufficiency, open reduction is required with exploration of the involved structures.

Supracondylar fractures in adults are often comminuted and have intra-articular extension; they are best managed by open reduction and internal fixation for allowing early range-of-motion exercises of the elbow.

The most serious complication is Volkmann's ischemia with subsequent contracture. Varus, valgus, and rotary malunion will not remodel and will persist. The most common malunion seen is that of cubitus varus (gunstock deformity), which may require corrective supracondylar valgus oseotomy.

Dislocations of the Elbow

Posterior dislocation by falling on an outstretched arm causes dislocation of the radius and ulna. Neurovascular structures are rarely affected, although arterial injury occurs occasionally. Anterior dislocations are caused by a blow on the flexed elbow. Dislocation of the radial head can occur as an isolated injury anteriorly or posteriorly. Dislocation of the ulna alone occurs rarely. Associated fractures of the coronoid process, medial epicondyle, or radial head can occur. Clinically, elbow motion is limited. There is deformity, and the neurovascular structures are usually intact. Median nerve injury occasionally occurs.

Gentle pull on the olecranon followed by flexion usually relocates the dislocation. After reduction, the elbow should be extended through a reasonable range of motion for testing stability. If the elbow is stable, temporary immobilization for comfort is recommended. Early range-of-motion exercises are instituted for avoidance of permanent stiffness. In simple dislocations, a functional range of motion usually results. Myositis ossificans, however, can produce mild or severe limitation of motion in a small percentage of patients.

Fractures of the Olecranon

Because of the subcutaneous location of the olecranon on the extensor surface of the arm, it is susceptible to direct trauma. In addition, avulsion fractures can occur as a result of a violent pull of the triceps muscle. Clinically, there is swelling and tenderness in the region of the proximal ulna. Crepitance may be noted at the fracture site. Ulnar nerve function should be carefully tested because contusion neurapraxia can be associated with this injury. Anteroposterior and lateral radiographs should be assessed for the size of the olecranon fragment, the degree of comminution, and the amount of displacement.

Undisplaced fractures are treated by splinting with the elbow in 60 degrees of flexion. Fractures that are significantly displaced should be treated by open reduction with anatomic realignment of the articular surface when possible. Avulsion fractures or comminuted fractures can be excised with primary repair of the triceps tendon. Achieving anatomic reduction with rigid internal fixation allows early active motion of the elbow and should diminish the delayed complications of limited motion and degenerative arthritis.

FRACTURES OF THE SHAFT OF THE RADIUS AND ULNA

The two bones of the forearm, the radius and ulna, share an intricate relationship that allows pronation and supination. As the radius rotates around the ulna, a smooth articulation at the proximal radial-ulnar joint is required. The interosseous membrane serves as a hinge during forearm rotation, and the distal radial-ulnar articulation is stabilized by the triangular fibrocartilage complex. Distortion by fracture or dislocation alters the biomechanics of the forearm and therefore limits forearm rotation. One or both bones of the forearm may be fractured. The fracture of the proximal third of the ulna associated with a radial head dislocation is termed a *Monteggia fracture*. A fracture of the distal third of the radius in conjunction with dislocation of the distal ulna is termed a *Galeazzi* or *Piedmont fracture*.

Clinically, pain and deformity of the forearm are present. Evaluation of the neurovascular condition of the extremity must be made as well as of the presence or absence of increased pressure within the muscle compartments of the forearm. Swelling within the tight muscle compartments of the forearm can cause occlusion of venous and arterial circulation with resultant Volkmann's ischemic contracture. Significant swelling of the forearm compartments associated with pain on passive extension of the fingers should alert one to this possibility. Radiographs should include both the elbow and wrist joints for identifying the location of the fractures and any associated dislocations. In adults, displaced fractures of the shaft of the radius and ulna, the Monteggia or Piedmont fractures, should be treated by open reduction and internal fixation with plates and screws. Conversely, most forearm fractures in children can be managed by closed means. The thick periosteum allows stable reduction, and the osteogenic potential in children allows excellent remodeling of angular deformities.

The most serious complication of forearm fractures, neurovascular compromise and subsequent ischemia contracture, must be avoided. Nonunion of forearm shaft fractures occurs in 5 to 10 per cent of cases in which closed treatment is used. Malunion is a frequent complication when open reduction with internal fixation is not utilized. Other complications include elbow stiffness, finger stiffness, and reflex sympathetic dystrophy.

FRACTURES OF THE DISTAL FOREARM

These are common in children and adults. The injury occurs by falling on the outstretched arm with forces transmitted through the carpus causing either volar or dorsal displacement. In children, displacement may occur through the metaphysis or through the growth plate. In adults, the fracture may be comminuted and have an intra-articular extension. In elderly patients, the dorsal cortex tends to become comminuted. The most common fracture pattern seen, *Colles' fracture,* is a fracture of the distal radius with dorsal displacement and volar angulation. Other fracture patterns have been described.

Clinically, pain, swelling, and deformity are present just proximal to the wrist. Often a "step-off" in the distal radius can be appreciated by palpation. The median nerve is at risk for compression by the displacement of the fragments.

Nondisplaced or minimally displaced fractures are treated by immobilization for 3 to 4 weeks in a cast or splint. Displaced fractures should be reduced under local or regional anesthesia. The wrist is generally immobilized in flexion and ulnar deviation. Intra-articular fractures, if displaced, require open reduction. Severely comminuted fractures may best be managed by external fixation with pins.

In children, physeal plate injuries may cause permanent growth disturbance. Comminuted fractures may cause shortening of the distal radius with incongruity of the distal radial-ulnar joint and subsequent limited motion and pain. Acute or late median nerve symptoms may occur. Other complications include rupture of the extensor pollicis longus and reflex sympathetic dystrophy.

IV

Fracture of the Carpal Scaphoid
Richard D. Goldner, M.D.,
and J. Leonard Goldner, M.D.

The initial physical examination comprises digital palpation, sensory assessment, and vascular patency. The patient's response to digital pressure is the most important clue to the existence and location of a carpal injury. Tenderness to pressure in the anatomic snuffbox is present with a fracture.

If a scaphoid fracture is suspected, the radiographic examination should include anteroposterior, lateral, and supination and pronation oblique views. A projection in ulnar deviation and pronation (posteroanterior, palm down) may show an undisplaced fracture. The lateral view shows the linear relationship between the distal radius, lunate, and capitate.

If the radiographs are negative at the time of the initial injury but clinical findings suggest a fracture, the radiographs are repeated 10 to 14 days after injury. Routine studies are made at that time, and if fracture is not noted but suspected, then special techniques are considered: (1) magnification radiograph, (2) anteroposterior and lateral tomograms or direct sagittal and transverse computed tomographic scan, (3) stress radiograph in ulnar deviation, (4) fluoroscopic examination, and (5) ^{99m}technetium bone scan.

TREATMENT. If a scaphoid fracture is suspected by history and clinical examination but is not demonstrated on radiographs, a cast is applied with the hand in radial deviation and 10 degrees of flexion for immobilization of the thumb, including the proximal phalanx and the forearm. This cast is removed 10 to 14 days later, and the radiographs are repeated. Thirty per cent of the middle third fractures and most proximal third fractures develop aseptic necrosis of the proximal fragment because of the blood flow pattern. The distal location with limitation of major blood supply is the

See the corresponding chapter or part in the *Textbook of Surgery*, 14th edition, pp. 1309–1313, for a more detailed discussion of this topic, including a comprehensive list of references.

etiologic factor of nonunion and aseptic necrosis of the proximal fragment. The blood vessels passing from distal to proximal are interrupted when the fracture occurs.

The average healing time of a scaphoid fracture depends on the location and obliquity of the fracture line. Fractures of the distal third (10 per cent) usually heal in about 8 weeks. For the middle third (70 per cent), the healing time is generally 8 to 12 weeks or longer. Fractures of the proximal third (20 per cent) heal more slowly (healing time 10 to 20 weeks). Most of the fractures of the proximal fifth of the scaphoid develop aseptic necrosis.

Nondisplaced, stable fractures of the scaphoid are adequately treated by external immobilization in a cast. The cast may be a well-molded short-arm cast that includes the thumb proximal phalanx and is changed every 10 to 14 days for the first 6 weeks, or it may be a long-arm cast that includes the thumb.

DIFFERENTIAL DIAGNOSIS OF CARPAL SCAPHOID FRACTURES. *Rotatory subluxation of the scaphoid* or scapholunate dissociation occurs after a tear of the complex ligaments between the radius, scaphoid, and lunate. The condition is not readily diagnosed unless it is suspected. Radiographs showing the spread between the scaphoid and lunate are suggestive of this pathologic lesion.

Rupture of the flexor carpi radialis tendon may occur from a fall on the outstretched hand and can occur in combination with ligamentous injury. This injury may also be spontaneous in older individuals.

Traumatic arthrosis occurs from cartilage damage during the original injury, incongruity of cartilage surfaces secondary to malposition or malunion, hypermobility from nonunion, or ligament injury.

In the management of nonunion, iliac crest bone grafting to bridge both proximal and distal segments of the scaphoid on the palmar surface has been 90 per cent successful. The Herbert screw has improved the fixation of the fragments, diminishes the length of time of external immobilization, and may increase the union rate.

V

Fractures and Dislocations of the Hand

*Richard D. Goldner, M.D.,
and J. Leonard Goldner, M.D.*

Hands are exposed to many forces that may cause bone or joint trauma. Fractures of the metacarpals and phalanges are

---

See the corresponding chapter or part in the *Textbook of Surgery*, 14th edition, pp. 1314–1326, for a more detailed discussion of this topic, including a comprehensive list of references.

estimated at 10 per cent of all fractures that occur; of these, fractures of the distal phalanx are the most common, followed in order by fractures of the metacarpals, the proximal phalanges, and then the middle phalanges.

TERMINOLOGY

Terminology providing description of alignment is as follows. *Dislocation* means that the articular surfaces are not apposed or congruous. *Subluxation* means a partial displacement of one side of the joint on the other, but with less severe distortion than in a dislocation. The term *reduction* refers to the action required for obtaining anatomic alignment.

Fractures are described as stable, unstable, displaced, nondisplaced, impacted, comminuted, intra-articular, extra-articular, transverse, oblique, or spiral. Angulation may occur in any direction: dorsal, volar, radial, ulnar, and combinations. Malrotation may also occur. If there is no wound, the fracture is referred to as *closed*, and if the skin is broken, the fracture is referred to as *open*.

RADIOGRAPHIC EXAMINATION

Radiographs determine the exact location of the fracture: articular surface, epiphysis, neck, metaphysis, shaft, or base of the digit. They indicate the type of fracture: complete, incomplete, transverse, oblique, spiral, or comminuted; they indicate the position of the fractured bones, the amount of displacement of one segment relative to the other, and the angulation of the segments compared with a straight line and with the apex of angulation either dorsal or volar. Correct rotation of the digit may be assessed radiographically by the relationship of the proximal to distal fractured segment but is best determined clinically by comparison with adjacent digits.

Multiple radiographic views of the involved hand or digit are essential for an accurate diagnosis. The usual views are posteroanterior, pronation and supination oblique, and true lateral. True lateral exposures must be obtained of the individual digits rather than of the entire hand, since in the latter case, the digits are overlapping. A 10-degree supination film for the ulnar side of the hand and a 10-degree pronation film at the radial side of the hand provide additional information.

ANATOMIC REGIONS OF FRACTURES

Distal Phalanx and Distal Interphalangeal Joint

DISTAL PHALANX FRACTURE. The fracture is splinted for 10 to 14 days to decrease discomfort and allow healing. The fingernail may be elevated by hematoma trapped between the nail plate and nail bed, which is very painful. The hematoma is released by making a hole in the center of the nail plate with the round end of an open paper clip that has been heated in a flame or by a disposable ophthalmic cautery. If the nail bed has been lacerated, the nail plate should be removed and the laceration repaired with fine, absorbable sutures.

DORSAL AVULSION FRACTURES. A dorsal segment of bone is elevated when the extensor digitorum communis is avulsed. After extensor tendon continuity is lost at the distal joint, a "drop finger" or "mallet finger" occurs. If the fragment is small (less than 40 per cent, displaced less than 2 mm.), slight hyperextension with a dorsal aluminum splint on the distal and middle phalanges produces sufficient apposition to allow healing. The splint is used for a total of 8 to 12 weeks. Similar treatment but longer protective splinting is used for the mallet finger of tendon origin in which no fracture or avulsion is noted.

AVULSION OF A FRAGMENT FROM THE FLEXOR SURFACE. This occurs when the flexor digitorum profundus is forcibly pulled from its distal phalangeal insertion, such as when the digit is hyperextended as a result of a forcible blow or fall or from catching the digit (usually the ring finger) in a football jersey. Physical findings are swelling, the patient's inability to flex the distal joint, and a palpable palmar mass at the base of the finger or in the palm. Radiographs may show the bone fragment in the digit. Operative treatment is required for reattaching the flexor tendon to the point of avulsion.

Middle Phalanx and Proximal Interphalangeal (PIP) Joint

The extrinsic muscles such as the extensor digitorum communis, flexor digitorum profundus, and flexor digitorum superficialis all affect the position of the fragments after phalangeal fractures. Active muscle contraction of the lumbricals and the interossei influences the position of the fragments and the deformity of the digit. Fractures through the distal portion (*neck*) of the middle phalanx are likely to have apex palmar angulation, because the proximal fragment is flexed by the superficialis tendon. A fracture through the proximal portion (*base*) of the middle phalanx is likely to have apex dorsal angulation caused by flexion of the distal fragment by the superficialis and extension of the proximal fragment by the central slip of the extensor. Fractures through the *middle* two thirds may be angulated in either direction or not at all. Rotary deformities and radial and ulnar deviation may also depend on the intrinsic tendon pull as well as the force of the original injury.

Stable fractures of the middle phalanx can be immobilized initially in a splint followed by adjacent digit taping (buddy taping). Fractures that are stable after closed reduction are immobilized for approximately 3 weeks. Although the fracture may be protected for 6 to 8 weeks, gentle motion should be initiated at 3 to 4 weeks. Displaced, unstable fracture of the middle phalanx that cannot be reduced or maintained by external immobilization requires fixation either by percutaneous pins or by open reduction and internal fixation. Spiral and long oblique fractures are well suited for internal lag screw fixation.

A *chip fracture* at the PIP joint indicates either a collateral ligament tear or marginal capsular avulsion. This radiographic finding may be a subtle suggestion of more extensive instability, but as long as the phalanx can be placed in anatomic alignment, in the position that decreases tension and stress on the collateral ligaments, adequate healing usually occurs. Large, displaced avulsion fractures with collateral ligament attached are repaired surgically.

A nondisplaced *condylar fracture* should be splinted for 2 to 3 weeks. These fractures are followed frequently because displacement may occur after motion has been initiated. Displaced condylar fractures often cannot be adequately reduced and held by closed methods. Open reduction corrects incongruity of the articular surfaces that if uncorrected would cause traumatic arthrosis.

DORSAL DISLOCATION OF THE PIP JOINT. Dislocations of the PIP joint are classified by the location of the middle phalanx in relation to the proximal phalanx (palmar, dorsal, lateral).

Dorsal dislocation of the middle phalanx with avulsion of the volar plate from the middle phalanx is a common injury. The PIP joint is swollen and may be mistaken for a "sprained finger." The lateral radiograph demonstrates displacement and often a small volar fragment from the proximal end of the middle phalanx. After reduction, a splint is applied with the PIP joint flexed 20 to 30 degrees for 2 to 3 weeks. If the joint is completely stable, taping the involved digit to the adjacent one provides assistive motion and protects the joint.

DORSAL FRACTURE-DISLOCATION OF THE PIP JOINT. Dorsal dislocation of the middle phalanx with displaced fracture of its volar portion is a serious injury. Fractures of greater than 40 per cent of the articular surface are usually unstable. If the fracture is reduced and is stable, it can be treated by a splint that blocks extension but allows flexion. If reduction is not maintained and if the alignment of the joint cannot be re-established, operative procedure is indicated.

PALMAR DISLOCATION OF THE PIP JOINT. Palmar dislocation of the middle phalanx may disrupt the central slip and dorsal capsule (palmar plate and one collateral ligament). This may produce a flexion deformity of the PIP joint and hyperextension of the distal interphalangeal joint (boutonnière deformity).

Proximal Phalanx

Fractures of the proximal phalanx are divided into oblique and transverse types.

TRANSVERSE FRACTURE OF THE PROXIMAL PHALANX. A fracture through the midportion of the proximal phalanx with volar angulation presses the long flexor tendons and causes a resulting flexion deformity at the PIP joint. Internal fixation, by percutaneous pins or after open reduction, is required if the alignment cannot be maintained by plaster splint.

OBLIQUE FRACTURE OF THE PROXIMAL PHALANX. For treatment of the oblique fracture, the distal fragment is derotated and the joints on either side of the phalanx are flexed. The wrist is held in dorsiflexion, the metacarpophalangeal joints are flexed about 70 degrees, and the proximal and distal interphalangeal joints are flexed slightly. This portion of metacarpophalangeal flexion and interphalangeal extension is termed the "intrinsic plus" portion.

INTERCONDYLAR FRACTURES OF THE PROXIMAL PHALANX. A condylar split fracture involving the distal end of the proximal phalanx is an intra-articular fracture. Collateral ligaments are attached to each of the condyles. If the condyles are malrotated and displaced greater than 2 mm, if adequate position cannot be obtained by manipulation, or if the reduction cannot be maintained, percutaneous pinning or open reduction and internal fixation of the condyles is performed.

METACARPOPHALANGEAL JOINT DISLOCATION. Metacarpophalangeal joint dislocation is due to a hyperextension force. The index is dislocated most frequently. If the palmar plate is avulsed from its origin and is trapped between the metacarpal head and the proximal phalanx, reduction is not possible by closed methods. Open reduction can be accomplished through either a palmar or dorsal approach.

THE METACARPALS

Metacarpal fractures are divided as follows: (1) fractures of the metacarpal *head*, with intra-articular involvement and dorsal or palmar angulation of the fragments; (2) fractures of the metacarpal *neck*, with dorsal or palmar angulation and with a rotary element; (3) *transverse* fractures through the shaft of the metacarpal; (4) *oblique* fractures through the shaft of the metacarpal; and (5) *dislocation* at the base of the metacarpals. Nondisplaced metacarpal fractures are treated closed and immobilized for 3 weeks followed by taping to the adjacent digit. Displaced fractures of the metacarpal head may require open reduction and internal fixation with small screws or wires. Severely comminuted fractures limited to the metacarpal head distal to the collateral ligament should be treated with early protective motion. Large articular fragments with collateral ligament avulsion may require open reduction and internal fixation.

A fracture of the neck of the fifth metacarpal is a common injury caused by a direct blow. This is known as a boxer's fracture and occurs from a dorsal force applied directly to the metacarpal head. Radiographs show the angulation on the oblique and lateral views. Up to 40 to 45 degrees of dorsal angulation is acceptable in the fifth metacarpal, approximately 30 degrees in the fourth metacarpal; in the index and long metacarpals, angulation greater than 15 degrees is unacceptable secondary to the lack of compensatory carpometacarpal motion. Rotation alignment should be restored in all fingers.

TRANSVERSE AND SHORT OBLIQUE METACARPAL SHAFT FRACTURES. *Transverse shaft fractures* are often caused by a direct blow with dorsal angulation secondary to exertion of palmar force by then interosseus muscles. The intermetacarpal ligaments prevent shortening, and the interossei stabilize the digits. If the fracture is minimally displaced, it can be controlled with a well-molded short-arm cast for 4 to 6 weeks with the metacarpophalangeal joints flexed 60 degrees.

Indications for internal fixation include any persistent rotational deformity, uncorrected dorsal angulation greater than 10 degrees in the second or third metacarpal, or uncorrected dorsal angulation greater than 20 degrees in the fourth or fifth metacarpals. Shortening more than 3 mm or multiple displaced fractures usually require treatment. Internal fixation of long oblique or spiral fractures with interfragmentary screw fixation controls excessive shortening and angulation and allows early motion of the digits.

Long, oblique, or spiral metacarpal fractures, minimally displaced, are treated by splinting. Displaced fractures that are not able to be reduced adequately or that are unstable after reduction are best treated by lag screw fixation.

THUMB METACARPAL FRACTURES. Fractures at the base of the thumb are classified as follows: (1) *intra-articular fracture* through the proximal end of the metacarpal, leaving a fragment held by the intermetacarpal ligament, and the base of the metacarpal displaced laterally out of the joint by pull of the abductor pollicis longus (Bennett's fracture); simultaneously, the adductor pollicis pulls the proximal phalanx and distal metacarpal toward the palm and the proximal metacarpal away from its base; (2) a *comminuted intra-articular fracture* of the proximal end of the metacarpal (Rolando's fracture); (3) *fracture through the metaphysis,* extra-articular, with angulation dorsal or volar. Other variations may occur.

Treatment of the displaced thumb fracture depends on the type of injury. The *intra-articular fracture* with two segments (Bennett's) is managed by closed reduction and pinning.

The *comminuted fracture* at the base of the metacarpal (Rolando's) may be treated by either percutaneous pin fixation or traction obtained by placing a transfixation pin through the base of the proximal phalanx or neck of the metacarpal.

The fracture at the proximal metaphysis of the thumb metacarpal, which does not include the joint, is managed by manipulation, realignment, and plaster fixation, with the thumb in wide abduction and the metacarpophalangeal joint in flexion.

Injuries to the *metacarpophalangeal joint of the thumb* include chip fractures of the ulnar collateral ligament, the fragment being avulsed from the proximal phalanx or from the distal metacarpal. The ligament can also rupture in its central portion or pull from bone without a fracture. In addition to the collateral ligament injury, the palmar plate and the dorsal capsule are usually torn, causing the phalanx to displace palmarward and radially. In most instances, these injuries are detected by clinical examination (carpometacarpal flexion, metacarpophalangeal flexion with stress). The stress radiograph is not essential, but if there is any question about the extent of soft tissue injury, the stress radiograph under local or regional block is helpful.

If there is less than 30 degrees difference between the injured and uninjured thumb, incomplete tear is diagnosed. Treatment of an incomplete tear can be managed satisfactorily by application of a plaster or fiberglass cast that holds the phalanx in the neutral adducted position and realigns the metacarpal and the phalanx. If there is greater than 30 degrees difference, complete tear is diagnosed, and operative repair is usually indicated.

Displaced intra-articular fractures involving more than 15 to 20 per cent of the articular surface and a small avulsion fracture displaced more than 5 mm are relative indications for open reduction.

VI

Fractures of the Pelvis, Femur, and Knee
Donald E. McCollum, M.D.

FRACTURES OF THE PELVIS

Pelvic fractures are classified into stable and unstable fractures. They may occur from lateral compression, from anterior blows from an automobile, or by vertical shear in a fall from a height. The pelvis is a rigid ring composed of pubic rami, ischium, acetabulum, ilium, and sacrum joined by heavy ligaments at the symphysis and the sacroiliac joints. Disruption at one point does not necessarily produce instability, but disruption of the ring anteriorly and posteriorly on the same side may allow displacement and produces an unstable fracture. These fractures are difficult to treat with prolonged skeletal traction, and open reduction with internal fixation of unstable fractures is most often necessary. Isolated fractures of the sacrum and coccyx are treated by bed rest until the patient is comfortable, after which the patient may be mobilized with crutches. Fibrosis may occur about the

See the corresponding chapter or part in the *Textbook of Surgery*, 14th edition, pp. 1326–1337, for a more detailed discussion of this topic, including a comprehensive list of references.

sacral nerve roots, and persistent pain may be present. Persistent coccygeal pain may be the result of traumatic arthritis of the sacrococcygeal joint. Surgery is seldom indicated and occasionally makes the problem worse.

Emergency evaluation of the patient with a pelvic fracture must include all organ systems that are frequently involved. Careful neurologic evaluation should include the obturator nerve, the sciatic nerve, and the lumbosacral plexus. The most common complication is retroperitoneal bleeding that may mimic gastrointestinal trauma, and peritoneal lavage may be necessary for excluding ruptured intraperitoneal organs. Careful examination of the rectum and vagina may reveal the presence of blood, which suggests that the fracture is compound.

Emergency management of a patient with a compound pelvic fracture includes wound packing for control of bleeding and application of a MAST suit for maintenance of blood pressure; in the event of a "wide open book" fracture, the volume of the pelvis may need to be decreased by use of an external fixator. Emergency radiographic evaluation should include an anteroposterior view and a 40-degree caudad and cephalad projection of the pelvis. When the acetabulum is involved, the 45-degree oblique view of the acetabulum demonstrates disruption of the acetabulum and the sacroiliac joint. After the patient is stabilized, a computed tomographic scan can show additional detail.

Complications of pelvic fracture include massive hemorrhage. If bleeding cannot be controlled by application of an external fixator, arteriography may be necessary to demonstrate bleeding points. These bleeding points can frequently be controlled by injection of Gelfoam emboli or emboli of autogenous blood clot. Lacerations of the pelvic arteries are best treated with ligation.

In fractures of the pelvis, injury to the urinary bladder is frequent. Injuries to the bladder and urethra occur in 14 per cent of all pelvic fractures and must be identified by a urethrogram, cystogram, and intravenous urogram. If the urethrogram shows the urethra to be intact, a retrograde cystogram should be done with a 14- or 16-French catheter and injection of 250 to 300 mm. of dye. Passage of a blind catheter without urethrography is condemned because it may enter and drain blood from the perivesical space, simulating extraperitoneal rupture of the bladder.

The rectum may be lacerated by either ischial or sacral fractures, and examination of the rectum for defects or bleeding should always be done in pelvic fractures. The sciatic nerve is the most frequently damaged nerve in fractures of the pelvis. Damage to the sciatic nerve can be recognized easily by failure to contract the hamstrings and dorsiflex or plantar flex the foot in the conscious patient or by failure to dorsiflex the foot in withdrawal in the semiconscious patient. Paralysis of the obturator nerve can be recognized by inability to contract the adductor muscles and by spotty hypalgesia over the medial aspect of the thigh. The femoral nerve is seldom damaged directly by fractures of the pelvis but may be damaged in anterior dislocation of the hip.

The most common cause of death following pelvic fractures is posttraumatic pulmonary insufficiency, often referred to as the adult respiratory distress syndrome. This syndrome is characterized by a decrease in oxygen saturation of the blood and rising carbon dioxide. It is best managed by mechanical ventilation and positive-pressure oxygen.

Fat embolism also occurs in fractures of the pelvis and is characterized by sudden confusion, a sudden fall in hemoglobin, and decrease in arterial oxygen saturation. Small petechiae appear on the conjunctiva and over the upper chest. A chest film may show hazy infiltrates through both lung fields. Prompt treatment with oxygen and intravenous human serum albumin is necessary for prevention of permanent damage.

The goal of treatment of fractures of the pelvis is achievement of bony union in a functional position as quickly as possible. Deformities of the pelvis may cause leg length inequality, difficulty in walking and sitting, and difficulty in subsequent pregnancy. Most fractures involving the pelvic ring are stable and can be treated by closed methods. Some fractures that are minimally displaced initially appear to be stable but are basically unstable fractures. Any fracture through the sacrum associated with disruption of the pubis must be considered an unstable fracture. The treatment of choice is an open posterior reduction with plate fixation. Unstable pelvic fractures are best treated by open reduction and internal fixation with plates or screws. Skeletal traction is not suitable for disruption of the sacroiliac joints because nonunion and malunion are common. Open reduction of pelvic fractures requires extensive specialized training and should not be attempted by surgeons who do not treat these injuries frequently. For details of open reduction of these fractures, the reader is referred to the main text chapter.

ACETABULAR FRACTURES

The radiographic evaluation of fractures of the acetabulum includes an anteroposterior view of the pelvis and 45-degree oblique views of the acetabulum. Computed tomography may be helpful in recognizing all the components of the fracture. The posterior wall, the anterior wall, the posterior column, and the anterior column or any combination of these elements may be involved. Open reduction is indicated in acetabular fractures if displacement of the articular surface is greater than 2 mm. For details of open reduction of the acetabular fracture, the reader is referred to the main text chapter.

FRACTURES OF THE HIP AND UPPER FEMUR

The classification of hip fractures is based on prognosis. In any fracture, healing depends not only on fixation but, more significantly, on blood supply. Intracapsular fractures of the hip include fractures of the head of the femur, impacted subcapital fractures, and displaced subcapital and neck fractures. The femoral head receives only a small amount of its blood supply from the pelvic side of the joint. The major blood supply arises from the vascular ring at the base of the neck, and fractures within the capsule damage this blood supply. Avascular necrosis frequently follows this type of fracture. Impacted subcapital fractures are relatively undisplaced and may be treated with multiple pin fixation without reduction. The impacted fracture is usually stable; but in the process of healing, the head frequently displaces from the neck, producing deformity and further damage to the blood supply. Displaced subcapital fractures in the elderly patient should be treated with prosthetic replacement since avascular necrosis occurs frequently in these patients.

In young patients with good bone density, the fracture should be reduced anatomically and fixed with multiple pins. In older patients with osteoporosis or when the fracture occurs lower in the femoral neck, fixation between the head and the shaft may require a side plate as used with the Richards' apparatus. For details of the technique, the reader is referred to the main text chapter.

Intertrochanteric fractures occur below the inferior attachment of the hip capsule; the blood supply is excellent. Nonunion seldom occurs if the fracture is fixed in a stable position. Stability in intertrochanteric fractures requires both support along the medial calcar and a lateral buttress for preventing the femoral shaft from shifting medially. Intertrochanteric fractures are classified as stable and unstable fractures. The unstable fracture requires an intramedullary rod in the femur for stability, whereas the stable fracture requires only a Richards' screw with a side plate.

Hip Fractures in Children

Intracapsular hip fractures in children may cause growth disturbance, avascular changes, nonunion, malunion, and partial ankylosis of the hip. For continuation of epiphyseal growth, reduction must be anatomic and fixation secure. These goals are best met by open reduction and internal fixation. The preferred method of treatment is reduction under general anesthesia and then fixation with multiple pins. Intertrochanteric and subtrochanteric fractures in children are best managed with traction followed by plaster cast. In very young children 2 to 6 years, the spica cast can be applied in the emergency room without admitting the child to the hospital.

FRACTURES OF THE FEMUR

Fractures of the femur can be divided into four areas: subtrochanteric, midshaft or diaphyseal, supracondylar, and condylar. Each level must be managed differently because the *deforming* forces acting on the fragments tend to produce different deformities and require different methods of fixation. The patient with a fractured femur has undergone severe trauma and must be evaluated carefully. The loss of two to three units of blood within the thigh may not be apparent, and shock may ensue without warning. The hip and knee joint must be viewed radiographically for exclusion of associated dislocation or fractures. Many fractures in the midshaft of the femur can be treated by traction for a week to 10 days followed by a cast brace. The fractures usually heal within 10 to 12 weeks, and knee motion can be started early in the brace. The most common complication of cast brace treatment of femoral fractures is shortening and limitation of knee motion.

OPEN REDUCTION OF FEMORAL SHAFT FRACTURES. The treatment of fractures of the shaft of the femur by skeletal traction and cast immobilization has largely been replaced by closed nailing of the fracture with an interlocking nail. Fractures between the lesser trochanter and the supracondylar area can be treated in this manner and patients can be walking on crutches within 4 or 5 days after fracture. In the more comminuted fractures, supplementary fixation with circumferential wires may be necessary.

SUPRACONDYLAR FEMORAL FRACTURES. In supracondylar fractures of the femur, the pull of the gastrocnemius causes rather marked displacement of the fracture fragments. Cast treatment does not allow early motion of the knee, and marked loss of motion of the knee frequently occurs. Open reduction of supracondylar fractures is usually indicated in order that early motion of the knee can be started and the fracture can be reduced anatomically. The most commonly used apparatus for fixation of supracondylar fractures is the condylar buttress plate, which fixes the plate to the shaft of the femur and fixes the condyles to the plate with multiple screws.

FRACTURES OF THE PATELLA

Fractures of the patella usually occur by direct injury but may occur with traction of the quadriceps against a knee fixed in flexion. The fractures may be comminuted and are frequently compound because of the subcutaneous position of the patella. Comminuted fractures are best treated by patellectomy and repair of the quadriceps tendon. Knee motion can be restored nearly to normal with this technique. If the fragments are undisplaced, simple treatment with a cylinder cast may produce normal function. In the transverse fracture in which the two fragments are the same size and the fragments are separated, the fracture is best treated with the tension band technique in which two Kirschner wires are placed longitudinally across the fracture site and a circumferential wire is placed about the Kirschner wires and tightened to release the fracture. The most common complication of fractures of the patella is chondromalacia, which may eventually require patellectomy or total knee replacement.

DISLOCATION OF THE KNEE

Dislocations of the knee occur primarily from motorcycle accidents, athletic injuries, or falls from a height. Most dislocated knees can be managed by closed reduction and cast immobilization. The most common complication and the most serious is that of nerve injury and vascular damage. The popliteal artery is firmly fixed to the femur just above the knee, and if the peripheral pulses are not palpable, immediate exploration is indicated without waiting for the results of arteriography. Because of the vascular damage, anterior and posterior compartment syndromes frequently follow knee dislocation and should be suspected when the patient continues to complain of severe pain in the leg following reduction. Pulses may be present, but tissue ischemia can still be present. Compartment syndromes must be suspected and identified by measuring compartment pressure with a Wick catheter or by the method of Whitesides.

VII

Fractures of the Tibia, Fibula, Ankle, and Foot

William G. Garrett, Jr., M.D., Ph.D.,
and L. Scott Levin, M.D.

FRACTURES OF THE TIBIA AND FIBULA

The tibia and fibula are two of the most frequently fractured long bones. High-speed motor vehicle accidents are responsible for a high proportion of these injuries. Open or compound fractures require treatment for the bone as well as soft tissue injury. The majority of the tibia is palpable along the medial lower leg as a subcutaneous structure. It bears the major portion of body weight. The lateral malleolus or distal fibula is also palpable through the subcutaneous tissue. The tibia and fibula are connected by a strong ligament, the interosseous ligament, which serves as an origin for muscles in the anterior and posterior compartment of the leg. The mechanism of injury is important in determining the prognosis of tibial fractures. The prognosis is directly related to the amount of energy absorption at the time of injury. Fractures of the fibula usually occur concomitantly with fractures of the tibia unless the fibula is struck by a direct blow. If the head of the fibula is fractured with an associated medial malleolus fracture, a Maisonneuve fracture results. Classification of tibial fractures is dependent on fracture

---

See the corresponding chapter or part in the *Textbook of Surgery,* 14th edition, pp. 1337–1344, for a more detailed discussion of this topic, including a comprehensive list of references.

location. Schatzker has classified the tibial plateau or tibial head fracture into six different types, Type VI being the most severe.

The decision to treat tibial plateau fractures is based on the amount of articular surface depression (usually greater than 5 mm.) and the degree of joint incongruity or comminution. Fractures of the tibial shaft are classified into proximal, middle, and distal thirds. Delays in healing are seen commonly in the middle third. Open fractures have been classified by Gustilo and Anderson: Type I fractures have perforation of the skin, usually within wounds less than or equal to 1 cm.; Type II open fractures have lacerations of the soft tissue greater than 1 cm.; Type III injuries are divided into three subclasses depending on whether there is periosteal stripping (Type IIIb) or vascular injury (Type IIIc). The most important aspect of the physical examination for tibial fractures is to ascertain whether there is an impending compartment syndrome. Pain on passive stretch of muscle compartments in the alert patient is suggestive of compartment syndrome. In the unconscious patient with a closed tibial fracture, compartment pressure of greater than 30 mm. Hg for prolonged periods is an indication for fasciotomy. A number of radiographic techniques can be used for evaluation of tibial fractures. Tomography is helpful in the tibial plateau fracture.

Treatment is based on the fracture pattern and the presence of soft tissue injury. Cast immobilization can be used for closed diaphyseal fractures that can be maintained in adequate alignment. When soft tissue injuries accompany the tibial fracture, the external fixator is the standard method used for stabilizing the bone while soft tissues heal. Closed fractures that are amenable to intramedullary nailing can be treated with reamed or unreamed nails; recently, locking the intramedullary device above and below the fracture creates more stability, which allows earlier weight-bearing. When there is a soft tissue defect of the tibia, the proximal third can usually be covered by a gastrocnemius rotational flap, the middle third by a soleus flap; the distal third usually requires free tissue transfer for healing of the soft tissue envelope. Complications of tibial fractures include delayed union, malunion, and nonunion. Methods such as electrical stimulation and bone grafting of various types have been used to achieve union. Despite major advances in bone and soft tissue care, there are patients whose wounds are so severely damaged that primary amputation is still the treatment of choice. For Type III injuries, indications for this include comminution of bone greater than 20 cm., disruption of posterior tibial nerve, and ischemia greater than 6 hours.

FRACTURES AND DISLOCATIONS OF THE ANKLE

Ankle injuries are among the most frequently treated conditions. Most ankle injuries involve external rotation of the foot in the ankle joint. The goal in treatment of ankle fractures is establishing and maintaining anatomic reduction. If this cannot be done by closed reduction and casting, then open reduction and internal fixation is performed. This is usually done with screws and plates.

FRACTURES OF THE FOOT

Fractures of the hindfoot are significant injuries in which functional disability often occurs. The talus has a delicate blood supply that may cause the bone to become avascular after injury. Fractures of the calcaneus are best defined by use of computed tomography. Open reduction and internal fixation of these fractures is difficult, and despite anatomic restoration, many patients develop hindfoot posttraumatic arthritis. Fractures of the midfoot include the Lisfranc fracture, which is a tarsometatarsal dislocation. This can be accompanied by severe soft tissue damage that may cause ischemia of the forefoot. Metatarsal fractures are usually treated with closed reduction and casting and usually do not produce any long-term ill effects. Stress fractures or fatigue fractures, which are not uncommon, should be suspected in anyone who presents with pain and puffiness in the foot following excessive activity. Fractures of the phalanges do not usually require reduction and can be treated by strapping the fractured toe to the adjacent toe or by the use of a cast shoe.

VIII

Amputations and Limb Substitutions

Frank N. Clippinger, M.D.

Amputation is a frequent result of trauma, neoplasm, and especially peripheral vascular disease, there being about 2 million amputees in the United States alone. The major disadvantage of amputation over other ablative surgical therapy is that the effect is immediately visible to the patient, and this produces a psychological sense of loss that is not present with other procedures. The emotional aspects can be a problem in rehabilitation even though this is one instance in which there is the possibility of restoring reasonable function with prosthetic replacement. Early rehabilitation is advantageous, and a team approach is important. The team

---

See the corresponding chapter or part in the *Textbook of Surgery*, 14th edition, pp. 1345–1350, for a more detailed discussion of this topic, including a comprehensive list of references.

consists of the patient, the surgeon, the prosthetist who fabricates and fits the artificial limb, and the therapist who trains the patient in its use. The family, vocational counselors, and others should also be involved.

LEVEL SELECTION

The level of amputation in both upper and lower extremities should be determined by physiologic, not prosthetic, criteria. The principle of saving all length that is viable is valid although there are some levels, such as supramalleolar, that are more difficult for the prosthetist to fit. In the upper limb, a very short residual ulna, even if not sufficient to allow the patient to be fitted as a below-elbow amputee, can be used for activating an elbow lock.

SURGICAL PRINCIPLES

SKIN. Flaps of equal length are used except for disarticulations, in which skin from the extensor surface is better, and below-knee amputations, in which a posterior flap is fashioned because it has better circulation than does the anterior skin.

MUSCLE. Muscle is divided without reattachment. The superficial layer of the deep fascia, however, is approximated from front to back.

NERVE. Nerves are pulled distally, sharply divided, and allowed to retract. Large accompanying vessels are cauterized. Special treatment of nerves in an attempt to prevent neuroma formation has not proved to be effective.

BLOOD VESSELS. Patent vessels are either ligated or cauterized, depending on their size. Major vessels such as the femoral or brachial arteries, however, should be doubly ligated individually and separated from their accompanying veins for preventing the formation of arteriovenous fistulas.

POSTOPERATIVE CARE AND REHABILITATION

All major amputation wounds should be drained because a large hematoma may create enough pressure to devascularize a skin flap. A plaster cast, or "rigid postoperative dressing," tends to decrease postoperative pain, control edema, and prevent joint deformity. Whether or not a rigid postoperative dressing is used, emphasis is on early ambulation and rehabilitation. A prosthesis can be fitted as soon as the patient tolerates manipulation of the stump and the wound begins healing. Ten to 14 days postoperatively is appropriate. Range-of-motion and isometric exercises are started in the first few postoperative days.

In the upper extremity, immediate postsurgical prosthetic fitting and training beginning the first postoperative day is definitely advantageous.

It is expected that the first prosthesis fitted in every

amputee, whether deliberately preparatory or definitive, will require replacement within a very few weeks because of shrinkage of the stump. Although compression wraps and elastic bandages may help, the stump changes size and shape when the first prosthetic socket is applied.

PROSTHETIC CONSIDERATIONS

Prostheses consist of several components that constitute a prescription. These are (1) socket, (2) appropriate joints, (3) type of foot or terminal device, and (4) suspension and, in the upper extremity, means of control, which is either body or external power. Prosthetics is a profession, and prosthetists are experts regarding components, techniques, and materials.

Amputation should not be catastrophic, since with proper prostheses, training, and support, most amputees can continue nearly all the normal activities they desire.

IX

Infections and Neoplasms of Bone
John J. Callaghan, M.D.

Infections and neoplasms of bone can be similar in both clinical presentation and radiographic appearance. For this reason, it is appropriate to discuss the two entities together and to remember that every suspected bone neoplasm should be cultured, and every suspected bone infection should be biopsied.

INFECTIONS OF BONE

Infections of bone—osteomyelitis—can be categorized into those caused by pus-forming organisms (such as *Staphylococcus aureus*), which are termed *pyogenic osteomyelitis,* and those caused by organisms that produce a less aggressive granulomatous type of infection, *nonpyogenic osteomyelitis.*

Pyogenic Osteomyelitis

The pus-forming suppurative infection of bone occurs by blood-borne bacteria lodging in bone (hematogenous osteomyelitis) or by bacteria reaching bone from the external

See the corresponding chapter or part in the *Textbook of Surgery,* 14th edition, pp. 1351–1361, for a more detailed discussion of this topic, including a comprehensive list of references.

environment (penetrating wounds, open fractures, surgical incisions) and establishing "exogenous osteomyelitis."

Hematogenous osteomyelitis is primarily a disease of childhood, occurring most frequently between the ages of 5 and 15 years. The sluggish blood flow in the metaphysis of long bones is thought to make them susceptible to hematogenous osteomyelitis. The physeal growth plate forms a barrier to the spread of infection from the metaphysis to the epiphysis. The most frequent sites of infection are the femur, tibia, and humerus, in that order. *Staphylococcus aureus* is the most common infecting organism. On radiographic examination, the infection may show necrosis of bone, and the residual dead bone called a *sequestrum* appears as an increase in radiodensity. The surrounding granulation tissue creates a radiolucency that becomes surrounded by new bone (radiodense) called an *involucrum*. Antibiotics have drastically reduced the long-term problems associated with hematogenous osteomyelitis including chronic osteomyelitis. Primary treatment of osteomyelitis includes obtaining blood cultures and elevating and immobilizing the extremity. If no pus is demonstrated on bone biopsy, then intravenous antibiotics with a later switch to oral antibiotics (using antistaphylococcal drugs) can be the definitive treatment. If a patient does not improve over the first 24 hours or if pus is obtained, surgical débridement followed by antibiotics is appropriate.

Exogenous pyogenic osteomyelitis from trauma and open fractures is best treated by prevention. When a patient presents with open musculoskeletal trauma, antibiotics are initiated immediately, and the patient is taken to the operating room for débridement of all dead tissue. Large amounts of irrigation (6000 ml.) are used after débridement. Wounds are packed open, and redébridement is performed in 2 days, at which time the wounds are closed or flap coverage is contemplated. Exogenous osteomyelitis from open trauma constitutes the majority of the chronic osteomyelitis that has been seen in the present era of antibiotic therapy. The tibia is the most common bone affected because it lacks surrounding soft tissue and is susceptible to injury in high-speed trauma.

Tuberculosis, Osteomyelitis, and Pyarthrosis

Skeletal tuberculosis is the result of hematogenous seeding of tubercle bacilli from a pre-existing pulmonary or gastrointestinal focus. The organism most frequently involves the joints and adjacent bone rather than the metaphyseal area of long bones. The intervertebral discs of the lower thoracic and upper lumbar spine and the adjacent vertebrae are the most frequent sites of skeletal tuberculosis (approximately 30 per cent of all cases), followed by the hip and knee joints. Children originally had a higher incidence than did adults, but recently adults have been more commonly affected. Tuberculosis has been on the rise in the last several years partially related to the increase in acquired immune deficiency syndrome. Caseous necrosis surrounded by a granulomatous inflammatory response constitutes the classic tubercle. The destruction of bone is usually slow in the non–weight-bearing area of joints and in the intervertebral discs initially, with the eventual development of large soft tissue abscesses in some cases.

The initial treatment of skeletal tuberculosis consists of appropriate antituberculous drugs (isoniazid, rifampin, PAS, streptomycin, ethambutol) and protection of the involved area, which usually requires bed rest and traction if the lower extremity is involved and bed rest or bracing in the spinal cases. If there is no significant evidence of healing after 6 to 8 weeks of antituberculous therapy, localized foci within the epiphysis or spine may be carefully removed by curettage. Arthrodesis of the joint may still be required for excessive joint destruction.

NEOPLASMS OF BONE

Primitive mesenchymal tissue produces cartilage, bone, fibrous tissue, and marrow elements, the four basic tissue components of the mature skeleton. From each of these tissue types, benign or malignant neoplasms may arise. However, metastases from sarcomas and carcinomas that include the breast, lung, thyroid, kidney, and prostate are the most common neoplasms present in bone.

Osteochondroma is the most common primary benign bone tumor. Others include enchondroma, chondroblastoma, osteoid osteoma, osteoblastoma, nonossifying fibroma, giant cell tumor, desmoplastic fibroma, and eosinophilic granuloma. Most benign bone neoplasms can be treated with curettage or resection, but local recurrence can occur.

Other than multiple myeloma, osteosarcoma is the most common primary malignant neoplasm of bone. Others include chondrosarcoma, fibrosarcoma, fibrous histiocytoma, Ewing's tumor, and lymphoma. Ablative surgery, usually amputation, was the treatment of choice for many bone sarcomas in the past, but presently preoperative chemotherapy and wide resections with limb salvage when resection margins are possible have produced similar survival rates. The Enneking staging system is commonly used to categorize musculoskeletal tumors. Stage I is low grade, Stage II is high grade, and Stage III is any grade with metastasis. Intracompartmental extent of a tumor is designated A, and extracompartmental extent of a tumor is designated B.

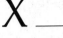

X

The Hand

1. COMPRESSION NEUROPATHIES OF THE HAND AND FOREARM

Richard D. Goldner, M.D., and J. Leonard Goldner, M.D.

The diagnosis of abnormal compression of the median, ulnar, or radial nerves may be easily overlooked although these syndromes occur relatively frequently.

DIFFERENTIAL DIAGNOSIS

A focal compression lesion must be differentiated from a neuropathy associated with systemic disease such as diabetes, hypothyroidism, rheumatoid arthritis, acromegaly, heavy metal intoxication, or paresthesias due to certain medications. Other more proximal lesions such as cervical root irritation, brachial plexitis, or a lesion associated with cerebral cortex disease may cause distal paresthesias. Conditions such as spinal cord tumor or syringomyelia may also cause distal symptoms and signs suggestive of a nerve compression lesion.

COMPRESSION OF THE MEDIAN NERVE AT THE WRIST (CARPAL TUNNEL SYNDROME)

The median nerve is compressed within the carpal canal, which is formed by the transverse carpal ligament on the palmar surface and the carpal bones on the dorsal side. The flexor tendons travel in the carpal canal with the median nerve. Hypertrophic synovium, edema fluid, dislocated carpal bones, or space-occupying lesions can compress the median nerve within this confined area. Women are affected more frequently than are men, and the age range is wide but generally 40 years or older. The usual complaints are weakness, clumsiness, hypesthesia, or paresthesias often aggravated by use of the hand. This syndrome encompasses a wide range of characteristics, such as nocturnal or early morning numbness that is quickly relieved by moving the hand, and finger tingling when a vibrating object such as an electric razor is held. Repetitive flexion and extension movements of the fingers and the hand may cause symptoms. Other conditions such as cold temperature, rapid weight gain, fluid retention associated with pregnancy, or compression from tight watchbands or rubber gloves may initiate or aggravate the original symptoms.

See the corresponding chapter or part in the *Textbook of Surgery*, 14th edition, pp. 1369–1376, for a more detailed discussion of this topic, including a comprehensive list of references.

Physical examination commonly shows a positive percussion test of the median nerve at the wrist either proximal to, under, or distal to the ligament. Wrist flexion (Phalen's test) often causes paresthesias in the median nerve distribution. Light touch is frequently decreased. A venous tourniquet applied to the arm for 20 to 30 seconds may reproduce the symptoms.

TREATMENT. Initial treatment is nonoperative and consists of splinting at night, weight reduction, decreased repetitive activities of the hand, and use of anti-inflammatory medications. Occasionally a soluble corticosteroid mixed with 1 per cent Xylocaine injected into the tendon sheaths of the flexor digitorum profundus, completely avoiding the ulnar and the median nerves, produces a remission of the median nerve compression symptoms. If symptoms and signs persist despite nonoperative treatment, operative decompression is considered. This procedure is performed by incision of the transverse carpal ligament at the wrist just proximal to the ligament extending to the midpalmar extension of the ligament at the superficial palmar arch. The palmar cutaneous branch of the median nerve is avoided. The motor branch is protected; the nerve is isolated carefully proximally and protected as the transverse carpal ligament is incised.

COMPRESSION OF THE ANTERIOR INTEROSSEOUS BRANCH OF THE MEDIAN NERVE

The anterior interosseous nerve is a motor branch of the median nerve that is present in the proximal third of the forearm. It supplies the flexor pollicis longus, the flexor digitorum profundus of the index and long fingers, and the pronator quadratus.

Anterior interosseous nerve compression causes a vague pain in the proximal forearm that is aggravated by exercise and relieved by rest. The pinch between thumb and index finger is weak. Individual testing of the flexor pollicis longus and the flexor digitorum profundus of the index demonstrates these muscle bellies to be weak. There is no sensory deficit. This syndrome must be differentiated from a rupture of the flexor pollicis longus or the index profundus tendons.

If symptoms persist after a reasonable period of observation, and depending on the other diagnostic studies, surgical therapy is performed by isolating the median nerve proximal to the lacertus fibrosus and dissecting it distally through the pronator teres and distally to where the branches enter the flexor pollicis longus and flexor profundus of the index and long fingers. Electrical stimulation of the nerve during this decompression is very helpful.

ULNAR NERVE COMPRESSION AT THE ELBOW

Ulnar nerve compression occurs within the cubital tunnel or proximal or distal to it: (1) a dense fascia over the flexor carpi ulnaris distally or the firm ridge of the interosseous membrane proximally may cause nerve irritation with repetitive motion; (2) synovium or osteophytes within the cubital tunnel may irritate the nerve as a result of repetitive acute elbow flexion; (3) a synovial cyst arising from the elbow joint and extending into the canal may compress the nerve; (4) repeated subluxation of the nerve as it moves across the medial epicondyle causes nerve compression; (5) positional stresses such as prolonged elbow flexion during sleep, external pressure on the elbow during general anesthesia, or repetitive use of the flexed elbow against the mattress by the patient's changing position while on bed rest can cause ulnar nerve compression; (6) other anatomic structures such as a fibrous arcade (arcade of Struthers) proximally or a combination of proximal tethering and distal muscle hypertrophy may irritate the nerve.

SYMPTOMS AND SIGNS. The patient complains of deep aching along the ulnar aspect of the proximal and mid forearm and intermittent numbness, tingling, and combinations of these sensations in the ring and little fingers. The heel of the hand and the little finger "are asleep." Percussion of the nerve should be performed distally and advanced proximally for detecting the site of compression. Forced voluntary flexion of the elbow with the forearm held in that position for 2 minutes should produce tingling if the nerve is tethered or hypermobile at the elbow. Early compression shows no intrinsic atrophy or overt cutaneous sensory changes. Late and prolonged compression causes atrophy of the hypothenar and first dorsal interosseous muscles along with dryness and diminished sensibility of the little and the ulnar half of the ring fingers.

TREATMENT. The nonoperative treatment depends on an accurate diagnosis. The patient is advised to avoid resting the elbow on chair arms, table surfaces, and airplane armrests. If the elbow is acutely flexed during sleep, a splint is applied for prevention. An elbow pad worn during the day may diminish direct contusion of the nerve and limit repetitive elbow flexion. Anti-inflammatory medications diminish connective tissue irritation and lessen the intensity of the complaints.

Surgical treatment is considered if one or more of the following is present: (1) hypesthesia and paresthesias persist for several months and are constantly uncomfortable; (2) rest, splinting, and other forms of treatment have not improved the persistent or progressive symptoms after 3 months of observation; (3) atrophy of the intrinsic muscles of the hand is evident; and (4) electrophysiologic studies are positive in either motor or sensory conduction tests and abnormal action potentials are observed.

One method of surgical treatment is subcutaneous transfer of the ulnar nerve anteriorly. Alternative approaches of managing the compressed ulnar nerve are (1) excision of the medial epicondyle of the humerus without transferring the nerve anteriorly; this can be successful in some instances; (2) placement of the nerve anterior to the ulnar groove and within the forearm flexor muscles; this may be as successful as subcutaneous transfer, but the muscle tissue may eventually constrict or compress the nerve; (3) placement of the nerve deep to the forearm muscles not only to warm the nerve as in the case of leprosy but also to protect the nerve during forceful exercise.

COMPRESSION NEUROPATHY OF THE RADIAL NERVE

Compression of the radial nerve high in the arm may cause total loss of function of the muscles extending the wrist, thumb, and fingers. A sensory defect also occurs along the course of the superficial radial nerve. The anatomic site of compression may be at the humeral midshaft near the radial groove or at the distal third of the humerus. A distal fracture may affect the nerve at this site.

Compression palsy (Saturday night palsy) or radial nerve injury after proximal or midshaft fracture of the humerus recovers spontaneously in 3 to 5 months in greater than 90 per cent of the patients. A distal oblique fracture of the humerus, however, may entrap the nerve, and operative decompression may be required.

POSTERIOR INTEROSSEOUS NERVE COMPRESSION

After innervating the brachioradialis, extensor carpi radialis longus, and extensor carpi radialis brevis, the radial nerve divides into the posterior interosseous branch (motor) and the superficial radial branch (sensory). The posterior interosseous nerve supplies the thumb extensors and the finger metacarpophalangeal extensors. These muscles are weak if the posterior interosseous nerve is compressed significantly. The posterior interosseous nerve enters the radial tunnel between the superficial and the deep heads of the supinator muscle. This nerve may be compressed if the hands of the patient are performing repetitive pronation and supination several hundred times a day for months or years, or the lesion may occur between the radial head and the supinator after a fracture or dislocation of the proximal radius.

The clinical findings in an extremity with a *complete* posterior interosseous nerve lesion are active dorsiflexion of the hand in radial deviation but loss of thumb and finger extension at the metacarpophalangeal joints.

An *incomplete* posterior interosseous nerve lesion may show lack of extension of one or two digits and weakness of extension of the abductor pollicis and/or the extensor pollicis longus.

TREATMENT. If the compression lesion is localized proximal to the supinator and caused by the extensor carpi radialis brevis, a posterior interosseous neurolysis is performed if the distal extensor muscles are weak and then the common radial nerve is isolated anterolaterally. If the distal extensor muscles are weak, the common radial nerve is isolated anterolaterally at the elbow and the nerve is followed into the supinator and distally. The vascular leash (radial recurrent) is ligated, the proximal fascial bands in the supinator are incised, and the arcade of Frohse is released. Electrical stimulation is attempted proximally and distally on the nerve for determining whether epineurial splitting is necessary at any location on the nerve.

Results of treatment depend on the duration of compression and the severity of the nerve injury. If decompression is performed relatively early and repetitive physical activities are not resumed, then improvement follows. Reinnervation of the affected muscles may be determined electrically 3 months after decompression, and clinical examination shows evidence of early regeneration by 5 months. At least a year is required before maximal recovery is expected. If improvement of muscle function does not occur within a year after nerve decompression, tendon transfer should be considered.

COMPRESSION OF THE SENSORY BRANCH OF THE RADIAL NERVE

Hypesthesia or hyperesthesia on the dorsum of the thumb and/or the index finger may be related to compression of the cutaneous branch of the radial nerve at the point at which the nerve exits beneath the brachioradialis and the shaft of the radius, or irritation occurs adjacent to an enlargement of the abductor pollicis longus annular ligament at the wrist. Also, direct trauma to the nerve at the wrist or at the base of the thumb may affect sensory conduction. A history is important in establishing diagnosis of proximal or distal irritation.

Clinical examination shows an area of hyperesthesia or hypesthesia along the course of the nerve slightly proximal and always distal to the point of compression. The condition usually improves in time with elimination of the abnormal external compressive forces, such as avoidance of cutting with a blunt large scissors or removal of a tight elastic watchband.

If sensory deficit persists, neurolysis is performed from the proximal point of compression under the brachioradialis tendon about 5 cm. proximal to the wrist joint to the distal area of compression as determined by skin sensitivity and percussion test.

43

REPLANTATION OF AMPUTATED LIMBS AND DIGITS

James R. Urbaniak, M.D.

The concepts of microsurgery and limb replantation originated in the early 1900s with the introduction of macrosurgical techniques for arterial and venous anastomoses in composite grafts and transplants. Hopfner and Carrel and Guthrie began early animal limb replantation before 1905. In 1922, Holmgren introduced the binocular operating microscope for middle ear surgery. The introduction of the operating microscope in 1960 by Jacobson and Suarez for the repair of small vessels had the greatest impact on the replantation of amputated hands and digits.

Microvascular surgery implies repair of small blood vessels (3 mm. or less in diameter) with use of an operating microscope, microsurgical instruments, and ultrafine suture material (usually about 20 μ in diameter).

Replantation is defined as reattachment of a part that has been completely severed, that is, there is no connection between the amputated part and the patient. *Revascularization* is the reattachment of a part of which some portion of the soft tissue (such as skin, nerves, or tendon) is still connected. Vascular repair is necessary to prevent necrosis of the partially severed distal limb. This may require repair of the arteries or the veins or both.

Malt in 1962 first successfully replanted a completely amputated arm in a 12-year-old boy. The first successful replantation of an amputated digit by microvascular technique was performed in 1965 by Komatsu and Tamai in Nara, Japan.

CARE OF THE AMPUTATED PART

Amputated or devascularized tissue will survive for about 6 hours if the part is not cooled. Because the digits essentially have no muscle tissue, they may be successfully replanted as long as 24 hours after amputation if they are cooled. The amputated part should be placed into a plastic bag containing Ringer's lactate or saline solution. The plastic bag is placed on ice. An alternative method of preserving the amputated part is to wrap it in a cloth or sponge moistened with Ringer's lactate or saline solution placed in a plastic bag, which is put on ice.

See the corresponding chapter or part in the *Textbook of Surgery*, 14th edition, pp. 1377–1381, for a more detailed discussion of this topic, including a comprehensive list of references.

PATIENT SELECTION

Guillotine-type amputations are ideally suited for replanting. Organs for replantation are selected according to the following priorities: (1) thumb, (2) multiple digits, (3) partial hand (amputation through the palm), (4) almost any part of a child, (5) wrist or forearm, (6) above-elbow amputation (only sharp or moderately avulsed), and (7) isolated digit distal to the superficialis insertion (distal to the proximal interphalangeal joint). The prime parts for replantation are thumbs, multiple digits, and the complete hand. Replantation of these parts provides the best results. In children, an attempt should be made to replant almost any part; if the replanted extremity survives, excellent function can be expected.

Types of injuries that are not favorable for replantation are (1) severely crushed or mangled parts, (2) amputations at multiple levels, (3) amputations in patients with other serious injuries or diseases, (4) amputations in which the vessels are arteriosclerotic, (5) amputations in mentally unstable patients, (6) injuries with more than 6 hours of ischemic time, (7) severely contaminated parts, and (8) an individual finger in the adult with the amputation proximal to the superficialis insertions (proximal to the proximal interphalangeal joint). Replantations of isolated fingers at the base (proximal to the superficialis insertion) generally result in a finger that "gets in the way" because of diminished tendon excursion. Often the final decision cannot be made until the status of the damaged blood vessels is determined under the operating microscope.

SURGICAL TECHNIQUE

Microscopic evaluation determines the feasibility of restoration by revascularization.

The sequence of replantation of amputated digits or hands is as follows: (1) locate and tag the vessels and nerves, (2) shorten and fix the bone with an intramedullary pin, (3) repair the extensor tendons, (4) repair the flexor tendons, (5) repair the arteries, (6) repair the nerves, (7) repair the veins, and (8) obtain loose skin coverage (split-thickness graft if necessary).

The bone is shortened to facilitate the vascular anastomoses. *The most important factors in achieving permanent microvascular patency are easy coaptation of vessels with normal intima and the skill and expertise of the microsurgeon.*

MAJOR LIMB REPLANTATION

Major limb replantation implies replantation of limbs proximal to the wrist or of the lower extremity proximal to the ankle.

Whereas amputated digits may be successfully replanted 24 hours after amputation, an amputated arm at the elbow is in jeopardy if it has been ischemic for 10 or 12 hours, even if it has been properly cooled. Extensive muscle débridement both on the detached part and on the stump is essential for prevention of myonecrosis and subsequent infection, which is the major problem in major limb replantation but is uncommon in digital reattachment.

In replantations proximal to the metacarpal level, immediate arterial inflow is necessary for preventing or diminishing myonecrosis. If the amputated part and the patient arrive in the operating room more than 4 hours after injury, initiation of immediate blood flow to the detached part is desirable. This is best accomplished by using some form of shunt, such as a Sundt or ventriculoperitoneal shunt, to obtain rapid arterial inflow to the detached part. Shunting should be performed before bone fixation unless the bone can be rapidly stabilized and early blood flow obtained. After the establishment of temporary blood flow, further débridement can be continued, the bone stabilized, the shunt removed, and a direct arterial repair or interposition vein grafting of the vessels performed.

Stable bone fixation is necessary for major limb replantation; however, the method should be rapid. In major limb replantation, it is critical to perform the arterial anastomosis before the venous anastomosis. This sequence allows a physiologic washout of noxious agents such as lactic acid in the distal part. The administration of intravenous sodium bicarbonate before venous anastomosis is beneficial.

Extensive fasciotomies are always indicated in major limb replantations. *The two most common causes of failure in major limb replantation are myonecrosis with subsequent infection and failure to provide adequate decompression of the restored vessels.*

In replantations of major limbs, the patients should be returned to the operating room within 48 to 72 hours for evaluation of the state of muscle tissue. In major limb replantations, the best replantation results are obtained at the wrist, followed by the arm and distal forearm. The poorest results occur in the proximal third of the forearm, an area where the motor branches of the radial, median, and ulnar nerves enter the extrinsic musculature of the hand.

There are few indications for replantation of the lower extremity. Upper extremity prostheses poorly duplicate hand function; however, lower limb prostheses provide a stable stance and a functional gait. With the currently available lower extremity prostheses, considerable thought should be given before replantation of the lower extremities is attempted, even with rather cleanly severed limbs.

POSTOPERATIVE MANAGEMENT

Most patients receive some type of anticoagulation. Intravenous heparin at 1000 units per hour for about 7 days is usually administered. Low-molecular-weight dextran, aspirin, chlorpromazine, and dipyridamole have been used in difficult cases. Skin color, pulp turgor, capillary refill, and skin temperature are the most useful indicators for monitoring. Seldom is it necessary to return the patient to the operating room for a revision; however, if re-exploration is to be successful, it must usually be done within 24 to 48 hours after the primary procedure.

RESULTS OF REPLANTATION

The Duke orthopaedic replantation team has attempted revascularization or replantation of more than 1200 partial or total amputations from 1973 to 1989. Ninety-two per cent of the partial amputations have been successfully revascularized, and 77 per cent of the complete amputations have remained viable. Most major replantation centers are obtaining about an 80 per cent viability rate in complete replantations.

Cold intolerance is a problem in most patients, but this subsides in 1 to 2 years. Replanted thumbs provide the best functional results. Strong pinch, adequate motion, excellent sensation, and almost normal appearance are to be expected. Replantations of multiple digits, partial hands (through the palm), or complete hands provide good sensibility and useful function. Although amputations through the wrist or distal forearm provide good function of the hand, amputations at a more proximal level have varied results.

44

THE SKIN: FUNCTIONAL, METABOLIC, AND SURGICAL CONSIDERATIONS

Donald Serafin, M.D.

The skin is a highly complex organ representing a barrier between the relatively closed system of the human body and the external environment. With glabrous skin on the prehensile surface, the human organism can communicate with its environment. The skin is tough and relatively impenetrable, providing protection from mechanical injury. Through its epithelial mesenchymal interaction, growth and regeneration of epithelium is made possible. The skin also serves as an important temperature-regulating mechanism. It has important immunologic functions related to keratinocytes and Langerhans cell interactions. In addition, the skin with its hair distribution patterns draped over an underlying bony skeleton serves as an organ of individual identification.

FUNCTIONS OF THE SKIN

The maintenance of an internal equilibrium and environment is made possible by the impenetrable stratum corneum of the skin. Both diffusion and water loss are inversely related to the thickness of this horny layer.

COMMUNICATION WITH THE ENVIRONMENT. Humans possess both glabrous and hairy skin, each with distinct features. Glabrous skin is highly specialized, being present on palms and soles of the feet and representing approximately 4 per cent of the total body surface area. The dermal-epidermal junction is corrugated, which permits firm attachment of the overlying epidermis to the underlying dermis. Multiple subcutaneous septae anchor the dermis to the underlying bony architecture, which minimizes sheer stresses. Papillary ridges, grooves, and collagen-anchoring fibers all stabilize overlying epidermis on the dermis. Glabrous skin contains a large concentration of non-neural mechanoreceptors that permit fine tactile discrimination. A complex interrelationship with the papillary ridges facilitates this discrimination. Hairy skin, in contrast to glabrous skin, contains fewer mechanoreceptors and a lower concentration of myelinated nerves. Hair functions to buffer the organism from tactile stimuli, thus protecting it from the environment.

PROTECTION FROM MECHANICAL INJURY. The skin is a tough, relatively impenetrable, resilient structure that can withstand considerable mechanical injury. This property

---

See the corresponding chapter or part in the *Textbook of Surgery*, 14th edition, pp. 1382–1398, for a more detailed discussion of this topic, including a comprehensive list of references.

resides in the dermis and is made possible by collagen fibers and the ground substance. The dermis varies considerably throughout the body in both its thickness and its composition. Viscoelastic properties characterize the dermis; these are attributed to both its collagen content and organization of its fibers and ground substance.

EPITHELIAL-MESENCHYMAL INTERACTION. Dermal mesenchyme has been demonstrated to be essential for the growth and regeneration of epithelium by a mechanism of inductive interreaction. In other experiments, epidermis has been demonstrated to differentiate according to the site of origin of the dermis.

TEMPERATURE REGULATION. One of the major functions of the skin is its ability to regulate body temperature. Heat is lost by radiation (60 per cent), evaporation (25 per cent), and conduction (15 per cent). Heat dissipation by both radiation and conduction is influenced by (1) the degree of cutaneous blood flow and (2) ambient temperature and humidity. If environmental temperature exceeds body core temperature, loss of heat by radiation and conduction becomes less effective. Convection, or the movement of cooler air to displace warm air surrounding the body, augments the effect of conduction. If heat cannot be dissipated by either conduction or convection, evaporative loss through sweating becomes the most efficient mechanism. It is estimated that 0.58 calorie of heat is lost for each gram of water that evaporates.

IMMUNOLOGIC FUNCTION. The skin has an important immunologic function, the importance of which has only recently been appreciated. Langerhans cells have been identified as being critical for the initiation of the cutaneous immune response. Antigen is taken up by Langerhans cells and processed. These immunologic moieties are then presented to T lymphocytes, which are activated. Keratinocytes are stimulated to release interleukin-1, which influences the production of interleukin-2, further amplifying the T cell response.

ORGAN OF INDIVIDUAL IDENTIFICATION. The underlying bony skeleton and subcutaneous tissue serves as a supporting framework for the overlying skin. Shape and contour thus achieved serve as an organ of individual identification. This is enhanced by varying patterns of hair distribution.

During aging, redundant skin with loss of elasticity causes alterations in form, contour, and aesthetic qualities.

SKIN METABOLISM

CARBOHYDRATE METABOLISM. The epidermis is metabolically more active than is the dermis. Qualitatively, pathways for glycolysis, oxidation, or other biosynthetic contributions do not differ from those in other tissues. The preferential selection of the glycolytic pathway for energy production, however, has been observed. Several explanations are possible. One explanation is related to the limitation of blood flow in extremely cold environments. Under such conditions, cell metabolism must be maintained despite limited oxygen availability in poorly perfused capillary beds. Another explanation may be related to ensuring cell maintenance and functioning in growth of epidermal cells at an increased distance from blood supply.

PROSTAGLANDINS. Prostaglandins are ubiquitous throughout the body and are formed from essential fatty acids within or adjacent to cellular membranes. Arachidonic acid in keratinocytes is metabolized to PGE_2 and $PGF_{2(alpha)}$, each with opposite effects. PGE_2 produces vasodilation and a loss of platelet adhesiveness. $PGF_{2(alpha)}$ has been demonstrated to promote cutaneous vasoconstriction as well as to stimulate dermal reparative processes such as ground substance biosynthesis.

PHOTOSYNTHESIS OF VITAMIN D. When 7-dehydrocholesterol, present in the stratum Malpighii, is exposed to ultraviolet rays of the sun (UVB, 295 nm.), previtamin D_3 is formed. This is then synthesized by thermal isomerization to vitamin D_3. Vitamin D_3 is then translocated by a vitamin D–binding protein into the circulation, where it is taken to gastrointestinal mucosa for regulating the absorption of calcium and phosphorus.

MELANIN PIGMENTATION. Skin color in humans is due largely to the content of melanin within keratinocytes. In the same species, there is the same number of melanocytes in any specific region of skin regardless of the color of the individual. Melanocytes, however, vary in numbers throughout the various regions of the body. In the skin, there appears to be a symbiotic relationship between the melanocytes and the keratinocytes. Ultraviolet light exposure causes the keratinocytes in the malpighian layer to approach the melanocytes, which then form dendritic processes that transfer melanosomes into the cytoplasm of the keratinocyte. Melanosomes contain the enzyme tyrosinase. This enzyme converts tyrosine to an intermediate dopa and subsequently to melanin.

MECHANISMS OF WOUND CLOSURE

AUTOGENOUS. When a wound is created, every attempt is made to close the wound and to restore the protective barrier function that the epidermis and dermis provide. This is accomplished by (1) epithelialization and (2) wound contraction. Within 24 hours following wounding, epithelial cells at the periphery of the wound margin begin multiplying and lose their cohesiveness to surrounding cells. When one migrating cell meets another, movement stops by contact inhibition. Epithelial migration continues until the wound is completely resurfaced. Extensive wounds provide physical limitation for epithelial migration and survival.

Wound contraction is mediated by myofibroblasts present in the 1 to 2 mm. of the wound margin. Wound contraction is a centripetal process that is apparent 72 hours after wounding. When the force of contraction becomes equal to forces resisting wound contraction, the process ceases. Thus, wounds overlying joints continue to contract, even at the expense of extreme flexion or extension of the joint.

WOUND CLOSURE OF SMALL DEFECTS

Excision and Primary Closure. Small wounds can usually be closed primarily, provided there is sufficient skin elasticity in the surrounding skin and joint function is not compromised. Wound closure should parallel, as much as possible, existing skin tension lines.

Local Skin Flaps. Local skin flaps adjacent to a tissue defect are often employed for wound closure. Local flaps provide skin with similar characteristics such as color, texture, and thickness as contrasted to distant flaps. Local flaps consist of two types: (1) flaps that are rotated about a pivot point, and (2) advancement flaps.

SKIN GRAFTS. Autogenous partial-thickness or full-thickness skin grafts can be employed for wound closure. These grafts are often harvested from a more distant donor site. Skin grafts may be either full-thickness or partial-thickness, depending on whether part or all of the dermis is included. A split-thickness skin graft consisting of epidermis and a portion of dermis may vary in thickness from (1) thin, 8 to 12/1000 inch, (2) medium, 12 to 16/1000 inch, to (3) thick, 16 to 20/1000 inch.

FLAPS. Exposed bone devoid of periosteum or tendon devoid of paratenon requires augmentation of existing blood supply, usually with a flap. Flaps are classified according to their blood supply.

Random Flaps. Random flaps are characterized by the absence of a direct cutaneous artery supplying the flap. Blood flow and perfusion pressure are limited, further limiting the dimensions of the flap. The length of a flap can be increased if a delay procedure is first performed 1 to 2 weeks before transfer.

Direct Axial Flaps. A direct axial pattern flap contains a dominant artery and vein that regionally supply the subdermal plexus.

Muscle/Musculocutaneous Flaps. Muscle flaps derive their blood supply from segmental arteries. Muscle flaps are classified I to V depending on the pattern and distribution of the blood supply. Muscles having a single dominant blood supply are classified as I. Muscles having multiple segmental blood supply are classified as IV. When a Class I muscle flap is employed, a portion of the muscle distal to the pedicle is detached and transferred to a recipient site. Circulation is maintained through the dominant pedicle.

In a musculocutaneous flap, blood supply to the overlying skin is derived from vessels perforating the muscle. Consequently, both skin and muscle can be transferred to a recipient site as a unit.

Fascial/Fasciocutaneous Flaps. Fascial/fasciocutaneous flaps can be classified according to the pattern of their blood supply. A Type B flap contains axial vessels usually coursing on the surface of the fascia and supplying a portion of that fascia. Contributions to the skin also exist. Consequently, a fasciocutaneous flap can be transferred in a manner similar to the musculocutaneous flap.

Microvascular Flaps. A microvascular flap consists of an island of composite tissue usually containing in its pedicle a single artery and vein. The pedicle is then transected, and the tissue is transplanted at a distant recipient site where circulation is restored with microvascular anastomoses. A variety of composite tissue can be transplanted in this manner for reconstruction of difficult recipient sites.

BENIGN TUMORS OF THE SKIN

SEBORRHEIC KERATOSES. These lesions are raised and pigmented and often contain a verrucous surface that is friable and easily removed. They occur everywhere except on the palm and on the soles of the feet. Rarely, differential diagnosis between pigmented basal cell epithelioma and melanoma must be made. Cryotherapy is the treatment of choice.

KERATOACANTHOMA. This benign lesion must be differentiated clinically and histologically from a squamous cell carcinoma. It easily occurs in an older individual as a single lesion. The lesion is raised to 2 cm. in diameter with a characteristic horn-filled center. Keratoacanthomas are characterized by rapid growth.

PREMALIGNANT TUMORS

SOLAR KERATOSIS. These lesions may be single or more often are multiple on sun-exposed areas in middle-aged, fair-complexioned individuals. Prolonged exposure to sunlight and environmental carcinogens are predisposing factors. These lesions are characterized by hyperkeratosis. It is estimated that squamous carcinoma develops from solar keratosis in 20 per cent of patients. These premalignant lesions can be successfully treated either with cryotherapy or with topical 5-fluorouracil.

LEUKOPLAKIA. Leukoplakia is a premalignant condition occurring on oral or rectal mucosa and on the vulva. It is manifested by a raised, whitish, single or confluent lesion that may be extensive. Leukoplakia must be distinguished from leukokeratosis, which reverts to normal when the irritant is removed. Treatment is directed to removal of the irritant and biopsy of residual areas of leukoplakia.

BOWEN'S DISEASE. The lesion is frequently solitary and is manifested by a slowly enlarging erythematous patch of skin with a sharp but irregular outline. Crusting is frequently noted in the center. On histologic examination, the lesion is an intraepithelial squamous cell carcinoma.

CARCINOMA

SQUAMOUS CELL CARCINOMA. Squamous cell carcinoma can arise from the skin or from the oral and rectal mucosa. A squamous cell carcinoma arising from a solar keratosis has a low propensity for metastasis (0.5 per cent).

This is compared with 2 per cent for all squamous cell carcinomas of the skin. Squamous cell carcinoma arising from the glans penis, oral mucosa, rectal mucosa, vulva, and lips has a high rate of metastasis. Treatment is dictated by the location, predisposing factors, and degree of differentiation.

TUMORS OF EPIDERMAL APPENDAGES

BASAL CELL CARCINOMA. Basal cell carcinomas are considered to be derivatives of pluripotential cells. Basal cell carcinomas usually occur on hair-bearing skin, almost never on glabrous skin. Metastasis is rare. Sufficient evidence exists that demonstrates the close relationship to sun exposure and subsequent development of basal cell carcinoma. Most basal cell carcinomas are undifferentiated. Histologic sections consist of palisading basal cells with uniform, elongated nuclei and very little cytoplasm. Clinically there are five common forms of basal cell carcinoma: (1) noduloulcerative, (2) pigmented, (3) sclerosing or morphea-like, (4) superficial, and (5) fibroepithelioma.

DECUBITUS ULCERS

Pressure ulceration results when excessive pressure is applied to a relatively small area over a prolonged period of time. Muscle is more susceptible to pressure necrosis than is skin. Pressure necrosis occurs when end-arterial pressure of 32 mm. Hg is exceeded for a prolonged period of time. Studies suggest that direct pressure (twice the end-capillary arteriolar pressure) of 70 mm. Hg applied for 2 hours' duration produces irreversible ischemia and tissue necrosis.

PROPHYLAXIS. Prophylaxis against pressure sores is directed toward: (1) patient education, (2) basic skin care, and (3) avoidance of excessive and prolonged pressure.

MANAGEMENT. Nonoperative management of pressure ulceration should be provided to those areas of superficial ulceration or in those select cases of contractile failures when all available flap options have been exhausted. The recurrence rate following nonsurgical management is quite high (32 to 77 per cent), with the majority recurring in the ischial area. Débridement of nonviable tissue and topical application of sulfadiazine (Silvadene) are important in the management of these patients.

SURGICAL MANAGEMENT. Surgical management usually consists of wound débridement and flap coverage. Local cutaneous flaps can be employed as well as musculocutaneous flaps.

44A

PILONIDAL CYSTS AND SINUSES

Onye E. Akwari, M.D., F.A.C.S., F.R.C.S.(C)

Hodges introduced the term *pilonidal* (*pilus*, hair, *nidus*, nest) in 1880 and proposed a theory of congenital origin of the disease. Most commonly, it occurs in the sacrococcygeal area, about 3 to 5 cm. posterior and superior to the anal orifice; the evidence weighs heavily in favor of an acquired nature for all but the rare case of pilonidal disease. Stretching of the integument at puberty associated with rapid growth, particularly of the gluteal muscles, produces distention of hair follicles, sebaceous glands, and apocrine glands and sufficient spreading of their cutaneous orifices to allow insinuation of foreign substances. The tiny midline holes or pits (sinuses) that are seen in the cleft of almost all patients with sacrococcygeal pilonidal disease represent distorted hair follicles, which may ingest hair or become filled with keratin and other debris. In time, they become infected and rupture into the deeper fat. That hair may be secondarily ingested by some of these existing cavities was cleverly demonstrated by Page in 1969. Hair is present in the cyst in only half of the patients.

Pilonidal disease has been reported in the umbilicus, the axilla, the clitoris, the interdigital webs of barbers' hands, the interdigital web of the foot of a worker in a hair mattress factory, the sole of the foot, and the anal canal. Pilonidal sinuses containing wool, grass, animal hair, and hair of a color different from that of the patient's have all been reported.

PRESENTATION. Patients with sacrococcygeal pilonidal disease may ask for advice about asymptomatic pits or pores in the natal cleft. Tenderness after physical activity or a long drive requiring the patient to sit for a prolonged duration is a common presentation. A tender or nontender nodule may be palpable. Twenty per cent of such patients seek care for the severe pain and tenderness of an acute abscess. The diagnosis is usually readily apparent, although other conditions should be considered, including perianal abscess arising from the posterior midline crypt, hidradenitis suppurativa, and a simple carbuncle or furuncle. Some other focus of infection such as osteomyelitis may rarely give rise to a sinus in this area. The abscess enlarges rapidly, but since it may be located deep to relatively thick skin, it rarely ruptures spontaneously. In general, there is minimal cellulitis and induration surrounding the pilonidal abscess, and systemic reaction to the abscess is infrequent. Occasionally fever, leukocytosis, and malaise are found.

See the corresponding chapter or part in the *Textbook of Surgery*, 14th edition, pp. 1399–1402, for a more detailed discussion of this topic, including a comprehensive list of references.

The inflammatory process may subside early or progress until relief is obtained—usually by surgical means. After drainage has occurred, the purulent discharge may cease completely, but more commonly it recurs intermittently with drainage from one or more sinuses as the disease enters its chronic phase. In this setting, care must be taken to exclude a complicated anal fistula, which may angulate posteriorly before passing into a retrorectal abscess. Thorough examination of the anal cavity usually discloses the point of origin, and a probe inserted into a pilonidal sinus follows a course away from the anus.

Eighty per cent of patients with pilonidal disease present with a chronic abscess and no history of a prior clinically apparent acute stage. Infection, particularly by anaerobic bacteria, has a central role in the extremely difficult problems of wound healing often associated with chronic pilonidal disease. *Staphylococcus aureus* and *Bacteroides* species are the most important offending organisms.

TREATMENT. There is a growing consensus that pilonidal disease should be managed conservatively. Treatment in an outpatient setting has gained acceptance and is widely practiced. Simple incision and drainage of first-episode acute pilonidal abscess may effect healing *per primam* within 10 weeks of treatment, especially in patients with few pits and lateral tracts. Definitive treatment, which includes evacuation of hair and curetting of granulation tissue with wide exposure of the posterior wall of the abscess cavity, should not be undertaken earlier than 10 weeks for those patients with pits and lateral tracts. With careful follow-up and local care, including shaving of hair, hot tub baths, and use of Water Pik irrigation, healing by secondary intention is generally completed in 2 weeks. Antibiotics are rarely indicated unless the patient has a medical condition such as rheumatic heart disease or is immunosuppressed.

However, because of the central role of bacterial infection in the perpetuation of chronic pilonidal disease, treatment of these patients is initiated with oral pain medication and an antibiotic regimen particularly directed against *Staphylococcus aureus* and *Bacteroides* species. Under local or regional anesthesia, the chronic abscess is opened widely by a long incision that lies parallel to and 2 cm. to one side of the midline. Avoidance of the midline "ditch" containing the pits and sinuses is increasingly advocated. The abscess cavity is scrubbed free of hair with push gauze, with removal of portions of the cyst wall impregnated with hair and debris. In the rare patient with long-standing disease, the abscess wall is covered with surface epithelium that has grown into the cavity. This is no longer a chronic abscess but an epithelial inclusion cyst, which is therefore excised. The lateral incision is left widely open to permit drainage; the small holes from the midline skin are excised, with minimal tissue loss, and closed with nonabsorbable suture material. The visible holes that represent enlarged follicles must be completely excised if recurrence is to be avoided. Multiple cavities may appear under insignificant-appearing follicles. Antibiotics are continued for 24 hours. The patient is instructed in local care of the wound.

Pilonidal disease recurring after formal conservative primary treatment as outlined is usually limited to the caudal portion of the scar. A blind cavity or sinus is frequently encountered through a midline opening. Local exposure of the posterior wall of the tract, scraping of the granulation tissue, and débridement of the edges of the tract produce complete healing in 3 to 4 weeks. Hot baths and Water Pik irrigation at least once daily keep the healing wound clean.

COMPLICATIONS. Very rarely, malignant degeneration occurs in these lesions. Verrucous carcinoma (giant condyloma acuminatum) has been reported in an established pilonidal sinus.

45

GYNECOLOGY (THE FEMALE REPRODUCTIVE ORGANS)

Charles B. Hammond, M.D.

Gynecology is that branch of medicine concerned with diseases of the female reproductive system. In practice, however, it includes multiple other areas of interest that are common to any surgical specialty. Of particular importance are the adjacent structures, such as the urinary system and the bowel, as well as remote, hormonally responsive structures such as the breast and even bone.

PATIENT EVALUATION

Adequate history remains a prerequisite for intelligent diagnosis and treatment of gynecologic disease. Additionally, a careful gynecologic examination is necessary for adequate assessment of women with possible gynecologic complaints. All elements of a general medical history are essential to evaluation of pelvic complaints. This gynecologic history should include present illness, menstrual pattern, history of vaginal discharge, obstetric history, marital history with specific reference to contraceptive use, and signs and symptoms of associated disease of the urinary or bowel systems, as well as a thorough general and endocrine systems review.

CONGENITAL ANOMALIES

There are a number of abnormalities of the pelvic structures that are dictated by the developmental embryology of the systems. Awareness of the underlying embryology is necessary for understanding these deficits.

Imperforate Hymen

Imperforate hymen may cause retention of mucus or blood, with resultant hematocolpos, hematometrium, hematosalpinx, and even hematoperitoneum. Diagnosis is based on careful examination of the external genitalia, which shows a bulging hymen without communication with the vagina and a fluctuant pelvic mass that lies anterior to the rectum. Pelvic ultrasonography may be particularly useful for diagnosis. With adequate surgical drainage, the distended structures promptly return to normal.

See the corresponding chapter or part in the *Textbook of Surgery*, 14th edition, pp. 1403–1432, for a more detailed discussion of this topic, including a comprehensive list of references.

Defects of Müllerian Fusion

A transverse vaginal septum is an unusual defect but may present in a manner similar to imperforate hymen. Defects of müllerian fusion may exist, causing duplication of part or all of the reproductive structures. The classic abnormality is the uterus didelphys, with two vaginas, cervices, and uteri, each with a separate tube and ovary. Such patients can present with pelvic pain due to obstruction or with a mass because of obstruction. Therapy, if indicated at all, is surgical excision or reconstruction.

Dysgenesis

There are a number of defects of the female genital tract due to hypoplasia or aplasia of the various components. Such defects may occur either primarily or as secondary underdevelopment due to lack of estrogen. Congenital absence of both ovaries is rare, but absence of one tube or ovary at birth is not unusual. There are cases of complete absence of the vagina, usually associated with absence of the uterus and a number of other abnormalities. Whereas dysgenesis of the müllerian system with absence of the structures is the most common problem, a few patients present with testicular feminizing syndromes (also known as androgen insensitivity), in which the gonads are testicular, yet secondary sex characteristics are feminine since the patient lacks the ability to respond to androgens. Usually, in patients with congenital absence of the pelvic structures, chromosomal studies are necessary for differentiation. If a testicular gonad is *in situ,* excision is necessary because of the risk of secondary malignancy. In all types of vaginal agenesis, a normally functioning vagina should be created surgically or by dilation. Other congenital anomalies of the urinary tract should be sought. There is a commonality of urologic and gynecologic anomalies, which approaches 50 per cent in patients with more severe defects.

THE VULVA

A number of problems may occur in the area of the female external genitalia. Trauma, allergy, inflammatory conditions, infections, degenerative changes, and neoplasia produce disorders ranging from minor annoyances to major hazards to life. An important precept in the evaluation and management of any noted abnormality of the vulva is to be absolutely sure to exclude neoplasia. Punch biopsy with local anesthesia should be done at any time a suspicious or unusual vulvar lesion is noted.

The vulva is rich in pigment, which increases in pregnancy. Vitiligo of the vulvar skin is the same as the lesion in other locations and does not require treatment. Vitiligo should not be confused with leukoplakia, in which the skin is whitish, but thickened and leathery. Various skin eruptions involving the body as a whole may affect the vulva and appear as do other lesions elsewhere on the body. Varicose veins of the vulva are often found in association with varicosities of the lower extremities, and pregnancy may cause further hypertrophy. Therapy consists of lower extremity and vulvar support and ligation or injection in the nonpregnant patient. A severe direct blow to the vulva may be complicated by subcutaneous hematoma formation. Such a hematoma may dissect widely beneath the fascia of the vulva, and surgical evacuation is often necessary. It is frequently difficult to isolate bleeding points, and packing may be required. Vulvar lacerations should be cleansed and sutured as are lacerations elsewhere on the body.

Glandular Lesions

The vulvar glands are subject to a number of disorders. Skenitis usually occurs as a consequence of gonococcal infection. A Bartholin's abscess should be treated with heat until fluctuant and then sharply incised on the mucocutaneous junction between the vagina and vulva. Often, a small inflatable Worde catheter may be inserted. If the abscess is drained by incision, the margins of the incision are marsupialized. The vulva is also a common site of sebaceous cysts. These may be removed if they become greatly enlarged or secondarily infected.

Vulvitis

The most common cause of vulvar irritation is an infectious vulvovaginitis caused by *Candida albicans* or *Trichomonas vaginalis* or both. The vulva appears swollen and red and may be excoriated and secondarily infected. Mycotic vulvovaginitis is a common problem among diabetics, oral contraceptive users, and those receiving systemic antibiotics. Diagnosis is based on fresh-preparation identification of yeast or *Trichomonas*. Therapy is with antimycotic agents such as nystatin or butaconazole or, in the case of trichomoniasis, metronidazole for the patient and consort. Immediate relief is obtained by the additional use of topical creams containing hydrocortisone or miconazole. Condylomata acuminata, or venereal warts, occur as a presumed infectious vulvitis of viral origin (HPV). Such lesions are associated with an irritating vaginal discharge. These benign epithelial neoplasms may be few or many, in some cases even covering the entire perineum and extending onto the vagina or cervix. Therapy is topical application of podophyllin or trichloroacetic acid. On occasion one may use 5-fluorouracil. Cautery or laser is used for the more extensive forms of the disease but requires an anesthetic.

Recently, there has been a near-epidemic of sexually transmitted vulvovaginitis caused by herpes progenitalis (herpes simplex, Type II). This infection is characterized by vesicular eruptions that are extremely painful and often are secondarily infected when the patient is seen. Current therapy includes warm baths in water containing potassium permanganate, drying, and systemic analgesics. The duration of this infection is usually limited, but it may recur. The antiviral agent acyclovir reduces the severity of primary herpetic infections. Other data suggest that chronic acyclovir use may reduce the frequency and severity of recurrences. To date, however, there is no permanent cure, and approximately 20 per cent of patients with a primary herpetic lesion have recurrent episodes.

Other sexually transmitted diseases may present as vulvar lesions. These include the primary chancre of syphilis or the moist, grayish patches (condylomata lata) of secondary syphilis. Lymphogranuloma venereum is a disease of viral origin, which may present with inguinal adenitis, multiple draining sinuses, and rectal stricture. Chancroid appears as a small papule 2 to 4 days after exposure and later becomes an indurated and punched-out lesion with soft edges and purulent surfaces.

Degenerative Diseases of the Vulva

There are three degenerative diseases of the vulva, all occurring most frequently after menopause. Kraurosis vulvae is a disease in which the vulva appears shrunken and dried. Leukoplakia presents initially as a hypertrophic lesion and later as an atrophic problem; the skin is whitened and leathery. Lichen sclerosus et atrophicus is the third form. It is a slowly changing, chronic, localized lesion but, unlike the other two problems, tends to involve the skin of the thighs. All cause itching, pain, dyspareunia, and frequent secondary infection. The incidence of vulvar carcinoma is increased with these lesions, and biopsy should be employed when necessary to exclude neoplasia. Treatment is symptomatic, with relief of pruritus a primary goal. Local excision may be necessary.

Carcinoma in situ of the Vulva

Carcinoma *in situ* of the vulva (VIN-III) may appear with leukoplakia, kraurosis vulvae, or lichen sclerosus et atrophicus, with or without pruritus. The diagnosis should be made only after adequate histologic study shows the criteria of intraepithelial changes characteristic of epidermoid carcinoma, but without invasion. Treatment should be surgical excision in most instances. In patients with carcinoma *in situ* of the vulva, up to 35 per cent may have a second malignant genital lesion elsewhere.

Carcinoma of the Vulva

Vulvar cancers constitute approximately 3.5 per cent of all genital malignancies, and the peak occurs in the seventh decade of life. In approximately half of the patients, the cancer develops in areas of pre-existing leukoplakia, kraurosis vulvae, or lichen sclerosus et atrophicus; others report a high incidence of syphilis and other vulvar venereal diseases among these patients. Most patients with vulvar carcinoma complain of a mass, ulceration or irritation, and pruritus. Bleeding and pain may be additional findings. Any firm tumor or ulceration must be biopsied and include the primary lesion as well as some adjacent normal tissue.

Carcinoma of the vulva is usually squamous (95 per cent), and most are rather well differentiated. Adenocarcinoma of the vulva usually arises from Bartholin's glands but may develop from paraurethral glands or embryonic cell rests. Melanocarcinoma, Paget's disease, and basal cell carcinoma all may be found on the vulva.

Vulvar cancer tends to spread by local extension and lymphatic metastasis. The primary lymphatic drainage of the vulva is via superficial inguinal lymph nodes ipsilateral and via Cloquet's node to the external iliac nodes and up the aortic chain. Contralateral vulvar drainage may occur, however, even from well-lateralized lesions. Vulvar lesions in the perineal, Bartholin, or posterior fourchette areas may involve the rectovaginal septum, rectum, or vagina and may metastasize via the deep pelvic nodes. Blood-borne metastases are unusual.

The treatment of vulvar cancer is surgical therapy. Radiotherapy has generally been of little use for primary or recurrent disease and is contraindicated. The prognosis is generally excellent for earlier lesions. *Operations such as local excision, hemivulvectomy, and simple vulvectomy have proved, in general, to be inadequate treatment of vulvar cancer.* Controversy exists as to whether all patients should also have a retroperitoneal node dissection. Certainly, if the inguinal nodes are sampled and positive or if the primary lesion is large, it should be performed. Overall, the 5-year cure rate after surgical therapy of cancer of the vulva is approximately 60 per cent. If the vulvar lesion involves the vagina, rectum, or urethra, pelvic exenteration may be the operation of choice.

THE VAGINA

The stratified squamous epithelium of the vagina is histologically similar to epithelium of the cervix and the skin of the vulva and responds to estrogen by proliferation. Vaginal inflammation can occur from protozoan, fungal, bacterial, or viral infection and also from deficiencies of estrogen. Nonspecific bacterial infections, now termed bacterial vaginosis and thought to be sexually transmitted, may also exist. Gonorrhea is an occasional cause of vaginitis in the child. In all of these categories, the cause of vaginal infection should be sought through wet preparation or culture, with appropriate treatment being instituted for the organism found. Often, there is vulvar inflammation that may require local therapy for immediate relief of symptoms.

Dysplasia and Intraepithelial Carcinoma of the Vagina

Dysplasia of the vaginal epithelium may be the source of abnormal genital smears even if the cervix is normal or absent. Intraepithelial carcinoma may also develop. These lesions may occur at the apex of the vagina in patients after hysterectomy or may be multifocal in areas remote from the vaginal apex. Diagnosis is suggested by genital cytologic and colposcopic examination and confirmed by biopsy. Therapy can be excision or partial or total colpectomy.

Carcinoma of the Vagina

Primary carcinoma of the vagina is a rare lesion, and most are epidermoid lesions. Postcontact bleeding is the usual presenting complaint. Many patients with invasive vaginal carcinoma have previously had other epidermoid lesions of the lower genital system. Exenterative surgery may be used as primary therapy or treatment for recurrence. After appropriate staging, therapy is either irradiation or surgery, with most favoring irradiation. Reasonable results are obtained with early stage disease.

DEFECTS OF PELVIC SUPPORT

Overdistention of the pelvic supporting structures may produce a number of defects in pelvic support. These problems include cystocele, urethrocele, rectocele, enterocele, and uterine prolapse. After hysterectomy, vaginal vault prolapse may occur. There may be attendant problems in urinary incontinence or exteriorization of pelvic structures. The common sensation of heavy pulling-down pressure in the pelvis is often documented. The proper assessment includes urodynamic investigation of urinary prolapse, careful search for occult enterocele, and surgical repair often combining abdominal and transvaginal approaches. Usually preservation of vaginal patency can be maintained with an excellent restoration of support.

BENIGN DISEASES OF THE CERVIX

The portio vaginalis of the normal cervix is covered with squamous epithelium and is subject to a number of problems. Cervical infection is one of the most frequently encountered gynecologic lesions. Acute cervicitis is rarely seen other than in gonorrhea or *Chlamydia* infection. Pain and tenderness are rarely prominent symptoms, but a purulent discharge is frequently seen. Diagnosis is made by appropriate smears and cultures, and therapy with topical or systemic antibiotics usually is curative.

In chronic cervicitis, the mucus is mucopurulent and often profuse. Erosions and eversions of the cervix are often observed. An erosion is a true ulcer of the cervix, whereas eversion is formed by proliferation downward of the columnar epithelium of the endocervical canal, forming a lowered squamocolumnar line. Diagnosis is based on cytologic examination and biopsy for exclusion of neoplasia, and these studies are more difficult when cervical infection is present.

Colposcopy may be of aid in localizing areas for biopsy. After exclusion of malignancy, chronic cervicitis is usually treated by electrodesiccation, laser desiccation, or cryosurgery.

CANCER OF THE CERVIX

Invasive carcinoma of the cervix is now the second most common pelvic malignancy and represents 15 per cent of cancers in women. In the past 2 decades, primarily through early detection, mortality from cervical cancer has declined significantly. Invasive carcinoma of the cervix should be a preventable disease, since regular examinations and frequent use of present technologies, particularly genital cytologic study, should enable detection of nearly all malignant lesions or preinvasive cervical carcinoma.

The average age of occurrence of carcinoma of the cervix is 49 years. However, many authors have reported cervical cancers in women as young as the teens and as old as the eighth decade. Epidemiologic relationships show peak occurrences among women of low socioeconomic status, those who begin coitus and childbearing at an early age, and those with multiple sexual partners. Cigarette smoking and heredity have a small role. The theory of a viral relationship has been advanced but not yet fully proved. Preinvasive carcinoma, or carcinoma *in situ* of the cervix, has been recognized for a number of years. It is suspected only on the basis of genital cytologic change, since *there are no gross lesions or symptoms of carcinoma in situ of the cervix*. The diagnosis of this lesion is made by histologic review of appropriate biopsy specimens.

Many patients with dysplasia or carcinoma *in situ* of the cervix are now being treated with electrocautery, cryosurgery, or cone biopsy. Close follow-up after therapy is warranted. The primary caution is to exclude invasive carcinoma before such treatments are done. Another treatment for extensive or recurrent carcinoma *in situ* of the cervix may be abdominal or vaginal hysterectomy with excision of 2 to 3 cm. of the upper vagina. Radical hysterectomy and pelvic lymph node dissection are not indicated, and results are generally good. Recurrence may occur, however.

Carcinoma of the Cervix

Approximately 95 per cent of cervical cancers are squamous; the remaining 5 per cent are usually adenocarcinomas. Microinvasive cancer of the cervix (Stage IA1 and above) denotes a minimal extent of invasion. A halo of carcinoma *in situ* is frequently found around an invasive cancer or on the vagina. There are few symptoms of early carcinoma of the cervix, the first symptom generally being bleeding. This may be postcontact or an irregular bloody discharge. More advanced cervical cancers cause symptoms referable to invasion of adjacent organs (bladder, rectum, or ureter) or to distant metastasis. Pain is a frequent symptom of advanced cervical cancer.

Although cytologic findings and clinical appearance may strongly suggest carcinoma of the cervix, the diagnosis can be made only on histopathologic study. Even in the presence of normal genital cytologic findings, cervical or vaginal ulcers or growths should be biopsied. False-negative genital cytologic study in the presence of ulcerative or exophytic cervical lesions is not uncommon.

The most common method of spread of cervical cancer and the most frequent cause of patient death is direct extension to involve the vagina, uterus, parametrium, pelvic sidewall, ureter, bladder, and rectum. Fistula formation is common, and bleeding may be a serious complication. Carcinoma of the cervix also has a propensity for lymphatic metastasis.

Treatment of cervical cancer can be effectively accomplished by surgical therapy or irradiation. Treatment, however, does not include simple hysterectomy or nonindividualized radiotherapy. No other major malignancy requires a more critical selection of technique or mode of therapy. The present operation for early cancer of the cervix (Stage I and Stage IIA) is an extended or radical hysterectomy (Wertheim) that removes the parametrial tissues, the upper third of the vagina, and perhaps the adnexa. Pelvic node dissection is usually performed. Radical irradiation may be used in early stage cancer of the cervix or in more extended disease. External irradiation followed by intracervical irradiation is the appropriate treatment. Results of treatment are generally good for earlier disease, 86.4 per cent for Stage I and only 8.8 per cent for Stage IV. Patients who have been treated for cancer of the cervix must be followed for many years, since late recurrence is reasonably common.

BENIGN UTERINE DISEASE

Various benign uterine diseases occur, including leiomyoma uteri, adenomyosis, endometrial hyperplasia, and polyps. Abnormal bleeding, uterine enlargement, and pain are the primary symptoms associated with these diseases, but the major difficulty is achieving an accurate diagnosis.

Leiomyoma Uteri

Uterine leiomyomas are the most common cause of benign uterine enlargement and are seen in 20 per cent of women with a higher incidence among blacks. Leiomyomas originate from the smooth muscle cells of the myometrium and vary in size from microscopic to large enough to fill the entire abdomen. Such tumors may be single but are more often multiple. Compressed peripheral fibers form a pseudocapsule. On microscopic examination, smooth muscle cells are arranged in interlacing muscle bundles, interspaced with varying amounts of connective tissue. Such tumors may be submucous, intramural, subserous, pedunculated, parasitic, cervical, or interligamentous.

The symptoms of leiomyoma vary according to location; some may produce severe complaints, others none at all. The three most common symptoms are abnormal bleeding, pain, and uterine enlargement. Abnormal bleeding, usually cyclic but possibly profuse and prolonged, is most frequently due to submucous tumors that distort the overlying endometrium and interfere with normal hemostatic mechanisms. Occasionally a submucous or cervical myoma may be extruded. Abnormal bleeding is the most common indication for hysterectomy for leiomyoma, but caution must be taken to exclude other causes, since a malignant lesion of the endometrium may coexist with myoma. Often a curettage may be mandatory for making this differentiation. Rapid enlargement is another symptom of concern in patients with leiomyoma, because 0.05 to 0.08 per cent may develop sarcomatous change. Estrogens, including the synthetic estrogens of oral contraceptives, may in some patients be associated with more rapid enlargement of leiomyomas. Myomas tend to regress after menopause, and any enlargement of these tumors after this age demands removal of the uterus. Slow enlargement of leiomyomas during the menstrual years frequently occurs with minimal symptoms, and surgical removal is not mandatory for slow growth or moderate size unless other symptoms occur. Pelvic pressure, frequency of urination, and sciatic or hip pain may be symptoms of uterine leiomyoma. Tenderness is usually caused by degeneration, and cystic changes and calcification can occur. Significant pain or tenderness may warrant hysterectomy. Infertility is uncommon in patients with myomas, as is abortion, but either may occur.

The treatment of leiomyoma is individualized for each patient. Some tumors require no treatment if small and asymptomatic, and only semiannual examination is warranted. If a young patient who desires further pregnancies has symptomatic leiomyomas, myomectomy may be a useful surgical procedure. In such patients, leiomyomas may recur, however. In larger or more symptomatic myomas in a woman who has completed reproduction, hysterectomy is the treatment of choice. Medical treatment of leiomyoma with gonadotropin-releasing analog has had limited success. Further information is required before its precise role is well defined.

Adenomyosis

Adenomyosis is an invasion of the myometrium by the endometrium. It is a frequent cause of uterine enlargement and pain. Grossly the uterus is enlarged, fibrotic, and thickened, and on cut section there are areas of endometrial growth and loculated menstruation within the myometrium. The classic signs and symptoms include acquired dysmenorrhea occurring in the 35- to 45-year-old patient; there often are menstrual irregularities with cyclic prolonged and profuse flow and an enlarged, tender uterus. Treatment is hysterectomy, although some types of hormonal suppression may provide temporary relief without removal of the uterus.

Endometrial Hyperplasia and Polyps

Hyperplasia of the endometrium, causing abnormal uterine bleeding, is a common problem of women in the perimenopausal years. It is occasionally seen in younger patients, particularly in adolescence. The basic problem is anovulation and failure of production of progesterone. Continued stimulation of the endometrium by estrogen produces proliferation, overgrowth, and hyperplasia. Areas of thickened endometrium may form polyps. Menstruation becomes irregular, with intervals of amenorrhea associated with other intervals of intermenstrual spotting or bleeding. Pelvic examination is usually not revealing, and biopsy or curettage is necessary to establish the diagnosis. Curettage also offers a therapeutic component. Because of the frequency of recurrence of hyperplasia, the administration of cyclic progesterone may limit recurrence. In various types of hyperplasias, notably the atypical adenomatous hyperplasias, there is a significant malignant potential, and consideration of hysterectomy is necessary.

MALIGNANT DISEASES OF THE UTERUS

Adenocarcinoma of the endometrium, now the most prevalent gynecologic cancer, is seen most commonly among postmenopausal women. The peak incidence occurs in the 50- to 70-year-old age group, but it must be suspected as early as the third decade if there is an irregularity of menstrual bleeding. Irregular or postmenopausal bleeding is the cardinal symptom of endometrial cancer. Papanicolaou cytologic study may yield negative results, since the exfoliated cells may not reach the vaginal pool. Fractional curettage is the diagnostic method of choice, although screening by endometrial biopsy may be performed. On histologic examination, adenocarcinoma of the endometrium has wide variations in differentiaton and in stromal invasion. The etiologic agent of endometrial cancer is unknown. There does appear to be a relationship to prolonged estrogen stimulation in some patients, as in patients with estrogen-producing ovarian tumors. Newer studies also suggest a higher incidence of endometrial adenocarcinoma in women given large-dose estrogen replacement therapy, without added progesterone, for menopausal symptoms.

Endometrial cancer is usually a polypoid lesion growing into the endometrial cavity, and only later in the disease does myometrial or cervical involvement occur. Uterine size is usually normal to slightly increased in women with early endometrial cancer. In addition to direct extension to adjacent structures, adenocarcinoma of the endometrium may spread through the lymphatic system at the upper uterus between the tube and ovary. When cervical lesions are present, lymphogenous dissemination may follow the pattern of cervical cancer.

After appropriate staging, the treatment of adenocarcinoma of the endometrium is primarily surgical. Survival in patients with early stage disease and well-differentiated lesions is very good. External pelvic radiotherapy or transvaginal irradiation may be used for palliation or recurrent disease. Rarely, hormonal manipulation may be of benefit for metastases.

Sarcomas of the uterus may arise from the endometrium, myometrium, cervix, or uterine blood vessels or from a leiomyoma. These diseases are most frequently seen in the fifth decade. Treatment is primarily surgical, although radiotherapy may offer benefit. The role of chemotherapy is being further investigated.

PELVIC INFECTION

Acute pelvic infection may occur after pelvic surgery or from other causes, but the most frequent etiologic factors are gonorrhea and chlamydial infection. The initial symptoms of acute pelvic infection usually occur within 3 to 6 days after inoculation, although they may be delayed until the onset of the next menses. Initial symptoms are referable to urethritis, skenitis, bartholinitis, or cervicitis, and consist of vaginal discharge. Tubal involvement is a later symptom, and at that time organisms spread rapidly from the endocervix, across the endometrium, and involve the endosalpinx. It is in the fallopian tubes that the major infection and damage occur. The tubes become acutely inflamed and edematous, and the lumen fills with a purulent exudate. The tubular, peritubular, ovarian, and pelvic peritoneal surfaces are rapidly involved. Secondary infection with anaerobic bacteria is common. Pelvic abscess may develop.

The signs and symptoms of acute pelvic infection are those of pelvic peritonitis with bilateral lower abdominal pain and tenderness, temperature of 38 to 39° C., and signs of peritoneal irritation with direct and rebound tenderness and muscle spasm. On pelvic examination, purulent exudate may be seen in the cervix, and exquisite tenderness is often present in both adnexal areas and with cervical manipulation. Bilaterality of pain is an important point in differentiating acute pelvic infection from appendicitis. Therapy is based on the degree of peritonitis and fever. If significant peritonitis is present or the temperature is greater than 38.5° C., hospitalization is indicated and intravenous antibiotic therapy recommended. For women with serious episodes of pelvic infection, a number of therapeutic regimens have been proposed, including doxycycline plus cefoxitan, clindamycin plus gentamicin, or doxycycline plus metronidazole. Aggressive antibiotic treatment, analgesia, elevation of the head for encouraging pelvic localization of purulent material, and parenteral fluid replacement, are continued until the acute symptoms have subsided, then oral therapy is begun and continued for at least a week. If the presenting symptoms are not severe, the patient can be treated as an outpatient, but close follow-up is warranted.

The patient with relatively asymptomatic gonococcal infection can be treated with aqueous procaine penicillin G, 4.8 million units intramuscularly in divided doses at two sites, preceded by probenecid, 1 gm. by mouth. Approximately a week after the therapy is completed, a follow-up culture for "test of cure" should be done. The patient should be examined twice weekly to follow her progress and exclude pelvic abscess. Surgical therapy is not generally indicated for acute pelvic infection unless pelvic abscess drainage is required or differentiation from appendicitis is needed.

Chronic Pelvic Infection

Included among chronic pelvic infections are chronic salpingo-oophoritis, pyosalpinx, hydrosalpinx, and tubercular salpingitis. Chronic salpingo-oophoritis is one of the major complications of gonococcal and probably chlamydial infections. The patient may have few complaints or be recurrently and acutely discomforted. The classic pattern of chronic pelvic infection is one of quiescent intervals interspaced with episodes of more acute inflammation. After the initial infection, anaerobic organisms invade and involve these tissues. These infections may be treated medically or surgically. The important elements of medical therapy are rest, heat, and antibiotic treatment. Analgesia may be required. Oral metronidazole, doxycycline, and tetracycline are the appropriate antibiotics utilized with modest increase of pain and symptoms from chronic pelvic infection. Symptoms in those patients who have recurrent pain or abnormal uterine bleeding from altered ovarian function caused by chronic pelvic infection are often difficult to relieve. In this instance surgical extirpation may be needed, although it should be delayed until maximal medical control has been obtained.

BENIGN DISEASES OF THE OVARY

Benign ovarian tumors may be solid or cystic and may represent a "functional" process or neoplasia. They on occasion may become massively enlarged, although they usually are modest in size. A number of authors report that more than 90 per cent of ovarian growths discovered in women under 30 years of age are benign. In the 30- to 50-year-old age group, 80 per cent are benign. After 50 years of age, approximately half of such ovarian growths are malignant. The various benign ovarian growths, excluding the frequently seen follicle and corpus luteum cysts, are endometrial cysts, simple cysts, serous and mucinous cystadenomas, and dermoids. Symptoms include slow abdominal enlargement, pain and tenderness from torsion of the pedicle, and, rarely, aberrations of menstrual bleeding.

The benign, non-neoplastic ovarian cysts are usually of "functional" origin. These represent failure of the normal development and regression of ovulatory cysts. Most usually regress over a 4- to 8-week period. Of the nonfunctional benign cysts, the most frequently seen is the endometrial or "chocolate" cyst of pelvic endometriosis; these may achieve large size. Serous and mucinous cystadenomas arise from neoplastic, nonmalignant changes in the germinal epithelium and often reach large size. These tumors are usually multilocular, have smooth capsules, and usually replace the entire ovary. The benign teratoma, or dermoid cyst, is a common ovarian tumor, benign in more than 99 per cent of patients. Approximately 15 per cent of dermoids are bilateral, and thus if one ovary is involved, the other should be carefully inspected.

The solid benign ovarian tumors include the Brenner tumor, which is thought to arise from Walthard's inclusion rests in the cortex of the ovary; ovarian fibromas; and a number of rare and unusual tumors that may have hormonal activity. The most important decision confronting the surgeon who finds a solid ovarian tumor is differentiation of benign from malignant.

The treatment of benign ovarian growths is primarily surgical removal with conservation of all normal ovarian tissue possible. The functional cysts should regress within a relatively short interval and do not require removal unless rupture and hemorrhage have occurred. Endometrial or "chocolate" cysts usually require resection of all involved ovarian tissue. In any event, bilateral oophorectomy is rarely indicated in young women with ovarian masses unless one is *certain* that malignancy is present. In general, the author believes that if an undiagnosed mass larger than 6 cm. is found in a cycling patient or, if smaller, it persists without diminution in size for longer than 3 months, exploration should be done. Acute torsion or significant hemorrhage may require immediate resection.

OVARIAN CANCER

Most series report that ovarian cancer represents 4 to 6 per cent of all cases of malignant disease in women. Most investigators include a number of types such as serous cystadenocarcinoma (60 per cent), pseudomucinous carcinoma (15 per cent), solid undifferentiated adenocarcinoma (10 per cent), granulosa cell carcinoma (6 per cent), and others at lesser percentages. The ratio of benign ovarian tumors to malignant ovarian tumors is 4:1 until the peak incidence of ovarian cancer at 40 to 60 years of age, when the ratio is 1:1.

Several factors need to be emphasized in regard to ovarian cancer. First, the delay in diagnosis is reprehensible: 50 per cent of ovarian cancers are neglected by the patient and 25 per cent by the physician, who does not examine the patient in more than 60 per cent of cases. Second, 30 to 50 per cent of ovarian cancers are inoperable at the time of diagnosis, and in only 20 per cent can the tumor be entirely removed surgically. Third, only 11 per cent of patients have suspicious or positive Papanicolaou cytologic findings. Fourth, as expected, the survival is greater the earlier the stage of the disease at the time of diagnosis. Since the overall survival of ovarian cancer has improved only slightly in the past 25 years, earlier diagnosis is mandatory.

The signs and symptoms of ovarian cancer may be only those of an enlarging tumor in the pelvis. Published reports include that half the patients complain of pain and abdominal swelling. A number of complaints include weight loss and abnormal bleeding. There may be ascites and even hydrothorax, and anemia is frequently found in advanced disease. Pelvic examination may reveal firm nodular implants. As noted, there are often no early symptoms of ovarian cancer. Annual bimanual examination is an important screening technique for this disease. Although no highly accurate for diagnosis, tumor "markers," if present, may be beneficial (CA 125, CEA).

The primary treatment of ovarian cancer is surgical. In general, this includes total abdominal hysterectomy, bilateral salpingo-oophorectomy, and omentectomy, although there may be residual tumor. The abdomen, including the diaphragms, should be carefully inspected and appropriate lymph node sampling performed. Peritoneal washings should be routinely obtained. Chemotherapy has been a primary adjunctive technology, although radiotherapy has had limited success. With such treatment, approximately half of the patients receive significant palliation, and the 5-year survival of Stage I ovarian cancer is only 66 per cent. Unfortunately, only 20 per cent of patients explored have disease limited to Stage I.

ECTOPIC PREGNANCY

An ectopic pregnancy is one in which the ovum implants and develops outside the normal location, the uterine cavity. Ninety-five per cent of ectopic pregnancies are tubal, with the greatest percentage of these occurring in the dilated ampulla. Less common sites of ectopic pregnancy are abdominal, ovarian, and interligamentary positions. Despite the fact that the ovum is implanted outside the uterine cavity, the uterine endometrium converts into a decidual structure similar to that of normal pregnancy. The size and consistency of the uterus also change in ectopic pregnancy, with the cervix and uterus softening and the corpus enlarging to 6 to 8 weeks' gestational size. All of these changes are due to the production of placental hormones from the ectopic pregnancy. As ectopic placental function declines, as usually occurs in tubal pregnancy, the hormonal support declines and irregular bleeding begins.

The duration and eventual outcome of tubal ectopic pregnancy are determined primarily by the area of the tube involved. If the ovum implants in the relatively large ampullary region of the tube, the pregnancy usually continues longer than does one in the narrow isthmus. The ovular sac may extrude from the end of the tube, or the tube may rupture, particularly in the more narrow areas. Intra-abdominal hemorrhage may occur. The classic symptoms of ectopic pregnancy are a history of infertility or pelvic disease, irregular vaginal bleeding within 2 to 4 weeks after the first missed menstrual period, and sharp and fleeting lower abdominal pain. Eventually the patient experiences sudden severe abdominal pain and shock as the tube ruptures. On examination, the signs of early pregnancy such as cyanosis and softening of the cervix and uterine enlargement are noted. There may be a unilateral tender mass. Fever is a rare finding, but progressive anemia is frequently observed. Newer, more sensitive pregnancy tests are usually positive in most patients with an unruptured tubal pregnancy.

The diagnosis of an unruptured tubal pregnancy is not difficult to make when classic symptoms are present, but unfortunately, the symptoms are frequently atypical and the pelvic findings misleading. A high index of suspicion is the most valuable adjunct. Culdocentesis may reveal considerable old dark blood, and laparoscopy may allow visualization of the ectopic pregnancy. Other confounding diagnoses include complete spontaneous abortion, incomplete spontaneous abortion, or threatened abortion. Salpingitis and appendicitis usually present with signs of infection without prior amenorrhea.

When this diagnosis is suspected, a sensitive pregnancy test should be done to determine if human chorionic gonadotropin (hCG) is elevated. If the test is positive, a quantified assay should be obtained. If the hCG titer is in excess of 4000 mIU per ml., an intrauterine pregnancy, if present, should be seen by ultrasound, preferably by the more sensitive vaginal probe techniques. The finding of an intrauterine pregnancy in such a setting likely excludes ectopic pregnancy in all but the very rare patient who might have simultaneous intrauterine and ectopic gestations. Failure to note an ectopically placed pregnancy with ultrasonography is not diagnostic but warrants follow-up, probably with laparoscopy. In patients in whom the initial value of hCG is less than 4000 mIU per ml., alternate-day hCG assays for quantified values should be obtained. In normal pregnancy, hCG doubles every 48 hours during that interval of pregnancy. Failure to show this rise supports the diagnosis of an abnormal pregnancy, either a missed abortion, an incomplete abortion, or possibly an ectopic pregnancy. All of these studies should be utilized in the subtle case.

46

THE URINARY SYSTEM
David F. Paulson, M.D.

SIGNS AND SYMPTOMS OF UROLOGIC DISEASE

Usually, pain or bleeding is the initial indicator of disease involving the urinary tract. Renal pain, ureteral pain, and bladder pain have distinct characteristics. Careful review of the presentation often suggests a diagnosis and directs attention to the specific anatomic site involved. Renal pain is usually dull and aching and localized to the flank. This is most common when the pain is due to inflammation; however, when produced by stone or acute bleeding, the pain may be sharp, localized to the flank, or radiate into the lower abdomen, the side, or the buttocks. The pain may be episodic, appearing in waves, and when so appearing is usually associated with ureteral obstruction. However, the pain may also be persistent, producing loss of appetite with nausea and vomiting. Renal pain, when dull in character, usually indicates a long-standing process, such as chronic infection or a slowly growing tumor. Severe renal pain may cause the patient to be restless and to hold the flank in an attempt to minimize the discomfort. Ureteral pain may cause flank discomfort and may be associated with severe abdominal pain, nausea, and vomiting. As the pain or calculus that produces the pain moves distally in the ureter, the pain radiates from the flank to the lower abdomen, occasionally radiating to the scrotum or labia majora and occasionally into the thigh. A calculus in the lower ureter or at the junction of ureter and bladder may cause urinary frequency with urgency and painful urination. Bladder pain is usually dull, aching, and localized to the suprapubic region.

DIAGNOSTIC STUDIES

Whereas the historic presentation may provide an accurate indication of the site of urologic disease, physical examination often predicts what subsequent imaging or other diagnostic studies will be confirmatory. Although inspection of the abdomen may disclose a lower abdominal mass when the bladder is full and unable to empty, in adults, neither the distended bladder nor the hydronephrotic obstructed kidney is easy to define. In the child, the bladder is an intra-abdominal organ and is easily palpated. In addition, because of the relative size differential in children and adults, the

---

See the corresponding chapter or part in the *Textbook of Surgery,* 14th edition, pp. 1433–1456, for a more detailed discussion of this topic, including a comprehensive list of references.

child's kidney is easily palpated and transilluminated. When the kidney is tense from intrarenal bleeding or inflammation, sudden pressure in the area of the kidney in both adults and children may produce pain.

Laboratory studies confirm the presence of urinary tract disease. Urinalysis that demonstrates white blood cells, red blood cells, or bacteria confirms the presence of infection or bleeding within the urinary tract. An assessment of renal function by evaluation of the blood urea nitrogen and creatinine determines whether the kidney is able to function adequately, such that exogenous waste products may be removed from the blood.

IMAGING OF THE URINARY TRACT

Multiple studies currently exist for imaging the urinary tract. Whereas many of the former imaging studies permitted only an anatomic evaluation of the urinary tract, many of the current imaging studies also provide an assessment of renal function. Current techniques include excretory urography with nephrotomography, retrograde ureteral pyelography, arteriography, venacavography, computed tomography, ultrasonography, and magnetic resonance imaging. The most commonly used imaging study is the excretory urogram. This study is dependent on renal function and visualizes the urinary tract by concentration of intravenous injection of organic iodine within the urinary tract. Retrograde ureteral pyelography and cystography involve the placement of the iodinated contrast agent directly into the ureter or bladder. These studies should be avoided during acute infection because instillation of the iodinated contrast material under pressure may precipitate a systemic infection by forcing bacteria into the lymphatics and venules of the bladder and kidney. Arteriography delineates the vascular pattern of the kidneys. Digital venous angiography and venacavography are alternative methods of observing the vascular supply of the kidneys. Computed tomography, magnetic resonance imaging, and ultrasonography plus radioactive renography are noninvasive methods that permit visualization of the kidneys and identification of pathologic processes that may involve either the kidney or ureter.

NONSURGICAL INFLAMMATORY DISEASES OF THE URINARY TRACT

The most frequent urinary tract infection is *cystitis*, an infection within the bladder associated with urinary frequency, painful urination, urgency, suprapubic pain, and hematuria. Pyelonephritis occurs when the infection involves the kidney. *Acute pyelonephritis* is accompanied by flank pain, fever, chills, and occasional nausea and vomiting. Acute pyelonephritis differs from acute cystitis in that patients with bacterial cystitis usually do not have fever and chills. The diagnosis of urinary tract infection is supported by urinalysis demonstrating white cells and bacteria and confirmed by a positive culture.

SURGICAL DISEASES OF THE URINARY TRACT

Surgical diseases of the urinary tract are most commonly calculi or malignancy. Congenital malformations are much less common, usually being diagnosed in infancy.

Urinary Tract Calculi

The symptoms of urinary tract calculi are flank pain, cramping, and abdominal discomfort radiating to the groin, scrotum, or labia with microscopic hematuria. A plain film of the abdomen usually identifies the location of the stone and directs a form of intervention. The intravenous pyelogram determines whether the stone is totally or partially obstructing and also identifies any other anatomic abnormality that may produce stasis causing stone formation. Whereas calculous disease was previously treated primarily by surgical removal, new techniques permit treatment without operative procedures. Currently, urinary tract calculi involving the kidney and/or ureter may be alternatively managed by extracorporeal shock wave lithotripsy to destroy calculi. These shock waves are generated either by an underwater spark discharge or by the focused simultaneous discharge of thousands of piezoelectrodes, similarly activated by an electrical discharge. The discharge produces a shock wave in the surrounding fluid, which then propagates concentrically in a manner similar to sound waves in air. These sound waves can be focused on the urinary tract calculus to destroy it and permit the passage of multiple stone fragments through the normal urinary tract. Percutaneous ultrasonic lithotripsy utilizes ultrasonic sound waves, transmitted down a hollow tube, to destroy calculi within the kidney or ureter. In addition, recent studies using laser discharges have demonstrated that these too pulverize stones within the ureter and/or kidney. Thus, with use of these noninvasive techniques, open surgical therapy for the management of renal calculous disease has become largely an item of historic interest.

Malignant Disease

Acquired diseases of the urinary tract consist primarily of malignant or traumatic disease. Malignant diseases of the urinary tract encompass carcinoma of the kidney, ureter, or bladder. Renal adenocarcinoma is the most common malignancy involving the kidney, occurring most often in the fifth decade of life, with an incidence three times higher in males than in females. Three histopathologic types of renal adenocarcinoma are identified: (1) clear cells, (2) granular cells, and (3) spindle-shaped cells. Renal carcinoma may present with a wide variety of symptom patterns.

EVALUATION OF RENAL LESIONS

Symptomatic or asymptomatic renal mass lesions may be evaluated by a series of sequential steps. By use of this systematic approach to the identification of renal mass lesions, approximately 85 per cent can be correctly identified by a combination of only two sequential examinations. The most frequent asymptomatic renal neoplasm is metastatic tumor, with carcinoma of the breast being the most common. Only 2.2 per cent of asymptomatic space-occupying lesions of the kidney are primary renal cell malignancy. Treatment of renal cell carcinoma is based on the anatomic extent of disease, and treatment is directed toward surgical removal of the kidney and the associated tumor, the adrenal gland, the surrounding perinephric fat, Gerota's fascia, and regional lymph nodes. Surgical therapy is less effective in controlling renal carcinoma when the disease is confined to the kidney or when it is extended minimally outside the renal capsule. Surgical therapy is not effective when the disease is extended to adjacent structures or regional lymph nodes or when it has invaded the renal vein or vena cava. Patients with a tumor confined to the renal substance beneath the capsule have a survival rate after resection of greater than 90 per cent at 10 years. The benefit of surgical removal of the renal primary tumor in patients with metastatic disease is controversial, since removal of the primary renal malignancy may provide temporary control of symptoms but it does not reduce further dissemination.

RENAL TRAUMA

Renal trauma may be classified as either blunt (nonpenetrating) or penetrating. Both can be divided into two groups, those that involve the parenchyma and those involving the renal pedicle. In patients with blunt trauma, fracture of the lower ribs, fracture of transverse processes, or scoliosis on the routine abdominal film, urologic evaluation is warranted, particularly in the presence of gross hematuria. It is thought that patients who have nonpenetrating injury with only microscopic hematuria are not candidates for intravenous pyelography, since the incidence of being able to identify an abnormality that requires treatment is so low. However, patients who have gross hematuria or penetrating injuries must be evaluated for determination of the extent of the genitourinary injury. Controversy continues concerning the optimal study, but intravenous pyelography has long been the standard screening study. Today, computed axial tomography with contrast is thought to be a much more accurate imaging study for determining the extent of the lesion and any associated perirenal bleeding. Computed axial tomography also allows the clinician to determine the bilaterality of renal function and the amount of gross urinary extravasation. In patients who have blunt renal trauma, the decision for exploration and repair is made only when the patient demonstrates hemodynamic instability. Even when major lacerations are identified, if the patient is hemodynamically stable, it is currently thought that conservative observation is the best form of treatment. However, when the patient has penetrating injury or is thought to have pedicle injury, exploration with attempted repair is warranted. Penetrating injuries are associated with other intra-abdominal injuries in four of five patients. Thus, with the exception of those patients who have superficial stab wounds, it is recommended that patients who have penetrating injuries near the kidney should have an intravenous pyelogram and should be considered for surgical exploration.

THE URETERS

The ureters are tubular structures that convey urine from the renal pelvis to the bladder. Generally they are protected by the fibrofatty tissue of the retroperitoneum, but their integrity can be threatened by a number of congenital and inflammatory or traumatic, iatrogenic, and neoplastic diseases. With the exception of malignant disease or congenital obstruction involving the ureter, acquired obstruction by calculous disease is usually managed by closed intervention with use of ultrasonic lithotripsy, extracorporeal shock wave lithotripsy, or laser lithotripsy. Malignant disease of the ureter may be intrinsic to the ureter itself or extrinsic. When extrinsic, it is usually associated with malignant disease of other origin and is manifested by progressive renal failure. Intrinsic malignant disease of the ureter is usually manifested by gross or microscopic hematuria and can be identified by intravenous pyelography.

Obstruction of the ureter can be relieved without open surgical intervention. In the patient with either unilateral or bilateral obstruction, internal drainage can be established by use of a "double J" Silastic catheter. These catheters may be inserted either transurethrally from below or percutaneously from above. The Silastic catheters may be left in place for 6 to 12 months with minimal encrustation. They may be removed percutaneously or transurethrally and replaced without difficulty.

Carcinoma of the renal pelvis constitutes approximately 5 per cent of all renal carcinomas and is of transitional cell origin, arising from the transitional epithelium that lines the calyceal system and renal pelvis. Ninety per cent of all carcinomas of the renal pelvis are transitional cell tumors. The malignant cells are shed into the urine where they can be identified by Papanicolaou smear. Eighty to 90 per cent of all patients with renal pelvic tumors have either gross or microscopic hematuria. Carcinoma of the ureter is usually a transitional cell tumor, and treatment has previously been nephroureterectomy with removal of the entire renal unit and ureter. Currently, preservation of the renal unit by local resection of the malignancy only has been advocated with the belief that salvage of patients with ureteral tumors depends more on the biologic aggressiveness of the tumor than on the aggressiveness of the chosen surgical therapy. Patients with high-grade lesions or lesions that have penetrated into the ureteral wall have little likelihood of cure, even with the most radical surgical procedures.

THE BLADDER

The normal bladder fills to a volume of 400 ml. with no increase in pressure, with no contraction of the bladder musculature, and without relaxation of the bladder sphincter. At approximately 400 ml., when the patient feels the necessity to void, the urodynamic study records a spiking increase in bladder pressure and a coincidental relaxation of the bladder sphincteric musculatures. When rising intravesical pressure overcomes falling urethral resistance, voiding begins and the bladder empties. Study of the coordinated filling of the bladder, relaxation and then contraction of the detrusor, and increase in intravesical pressure during the relaxed and voiding phase with simultaneous examination of the electrical activity of the urinary sphincters is of extreme value in determining the nature of neuromuscular disorders affecting either emptying or storage. Whereas absolute recommendations cannot be made as to the appropriate management of the various disorders of storage and emptying, when no specific anatomic defect or required surgical correction is identified, it is often possible to enhance either emptying or facilitate storage by the use of various pharmaceutical agents.

Nonmalignant Surgical Disease of the Bladder

The common nonmalignant surgical diseases of the bladder are bladder fistulas, disorders of storage, and vesical trauma.

BLADDER FISTULAS. Bladder fistulas produce disorders of storage since the urine is not retained within the bladder. The defect is between the bladder and the small or large bowel (enteric fistula), the vagina, the uterus, or the skin. They usually are of inflammatory, neoplastic, iatrogenic, or traumatic origin. Fifty per cent of all vesicoenteric fistulas are secondary to sigmoid diverticulitis. Malignancy is responsible for approximately 16 to 20 per cent of all enteric fistulas, with 12 to 15 per cent associated with Crohn's disease. Pneumaturia and fecaluria are the classic signs of vesicoenteric fistula. Pneumaturia is not pathognomonic of an enteric fistula, since gas per urethra may follow fermentation of diabetic urine, urinary tract infection by gas-producing organisms, or urinary tract instrumentation. However, pneumaturia is the presenting sign in two thirds of patients with vesicoenteric fistula. Although fecaluria is diagnostic of vesicoenteric fistula, it occurs in only 20 to 50 per cent of all patients. When a fistula is suspected, contrast studies, such as intravenous pyelography, upper gastrointestinal studies, or a barium enema, may be necessary to identify the fistula. Surgical repair usually requires resection of the affected bowel segment and bladder *en bloc* with primary restitution of bowel and a primary bladder closure. Approximately 90 per cent of all vesicovaginal fistulas are secondary to gynecologic procedures. The remaining 10 per cent are a consequence of urologic surgery, extensive pelvic trauma, complications of internal/external radiotherapy, or direct extension of malignant disease processes.

DISORDERS OF STORAGE. One disorder of storage occurs when the bladder may not distend owing to chronic inflammatory disease involving the bladder wall. In such instances, bladder augmentation by use of ileum, cecum, or sigmoid may increase the bladder capacity and facilitate storage. Urinary incontinence is another disorder of storage, occurring most frequently in the aging female. Total incontinence is the continuous leakage of urine with the bladder functioning only as a urinary conduit. However, the most frequently encountered form of urinary incontinence is that of *stress* urinary incontinence. This occurs in females through a loss of closing urethral pressure secondary to loss of pelvic floor support and shortening of the urethral length. Stress incontinence is evidenced by leakage of urine during cough or straining and must be distinguished from urge incontinence, in which the patient has spasm of the bladder musculature as a result of unrecognized stimuli that cause the necessity to void immediately. Techniques devised for the control of stress urinary incontinence in the female consist primarily of urethral lengthening procedures. These may be done either transvaginally or suprapubically. When there is damage to the sphincteric muscle in males, due either to previous operative procedure or to trauma, artificial inflatable urinary sphincters that are under volitional control can be used to restore continence.

VESICAL TRAUMA. Vesical trauma can be divided into (1) trauma with and without pelvic fracture, (2) penetrating injuries, either high- or low-velocity, and (3) iatrogenic trauma. Each requires identification and repair. Cystography is employed in the patient who is suspected of having vesical trauma; retrograde urethrography and cystography should be used to determine the nature and extent of the bladder rupture. When a bladder rupture has been identified, surgical exploration, identification of the defect, sharp excision of the devitalized tissue, and primary repair are appropriate.

Carcinoma of the Bladder

Approximately 90 per cent of all bladder malignancies are transitional cell tumors; hematuria occurs in approximately 75 per cent of these patients. The disease may be confused with urinary tract infection, since hematuria also occurs in acute urinary tract infection. Bladder irritability is a presenting symptom in 30 per cent of patients and is thought to be associated with muscular invasion of the bladder. The treatment is removal of all offending malignancy. Tumor that has not invaded the basement membrane of the epithelial surface may be controlled by transurethral resection, by fulguration, or by use of intravesical agents that promote sloughing of the superficial mucosa. When the disease invades the basement membrane, the disease must be treated by complete resection. This is best accomplished transurethrally, and radical cystectomy is advised for tumor invasion of the muscular layer. Radical cystectomy in the male includes removal of the bladder, prostate, seminal vesicles, and all adjacent perivesical tissues; in the female, radical cystectomy includes the bladder, uterus, tubes, ovaries, anterior vagina, and urethra.

When it is necessary to remove the bladder, the bladder may be replaced by either conduit or continent diversion. In conduit diversion, a segment of either large or small bowel is used merely as a conduit for establishing rapid transit of the urine to the body surface where the urine is collected.

47

THE MALE GENITAL SYSTEM

John L. Weinerth, M.D.

ANATOMY

Unlike the female genital system, parts of the male genital system are conjoined with regard to sexual and excretory functions, specifically, the prostate and the urethra. The components of the male genital tract are the prostate gland, seminal vesicles, Cowper's glands, glands of Littre, the penis with its incorporated urethra, and the scrotum containing the testes, epididymides, vasa deferentia, and spermatic vessels. The male genitourinary system functions for the purposes of copulation, reproduction, hormone production, and urinary excretion.

The prostate gland, seminal vesicles, Cowper's glands, and glands of Littre produce secretions that serve to lubricate the system and provide a vehicle for storage and passage of spermatozoa. In addition, secretions of the seminal vesicles as a base and enzymes from the prostate gland and Cowper's glands conjoin to produce coagulation and subsequent liquefaction of the ejaculate. The penis is composed of two vascular erectile bodies. The corpora cavernosa also incorporate the corpus spongiosum, which contains the male urethra. The paired testes produce both male hormones, predominantly testosterone, and spermatozoa, the former in the interstitial cells and the latter in the seminiferous tubules. The epididymides, lying in intimate contact with the testes, serve as an area of maturation and storage of sperm, which are further transported along the efferent tract composed of the vasa deferentia and the ejaculatory ducts, emptying into the posterior urethra at the verumontanum of the prostate.

The testes are the central organs of male reproduction, two in number, ovoid in form, averaging 4 to 5 cm. in length and 2.5 to 3.5 cm. in width in the normal adult male. The factors that control the descent of the testes from the abdominal cavity into the scrotum are probably mainly hormonal, but there may be some anatomic considerations associated with the poorly defined gubernaculum testis. The descent occurs predominantly during the later phase of gestation but may continue into early childhood.

Since the testes arise from portions of the wolffian body on the genital ridge in proximity to the kidney, it is not surprising that the major blood supply of the testis arises from the aorta just below the renal arteries. Venous drainage of the testis is through multiple veins of the pampiniform plexus to the spermatic vein, usually single, emerging from the upper end of the cord, then following the internal

See the corresponding chapter or part in the *Textbook of Surgery*, 14th edition, pp. 1457–1478, for a more detailed discussion of this topic, including a comprehensive list of references.

spermatic artery through the retroperitoneum. On the right, the spermatic vein empties into the vena cava below the right renal vein; whereas on the left, the spermatic vein empties into the left renal vein. Increased hydrostatic pressure, particularly on the left, may cause dilation of the pampiniform venous plexus, producing a varicocele.

On histologic examination, there are two principal portions of the testis: the seminiferous tubules, which are responsible along with the Sertoli cells for spermatogenesis; and the interstitial or Leydig cells, which elaborate androgenic hormones, predominantly testosterone. Spermatogenesis appears to require relative hypothermia and seminiferous tubule function may be impaired in the cryptorchid or maldescended testis, whereas hormonal function may be unimpaired even in the intra-abdominal undescended testicle.

The epididymides are coiled structures, each containing a single epididymal tubule 12 to 19 feet long and attached to the posterior lateral surface of each testis. The medial surface of each epididymis attaches to the terminal portions of the spermatic cord through which the blood, nerve, and lymphatic supply are received. After the spermatozoa pass from the rete testis via the dozen or more tiny tubular efferent ducts into the epididymis, they progressively pass through the entire length of the epididymis, undergoing maturation and finally storage in the more distal portions. From the tails of the epididymides, sperm are transmitted into the vasa deferentia, which are direct continuations of the duct of the epididymides passing up the spermatic cord, across the inguinal canal, and then retroperitoneally to the ampulla of the seminal vesicles with which they conjoin to form an ejaculatory duct on each side.

The scrotal sac, consisting of two lateral compartments fused in the midline, denoted by the median raphe, encloses the testes, epididymides, and terminal portions of the spermatic cords. The dartos, consisting of elastic fibers, connective tissue, and smooth muscle fibers, is intimately attached to the corrugated skin of the scrotum, rich in sebaceous glands, and provides muscular contraction of the scrotal sac in response to temperature changes or sexual excitation. The blood supply of the scrotum is derived from the deep pudendal branches of the femoral artery and branches of the internal pudendal artery. The lymphatics of the scrotal halves anastomose freely, surround the penis, and drain to the inguinal and femoral nodes.

The seminal vesicles are paired, monotubular, convoluted structures lying beneath the base of the bladder and trigone. The seminal vesicles secrete a mucoid vehicle for the spermatozoa and also elaborate the body's only source of fructose, used as an essential nutrient for maintenance of spermatozoal viability.

The prostate is a fibromuscular glandular organ that surrounds the vesicle neck and the proximal portion of the male urethra. The prostate of a normal young adult male is approximately 20 gm. consisting of two portions, an anterior (inner) group of glands intimately associated with the urethra, and a posterior (outer) portion of more fibromuscular character. Normal prostatic function is dependent on androgens, principally testosterone, which is metabolized to dihydrotestosterone and other substances of similar androgenicity within the prostate.

The anterior (inner) portion, consisting of the periurethral glandular structures, produces the hyperplasia and hypertrophy of benign enlargement in bladder neck obstruction in older men. The posterior segment, however, a musculoglandular structure, is the most frequent origin of prostatic carcinoma. Operations that involve benign hyperplasia and hypertrophy leave the posterior (outer) portion of the gland.

The male urethra consists of two major portions, the posterior urethra and the anterior urethra, each with two subdivisions. Beginning most proximally at the bladder neck, the posterior urethra consists of the prostatic portion and the membranous urethra. The membranous urethra lacks periurethral glands, although Cowper's glands are located in the urogenital diaphragm lateral to the membranous urethra, the site of external or voluntary sphincteric action. The prostatic and membranous portions of the urethra are relatively fixed by the puboprostatic ligaments and the inherent stability of the urogenital diaphragm, whereas the urethra distal to the urogenital diaphragm is relatively mobile.

The penis serves the dual function of copulation and excretion of urine. It consists of two parallel erectile compartments known as the corpora cavernosa, which are situated dorsolaterally, and the corpus spongiosum, which invests the urethra ventrally, terminating distally in the erectile glans penis. The principal blood supply of the penis is through the dorsal arteries that course over the superior portion of the corpora cavernosa, lying deep to Buck's fascia, and being derived initially from the internal pudendal arteries, branches of the internal iliac artery. The venous drainage is through the dorsal veins, the superficial dorsal vein emptying into the saphenous vein, and the deep dorsal vein emptying into the prostatic plexus known as the plexus of Santorini.

Lymphatic drainage of the penis is abundant. The lymphatics from the shaft of the penis, the corpora cavernosa, and the skin pass through the superficial and deep inguinal nodes communicating with the iliac nodes. Lymphatic drainage of the glans penis parallels that of the urethra to the subinguinal, external iliac, and deep pelvic nodes; lymphatics from the urethral mucosa drain to the hypogastric nodes.

TESTES

INFERTILITY. The testes have two primary functions: the production of the major male sex hormone, testosterone, and the production of spermatozoa. Infertility, therefore, can be the consequence of disturbance in either one or both of the primary testicular functions. The inability of a couple to produce offspring is termed infertility or sterility. It is estimated that up to 10 to 15 per cent of marriages in this country are initially barren, approximately half of this number responding to various therapeutic measures.

Infertility may be attributed to the male in as many as 50 per cent of these barren marriages. The principal cause of male infertility is a spermatogenic defect estimated to cause 95 per cent of cases of male infertility or sterility. Most males with such spermatogenic defects produce sperm in some quantity, although there are usually diminished numbers of sperm and those produced are of inadequate quality, exhibiting malformations and diminished motility. Oligospermia, by definition, indicates a sperm count of less than 20 million per ml., and under such circumstances fertility is difficult. Azospermia, complete absence of spermatozoa in the ejaculate, may be the result of total occlusion of the sperm transport system, vasa, seminal vesicles, or ejaculatory ducts.

In some cases, infertility may be due to mechanical factors with no defects in spermatogenesis or delivery of spermatozoa. Operations on the vesicle neck, particularly transurethral resection, open wedge resection, or plastic reconstruction, or treatment of a congenital contracture may cause inability of the vesical neck to close with ejaculation, causing the ejaculate to pass in a retrograde manner into the bladder rather than through the urethra.

CONGENITAL ANOMALIES. The most common congenital anomalies of the testes relate to anomalous location, although congenital absence of one or both testes may be observed. The term *cryptorchidism,* derived from the Greek *cryptos* or hidden, should be reserved for those testes that are truly obscure, usually within the abdominal cavity and not palpable on examination. Cryptorchid or intra-abdominal testes are observed unilaterally or bilaterally in 1 to 10 per cent of male infants. Spermatogenic failure is progressive, and transposition of an intra-abdominal testis to the scrotum should be accomplished before the age of 2 years for ensuring production of normal quantity and quality of spermatozoa.

When it is impossible to bring the testis to a palpable location within the scrotum or low in the inguinal canal, it is generally thought best to remove the testis, since there is a very high incidence of carcinoma in abdominal testes, the incidence perhaps being as much as twenty times greater than that of carcinoma in a normally undescended testis.

Occasionally, one or both testes may undergo excursion in the course of descent, coming to lodge in ectopic positions. The exact cause of such ectopia is obscure but must relate to mechanical factors. Sites of testicular ectopia are symphyseal, prepubic, femoral, crural, penile, or perineal positions. Surgical correction should be accomplished for cosmetic reasons as well as for ensuring normal testicular function and patient comfort.

INFECTIONS. Pyogenic infections of the testis are usually secondary to spread of infection through the male ductal system, the vas deferens, and the epididymis. In rare instances, systemic bacteremia may cause embolic metastatic foci of infection within the testis. Orchitis may follow viral infection in association with mumps, usually after the patient has reached pubescence. Tuberculous orchitis is usually secondary to tuberculosis epididymitis, the primary focus within the urinary tract generally being within the kidneys, sometimes in the prostate.

The patient with an acute testicular infection quickly appears for examination and treatment, since the condition is exquisitely painful. Orchitis must be differentiated from testicular tumor with hemorrhage and from torsion of the spermatic cord, both conditions demanding immediate surgical intervention.

TESTICULAR TUMORS. Neoplasms of the testis are generally malignant, with exceptions being rare fibromas of the tunica vaginalis and pure Leydig cell tumors, which are usually benign. In contrast, extratesticular tumors within the scrotum are usually benign, such as the adenomatoid tumors of the epididymis and cord. Because of this sharp distinction in the potential of neoplasms within the scrotum, diligent physical examination is necessary in distinguishing the site of origin of a scrotal mass.

The malignant germinal tumors of the testis arise from the totipotential cells of seminiferous tubules and constitute a serious threat to the male population, representing 2 per cent of all malignant tumors, the dominant cause of death from genitourinary malignant disease in the younger adult male population. Testicular tumors occur in all ages but predominate in those between the ages of 20 and 35 years. Germinal testicular tumors are categorized according to degree of cellular differentiation, which parallels malignant potential.

The earliest symptom of testicular tumor is a mass in the testicle, unfortunately unrecognized by most patients until there is associated pain, usually of a dull, aching character. The successful treatment of testicular tumors demands scrupulous physical examination, a high index of suspicion, and the willingness to accomplish prompt inguinal exploration when the diagnosis is suggested.

SPERMATIC CORD

TORSION. Torsion of the spermatic cord is probably the result of an abnormally high attachment of the tunica vaginalis around the terminal cord, allowing the testicle to twist freely within the compartment, the bell clapper deformity. Incomplete torsion may cause partial strangulation, the effects of which may be overcome if surgical intervention is accomplished within approximately 12 hours, whereas severe torsion with total compromise of the blood supply is responsible for the loss of testes unless operation is effected within approximately 4 hours.

When torsion is treated on one side, the contralateral scrotum should also be explored; the tunica vaginalis should be opened and inverted around the testis as with hydrocele repair, and any additional defect such as deficient attachment of the epididymis to the testis should be corrected.

EPIDIDYMIDES

EPIDIDYMITIS. Acute nonspecific epididymitis is nongonococcal and nontuberculous, secondary to suppurative infection that usually has its origin in the prostate and seminal vesicles and then spreads in a retrograde manner to the epididymis. It is important to differentiate testicular swelling from epididymitis, since a mass in the testicle always suggests testicular tumor, and to differentiate acute epididymitis from torsion of the spermatic cord. Torsion demands immediate surgical exploration, whereas epididymitis is treated by conservative measures.

Treatment of epididymitis consists of bed rest, elevation and support of the scrotum, application of cold packs, antipyretics, anti-inflammatory agents, and appropriate antimicrobial agents, sometimes administered intravenously. Occasionally, suppurative epididymitis may localize into an abscess and drain spontaneously; usually surgical intervention should be avoided unless testicular abscess develops.

TUNICA VAGINALIS

The tunica vaginalis, derived from the peritoneum as the processus vaginalis at the time of testicular descent, is a secretory membrane. Fluid is generated by the serous surface of the tunica vaginalis, fluid formation being enhanced by inflammation or trauma. Fluid within the tunica vaginalis is resorbed at a constant rate through the extensive venous and lymphatic systems of the spermatic cord. Hydrocele, the excessive accumulation of this serous fluid, results when there is increased production or decreased resorption, the latter condition usually being idiopathic. Congenital hydrocele, particularly with associated hernia, demands surgical repair, accomplished through a high inguinal incision giving access to the internal inguinal ring, at which point the hernia sac or processus vaginalis is ligated. In older patients, a hydrocele is frequently secondary to epididymo-orchitis or trauma. If active pyogenic infection is present, the hydrocele may become infected, demanding surgical incision and drainage.

PROSTATE GLAND

PROSTATIC INFECTION. Prostatic infections constitute a significant fraction of urologic practice. Infectious agents that may involve the prostate gland include the spectrum of gram-negative organisms, gram-positive cocci, gonococci, various mycotic organisms, mycobacteria, trichomonads, and *Chlamydia* and *Candida* species. The ascending transurethral route of infection is usual, and exogenous infection is enhanced by urethral abnormalities. Hematogenous and lymphatic routes of access to the prostate as well as descending infection from the upper urinary tract have been described, especially with tuberculosis.

Before antibiotic therapy, prostatic abscesses were frequent sequelae of acute prostatitis, but they are encountered less frequently today. Surgical drainage of prostatic abscesses is required and may be accomplished by transurethral incision and resection, perineal incision and drainage, aspiration, or massage.

BENIGN PROSTATIC HYPERPLASIA. Benign prostatic overgrowth is the most common cause of bladder outlet obstruction in males over 50 years of age. Whereas exact mechanisms of prostatic hyperplasia are incompletely understood, it is recognized that adolescent development of the glandular acini and the fibromuscular matrix of the prostate is stimulated by gonadotropins and the androgens of the interstitial cells of the testes. As the enlargement progresses, the prostatic urethra may become elongated, and the caliber of the prostatic portion of the urethra may actually increase. However, the adenomatous process causes compression of the prostatic urethra, restricting the free flow of urine, sometimes associated with actual mechanical intrusion of a median lobe at the vesical outlet.

The symptoms of benign prostatic hyperplasia are those of mechanical obstruction and the consequences of urinary stasis. Urinary bleeding may first bring the patient to the attention of the physician. Hematuria may follow prostatic enlargement with engorgement of the small mucosal vessels covering the adenomatous gland, ruptured as a consequence of straining to urinate. With progressive amounts of residual urine, infection may occur with purulent cystitis. Similarly, vesical stasis of urine can predispose to the formation of bladder calculi with severe symptoms of dysuria and strangury.

Conservative and medical measures of managing benign prostatic enlargement with bladder outlet obstruction are generally unsuccessful. Prostatic massage and urethral dilation are of little value unless there is demonstrated substantial congestion and stricture formation, respectively.

There are standard surgical procedures for removal of the obstructing enlarged portion of the prostate gland. None of these procedures constitutes total prostatectomy, all being designed for removal of the adenomatous hyperplastic portion of the gland lying centrally and periurethrally. These procedures should most properly be termed prostatic adenectomy rather than prostatectomy, since the true prostate, compressed laterally into a fibromuscular and acinar surgical capsule, is retained after removal of the central adenomatous elements and may be the source of later carcinoma of the prostate.

CARCINOMA OF THE PROSTATE. Adenocarcinoma of the prostate is the most common malignant disease of males, and the incidence has increased. Cancer of the prostate is now the most prevalent cancer in males by the most recent American Cancer Society statistics. It barely exceeds cancer of the lung with 21 per cent of all male cancers. Autopsy studies have established the fact that prostatic carcinoma, occult or overt, is present in about 15 per cent of men over the age of 50 years. It is estimated that the prevalence of prostatic carcinoma may be as high as 48 cases per 100,000 population at present. As the geriatric population increases, an increase may be expected.

Prostatic carcinoma most often arises in glandular acini of

the peripheral group of glands located in the posterior and posterolateral regions of the prostate. One of the unique qualities of prostatic carcinoma is that many tumors produce an enzyme, acid phosphatase, that can be detected in the serum of patients with metastatic disease. Serum acid phosphatase has many sources, but the addition of tartrate to the serum inhibits over 90 per cent of the prostatic contribution and thereby separates the prostatic acid phosphatase from the total acid phosphatase.

The prostate gland is also known to be the source of fibrinolytic factors. Normal seminal fluid has significant fibrinolytic activity, possibly enhancing motility of the sperm, attributed to the release of fibrinolytic activators from prostatic epithelium.

Unfortunately, early symptoms of prostatic carcinoma are infrequent. Since the majority of prostatic tumors occur in the periphery of the gland, encroachment on the urethra is a late manifestation of the disease. In essence, the diagnosis of prostatic carcinoma must be based on suspicion. Every male over the age of 50 should have a regular rectal examination, and the findings of areas of induration and irregularity should suggest the diagnosis. In advanced cases of local disease, there is usually little doubt as to the diagnosis. The prostate becomes nodular and irregular with extension of the indurated process beyond the confines of the gland, culminating in fixation of the prostate to the surrounding pelvic structures.

Prostatic carcinoma can metastasize by local extension, by hematologic dissemination, or by lymphatic invasion and may occur early even with a very small lesion, although generally the size of the primary lesion correlates with degree of metastatic extent of the disease. The current treatment of prostatic carcinoma is selected on the basis of accurate anatomic definition of the stage of the disease. It is the general view that local disease that has not extended beyond the confines of the prostate is best treated by surgical extirpation.

Radical prostatectomy involving removal of the entire prostate and the seminal vesicles can constitute cure only when the malignant process is confined to the prostate with no contiguous or distant spread. Prostatectomy can be accomplished in the classic perineal operation or by the retropubic approach during which both pelvic lymphadenectomy and radical prostatectomy can be performed simultaneously if the surgeon is willing to base surgical decisions on a frozen section of the lesion.

Observations by Huggins and associates more than 40 years ago led to the recognition of the androgen dependency of a large percentage of prostatic tumors and the therapeutic response of these tumors to estrogen administration. These observations and subsequent investigations demonstrated the efficacy of hormonal management and provided the basis for the first genuinely effective chemotherapeutic approach to malignant disease. Whereas hormonal manipulation cannot effect cure of prostatic carcinoma, excellent prolonged tumor control can be achieved. A new area of adjunctive therapy is the use of multiple chemotherapeutic agents. A number of agents including 5-fluorouracil, estramustine phosphate, and *cis*-platinum have been used in various protocols with some success in terms of partial objective and subjective responses. Considering the rapid development of new chemotherapeutic agents, this is an area that may have the greatest impact over the next 10 years on the treatment of metastatic prostatic carcinoma and even as an adjunctive treatment for localized disease.

MALE URETHRA

CONGENITAL ABNORMALITIES. Congenital abnormalities in the male urethra occur in the bladder neck, prostatic urethra, membranous urethra, bulbous urethra, pendulous urethra, or meatus. The most common distal abnormality is urethral meatal stenosis, which can usually be diagnosed by inspection and suspected when the urinary stream is of poor caliber.

In the area of the prostatic urethra, congenital valves occur, usually causing severe obstructive uropathy with decompensation of the urinary bladder, hydroureteronephrosis, infection, and renal insufficiency unless prompt and adequate treatment is instituted.

Hypospadias is another anomaly of the urethra that involves varying degrees of failure of complete development of the distal urethra. The urethra may terminate just proximal to the glans (glandular hypospadias), at some point along the penile shaft (penile hypospadias), at the anterior margin of the scrotum (penoscrotal hypospadias), or in the perineum with a bifid scrotum (perineal hypospadias). Associated with this defect is a severe ventral curvature of the penis, or chordee, which is produced by a fibrous band occurring in the projected course of the urethra.

Epispadias is the failure of development of the anterior wall of the urethra and concomitant failure of dorsal fusion of the penile corpora. Complete vesical exstrophy, a rare condition, is always associated with epispadias. Epispadias alone with some degree of urinary continence is more commonly seen although still infrequently.

Traumatic injury of the urethra commonly occurs in association with pelvic fractures but also can occur with injuries to the perineum, gunshot or stab wounds, or iatrogenic injury from instrumentation. Shearing injuries induced by external forces during blunt trauma cause rupture at the urogenital diaphragm in the region of the membranous urethra. Urinary extravasation is noted, often with extensive pelvic hemorrhage. The prostate and bladder may be displaced superiorly, away from the distal urethra. Depending on the circumstances, either open surgical repair or temporizing suprapubic urinary diversion should be accomplished promptly. The diagnosis of urethral rupture must be suspected in every instance of pelvic injury, and unless the patient is able to void clear urine normally, retrograde urethrography should be performed in an aseptic manner to determine the patency and competence of the urethra.

TRAUMA. Penetrating injuries of the urethra are also observed, most commonly due to shotgun or stab wounds. Immediate urethral reconstruction and urinary diversion by suprapubic cystostomy is appropriate. Iatrogenic perforation or rupture of the urethra may occur in the course of instrumentation, cystoscopy, or urethral dilation. Pre-existing urethral strictures due to trauma or gonococcal urethritis predispose to difficult instrumentation and potential perforation of the urethra, often followed by the establishment of a urethral diverticulum or false urinary passage. Periurethral abscesses and attendant complications may ensue unless urethral injury of this type is recognized and promptly treated.

URETHRAL MALIGNANT DISEASE. Carcinoma of the male urethra is rare, with less than 1000 cases being documented in the English literature. Those malignant lesions occurring in the distal penile portion of the urethra are most often squamous cell carcinoma, whereas the more proximal tumors are transitional cell lesions. Spread of malignancy is by lymphatics of the corpus spongiosum into the deep pelvic nodes and by venous channels. Depending on the location of the lesion, partial urethrectomy with or without penectomy may be effective, as well as possible anterior exenteration and lymphadenectomy.

PENIS

PENILE MALIGNANT DISEASE. Cancer of the penis is a rare tumor in the United States. It has a much higher proportion in populations where circumcision and personal hygiene are not well established. The most common form of cancer of the penis is squamous cell carcinoma, although basal cell carcinoma and melanoma have been described. Squamous cell carcinoma constitutes a more difficult challenge and is generally associated with chronic balanoposthitis from lack of circumcision, although occasional cases of penile carcinoma have been reported in circumcised individuals.

The diagnosis is established by biopsy, and treatment consists of partial or total penectomy. A proximal margin free of tumor of at least 1.5 cm. is desirable. Inguinal node dissection with excision of both superficial and deep inguinal nodes is advocated when clinically palpable nodes persist after amputation. Chemotherapeutic efforts have been attempted with bleomycin either locally or systemically, or in conjunction with other agents for very small lesions and carcinoma *in situ*, or as an adjunct to systemic disease.

SPECIAL CONDITIONS. Certain peculiar disorders of the penis or of penile function deserve special consideration, particularly since etiologic factors remain obscure in these disorders. A localized induration of the fibrous investments of the penile shaft was first described by Peyronie more than 100 years ago. Despite adequate description and an abundance of clinical observation, the cause of the condition is unknown. A firm fibrotic thickening of the fascia of the corpora cavernosa is present, usually involving the dorsolateral aspects of the penile shaft or the intracavernous septum between the corpora cavernosa, histologically similar to keloid or Dupuytren's contracture.

Patients usually note the lesion by self-examination, and they may have experienced significant deviation of the penis that interferes with intromission and coitus. If the patient is totally disabled and has long-term resistant disease, excision of the plaque with skin grafting with or without the insertion of penile prostheses has been advocated.

Prolonged pathologic and painful erection of the penis is termed priapism, in recognition of the Greek god of sexual excess, Priapus. Pelvic venous thrombosis predisposes to priapism, and such thrombosis is observed with metastatic malignant diseases of various types, leukemia, pelvic trauma, sickle cell disease or trait, trauma to the corpora, or spinal cord injury. In the majority of patients, no definite etiologic factor can be identified, and both local and neurovascular abnormalities have been incriminated as possible causes. Prompt recognition and therapy is essential, since prolonged unrelieved priapism almost inevitably causes subsequent permanent impotence from fibrosis of the corpora cavernosa.

Although it is recognized that the aging process diminishes not only the libido but the capacity of erection as well, many males remain potent throughout their lifetime. Disease may well affect the ability of a male to be potent, and such should be carefully sought. Arteriosclerotic cardiovascular disease may compromise circulation to the corpora, and in addition, many drugs used to treat hypertension and cardiovascular disease may have a secondary effect on the ability to maintain an erection. Diabetes and other systemic disorders producing generalized neuropathies may diminish ability for erection.

Psychological consultation is mandatory when the various physical causes of impotence have been eliminated. The use of nocturnal penile tumescence studies has been helpful in distinguishing some patients with purely psychological reasons for impotence from physiologic causes.

INTERSEX STATES

The intersex state is that congenital condition in which there is ambiguity of the external genitalia or inadequate and incomplete differentiation in gonadal and ductal structures. The most common mode of presentation of the intersex patient is by request for sexual differentiation in the neonatal nursery. Ambiguity of the external genitalia necessitates prompt and definitive assignment of sex, reassurance of parents, and early mobilization of medical and surgical measures required for establishing the appropriate sex of the child. On occasion, the intersex patient may be seen rather late, often because of microphallus, undescended testes, labial fusion, or clitoral hypertrophy seen as late as pubescence. There are a number of definitive texts and monographs that discuss the various types of intersex.

48

DISORDERS OF THE LYMPHATIC SYSTEM

Ralph G. DePalma, M.D.

Primary disorders of the lymphatic system amenable to direct surgical correction are uncommon, yet effective treatment exists for certain patients with particularly challenging problems.

LYMPHEDEMA

Primary lymphedema occurs in the absence of acquired diseases damaging the lymphatic system and usually affects the lower limbs. Edema may be present at birth or begin later in life. Lymphedema usually begins at puberty. Most patients are female. Lymphedema presenting at birth is *lymphedema congenita*. When, as is most common, edema begins before the age of 35 years, the term *lymphedema praecox* is used. Lymphedema beginning after the age of 35 years is termed *lymphedema tarda*. Milroy's disease, a congenital familial lymphedema, follows vertical autosomal inheritance of a single gene. Males are affected as frequently as are females. Milroy's disease comprises less than 2 per cent of primary lymphedemas. When lymphedema appears in a single limb, the most important differential diagnoses include lymphoma, malignancy involving iliac and lumbar lymph nodes, and venous occlusion. In primary lymphedemas, lymphangiography usually documents defective lymphatic development. Swelling often begins spontaneously but can be precipitated by trauma, pregnancy, infection, insect bites, or episodes of cellulitis.

Primary lymphedema is sometimes associated with developmental deformities including gonadal dysgeneses such as Turner's syndrome. Certain individuals with megalymphatics exhibit patches of blood capillary angiomas of the skin and some exhibit overgrowth of bones of the involved limb. However, hypoplasia of the lymphatics exists in 90 per cent of patients with primary lymphedema. Most involve the distal rather than the proximal lymphatics. A diffuse increase in the size and number of the lymphatics of both lower limbs, that is, megalymphatics associated with hyperplasia of the abdominal vessels and nodes, causes chylous reflux lymphedema.

Secondary lymphedema is due to trauma and wounds involving the lymph pathways, malignant disease, filariasis, infections and inflammations, and radiation. Ulceration is rare in lymphedema; however, a common cause of lymphedema is chronic venous ulceration causing episodes of

---

See the corresponding chapter or part in the *Textbook of Surgery*, 14th edition, pp. 1479–1489, for a more detailed discussion of this topic, including a comprehensive list of references.

lymphangitis that obliterate normal lymph channels. Patients prone to recurrent attacks of lymphangitis are best treated with intermittent long-term antibiotic therapy used at the first sign of infection. Lymphedema of the upper extremity was commonly secondary to radical mastectomy, which removes the axillary nodes *en bloc*. Defects in healing and concomitant infection and fibrosis obliterate remaining lymphatics. A lesser incidence of lymphedema now occurs with modified radical mastectomy.

TREATMENT. Treatment is usually conservative. Overall, only 15 per cent of patients eventually require surgical therapy. Late prognosis is determined by the location of hypoplastic lymphatics. Severe lymphedema seldom develops in patients with distal hypoplasia and adequate pelvic lymph nodes. Nonoperative measures have the goals of minimizing the risk of infection and reducing the subcutaneous fluid volume. The most trivial skin complications are treated for preventing infection that might further damage lymph channels. The patient should be fitted with graduated compression support stockings (40 to 60 mm. Hg pressure at ankle) after the limb has achieved maximal reduction by use of elevation and sequential pneumatic compression. The support stockings are removed at night, and the bed is raised to maintain the legs above the level of the right atrium.

Sequential pneumatic compression devices are particularly useful for control of lymphedema; although home use is possible, initial treatment may require 1 to 3 days of hospitalization. Diuretics are not prescribed unless in women excess fluid is retained in the premenstrual period. Eczema is treated with triamcinolone 0.05 to 0.1 per cent while fungal lesions are treated with specific agents. Occasionally, lymph-producing fistulas and vesicles appear which sometimes require excision. Secondary lymphedema requires specific therapy for the underlying disease process.

Operations for treatment of lymphedema are excisional or physiologic. Excisional operations remove excess skin and subcutaneous tissue and are based on the principle that the subfascial tissues are unaffected by lymphedema. Currently, these operations offer one solution to the problem of massive limb enlargement. An alternative to surgical therapy is hospitalization and intensive therapy with sequential compression. Among excisional operations, free skin grafts are employed to cover the lower leg after excision of lymphedematous tissue. This operation is applicable when local skin is in poor condition and not, as is common in topical lymphedemas, suitable for flaps. Other reducing operations elevate thick flaps with good blood supply, then underlying lymphedematous tissue is excised. Servelle emphasizes the need for preoperative venography for assuring normal venous drainage. Kinmonth's modification of Homan's procedure is most commonly used.

LYMPHANGITIS AND LYMPHADENITIS

Lymphangitis, an inflammation of the peripheral lymphatics, appears as erythematous streaks progressively coursing toward regional lymph nodes. Brawny distal edema develops owing to coagulation of lymph within the vessels. Lymphangitis is most frequently caused by hemolytic streptococci but can also occur with staphylococcal infections. With ascending lymphangitis, there is usually little pus and incision is contraindicated unless a distal purulent accumulation such as a paronychia or an infected blister exists. Lymphangitis is treated with rest for decreasing lymph flow, local heat, elevation, and specific antibiotics. Since *beta-hemolytic streptococci* are the common infecting organisms, penicillin is usually first employed.

Enlargement of the regional lymph nodes draining areas of infection is the usual reaction to sepsis. Common regional viral lymphadenopathies include lymphogranuloma venereum, cat scratch fever, and cytomegalovirus infections. Human immunodeficiency virus infection has emerged as a common cause of lymphadenopathy. Among the chronic indolent adenopathies are tuberculosis and fungal infections such as sporotrichosis or toxoplasmosis. With suppuration of lymph nodes, the infecting agent must be sought from among a vast number of organisms.

Before excision of lymph nodes, the patient must be examined completely for the detection of foci of infection or tumors. Computed axial tomography is quite useful. If a focus of infection is detected, antibiotic therapy and the observation of regression of adenopathy suffice. There has been a trend toward delayed use of cervical lymph node biopsy when malignancy is improbable because so many of these nodes simply exhibit reactive hyperplasia. When the abnormal nodes are supraclavicular in location, prompt excisional biopsy is recommended. Persistent generalized adenopathy due to human immunodeficiency virus is a prodrome of acquired immunodeficiency syndrome. The syndrome is defined as lymphadenopathy of at least 3 months' duration involving two or more extrainguinal sites and absence of other illness or drug use causing lymphadenopathy. Serologic testing for human immunodeficiency virus infection should be done if indicated.

Fine-needle aspiration is often preferable to biopsy for initial diagnosis of cervical lymphadenopathy and often averts the need for open biopsies. Whenever there is a need for lymph node excision, the involved nodes should be excised by an incision in the skin lines. When anterior cervical nodes appear to be matted, extensive or adherent to vessels and deep structures, excision is more safely done under general anesthesia. Posterior cervical nodes can be more easily removed under local anesthesia.

LYMPHATIC TUMORS

Benign lymphatic tumors of childhood appear in the axilla, shoulders, and groin. Most are of developmental origin and are noted at birth. These are classified as (1) simple and capillary lymphangiomas, (2) cavernous lymphangiomas, and (3) cystic hygromas, which are most common.

Diffuse or localized lymphangiomas of the skin appear as vesicles localizing on the inner side of the thigh, on the axilla, or on the shoulder. If lymphangiography reveals that the lesion is separate from the main lymphatic system, these can be excised. Diffuse and cavernous lymphangiomas often involve the face and mouth to cause enlargement of the lips and alarming swelling of the tongue. On occasion, these tumors in children demand emergency surgical intervention for maintenance of the airway.

The most common lymphangioma, cystic hygroma, exhibits large cystlike cavities containing clear, watery fluid. The lesion usually transilluminates. Occasionally, hemorrhage within the cyst renders the mass tense and opaque. Most cystic hygromas present in the neck; 20 per cent are observed in the axillary region, and the remaining 5 per cent are seen in the mediastinum, retroperitoneum, pelvis, and groin. Two or 3 per cent of the cervical hygromas have mediastinal extensions extending as far as the diaphragm. Cystic hygromas are treated by operative excision. Cyst walls appear in juxtaposition to the carotid artery, jugular vein, brachial plexus, vagus nerves, and other deep structures. Cystic hygroma is not a malignant neoplasm, and normal anatomy need not be sacrificed.

LYMPHANGIOSARCOMA

Lymphangiosarcoma is a rare malignant tumor occurring in long-standing cases of primary or acquired lymphedema of the extremities. The classic description of Stewart and Treves emphasized its usual occurrence in postmastectomy arm lymphedema, but the tumor also occurs in the legs. The malignancy first appears as a bruise mark, a purplish discoloration, or a tender skin nodule in the chronically lymphedematous extremity. Early lesions appear first on the anterior surface of the extremity, progressing to ulcers with crusting and then to necrosis that extends to involve the skin and subcutaneous tissue. The lesion progresses and metastasizes widely and is uniformly fatal.

CHYLOUS EFFUSIONS AND LYMPHATIC LEAKS

The most common causes of lymphatic leaks are trauma, malignant disease, primary hyperplastic lymphatic deformities, and filariasis. Chronic chyle loss threatens nutrition and immune competence. Intravenous alimentation and oral feeding with medium-chain triglycerides are required until the chyle leaks can be controlled.

Lymph also leaks through vesicles of the extremities and scrotum in rare instances of developmental lymphangiomas. When megalymphatics continue to drain, dilated incompetent lymph pathways are located proximal to the leak. Abnormal thoracic duct anatomy appears to be a factor in some cases. Surgical operations for dividing and ligating incompetent lymph pathways are facilitated by preoperative milk ingestion on the day before operation or by preoperative injection of dye into the extremity.

Lymphoceles rarely present in the groin as primary complications of developmental lymphatic disease and should not be excised. Postoperative lymphoceles in the femoral triangle are due to disruption of nodes and lymphatics when a vascular graft has been placed in this area. Lymphoceles also occur in the subclavian and supraclavicular areas. Sterile lymph effusion does not require open drainage; open drainage is contraindicated because this will cause infection of the vascular graft. Repeated aspirations and application of pressure dressings for several weeks generally resolve this problem.

49

VENOUS DISORDERS
M. Wayne Flye, M.D., Ph.D.

The pathophysiology of venous disease is in some respects more complex than that of arterial disease. With the exception of aneurysm formation, obstruction is responsible for almost all the physiologic aberrations characteristic of arterial disease. On the other hand, venous disorders involve both obstruction and valvular insufficiency. Moreover, the disability from venous disease includes not only regional problems but also those that are caused by the escape of thrombi into the pulmonary circulation. Varicose veins with their associated symptoms and complications constitute the most common vascular disorder of the lower extremities. More than 20 million people in the United States alone are significantly affected. Most of these have either symptoms or complications from chronic venous insufficiency, and a substantial number suffer from the resulting economic hardship.

ANATOMIC AND PHYSIOLOGIC CONSIDERATIONS

Unlike arteries, veins are divided into a superficial and a deep system. Among the thick-walled superficial veins are the greater and lesser saphenous veins of the leg, the cephalic and basilic veins of the arm, and the external jugular veins of the neck. The deep veins, in contrast, are thin-walled, less muscular, and protected by the muscles and deep fascia. Perforating veins connect the deep and superficial systems by passing through the fascial layer that invests the deep system. Normally, the delicate valves in the venous system partition the column of blood from ankle to atrium that, if unopposed, would potentially exert a gravitation force at the ankle of 110 to 120 mm. Hg. Even modest motion, such as shifting weight, however, contracts the calf muscles and forces blood toward the heart in the valved venous system. When venous valves are incompetent, the resulting hydrostatic column of blood is longer and there is immediate retrograde venous filling with muscle contraction. The venous pressure of the lower leg therefore remains abnormally high, and encourages the development of dependent edema. According to the Starling concept, return of fluid escaping from the arteriolar end of a capillary to the circulation at the venular end is facilitated by lower venous pressures. Normally, the little swelling that accumulates during the day disappears overnight when the body is horizontal. In the abnormal state, greater edema formation resolves more slowly and predisposes to chronic venous stasis changes.

See the corresponding chapter or part in the *Textbook of Surgery*, 14th edition, pp. 1490–1501, for a more detailed discussion of this topic, including a comprehensive list of references.

CLINICAL MANIFESTATIONS

Varicose veins, venous thrombosis, and venous valvular incompetence with venous stasis are the most common venous disorders seen in clinical practice. *Varicose veins* are dilated, elongated veins in the superficial regions of the legs. Dilations of the smaller, cutaneous venules are somewhat different and are called spider veins. Some degree of varicose vein formation is present in half the adult population. The precise etiology of varicose veins is unclear, but the following factors contribute to their development: heredity, congenitally defective venous valves, trauma, hormonal factors in women, increased abdominal pressure in pregnancy, and arteriovenous fistulas.

The patient's complaints vary with the type and size of the varicose veins. Symptoms range from cosmetic dissatisfaction to intractable pain. The pain and aching are characteristically dull, never occur in bed or early in the morning, usually begin in the afternoon after a long period of standing, and are promptly relieved by leg elevation. Nocturnal cramps may be associated with edema, which recedes at night when the patient is recumbent. Itching is a manifestation of local cutaneous stasis and precedes the onset of dermatitis. A burning sensation over the varicose veins is probably caused by local pressure on cutaneous sensory nerves (Table 1).

Thrombosis of the deep veins is the common pathway to both the immediate problem of pulmonary embolism and the chronic insidious disability produced by venous stasis disease. Factors predisposing to venous thrombosis include (1) stasis of blood, (2) local venous trauma, and (3) systemic coagulation abnormalities (Virchow's triad).

The diagnosis of *superficial thrombophlebitis* is usually easily made. It presents with pain and red linear streaks over the distribution of a tender venous cord. The pain increases with extremity dependency and palpation. This type of thrombophlebitis most commonly occurs at the site of an intravenous infusion but also occurs frequently in the greater saphenous system below the knee in patients with varicose veins. In contrast, the diagnosis of *deep venous thrombosis* is more difficult. An accurate clinical diagnosis is made only in about half the cases. Positive physical findings may include (1) unilateral ankle edema, (2) pretibial venous distention or an increased venous pattern of collateral veins over the upper thigh and groin, (3) increased circumference of the calf or thigh, (4) tenderness over the femoral vein or behind the knee, and (5) discomfort with forceful dorsiflexion of the foot (Homan's sign).

Deep venous thrombosis causes significant swelling of the affected extremity by partially occluding venous outflow. When more complete venous occlusion occurs, phlegmasia alba dolens or phlegmasia cerulea dolens may result. *Phlegmasia alba dolens* ("milk leg") usually occurs in postpartum women and produces a cool, pale, and swollen limb with nonpalpable pulses. Therapy for venous thrombosis will generally produce the return of arterial perfusion. In contrast, the near-total venous occlusion of *phlegmasia cerulea dolens*

TABLE 1. Venous Disorders

Disorder	Symptoms and Signs	Tests	Treatment	Morbidity
Varicose veins	Dilated tortuous superficial veins Tired, aching legs relieved by elevation	Clinical examination	Elastic support hose Injection sclerotherapy Ligation and stripping of superficial veins	Pain Cosmetic Chronic venous insufficiency
Superficial venous thrombosis	Tender, erythematous, warm cord with local swelling	Clinical examination	Leg elevation Hot compresses Analgesics Excision of purulent phlebitis	Recurrent phlebitis Propagation to deep system Chronic venous valvular insufficiency
Deep venous thrombosis	May be asymptomatic; otherwise, swelling, tenderness, aching, positive Homan's sign	Perthes' test Ascending venography (phlebography) Duplex Doppler Impedance plethysmography ^{125}I-labeled fibrinogen	Absolute bed rest Heparin until asymptomatic, 7–14 days, then Coumadin for 3–6 months Elastic compressive hose Vena caval filter if anticoagulation ineffective or contraindicated Venous thrombectomy for phlegmasia cerulea dolens	Pulmonary embolus Phlegmasia alba dolens ("milk leg") Phlegmasia cerulea dolens (venous gangrene) Postphlebitic syndrome

688

Postthrombotic venous insufficiency (postphlebitic syndrome)	Venous hypertension Brownish, atrophic, indurated, often ulcerated skin—most commonly around ankle Heavy feeling to severe chronic pain	Brodie-Trendelenburg test Venous pressure at rest and at exercise Duplex Doppler ultrasound imaging Descending venography	For edema: Fitted compressive stockings Leg elevation often Meticulous skin care For ulceration: Compressive zinc oxide boot (Unna's boot) Bed rest Ligation of incompetent venous perforators Modified Linton procedure Venous valve reconstruction	Limb disability Nonhealing ulcers Chronic infection

(venous gangrene) produces rapidly rising pressure within the affected extremity and eventual obstruction of arterial inflow. This condition is diagnosed by sudden intense pain, massive edema, and cyanosis. Amputation may be necessary in about 50 per cent of untreated cases. If there is no immediate response to elevation of the extremity and heparinization, venous thrombectomy should be considered.

CHRONIC VENOUS INSUFFICIENCY. The edema that immediately follows deep venous thrombosis is purely obstructive in origin and quickly subsides with bed rest and anticoagulants, allowing recanalization and the development of venous collaterals. However, if recanalization traps the delicate venous valves, the valveless deep venous system transmits the gravitational pressure of the blood column unimpeded from the level of the heart to the ankles. This increased pressure is the central predisposing feature in the pathophysiology of the postphlebitic state.

Valvular incompetence alone is not enough to produce serious stasis sequelae. Instead, it must occur with incompetent perforator veins through which the high deep venous pressure in the ambulatory state is transmitted to the superficial tissues. The location of these perforating veins determines the predilection of stasis changes and ulcers to the area extending from the malleoli up the lower half of the leg. These perforators may have been involved in the initial thrombosis or may become incompetent by dilation caused by the back pressure of the valveless deep venous system. Within 10 years of untreated thrombophlebitis, 75 per cent of patients will develop advanced stasis changes, and 50 per cent will have had stasis ulcers.

In chronic venous insufficiency, when the deep venous hypertension is finally transmitted into the superficial veins and tissues, edema recurs when the patient is upright for any significant period of time. The edema associated with peripheral venous disease, even in the acute stage, does not "pit" readily. In the chronic stage, it is frankly "brawny" and associated with characteristic skin changes caused by chronic venous hypertension. Unfortunately, these changes are subtle and gradual at first, and the patient comes to accept a degree of swelling, discoloration, and aching in the involved leg. It is often not until after some minor trauma leading to a skin break that an actual stasis ulcer develops.

DIAGNOSIS

Whereas superficial varicosities are apparent on physical examination, additional studies are necessary for evaluating the patency of the deep venous system and valvular competency. In fact, the deep system is usually patent if there is no history of deep venous thrombosis. Historically, the *Perthes' test*, total compression of the superficial varicosities, caused increasingly severe crampy pain when a deep venous obstruction was present. Currently, venous plethysmography and Doppler flow studies can be used to detect deep venous thrombosis. Doppler flow studies are preferable because they can detect not only deep venous thrombosis but also post-thrombotic venous collateral veins and postphlebitic valvular insufficiency. However, the accuracy of Doppler studies is best in the thigh and is not as reliable in the calf.

The *Brodie-Trendelenburg test* was the first scientific attempt at evaluation of valve function. After the veins of the leg are emptied, an elastic tourniquet is adjusted around the thigh just below the saphenofemoral junction to occlude the superficial veins. Upon standing, rapid venous refilling after release of the tourniquet suggests incompetent valves in the saphenous system. Filling of the superficial veins before release of the tourniquet indicates that incompetent valves are also present in some of the perforating veins.

Currently, there are several noninvasive tests available for identifying deep venous occlusion including Doppler ultrasound, venous outflow plethysmography, venous volume plethysmography (phleborheography), and B-mode scanning (Table 2). The simplest and most available method is the venous Doppler examination. Absence of a normal respiratory pattern suggests a venous obstruction. This test is very accurate in evaluating the popliteal veins and those more proximal. The anatomic positions of the deep femoral vein, the internal iliac vein, and the soleal sinuses are not easily evaluated by the Doppler. Addition of B-mode scanning to Doppler ultrasonography allows visualization of the veins with duplex scanning.

By use of the directional Doppler, valvular incompetence is indicated by reverse venous flow. However, the degree of venous insufficiency cannot be quantitated. The initial evaluation of a patient with suspected deep venous thrombosis or chronic venous insufficiency should be by noninvasive tests, but venography may be required to resolve confusing noninvasive results or to delineate the precise location of valvular incompetence. Whereas ascending venography is the most reliable method of documenting the presence and extent of venous thrombosis, descending venography is useful in identifying incompetent valves.

TREATMENT OF VARICOSE VEINS

Both surgical and nonsurgical methods are used in the management of superficial varicose veins. In general, the surgical removal of incompetent veins is the more definitive treatment, and the results are more satisfactory and lasting. However, excision of varicose veins has decreased in frequency in order to preserve the saphenous vein for reconstructive vascular procedures. Nonsurgical methods are reserved for patients who have medical contraindications to surgical treatment, deep venous insufficiency, or very minimal varicosities. These nonsurgical methods include sclerotherapy, elastic support, periodic elevation of the lower extremity, and exercise of the leg muscles. Normal prominent superficial veins should not be disturbed or destroyed. Before any treatment is advised, the severity of the varicose problem must be carefully assessed.

TABLE 2. Diagnostic Venous Tests

Test	Positive Finding	Limitation
Noninvasive Tests—Deep Venous Thrombosis		
Doppler ultrasound	Absence of normal respiratory pattern	Most accurate in veins proximal to popliteal veins Can miss nonocclusive thrombosis
Impedance venous outflow plethysmography (increased blood volume, decreased electrical resistance)	Decreased rate of leg venous volume emptying	Decreased sensitivity with calf vein thrombosis alone and without proximal obstruction
Venous volume plethysmography (phleborheography)	Absence of limb volume changes to respiration and compression maneuvers	Recanalization or collateral flow gives approx. 5% false-negative and 15% false-positive exams
Noninvasive Tests—Chronic Venous Valvular Insufficiency		
Bidirectional Doppler	Reversed flow in femoral and popliteal veins and at saphenofemoral junction	Cannot quantitate degree of venous insufficiency

Photoplethysmography	Incompetent venous valves result in shorter capillary refilling time	Accurate tourniquet placement is necessary for differentiating superficial from deep venous valvular insufficiency Requires experienced examiner
Duplex scan (B-mode scan and Doppler ultrasound)	Provides direct anatomic and flow evaluation of venous thrombosis and chronic venous insufficiency Most frequently used test	
^{125}I-labeled fibrinogen	Increased localized radioactivity indicates fresh thrombus formation	Requires re-evaluation over 2–4 days
Invasive Testing		
Ascending venography (phlebography)	Most reliable method for documenting presence and extent of venous thrombosis Identifies incompetent venous valves	Does not visualize pelvic veins well
Descending venography ^{125}I-radiolabeled fibrinogen	Detects actively forming deep vein thrombosis	Requires an experienced radiologist Costly and requires 48- to 72-hour delay in establishing diagnosis Only 60–80% of pelvic and groin thrombi detected

Surgical therapy may be performed for cosmetic reasons or for relief of symptoms but should be designed to correct abnormal venous hemodynamics. Little more than visual inspection is required to diagnose varicose veins. Before they can be treated intelligently, however, the surgeon should be aware of the functional status of the deep iliofemoral vein and perforating vein valves. The ideal patient for varicose vein surgery is one who has patent deep veins and competent valves in the deep and perforator systems. The next most suitable patient is one who has a patent deep venous system with competent deep valves but incompetent perforator valves. When the perforating veins are ablated along with the superficial venous stripping, good results can be expected. Patients with incompetence of all or most deep and perforator venous valves should not be considered for simple vein stripping because recurrence of varicosities is likely. Venous valve reconstruction or transposition may prove to be a logical choice for these patients as an effort to restore deep venous valvular competency. Finally, patients with deep vein obstruction, regardless of the condition of their venous valves, are the worst candidates for superficial ligation and stripping because stripping of the superficial veins in such a patient may remove the major patent collateral network and cause a precipitous worsening of the venous outflow problem.

SURGICAL TREATMENT. General indications for surgical treatment are (1) symptoms of aching, heaviness, and cramps; (2) complications of venous stasis such as pigmentation, dermatitis, induration, superficial ulceration, and thrombosis of varicosities; (3) large varicosities subject to trauma; (4) cosmetic concern; and (5) need for prophylaxis in younger patients. Surgery is not required for patients who obtain relief by elastic stocking support, and it should be recommended only for those patients in whom nonsurgical treatment is not satisfactory. All incompetent superficial veins and perforators should be thoroughly removed to prevent the tendency toward recurrence.

NONSURGICAL TREATMENT. The aim of sclerotherapy is to inject a small volume of an effective sclerosant into the vein's lumen in order to destroy the venous intima. If compression is not applied at that time, a large thrombus forms that soon recanalizes. This process may cause destruction of valves so that the venous disorder is actually worsened. However, if the sclerosant is injected into an empty vein and external compression is maintained until permanent fibrosis has obliterated the lumen, good results may be obtained.

The enthusiasm for sclerotherapy varies, but many authorities do not use it as the primary treatment for incompetent varicose veins. The recurrence rate is high even after relatively few years. Hobbs reported a recurrence rate of 29.5 per cent with sclerotherapy versus 7 per cent with surgery at 3 years. This is a problem particularly when sclerotherapy is used for large-caliber veins.

TREATMENT OF VENOUS THROMBOSIS

Whereas superficial venous thrombosis is usually a benign self-limiting disease, involvement of the deep venous system is a major cause of morbidity and mortality. Any venous system may be involved. The incidence of venous thrombosis is between 40 and 50 per cent in older patients undergoing surgery. In the United States alone, Hume and associates estimated that at least 140,000 fatal and 400,000 nonfatal cases of pulmonary embolism occur each year.

SUPERFICIAL VENOUS THROMBOSIS. The treatment of superficial venous thrombosis depends on its etiology, extent, and symptoms. Localized thrombophlebitis usually requires a mild analgesic such as aspirin, and activity may be continued. Severe thrombophlebitis with increased pain and redness should be treated with bed rest, elevation, and hot compresses. Purulence within the vein or suppurative thrombophlebitis is a more serious condition often associated with generalized septicemia. Treatment requires immediate and complete excision of the involved vein and appropriate systemic antibiotics. Upon resolution of symptoms, ambulation is initiated with elastic stockings. Antibiotic treatment is usually not necessary unless the process is suppurative and may require both antibiotics and surgical drainage. Pulmonary emboli rarely originate from superficial thrombi. Also, deep venous thrombosis rarely develops in association with superficial venous thrombosis, but superficial involvement frequently occurs in patients with deep venous disease, especially in those with ankle ulceration.

DEEP VENOUS THROMBOSIS. Since deep venous thrombosis generally begins in the soleus venous plexus of the calf and ascends to the level of the groin, those patients who initially present with iliofemoral venous thrombosis are likely to have proximal venous narrowing as a primary or contributing pathogenic factor. Absolute bed rest is mandatory until symptoms have subsided. Intravenous heparin in a dose maintaining a partial thromboplastin time at 70 to 80 seconds for 7 to 14 days will prevent thrombus propagation and possible pulmonary embolism while natural fibrinolysis occurs. Anticoagulation with Coumadin should be continued for 3 to 6 months.

Treatment of chronic venous insufficiency should begin as soon as the diagnosis of deep vein thrombosis has been made. It is important for patients to understand that the damage to the leg is directly proportional to the swelling that they allow to occur. They must also understand that good custom-fitted elastic stockings worn whenever they are out of bed are not sufficient and must be combined with periods of elevation of the ankles above heart level during the day. It is rarely necessary for a patient to wear the stockings above the knee since ulceration does not occur above the knee, and higher stockings are so uncomfortable that most patients will not wear them for any extended period of time. The frequency of daily leg elevation must be individualized according to the rapidity of edema formation. These measures will control stasis sequelae in 100 per cent of patients if they are scrupulously followed. Unfortunately, when patients think that they are doing well, they are less attentive to this chronic problem.

In those patients who develop postphlebitic stasis ulcers, periodic application of Unna's paste boots is the primary ambulatory treatment. This consists of a gauze dressing impregnated with gelatin, zinc oxide, and Caladryl, which is applied from the toes to knee after the ulcer has initially been cleansed and wrapped with an Ace bandage. Weekly reapplication of these compressive "boots" combined with elevation of the legs for at least 20 minutes several times each day will allow healing of the stasis ulcer. Whereas 90 per cent of venous stasis ulcers can be managed nonoperatively, those patients who cannot or will not follow this postphlebitic routine should be evaluated for an operative procedure. Removal of all superficial varicosities and complete subfascial ligation of all incompetent perforating veins has produced ulcer recurrence rates ranging from 2 to 43 per cent. When proximal deep venous occlusion is present, it must be relieved before the incompetent perforators are ligated. Only if there is marked deep venous reflux will venous valvular reconstruction improve the abnormal venous hemodynamics. This may be accomplished by venous valvuloplasty or valve transplantation.

50

PULMONARY EMBOLISM

David C. Sabiston, Jr., M.D.

Pulmonary embolism is a common complication of a number of medical and surgical disorders. Its incidence continues to increase, and it is estimated that in the United States more than 600,000 patients develop this complication annually with approximately 200,000 deaths. A greater number of the population now live longer and are subject to many medical problems that predispose to the development of thromboembolism. The pathogenesis of venous thrombosis is best conceptualized by *Virchow's triad:* (1) *stasis* due to reduced venous flow, (2) *intimal injury* predisposing to thrombosis, and (3) a state of *hypercoagulability*. Venous thrombosis occurs primarily in the iliofemoral and pelvic veins as well as the inferior vena cava. Surgical conditions that are especially apt to be complicated by pulmonary embolism include fractures of the hip, prostate operations, procedures on the lower extremities including amputation, and soft tissue injuries of the legs and thighs. Whereas pulmonary embolism clearly has a tendency to occur postoperatively, most series have shown that the majority of cases are *nonsurgical* in origin and develop as a complication of a serious underlying *medical* disorder. These include congestive heart failure, pulmonary disease, cerebrovascular accidents, carcinomatosis, hypercoagulable states, and many other conditions (Table 1).

CLINICAL MANIFESTATIONS

The clinical manifestations of pulmonary embolism include three major features: (1) dyspnea, (2) pleural pain, and (3) hemoptysis. The primary clinical signs are tachycardia, tachypnea, fever, rales, clinical evidence of thrombophlebitis, shock, and cyanosis. It should be emphasized that only a third of patients demonstrate clinical evidence of thrombophlebitis and the remainder are *silent* with no abnormal physical findings in the legs. *Asymptomatic* pulmonary embolism is quite common as has been repeatedly documented in postoperative patients undergoing routine pulmonary scans.

It is useful to assess each *patient's risk* of thromboembolism before major operations. *Low-risk* patients are those undergoing major surgical procedures who are under the age of 40 years and all patients undergoing minor surgical procedures. *Moderate-risk* patients are those 40 years of age or over undergoing surgical procedures of a duration of less than 30 minutes. *High-risk* patients are those over 40 years of age undergoing longer operative procedures and those with a

---

See the corresponding chapter or part in the *Textbook of Surgery,* 14th edition, pp. 1502–1512, for a more detailed discussion of this topic, including a comprehensive list of references.

TABLE 1. Risk Factors in Pulmonary Embolism

Venous Stasis	Vascular Injury		Hypercoagulability
Congestive heart failure	Surgical procedure on	Cancer	Nephrotic syndrome
Postoperative state	extremities	Pregnancy	Other drugs (heparin-induced disseminated
Immobilization	Trauma	Oral contraceptives and estrogens	intravascular coagulation syndrome; EACA;
Postpartum state	Burns	Antithrombin III deficiencies	prothrombin complex concentrate (Proplex,
Obesity	History of phlebitis	Protein C deficiencies	Konyne)
Varicose veins		Abnormal fibrinogen	"Lupus-like" anticoagulant
		Decreased or abnormal plasminogen	Disorders of platelets (myeloproliferative,
		Vascular plasminogen-activated deficiency	paroxysmal nocturnal hemoglobinuria, diabetes
		Plasminogen activator inhibitor	mellitus)
		Homocystinuria	Polycythemia
			Prosthetic devices in the venous system

history of deep venous thrombosis or pulmonary embolism, extensive malignant disease, prostatic operations, and orthopedic and other procedures on the extremities.

DIAGNOSIS

The plain chest film may show evidence of diminished vascular markings of the involved pulmonary vessels (Westermark's sign). However, this finding is seldom of sufficient prominence to be diagnostic. The electrocardiogram is usually nonspecific with only 20 per cent of patients with proven emboli showing any significant electrocardiographic changes. When present, the electrocardiographic alterations include atrial fibrillation, ectopic beats or heart block and enlargement of the T waves, ST segment depression, and T wave inversion. Right axis deviation suggests the presence of massive embolism.

Of particular importance is the measurement of arterial blood gases. In nearly all patients with significant pulmonary embolism, the arterial PO_2 is reduced, usually in the range of 50 to 70 mm. Hg, but it may be lower. In perhaps 10 per cent of patients, the PO_2 is greater than 80 mm. Hg. Retention of carbon dioxide is also common, causing an increase in PCO_2. *Pulmonary scanning* (ventilation-perfusion) is a very useful screening examination, particularly if the plain chest film is otherwise *completely normal.* Great caution must be exercised in interpreting any pulmonary scan on which there are changes in the plain chest film, since suspicious areas may be caused not only by embolism but by atelectasis, pneumonitis, neoplasm, fluid, emphysematous blebs, or pneumothorax.

There are numerous *specific* tests available for laboratory evaluation in the presence of a suspected hypercoagulable state (Table 2). In addition there are a series of nonspecific but helpful laboratory tests that provide additional data (Table 3). Ventilation-perfusion scan mismatch and intrapulmonary shunting are important features of pulmonary embolism and are caused primarily by regional atelectasis, bronchoconstriction, and pulmonary edema. A combination of ventilation-perfusion scan mismatch together with shunting produces hypoxemia, hyperventilation, increased pulmonary dead space, and an elevated alveolar-arterial gradient. If the perfusion scan is *normal,* clinically significant pulmonary embolism is excluded.

Pulmonary angiography is the most objective test for the diagnosis of pulmonary embolism and should be performed if the perfusion scan is not conclusive. In general, all patients with an abnormal pulmonary perfusion scan are candidates for pulmonary angiography. This is particularly important if the patient is to be given intravenous heparin, since a definite diagnosis of pulmonary embolism should be established in view of the complications that may follow heparinization. Contraindications include surgical procedures, gastrointestinal bleeding, blood dyscrasias, and many other conditions.

Venography is useful in establishing a firm diagnosis of

TABLE 2. Specific Tests Available for Laboratory Evaluation of the Suspected Hypercoagulable Patient

Condition	Assay	Comments
Abnormal or deficient inhibitors of coagulation		
AT-III deficiency	Immunologic	Assay widely commercially available; warfarin may elevate levels, and
	Functional	heparin may decrease levels
Protein C deficiency	Immunologic	Depressed levels may be associated with secondary hypercoagulable state
	Functional	Assay not readily available; must be measured off anticoagulants or normalized for anticoagulant effect
Defective fibrinolysis		
Defective release of plasminogen activator	Functional	Assay not widely available
Factor XII deficiency	Functional	PTT prolonged; assay widely available
Plasminogen activator inhibitor	Functional	Impaired fibrinolysis
Abnormal fibrinogen (dysfibrinogenemia)	Functional	Usually associated with bleeding but may be associated with thrombosis
Abnormal plasminogen	Immunologic	Assay not widely available
	Functional	
Other		
Homocystinuria	Biochemical	Arterial and venous events commonly associated with endothelial damage
Myeloproliferative disease		Usually associated with bleeding, but may be associated with thrombosis; no assay available, clinical features of myeloproliferative disease apparent (e.g., splenomegaly, abnormal CBC, platelet count, karyotype, LAP score)
"Lupus-like anticoagulant"	Functional	PTT prolonged; assay widely available; may be associated with a secondary hypercoagulable state

*From Stead, R. B.: The hypercoagulable state. *In* Goldhaber, S. Z. (Ed.): Pulmonary Embolism and Deep Venous Thrombosis. Philadelphia, W. B. Saunders Company, 1985.

TABLE 3. Nonspecific Tests Available for the Laboratory Evaluation of the Suspected Hypercoagulable Patient

Tests that detect transient responses to trauma and inflammation.
  Elevated levels of "unactivated" clotting factors: fibrinogen, factors V, VII, VIII
  Elevated platelet count
  Reduced levels of antithrombin III
  Reduced fibrinolytic activity
    Prolonged euglobulin lysis time
    Elevated antiplasmin time

Tests that detect clinical or subclinical thrombosis
  Platelet activation or release
    Shortened platelet survival
    Elevated thromboxane B_2 (TxB_2)
    Elevated platelet factor 4 (PF4)
    Elevated beta-thromboglobulin (βTG)
    Elevated circulating platelet aggregates
    Spontaneous or hyperreactive platelet aggregation
  Activation of coagulation enzymes
  Fibrin formation
  Elevated fibrin split products (FSPs)
  Elevated fibrin monomer complexes
  Increased fibrinogen turnover
  Elevated fibrinopeptide A (FPA)
  Elevated fibrin (fibrinogen fragment E)
  Thrombin generation
    Elevated F_{1+2} fragment
    Elevated thrombin:antithrombin complex
  Plasmin:antiplasmin complex

*From Stead, R. B.: The hypercoagulable state. *In* Goldhaber, S. Z. (Ed.): Pulmonary Embolism and Deep Venous Thrombosis. Philadelphia, W. B. Saunders Company, 1985.

thrombophlebitis in the legs with localization of the thrombi. It is of particular significance in those patients in whom the diagnosis is in doubt or if interruption of the inferior vena cava is being considered. Radioactive fibrinogen scans of the legs can also be useful in the detection of developing thrombi, but the technique is less accurate in the iliofemoral region because of the background activity of the urinary bladder. Doppler flow studies are relatively simple and may be helpful. Recently, *magnetic resonance scanning* has been demonstrated to be quite sensitive in detecting venous thrombi and is quite reliable. It is especially helpful in demonstrating the pelvic veins, which are known to be difficult to visualize by venography.

An algorithm depicting the stepwise establishment of the diagnosis and the treatment indicated is depicted in Figure 1.

PROPHYLAXIS

Prophylaxis of pulmonary embolism is important, especially in those patients in high-risk groups. Many prophylactic measures have been recommended, but few have been convincingly supported by randomized studies. The simplest and safest method of prevention is simple *elevation* of the

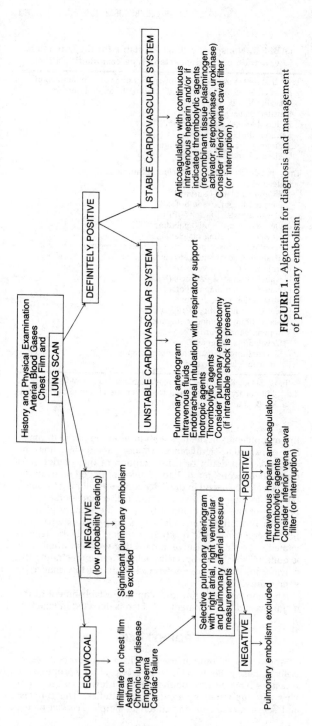

FIGURE 1. Algorithm for diagnosis and management of pulmonary embolism

History and Physical Examination
Arterial Blood Gases
Chest Film and
LUNG SCAN

EQUIVOCAL

Infiltrate on chest film
Asthma
Chronic lung disease
Emphysema
Cardiac failure

Selective pulmonary arteriogram with right atrial, right ventricular and pulmonary arterial pressure measurements

NEGATIVE

Pulmonary embolism excluded

POSITIVE

Intravenous heparin anticoagulation
Thrombolytic agents
Consider inferior vena caval filter (or interruption)

NEGATIVE (low probability reading)

Significant pulmonary embolism is excluded

DEFINITELY POSITIVE

UNSTABLE CARDIOVASCULAR SYSTEM

Pulmonary arteriogram
Intravenous fluids
Endotracheal intubation with respiratory support
Inotropic agents
Thrombolytic agents
Consider pulmonary embolectomy (if intractable shock is present)

STABLE CARDIOVASCULAR SYSTEM

Anticoagulation with continuous intravenous heparin and/or if indicated thrombolytic agents (recombinant tissue plasminogen activator, streptokinase, urokinase)
Consider inferior vena caval filter (or interruption)

legs. Here gravity is quite effective in rapidly draining blood from the legs to prevent venous stasis. This can be easily shown by inspection of the legs elevated to 20 to 25 degrees and noting the complete collapse of the superficial veins. It has been used quite effectively, particularly when it is made certain that *constant elevation of the legs* is maintained throughout the postoperative course. This is best done in the conscious patient by explaining the necessity and reasons as well as the position directly with the patient. Leg exercises, elastic stockings, and compression devices have each been recommended but remain controversial concerning their efficacy. Considerable discussion continues to surround the role of prophylactic *low-dose heparin*. Whereas some studies indicate successful prevention, others have been equivocal or negative. In postoperative patients, it may cause increased bleeding. Moreover, the recent recognition that it may induce heparin sensitivity with disastrous consequences of the *heparin-associated thrombotic thrombocytopenia syndrome* has discouraged many from the use of low-dose heparin as a prophylactic measure.

PROPHYLACTIC REGIMENS

The *low-dose heparin* regimen consists of 5000 units of heparin administered subcutaneously each 12 hours and 2 hours before the surgical procedure. This dosage is continued until the risk of thromboembolism has significantly decreased. Care should be taken to observe postoperative bleeding. *Low-dose warfarin* can be administered preoperatively with maintenance of the prothrombin time 1.2 to 1.5 seconds longer than the control value. Postoperatively the dose should be increased to maintain the prothrombin time 1.5 to 2 times the control value. Abnormal bleeding should be noted in the postoperative period. Antiplatelet agents including aspirin and dipyridamole (Persantine) have been used in prophylaxis with reports of success compared with placebos, but certainty concerning the value of their use has not been established.

ANTICOAGULANT MANAGEMENT OF PROVEN PULMONARY EMBOLISM

Many patients with proven pulmonary embolism and a *stable* cardiovascular status are preferably managed by intravenous heparin by continuous pump-driven delivery. An initial intravenous bolus of 10,000 to 20,000 units should be given with maintenance infusion of 800 to 1200 units per hour. The partial thromboplastin time should be evaluated at 4 to 6 hours and maintained between 1.5 and 2 times control. With partial thromboplastin times 2.5 times greater than normal, bleeding is apt to become a complication. Therapy is maintained for 7 to 10 days with a gradual shift to warfarin therapy.

Warfarin (Coumadin) anticoagulation can be achieved with the goal of maintaining the prothrombin time at 1.2 to 1.5

times control. This generally requires a loading dose of 15 to
30 mg. on the first day and 10 to 20 mg. on the second day.
The maximal effect is usually reached in 1½ to 2 days, and
the average daily maintenance dose is between 5 and 10 mg.
(range from 2 to 20 mg.). Although the recommended duration of warfarin therapy is controversial, most advise a
minimum of 6 weeks or continuance for 3 to 6 months. If
thrombophlebitis persists, long-term anticoagulation is advisable. Should bleeding complications occur, vitamin K counteracts the effects of warfarin.

If the patient is in stable cardiovascular condition, the
therapy is primarily directed toward continuous intravenous
heparin, oxygen, and minimal amounts of inotropic agents
and vasopressors as necessary. Surveillance is achieved on
an intensive care unit. If the patient becomes unstable with
hypotension, tachycardia, cardiac arrhythmias, cyanosis, low
arterial oxygen saturation, and reduced urinary output, more
intensive inotropic agents may be required as well as tracheal
intubation and placement on a ventilator.

THROMBOLYTIC AGENTS

Although several thrombolytic agents have been available
for many years, only recently has interest been renewed in
the role of thrombolytic therapy in the management of
pulmonary embolism. Three thrombolytic enzymes are being
used—streptokinase, urokinase, and recombinant tissue plasminogen activator (rtPA)—and may be especially indicated
in patients with *massive* pulmonary embolism. Since this is a
developing field, specific series and the results are cited. In
a multi-trial evaluation at eight centers, administration of
rtPA was evaluated in 34 patients with acute massive pulmonary embolism. All patients received a bolus of intravenous heparin (5000 IU) followed by 1000 IU per hour. After
50 mg. of rtPA was given during a 2-hour period, the severity
of the embolism as determined by pulmonary arteriograms
declined. The mean pulmonary arterial pressures fell, and
following an additional dose of 50 mg. of rtPA, the severity
of the embolism decreased by 38 per cent with a further
reduction in mean pulmonary arterial pressure.

Streptokinase therapy may also be appropriate both in the
management of deep venous thrombosis and in thromboembolism. Among 108 patients with phlebographically verified deep venous thrombosis treated with streptokinase, total
or partial thrombolysis was demonstrated angiographically
in 60 (55.6 per cent). Twenty-two patients showed evidence
of allergic reactions due to the foreign protein in streptokinase, and anaphylactic shock was observed in one patient.
The dose of streptokinase is 250,000 units intravenously over
a 30-minute period followed by 100,000 units hourly for 24
hours. Conventional heparin therapy is then administered
intravenously. Whereas the incidence of bleeding is slightly
higher with thrombolytic therapy compared with heparin or
warfarin anticoagulation, nevertheless its thrombolytic effect
is often desirable or urgently needed. In one study using
both agents, the results appeared more rapid and safer.

In a multicenter study of 2539 patients with pulmonary embolism, it was determined that 1345 (53.5 per cent) surveyed would have been acceptable for treatment with thrombolytic therapy. Risks of major blood loss were the most frequent contraindications to thrombolytic therapy and were found in 838 patients (33.3 per cent). Potential risk to the central nervous system was found to contraindicate thrombolytic therapy in 453 (17.9 per cent). Similarly, risks of bleeding into special compartments were found to contraindicate thrombolytic therapy in 76 (3 per cent).

SURGICAL THERAPY

Although anticoagulant therapy is usually successful in preventing further pulmonary emboli, occasionally absolute contraindication to anticoagulation or recurrent emboli may occur and raise the possibility of surgical management for preventing further embolization. Although various forms of interruption of the inferior vena cava have been advocated including complete ligation and application of clips and other devices for partial or complete occlusion, the most frequently utilized approach is the transvenous insertion of a conelike umbrella filter designed to prevent large emboli from passing into the upper inferior vena cava. This filter is relatively easily placed; indications for its use include patients in whom anticoagulation therapy is not appropriate or those in whom fear of repeated embolism is sufficiently great. Although this technique has a low morbidity and mortality, the filters can migrate into the right atrium, right ventricle, and pulmonary artery. They may also perforate the vena cava and migrate to the iliac veins.

In patients with massive pulmonary embolism associated with cardiovascular instability and intractable shock, pulmonary embolectomy with extracorporeal circulation may be indicated. Under these circumstances, a proven diagnosis of pulmonary embolism by arteriography is highly desirable if not mandatory. Occasionally pulmonary embolectomy can be performed unilaterally without the use of the heart-lung machine. The mortality of the procedure ranges as high as 50 per cent; nevertheless, it can be lifesaving.

CHRONIC PULMONARY EMBOLISM

Whereas the majority of patients with pulmonary thromboembolism demonstrate resolution of the thrombi with the passage of time, nevertheless a small per cent of emboli do not undergo thrombolysis and chronic embolism ensues. Ultimately these emboli may become so extensive that right ventricular and pulmonary arterial hypertension occurs. The disorder may progress to chronic cor pulmonale with severe dyspnea, cyanosis, and right ventricular failure with a fatal outcome. Fortunately, in those with emboli in the primary and secondary branches of the pulmonary arteries and in the presence of a *patent distal arterial* circulation, great improvement can be achieved by embolectomy. Distal pulmonary arterial patency can be demonstrated by selective *retrograde* bronchial arteriography in which the contrast medium fills the bronchial vessels and passes through the pulmonary capillary circulation into the distal small pulmonary arteries. Postoperatively patients demonstrate a decrease in pulmonary arterial pressure, increase in pulmonary arterial oxygen saturation, and relief of symptoms. In symptomatic patients, the natural history of this disorder is dismal, with only 20 per cent of those with a mean pulmonary artery pressure greater than 50 mm. Hg alive at 2 years.

I

Chronic Pulmonary Embolism
H. Kim Lyerly, M.D.

Pulmonary embolism usually presents as an acute clinical problem but may occur with chronic manifestations as a characteristic syndrome. Most pulmonary emboli eventually resolve spontaneously as a result of naturally occurring fibrinolytic systems in the body. In some patients, because of inadequate fibrinolysis or recurrent episodes of embolism, emboli gradually accumulate in the pulmonary arterial system. This may ultimately cause pulmonary hypertension and produce symptoms of progressive respiratory insufficiency, hypoxemia, and right ventricular failure. In most patients, medical management of these disorders is unsatisfactory, and clinical studies in this group have revealed a poor prognosis.

CLINICAL PRESENTATION. Patients with the syndrome of chronic pulmonary embolism have exertional dyspnea progressing to severe respiratory insufficiency over several months to years. They may also complain of recurrent episodes of thrombophlebitis, hemoptysis due to the presence of large bronchial collaterals, and chest pain. Physical findings include signs of severe pulmonary hypertension, often combined with evidence of right ventricular failure, and may be manifested as an increased pulmonary second sound, a systolic murmur, hepatomegaly, and an S3 or S4 gallop.

Chest films show a dilated pulmonary artery and oligemic pulmonary fields in approximately 50 per cent of patients. Right ventricular enlargement is present in 68 per cent and pleural effusion in approximately one third of patients. Arterial blood gas analyses at room air reveal evidence of severe respiratory insufficiency, with hypoxemia and arterial oxygen tension (Pao_2) values of 55 to 60 mm. Hg and an arterial

---

See the corresponding chapter or part in the *Textbook of Surgery,* 14th edition, pp. 1513–1519, for a more detailed discussion of this topic, including a comprehensive list of references.

carbon dioxide tension (Paco$_2$) of approximately 30 mm. Hg. The electrocardiogram usually suggests the presence of chronic cor pulmonale and includes right-axis deviation and right ventricular hypertrophy. Peripheral venography demonstrates venous thrombosis in patients and indicates the source of the emboli. Magnetic resonance imaging provides more accurate delineation of pelvic vein thrombosis than does venography and is more reliable as well as noninvasive. Ventilation and perfusion radionuclide scans obtained during evaluation are consistent with pulmonary emboli, and perfusion defects correspond to oligemic regions on the plain film and arteriogram. Perfusion defects are usually noted bilaterally. Pulmonary arteriography allows documentation of emboli, determination of anatomic distribution of emboli, and recording of pulmonary artery pressures.

Determining the presence of elevated pulmonary artery pressures is important because it has been demonstrated that the natural history of this syndrome is related to the magnitude of the pulmonary arterial hypertension. If the mean pulmonary artery pressure is more than 30 mm. Hg, survival at 5 years is only 30 per cent. In those patients with a mean pressure greater than 50 mm. Hg, only 10 per cent were alive at 5 years. Arteriography usually shows emboli in both lungs, with 55 to 75 per cent of the total pulmonary blood flow obstructed. Further preoperative studies include a thoracic aortogram or selective bronchial arteriography for demonstration of dilated and tortuous bronchial vessels. The bronchial circulation is often considerably dilated and communicated by collaterals with the distal pulmonary arteries.

SURGICAL MANAGEMENT. Pulmonary embolectomy may be performed on one or both pulmonary arteries. In patients who have primarily unilateral involvement, either a right or left anterior thoracotomy can be performed when there is proximal occlusion of the vessel. In those with bilateral pulmonary emboli or in those with involvement of the main pulmonary artery, extracorporeal circulation is generally indicated. These emboli are densely adherent to the wall of the pulmonary artery, and great care must be taken in the dissection. All distal emboli should be removed until there is adequate back-bleeding of bright red blood.

Satisfactory distal back-bleeding can usually be predicted in advance from the information gained by the thoracic aortogram with selective injection of the bronchial arteries. Postoperative complications include right ventricular failure in patients with long-standing cor pulmonale and pulmonary hypertension. One patient in the author's series died of this cause 3 days after operation despite removal of the chronic pulmonary emboli. Another complication that has been described is the hemorrhagic lung syndrome. Successful management of this complication can be achieved by the use of a Carlens (Broncho-Cath) catheter for tracheal intubation. Other postoperative complications include phrenic nerve paresis after the use of deep hypothermia and psychiatric disturbances that are usually transient.

Embolectomy for chronic pulmonary embolism generally causes a decrease in pulmonary artery pressures along with an increase in Pao₂ toward normal. These data, combined with those of other similar series in the literature, indicate favorable results. It is now established that pulmonary embolectomy in patients with proximal pulmonary arterial obstruction is likely to produce relief of respiratory insufficiency, with reduction in pulmonary hypertension and improvement of right-sided heart failure.

51

FAT EMBOLISM SYNDROME

Joseph A. Moylan, M.D.

Fat embolism continues as a major cause of pulmonary decompensation after injury. The incidence of this syndrome remains 35 per cent in patients involved in multisystem trauma, particularly that secondary to motor vehicle accidentsreas there are two major theories describing the pathophysiologic mechanism of fat embolization, the mechanical theory and the physiochemical theory, recent data support the latter as the primary cause. Free fatty acids that arise from either the hydrolysis of neutral fats or the mobilization of fat stores by catecholamines produce alterations in the capillary alveolar membrane as well as in surfactant production. The result of this phenomenon is hemorrhage, edema, and alveolar collapse. Clinical investigation has shown the correlation between elevated free fatty acids and severity of the fat embolism syndrome.

Clinically, the syndrome can be classified by using the respiratory distress index: $RDI = PaO_2/FiO_2 (VF + PF)$, where VF equals 1 without mechanical ventilation or 1.5 with mechanical ventilation and PF equals 0 when positive end-expiratory pressure (PEEP) is less than 5 cm. H_2O or 0.5 when PEEP is greater than 5 cm. H_2O. The severity of pulmonary dysfunction estimated by this formula correlates with increasing levels of free fatty acids. Clinical studies have been supported by a number of animal experiments. The binding of free fatty acids by albumin has also been demonstrated experimentally as well as clinically to decrease the risk and incidence of fat embolism syndrome.

DIAGNOSIS. The fat embolism syndrome consists of changes in the cerebral, pulmonary, and cutaneous organ systems. Patients exhibit hypoxia, confusion, and petechiae as well as agitation, stupor, and tachypnea with progressive hypoxia. The peak incidence of this syndrome occurs from the second to fourth day following injury, and the diagnosis is usually made by a combination of laboratory and clinical parameters including a history of multisystem injury, presence of post-traumatic shock, changes in respiratory and cerebral function, and the presence of petechiae. Radiologic changes may be initially present in only 30 per cent of patients with the fat embolism syndrome, but over the subsequent 24 hours almost all develop radiologic abnormalities. Another important laboratory test is arterial Po_2, which frequently falls to less than 60 mm. Hg on room air. Other studies include the presence of fat emboli, fat globules in the urine, and elevated free fatty acid levels.

PREVENTION AND TREATMENT. The syndrome can be

See the corresponding chapter or part in the *Textbook of Surgery*, 14th edition, pp. 1520–1522, for a more detailed discussion of this topic, including a comprehensive list of references.

prevented by careful attention to risk factors following multisystem injuries, particularly the presence of a low circulating albumin. Since albumin binds circulating free fatty acids, preventive treatment with albumin to maintain a circulating level of 3 gm. per 100 ml. is important. The role of steroids is controversial. Double-blind studies have failed to demonstrate any specific advantage on the outcome of the fat embolism syndrome. Therefore, steroids should not be routinely used, since they increase the risk of infection in a severely injured patient.

Ventilatory support with endotracheal intubation and a volume cycled respirator with PEEP remains the primary therapy. PEEP increases functional residual capacity and directly decreases pulmonary shunting.

In summary, the fat embolism syndrome is a frequent sequela of multisystem trauma producing confusion, tachypnea, and petechiae. This syndrome is caused by the vascular and membrane toxicity of unbound free fatty acids. Maintenance of an adequate serum albumin level in the early postinjury period is preventive. When the fat embolism syndrome develops, treatment includes careful attention to maintaining the PaO_2 by using early endotracheal intubation and volume cycled ventilator with PEEP.

52

DISORDERS OF THE ARTERIAL SYSTEM

I

Introduction*
David C. Sabiston, Jr., M.D.

The history of surgery is a combination of its scientific and technical advances, and prime examples of these are control of the arterial system and introduction of techniques to relieve arterial obstruction. During the past few decades, several quite significant developments have occurred including the use of vascular autografts, arterial prostheses, extracorporeal circulation, and an improved understanding of the factors that affect endothelium and thrombosis. Considered together, these comprise brilliant accomplishments.

Whereas hemostasis was achieved by the ancient Chinese with use of bandages and styptics, extremities could be amputated only at the site of gangrene where the blood vessels had thrombosed and would not be subject to hemorrhage when divided. Celsus advocated limited use of the suture to prevent bleeding, but this fell into disuse and was rediscovered by Paré in 1552 when he used ligature instead of the hot cautery in controlling hemorrhage. Carrel was the first to place the direct suture of blood vessels on a firm basis in a study published in 1906, work for which he later won the Nobel Prize. The use of saphenous vein as an autograft was first performed by Goyanes in Madrid in 1906. Arteriography of the femoral arteries was introduced by Brooks in 1923; in 1927 Moniz performed carotid arteriography, and in 1929 an abdominal aortogram was first done by dos Santos. This was followed by the use of vascular grafts composed of plastic materials in the early 1950s and by development of extracorporeal circulation in 1953 by Gibbon.

II

Anatomy†
David C. Sabiston, Jr., M.D.

The arterial system delivers blood from the heart to the tissues, and the arteries are classified as being large, medium-

---

*See the corresponding chapter or part in the *Textbook of Surgery*, 14th edition, pp. 1523–1524, for a more detailed discussion of this topic, including a comprehensive list of references.

†See the corresponding chapter or part in the *Textbook of Surgery*, 14th edition, p. 1524, for a more detailed discussion of this topic, including a comprehensive list of references.

sized, and small vessels. Arteries less than 100 microns in diameter are *arterioles*. The histologic characteristics of the arterial wall are largely dependent on the size of the vessel. For example, large arteries, which must withstand the greatest pressure, contain considerable elastic tissue for appropriately controlling differentials in pressure. Medium-sized arteries have less elastic tissue and more smooth muscle, and at the arteriolar level the elastic tissue is either scant or absent. Collagen is present in all three arterial systems and forms the strongest layer of the vascular wall for the larger vessels as well as the smaller arteries.

The *natural collateral circulation* of tissues and organs is important, especially in the sequence of events that follow *acute arterial occlusion*. In addition, the duration of occlusion of an artery is of considerable significance. For example, with slow, progressive arterial occlusion there is sufficient time for collateral vessels to develop and become larger. Generally, as a smaller vessel is subjected to the need for increased flow (primarily due to the pressure gradient), the vessel is apt to become thin-walled and tortuous. This characteristic is easily demonstrated by arteriography, as in chronic occlusion of the abdominal aorta (Leriche's syndrome). Under these circumstances, adequate arterial collaterals develop that join the branches above the occlusion with distal vessels. It is surprising that slowly progressive occlusion of the entire abdominal aorta occurring over a period of time may produce minimal symptoms in some patients, whereas in others it produces the characteristic symptoms of intermittent claudication and impotence. Nevertheless, gangrene of the extremities is rare until late in Leriche's syndrome. However, sudden *acute* occlusion of the abdominal aorta usually produces disastrous effects with immediate appearance of severe ischemia; if this is untreated, gangrene of the lower extremities ensues.

The principles of collateral circulation are of primary importance in all aspects of medicine, especially in surgical procedures. All vascular circuits have some natural collateral circulation, although it may vary greatly in different tissues and organs. The subclavian artery can usually be ligated safely in the first portion, as in the performance of a subclavian-pulmonary anastomosis for congenital cyanotic heart disease (Blalock operation), since the collateral circulation around the shoulder is excellent. It is rare for ischemic symptoms to follow ligation of the subclavian at this site; indeed, with the passage of time, a pulse frequently reappears in the affected radial artery as additional collateral circulation develops. Moreover, three of the four major arteries of the stomach (the left and right gastric and left and right gastric epiploic) can be ligated without significant ischemia. In a number of other arteries the extensiveness of collaterals varies considerably, with ligation producing no ill effects in some patients and ischemic symptoms in others. Some arteries, such as the coronary, renal, and retinal arteries, have very inadequate natural collateral circulations. Acute occlusion of these vessels is usually followed by serious changes of ischemia and infarction.

III

Physiology of the Arterial System
Richard L. McCann, M.D.

The proximal arterial system encompasses the main elastic vessels, principally the aorta and its major branches, which have a high proportion of elastin fibers and function to store kinetic energy generated by the heart during systole. The elastic recoil of these vessels assists in promoting continued distribution of blood during diastole. These vessels branch into the muscular arteries, which contain a higher proportion of vascular smooth muscle cells in their walls. This muscular tissue is important for the function of these vessels in regulating the relative distribution of blood flow to various vascular beds. The greatest degree of regulation occurs at the level of the arterioles, which are 20 to 50 μ in diameter and have a single layer of vascular smooth muscle cells. Small changes in the caliber of these vessels cause large changes in total peripheral resistance.

The motion of the blood in the arterial system is best understood by considering the total energy involved. The pumping action of the heart imparts potential and kinetic energy to the blood through several mechanisms. The most important of these is the potential energy stored as the intravascular pressure and the pressure due to the volume of blood contained within the elastic confines of the vascular tree. Second, there is potential energy that is due to hydrostatic forces associated with gravity, that is, the weight of the blood. Because there are no valves in the peripheral arterial system, the pressure at any point is influenced by the height of the column of blood between it and the reference point that is usually taken to be the level of the right atrium. As an example, in an erect 6-foot human, the hydrostatic pressure is equivalent to 93 mm. Hg, and the ankle pressure is increased by that amount when the subject changes from a recumbent to a standing position.

As the blood is propelled through the arterial system, energy is dissipated by both viscous and inertial factors. Viscous losses are the result of friction within the flowing blood due to the intermolecular attractions between fluid layers. Viscous energy losses are expressed by Poiseuille's law, which states that the pressure gradient across a uniform cylinder is related to the fluid flow, the cylinder length, and the fluid viscosity and is inversely proportional to the fourth power of the radius. This can be expressed as

$$P_1 - P_2 = Q \cdot \frac{8L\eta}{r^4}$$

where P_x equals pressure at any point, Q is flow, L is length,

See the corresponding chapter or part in the *Textbook of Surgery*, 14th edition, pp. 1524–1528, for a more detailed discussion of this topic, including a comprehensive list of references.

η is viscosity, and r is radius. Because flow varies as the fourth power of the radius and linearly with length, it is the radius of a stenosis that primarily influences flow at the site of an arterial obstruction. It follows that for a progressive arterial stenosis, flow changes will be small until the stenosis approaches 70 to 80 per cent narrowing of the cross-sectional area (corresponding to 50 per cent diameter).

In addition to viscous energy losses, additional energy is lost owing to inertial factors. These are related to changes in velocity and direction associated with the turbulent flow that occurs at the site of a stenosis. These energy losses are dissipated as heat and are described by Reynolds number, which is defined as

$$RE = \frac{\rho \, \bar{v} d}{\eta}$$

where ρ_x is density, v is kinetic viscosity, d is diameter, and η is viscosity.

A critical stenosis is defined as the degree of narrowing of a vessel that is required to produce a measurable reduction in pressure or reduction in flow of the blood through it. This is generally accepted to occur when a diameter reduction of 50 per cent occurs. This corresponds to a reduction in vessel cross-sectional area of 75 per cent. However, this does not consider the pulsatile nature of blood flow or the fact that many vascular stenoses are not isolated but serial in nature. However, it is clear that short stenoses with marked reduction in diameter are more physiologically important than is a lesser degree of stenosis that exists over a longer vessel segment. Also, two stenoses in tandem have a greater effect than does a single stenosis the length of which is the sum of the length of the tandem stenoses. Therefore, multiple stenoses in series are additive, and several subcritical stenoses may become the equivalent of a critical stenosis and produce a significant decrease in flow.

The concept of hemodynamic resistance is helpful in understanding the physiology of arterial disease. In the normal limb, resistance is very low in the large axial vessels. The major site of peripheral resistance exists in the muscular run-off bed. This high resistance is remarkably variable and is used to control blood flow to muscular beds during exercise. When obstruction occurs in the major axial vessels, in the course of the development of atherosclerosis, flow is forced to proceed through smaller collateral vessels. These collateral vessels characteristically have a diameter of 1 to 2 mm., and recalling the Poiseuille relationship, it can be seen that it would require thousands of these collaterals to reduce the segmental resistance to the same level as a major unobstructed axial vessel with the diameter of 8 to 10 mm. Resistance in the collateral vessels is relatively fixed compared with that in the vascular run-off bed. Under the demands of exercise, the resistance in the muscular run-off bed is sharply reduced. Because of the fixed obstruction proximally, flow cannot increase to maintain pressure, and thus the pressure measured distally in the limb falls precipitously. This corresponds to the decrease in ankle pressure that is observed with the onset of intermittent claudication or pain in the muscular bed associated with vascular insufficiency. This decrease in ankle pressure with exercise is a hallmark of peripheral vascular obstructive disease.

IV

Arterial Substitutes

Gregory L. Moneta, M.D., and John M. Porter, M.D.

The ideal arterial substitute has not yet been developed. Intensive laboratory and clinical investigations over the last 80 years, however, have produced reasonably satisfactory arterial substitutes that have in large part been responsible for the increased growth of arterial surgery.

BACKGROUND

Since the first implantation of experimental venous autografts by Carrel and Guthrie in 1906, a large number of arterial substitutes have been used experimentally and clinically, including arterial and saphenous vein allografts, umbilical vein allografts, arterial and venous autografts, xenografts, and various prosthetic grafts. Allografts and xenografts are antigenic and, unless modified, incite a prominent rejection reaction. Because of problems with rejection, degeneration, aneurysm formation, and rupture and infection, xenografts and allografts currently have very few clinical applications. The exceptions include limited use of bovine carotid xenografts for dialysis access and occasional but diminishing use of modified umbilical vein allografts for infrainguinal arterial reconstructions.

ARTERIAL AUTOGRAFTS

Arterial autografts have limited but well-defined clinical applications. Currently, internal mammary autografts provide patency results superior to saphenous vein autografts in coronary artery bypass grafting. Internal iliac artery autografts are the preferred grafts for renal artery reconstruction in children. Such grafts do not have the propensity demonstrated by saphenous vein autografts to undergo late aneurysmal dilation in pediatric renovascular reconstructions. The

---

See the corresponding chapter or part in the *Textbook of Surgery*, 14th edition, pp. 1528–1539, for a more detailed discussion of this topic, including a comprehensive list of references.

obvious disadvantage of arterial autografts is lack of availability and length of sacrificible arteries.

VENOUS AUTOGRAFTS

Venous autografts are the most versatile and clinically important small-caliber arterial substitutes. Greater saphenous vein, lesser saphenous vein, and cephalic and brachial veins as well as superficial femoral and internal jugular veins have all been used as bypass conduits.

Although many sources of autogenous vein give satisfactory results, the greater saphenous vein is the most frequently used venous autograft for infrainguinal arterial reconstruction. Over 200,000 such operations are performed each year in the United States. Lower extremity bypasses using autogenous saphenous vein may be performed with one of two basic techniques. An appropriate length of vein may be removed from either the ipsilateral or contralateral lower extremity, reversed in direction to permit arterial flow in the direction of the venous valves, and then sutured in place. Alternatively, in the "in situ" saphenous vein bypass, an intact ipsilateral vein of adequate quality may largely be left in its anatomic position and the valves mechanically disrupted by one of a number of intraluminal devices. Both techniques are currently widely employed.

Reversed femoropopliteal saphenous vein autograft patency has ranged from 80 to 90 per cent at 1 year, to 55 to 86 per cent at 5 years, to 38 to 46 per cent at 10 years. Reversed saphenous vein grafting to tibial arteries produces patency approximately 10 to 15 per cent lower than that of femoropopliteal grafting at all time intervals. Exhaustive analyses of variables affecting femoropopliteal patency indicate that patency is higher when bypass surgery is performed for claudication rather than limb salvage, and that it is generally higher with a widely patent popliteal and tibial artery outflow tract. A patent outflow tract, however, is not an absolute requirement for long-term patency, since Mannick has reported an intermediate-term patency rate of 65 per cent when bypassing to an isolated popliteal segment without demonstrated angiographic patency of the popliteal artery trifurcation vessels. Both continued cigarette smoking and the use of a small vein (less than 4 mm. after gentle distention) have adverse effects on long-term patency. Postoperative antiplatelet drugs may improve graft patency, but the evidence is inconclusive.

Large modern series of in situ vein bypasses initially suggested superior patency rates with use of this technique in comparison with the reversed vein technique. Modern series of reversed vein bypasses, however, have proved to have similar cumulative patency rates. Since in situ bypasses frequently require secondary operations for maintaining graft patency, primary patency may actually be better with reversed rather than in situ grafts. Clearly, reversed vein grafting is applicable to larger numbers of patients, since many patients do not have the intact ipsilateral saphenous vein available that is required for in situ bypass.

PATHOLOGY OF VENOUS AUTOGRAFTS. Perioperative vein graft failure (up to 30 days) is usually attributed to technical flaws in the performance of the operation or the presence of an unrecognized hypercoagulable state. Late failures (beyond 12 months) typically follow progression of atherosclerotic disease above or below the vein graft. It is quite clear, however, that vein grafts are subject to a number of pathologic alterations that may cause eventual occlusion of the graft. These include localized stenoses associated with clamp application, fibrosis of venous valves, and late vein graft atherosclerosis. Fibrointimal hyperplasia, however, is the most significant pathologic process affecting autogenous vein grafts. It occurs in at least 10 per cent of saphenous vein grafts and has been implicated as the cause of failure in 15 to 30 per cent of occlusions of aortocoronary grafts during the first year.

Fibrointimal hyperplasia is a myoproliferative process that appears to produce stimulation of normally quiescent myointimal and medial smooth muscle cells into actively proliferating secretory myofibroblasts. Endothelial cell damage appears to be essential in the production of fibrointimal hyperplasia. Such damage may occur at the time of graft harvest or implantation or may result from changes in shear forces or from compliance mismatch between the host artery and the vein graft. The process undoubtedly involves a series of complex cellular interactions including mitogen production by endothelial cells, platelets, smooth muscle, and macrophages. In addition, endothelial cells can also produce growth-inhibiting factors. The precise mechanism by which these derangements in cellular interactions and growth factor production combine to produce a failed vascular graft is unknown but obviously is an area of great interest with important clinical implications.

PROSTHETIC GRAFTS

The most widely used prosthetic grafts currently in clinical use are fabricated from Dacron or polytetrafluoroethylene.

DACRON GRAFTS. Dacron grafts are manufactured by weaving or knitting multifilament texturized yarns. Woven grafts are tightly interlaced with small interstices and low porosity. Standard woven grafts leak minimally at implantation but are somewhat stiff and moderately difficult to handle. Knitted grafts are softer with larger interstices and must be preclotted before implantation. A large percentage of modern Dacron grafts have velour surfaces added to either the luminal or external surface or both surfaces. Velour surfaces have loops of yarn extending almost perpendicular to the fabric surface. Velour improves the handling characteristics of woven grafts and provides a scaffold for fibroblast ingrowth for firm graft adherence to surrounding tissue.

POLYTETRAFLUOROETHYLENE (PTFE) GRAFTS. PTFE is a semi-inert polymer composed of solid nodes of PTFE with interconnecting fibrils. The graft has an electronegative surface charge and is thus hydrophobic and theoretically more resistant to thrombosis. Grafts must be coated with a thin outer wrap of PTFE for avoidance of aneurysm formation associated with clinical use of unwrapped grafts.

CLINICAL USE OF PROSTHETIC GRAFTS. Dacron grafts function extremely well in arterial reconstructions proximal to the inguinal ligament. Such grafts yield 5- and 10-year patencies of 91 and 66 per cent, respectively, for aortofemoral bypass. Axillofemoral bypass patency has been 75 per cent at 5 years, and femorofemoral bypass patency at 5 years has similarly been 75 to 80 per cent. Because of decreased patency compared with venous autografts, Dacron grafts are infrequently employed in infrainguinal reconstructions.

PTFE grafts give results similar to Dacron in aortic reconstructions. However, they have received the most interest as an alternative to autogenous vein in infrainguinal reconstructions. When used in the above-knee femoropopliteal position, PTFE grafts provide patency results that approach but do not equal those for autogenous vein. They remain distinctly inferior to autogenous vein in infrapopliteal reconstructions.

PROSTHETIC GRAFT HEALING. Unfortunately, prosthetic grafts in humans, unlike in experimental animals, never achieve complete healing with the development of a living neointima. With the exception of the para-anastomotic areas, they remain covered on their luminal surface, even after many years, with a compacted layer of fibrin. Much of the current focus of prosthetic graft research concerns means of improving graft healing. Well-healed grafts offer the potential for decreased thrombogenicity and increased resistance to infection.

COMPLICATIONS OF PROSTHETIC GRAFTING. The most frequent complications of prosthetic grafting are neointimal hyperplasia that may cause graft occlusion, anastomotic false aneurysms, and infection. Para-anastomotic prosthetic graft neointimal hyperplasia is similar to that described for autogenous vein with the same postulated etiologic factors. Both Dacron and PTFE grafts are equally affected. As with saphenous vein grafts, antiplatelet drugs are frequently prescribed to patients with prosthetic grafts in an effort to reduce anastomotic fibroplasia. However, the evidence for efficacy of this treatment is inconclusive.

Anastomotic false aneurysms are of uncertain cause. Improper suture technique, arterial degeneration, infection, and compliance mismatch may all be important. With rare exception, anastomotic aneurysms should be repaired when discovered.

Infection occurs in about 1 to 2 per cent of prosthetic grafts. Standard treatment is graft excision with revascularization, if necessary, through clean tissue planes. Morbidity and mortality of prosthetic infection can be reduced by performing revascularization before graft excision. Such an approach limits the complications of prolonged distal ischemia.

FUTURE CONSIDERATIONS

Much current research activity in graft design and fabrication is directed toward the development of a satisfactory prosthetic graft for small artery bypass. Most investigators believe that a satisfactory small artery prosthesis requires improved luminal healing and compliance characteristics compared with available prosthetic arterial grafts.

Vascular surgeons appear to be approaching the limits of technical competence. Further improvement in the results of vascular grafting requires better prostheses than any currently available and, perhaps more significantly, improved understanding and ultimate modifications of the processes of atherosclerosis, thrombosis, and arterial healing.

Aneurysms*

David C. Sabiston, Jr., M.D.

Aneurysms are localized or diffuse dilations of blood vessels. Most aneurysms involve arteries and are *true* aneurysms containing all components of the arterial wall (intima, media, and adventitia). A *false* aneurysm ("pulsating hematoma") is the term applied when the aneurysmal sac is composed only of adventitia. Aneurysms may be either *saccular* or *fusiform;* the saccular aneurysm arises from a distinct portion of the arterial wall with a *stoma*, whereas the fusiform aneurysm is a generalized dilation of the entire circumference of the vessel. Aneurysms tend to form at specific sites and are either *congenital* or *acquired* in origin. Acquired aneurysms may be caused by arteriosclerosis, trauma, infection (mycotic), syphilis, or medial cystic necrosis. Most aneurysms can be managed surgically with excellent results.

1. ANEURYSMS OF THE SINUS OF VALSALVA†

Frederick L. Grover, M.D., and John H. Calhoon, M.D.

Sinus of Valsalva aneurysms are dilations of the aortic sinuses of Valsalva that may rupture into cardiac chambers

---

*See the corresponding chapter or part in the *Textbook of Surgery*, 14th edition, pp. 1539–1540, for a more detailed discussion of this topic, including a comprehensive list of references.

†See the corresponding chapter or part in the *Textbook of Surgery*, 14th edition, pp. 1540–1543, for a more detailed discussion of this topic, including a comprehensive list of references.

or the pericardium. These aneurysms occur secondary to acquired or congenital disease.

ACQUIRED ANEURYSMS OF THE SINUS OF VALSALVA

Acquired sinus of Valsalva aneurysms occur secondary to subacute bacterial endocarditis, Marfan's syndrome, chronic dissection of the aorta and other degenerative lesions of the aortic root, atherosclerosis, and syphilis. Those associated with endocarditis are repaired usually at the time of aortic valve replacement by obliterating the orifice of the aneurysm. Atherosclerotic aneurysms are usually repaired with a Dacron patch. Those aneurysms caused by cystic medial necrosis or degenerative lesions of the aortic root usually require total replacement of the aortic root and valve with a composite graft with implantation of the coronary arteries. This can now be accomplished with a 5 per cent operative mortality.

CONGENITAL ANEURYSMS OF THE SINUS OF VALSALVA

ETIOLOGY AND PATHOPHYSIOLOGY. The pathologic process of congenital aneurysms is a separation between the aortic media and the heart at the anulus fibrosus of the aortic valve above the valve. The incidence varies from 0.23 to 0.69 per cent of all cardiac procedures. These aneurysms frequently rupture into an intracardiac chamber, producing a sudden left to right shunt. The most common sinus involved is the right sinus, which most commonly ruptures into the right ventricle and less frequently into the right atrium. The noncoronary sinus is the next most frequent site, and it usually ruptures into the right atrium. There have been unusual reports of rupture of the left sinus into all four chambers and the pulmonary artery. Associated intracardiac defects are frequently present, the most common of which are ventricular septal defect and aortic regurgitation.

CLINICAL PRESENTATION. The majority of patients are asymptomatic until the fistula ruptures. With rupture, the usual symptoms are dyspnea, palpitation, and chest pain. The symptoms are sometimes associated with dizziness, peripheral edema, and orthopnea and are usually accompanied by a precordial thrill with a continuous murmur heard loudest over the second to fourth intercostal spaces to the left of the sternal border for those that communicate with the right ventricle, and over the right third and fourth intercostal spaces for those that rupture into the right atrium. Pulse pressures are increased, and the murmur of aortic regurgitation may be present. Approximately one third of patients have a sudden onset of symptoms, sometimes associated with strenuous activity. Patients whose fistulas rupture into the pericardium present in cardiogenic shock with signs of cardiac tamponade.

Nonruptured aneurysms rarely cause symptoms due to compression of adjacent structures. Obstruction of the right ventricular outflow tract produces signs of right heart failure. Aneurysms can cause acute myocardial infarction or unstable angina by compressing a coronary artery. Left ventricular obstruction has occurred when an aneurysm protrudes into the left ventricle. Ventricular tachycardia and heart block have also been reported.

Chest roentgenograms usually reveal increased pulmonary vascular markings with enlargement of the right side of the heart and prominence of the main pulmonary arteries. Common electrocardiographic changes are left ventricular hypertrophy, right ventricular strain, axis shift, and biventricular hypertrophy. By use of two-dimensional and Doppler echocardiography techniques, it is possible to visualize the aneurysm and to identify a fistula, if present, in more than 80 per cent of patients. Cardiac catheterization is also helpful in delineating the anatomy of the aneurysm and identifying and quantitating the shunt.

TREATMENT. The presence of a fistula involving the sinus of Valsalva is considered an indication for operation because of progressive heart failure that can cause death. Those patients who have a nonruptured aneurysm of the sinus of Valsalva should be managed conservatively if they are asymptomatic but followed closely.

The fistula can be approached via the chamber into which it ruptures, through the aorta, or by a dual approach via the aorta and the chamber of entry of the fistula. Right ventricular fistulas can also be approached through the pulmonary artery. The advantage of the aorta-cameral approach is that the fistula can be probed from the aorta into the chamber involved and closed at both its origin and termination with an apparent decrease in recurrent fistula. The aortic valve can be inspected and protected from improperly placed sutures and repaired or replaced if significant insufficiency is present. The ventricular septum can be carefully inspected for the presence of a ventricular septal defect, which, if present, is closed.

RESULTS. In one review, the operative mortality was 12.7 per cent, with failure to close the fistula in 1.6 per cent and a favorable result in 85.7 per cent of patients. Seventy per cent of the patients who died had an associated cardiac abnormality. More recent series report an operative mortality of 0 to 13 per cent with an almost negligible reoperation rate. Actuarial survival at 25 years has been reported at 86 per cent.

2. TRAUMATIC ANEURYSMS OF THE AORTA

Walter G. Wolfe, M.D.

The incidence of traumatic rupture of the aorta has increased markedly with the development of high-speed motor

---

See the corresponding chapter or part in the *Textbook of Surgery*, 14th edition, pp. 1543–1548, for a more detailed discussion of this topic, including a comprehensive list of references.

vehicle accidents. The method of injury is trauma of the chest, which may produce rib or sternal fractures, pulmonary contusion, and/or pulmonary lacerations. The high-speed automobile accident produces a deceleration injury that appears to be tearing of the aorta, which is also seen in patients who fall from appreciable heights. In sudden deceleration of the body at the time of impact with differential rates of deceleration of the thoracic organs, the thoracic aorta and the great vessels can cause a tear that involves the intima and the media. The tear may be partial or complete. Eighty per cent of patients with rupture of the aorta into the pleural space die at the scene of the accident. Associated injuries are an important component of high-speed motor vehicle accidents and include head injuries, closed and compound long bone fractures, and injury to the viscera including the liver and spleen.

The diagnosis should be suspected in an individual who has had a sudden decelerating accident, especially if there is a widened mediastinum and/or fracture of the first rib. In these patients, aortography should be done to establish the diagnosis of a traumatic rupture of the aorta. In acute transection, when the diagnosis is established, the patient is resuscitated and other critical injuries are assessed and treated.

Immediate repair of the aorta is recommended. Generally, the operation is done through the left chest with repair and/ or grafting of the transected aorta. Bypass or shunting procedures may be used, with avoidance of systemic heparinization because of problems with associated injuries and bleeding.

MANAGEMENT OF CHRONIC TRANSECTION. A group of patients survive transected aorta and present with an enlarging aneurysm, which is considered a chronic transected aortic aneurysm. Usually the finding of this lesion is an indication for surgical therapy, since over time it increases in size and ruptures later. The results and mortality for managing future transections are usually less than 10 per cent, and death is usually related to associated injuries. Complications include bleeding and paraplegia, which may be associated with spinal injury at the time of the accident. On rare occasions, the ascending aorta may be injured, and the approach is through a median sternotomy with cardiopulmonary bypass and repair of the transected ascending aorta. Occasionally there may be associated valvular injuries also, which must be corrected.

3. DISSECTING ANEURYSMS OF THE AORTA

Walter G. Wolfe, M.D.

Dissecting aortic aneurysms are classified as DeBakey Type I, Type II, or Type III; Type I or Type II originates in the ascending aorta, and Type III originates in the distal subclavian. Other classifications divide these into ascending and descending dissecting aneurysms. They also may be acute or chronic. Aortic dissection is one of the most common catastrophic events involving the aorta and is a common cause of sudden death that may go undiagnosed without an autopsy. Acute dissection of the ascending aorta usually produces aortic insufficiency and may rupture into the mediastinum and/or pericardium, producing tamponade. Varying degrees of coronary as well as cerebral insufficiency may be seen. Dissection of the descending aorta may rupture into the left chest and commonly involve the entire length of the distal aorta, thereby involving the viscera at varying degrees.

CLINICAL PRESENTATION. Pain is the most frequent symptom in patients presenting with acute aortic dissection located in either the ascending or descending aorta. The patients are usually seriously ill and may have severe aortic insufficiency with pulmonary edema as well as diminished pulses. Differential diagnosis is myocardial infarction, rupture of sinus of Valsalva, aneurysm, cerebral vascular accident, acute surgical abdomen, pulmonary embolism, or arterial thrombosis at the bifurcation of the aorta. A high index of suspicion is necessary. The chest film usually reveals a widened mediastinum. The diagnosis is made by aortography, computed tomography, or, on occasion, transesophageal Doppler echocardiography. Survival of undiagnosed, untreated dissection is extremely low. By 48 hours, only 50 per cent of the patients are alive. Management of this condition is control of hypertension if it is present.

If aortic dissection originates in the ascending aorta, immediate operation with grafting of the ascending aorta with correction of the aortic insufficiency is the main operative intervention. In those patients with descending dissection, if the blood pressure is controlled and the patient is pain-free and there is no evidence of rupture or leak in the pleural space, continued observation with medical management and control of hypertension can be the primary therapy. If there is evidence of expansion or leak, left lateral thoracotomy with partial cardiopulmonary bypass and grafting of the descending thoracic aorta should be done.

Treatment of chronic dissections is similar, with resection and grafting of the aneurysm with use of Dacron in both the ascending and descending thoracic aorta. Usually, in the chronic state in the ascending aorta, if there is aortic insuffi-

See the corresponding chapter or part in the *Textbook of Surgery,* 14th edition, pp. 1548–1556, for a more detailed discussion of this topic, including a comprehensive list of references.

ciency, a valve replacement is necessary. Long-term follow-up has been excellent in those patients treated appropriately. Surgical mortality for acute ascending dissections is between 10 and 20 per cent, and the long-term survival approaches 50 per cent. In patients with descending aortic dissections, the mortality again is 10 per cent or less with excellent long-term outlook.

4. ANEURYSMS OF THE THORACIC AORTA

Walter G. Wolfe, M.D.

The thoracic aorta is composed of the ascending aorta, aortic arch, and descending thoracic aorta. The etiologic factor of thoracic aortic aneurysms today is most commonly atherosclerosis. However, cystic medial degeneration, myxomatous degeneration, and dissection trauma with a false aneurysm occurring most commonly at the ligamentum may be seen. Syphilitic aortitis is unusual today, but formerly it was a common cause. The incidence of thoracic aortic aneurysms increases with age, at which time cystic medial necrosis may accompany degenerative changes seen with atherosclerosis. Marfan's syndrome is best known through the finding of cystic medial necrosis as the etiologic basis for its degenerative nature and aneurysm formation in these patients.

Thoracic aneurysms present as an asymptomatic finding on chest film or perhaps with chest pain or pressure as a presenting symptom. Patients may experience hoarseness, superior vena caval syndrome, and tracheobronchial obstruction. Aneurysms of the ascending aorta may present with aortic insufficiency and cardiac failure. Diagnosis is made by use of the chest film, computed axial tomography, or arteriography. Surgical therapy for thoracic aneurysms began in 1953 with the method of local excision. Today the techniques are well established with use of cardiopulmonary bypass, deep hypothermia where necessary with resection and grafting of the aneurysm, and repair of the associated structures. The mortality is approximately 10 per cent.

ASCENDING AORTIC ANEURYSMS. These aneurysms are usually degenerative and include the aortic root, anulus, and leaflets. Certain aneurysms may be seen at the sinus of Valsalva, which may rupture into one of the chambers of the heart. Anuloaortic ectasia, another commonly presenting condition, also involves the sinuses and the anulus; it is usually accompanied by aortic insufficiency and commonly seen in Marfan's disease. Usually, the operation of choice is the Bental operation with replacement of the aortic valve and ascending aorta with a composite graft with reimplantation of the coronary arteries.

See the corresponding chapter or part in the *Textbook of Surgery*, 14th edition, pp. 1556–1559, for a more detailed discussion of this topic, including a comprehensive list of references.

TRANSVERSE AORTIC ARCH. The transverse aortic arch constitutes that portion of the aorta including the innominate, carotid, and subclavian vessels. Patients with this disorder are difficult to manage, and the operation performed is usually through a median sternotomy on cardiopulmonary bypass and deep hypothermic circulatory arrest. The aneurysm is replaced, and reconstruction of the arch vessels is done with use of a Dacron graft. This treatment has a mortality of 10 to 15 per cent with occasional significant neurologic complications occurring because of prolonged circulatory arrest.

DESCENDING THORACIC AORTA. The descending thoracic aorta is that segment from the left subclavian to the diaphragm. The incidence of aneurysms is second only to those seen in the infrarenal abdominal aorta. The etiologic factor is most commonly atherosclerosis. The patient may present with chest pain, hoarseness, cough, and occasionally hemoptysis or dysphagia. The treatment is resection and grafting of the aneurysm, usually with use of a synthetic woven Dacron graft. The operation is done through the left chest with the use of femorofemoral bypass, heparin-bonded shunts, or left atrial aortic bypass. These techniques are used to reduce left ventricular strain as well as to maintain good flow to the viscera and spinal cord. The most serious complication of operation on the descending thoracic aorta is paraplegia. Today, aneurysms of the descending thoracic aorta can usually be treated with a mortality of less than 10 per cent. The long-term survival has been excellent, with 5-year survival approaching 70 per cent.

5. ANEURYSMS OF THE CAROTID ARTERY

Richard H. Dean, M.D.

The most frequent site of carotid artery aneurysms is the common carotid artery, particularly its bifurcation. The mid and distal portions of the internal carotid artery are the next most common sites. Aneurysms at the bifurcation are usually fusiform, whereas those located in the internal carotid artery are usually saccular. Atherosclerosis is responsible for 46 to 70 per cent of all carotid artery aneurysms. Trauma and previous carotid artery surgery are less common causes.

The most common serious risk associated with carotid artery aneurysms is transient ischemic attacks and stroke. Most such central nervous system defects are caused by embolization of laminated thrombus lining the wall of the aneurysm. Less commonly, cerebral symptoms are caused by diminished flow through the carotid artery secondary to its compression by the mass of an adjacent saccular aneurysm.

See the corresponding chapter or part in the *Textbook of Surgery*, 14th edition, pp. 1560–1562, for a more detailed discussion of this topic, including a comprehensive list of references.

Although common in reports during the late nineteenth and early twentieth centuries, rupture of carotid artery aneurysms is rare today. When rupture occurs, it is manifested by hemorrhage from the pharynx, ear, or nose and may cause death by suffocation.

Elongation with kinking of the carotid artery is the most frequently found lesion masking as a carotid artery aneurysm. Usually, this lesion presents as a pulsatile mass at the base of the right neck, typically in hypertensive elderly women. This mass is easily distinguished from an aneurysm by the fact that the pulsation is along the long axis of the vessel. A prominent carotid artery bifurcation in a patient with a thin neck, a carotid body tumor, enlarged lymph nodes, branchial cleft cysts, or other masses that overlie and transmit the carotid pulse can be mistaken for an aneurysm.

Duplex sonography with B-mode imaging usually confirms or excludes the presence of an aneurysm of the extracranial carotid artery. However, high internal carotid artery aneurysms cannot be assessed accurately by this method owing to the limitations in visualizing that region. Computed tomography or magnetic resonance imaging is a useful substitute for B-mode imaging for the diagnosis of such lesions when they are located high in the neck. Angiography remains the definitive diagnostic test on which to base therapy, even when the diagnosis has been established by one of the noninvasive methods. Visualization of the entire length of both extracranial and intracranial components of the carotid artery and the vertebrobasilar system is required for any treatment strategies to be adequate.

Because most carotid bifurcation aneurysms are associated with a redundant internal carotid artery, resection of the aneurysm and reanastomosis of the internal carotid artery are employed in about 50 per cent of cases. Most of the other aneurysms are treated by resection and interpositional placement of either a saphenous vein graft or a polytetrafluoroethylene graft. Occasionally, a saccular aneurysm can be treated by resection and lateral arteriorrhaphy or patch angioplasty.

Occasionally, resection of the aneurysm is impossible owing to aneurysmal distal location at the base of the skull. In this instance, ligation of the internal carotid artery remains the only therapeutic option. If test clamping of the vessel is tolerated, ligation can be performed at a single stage. If crossclamping cannot be tolerated, extracranial-to-intracranial bypass with use of a microvascular technique can provide improved collateral perfusion to allow ligation. Gradual occlusion (over several days) with a Crutchfield clamp also continues to be useful. With either technique, anticoagulation for 10 days to 2 weeks is necessary to reduce the frequency of propagation of the distal clot into the collateral cerebral circulation.

6. CAROTID BODY TUMORS*

Richard H. Dean, M.D.

Carotid body tumors are uncommon paragangliomas located at the carotid bifurcation. Most are benign, but approximately 5 per cent metastasize. Cells of the carotid body producing such tumors are of mesodermal and third branchial arch and neural crest ectodermal origin. Although most are found as single tumors without association with tumors at other sites, occasionally they may have an autosomal dominant pattern of familial occurrence.

Most commonly, a carotid body tumor presents as a painless mass that is palpable at the carotid bifurcation. Large tumors may become painful and produce dysphagia, hoarseness, or even disturbance of tongue function by pressure or involvement of adjacent cranial nerves. Diagnostic studies may include computed tomography of the neck, but the definitive diagnostic study remains selective cerebral arteriography. The characteristic arteriographic appearance is that of an oval, hypervascular mass located between and widening the angle between the origins of the internal and external carotid arteries.

The preferred *treatment* of carotid body tumors is resection. Most small tumors can be removed without entering or resecting the carotid bifurcation. Since the cells producing the tumor are located in the outer region of the media, the tumor can usually be resected by entering and developing a subadventitial plane in the respective vessels of the carotid bifurcation. Large tumors may require resection of the bifurcation area and either patch closure of the defect or placement of an interposition graft. A few tumors are unresectable, and in these instances, radiation therapy may have some value. Resection can be achieved with minimal morbidity and mortality. Current results should include a combined incidence of major neurologic deficits and operative deaths that is less than 2 per cent.

7. SUBCLAVIAN ARTERY ANEURYSMS†

David C. Sabiston, Jr., M.D.

Subclavian arterial aneurysms are most often the result of atherosclerosis or trauma, and they may develop with the thoracic outlet syndrome as post-stenotic dilation of the

---

*See the corresponding chapter or part in the *Textbook of Surgery*, 14th edition, pp. 1562–1563, for a more detailed discussion of this topic, including a comprehensive list of references.
†See the corresponding chapter or part in the *Textbook of Surgery*, 14th edition, p. 1563, for a more detailed discussion of this topic, including a comprehensive list of references.

subclavian artery. A common complication of these aneurysms is the presence of mural thrombi, and thromboembolism of the upper extremity may be a serious problem. Rupture of the aneurysm may also occur. Appropriate treatment is excision of the aneurysm with restoration of arterial continuity, which may require the use of a graft.

8. VISCERAL ARTERIAL ANEURYSMS

David C. Sabiston, Jr., M.D.

More frequent than is often thought, visceral arterial aneurysms include those of the splenic, celiac, gastroduodenal, pancreaticoduodenal, and gastroepiploic arteries. *Splenic artery* aneurysms are the most common, particularly in females during pregnancy, and rupture is a recognized complication. Approximately half of the women with these aneurysms have had six or more pregnancies. Whereas most are due to medial degeneration of the arterial wall, fibromuscular dysplasia is also an etiologic factor. Mycotic aneurysms usually follow sepsis and are often the result of splenic emboli caused by subacute bacterial endocarditis. *Pain* in the left upper quadrant that may radiate to the left subscapular region is the most common symptom. Rupture is the most serious complication. A diagnosis can be made at times by the presence of a calcified lesion on the abdominal film and confirmed by arteriography. In one series of 40 ruptured splenic artery aneurysms, 10 were fatal. Operation is generally recommended when the aneurysm is discovered, especially those that are 2 cm. or greater in diameter. The procedure is excision of the aneurysm with ligation of the artery proximally and distally. Splenectomy is not necessary, since there is adequate collateral circulation for preservation of the spleen.

Celiac artery aneurysms are relatively uncommon with clinical manifestations being primarily vague abdominal discomfort with rupture as the most serious complication. These aneurysms should generally be excised when diagnosed.

Hepatic artery aneurysms usually present with signs and symptoms similar to those of gallbladder disease. Occasionally, hematemesis or melena may follow erosion of the aneurysm into the gastrointestinal tract. Free rupture into the peritoneal cavity is the most serious complication and is frequently fatal because of massive blood loss. Surgical extirpation is recommended when the diagnosis is made. About 20 per cent of these lesions are located within the liver and may be difficult to excise. Resection with use of a venous graft for preserving arterial continuity for prevention of hepatic ischemia is the operation of choice. Gastroduodenal, superior mesenteric, and pancreaticoduodenal artery aneurysms are uncommon; most present with rupture as the first

See the corresponding chapter or part in the *Textbook of Surgery*, 14th edition, pp. 1564–1566, for a more detailed discussion of this topic, including a comprehensive list of references.

indication of a problem. Resection is the procedure of choice, and in some instances multiple exclusion ligation can be performed.

Renal artery aneurysms are not uncommon and are generally located in the main renal artery or the bifurcation of the primary branches. A few are intrarenal and may be difficult to expose. Saccular aneurysms are more frequent than are fusiform, and the primary risk is free rupture into the peritoneal cavity. Clinical manifestations include symptoms of hypertension and upper abdominal pain. Multiple aneurysms also occur. The diagnosis is established by arteriography, and the management is excision of the aneurysm following diagnosis.

9. AORTIC ABDOMINAL ANEURYSMS

David C. Sabiston, Jr., M.D.

Aortic abdominal aneurysms are common and are dangerous if not treated appropriately. Dubost excised the first aortic abdominal aneurysm in 1951 and replaced it with an aortic homograft from a cadaver. Since then, thousands of patients have had successful corrections, and today the aorta is generally replaced with a Dacron graft.

The *natural history* of untreated abdominal aortic aneurysms is dismal, and for this reason nearly all aneurysms 5 to 6 cm. or more in diameter should be corrected soon after diagnosis. Prior to correction of aortic abdominal aneurysms, 102 patients seen at the Mayo Clinic before 1950 were followed with 67 per cent surviving 1 year, 49 per cent 3 years, and 19 per cent 4 years with similar findings reported by others. If an aortic abdominal aneurysm is *symptomatic*, approximately 30 per cent of these patients succumb within 1 month, and 75 per cent are dead by 6 months. These statistics indicate the importance of early operative correction.

The *clinical manifestations* of aortic abdominal aneurysm vary from the majority, which are *asymptomatic*, to those with sudden rupture with excruciating pain and profound shock due to blood loss retroperitoneally or into the peritoneal cavity. The *physical examination* of those patients with asymptomatic aneurysms reveals the presence of a pulsating mass generally located between the xiphoid process and the umbilicus. About 95 per cent of these aneurysms arise *distal* to the renal arteries. The inferior mesenteric artery arises from the abdominal aorta, usually at the site of the aneurysm, and is frequently severely stenotic or totally occluded owing to atherosclerosis in the aortic wall. This causes prominent development of collateral vessels, which anastomose with the inferior mesenteric artery distal to the obstruction. The iliac arteries may also be involved with aneurysms either

---

See the corresponding chapter or part in the *Textbook of Surgery,* 14th edition, pp. 1566–1574, for a more detailed discussion of this topic, including a comprehensive list of references.

unilaterally or bilaterally, and the femoral arterial system may show evidence of atherosclerotic disease with diminished or absent pulses in the groin and in the popliteal, posterior tibial, and anterior tibial arteries. Increased attention has been given the occurrence of inflammatory aortic abdominal aneurysms. These are characterized by aneurysms surrounded by dense periaortic inflammation and at times involvement of surrounding structures such as the duodenum, renal vein, and ureter. This problem occurs in about 7 to 10 per cent of patients undergoing aneurysmectomy.

Diagnostic studies usually reveal the size of the aneurysm together with its exact anatomic location. The wall of the aneurysm may be calcified, showing the "eggshell" appearance on the abdominal film, and the lateral film is quite helpful in confirming this point. Ultrasonography is a useful diagnostic procedure and provides objective information concerning the diameter of the aneurysm. Computed tomography is also helpful and permits delineation of the aortic lumen and aneurysmal thrombus with contrast enhancement. Aortography is the most definitive diagnostic technique and reveals the luminal size and extent of the aneurysm, the site of its anatomic location, and its relationship to the renal arteries and lesions within them as well as the distal circulation including the presence of aneurysms, stenoses, and arterial occlusion. It is important to recognize the presence of *suprarenal* involvement of the aneurysm, because this is likely to change the surgical approach and increase the risk factors of operation. Although aortography is not essential, it is quite helpful, especially in localizing sites of renal and peripheral vascular disease.

The complications of aortic abdominal aneurysms comprise the most significant problems. Since size is known to be related to rupture, it is important to recognize that with aneurysms greater than 7 cm. in diameter the mortality ranges between 72 and 83 per cent if such lesions are simply followed. Other complications include distal embolization of the iliofemoral arterial system with thrombi from the aneurysm, sudden thrombosis of the terminal aorta, infection, chronic consumptive coagulopathy, development of an aortic-intestinal fistula, and an aortic–vena caval arteriovenous fistula. In the preoperative assessment, careful attention should be given to cardiac function with a Holter monitor recording for 24 hours if there is concern regarding the presence of ischemic myocardial disease. In some patients, the extent and effects of coronary atherosclerosis may warrant myocardial revascularization before resection of the aortic aneurysms. The treatment of aortic abdominal aneurysms is surgical with correction of the aneurysm and replacement with a prosthetic Dacron graft. The operation is usually performed through a midline incision extending from the xiphoid process to the symphysis pubis. An incision in the left flank with a retroperitoneal approach has also been recommended for patients who have had previous abdominal procedures when dense adhesions might represent a serious technical problem. In these circumstances, the retroperitoneal approach can be preferable in the management of smaller aneurysms and those located in the midportion of the abdominal aorta between the renal arteries and bifurcation. However, prolonged postoperative incisional pain may be a complication in some patients with use of this approach. The intestines are drawn toward the right and carefully protected while the retroperitoneum is incised over the aneurysm. After thorough identification of the site of the aneurysm and its relationship to the renal arteries, the aorta proximal to the aneurysm is occluded as are the iliac vessels distally. The aneurysm is incised, and a Dacron graft is then inserted with an end-to-end anastomosis. A bifurcation graft is used when there is aneurysmal involvement of iliac arteries. The excess aneurysmal sac is excised, and the remainder is used to close over the graft for protecting it from adherence to the duodenum and small intestine postoperatively. Prophylactic antibiotics are administered several hours preoperatively and for several days after operation.

For the patient presenting with a ruptured aortic abdominal aneurysm, *emergency* operation must be performed immediately. Blood loss should be rapidly replaced with restoration of a normal blood pressure and blood volume. A Swan-Ganz catheter should be inserted to monitor pulmonary arterial wedge pressure such that volume replacement fluids and blood can be administered appropriately. If the patient has been resuscitated, the ruptured aneurysm can be managed successfully. Renal failure and cardiac problems often complicate the postoperative course and are related to the severity and length of preoperative hypotension and shock. Aggressive postoperative management including careful monitoring of cardiovascular dynamics is helpful in achieving a favorable result. In most series, the mortality of ruptured aneurysms varies between 30 and 50 per cent.

Myocardial insufficiency is the most common serious associated problem, and careful monitoring is necessary particularly in patients with a known history of coronary artery disease. Paralytic ileus is a common complication and should be managed by the use of a nasogastric tube. Occasionally bleeding may occur from the graft and require blood replacement or reoperation for control. Infection of the graft, usually at the suture lines, is another postoperative problem that occurs in approximately 1 to 2 per cent of patients. The treatment is quite extensive and usually requires reoperation with removal of the original graft and insertion of an axillobifemoral graft in a subcutaneous tunnel away from the previous graft site. If a new arterial prosthetic graft is placed at the site of the former graft, it usually becomes infected and necessitates another procedure. Other postoperative problems include changes in *sexual function* such as retrograde ejaculation and reduction or loss of sexual potency. These facts should be made known to the patients preoperatively. Spinal cord paralysis is uncommon with aortic abdominal aneurysm since the circulation to the spinal cord is rarely involved with lesions of the abdominal aorta in contrast with those in the thorax.

The results of aortic aneurysmectomy are quite favorable, and the mortality is less than 5 per cent for elective procedures. Fatalities are usually due to associated atherosclerotic lesions including myocardial infarction, cerebrovascular disease, and renal disease. In a recent study, the 5-year survival was 72 per cent for those patients less than age 70 years at the time of operation. Thus, nearly all patients with aneurysms 5 cm. or more should undergo elective operation in order to reduce the morbidity and mortality. For ruptured aneurysms, an emergency operation is the only hope for survival.

10.   FEMORAL ARTERY ANEURYSMS

William J. Fry, M.D.

The most common etiologic factor in the development of femoral artery aneurysm is atherosclerosis. With the advent of peripheral vascular reconstructive surgical techniques, an increased incidence of false aneurysms associated with aortofemoral bypass has been seen. The third most common type of femoral artery aneurysm is that associated with trauma, secondary to either penetrating or blunt injury. The common sequela of penetrating trauma in the femoral area is disruption of the femoral artery. A high incidence of false aneurysm and arteriovenous fistula formation is seen after penetrating wounds of the groin. Bacterial aneurysms are increasing. These are generally due to bacteria resistant to the usual antibiotics. In the past, they were almost always the result of *Salmonella* infection. Recently, bacterial aneurysms are being seen secondary to coagulase-positive *Staphylococcus* infections that are methacillin-resistant. Sepsis associated with femoral artery aneurysms has become more common. This is related to the increase in the drug culture. Not only are these difficult to treat, but the risks of associated AIDS infection must be borne in mind. The infection may be so extensive and the patient so debilitated that ligation and débridement may be the therapy of choice.

False aneurysms of the femoral artery and its branches may occur after cardiac catheterization or after angiography. These lesions, if left unattended, may pose a severe problem with distal embolization, occlusion of the femoral vein, or femoral nerve compression. They should be repaired as soon as the diagnosis is made. Duplex scanning can be very helpful in differentiating a false aneurysm from a hematoma. The palpation of a smooth, dilated femoral artery with expansile pulsations is, in most instances, sufficient to make the diagnosis of femoral artery aneurysm. In an occasional patient because of obesity, scar tissue formation, or heavy musculature, some doubt may be present after careful physical examination. In such instances, the use of ultrasound scan-

---

See the corresponding chapter or part in the *Textbook of Surgery*, 14th edition, pp. 1574–1575, for a more detailed discussion of this topic, including a comprehensive list of references.

ning is helpful in making the diagnosis and delineating the size of the femoral artery aneurysm.

When a femoral artery aneurysm is suspected or diagnosed on physical examination, an arteriogram of the abdominal aorta and iliac, femoral, and tibial vessels should be obtained. It has been found that 85 per cent of patients with a femoral artery aneurysm have some other associated aneurysm within the arterial tree. The majority were associated aortoiliac artery aneurysms, and 72 per cent of atherosclerotic aneurysms were found to be bilateral.

In bland femoral artery aneurysms, serious limb-threatening complications occur in only 3 per cent of the aneurysms when followed an average of 52 months. Symptomatic aneurysms may occlude or embolize, with resulting ischemia of the lower extremity. Spontaneous rupture of an atherosclerotic femoral artery aneurysm is a rare event. Because of the musculofascial compartment surrounding the common femoral artery, exsanguination is an unusual sequela. Tamponade usually occurs with marked ischemia of the distal portion of the involved extremity. Most femoral artery aneurysms are lined with laminated thrombus. The thrombus may lyse, with portions washed downstream, forming embolic occlusion in the popliteal or tibial vessels. Careful examination of the patient with a femoral artery aneurysm usually demonstrates the presence of multiple, small petechial hemorrhages in the distal portion of the extremity. These are secondary to microemboli from the interior of the aneurysmal sac.

The results of arterial reconstruction of the femoral artery are excellent, with mortality approaching zero. Saphenous vein grafts are regarded as being preferable to prosthetic grafts.

All patients should be followed closely because of the propensity of arterial aneurysms to develop at other sites.

11. POPLITEAL ARTERY ANEURYSMS

William J. Fry, M.D.

The majority of popliteal aneurysms seen are secondary to atherosclerosis. The incidence of aneurysm secondary to bacterial invasion of the arterial wall is slightly higher in the popliteal area than it is in the femoral artery. As with infected femoral aneurysms, the methacillin-resistant *Staphylococcus* organism has an important role. The diagnosis of a popliteal artery aneurysm is most commonly made by physical examination. The findings of an aneurysm in the popliteal space are sometimes subtle and may be overlooked by the inexperienced. Popliteal artery aneurysms seldom involve the distal popliteal artery. They more commonly present opposite the joint space. Physical findings may be masked in the heavily

See the corresponding chapter or part in the *Textbook of Surgery*, 14th edition, pp. 1575–1577, for a more detailed discussion of this topic, including a comprehensive list of references.

muscled lower extremity. Ultrasound scanning is a readily available, noninvasive diagnostic procedure that serves as a good screening technique for making the diagnosis of popliteal aneurysm when there is some question on physical examination.

Arteriography is mandatory. Popliteal aneurysms are bilateral in 47 per cent of patients. In addition, 78 per cent of patients with popliteal aneurysms have another aneurysm somewhere in the arterial tree. The majority, 64 per cent, are located in the abdominal aorta or iliac arteries. Popliteal artery aneurysms are often associated with distal occlusive disease. The laminated thrombus within the wall of the aneurysm forms the nidus for distal embolization. Constant trauma secondary to motion of the knee joint adds to fragmentation of the intraluminal thrombus. Accurate arteriography for delineation of the outflow tract is always necessary before any operative approach in the treatment of a popliteal artery aneurysm.

The most common sequela of the untreated popliteal artery aneurysm is distal arterial occlusion. Careful examination of the distal extremity in the patient with a popliteal artery aneurysm usually reveals areas of petechial hemorrhage secondary to small emboli. As the laminated thrombus collection progresses within the aneurysmal sac, three events occur: (1) extensive embolization, which may occlude the outflow tract; (2) laminated thrombus, which may occlude the orifices of the popliteal trifurcation; and (3) complete thrombosis of the aneurysm. These possibilities are limb-threatening, and the possibility of arterial reconstruction for maintaining viability of the extremity may be compromised.

Popliteal aneurysm rupture is not a common occurrence. As with femoral artery aneurysms, the patient is not likely to exsanguinate because of the strong musculofascial compartment surrounding the popliteal artery. Rupture usually tamponades, and the resulting ischemia to the distal leg is severe. Attempts at arterial reconstruction after rupture are difficult, and the ability to restore viability may be difficult. Large popliteal aneurysms may cause chronic or acute venous obstruction, and thrombophlebitis is not an uncommon finding with the acutely expanding popliteal artery aneurysm.

The author has used the *medial* approach to popliteal artery aneurysms, and use of an autogenous saphenous vein is preferred. It is important not to excise the popliteal artery aneurysm because damage to the popliteal vein invariably occurs. Experience in the therapy of popliteal aneurysms reveals the continued preference for the use of autogenous saphenous vein as a replacement for the popliteal artery aneurysm. Experience shows a continued lower failure rate with saphenous vein over either polytetrafluoroethylene or Dacron. The long-term amputation rate with all forms of therapy was 6 per cent. Emphasis should be placed on the danger of concomitant heart disease in patients with popliteal aneurysms, there being 15 per cent better survival in patients without aneurysms and those with successfully repaired popliteal aneurysms. Szilagyi has reported a long-term follow-up with 50 popliteal aneurysms treated by surgical therapy. He has treated 30 patients with an autologous saphenous vein and 20 with a Dacron prosthesis and has a cumulative patency rate of 60 per cent at 5 years and 28 per cent at 10 years. In this series, there were no late amputations secondary to graft failure. These results emphasized that atherosclerotic popliteal artery aneurysms are part of the pathologic process of systemic atherosclerosis and that continued progression of the disease ultimately may cause graft occlusion.

The patient who has had repair of a popliteal artery aneurysm should be followed indefinitely, since the multiplicity of aneurysms as well as the ever-present hazard of the replacement graft makes it mandatory to follow these patients very carefully.

VI

Thrombo-obliterative Disease of the Aorta and Its Branches*

David C. Sabiston, Jr., M.D.

Atherosclerosis is the most frequent cause of occlusive disease of the major branches of the aorta. The most susceptible site for stenosis or occlusion is at the *origin* of vessels where the *turbulence* is maximal. When branches of the aortic arch such as the innominate, carotid, and subclavian vessels become stenotic or occluded, the symptoms produced are caused by ischemic disturbances due to reduction in blood flow.

The surgical management is prosthetic bypass grafts. More specific indications such as those involving the carotid, subclavian, and axillary arteries are separately described.

1. TAKAYASU'S ARTERITIS†

David C. Sabiston, Jr., M.D.

In 1908 a Japanese ophthalmologist, Takayasu, described a nonspecific arteritis that affects the thoracic and abdominal aorta and its major branches. Although uncommon in the United States, it is often seen in the Orient and occurs

*See the corresponding chapter or part in the *Textbook of Surgery*, 14th edition, p. 1577, for a more detailed discussion of this topic, including a comprehensive list of references.

†See the corresponding chapter or part in the *Textbook of Surgery*, 14th edition, p. 1580, for a more detailed discussion of this topic, including a comprehensive list of references.

predominantly in young females but also in older women and men as well. The arteritis involves all layers of the arterial wall with proliferation of connective tissue and degeneration of elastic fibers. Granulomatous lesions may be present with associated fusiform or saccular aneurysms. This arteritis may be localized to the aortic arch and great vessels (Group I), to the distal thoracic and abdominal aorta (Group III), or to the entire aorta (Group II).

The clinical manifestations include those that are systemic with production of fever, malaise, and arthritis. Pericardial pain, tachycardia, and vomiting may also occur. Some believe this disorder to be an autoimmune disease, and steroids may be beneficial. The late manifestations of the disorder are those of ischemia to the arterial circulation of the brain and upper extremities. Surgical treatment has often proved disappointing because the site of endarterectomy or bypass may subsequently be involved in recurrent disease. Operation is occasionally recommended for patients with disabling symptoms.

2. CAROTID ARTERY OCCLUSIVE DISEASE

Richard H. Dean, M.D.

Although the association of carotid artery disease and stroke had been suggested for over 130 years, intensity of interest developed with the introduction of reliable, safe arteriography and techniques of operative correction.

Three causes of transient ischemic attacks (TIAs) and stroke stem from occlusive disease of the extracranial carotid artery. These are thrombosis and propagation of distal clot, low flow–related ischemic events, and embolization from the atherosclerotic lesions at the carotid bifurcation. The most frequent cause is embolization from the atherosclerotic lesion with occlusion of an intracerebral branch. The clinical presentations of carotid artery occlusive disease can be categorized into three general groups: asymptomatic lesions, lesions producing TIAs, and those lesions that have produced cerebral infarction.

Asymptomatic patients are those who have a hemodynamically significant lesion or nonocclusive ulcerated lesion of the carotid artery but no history of cerebral symptoms. The presence of a bruit in an asymptomatic patient does not define this group, Kartchner and McRae finding that less than one third of patients with a cervical bruit had a hemodynamically significant lesion of the carotid artery by noninvasive criteria.

The importance of an asymptomatic carotid artery stenosis should be emphasized, since serial studies using serial duplex

---

See the corresponding chapter or part in the *Textbook of Surgery*, 14th edition, pp. 1580–1583, for a more detailed discussion of this topic, including a comprehensive list of references.

scanning show an annual 4 per cent rate of recurrent symptoms. Progression of a lesion to more than an 80 per cent stenosis, however, has a 35 per cent risk of ischemic events or total occlusion within 6 months.

By definition, TIAs are temporary neurologic deficits lasting less than 24 hours and followed by complete recovery. When in the area supplied by the carotid artery, they are usually discrete motor and/or sensory dysfunctions. Contralateral facial, arm, and/or leg motor weakness or sensory loss is the classic presentation. Since the left hemisphere is dominant in 95 per cent of the population, left hemispheric TIAs may also cause either receptive or expressive aphasia. Probably the most classic TIA of carotid artery origin is transient loss or blurred vision (amaurosis fugax) in the ipsilateral eye. It is classically described as a curtain being drawn down over the eye or as a quadrant field defect and is caused by embolization to the retinal branches of the ophthalmic artery, the first major intracranial branch of the internal carotid artery. In addition, the first clinical manifestation of carotid artery disease may be a permanent neurologic deficit or stroke. Depending on the area of cerebral cortex affected, the defect may range from minimal, with ultimate recovery of the lost function, to massive, causing death.

Initial evaluation of an asymptomatic cervical bruit is best achieved with duplex scanning. Cerebral arteriography is required if a severe lesion is found and in all patients evaluated following the onset of TIAs or stroke. In the last two groups, computed tomographic scanning of the head also is required to assess the cerebrum for the presence and size of infarcts and to exclude other pathologic intracranial processes.

Carotid *endarterectomy* is indicated for treatment of patients with hemispheric TIAs and of patients with either retained or regained significant residual functioning cortex after a completed stroke associated with carotid bifurcation occlusive disease. Although use of prophylactic carotid endarterectomy for asymptomatic patients remains debatable, it is probably indicated for patients with severe (more than 80 per cent) stenosis and complex, ulcerated plaques. The technique of carotid endarterectomy is relatively simple but requires precision if the results are to be good.

Current results of carotid endarterectomy should include less than a 5 per cent combined cerebrovascular morbidity and operative mortality. Most current series have combined morbidity and mortality in the asymptomatic patient group of less than 3 per cent. Obviously, the preoperative neurologic status of the patient affects the incidence of immediate perioperative events as well as the late results. Many issues regarding the necessity for evaluation and intervention in patients with cerebrovascular disease remain controversial. The role of intervention for asymptomatic lesions is currently being investigated with a prospective randomized multicenter trial. Until proven otherwise, however, carotid endarterectomy remains the treatment of choice for symptomatic carotid artery disease and severe asymptomatic lesions.

3. SUBCLAVIAN STEAL SYNDROME

John A. Mannick, M.D.

The subclavian steal syndrome occurs when there is reversal of flow in the ipsilateral vertebral artery distal to a stenosis or occlusion of the proximal subclavian or, more rarely, of the innominate artery. Because of the lowering of pressure in the subclavian artery distal to the obstruction, blood flows up the vertebral artery on the unaffected side into the basilar artery and down the vertebral artery on the affected side to supply collateral circulation to the subclavian artery and its subsidiary arterial systems. Thus, blood supply is presumably "stolen" from the basilar artery, and, at least theoretically, blood supply to the brain stem may be compromised.

CLINICAL EVALUATION. Classically, the subclavian steal syndrome should be suspected in a patient who manifests symptoms of vertebrobasilar arterial insufficiency and is found on examination to have a difference in brachial systolic blood pressure of at least 30 mm. Hg between the two arms and in whom there is a *bruit* at the base of the neck or in the supraclavicular area on the affected side. The cause of proximal subclavian obstruction is arteriosclerosis in the majority of instances. The left subclavian artery is involved in a much greater percentage of cases (about 70 per cent) than is the right. The neurologic symptoms reported in patients with this syndrome most commonly include vertigo, limb paresis, and paresthesias. Bilateral cortical visual disturbances, ataxia, syncope, and dysarthria occur somewhat less frequently. The symptoms are encountered initially as transient ischemic attacks in the majority of patients. The diagnosis of subclavian steal is made by retrograde catheter angiography with injection of contrast into the aortic arch.

Early reports suggested that the subclavian steal was associated with disabling neurologic symptoms in the majority of patients in whom it was encountered, whereas increasing clinical experience has demonstrated that the subclavian steal phenomenon is probably an asymptomatic lesion in most patients. In the report of the Joint Study of Extracranial Arterial Occlusion in which 168 patients with the subclavian steal syndrome were evaluated, patients with subclavian artery disease alone did not have strokes during the follow-up period whether they were treated medically, surgically, or not at all. It appears reasonable to conclude, therefore, that the subclavian steal phenomenon may frequently be an asymptomatic lesion but can produce or contribute to symptoms of cerebrovascular insufficiency when it exists in conjunction with other lesions of the extracranial cerebral arterial supply, particularly carotid bifurcation lesions. Whether the subclavian steal phenomenon produces symptoms in a specific individual is probably dependent on (1) the size of the

---

See the corresponding chapter or part in the *Textbook of Surgery*, 14th edition, pp. 1584–1588, for a more detailed discussion of this topic, including a comprehensive list of references.

vertebral artery on the uninvolved side and whether it is free from disease, (2) the anatomy of the circle of Willis, (3) the amount of collateral circulation from other sources that develops to supply the arm on the affected side, and (4) most significantly, the presence of other lesions in the cerebral arterial supply.

SURGICAL CORRECTION. In patients in whom the subclavian steal syndrome appears to be responsible for symptoms of vertebrobasilar insufficiency, in the absence of other lesions in the extracranial cerebral arterial circulation, surgical correction of the subclavian steal appears warranted and can ameliorate symptoms. However, surgical therapy cannot justifiably be urged for the prevention of stroke, since subclavian steal does not appear to cause stroke in the majority of patients. When the subclavian steal syndrome occurs in association with other extracranial arterial lesions, it is evident that the other significant lesions should be repaired as well, since there are a number of reports of symptomatic relief in patients with subclavian steal in whom only the other arterial lesions were corrected. Whereas a number of surgical procedures have been recommended for correction of subclavian steal, the most commonly applied operation today is probably the common carotid to subclavian artery bypass graft performed through a cervical incision. When it is normally patent, the common carotid artery in man has the capacity to supply both the brain and the arm with blood without any drop in pressure distal to the origin of the carotid to subclavian bypass graft. An equally effective means of correcting subclavian steal is the subclavian-carotid transposition in which the subclavian artery is divided just distal to its proximal stenosis or occlusion. The distal end of the artery is sutured end-to-side to the common carotid artery, which thus serves as a new innominate artery trunk perfusing the subclavian and vertebral arterial systems.

The results of surgical correction have been excellent in terms of reversal of the hemodynamic abnormalities of the subclavian steal. Relief of the associated cerebral symptoms has been achieved in a high percentage of those patients operated upon as well. Recent publications suggest that mortality from carotid subclavian bypass by experienced surgeons is nearly nonexistent and that the risk of associated stroke is also very low.

4. THROMBOTIC OBLITERATION OF THE ABDOMINAL AORTA AND ILIAC ARTERIES (LERICHE'S SYNDROME)

David C. Sabiston, Jr., M.D.

Thrombotic obliteration of the terminal abdominal aorta, often involving the iliac vessels, is due to underlying athero-

See the corresponding chapter or part in the *Textbook of Surgery*, 14th edition, pp. 1588–1590, for a more detailed discussion of this topic, including a comprehensive list of references.

sclerosis superimposed by thrombus. The process is usually one of slow but progressive involvement. The duration of the pathologic process provides ample time for multiple collateral vessels to develop between the aorta proximally and the iliofemoral system distally, thus allowing reasonable circulation to the lower extremities. However, with the passage of time and continuously increasing obstruction, symptoms appear.

CLINICAL MANIFESTATIONS. Symptoms characteristic of Leriche's syndrome include (1) fatigue in both lower limbs and thighs, which has often been described as a weariness rather than typical intermittent claudication, (2) atrophy of both lower limbs without atrophic changes in the skin or nails, (3) pallor of the legs and feet, and (4) inability of males to maintain a stable erection owing to inadequate arterial flow to the penis.

The positive physical findings include absence of pulsations in the abdominal aorta and in the distal arteries. This disorder is often well tolerated for 5 or even 10 years, but ultimately ischemia and gangrene ensue. Therefore, surgical therapy should be performed when symptoms are marked and before severe ischemic changes in the legs.

The *diagnosis* is made by clinical examination and confirmed by arteriography, which reveals occlusion of the terminal aorta and often of one or both iliac arteries. Extensive collateral circulation is usually apparent. An arterial bypass graft is the treatment of choice from the proximal aorta to the distal aorta with an end-to-end anastomosis. If one or both iliac vessels are involved, a *bifurcation* graft is employed. The results are usually quite good. Patients should be strongly advised to cease smoking postoperatively because occlusion of the prosthetic graft is much more apt to occur if smoking continues.

5.   ILIAC ARTERIAL OCCLUSION

David C. Sabiston, Jr., M.D.

The iliac arteries may be the site of stenosis or occlusion that causes symptoms or claudication of the hips and thighs. The distal pulses are usually diminished or absent in the involved extremity. Arteriography is diagnostic for both the site and magnitude of arterial obstruction. Even when the symptoms are unilateral, the arteriogram often demonstrates disease in the asymptomatic limb. Bypass grafting with a plastic prosthesis is the operation of choice and should be performed when symptoms are sufficiently severe to interfere with the patient's life-style.

See the corresponding chapter or part in the *Textbook of Surgery*, 14th edition, p. 1590, for a more detailed discussion of this topic, including a comprehensive list of references.

6. FEMOROPOPLITEAL AND FEMOROINFRAPOPLITEAL BYPASS

Richard L. McCann, M.D.

Patients with peripheral vascular obstructive disease in the lower extremities usually present with *pain*. A careful analysis of the location, quality, and intensity of the pain and factors that aggravate and relieve the pain yields important clinical information. The term *claudication* is applied to the cramping pain felt in specific muscle groups when blood flow is inadequate for meeting the metabolic demands of exercise. The distance walked before onset of this pain is strikingly reproducible, and the pain is promptly relieved simply by cessation of ambulation. The site of the claudication is related to the site of principal arterial obstruction. Claudication in the buttock and thigh muscles is indicative of proximal aortoiliac obstruction, whereas calf claudication usually indicates femoral artery disease. When blood flow is inadequate for meeting the metabolic requirements at rest, continuous pain may be described. This pain, in contrast to claudication, is usually felt in the toes and forefoot. Rest pain is an ominous symptom and demands prompt evaluation not only because of the considerable discomfort but because it indicates such severe vascular compromise that the involved limb may soon progress to frank gangrene in the absence of intervention.

It is important to recognize that atherosclerosis is a systemic metabolic disorder, and overt manifestations of concomitant cerebrovascular or coronary artery disease are often present in patients with lower extremity ischemia. The importance of associated coronary and cerebrovascular disease is emphasized by the fact that in most long-term studies, 75 per cent of the patients requiring lower extremity revascularization were dead by 10 years, and almost all of the deaths were from myocardial infarction or cerebrovascular accident.

Physical examination often confirms suspicions elicited by the clinical history. Pallor of the skin may be present, particularly with elevation of the legs, and this is often associated with rubor of dependency, which is thought to be due to cutaneous reactive vasodilation in response to chronic ischemia. Proximal obstruction not only decreases mean arterial pressure but also decreases the perceived pulse amplitude because the pulse pressure is diminished distal to a site of obstruction. Dorsalis pedis and posterior tibial pulses are usually not palpable in patients with lower extremity ischemia. Noninvasive vascular laboratory examinations are useful in providing a quantitative description of the vascular status of the lower extremities. The most useful examinations include determination of segmental blood pressures by use of a Doppler velocity detector, the use of pulse volume recordings, and the response of these indices to a standardized

---

See the corresponding chapter or part in the *Textbook of Surgery*, 14th edition, pp. 1590–1597, for a more detailed discussion of this topic, including a comprehensive list of references.

exercise regimen. However, the noninvasive vascular study should not be used alone; rather, it is used to complement the information obtained from the history and physical examination. These help to establish a baseline for longitudinal comparisons, particularly before and after active interventions.

Studies of the natural history of intermittent claudication have shown that patients with this as the sole manifestation of lower limb ischemia have a low risk of limb loss. More than 75 per cent of patients remain stable or even improve with conservative management alone. Medical treatment includes complete abstinence from the use of tobacco, control of weight, and a program of graduated exercise. Patients who cease smoking, even at this late stage, improve their prognosis for limb retention significantly. Regular walking exercise also produces a measurable improvement in walking distance in patients with intermittent claudication. The mechanism responsible for this improvement is not fully understood but may be due to adaptive changes in the muscle enzyme systems producing more efficient oxygen extraction and utilization. Strict compliance with these nonsurgical treatments often yields double or more claudication distance and may be the only treatment required. However, in patients in whom nonsurgical treatment fails to alleviate the disability imposed by intermittent claudication and in whom symptoms interfere with gaining a livelihood or impose an intolerable limitation of life-style, surgical treatment can be offered if it is understood that the goal is improvement in exercise capacity rather than limb salvage. In contrast, patients with rest pain, ischemic ulcerations, or limited gangrene are usually candidates for vascular reconstruction because the threat of limb loss is much greater.

Arteriography is necessary only if it has been decided that revascularization is indicated. The entire vascular tree from the aorta to the foot should be visualized to ensure that all significant stenoses and occlusions are corrected.

A number of catheter-based treatment options are now available for the treatment of patients with peripheral vascular disease. Balloon dilation, with and without the assistance of laser energy, and the use of miniature cutting devices (atherectomy catheters) have been found to be successful in treating short stenoses and occlusions but are much less successful in treating long occlusions or long stenoses with multiple sites of disease in the femoral artery, which continue to be better treated by surgical bypass. For patients treated surgically, most undergo vein bypass grafting. Endarterectomy is occasionally useful, as is enlargement of the orifice of the profunda femoris when it has been severely restricted by atherosclerotic disease. There has been considerable debate regarding the most appropriate graft material used in lower extremity bypass operations. It has now been clearly demonstrated that autogenous venous reconstructions are significantly more durable than are reconstructions performed with use of a synthetic vascular conduit. Results with synthetic grafts become progressively worse compared with autogenous venous grafts, the closer to the foot is the distal anastomosis and the longer the period of time over which they are studied.

With respect to the saphenous vein, two opposing camps have been established. In the *in situ* technique, the saphenous vein is not dissected from its bed except for the proximal and distal limbs, which are mobilized and used to create the proximal and distal end-to-side anastomoses of the bypass. The intervening side branches must be ligated to prevent occurrence of hemodynamically significant arteriovenous fistula. The valves must be destroyed or cut with a specially designed valvulotome in order to allow flow toward the foot. Advocates of this technique claim it allows the use of smaller grafts because the small end of the vessel is attached to the smaller artery and the large end of the graft to the larger artery. With use of this technique, excellent patency and limb salvage rates have been achieved.

However, comparable concurrent series using the more traditional reversed saphenous vein graft have also shown improved results in the last decade. Proponents of this technique also claim improved vein utilization rates and avoidance of reliance on synthetic grafts because in patients who do not possess an intact ipsilateral vein, a satisfactory graft can be constructed by use of the contralateral limb or fragments of large veins from either leg or even the arm.

Improvement in patency and limb salvage rates in patients treated for lower extremity peripheral vascular obstructive disease has been one of the most dramatic improvements in vascular surgery in the last decade. Compared with 75 and 50 per cent, 1- and 5-year patency rates 10 years ago, current results show 90 per cent 1-year and 70 per cent multiyear patency rates with limb salvage 5 to 10 per cent higher. These improvements have been achieved by an increased appreciation of the fragility of the saphenous vein and the importance of gentle technique in its preparation for use by either the *in situ* or the reversed technique. In addition, the increased appreciation of the clear superiority of autogenous venous grafting over synthetic or modified biologic grafts has also had a role in this improvement.

7. PERCUTANEOUS TRANSLUMINAL ANGIOPLASTY

R. Duane Davis, M. D.

Since its introduction in 1964, percutaneous transluminal angioplasty (PTA) has been applied to the treatment of a large number of vaso-occlusive disorders, most frequently those involving the peripheral vasculature, renal arteries, subclavian arteries, hemodialysis fistulas, and coronary arteries. Although PTA may be the modality of choice in certain

See the corresponding chapter or part in the *Textbook of Surgery*, 14th edition, pp. 1597–1611, for a more detailed discussion of this topic, including a comprehensive list of references.

clinical settings, it is more often an adjunctive technique to existing vascular surgical techniques.

COMPARISON OF SURGICAL MANAGEMENT WITH PTA. PTA has inherent advantages compared with surgical revascularization—the use of local anesthesia and mild sedation, shorter hospitalization, lower cost per procedure, less morbidity, and less lost productivity. PTA can be applied to patients whose medical condition contraindicates surgical therapy, and it avoids the disruption of local nerves, lymphatics, and blood vessels intrinsic to adequate surgical exposure. PTA can be repeated without loss of efficacy, and when unsuccessful, usually the patient's condition is not worsened.

However, the majority of patients with vascular occlusive disease are not optimally treated with PTA. Lesions that are best treated by PTA are short stenoses less than 5 cm. in length. Occlusions in the superficial femoral arteries often can be treated by angioplasty; however, treatment of occlusions in most other vessels is less successful. Multiple lesions are associated with poorer clinical results and patency rates. Restenosis occurs in 30 per cent of coronary vessels after 6 months. Larger vessels have lower restenosis rates.

COMPLICATIONS. Complications occur, on the average, in 5 to 10 per cent of patients undergoing PTA, but rates as high as 33 per cent have been reported. Mortality is 0 to 2 per cent, reflecting the presence of generalized atherosclerosis involving other vascular beds. Complications of PTA can be categorized as those occurring at the puncture site, at the angioplasty site, distal to the angioplasty site, and those systemic in nature.

Systemic complications include renal insufficiency or allergic reactions due to the contrast agent, hypotension due to hemorrhage or renal artery PTA, and anemia associated with hemorrhage.

PERIPHERAL VASCULAR PTA. Occlusive lesions of the iliac, femoral, popliteal, and infrapopliteal arteries as well as of the terminal aorta have been successfully treated with PTA. The best results have been in the treatment of iliac artery stenosis, with technical success in 85 to 95 per cent of patients and patency of successful dilations of 86 to 100 per cent, 78 to 89 per cent, and 47 to 85 per cent at 1, 3, and 5 years, respectively. Clinical success is somewhat lower, 50 to 65 per cent and 48 to 60 per cent at 3 and 5 years, respectively. PTA of iliac occlusions has a higher incidence of embolic complications, a lower rate of technical success (33 to 88 per cent), and a lower patency rate (50 to 100 per cent at 3 to 5 years). Surgical revascularization by use of aortofemoral bypass has been associated with a primary success rate of 92 to 100 per cent; cumulative patency rates are reported to be 94 to 98 per cent after 1 year, 90 to 97 per cent after 2 years, and 80 to 90 per cent after 5 years (mortality between 3 and 6 per cent). PTA provides a much less invasive modality of therapy but is less durable owing to restenosis and progression of the disease within the iliac vessels. For optimal short stenoses, PTA is a good initial modality of therapy.

PTA of the femoropopliteal system has an initial technical

success between 70 and 96 per cent, with 1-year patency rates of 54 to 90 per cent and 3-year patency rates of 43 to 84 per cent. Because of the straighter course of the femoral artery, treatment of femoral artery occlusions is more effective than is treatment of iliac artery occlusions. Although the technical success rate of dilating occlusions is only mildly less than that of treating stenoses, the long-term patency rates are poor (57 per cent at 2 years). Clinical success is lower, 50 and 40 per cent at 3 and 5 years, respectively. Predictors of success include (1) short, singular lesions, (2) good outflow, (3) claudication versus limb salvage, and (4) absence of tobacco use and diabetes mellitus. Femoropopliteal bypass with use of saphenous vein provides better long-term patency and clinical benefit; however, PTA results are comparable to or better than results obtained with use of synthetic material for bypass.

PTA of infrapopliteal vessels produces clinical successes in approximately 50 to 60 per cent of patients. However, more recently, with utilization of an aggressive pharmacologic regimen for prevention of vasospasm, technical successes in 97 per cent of patients and limb salvage in 86 per cent at 2 years have been reported.

Hypertension and renal insufficiency due to renal artery stenosis have been successfully treated by PTA, particularly when the etiologic factor is fibromuscular dysplasia. Ideal lesions treated by PTA include atherosclerotic lesions that are short, located in the main renal artery and not contiguous with the renal artery ostium, and stenoses due to fibromuscular dysplasia that do not involve the branch vessels. In contrast, renal artery PTA of atherosclerotic ostial lesions is less often technically successful, is more prone to restenosis, and provides less clinical benefit. PTA of stenoses due to fibromuscular dysplasia is technically successful in 87 to 100 per cent of patients, which is clinically beneficial in approximately 84 per cent. Cure of hypertension occurs in 57 per cent, and improvement occurs in 27 per cent. Technical success in the treatment of nonostial atherosclerotic lesions occurs in 72 to 79 per cent of patients, and in only 62 to 66 per cent of patients with ostial lesions. Treatment of atherosclerotic renovascular hypertension provides cure in 22 per cent and improvement in 39 per cent, for an overall benefit of 61 per cent. Restenosis occurs in approximately 5 per cent of fibromuscular dysplasia PTAs, 15 to 25 per cent of PTAs of atherosclerotic lesions, and up to 74 per cent of ostial lesions.

Complications are more common following renal artery PTA, averaging 7 to 10 per cent but occurring in as many as 33 per cent. The most common complication is renal insufficiency, which is usually reversible. Other common complications include renal artery dissection and perforation, renal artery emboli as well as other atheromatous emboli, myocardial infarction, and local complications at the femoral artery puncture site. Approximately 2 to 5 per cent of patients require operative intervention, sometimes as an emergency. Mortality, most commonly due to myocardial infarction or diffuse atherosclerotic emboli, averages 1 per cent but ranges up to 7 per cent.

Treatment of renovascular hypertension occurring in the 5 to 7 per cent of renal transplant patients with use of PTA is technically successful in 84 to 90 per cent. Improvement in blood pressure control occurs in 75 per cent of patients. PTA is the initial invasive modality for treatment of these patients. PTA of coarctation of the aorta is usually technically successful with significant gradient reduction and enlargement of the aorta at the coarctation site, usually without the paradoxical hypertension that can complicate surgical repairs. However, approximately 30 per cent of patients have recoarctation. A significant incidence of aneurysm formation occurs at the PTA site. PTA of recurrent coarctation after surgical repair does not appear to be complicated by aneurysm formation or a high rate of restenosis.

Occlusive vascular disease in many other vascular beds has been successfully treated with use of PTA, including visceral arteries, subclavian arteries (subclavian steal), superior vena cava (superior vena caval syndrome), hepatic veins (Budd-Chiari syndrome), hemodialysis fistulas, and portal-systemic venous shunts. Cerebrovascular lesions not due to atherosclerosis have been treated without significant complications. However, PTA of atherosclerotic stenoses of the cerebral vessels has been cautiously pursued because of the risk of cerebral emboli.

Although the majority of patients with vascular disease have obstructions better treated with surgical revascularization because of the presence of diffuse, long, or multiple lesions, PTA is an effective therapy for a number of patients with vascular occlusive disease, particularly when the obstructing lesion is anatomically favorable. In addition, PTA can be applied to patients whose attendant risk with operation is great. Angioplasty can be used in a number of clinical settings as an adjunct to surgical techniques to simplify arterial reconstruction or salvage existing grafts with occlusive lesions. Optimal care of the patient with vaso-occlusive disease requires close cooperation between the angiographer and surgeon for the proper treatment selection and management of the potentially catastrophic complications that may occur following angioplasty.

8.   ARTERIAL INJURIES

Robert J. Freeark, M. D., William H. Baker, M. D., and John J. Klosak, M. D.

In the late nineteenth and early twentieth centuries, suture techniques were developed for the repair and reconstruction of blood vessels. These techniques were first applied in the

See the corresponding chapter or part in the *Textbook of Surgery*, 14th edition, pp. 1612–1623, for a more detailed discussion of this topic, including a comprehensive list of references.

Korean Conflict when rapid evacuation of the wounded allowed prompt care of these injuries. Currently, the automobile and urban violence are the common etiologic agents of injury. Penetrating injuries are increasingly due to gunshot wounds.

MECHANISMS OF INJURY. Arteries and veins can be injured by penetrating or blunt trauma. Knife wounds transect arteries much as a surgical scalpel does, leaving little devitalized tissue on either side of the wound. Contrariwise, gunshot wounds involving high-velocity missiles may produce tissue damage for some distance on either side of the obvious wound and require extensive débridement.

Blunt trauma directly compresses and damages the vessel. For example, an artery that is crushed may be intact but have a damaged intima that will cause thrombosis. Rapid deceleration, as occurs when an automobile inpacts on a stationary object, can stretch an artery. This stretching produces an intimal tear that will cause either immediate or delayed thrombosis. If the artery is torn sufficiently to weaken the entire blood vessel, severe hemorrhaging may occur. The adventitia of the artery usually contains the flow of blood, albeit temporarily.

PATHOPHYSIOLOGY. When an artery is completely severed, the ends characteristically constrict and retract into the adjacent tissue. The bleeding usually arrests spontaneously, since there is circumferential arterial constriction, perhaps some hypotension, and the formation of a thrombus in the open vessel. A partially severed artery cannot retract and constrict. Hemorrhage under these circumstances may be greater than the hemorrhage encountered with a completely severed artery. A partially severed artery may or may not develop a thrombus that obstructs flow. Thus, in this injury, distal pulses may be palpable. Blunt injury to arteries and veins produces intimal damage. These patients may present with palpable pulses because thrombosis may be delayed for hours.

RECOGNITION OF ARTERIAL INJURY. The diagnosis of arterial injury is directly related to the awareness of such injuries by the examining physician. Is the direction of the penetration in the anatomic area of an important vessel? Was there extensive hemorrhage noted at the site of injury? Is there a possibility of a decelerating injury? In the case of other (usually orthopedic) injuries, are these injuries associated with arterial trauma?

Hemorrhage is controlled emergently while the airway is being secured and fluid resuscitation is initiated. Direct pressure is the best method for controlling arterial bleeding. Tourniquets are usually ineffective. If the patient has a low blood pressure, palpation of all pulses is difficult. When vital signs have been restored toward normal, there should be a palpable pulse in all four extremities. If the injured extremity is pulseless, an arterial injury must be assumed. A handheld Doppler and blood pressure cuff can be used to compare pressures in all extremities. If the injured extremity has a reduced systolic pressure, this verifies the diagnosis of arterial injury. Doppler flow will still be audible even with a completely occluded axial artery if collateral circulation is present. This flow bodes well for the viability of the extremity but does not predict an asymptomatic extremity when the patient resumes full activity.

Critical ischemia of an extremity is noted by the five Ps: pulselessness, pallor, pain, paresthesia, and paralysis. A painful extremity that has reduced sensation and motion requires urgent arterial repair. Extremities with intact sensation and motion may have arterial repair triaged until later in the patient's total treatment plan. Patients with carotid injuries who present with a stroke and patients with renal injuries require special consideration.

ANGIOGRAMS. Angiograms are rarely necessary for the diagnosis of a completely occluded artery but are extremely helpful in the diagnosis of partially severed or bluntly injured arteries. A patient with a single wound and no pulses distal to this wound does not require angiography for diagnosis. The patient with multiple gunshot wounds in a pulseless extremity requires angiography for localization of the exact site(s) of injury. Patients with multiple long bone fractures form the same category. These angiograms may be obtained as "one shot" studies in the emergency room or formal catheter angiograms in the radiology suite. Performance of an angiogram requires approximately an hour in the radiology suite, and this hour of delay should be factored into the total treatment plan of the multiply injured patient.

OPERATIVE TREATMENT. All major arterial and venous injuries are optimally treated with vascular reconstruction. This dictum is true especially when the tissues they supply are viable, the general condition of the patient is satisfactory, and the risks of infection are not great. Operative repair should be undertaken promptly by a surgeon skilled in techniques of emergency vascular surgery. Patients who are hemorrhaging are rushed to the operating room. Patients with critical ischemia should have these injuries repaired within hours of injury. Patients without either hemorrhage or critical ischemia may have the repair of injury triaged until later in the patient's total care.

The incision should be planned to allow prompt proximal and distal control of potential arterial injury. For example, the thorax is prepared and draped with injuries that may involve the abdominal aorta. This will allow clamping of the thoracic aorta should tamponade of the retroperitoneum be lost during exploration. In some extremity explorations, a tourniquet is placed but not inflated proximal to the site of injury as a precaution. When the arterial injury is identified and controlled, all devitalized artery is débrided. The artery is then preferentially sutured end-to-end. If a graft replacement is required, autogenous vein, preferably from an uninjured extremity, is used to bridge the gap. Prosthetic material is seldom used except in repair of the abdominal or thoracic aorta. If there has been extensive soilage of the wound, the risk of infection is obviously greater. In patients with critical ischemia of the extremity, a fasciotomy must be considered. If there is tense muscle in the operating room, this is done prophylactically. If a four-compartment fasciotomy is not performed immediately, the patient must be constantly observed for evidence of a compartment syndrome. Any loss of motion or development of hypesthesia, pain, or myoglobinuria should prompt immediate decompression. In questionable cases, compartmental pressures can be measured.

POSTOPERATIVE CARE. The pulses distal to the site of arterial repair should be evaluated at hourly intervals by trained personnel. Should any question arise, Doppler pressures can be followed. Decreasing pulses or pressures should prompt either a return to the operating room or an angiographic exploration of the operative site.

SPECIAL PROBLEMS

IATROGENIC. Cardiologists and radiologists alike use the arterial system for diagnostic and therapeutic access to patients. These arterial punctures are usually well tolerated, but in a rare instance, bleeding after angiographic study may require operative control. Thrombosis at the site of arterial puncture may produce an occluded artery. Because these complications are so infrequent, recognition may be delayed because of lack of awareness by medical personnel. Hemorrhage from an axillary artery puncture may cause compression of the nerves in the axillary sheath. Operative decompression of this syndrome is urgently required.

ORTHOPEDIC. Many orthopedic injuries such as knee dislocations cause secondary trauma to an artery. Whereas fractures may directly puncture and damage the artery, dislocated bones usually stretch the arteries so that the intima alone is damaged. In instances of either partial severance or blunt injury, the pulses are palpable immediately after the injury, and the physician is lulled into a false sense of security. These arteries then occlude later, but nonetheless critical ischemia may develop. These patients should be managed by either early routine angiography or close observation.

VEINS. Venous injuries are repaired whenever possible. An end-to-end interrupted anastomosis is preferred. Although flow is slower and the incidence of thrombosis is increased, most authors agree that the long-term results of such extremities are superior to extremities in which the injured veins have been ligated. Pulmonary embolism occurs infrequently in these patients.

RENAL ARTERY. The kidney tolerates but an hour or two of warm ischemia time. Injuries of the renal artery that are repaired after several hours may or may not produce a functioning kidney. Nonetheless, in a young patient, repair is usually undertaken.

CAROTID. The patient with a carotid artery injury who presents with a severe stroke is usually not reconstructed because restoration of a normal pressure to the damaged brain may cause worsening of the neurologic deficit. Patients with either no or mild deficits are reconstructed, since most authors believe the results merit such action. The management of patients with "moderate" neurologic findings is controversial.

LATE SEQUELAE. If an arterial injury is not recognized or is improperly treated, the patient may develop chronic ischemia. In the extremity, this may require amputation, or Raynaud's phenomenon, intolerance to cold, or intermittent claudication may develop. Late reconstruction is indeed possible if the extremity is viable and potentially may be returned to useful function. The partially severed artery may develop a pulsating hematoma or false aneurysm. These false aneurysms by their very nature continue to grow until they compress the adjacent organs or rupture. Partial injuries that involve both the artery and vein may cause formation of an arterial venous fistula. Not only will they have all the complications of a false aneurysm, but these patients will also have an increase in venous return and potentially may develop congestive heart failure. This increase in venous return may give signs and symptoms of venous hypertension in the affected extremity.

SUMMARY

Arterial injuries are some of the most dramatic injuries encountered by the trauma surgeon. After potentially exsanguinating hemorrhage is controlled, arterial repair is necessary for ensuring function of the end organ. Delayed recognition in patients with critical ischemia may cause loss of limb. All practitioners of medicine must have an acute awareness of the potential of these injuries.

9.   ACUTE ARTERIAL OCCLUSION

Thomas J. Fogarty, M.D.

ETIOLOGY

Most arterial emboli arise in the heart owing to underlying cardiac disease. The primary cardiac disorder is atherosclerotic heart disease causing myocardial infarction, atrial fibrillation, congestive heart failure, and ventricular aneurysm. Embolization from mitral stenosis is less prevalent today because of a decreased incidence of rheumatic heart disease. Occlusions may also be of thrombotic origin, prompted by chronic degenerative atherosclerotic disease in the arterial wall.

PATHOLOGY

The majority of surgically treatable emboli lodge in the lower extremities. The highest incidence is in the femoral

---

See the corresponding chapter or part in the *Textbook of Surgery,* 14th edition, pp. 1623–1630, for a more detailed discussion of this topic, including a comprehensive list of references.

artery followed by the iliac, aortic, and popliteal vessels; embolism of the renal, mesenteric, brachial, and cerebral arteries is less common. Regardless of the source or histologic structure of an embolus, it is the location and sequelae following occlusion that determine the viability of an extremity. After occlusion, a softer coagulum of blood forms in areas of decreased flow, and thrombus can propagate both proximal and distal to the embolus. Compromised tissue oxygenation at the site of the occlusion causes acidosis, and potassium, lactic acid, carbon dioxide, creatinine phosphokinase, and lysozymes are released into the blood and interstitial tissues. The ischemia state induces localized pain and paresthesia; if it is uncontrolled, muscle swelling and rigor follow. Tissue necrosis typically occurs after 6 to 12 hours of significant ischemia. Further propagation of the distal thrombus can eventually cause venous thrombosis.

It is important to remove all distal thrombus and to recognize that discontinuous thrombus is present in approximately a third of patients. Under these circumstances, back-bleeding from collaterals may be quite forceful despite the presence of additional distal thrombus. If this is not recognized, suboptimal restoration of the circulation follows. Routine distal exploration with balloon catheters should be done independently of the status of the back-bleeding.

Arterial emboli most commonly occur in the *elderly* and *seriously* ill patient with multiple systemic disease.

PREOPERATIVE EVALUATION AND CARE

Patients with acute embolic occlusion should be assumed to have significant underlying heart disease. Sources of arterial emboli in a series of 300 patients are shown in Table 1. Evaluation of cardiac function should proceed simultaneously with examination of the peripheral vessels. Noninvasive Doppler ultrasound techniques and pressure and waveform measurements can usually be performed within 10 minutes and are helpful in differentiating occlusion of embolic origin from occlusion of thrombotic origin in patients with underlying vascular disease. They also provide a useful preoperative standard against which postoperative results may be compared.

Appropriate therapy is initiated while emergency preparation for operation is being made. The presence of congestive heart failure, cardiogenic shock, and significant arrhythmias requires intensive care unit monitoring. Digitalis, antiar-

TABLE 1. Predisposing Factors in Arterial Emboli in 300 Consecutive Patients

Atrial fibrillation	231
Atherosclerotic heart disease	183
Rheumatic heart disease	48
Acute myocardial infarction	50
Atherosclerotic plaque	7
Unknown	12

rhythmic agents, morphine, diuretics, and heparin can be administered as needed without delaying surgical intervention. Placement of a central venous catheter (e.g., via the internal jugular vein) is usually required. This permits rapid administration of drugs and fluids (including heparin) with monitoring of central venous pressures. Pulmonary artery pressure should be monitored in patients who are hemodynamically unstable.

In the presence of an embolus to a lower extremity, the possibility of simultaneous emboli to mesenteric or renal arteries should always be considered. Hematuria or abdominal complaints may raise the consideration of preoperative visualization of the visceral vessels. Involvement in other extremities should also be considered. When the diagnosis of an acute arterial occlusion has been made, heparin should be administered immediately with preparation for operation.

INSTRUMENTATION

The balloon embolectomy catheter is flexible and available in graduated sizes for use in major vessels of any caliber. At its proximal portion the syringe fitting provides the means for fluid exchange into a soft, distensible balloon located at the distal tip of the instrument. The catheter is inserted into the acutely occluded vessel as far as possible. The balloon is inflated and withdrawn in the inflated position while the surgeon manipulates both the syringe and the catheter during withdrawal. Alternatives to the conventional balloon catheter, such as the spiral balloon embolectomy catheter and the wire loop graft thrombectomy catheter, can be used to remove particularly adherent thrombus in grafts and native vessels. Complications include plaque dissection, separation of the catheter tip, and perforation. Experience is the most significant factor in reducing the incidence of complications.

OPERATIVE PROCEDURE

The procedure is initiated with local anesthesia, and an anesthetist should be present to monitor vital signs and administer a general anesthetic if necessary. The field should be surgically prepared from the toes to the nipple line, and aortic iliac emboli require preparation of both extremities. Intraoperative arteriographic equipment should be readily available for visualization during the procedure. Regardless of anatomic location, the approach to embolic occlusion is through a femoral incision at the origin of the superficial femoral artery and the profunda. A distal exploration is conducted with routine passage in the superficial femoral artery (3- or 4-French catheter) and in the profunda (2- or 3-French). Any uncertainty about adequate removal of thrombi should be resolved by operative arteriography. Angioscopy is also useful and can be a valuable complement to operative arteriography for documenting complete removal. Angioscopy also allows directional access to the tibial vessels and minimizes the need for distal incisions. After removal of the thrombotic material, the distal arterial system should be irrigated copiously with heparinized saline solution.

In patients with *advanced* ischemia, concomitant major venous occlusion may also be present and may require venous thrombectomy. After removal of the arterial emboli, the distal arteries and veins are irrigated with heparinized saline. The artery is closed first, followed by venotomy closure. Advanced ischemia secondary to acute embolic occlusion is a surgical emergency. Heparin is administered at operation and in the immediate postoperative period. When postoperative heparin is used, vacuum drainage of the wound is indicated.

Massive swelling that may embarrass arterial inflow is most common in cases of advanced ischemia before surgical intervention. It may require treatment for prevention of arterial reocclusion. Capillary damage and compromised venous outflow are factors in this swelling, and fasciotomy is useful in these situations. Initial decompression is accomplished by a limited fasciotomy. If immediate improvement is not obtained, the skin incisions should be extended and the deeper fascial compartments opened widely.

Immediately following restoration of arterial continuity in extremities with advanced ischemia, significant alterations in electrolytes and acid balance may occur, which can produce electrocardiographic changes and hypotension. Buffering agents and antiarrhythmic agents can be employed at the time of clamp release. Electrolytes should be followed closely in the postoperative period, and an elevated creatine phosphokinase in the venous efflux indicates significant muscle damage.

EMBOLIC OCCLUSION IN THE PRESENCE OF SIGNIFICANT CHRONIC OCCLUSIVE DISEASE

A careful history and examination of the uninvolved extremity often provide a reliable assessment of the peripheral circulation before the acute episode. Initially, it is advisable only to attempt to return the circulation to the acute preocclusive state. However, definitive procedures may be performed adjunctively, particularly if there is concern about the viability of the extremity and if the patient had been active before the acute occlusion. Reconstructive procedures such as localized endarterectomy or femorofemoral grafts can be done under local anesthesia. Catheter therapy, such as adjunctive dilation and atherectomy, can be employed at the time of thrombectomy or embolectomy and is being utilized with increasing frequency.

UPPER EXTREMITY, RENAL, MESENTERIC, AND CAROTID ARTERY EMBOLI

The management of emboli to these areas is similar to that described for the lower extremity. When thrombus is being extracted from the proximal subclavian artery, care should be taken for avoiding fragmentation and migration to the carotid and vertebral vessels. The vessels supplying the viscera and the brain are less well supported by adjacent tissue and therefore require considerable care during catheter manipulation. Unless emboli are observed within the first few hours of onset, surgical intervention in the internal carotid system should not be considered because of the risk of potentially fatal hemorrhagic infarction. The possible presence of simultaneous venous thrombosis and embolization after acute myocardial infarction is an indication for postoperative heparin.

MORBIDITY AND MORTALITY

The aim of surgical intervention for arterial emboli is restoration of the peripheral circulation to its preocclusive state. Evaluation of results is based on restoration of pulses, relief of symptoms, and return of normal color and temperature. The possibility of maintaining a viable, functional extremity after acute arterial occlusion should exceed 90 per cent. The condition of the extremity rather than the duration of occlusion represents the primary determinant of operability. Failure of the initial exploration after an apparent success is an indication for re-exploration. The most common cause for failure concerns technical factors, which can often be corrected if they are recognized.

The presence of a stronger than normal "water-hammer" pulse after an apparently successful embolectomy has been associated with a high incidence of reocclusion; this indicates obstruction at the level of small arteries and requires arterial and venous exploration with copious distal irrigation. The mortality associated with arterial embolism primarily concerns the underlying cause, and prompt recognition and treatment of the cause for embolism is the key to decreasing mortality. Coronary arteriography should be performed in accordance with the general condition of the patient. Revascularization or aneurysmectomy, if indicated, should be performed as soon as possible. Of 300 cardiac procedures associated with peripheral arterial emboli, half were emergencies, and treatment of the cardiac disorder was accomplished at the time of arterial embolectomy. The remainder were semiurgent, and all were performed within 1 month of acute occlusion.

THROMBOLYTIC AGENTS

Thrombolytic agents are also useful in the treatment of acute arterial occlusion. Streptokinase, a foreign bacterial protein, combines with plasminogen through an intermediary complex to form plasmin, which degrades fibrin. It is antigenic and hence requires high dosage levels. Urokinase is a naturally occurring nonantigenic enzyme that forms plasmin without intermediary steps and, as a result, requires smaller doses than of streptokinase. Urokinase has been shown to produce lower complication rates and improved efficacy over streptokinase but is more expensive. Lytic agents are delivered locally to reduce systemic exposure. Systemic complications from streptokinase and urokinase have prompted development of lytic agents that convert plasminogen to plasmin specifically at the site of the obstruction rather than elsewhere in the circulation. Two such fibrin-specific lytic agents are tissue plasminogen activator (tPA) and pro-urokinase. Both agents are currently under investigation for peripheral arterial occlusion. Time delay to reperfusion, cost, multiple angiograms, and the potential for hemorrhage have limited their use. Heparinization with surgical balloon embolectomy remains the most effective form of treatment for acute arterial occlusion.

10. ARTERIOVENOUS FISTULAS

H. Kim Lyerly, M.D.

Arteriovenous fistulas form a fascinating group of congenital and acquired lesions of variable etiology, anatomic distribution, and clinical presentation. They are associated with numerous pathophysiologic changes at the local site and systemically. An arteriovenous fistula can be defined as a connection, other than the capillary bed, between the arterial and venous systems. This definition encompasses a vast array of conditions including some occurring in the normal development of the circulation, congenital malformations, acquired lesions, and iatrogenic shunts. A classification based on the etiology of the fistula is helpful and is shown in Table 1.

The two major types of arteriovenous fistulas are *congenital*

TABLE 1. Classification of Abnormal Arteriovenous Communication

Congenital	Acquired
Single fistula	Single fistula
Multiple fistula—	Surgical
arteriovenous malformation	Pathologic
Hemangiomas	Aneurysm
	Iatrogenic
	Infection
	Neoplasia
	Spontaneous
	Traumatic
	Tumor-associated
	communications
	Vascular tumors
	Tumors associated with
	shunting

See the corresponding chapter or part in the *Textbook of Surgery*, 14th edition, pp. 1630–1637, for a more detailed discussion of this topic, including a comprehensive list of references.

and *acquired*. Congenital lesions may have single or multiple communications and are respectively denoted as arteriovenous fistulas or arteriovenous malformations. Lesions with a single communication usually represent either a normal fetal communication that fails to resolve or a developmental abnormality. Lesions with multiple communications usually represent persistent communications that normally exist during the early phase of the development of the arterial and venous systems. Hemangiomas are multiple abnormal venous communications.

Acquired lesions usually have a single communication and are termed arteriovenous fistulas; frequently they consist of a distinct communication between an artery and a vein bypassing the capillary bed. The causes of acquired arteriovenous fistula are shown in Table 1.

PATHOPHYSIOLOGY

Changes are maximal in fistulas involving a large artery that conducts massive amounts of blood flow. Under these circumstances, much blood is shunted through the fistula because the venous side offers very little resistance. With large volumes of blood shunted directly into the venous circulation, a sequence of events follows that is directly related to the volume of blood flowing through the fistula. Cardiac output may be increased in patients with arteriovenous fistulas, and compression of the fistulas, which diminishes the flow through the fistulas, is followed by a diminished heart rate (Branham's or Nicoladoni's sign) and a lower cardiac output. If the fistula is acute with a large volume of blood flowing through it, the heart may not be able to compensate adequately.

Structural changes in the vascular wall are also created by hemodynamic disturbances associated with arteriovenous fistulas. The venous wall of large fistulas becomes thin, closely simulating the sac of a false aneurysm. The walls of small fistulas may become thickened and assume the appearance of an artery. Thrombi are also apt to form in the dilated parts of these fistulas and may harbor bacterial organisms.

CLINICAL FEATURES

Aneurysmal dilation is usually present at the site of the fistula with involvement of both the artery and vein caused by turbulence due to the high to low pressure interface within the fistula. In response to the low arterial pressure distal to the site of the fistula, an extensive collateral circulation develops that connects the arteries proximal to the fistula with those distal. This collateral circulation can become massive and often causes an increase in temperature in both skin and muscle. When the fistulas occur in an extremity, the limb may increase in length. Other local features are demonstrated by the presence of a thrill at the site of the lesion, especially if it is located near the surface. On auscultation, a bruit that continues through most if not all of the cardiac cycle is audible.

Angiography is the standard diagnostic study in the evaluation of an arteriovenous fistula. In acquired fistulas, a single communication often occurs at the site of the fistula and can be localized either by direct visualization of the communication or by the initial venous opacification at the site of the fistula. Congenital lesions with multiple communications often have a radiologic appearance that is much more complicated. Indirect signs of an abnormal arteriovenous communication, including increased flow in the afferent arteries, decreased flow in the peripheral arteries, and rapid venous filling, are usually present. However, the multiple communications may not be visible because they are often of microscopic size, and overlying opacified arteries and veins add to the complexity of the radiographic pattern. Selective angiography of the afferent artery or arteries may be helpful in delineating the extent of the fistula. Sometimes localized dilated contrast-filled spaces indicate the site of the fistula with some precision. On other occasions, small fistulas are revealed as faint, diffuse opacifications between major arterial and venous channels. Other indications may include abnormal vessels arising from the parent artery, horizontal branches connecting parallel veins, and venous retia.

Ultrasonic imaging has also been used to identify arteriovenous fistulas. Although ultrasonography may not be expected to reveal the actual fistula, the detection of aneurysms may call attention to a previously unsuspected fistula as well as determine the diameter and morphologic features of the proximal vessels. Color-flow imaging may also reveal patterns suggestive of increased turbulence at sites of increased flow.

Computed tomography and magnetic resonance imaging may be used to demonstrate the location and extent of arteriovenous communications, including the involvement of specific muscle groups and bone.

TYPES OF FISTULAS

Congenital arteriovenous communications of the extremities are quite common, especially in the legs, and varicose veins often result. Congenital arteriovenous communications have been reported in all organs of the body and are frequently difficult to manage because multiple communications exist between arteries and veins.

Congenital pulmonary arteriovenous fistulas are common and are often multiple. These are usually seen as well-circumscribed lesions on the chest film; if large, they may be accompanied by cyanosis due to the right-to-left shunting. The symptoms include exertional dyspnea, easy fatigability, cyanosis, and clubbing of the fingers. Approximately 10 to 15 per cent occur in children. Complications of these lesions include cerebrovascular accidents, brain abscesses, hemoptysis, and intrapleural rupture. A continuous bruit with systolic accentuation during deep inspiration is heard in approximately two thirds of patients. Pulmonary arteriography confirms the diagnosis. Hereditary telangiectasis (Rendu-Osler-Weber disease) is quite common and may be familial in origin.

Venous malformations commonly referred to as hemangiomas represent a specific type of lesion composed of large venous spaces under low pressure with no clinical or angiographic evidence of significant arteriovenous shunting. They may occur anywhere in the body. Venous lesions are often asymptomatic but may be disfiguring in a large exposed area. Localized symptomatic lesions may be treated by excision, although, as previously mentioned, they may be more extensive than is evident clinically.

Acquired fistulas are most frequently found in the extremities and are often secondary to penetrating trauma with accompanying varices, edema, and pigmentation. Unlike congenital communications, a single or limited number of abnormal communications occur that can be demonstrated by angiography or color-flow Doppler. Vascular insufficiency of digits and ulceration may also be present in the more severe forms. A palpable thrill and an audible coarse machinery-like bruit are usually present at the site of the fistula.

Iatrogenic fistulas may follow a number of surgical procedures including operations on the kidney and intervertebral discs. Disc procedures may be associated with fistulas in the iliac vessels or with aortocaval fistulas. Iatrogenic fistulas following thyroid procedures, coronary artery bypass grafting, distal splenorenal shunts, small bowel resection, Fontan's operation, and pelvic surgery have each been described.

Atherosclerosis of the wall of an aneurysm can also erode into accompanying veins, the prominent example being that of an aortocaval fistula from an abdominal aortic aneurysm. Such a lesion may place a patient precipitously in congestive heart failure and require an emergent surgical procedure. Proximal and distal control of the aorta allows the artery to be opened and the fistula controlled by a finger placed on the communication. Compression with sponge sticks proximal and distal to the fistula allows repair of the vein. After the vein is repaired, the preferred method for restoring arterial continuity is with a graft. Aortocaval fistulas of neoplastic origin have also been reported.

In current practice, the *most common* acquired arteriovenous fistula is that associated with vascular access for permitting renal dialysis in the management of renal insufficiency. Arteriovenous fistulas have also been surgically constructed to increase blood flow and patency to a vascular anastomosis, such as venous reconstruction procedures.

MANAGEMENT OF ARTERIOVENOUS COMMUNICATIONS

Since most arteriovenous fistulas are potentially symptomatic, closure of the communication is generally recommended. Early surgical attempts to correct these lesions consisted primarily of ligation of the involved artery proximal to the fistula. Gangrene can result because blood reaching the distal extremity by arterial collaterals is apt to drain retrograde through the fistula directly into the venous system, thus depriving the limb of adequate distal arterial blood flow. The first successful treatment of an arteriovenous fistula was proximal and distal ligation of both the artery and the vein.

Currently, management includes accurate diagnosis and determination of the extent of the lesions. Acute fistulas with high flow causing cardiovascular collapse or distal ischemia require immediate repair, whereas long-standing lesions with extensive involvement of surrounding tissue require thoughtful preoperative planning. The site of the communication should always be carefully localized by arteriography; however, computed tomographic scanning, magnetic resonance imaging, and color-flow Doppler imaging are becoming increasingly utilized to diagnose arteriovenous communications. The ideal surgical management usually includes direct closure of the fistula with restoration of arterial and venous continuity. However, when this is not possible, quadripolar ligation is acceptable when sufficient arterial collateral circulation for adequately supplying the tissues distally exists. Complete excision is reserved for fistulas involving small nonessential arteries, such as the radial or ulnar arteries when adequate collaterals are present. Rarely, small fistulas have closed spontaneously.

Although surgical excision has a role in specific types of arteriovenous communications, especially in localized lesions, some are too extensive for appropriate and complete surgical excision. For these, palliative surgical procedures are used to control disabling ulceration and infection or life-threatening hemorrhage. Ligation of major feeding arteries is not recommended because distal ischemia may result and the intravascular access required to allow embolization becomes limited. Staged treatment with intervals between embolization allows portions of major malformations to be obliterated and repeated treatments in persistent areas. Often this combination of embolization followed by surgical excision is effective in managing these difficult malformations. Other types of therapy include injection of sclerosing solutions or irradiation. The complex communications seen with congenital arteriovenous malformation often require a multidisciplinary approach including selective intra-arterial embolization in conjunction with surgical therapy. Asymptomatic lesions may not require treatment; nevertheless, a fistula represents a hazard. Absolute indications for treatment include hemorrhage, secondary ischemic complications, and congestive heart failure from arteriovenous shunting; relative indications include pain, nonhealing ulcers, functional impairment, and cosmetic deformity. If treatment is required, careful planning is mandatory.

11. THROMBOANGIITIS OBLITERANS (BUERGER'S DISEASE)

H. Brownell Wheeler, M.D.

In 1908, Leo Buerger published clinical and pathologic observations on young male smokers with severe ischemia of the extremities. Buerger termed the syndrome *thromboangiitis obliterans* because the acute histologic pattern was characterized by thrombosis in both arteries and veins and was associated with a marked inflammatory response. The classic syndrome described by Buerger is an uncommon but dramatic form of peripheral vascular disease.

CLINICAL MANIFESTATIONS. Thromboangiitis obliterans typically occurs in heavy smokers, usually presenting between 20 and 35 years of age. Thromboangiitis obliterans was formerly thought to occur only in men, but several cases in women have been reported in recent years associated with the increase in female smokers. The diagnosis of thromboangiitis obliterans should be considered in any young smoker with peripheral ischemia, particularly if the upper extremities are involved or if there is a history of migratory superficial phlebitis. Small vessel occlusions are characteristic of thromboangiitis obliterans but atypical for atherosclerosis. Exacerbations with smoking and remissions following abstinence from tobacco are also typical of thromboangiitis obliterans. Careful clinical evaluation is necessary to exclude other causes of peripheral ischemia, especially atherosclerosis. Serologic tests should be obtained to exclude autoimmune diseases, such as lupus erythematosus, which are sometimes associated with peripheral arterial thrombosis. Arteriography early in the disease usually reveals segmental obliteration of arteries, especially the medium-sized arteries of the forearm and calf, with a strikingly normal appearance of the uninvolved vessels. Digital arteries are frequently involved. Collateral circulation in chronic cases is unusually well developed.

The clinical course of Buerger's disease is protracted and painful but relatively benign. If a patient ceases smoking, prolonged remission usually occurs. Most patients appear addicted to tobacco and continue to smoke despite all advice. They have repeated attacks and may require multiple amputations, but life-endangering complications are infrequent. Long-term life expectancy is only slightly less than that of the general population, unlike patients with comparable degrees of peripheral ischemia due to atherosclerosis.

ETIOLOGY. The striking association with cigarette smoking suggests a strong etiologic relationship, but a specific cause for thromboangiitis obliterans has never been demonstrated. Autonomic overactivity is suggested by the association with severe peripheral vasospasm and hyperhidrosis. Any factor that causes vasospasm, thrombosis, or local in-

---

See the corresponding chapter or part in the *Textbook of Surgery*, 14th edition, pp. 1637–1640, for a more detailed discussion of this topic, including a comprehensive list of references.

flammation may contribute to the development of the syndrome in a susceptible individual. It appears increasingly likely that some immunologic process, typically initiated in response to cigarette smoking, has a major role in Buerger's disease.

INCIDENCE. At present in the United States, thromboangiitis obliterans comprises less than 1 per cent of all patients presenting initially with severe peripheral ischemia. In Israel and Eastern Europe, the corresponding incidence is approximately 5 per cent, whereas in Japan it has been reported to be 16 per cent. Patients with Buerger's disease are observed much more frequently in Asia than in the United States, even in populations in which atherosclerosis is rare.

MANAGEMENT. The major problem in Buerger's disease is pain, which is often excruciating. Narcotics are usually necessary but must be used cautiously because of the frequency of drug addiction. Peripheral or sympathetic nerve blocks may provide temporary pain relief, especially when the disease is accompanied by severe vasospasm. Cervical or lumbar sympathectomy may also benefit such patients. Every effort should be made to have the patient cease smoking, since indefinite remissions often follow abstinence from cigarettes. No specific medication has found wide acceptance. Arterial reconstruction is usually impossible because of the distal nature of the disease, but it should be considered in segmental proximal occlusions. Amputation at the lowest possible level is indicated for intractable pain or gangrene. Unlike atherosclerosis, it is often possible to do digital amputations with satisfactory healing.

12. RAYNAUD'S SYNDROME

James M. Edwards, M.D., and John M. Porter, M.D.

Raynaud's syndrome defines a condition characterized by episodic attacks of vasospasm that cause closure of the small arteries and arterioles of the distal parts of the extremities in response to cold exposure or emotional stimuli. Classically, the attacks consist of intense pallor of the distal extremities followed by cyanosis and rubor upon rewarming, with full recovery requiring 15 to 45 minutes.

The pallor in the early stage of Raynaud's attacks is caused by severe spasm of the arteries and arterioles, which causes cessation of capillary perfusion. After some minutes, the capillaries and probably the venules dilate. This is followed by a relaxation of the arteriolar spasm with the entry of a trickle of blood into the dilated capillaries where it rapidly

See the corresponding chapter or part in the *Textbook of Surgery*, 14th edition, pp. 1640–1648, for a more detailed discussion of this topic, including a comprehensive list of references.

Supported by Grant RR00334 from the General Clinical Research Centers branch of the Division of Research Resources, National Institutes of Health, and Grant 8839 from the Medical Research Foundation of Oregon.

becomes desaturated, producing cyanosis. Rubor follows the entry of increasing amounts of blood into dilated capillaries. The attack terminates with the entry of a normal volume of blood through the relaxed arterioles.

Patients with Raynaud's syndrome may be divided into two distinct pathophysiologic groups, obstructive and spastic. Patients with obstructive Raynaud's syndrome must have sufficiently severe arterial obstruction to cause significant reduction in resting digital artery pressure. In such patients, a normal vasoconstrictive response to cold is sufficient to overcome the diminished intraluminal distending pressure and cause arterial closure. Patients with spastic Raynaud's syndrome do not have significant palmar-digital artery obstruction and have normal digital artery pressure at room temperature. Arterial closure in these patients is caused by the markedly increased force of cold-induced arterial spasm. A number of studies have suggested altered adrenoceptor activity in patients with spastic Raynaud's syndrome. Although conclusive data are lacking, abnormalities in both alpha$_2$-adrenoceptors and presynaptic beta-receptors have been implicated in the cause of Raynaud's syndrome.

CLINICAL DESCRIPTION. In spastic Raynaud's syndrome, both hands are affected equally, and frequently the thumbs are spared. About 10 per cent of patients have a primary lower extremity involvement. Obstructive Raynaud's syndrome appears to be about equally distributed between males and females; the symptomatic onset occurs after the age of 40 years, and the area of involvement is frequently limited to one or several fingers. Typically, younger women present with spastic Raynaud's syndrome, and idiopathic Raynaud's without associated disease is most common in this age and sex group. Older males who develop Raynaud's usually have the obstructive type associated with digital artery occlusion, usually from atherosclerosis. Most episodes of digital vasospasm are induced by environmental cold exposure, although emotional stimuli such as fear or anger may also produce attacks. Fingertip ulceration occurs only in the presence of widespread palmar or digital artery obstruction. Ischemic ulceration is never caused by vasospasm alone.

EVALUATION. Historic information should be sought regarding symptoms of connective tissue disease including arthralgia, dysphagia, skin tightening, xerophthalmia, or xerostomia. Symptoms of large vessel occlusive disease, exposure to trauma or frostbite, drug history, and history of malignancy should also be sought. The skin of the hands and fingers should be inspected for ulceration or fingertip hyperkeratotic areas suggesting healed ulcers. The hand and fingers should be examined for evidence of an associated autoimmune disease. It should be noted that the physical examination is frequently completely normal in patients with Raynaud's syndrome. The diagnosis is made primarily from the history.

Although the diagnosis is usually established by the clinical history, increasingly sophisticated vascular laboratory techniques have been used to diagnose Raynaud's syndrome. Arteriography is recommended only in patients presenting with ischemic digital ulceration, because a small percentage of these patients develop these ulcers as a result of embolization from a surgically correctable proximal lesion. The vascular laboratory allows a separation of spastic from obstructive Raynaud's syndrome. Hand ice water exposure with timing of digital temperature recovery is used in some laboratories. Whereas this test is 100 per cent specific, it is only about 50 per cent sensitive and thus is insufficiently accurate for clinical use. A more accurate test is digital blood pressure response to 5 minutes of digital occlusive hypothermia, which has proved to be 87 per cent specific and 90 per cent sensitive, yielding an overall accuracy of 92 per cent. Digital photoplethysmography with digital blood pressure determination has become as accurate as arteriography in the detection of significant digital artery obstruction. The extent of laboratory evaluation varies somewhat depending on the findings of the history and physical examination. Minimal evaluation should include a hand radiograph for calcinosis or tuft resorption, hemogram, sedimentation rate, rheumatoid factor, and antinuclear antibody for aiding in the detection of any associated autoimmune disease.

TREATMENT. Most patients with Raynaud's syndrome have only mild symptoms that respond well to simple cold and tobacco avoidance. Patients who work in cold areas may not respond to any treatment until their occupational exposure is reduced. At the present time, nifedipine is the first-line drug for Raynaud's syndrome. Patients with spastic Raynaud's syndrome are more likely to respond to medication than are those with obstructive Raynaud's syndrome.

In a very small number of patients with Raynaud's syndrome, there is a proximal cause of upper extremity arterial insufficiency, sometimes associated with distal emboli to the palmar and digital arteries. The occasional appropriate patient for vascular surgery may generally expect satisfactory results. For the past 75 years, upper extremity sympathectomy has been used sporadically as a treatment for Raynaud's syndrome. The typical history of the procedure is that the patient experiences a few months of good results followed by a gradual recurrence of symptoms. At the present time, the modest surgical risk, expense, and mediocre long-term results of thoracic sympathectomy for Raynaud's syndrome constitute overwhelming arguments against its use, and the procedure is not recommended. In the treatment of patients with Raynaud's syndrome, occasionally patients are encountered with painful digital ulceration, which always implies widespread palmar and digital arterial occlusions. The healing rate with conservative therapy is 85 per cent, which is the same reported after sympathectomy; thus, sympathectomy confers no added advantages and is not recommended.

13. CIRCULATORY PROBLEMS OF THE UPPER EXTREMITY

Donald Silver, M.D.

ARTERIAL INSUFFICIENCY

Arterial flow to the upper extremity may be reduced by atherosclerotic stenoses or occlusions, thromboembolism, trauma, tumor, inflammatory processes, or compression of the subclavian-axillary arteries in the region of the thoracic outlet. Penetrating arterial injuries are more common in the upper extremities (53 per cent), whereas blunt traumatic vascular injuries occur most often in the lower extremities (89 per cent). Three to 5 per cent of all arterial emboli lodge in the arteries of the upper extremities. Brachial and axillary catheterizations cause thrombotic occlusions of the respective arteries in approximately 0.5 to 10 per cent of the cases. Arteritis is an increasingly frequent cause of upper extremity and hand ischemia. The larger proximal arteries may be obstructed by giant cell arteritis or idiopathic arteritis, whereas the palmar and digital arteries are more frequently affected by collagen-related vasculitis—especially sclero-derma.

Management of the upper extremity ischemia includes treatment of an arteritis with steroids and, at times, immu-nosuppression. If bypass grafting is required, the inflamma-tory process should be controlled before grafting. Arterial occlusions are treated according to the etiologic basis: dam-aged arteries can be repaired or replaced with vein grafts; thromboembolic occlusions can be extracted with an embo-lectomy catheter, usually with local anesthesia, or lysed with fibrinolytic agents followed, when necessary, with throm-boendarterectomy or bypass grafting.

VENOUS INSUFFICIENCY

The manifestations of venous insufficiency include edema, distention of superficial veins, tightness, aching, and a reddish-blue discoloration, and pain. Most of these symptoms are caused by occlusions of the axillary, subclavian, or innomi-nate veins. More distal venous occlusions rarely produce significant edema or chronic symptoms. Tumors, mediastinal fibrosis, trauma, and indwelling catheters for central cardio-vascular monitoring are the common causes of thrombosis in the large central veins.

The extent of the venous thrombosis should be docu-mented by phlebography. Management of the patient with symptomatic upper extremity venous obstruction varies ac-cording to the cause of the obstruction. If there is obstruction

---

See the corresponding chapter or part in the *Textbook of Surgery*, 14th edition, pp. 1648–1650, for a more detailed discussion of this topic, including a comprehensive list of references.

of venous outflow, but no thrombosis, the sites of obstruction should be eliminated; for example, the thoracic space is decompressed, tumors are resected or irradiated, abscesses are drained. If there is acute thrombotic occlusion, the thrombus can be lysed with fibrinolytic agents or can be contained with heparin. The cause of the thrombosis should be eliminated. If restoration of patency of the venous system cannot be achieved with fibrinolytic agents and/or operative decompression, symptoms caused by the thrombotic compression can be relieved with saphenous vein bypasses of the obstruction, for example, axillary-jugular bypass, brachial-subclavian bypass, and the like.

LYMPHEDEMA

Primary lymphedema of an upper extremity is rare. Secondary lymphedema occurs in up to 10 per cent of women who have had radical mastectomies, usually followed by radiation therapy, for breast cancer. Secondary lymphedema is a potential complication of any axillary dissection. Most often the lymphedema can be controlled with elevation of the arm, elastic sleeves, salt restriction, good skin care, and prompt management of infection. Resistant lymphedema may require the use of a lymphedema pump. Uncontrollable edema usually requires operative procedures for improvement of lymph flow and/or reduction in the size of the extremity.

ASSOCIATED CIRCULATORY PROBLEMS

Causalgia describes the burning, agonizing pain and vasomotor disturbances that occur in 2 to 5 per cent of patients after peripheral nerve injuries. Sympathetic blockade is an excellent diagnostic and therapeutic procedure. If sympathetic blocks provide relief for only short periods, operative sympathetic denervation may be required. Active physical therapy is an important part of the postsympathectomy management.

Causalgia-like pain may also occur after an injury to an extremity in which there is no demonstrable nerve damage. These patients have pain, edema, vasomotor disturbances, soft tissue dystrophy, and atrophy of bone. This disorder has been termed posttraumatic reflex sympathetic dystrophy. Management consists of treating the local injury with supportive measures, controlling, if necessary, the pain with sympathetic blockade, and physical therapy.

Acrocyanosis is characterized by painless coldness and cyanosis of the distal portions of the extremities caused by spasm of the small arteries. This symptom complex does not cause any serious disability, and management consists only of protection from cold and trauma.

14.   VISCERAL ISCHEMIC SYNDROMES: OBSTRUCTION OF THE SUPERIOR MESENTERIC ARTERY, CELIAC AXIS, AND INFERIOR MESENTERIC ARTERY

John J. Bergan, M.D., F.A.C.S., Hon. F.R.C.S. (Eng.)

Syndromes of obstruction of intestinal blood vessels may be acute or chronic. Because collateral blood flow to intestinal arteries is exceedingly profuse, symptomatic visceral ischemia occurs uncommonly. When it does, blockage of the superior mesenteric artery and celiac axis as well as of the inferior mesenteric artery is largely due to atherosclerosis. Much more rare conditions are polyarteritis nodosa, Kawasaki's disease, drug abuse arteritis, Cogan's syndrome, allergic vasculitis, rheumatoid arteritis, systemic sclerosis, and lupus erythematosus.

The mechanism for production of symptoms is under-perfusion of the visceral vascular bed, complicated by peristalsis. During peristalsis, induced by food intake, extramural pressure exceeds intramural perfusion pressure, and arterial blood flow ceases. The intestinal response to such ischemia is a more violent spasm that is perceived by the patient as a nauseating cramp. This causes weight loss, and the entire syndrome is typified by the phrase *food fear*. The designation *small meal syndrome* has also been applied to this condition, which is referred to in medical terms as postprandial pain.

The clinical suspicion of chronic visceral ischemia depends on the observation of severe weight loss in the absence of diagnosable malignancy. Noninvasive evaluation of the visceral arteries is then performed by ultrasound duplex scanning. Ultimately, angiography confirms the clinical diagnosis and the findings of ultrasound duplex scanning and provides information for reconstruction. Surgical treatment consists of revascularization of the main trunks to the intestinal arborization. Current approaches favor use of the supraceliac aorta as a bypass inflow source.

Special mention must be made of the entity of celiac artery compression. A large number of patients, frequently women, often under 35 years of age, demonstrate severe compression of the origin of the celiac axis by an arcuate ligament or low-lying crus of the diaphragm. Symptoms are rarely encountered. Nevertheless, an occasional patient is found in whom weight loss is predominant and in whom food fear is the cause of the weight loss. Selective angiography in such cases demonstrates a paucity of collateral vessels from the superior mesenteric circulation to the celiac territory.

Acute visceral ischemia is a devastating, lethal, and severe, life-threatening illness. Resectional therapy as the only form

See the corresponding chapter or part in the *Textbook of Surgery*, 14th edition, pp. 1650–1656, for a more detailed discussion of this topic, including a comprehensive list of references.

of treatment is attended by a 90 to 95 per cent mortality. Revascularization before intestinal resection has lowered the mortality, but results remain unacceptable. Future advances in patient care may lower mortality satisfactorily.

The most frequent cause of acute intestinal ischemia is embolization to the superior mesenteric artery. When it occurs, the symptoms are characteristic. A clinical diagnosis can be made immediately. No prior history of food fear is obtained. Atherosclerotic occlusive disease of the celiac axis and superior mesenteric artery is also important. When thrombosis occurs, acute intestinal infarction supervenes. In such patients, a history of food fear, weight loss, and post-prandial pain may be obtained. Third most important as a cause of acute intestinal infarction is a hypoperfusion or nonorganic visceral ischemia produced by cardiac failure.

Clinically, all forms of acute mesenteric arterial occlusion produce the same effects. These are severe abdominal pain out of proportion to physical findings, profound leukocytosis in excess of 14,000, and gut emptying characterized by vomiting and defecation. All patients manifest melena coincident with peritonitis and its findings, often ending fatally. In the later stages, profound acidosis, anuria, dehydration, and some cyanosis appear. Multiorgan failure follows. No specific serum diagnostic studies are present at this stage, only the profound acidosis and secondary serum alterations characteristic of renal failure.

Reperfusion injury may have a strong part in failure of intestinal revascularization in such patients. However, this is a hypothesis depending on the observation that toxic-free radical metabolites of oxygen appear to be responsible for much of the injury that follows ischemia in the experimental animal. In the future, treatment directed to this entity may contribute to therapy.

15. RENOVASCULAR HYPERTENSION

J. Caulie Gunnells, Jr., M.D.,
and Richard L. McCann, M.D.

Hypertension produced by obstructive lesions in the renal arteries is termed *renovascular hypertension* and is the most common form of potentially curable high blood pressure. The importance of renovascular disease as a cause of hypertension is further emphasized by the fact that it is often progressive and thus jeopardizes long-term renal function. Both the hypertension and potential renal insufficiency can be prevented by appropriate mechanical intervention with the utilization of modern revascularization techniques.

Estimates of the prevalence of renovascular hypertension vary from less than 5 to more than 20 per cent of the adult

---

See the corresponding chapter or part in the *Textbook of Surgery*, 14th edition, pp. 1656–1664, for a more detailed discussion of this topic, including a comprehensive list of references.

hypertensive population in the United States. The true incidence is difficult to determine accurately owing to wide variability in criteria for patient selection for clinical investigation. That renal ischemia can cause hypertension was demonstrated experimentally more than 50 years ago by Goldblatt. Renal ischemia stimulates secretion of the enzyme renin, which acts upon renin substrate, a plasma protein synthesized in the liver. This reaction cleaves an octapeptide, angiotensin I, a substance with little physiologic activity. Angiotensin I is acted upon by another enzyme, angiotensin-converting enzyme, causing the production of angiotensin II. This substance has two major physiologic activities, namely, direct vasoconstriction and stimulation of aldosterone. Aldosterone, a product of the adrenal cortex, produces sodium retention and increased intravascular volume. Thus, hypertension is produced by two complementary mechanisms of vasoconstriction and augmentation of vascular volume.

In man, the most common cause of renal artery stenosis is atherosclerosis; these obstructive lesions are most apt to occur near the origin of the renal arteries from the aorta and are often segmental and frequently short. The second most frequent cause of renovascular hypertension is fibromuscular dysplasia of the renal arteries. This group of lesions may involve disease of any of the vascular coats, but the most common is fibrous dysplasia of the medial layer. This lesion usually occurs in young women and causes serial constrictions alternating with areas of increased diameter, which on angiography produce a corrugated effect termed the *string of beads*. A third group of vascular lesions has recently been identified as an important cause of renovascular disease. This refers to atheroembolic renal artery disease. The concomitant development of emboli involving the renal circulation may contribute to hypertension as well as compromise renal function.

Considerable disagreement continues regarding which patients within the larger population with hypertension should be evaluated for renovascular disease. Patients with renovascular disease tend to have sudden or abrupt onset of hypertension, often before age 35 years or subsequent to age 55 years. Patients with renovascular hypertension often have sustained severe diastolic blood pressures (greater than 115 mm. Hg) or accelerated or malignant hypertensive disease. Patients who exhibit failure of antihypertensive drug therapy or who lose previous control and those with deteriorating function despite adequate blood pressure control should be considered for investigation of renovascular disease. In patients with renovascular disease, physical examination may reveal an abdominal or epigastric bruit. Patients with all of these findings are relatively rare, but when several of these findings are present, they demand strong consideration for further investigation for establishing a diagnosis of functionally significant renovascular hypertension.

The *sine qua non* for diagnosis of renovascular disease is contrast arteriography. Since not all hypertensive patients can undergo this examination, it is necessary to select patients from the larger hypertensive population who have a higher probability of harboring renovascular disease as a contributing etiologic factor to their hypertension. A number of screening evaluations have been proposed with variable utility. The value of the measurement of plasma renin activity has been enhanced recently by the finding that plasma renin activity can be increased in patients with renovascular hypertension by acute inhibition of angiotensin-converting enzyme by inhibitors such as captopril. The predictive value of both peripheral plasma renin activity and renal vein renin ratio determinations can be significantly enhanced by acute administration of captopril. Similarly, the utility of radioisotope renography is increased by concomitant administration of angiotensin-converting enzyme inhibitors.

The treatment of patients with renovascular disease is amelioration of the high blood pressure together with preservation and occasionally improvement of renal function. Whereas medical therapy of hypertension of renovascular origin may obviate the risk of operation, it requires a high degree of patient compliance, constant medical supervision, and lifelong administration of antihypertensive medication. Medical therapy has also been demonstrated to be less effective than is restoration of renal blood flow in terms of long-term preservation of renal function.

Balloon catheter dilation of renal artery stenoses can be used in some patients. In patients with fibromuscular disease, particularly of the medial fibroplasia type, balloon angioplasty has a high rate of success, and recurrence is unusual. The experience with atherosclerotic disease has not been as favorable, and recent studies suggest less than half of patients with atherosclerotic obstruction of the renal artery are improved after a follow-up of less than 2 years. Ostial lesions of the renal artery, in particular, respond poorly to attempted balloon dilation.

If the affected kidney has been so severely damaged by ischemia that it contributes little to total renal function, the most appropriate procedure may be nephrectomy. A renal length of 7 cm. and severe arteriolar nephrosclerosis with hyalinization of all or most glomeruli on biopsy suggest an unsalvageable kidney, the removal of which may ameliorate hypertension and improve prognosis for maintenance of renal function in the contralateral kidney. Aortorenal bypass, by use of an autogenous saphenous vein graft, is the most frequently selected surgical procedure for renal artery stenosis. When there is severe disease of the aortic wall, however, it may be difficult to attach a graft at this location, and a more peripheral origin such as the splenic or hepatic artery may be used to revascularize the left and right kidneys, respectfully. Severe branch vessel disease may be surgically corrected through "bench work" surgery after the kidney has been cooled and temporarily removed from the body, with replacement after the arterial obstructions have been corrected.

Good long-term results with 70 to 90 per cent improvement in hypertension have been reported in recent series. The effect of revascularization on preservation of renal function is less certain but clearly of major importance. Mortality occurs almost exclusively in patients with widespread systemic atherosclerotic disease.

VII

Venous Injuries
Norman M. Rich, M.D.

In contrast to the management of injured arteries, in which repair rather than ligation has been widely and enthusiastically practiced in the years since the Korean Conflict, the management of venous injuries has not been widely developed with the same approach. It is ironic that Murphy made the following statement in 1897 when he described the first successful clinical end-to-end anastomosis of an artery: ". . . closure of wounds in the veins by suture is now an acceptable surgical practice."

Two major concerns prevented the development of repair of injured veins: (1) belief that there would be an increased incidence of thrombophlebitis and (2) fear of pulmonary embolism. It is recognized that many injured veins can be ligated with few or no immediate problems and no recognized long-term disability. Until the last 25 years, the effectiveness of venous repair remained uncertain. Thrombosis was recognized to be much more common in the lower pressure venous system, compared with the good results achieved following repair of arterial injuries. Also, in contrast to arterial repair, in which simple palpation of a peripheral pulse is usually adequate for determining success or failure, effectiveness of venous repair is more difficult to evaluate because there is no simple method for determining patency of venous reconstruction.

Acute venous hypertension in the extremities following ligation of major extremity veins, particularly in the lower extremities, may contribute to an increased amputation rate. In addition, the degree of disability from chronic venous insufficiency is not recognized by many. This disability may not become evident for months or even 5 to 10 years following injury. It has been recognized and documented throughout history that important surgical progress has occurred during periods of armed conflict when surgeons are required to treat large numbers of patients with similar injuries within a relatively short period of time. This corollary between military surgery and vascular surgery has been particularly noteworthy in the twentieth century. An analysis that included the

See the corresponding chapter or part in the *Textbook of Surgery*, 14th edition, pp. 1664–1672, for a more detailed discussion of this topic, including a comprehensive list of references.

importance and effectiveness of repair of venous injuries during the American experience in Southeast Asia was started at Walter Reed Army Medical Center in 1966 as the Vietnam Vascular Registry. A preliminary report from the Vietnam Vascular Registry demonstrated a significant incidence of venous injuries: 27 per cent. An early report emphasized the need for the repair of injured veins, and a more aggressive approach for the repair of injured veins, particularly in lower extremity venous trauma, was advocated in 1974.

Venous repair may be particularly important in large-caliber lower extremity veins, specifically the popliteal vein. Venous repair may be necessary in the presence of massive soft tissue injury and is mandatory in replantation of extremities. Repair of injured veins should be considered routinely with large-caliber veins in an attempt to prevent acute or chronic venous insufficiency. Important central veins such as the portal vein, the superior mesenteric vein, and the vena cava should be included. Lateral suture repair of a lacerated vein is frequently the most rapid and safest method of halting hemorrhage from an injured vein. Although the general status of the patient with multiple injuries must be considered, it is often possible to also repair veins by end-to-end anastomosis and by interposition grafts, including compilation venous grafts and spiral venous grafts. The challenge of obtaining successful venous reconstruction remains, a major obstacle being identification of the ideal substitute that will have a high degree of success with long-term patency in the venous system where pressure is lower than in the arterial system.

Recent studies have provided data that refute the fear of producing a higher incidence of venous thrombosis and pulmonary embolization following repair of injured veins. Although this is a possible hazard, the dangerous sequence has been surprisingly absent. It is conceivable that small emboli may not be recognized clinically; however, the absence of clinically detectable pulmonary emboli has been uniformly documented both in the Vietnam Vascular Registry and in previous reports by others. Civilian experience in the past decade has corroborated the previous military experience cited in some aspects; however, the difference in wounds in civilian practice has also been emphasized with a number of experiences and results.

INCIDENCE OF VENOUS INJURIES. Because many surgeons have considered venous injuries to be unimportant and have not reported many of them, their true incidence is undetermined. There is one notable exception in the report by Gaspar and Treiman of a group of 228 patients with vascular injuries at the Los Angeles County General Hospital over a 10-year period with 51 patients (about 22 per cent) who had venous injuries. There are recent reviews, including the report of Meyer (1987), who identified 36 patients with major extremity venous injuries with 34 also having major arterial injury. Aitken (1989) reviewed the cases of 26 patients with lower limb venous trauma.

ETIOLOGY. Although an endless number of wounding agents have been identified as the etiologic factor in venous trauma, specific documentation in published reports is very limited. The number of iatrogenic injuries to the venous system has increased during the past 20 years as a result of the rapid development of vascular and cardiac angiography and catheterization. Fractures have been associated with venous injuries.

DIAGNOSTIC CONSIDERATIONS. Doppler ultrasound may be useful as a diagnostic technique in the management of venous disease. Impedance plethysmography, phlebography, and radionuclide studies have also had a degree of success in diagnosing venous occlusions.

SURGICAL MANAGEMENT. General considerations for management of the injured patient should be of primary concern. The principles of elective surgical procedures should be followed in the management of the injured patient who has sustained venous trauma. The venous injury can be managed by at least five different methods. These are listed in order of popularity: (1) ligation, (2) lateral suture repair, (3) end-to-end anastomosis, (4) venous patch graft, and (5) venous replacement graft.

POSTOPERATIVE CARE. Specific attempts should be made after the operation to minimize or eliminate edema of the involved extremity.

53

DISORDERS OF THE LUNGS, PLEURA, AND CHEST WALL

I

Anatomy
Walter G. Wolfe, M.D.

Knowledge of the anatomy of the lung is fundamental in understanding and management of difficult clinical problems involving the pulmonary system. The lung is of additional importance because of its position as a target organ for many complications that occur following surgical procedures in any specialty. Complications occur with passage of tubes through the nasal pharynx. Vocal cord injury and injury to the larynx and trachea occur with intubation and may be involved in traumatic injuries of the neck and thorax. Consequently, knowledge of this anatomy is essential because of the seriousness of overlooked injury in this area and the surrounding structures including the great vessels and esophagus. The interruption or loss of function of the laryngeal mechanism that protects patients from the dangers of aspiration may be the most serious pulmonary complication occurring in surgical patients. Contamination of the airway by either aspiration or bacteria produces pneumonia and sepsis.

Knowledge of the airways and their hyperreactivity, such as seen in patients with asthma, as well as of fluid overload and sudden mucosal edema producing small airway obstruction is extremely important. The mucociliary blanket protects the alveoli by moving mucus and particles from the conducting airways so that they can be expelled by cough. Interference with this mechanism subjects the patient to pulmonary complications. Consequently, loss of ciliated cells and the increased production by mucus cells have a significant role in the ability of these surgical patients, especially smokers, to clear secretions in the postoperative period.

Alveolar epithelium and the endothelium of the capillaries are susceptible to toxic substances, the most common used in the intensive care unit being oxygen. Therefore, protecting patients on long-term ventilation from oxygen toxicity is mandatory.

The blood supply to the lung, including the pulmonary circulation and the bronchial circulation, is of utmost importance. Obliteration of pulmonary arteries through either pulmonary emboli or inflammatory processes may have serious consequence to the alveoli and gas exchange. In inflammatory

---

See the corresponding chapter or part in the *Textbook of Surgery*, 14th edition, pp. 1673–1682, for a more detailed discussion of this topic, including a comprehensive list of references.

situations or in cyanotic conditions in which there is a prominent bronchial circulation, significant hemoptysis may occur. Also, the blood supply of primary bronchogenic tumors of the lung is usually via the bronchial circulation. Knowledge of the bronchial circulation as well as of the pulmonary artery circulation is important because of resurgence of lung transplantation and problems that occur with healing of the bronchial anastomosis.

In summary, the anatomy of the lung and its metabolic functions continue to be essential in surgical therapy, not only for the management of the conditions that occur primarily in the lung, such as inflammation, abscess, and carcinoma, but because the pulmonary system remains a significant target organ for morbidity and mortality in patients who undergo operations in all surgical disciplines.

II

Clinical and Physiologic Evaluation of Respiratory Function

Richard A. Hopkins, M.D., and Walter G. Wolfe, M.D.

PULMONARY FUNCTION

Understanding of the factors that contribute to and alter pulmonary ventilation and gas exchange requires a detailed knowledge of lung function at the alveolar level. Ventilation serves to replenish the gas in the lungs for maintenance of the high oxygen–low carbon dioxide pressure, with production of maximal gradients. Distribution of gas is the delivery of air to the alveolar units by way of the bifurcating tracheobronchial tree. Diffusion is the transfer of gas molecules across the alveolar membranes in the region of high concentration. The blood-air surface of over 90 square meters in adult humans is condensed in a lung volume of only 5 liters. This is made possible by the small radius and the large number (300 million) of alveoli. Perfusion is the means by which desaturated blood is brought into intimate contact with the alveolar-capillary bed.

The necessity for measurement of lung function in a specific patient is usually obvious from the clinical evaluation. Initial tests are done to determine if there is functional impairment. When the history and physical examination do not suggest

---

See the corresponding chapter or part in the *Textbook of Surgery*, 14th edition, pp. 1682–1694, for a more detailed discussion of this topic, including a comprehensive list of references.

any evidence of lung disease, measurement of the vital capacity and forced expiratory volume in 1 second combined with a normal chest film and normal blood gas determination is sufficient to screen the patient to support the clinical impression that there is no underlying pulmonary disease. However, in patients with obvious or suspected lung disease, more detailed studies are necessary.

LUNG VOLUMES. Respiratory excursion is the amount of air inspired and expired; this is termed tidal volume (V_T). The amount of gas contained in the lung at the end of quiet expiration is termed the functional residual capacity (FRC). When the patient makes a maximal inspiration and increases the lung volume compared with that contained at the peak tidal volume, the inspiratory reserve capacity or volume (RV) is reached. With forcible expiration, with exhalation of as much air as possible from the lung, the volume expired from the maximal inspiration to maximal expiration is the vital capacity (VC). The amount of air remaining in the lungs after maximal expiration is the residual volume (RV). These lung volumes may be measured in the spirometer, except for the RV and the FRC. The FRC must be measured by other techniques. One of three different methods—inert gas dilution and washout, whole body plethysmography, or radioisotope techniques—may be employed.

MAXIMAL BREATHING CAPACITY. Maximal breathing capacity (MBC) is defined as the largest volume of air that can be moved in and out of the chest per minute. The term MBC is reserved for the maximal breathing capacity of an individual, whereas the term maximal voluntary ventilation (MVV) indicates the maximal volume of gas breathed per minute under specific testing conditions. The analysis of VC and of MBC permits differentiation of ventilatory abnormality into obstructive versus restrictive disease, since MBC is markedly decreased in obstructive disease.

FLOW RATES. Measurement of dynamic properties of the lungs, that is, flow rates, is extremely important. The patient inhales maximally and then exhales forcibly into the spirometer while the device records the volume versus the time. A common test of maximal expiratory airflow is the volume of air expired in 1 second (FEV_1). This number is decreased in the presence of bronchial obstruction, but the value may also be decreased in restrictive disease. For this reason, the FEV_1 is usually related to the total exhaled VC. This ratio of FEV_1 to VC may be decreased in the presence of airway obstruction but normal in restrictive lung disease.

GAS DIFFUSION. A single-breath carbon monoxide ($D_{L_{CO}}$) diffusion capacity should be considered a screening test. In this test, the patient is required to inhale low, nontoxic concentrations of carbon monoxide, hold the breath for 10 seconds, and then exhale. This test is rapid, simple, safe, and painless. $D_{L_{CO}}$ is an estimate of the pulmonary capillary surface area. There are several factors that affect diffusion in a single alveolus. The thickness of the alveolar lining membrane is important as well as the thickness of the layer of plasma between the capillary wall and the red blood cell. In addition, the permeability of the erythrocyte to carbon monoxide or oxygen must be considered along with the reaction rate of hemoglobin with carbon monoxide or oxygen. In a single-breath diffusion capacity with use of carbon monoxide, the presence of carbon monoxide hemoglobin in the pulmonary arterial blood diminishes the rate of carbon monoxide transfer.

The measurement of arterial blood gases is probably the most frequently used pulmonary function test. The interpretation of Pa_{O_2} depends on the oxygen tension in the inspired air. One can then calculate first the alveolar oxygen tension and then the alveolar-arterial oxygen tension gradient; if the Pa_{O_2} and the A-aDO_2 are normal, there is no disturbance in oxygen transport.

The measurements of Pa_{CO_2} provide an immediate indication of the patient's alveolar ventilation. A Pa_{CO_2} of less than 37 mm. Hg indicates hypocapnia, whereas hypercapnia is defined as greater than 43 mm. Hg (i.e., normal range, 38 to 42 mm. Hg). Any level of hypercapnia indicates severe disease representing functional loss of perhaps more than 50 per cent of the lung. Acidosis is defined as a pH of less than 7.37, and alkalosis indicates a pH of greater than 7.43. Evaluation of acid-base requires interpretation of both respiratory and metabolic determinants of pH; potential aberrations include respiratory acidosis, respiratory alkalosis, metabolic acidosis, and metabolic alkalosis.

CLOSING VOLUMES. The closing volume is the remaining lung volume at the end of expiration below which alveolar collapse begins to occur, with production of "physiologic" shunting. In the normal young individual, this closing volume is well below the FRC. Age alone is associated with a decrease in the elastic properties of the lung such that although FRC gradually increases with age, so does the effective closing volume. At some point these lines cross, and at end expiration, portions of alveoli are being underventilated so that a physiologic right-to-left shunt occurs and the total oxygen saturation decreases. This is the reason why the partial pressure of oxygen in the arterial blood gradually decreases with age. This process is accelerated by smoking and other causes of chronic pulmonary disease, which produces hypoxemia at a younger age. In addition, placing a patient supine, even at a young age, or other mechanical factors such as obesity may produce an elevation in closing volume and relative hypoxemia. Hypoxemia is common postoperatively because of this "closing volume effect." The presence of interstitial pulmonary edema accentuates this effect. When end-expiratory pressure is applied, FRC returns to normal and corrects the closing volume abnormality.

PREOPERATIVE EVALUATION

Pulmonary complications are not infrequent following major operative procedures. Age, obesity, type of surgical procedure, cigarette smoking, and anesthesia impair pulmonary function and are preoperative risk factors. With age, the lungs show gradual deterioration both in performance of the airways and in gas exchange. Both flow-volume curves and position as well as blood gases change with age. Although a nonsmoker's pulmonary function deteriorates only slightly with time, age still remains a relative factor. The older patient with obstructive airway disease has a markedly increased risk. Obesity impairs lung and chest wall compliance. There may be a component of restrictive lung disease, and the work of breathing is increased. When abnormal closure of small airways occurs, this produces significant ventilation-perfusion mismatches. These changes become worse in the supine position, in which the weight of the abdomen and chest wall contributes to the impairment of pulmonary function. These changes may be even more apparent if the patient is placed in a lateral position with one lung partially deflated. More effort is required for each breath, and the Pa_{CO_2} usually falls.

Pulmonary function should be evaluated in relation to the operative procedure planned. Patients can be divided into the following groups: (1) those undergoing thoracotomy for removal of lung tissue, (2) those undergoing thoracotomy without excision of pulmonary tissue, (3) those undergoing abdominal surgery, and (4) those undergoing procedures on extremities or elsewhere. It is apparent that each group responds somewhat differently to the effects of the operation, anesthesia, and pulmonary function. Every effort should be made postoperatively to obtain maximal pulmonary function as soon as possible for ensuring rapid return of the FRC to the preoperative level. Supplemental oxygen should be used as necessary for prevention of hypoxemia. In general, if the VC and the FRC are returned to the preoperative level and hypoxemia is prevented, the ventilation-perfusion ratio will be corrected.

RISK IN PATIENTS WITH PRE-EXISTING PULMONARY DISEASE. Obstructive pulmonary disease is the most important risk factor in the patient undergoing operation. The more severe the disease, the greater the risk of postoperative complications. Restrictive lung disease is usually better tolerated; however, these patients cannot afford to lose much functioning lung. Because of better expiratory flow rates, cough is better preserved than with obstructive disease. In general, an FEV_1 of 1 to 2 liters is not associated with an increased operative risk; with an FEV_1 less than 800 ml., there is clearly increased risk for severe pulmonary complications; those with less than 500 ml. have the greatest risk. The presence of carbon dioxide retention is a marker for the patient at dramatically increased risk.

Thoracotomy and pulmonary resection are not well tolerated in patients with obstructive airway disease. Not only is there a loss of functional tissue in a patient with pulmonary disease, but the thoracotomy alters the mechanical and gas exchange properties of the lung. This may be accentuated if lung tissue is removed during operation. Thoracotomy produces pain in the postoperative period, which reduces the patient's ability to cough for clearance of secretions. If the airway disease is severe, the patient may not be able to tolerate the loss of even a single pulmonary segment. Thus, in these patients, preoperative evaluation is extremely important, and preparation of the patient by cessation of smoking and the use of a number of drugs for improvement of airway function and ventilation is extremely helpful in decreasing operative risk.

In individuals with pulmonary hypertension and carbon dioxide retention, resective procedures may be contraindicated. For example, if FEV_1 is less than 2 liters and the MVV or MBC less than 50 per cent, patients usually do not tolerate pneumonectomy. Therefore, predicting postresection lung function can be helpful in preventing a surgically cured but pulmonary-crippled patient. A good estimate of postoperative pulmonary function can be obtained by comparing the quantitative perfusion lung scan with the patient's preoperative FEV_1. Ferguson and colleagues have demonstrated that measurement of $D_{L_{CO}}$ is an important discriminator for postoperative morbidity and mortality following pulmonary resection; they reason that the $D_{L_{CO}}$ is a sensitive indicator of both structural and functional abnormalities, since it is a measure of functional alveolar microarchitecture and can be an independent measure of physiologic capability apart from FEV_1 and forced vital capacity (FVC).

OPERATIVE AND POSTOPERATIVE CHANGES. The effects of anesthesia may increase venous admixture, increase ventilation and perfusion mismatching, change the cardiac output, and alter the mechanical properties of the chest wall or the lung itself, whether or not paralysis is used during anesthesia. Mucociliary transport may be decreased, and the hemoglobin concentration and function may change. Diaphragmatic function may be impaired, and the position of the patient during operation may compound some of these difficulties. The dependent basilar segments, for example, are usually underventilated and therefore have a greater tendency to develop atelectasis. In general, the patient is ventilated with positive pressure, and the dependent areas of the lung, which have the smallest airway diameters and are the least compliant, are poorly ventilated. The more compliant and less perfused areas receive the greatest ventilation. This produces ventilation-perfusion mismatching and hypoxemia and atelectasis. The FRC decreases in almost all anesthetized surgical patients as well as in injured patients regardless of whether the injury is a result of the operation or of trauma. It follows, therefore, that the FEV_1 and VC are also reduced. These changes are maximal in the first and second postoperative days but remain abnormal for a week following operation. Decrease in the FRC causes airway closure and ventilation-perfusion mismatching with resulting hypoxemia, which may be accentuated in the older patient.

The patient should be encouraged to sit upright as soon as possible. Lung function is clearly improved with early ambulation. This is especially important in the obese and elderly. Early ambulation increases FRC and also helps to reduce the risk of pulmonary embolism. Pulmonary embolism in the postoperative period is a dangerous postoperative complication in these higher risk patients with impaired pulmonary functions. Care must be taken to prevent aspiration.

III

Bronchoscopy
Ross M. Ungerleider, M.D.

Bronchoscopes are either *rigid* or *flexible*. Each type has specific advantages and disadvantages, and the use of each requires specific training.

RIGID BRONCHOSCOPES. These hollow metal tubes are similar to the first bronchoscope developed. They usually have illumination at the tip as well as side holes near the tip for facilitating ventilation; they are always inserted transorally. Insertion can be under topical anesthesia if the patient is cooperative, but general anesthesia is recommended for combative or pediatric patients.

The view through these instruments is limited, and as can be expected, the longer the bronchoscope and the smaller its diameter, the more limited the view. Specially designed telescopes can be inserted into these tubes for enhancement of the view without substantially reducing the airway.

The primary advantage of the rigid bronchoscope is that it provides a large controlled airway that is valuable in patients with excessive secretions or massive hemoptysis. This is the instrument of choice for removal of foreign bodies. These rigid tube bronchoscopes are also utilized during endobronchial surgery because they provide a large lumen for the insertion of instruments or for the control of significant bleeding.

FLEXIBLE BRONCHOSCOPES. These instruments are flexible and incorporate a bending tip that can be controlled by a unit held in the physician's hand. The bronchoscopes range in outside diameter from 1.8 to 6 mm. with innerchannels to provide light (via fiberoptics). The larger models also contain separate channels for suction as well as for insertion of specially constructed instruments. Because these instruments are highly maneuverable and smaller in size than most rigid bronchoscopes, they can be used to reach areas in the endobronchial tree not accessible to their rigid counterparts. These instruments are easy to use, are well tolerated by the awake patient, and can be inserted either transorally or transnasally. Because of their unique design, these instruments can provide visualization of lobar and segmental bronchi and allow the physician to diagnose lesions beyond the view of the rigid bronchoscopes. The major disadvantage of the flexible instrument is that unlike the open rigid tube, it is a *closed* system that does not provide an airway, and the relatively small innerchannel is considered by many to be incapable of allowing adequate suction in the presence of copious secretions or massive hemoptysis.

INDICATIONS, USES, AND COMPLICATIONS. The indications for bronchoscopy range from diagnosis to treat-

---

See the corresponding chapter or part in the *Textbook of Surgery,* 14th edition, pp. 1695–1701, for a more detailed discussion of this topic, including a comprehensive list of references.

ment. The most common diagnostic use is for the evaluation of endobronchial and parenchymal lung tumors. Bronchoscopy can be utilized not only to demonstrate the presence of radiologically unapparent endobronchial lesions but also to permit evaluation of masses within the tracheobronchial tree that are first disclosed by radiographs. The flexible bronchoscope is capable of detecting more peripheral lesions than can be viewed through the rigid instrument. Brushings and washings for cytologic study as well as direct biopsies in some instances guided by fluoroscopic control can be obtained for further diagnostic evaluation. In addition, transthoracic needle aspiration of the subcarinal area can be easily accomplished through bronchoscopy. Proper bronchoscopic evaluation enables the diagnosis of 95 per cent of lung cancers and is a crucial part of the evaluation for resectability of the tumor. Bronchoscopy is also useful in the diagnosis of hemoptysis, although it is recommended in massive hemoptysis (greater than 600 ml. in 24 hours) that the rigid bronchoscope be used, since it provides a more secure and controlled airway with the ability to provide better suctioning. Bronchoscopy has also proved useful in the diagnosis of pulmonary infections and diffuse interstitial pneumonitis. It is valuable for use in emergency departments for evaluation of smoke inhalation or acute airway obstruction and is a useful addition to radiology departments for the performance of bronchography.

From a therapeutic standpoint, bronchoscopy is essential for removal of foreign bodies. Since, in many instances, foreign body aspiration requires bronchoscopy for establishing the diagnosis, the patient can be examined with flexible bronchoscopy for demonstration of the nature of the foreign body, which can then be safely removed through a rigid bronchoscope. Other uses for bronchoscopy include directed suctioning for patients with atelectasis. Moreover, rigid bronchoscopes are useful for the application of endobronchial laser therapy, and the flexible instruments can be a valuable visually guided stylet for patients who are otherwise difficult to intubate. Recent advances in the technology have extended the uses of bronchoscopy to the pediatric population; several excellent articles have appeared outlining indications for bronchoscopy in children, which are not dissimilar from those in adults.

Bronchoscopy is safe with a complication rate of less than 0.08 per cent and a mortality of less than 0.01 per cent. Most complications are related to premedication and not to the procedure itself. However, a number of problems have been reported including pneumothorax, bronchospasm, hemorrhage, bronchial perforation (after biopsy), subglottic edema, infections, arrhythmias, and, rarely, cardiopulmonary arrest. Rigid bronchoscopy should be avoided in the presence of cervical spine injury and in patients with aneurysms of the thoracic aorta. Flexible bronchoscopy is avoided in patients with massive hemoptysis.

IV

Diagnostic Thoracoscopy

James W. Mackenzie, M.D.

The correct diagnosis in most patients with pleural or tracheobronchial disease is usually established by appropriate cultures, cytologic studies of sputum, bronchoscopy, or mediastinoscopy. Thoracentesis and needle aspiration of pleural or parenchymal lesions complete the usual diagnostic armamentarium. Frequently, pleural disease and, more uncommonly, parenchymal disease cannot be diagnosed by these methods. For these patients, thoracoscopy provides an excellent means for establishing the diagnosis without resorting to diagnostic thoracotomy with its attendant morbidity and mortality.

General, regional, or local anesthesia may be used. With the greater availability of competent anesthesiologists, general anesthesia is recommended in all but the most severely compromised patient. This technique is more acceptable to patients and, combined with selected ventilation of the lung, provides excellent conditions for careful inspection of the intrapleural contents. Intermittent sampling of the arterial blood gases or measurement of end-tidal carbon dioxide and transcutaneous oxygen provides an added measure of safety. Patients with undiagnosed pleural disease comprise the most frequent indication for this procedure. Mesothelioma, in particular, resists diagnosis by needle biospy and pleural fluid analysis.

There are a number of other uses for thoracoscopy as a diagnostic means, such as obtaining material for estrogen binding studies in patients with metastatic carcinoma of the breast. *It should be emphasized that most patients with known or suspected lung cancer need not be subjected to thoracoscopy for diagnosis or staging.*

TECHNIQUE. Techniques have been described with utilization of a flexible bronchoscope or a rigid two-trocar system that allows vision through one site and manipulation of instruments through the other site. The mediastinoscope, available in most hospitals, or a specially designed thoracoscope provides excellent visualization and is preferred by most. This procedure may be combined with bronchoscopy and mediastinoscopy. Although thoracoscopy by entry into the pleural cavity through the cervical mediastinoscopy incision has been described, access to the inferior reaches of the pleural cavity is not easy. The best exposure is provided with the patient in the true lateral position with entry into the pleural cavity through the fifth intercostal space in the mid-axillary line.

After the extracostal muscles are separated in the direction of their fibers, the intercostal muscles are incised with a

---

See the corresponding chapter or part in the *Textbook of Surgery*, 14th edition, pp. 1701–1703, for a more detailed discussion of this topic, including a comprehensive list of references.

cautery. Care is taken to aspirate all the fluid within the pleural space and to send aliquots for the appropriate cytologic, bacteriologic, or biochemical studies. Any adhesions are carefully divided by blunt dissection, and the instrument is then inserted. Obvious abnormalities on the pleural surface are sampled.

Occasionally, a rigid bronchoscope provides better visualization of the apex. A flexible bronchoscope may be inserted through this rigid bronchoscope. Antituberculosis drugs are administered the day of operation if frozen section suggests the possibility of active tuberculosis; otherwise, no antibiotics are given. If biopsy of a lesion on the visceral pleura is performed, care should be taken to control the surface with cryotherapy or electrocautery. The pleural cavity is drained by a tube attached to an underwater seal; this tube is usually removed the next day. Obviously, the chest tube should not be removed until all air leakage is controlled and the fluid drainage is minimal.

The therapeutic uses of thoracoscopy are beyond the discussion for this section. There are a number of obvious uses, and thoracoscopy remains an underutilized diagnostic technique for patients with thoracic disease. It is safer than and at least as accurate as limited diagnostic thoracotomy.

V

Tracheostomy and its Complications

Hermes C. Grillo, M.D., and Douglas J. Mathisen, M.D.

The indications for tracheostomy are relief of upper airway obstruction, control of secretions, and, in patients requiring mechanical ventilation, support for respiratory failure. The use of rigid bronchoscopes or the laser to dilate or core-out benign and malignant strictures of the airway and flexible bronchoscopy and mini-tracheostomy for pulmonary toilet may diminish the frequency of tracheostomy for the first two indications.

The timing of tracheostomy for long-term mechanical ventilation is controversial. The authors' policy has been to perform tracheostomy *early* if long-term ventilation can be predicted or if, after 7 to 10 days, it appears extubation is not likely in the next 3 to 4 days. Critical to this policy is the reversibility of most complications of tracheostomy versus

See the corresponding chapter or part in the *Textbook of Surgery*, 14th edition, pp. 1704–1709, for a more detailed discussion of this topic, including a comprehensive list of references.

irreparable injury to the glottis from prolonged endotracheal intubation. This is especially true of glottic injuries from an endotracheal tube too large for the glottis or pressure necrosis posteriorly by the tube. This concern is substantiated in a study that showed an increasing incidence of complex laryngeal injuries the longer oral endotracheal intubation was utilized (especially with large tubes).

There are many techniques of tracheostomy. The technique the authors prefer involves a horizontal skin incision, separation of the strap muscles in the midline, and division of the thyroid isthmus to allow accurate identification of the second and third tracheal rings. A longitudinal incision is then made through these cartilages. The trachea is spread, and a tracheostomy tube is inserted, secured to the skin, and tied around the neck. The tracheostomy tube should be the smallest size compatible with the patient's trachea and utilize a low-pressure, high-volume cuff.

Many authors refer to a high incidence of complications from tracheostomy. Usually, these statements are made in reference to the emergent procedure, performed under less than ideal conditions, and possibly with tubes of inferior design and quality. A precise, carefully performed tracheostomy should be associated with few complications. Careful identification of anatomic landmarks should avoid injury to recurrent nerves, esophagus, and nearby vascular structures. By use of the second and third rings, the risk of subglottic stenosis from injury of the cricoid cartilage or innominate artery hemorrhage from the tube's pressing against this structure, which can occur if the tracheostomy is placed too low, can be minimized. High-volume, low-pressure cuffs have markedly reduced cuff stenosis, but constant vigilance must be exercised to not overinflate low-pressure cuffs, thereby converting them into high-pressure cuffs. Avoidance of excessively large tubes, large openings in the trachea, and excessive leverage on the tubes by heavy rigid connecting tubing should minimize stomal stenosis. Conscientious nursing care will prevent many potential problems by ensuring that tubes are tightly secured for avoidance of dislodgment; that proper levels of humidification are provided for avoidance of drying and crusting of secretions; and that cuffs are not overinflated, thus risking herniation and obstruction by the cuff. Tracheoesophageal fistula is avoided by eliminating the use of large, hard nasogastric tubes and cuffed airway tubes. The combination acts in a pincer manner, eroding the tracheoesophageal walls. Gastrostomy tubes or soft, small Silastic feeding tubes are preferable.

Despite improvements in tube and cuff design and attention to surgical technique, postintubation tracheal stenosis still occurs. *Every patient with signs of upper airway obstruction—wheezing or stridor, dyspnea on effort, or episodes of obstruction from secretions—who has been previously intubated with either an endotracheal tube or tracheostomy tube must be considered to have obstruction until it is proved otherwise.* These patients are often treated for asthma with steroids because of wheezing despite a clear chest film.

Patients too ill or inappropriate for resection and reconstruction are best managed by tracheostomy or a T-tube placed *through the old stoma or stenotic segment—never through viable trachea, which may preclude future repair*. Tracheal dilation by rigid bronchoscopes or use of the laser is only a temporary measure, since restenosis usually occurs.

Resection and reconstruction is preferred for the management of postintubation stenosis. At the Massachusetts General Hospital, 279 patients have been treated for postintubation stenosis (etiologic basis of stenosis: stomal, 32 per cent; cuff, 53 per cent; both, 9 per cent; uncertain, 6 per cent). Good to excellent results were attained in 225 patients (81 per cent); 25 (9 per cent) had satisfactory results; there were 20 failures (9 good results with reoperation) and 5 deaths, and 4 were lost to follow-up.

Subglottic stenosis and acquired tracheoesophageal fistulas are best managed by single staged operation but represent challenging problems.

VI

Pulmonary Infections
Stewart M. Scott, M.D.

PYOGENIC LUNG ABSCESS

A lung abscess is a localized area of pulmonary suppuration with cavitation and it occurs in a number of diseases: tuberculosis, fungus or parasitic infections, bronchiectasis, infected cysts, pulmonary infarction, and cavitating lung tumors. A pyogenic lung abscess, however, is one that occurs with aspiration pneumonitis.

PATHOGENESIS. Pyogenic lung abscess occurs when septic debris is aspirated from the oropharynx of a patient whose cough reflex is suppressed. Aspiration is more likely to occur in patients unconscious from alcoholism, general anesthesia, epilepsy, cerebrovascular accidents, or drowning. Also, patients with esophageal disease are prone to regurgitation and aspiration. The patient is usually supine when aspiration occurs, and the aspirated material enters the most dependent bronchi. These are the superior segment of the right lower lobe and the posterior segment of the right upper lobe.

The microorganisms commonly responsible for pyogenic lung abscess are anaerobic bacteria, alpha- and beta-hemolytic streptococci, staphylococci, nonhemolytic streptococci, and

---

See the corresponding chapter or part in the *Textbook of Surgery,* 14th edition, pp. 1709–1718, for a more detailed discussion of this topic, including a comprehensive list of references.

Escherichia coli. Septic debris aspirated into the lung causes a localized pneumonitis that is followed by liquefaction necrosis. Some of the necrotic material empties through a draining bronchus, leaving a cavity containing air and pus. The clinical features of lung abscess typically include cough, foul-smelling sputum, fever, pleuritic chest pain, weight loss, and night sweats. An upright thoracic roentgenogram demonstrates a cavity with an air-fluid level unless the cavity is obscured by pleural thickening, pneumothorax, or atelectasis. The staphylococcic pneumoceles seen in infants are different in that they appear as thin-walled cystlike lesions that are often accompanied by pleural effusion, empyema, or pyopneumothorax. The toxic symptoms of staphylococcic pneumonia may overshadow the symptoms of lung abscess.

Lung abscesses in immunosuppressed patients are frequently multiple, occur in all the lung segments, and are usually the result of hospital-acquired organisms. *Staphylococcus aureus* is most frequent, but alpha-streptococci, *Neisseria catarrhalis*, pneumococci, *Pseudomonas*, *Proteus*, *E. coli*, and *Klebsiella* are common. Suppressed immunity may be present in the very young, in the very old, in patients receiving corticosteroids or immunosuppressive or radiation therapy, and in patients with malignancies and other systemic diseases such as acquired immunodeficiency syndrome (AIDS). Identification of the organisms in these patients is especially important for ensuring effective treatment.

TREATMENT. The management of aspiration lung abscess is prolonged administration of penicillin G or clindamycin. Bronchoscopy is indicated to exclude cancer, to aid in identifying causative organisms, to remove any foreign body present, and to drain the abscess through the bronchus. *Surgical therapy* is indicated if a large thick-walled abscess fails to respond to antibiotics or if a malignant lesion is suspected. Surgical resection may be necessary for massive hemoptysis or empyema. Occasionally, percutaneous drainage is necessary for the poor-risk patient. Mortality for pyogenic lung abscess in immunocompetent patients is 5 to 6 per cent; mortality in immunosuppressed patients and patients with debilitating disease is much higher.

ACTINOMYCETIC INFECTIONS OF THE LUNG

Actinomycosis and nocardiosis are diseases caused by bacteria of the Actinomycetaceae.

Actinomycosis

Actinomycosis in man is most often caused by *Actinomyces israelii*. *Actinomyces* are anaerobic or microaerophilic bacteria with characteristic branching filaments. Clusters of these organisms in sinuses and abscesses have the appearance of "sulfur granules." Actinomycosis may be cervicofacial, thoracic, or abdominal. Thoracic actinomycosis is the result of invasion by the organism from the oropharynx, where it is a normal inhabitant. Empyema and chronic chest wall draining sinuses are typically present. The pulmonary lesion appears as an infiltration or a hilar mass and resembles bronchogenic carcinoma.

Treatment requires large doses of penicillin G for a prolonged time and radical surgical excision when possible.

Nocardiosis

Nocardia asteroides, the most common cause of nocardiosis in man, is an aerobic, gram-positive, acid-fast organism that is sometimes mistaken for *Mycobacterium tuberculosis*. Nocardiosis mimics tuberculosis, actinomycosis, pneumonia, and lung abscess. It is an opportunistic infection often associated with malignancy, organ transplantation, immunosuppressive therapy, and AIDS. Treatment requires long-term administration of trimethoprim-sulfamethoxazole or minocycline.

FUNGUS INFECTIONS OF THE LUNGS

The normally pathogenic fungi are *Histoplasma, Blastomyces, Coccidioides, Paracoccidioides,* and *Sporothrix*. These fungi are dimorphic, occurring in nature as molds that are not susceptible to phagocytosis by human leukocytes. In hosts, however, these fungi change into yeast forms or spherules that are susceptible to phagocytosis. *Aspergillus, Candida,* and *Mucor* are human saprophytes that cause opportunistic fungal infections. Most fungi causing human infections are inhabitants of the soil. Most infections are thought to follow inhalation of organisms in contaminated dust. *Histoplasma capsulatum, Coccidioides immitis,* and *Blastomyces dermatitidis* have been shown to be endemic and present in the soil of specific geographic areas.

Histoplasmosis

Histoplasmosis is the most common of pathogenic fungal infections. It is caused by *Histoplasma capsulatum*, which is endemic along the Mississippi river and its tributaries. An acute infection produces a diffuse pulmonary infiltration or scattered nodules. Most infected individuals are asymptomatic. However, in patients with AIDS, the infection can be severe and should be aggressively treated.

The most common clinical presentation of histoplasmosis is that of an asymptomatic granuloma appearing as a solitary nodule with concentric rings of calcium on thoracic roentgenogram. Chronic cavitary histoplasmosis occurs and resembles tuberculosis. Identification of the organism from sputum or tissue specimens is required for diagnosis.

Acute histoplasmosis is treated with amphotericin B. Chronic cavitary histoplasmosis may be treated with amphotericin B or ketoconazole. Surgical therapy is reserved for chronic thick-walled cavities that do not respond to amphotericin B. Occasionally, the diagnosis of a chronic granuloma may be made only after surgical excision.

Coccidioidomycosis

Coccidioidomycosis is caused by *Coccidioides immitis*, which is found in the desert areas of southern California, Nevada, Arizona, and New Mexico. More than 10 million people in the United States have been infected with this fungus. The organism appears in tissue as a large spherule packed with endospores. Pulmonary lesions vary from the highly characteristic "thin-walled cavities" to suppuration, infiltration, and chronic granulomas, which makes coccidioidomycosis sometimes difficult to distinguish from tuberculosis and histoplasmosis. Hemoptysis occurs in patients with chronic infection. Cough, weight loss, fever, and chest pain accompany acute infection. Skin tests and complement fixation are usually positive, and organisms can be found in the sputum.

Only acutely ill patients require therapy with amphotericin B or ketoconazole. Surgical therapy may be necessary for some patients with severe recurrent hemoptysis or enlarging thick-walled cavities (greater than 2 cm.).

North American Blastomycosis

North American blastomycosis is caused by the round, thick-walled, single-budding yeast *Blastomyces dermatitidis*, which is endemic to the central United States and Canada. Ulcerating cutaneous lesions are common. Symptoms due to pulmonary involvement are nonspecific. Lesions appearing in the thoracic roentgenogram may be cavitary, nodular, fibrotic, or disseminated. The diagnosis is often made from sputum or serologic testing. Treatment consists of amphotericin B or ketoconazole. Surgical therapy is performed only if bronchogenic carcinoma is suspected.

Cryptococcosis

Cryptococcosis is primarily an opportunistic infection caused by *Cryptococcus neoformans*. The organism is a round budding yeast cell with a characteristic thick gelatinous capsule. The pigeon is its vector. Benign and subclinical bronchopulmonary infections occur. Roentgenographic features are nonspecific and may include pleural effusion. The disease may signify an underlying cancer or significant systemic disease. It is the most common fungus infection in renal transplant patients and is a frequent cause of pulmonary infection in patients with AIDS. Treatment consists of 5-fluorocytosine or amphotericin B and is indicated if there is active progression of a pulmonary lesion or if there is associated meningeal involvement.

Aspergillosis

Aspergillus fumigatus, the most common cause of aspergillosis in man, is an ubiquitous fungus that colonizes pre-existing lung cavities, forming fungus balls. Aspergillomas are masses of necrotic hyphae and have a typical roentgen-ographic appearance. A crescent-shaped radiolucency out-lines the fungus ball, which moves freely within the cavity. Hemorrhage is a common complication for which surgical excision is often necessary. Antimycotic drug therapy is very unsatisfactory. Aspergillosis is an opportunistic infection in transplant patients and in patients with leukemia and lymphoma, but not in patients with AIDS.

Candidiasis

Candidiasis is an opportunistic infection caused by *Candida albicans*, a normal inhabitant of the gastrointestinal tract and the female genital tract. It occurs when host defenses are altered as from diabetes, prolonged use of antibiotics or other drugs, and debilitating disease. Colonization occurs from indwelling catheters used for hyperalimentation or dialysis. *Candida* endocarditis is a complication of intravenous drug abuse. Both *Candida* and *Aspergillus* prosthetic valve endocar-ditis are reported. Amphotericin B alone or in combination with 5-fluorocytosine is the most effective treatment available. Surgical intervention is necessary for eradication of large vegetations that may occur on natural or prosthetic heart valves.

Miscellaneous Fungal Infections

Approximately 150 cases of pulmonary sporotrichosis have been reported. Both iodides and amphotericin B are recom-mended for this rare disease, but surgical excision may be required. Zygomycosis (mucormycosis), another rare and serious infection, occurs primarily in debilitated patients. Treatment consists of amphotericin B and sometimes surgical excision. *Pseudallescheria boydii* is a secondary invader of damaged lung tissue (monosporosis). It is resistant to am-photericin B. Surgical resection is necessary for cavitating lesions. South American blastomycosis (paracoccidioidomy-cosis) begins as a subclinical pulmonary infection. Later, pulmonary granulomas and cavities form along with muco-cutaneous lesions of the hypopharynx. It responds to am-photericin B and ketoconazole.

AIDS-ASSOCIATED PULMONARY INFECTIONS

Opportunistic infections that most often occur in patients with AIDS are those due to *Pneumocystis carinii*, cytomegalo-virus, atypical mycobacteria, *Toxoplasma gondii*, *Candida*, herpes simplex virus, *Cryptococcus neoformans*, and *Cryptospo-ridium*. *Pneumocystis* pneumonia occurs in 80 per cent of patients with AIDS. *Pneumocystis carinii* is a protozoan that stains with silver methenamine and can be identified in sputum or lung tissue obtained by needle or open biopsy. Trimethoprim-sulfamethoxazole and pentamidine isethionate are equally effective for *Pneumocystis* pneumonia. Kaposi's sarcoma, a hallmark of AIDS, is a virus-induced tumor that occurs as a painless purple nodule in the lungs and airway.

VII

The Pleura and Empyema
Stewart M. Scott, M.D.

The pleura is a serous membrane that lines two independent pleural spaces. These spaces extend into the neck, the retrosternal areas, the costophrenic sinuses, and the interlobar fissures. The pleural surface consists of a uniform layer of flattened mesothelial cells beneath which are layers of areolar connective tissue containing blood vessels, nerves, and lymphatics. The visceral pleura is thin, elastic, and intimately attached to underlying lung by intrapulmonary fibrous extensions of connective tissue. The parietal pleura is thicker and easily separated from the endothoracic fascia of the chest wall. It is supplied by the intercostal arteries. The visceral pleura is supplied by the bronchial arteries. Sensory nerve endings are present in the costal and diaphragmatic parietal pleura. Sensory fibers are absent in the visceral pleura.

The secreting and absorbing properties of the pleura are substantial. Increased capillary hydrostatic pressure and increased negative intrapleural pressure increase transudation into the pleural space. As much as a liter a day may form. Loss of intrapleural pressure diminishes transudation, and increased diaphragmatic and intercostal activity increases absorption. Resorption is made possible by the numerous microvilli present on the mesothelial cells lining the visceral and parietal pleura.

The visceral and parietal pleurae are normally 10 to 27 μ apart. The elastic recoil of the lungs causes intrapleural negative pressures of -6 to -12 cm. H_2O during inspiration and -4 to -8 cm. during expiration. Extremes of $+40$ cm. H_2O occur during a Valsalva maneuver and -40 cm. H_2O during inspiratory effort against a closed glottis.

PLEURAL EFFUSIONS

Pleural effusions are usually secondary to some primary disease and often are the first manifestation of disease. The classic signs of pleural effusion are dullness, diminished

---

See the corresponding chapter or part in the *Textbook of Surgery*, 14th edition, pp. 1718–1726, for a more detailed discussion of this topic, including a comprehensive list of references.

breath sounds, and mediastinal displacement. An effusion of 500 ml. or less may not be clinically or roentgenographically apparent in an adult.

Infections, tumor, and congestive failure are responsible for 75 per cent of effusions in most populations. The diagnosis may depend on obtaining a sample of the fluid or a biopsy of pleura or lung. If the pleural fluid is a transudate, that is, fluid low in protein and lactic acid dehydrogenase, it is probably due to systemic disease such as congestive heart failure, cirrhosis, or renal insufficiency. An exudative effusion is more likely to be associated with a diseased pleura, which causes increased permeability of the pleura to proteins and decreased lymphatic clearance, as seen with malignancies and infections. When the diagnosis is not clear from bacteriologic or cytologic examinations, pleural fluid analysis is helpful. Normal pleural fluid pH is 7.64. A pH less than 7.20 is found only in parapneumonic effusions, tuberculosis, rheumatoid pleuritis, esophageal rupture, malignancy, hemothorax, and systemic acidosis. Pleural fluid glucose less than 60 mg. per 100 ml. is found in tuberculosis, malignancy, rheumatoid disease, or parapneumonic effusion. Other pleural fluid measurements indicated at times are white blood cell count, amylase content, chromosome analysis, lupus erythematosus cells, complement, rheumatoid factor, and lipid analysis. When the diagnosis cannot be made from pleural fluid analysis, a pleural or pulmonary tissue biopsy may be indicated. Fluid is obtained by thoracentesis, which is best performed with use of local anesthesia, a 20 ml. syringe, and a three-way stopcock after careful localization of the effusion by roentgenograms.

SPONTANEOUS PNEUMOTHORAX

Spontaneous pneumothorax is usually due to rupture of a subpleural cyst or bulla. It occurs in the healthy young adult, in older patients with emphysema, and even in the newborn and requires vigorous resuscitation. The patient may be asymptomatic or extremely dyspneic. Chest pain may be present. Breath sounds are diminished or absent. The diagnosis is confirmed by chest roentgenogram.

A small (20 per cent or less) asymptomatic pneumothorax will absorb. This is facilitated by supplemental oxygen, which lowers the pN_2 of capillary blood and increases the partial pressure difference between the pleural space and the pleural capillary. Closed thoracostomy is adequate for most large pneumothoraces. If the air leak persists after a reasonable trial, thoracotomy and ligation or excision of the ruptured bulla is indicated.

Tension pneumothorax is the result of a valvelike mechanism that allows air to enter the pleural space from the lung parenchyma when airway pressure is elevated. This occurs during episodes of coughing and in patients on respirators. Severe respiratory distress results when the lung collapses and increased intrapleural pressure causes the mediastinum to shift. Emergency needle aspiration is necessary followed by closed thoracotomy. A drainage system used with closed thoracostomy must provide an underwater seal to allow air and fluid to escape from the pleural space while normal negative intrapleural pressure is maintained. The chest tube is attached to a glass or plastic tube, the tip of which is 2 cm. below the surface of a water reservoir. If blood or fluid is to be drained from the chest, a collecting chamber is interposed between the underwater seal and the chest tube. If an air leak is present, a third chamber to which a vacuum source is attached is required for regulation of the negative pressure. The amount of negative pressure is determined by the depth to which a tube open to air extends beneath a water reservoir, usually 20 cm. Most commercial drainage sets have all three chambers.

HEMOTHORAX

Trauma is the most frequent cause of blood within the pleural cavities, but hemothorax occurs also with pulmonary infarction, pleural and pulmonary neoplasms, torn pleural adhesions accompanying pneumothorax, and anticoagulant therapy.

Blood within the pleural and pericardial cavities is partly defibrinated. It is absorbed unless it becomes infected, at which time a fibrothorax may develop, which can compromise pulmonary function. A small, self-limited hemothorax, therefore, requires only observation. For moderate blood loss (500 ml. or greater), the pleural cavity should be completely drained by closed thoracostomy. If active bleeding persists (200 ml. per hour or more), a thoracotomy for control of bleeding is necessary. Massive bleeding may require vigorous blood volume replacement, which can be augmented by reinfusion of the partially defibrinated blood collected from the chest tubes.

CHYLOTHORAX

Chylothorax is the accumulation of lymph in the pleural space and is usually the result of trauma to the thoracic duct or tumor. Gunshot wounds, stab wounds, and automobile injuries represent 80 per cent of occurrences due to trauma, but 20 per cent are iatrogenic, usually following congenital heart surgery. Spontaneous chylothorax in an adult is ominous and suggests a malignancy. The diagnosis of chylothorax is made by examining the milky white pleural fluid for its high fat and protein content and may be confirmed by lymphangiography. Considerable fluid can escape from the thoracic duct, and symptoms may be due to impaired nutrition or compression of the lung. Conservative treatment includes decompression of the thoracic lymphatics by hyperalimentation or oral medium-chain triglycerides and drainage of the pleural space. If chylothorax persists after 3 to 4 weeks, an attempt to ligate the thoracic duct can be made, or talc pleurodesis can be tried. A pleuroperitoneal shunt has been suggested for infants.

EMPYEMA

Pleural empyema is a collection of pus in the pleural cavity. It is generally secondary to some underlying disease, usually pneumonia, but it occurs with lung abscess, ruptured bullae, bronchopleural fistulas, esophageal rupture, and abscessed lymph nodes. It also occurs when infection is introduced by trauma, surgical procedures, or needle aspiration. The diagnosis is made by aspiration of the empyema and identification of bacteria. The most common bacteria are Staphylococcus aureus, Streptococcus, and a number of gram-negative organisms including anaerobic flora.

Treatment consists of (1) control of the underlying disease, (2) evacuation of the empyema and eradication of the empyema sac, and (3) re-expansion of the lung. Regardless of the underlying condition, adequate drainage is necessary. Occasionally, evacuation of the empyema by thoracentesis is sufficient, but usually an intercostal tube of generous caliber is necessary. The tube should be placed in the most dependent portion of the empyema space. This may require resection of a short segment of rib for identifying the extent of the cavity and for disruption of adhesions. A chronic empyema may need open drainage with a wide-bore tube or a modified Eloesser skin flap. Perhaps 25 per cent of today's empyemas follow thoracic surgical procedures, usually pneumonectomies. If a bronchopleural fistula is present and develops early following operation, an attempt can be made to close the fistula with a muscle flap. Fistulas late in onset are likely to be associated with residual tumor or disease and should be treated with open drainage. If no bronchopleural fistula is present, instillation of antibiotics is sometimes successful in sterilizing the thoracic cavity.

PLEURAL TUMORS

Primary pleural tumors are essentially mesotheliomas, of which there are localized benign and diffuse malignant types. Both may contain fibrous and epithelioid elements, making it difficult at times to distinguish benign from malignant and mesothelioma from carcinoma. Patients with benign localized fibrous mesotheliomas may be asymptomatic or they may have arthralgia, clubbing of the fingers, or fever. The tumor, which ordinarily arises from the visceral pleura, is easily excised, after which symptoms usually disappear.

Diffuse malignant mesotheliomas cause chest pain and bloody pleural effusion. Both visceral and parietal pleura are involved, and the extent of the tumor varies. Metastases are uncommon, but prognosis is poor, and death usually occurs within 2 years regardless of treatment used. The causal relationship between exposure to asbestos dust and malignant mesothelioma is strong. Metastatic tumors are far more common than are primary pleural tumors. The most frequent are tumors of the lung, breast, pancreas, and stomach. As with malignant mesothelioma, bloody pleural fluid containing malignant cells is usually present. Treatment is palliative. Radiation, thoracostomy, and instillation of talc, quinacrine, or tetracycline are sometimes helpful, and pleurectomy may be tried in selected patients.

VIII

Bronchiectasis
Donald D. Glower, M.D.

Bronchiectasis today remains an important but far less common disease than in earlier years and occasionally requires surgical intervention.

PATHOPHYSIOLOGY. Bronchiectasis is defined as persistent, abnormal dilatation of the bronchi, generally beyond the subsegmental level. The gross appearance of bronchiectasis has been described as cylindrical, varicose, or saccular with relative frequencies of 27, 62, and 11 per cent, respectively. The left lung is more frequently involved than the right, and the lower lobes and right middle lobe are more commonly affected than the upper lobes. The anatomic distribution of bronchiectasis may be limited to several isolated segments or may be more diffuse and multisegmental.

In at least 75 per cent of patients, bronchiectasis can be attributed to acquired causes with airway infection and impaired clearance of bronchial secretions producing bronchial injury and subsequent bronchiectasis. The initial insult may be either primary pulmonary infection or bronchial obstruction by mucous plugging, foreign body, neoplasm, or enlarged peribronchial lymph nodes. Truly congenital bronchiectasis is considered to be quite rare in the form of congenital cystic bronchiectasis with incomplete terminal airways, lack of alveolar tissue, and saccular bronchi. A number of congenital disorders can, however, contribute to bronchiectasis. These include Kartagener's syndrome (bronchiectasis, situs inversus, and sinusitis) with abnormal ciliary motility, alpha$_1$-antitrypsin deficiency with impaired clearance of sputum elastase, cystic fibrosis with poor clearance of viscid bronchial secretions, intralobar pulmonary sequestration, panhypogammaglobulinemia, and the Williams-Campbell, Ehlers-Danlos, and Mounier-Kuhn syndromes in which deficient supporting tissue in the bronchial airways may produce bronchiectasis.

CLINICAL PRESENTATION. The onset of symptoms from bronchiectasis generally occurs in childhood or early adult life with a female to male predominance of up to 2.5 to 1. Three quarters of patients have a persistent cough

---

See the corresponding chapter or part in the *Textbook of Surgery*, 14th edition, pp. 1726–1729, for a more detailed discussion of this topic, including a comprehensive list of references.

productive of purulent sputum with disabling fetor oris being present in up to one half of the patients. Hemoptysis or repeated pulmonary infections may also occur in up to 50 per cent of patients. Physical findings are generally limited to audible rales over the involved lung fields, although osteoarthropathy and clubbing may occasionally be present, particularly in severely affected children.

DIAGNOSIS. The diagnosis is by bronchography, and either topical or general anesthesia may be used. Bronchography may be performed bilaterally or unilaterally at two different times. All candidates for operation should undergo bronchography for defining the bronchial anatomy. Computed tomography of the chest using thin, contiguous slices has a sensitivity and specificity of 95 per cent and may have an increasing role as a noninvasive means of diagnosing bronchiectasis. Bronchoscopy should be performed in search of bronchial obstruction or endobronchial disease but is generally nondiagnostic of bronchiectasis. Sinus radiographs, lung ventilation and perfusion scans, quantitative immunoglobulins, and sweat chloride determinations may be useful in selected patients.

TREATMENT. Conservative medical treatment is the primary therapy for bronchiectasis. A 2-week course of antibiotics such as amoxicillin has been shown to be effective for acute exacerbations, and chronic antibiotic therapy may decrease morbidity in selected patients. Chest physiotherapy and postural drainage are generally beneficial but may involve difficulty in long-term compliance. Surgical resection of the most severely involved lung segments is reserved for patients with significant symptoms despite a prolonged medical trial and may be performed by segmentectomy, lobectomy, or pneumonectomy as indicated by anatomic involvement. Preservation of lung tissue is a priority in surgical treatment for bronchiectasis. In patients with bilateral disease, staged bilateral resection may be performed but is indicated only if symptoms persist after the initial resection of the more severely involved side.

Whereas life expectancy after the onset of bronchiectasis was 10 years before the use of antibiotics, patients dying from bronchiectasis today have a mean age of greater than 50 years. The majority of patients treated with either medical or surgical therapy experience improvement in symptoms, and up to 95 per cent of patients undergoing surgical resection are either improved or asymptomatic at follow-up. Patients with multisegmental disease are more likely to have persistent symptoms with either medical or surgical therapy but do benefit from treatment. In the minority of patients presenting with severe disease, however, chronic lung disease and cor pulmonale remain predominant causes of death. Today, most patients with bronchiectasis have an opportunity for significant longevity and reduction in symptoms with current medical and surgical therapy.

IX

Surgical Treatment of Pulmonary Tuberculosis

Jon F. Moran, M.D.

It is estimated that 5 million new cases of active tuberculosis and 3.5 million tuberculosis deaths occur worldwide each year. Pulmonary tuberculosis represents 90 per cent of all cases of tuberculosis today. *Mycobacterium tuberculosis,* an aerobic nonmotile slow-growing bacillus, is responsible for the majority of pulmonary mycobacterial disease. Several other species of mycobacteria can cause pulmonary infection, and these are referred to as *atypical mycobacteria* (Table 1). Atypical mycobacteria are more frequently resistant to chemotherapy. *Mycobacterium avium–intracellulare* and *Mycobacterium kansasii* are the two atypical organisms that most often cause clinical pulmonary infection. Surgical treatment of pulmonary mycobacterial infection is rarely required because current antituberculous chemotherapy is so effective. Operations for pulmonary mycobacterial infection are required only for catastrophic complications such as massive hemoptysis or for treatment of drug-resistant infections.

PATHOLOGY. The pathologic response within the lung to the various mycobacteria is identical. *M. tuberculosis* is a virulent organism requiring a minimal airborne inoculum for occurrence of infection in normal tissue. Atypical mycobacteria more often invade abnormal lung tissue or compromised individuals. The pneumonic process caused by mycobacteria is characterized by caseous necrosis with formation of a granuloma containing the mycobacteria within a rim of granulation tissue. The peripheral pneumonic lesion accompanied by hilar nodal enlargement is termed a primary Ghon complex. Most mycobacterial infections are contained at this early stage by the body's own immune response. Occasionally, in children, primary tuberculosis progresses locally or by hematogenous spread. Miliary tuberculosis arises from massive hematogenous spread with thousands of 1- to 2-mm. (millet seed–sized) tubercles throughout the body.

Adult pulmonary tuberculosis is the most common pattern of mycobacterial infection and is termed *reinfection* or *postpri-*

TABLE 1. Classification of Mycobacterial Species (Runyon)

Group I	Photochromogens	*M. kansasii*
Group II	Scotochromogens	*M. scrofulaceum*
Group III	Nonchromogens	*M. tuberculosis*
		M. avium–intracellulare
Group IV	Rapid growers	*M. fortuitum*
		M. chelonei

See the corresponding chapter or part in the *Textbook of Surgery,* 14th edition, pp. 1729–1737, for a more detailed discussion of this topic, including a comprehensive list of references.

mary tuberculosis. Adult tuberculosis begins as a segmental pneumonia in the apical or posterior segment of an upper lobe or the superior segment of a lower lobe. Bilateral disease is common. The pneumonic infiltrates progress to caseous necrosis with cavity formation when the necrotic area erodes into an adjacent bronchus. Erosion of a cavity into a bronchial vessel may cause severe hemoptysis. A Rasmussen aneurysm, a pulmonary artery aneurysm within or adjacent to a cavity, is found in about 4 per cent of advanced cavitary mycobacterial disease. The visceral and parietal pleura adjacent to the disease are involved by intense inflammatory reaction with obliteration of the pleural space. Endobronchial tuberculosis may cause bronchostenosis with distal bacterial or fungal infection. Tuberculous empyema may occur from hematogenous or lymphatic seeding of the pleural space or rupture of a cavity into the pleural space.

DIAGNOSIS. An important distinction is made between mycobacterial infection and mycobacterial disease. Infection implies the entrance of an organism into the body without symptoms. The diagnosis of mycobacterial disease depends on the confirmation of active disease by radiographic and bacteriologic studies. Approximately 10 per cent of individuals infected with *M. tuberculosis* develop disease. Symptoms of pulmonary tuberculosis are a chronic cough, easy fatigability, weight loss, hemoptysis, and fever with night sweats. Pulmonary mycobacterial infection is more common in the immunosuppressed, in diabetics, or after gastrectomy.

The most frequent radiographic findings in pulmonary tuberculosis are apical infiltrates with frequent cavitation. Current standard tuberculosis skin testing involves the intracutaneous injection of 5 tuberculin units of purified protein derivative (PPD) on the volar aspect of the forearm. This is termed an intermediate PPD, and greater than 10 mm. of induration after 48 to 72 hours defines a positive test. The intermediate PPD is positive in at least 90 per cent of cases of tuberculosis. The isolation of mycobacterial organisms from the sputum is required to confirm the diagnosis of mycobacterial disease. The presence of acid-fast organisms on smear allows rapid presumptive diagnosis, although cultures are necessary to document the species of mycobacteria. Approximately 10,000 organisms per milliliter of sputum are required for smear positivity. Mycobacterial cultures require 3 to 6 weeks to grow, and it may be necessary to obtain multiple samples before a positive smear or culture is obtained. Antimycobacterial chemotherapy is often initiated as a therapeutic trial while final cultures are awaited. Patients referred for surgical treatment are frequently infected with organisms that are resistant to most antituberculous drugs. Sensitivity testing for a number of antituberculous drugs is particularly important in patients being considered for surgical therapy.

CHEMOTHERAPY. Chemotherapy for pulmonary mycobacterial infection requires administration of two or three drugs simultaneously for avoiding the emergence of drug-resistant organisms. Mycobacteria react differently to drugs depending on whether the organisms are extracellular or intracellular. Extracellular organisms tend to multiply rapidly in the hyperoxic neutral pH environment of the pulmonary cavity. In the acidic environment within activated macrophages, organisms grow slowly. An effective treatment program halts mycobacterial growth, both intracellularly and extracellularly, with conversion of the patient to a sputum-negative status within 6 weeks. The five most commonly employed antimycobacterial drugs are listed in Table 2. Atypical mycobacterial infections may require the use of other antibiotics.

Until recently it was recommended that chemotherapy be administered continuously for 18 to 24 months. Short-course therapy (6 to 9 months) has recently been shown to be equally effective. The two currently recommended regimens for treatment of pulmonary tuberculosis are (1) a 6-month course of isoniazid and rifampin with pyrazinamide during the first 2 months, or (2) a 9-month course of isoniazid and rifampin. The primary drug resistance rate for *M. tuberculosis* in the United States is generally 7 to 10 per cent. Although atypical mycobacteria are frequently resistant *in vitro* to many drugs, four- and five-drug regimens may still be effective. Coordination of chemotherapy for pulmonary mycobacterial infections and surgical intervention requires careful planning. Complications of resectional surgery are reduced in patients who have been converted to sputum-negative status. In the treatment of drug-resistant organisms, two or three chemotherapeutic agents to which the infecting organism is sensitive should be given perioperatively and for 6 to 9 months postoperatively.

SURGICAL TREATMENT. When an operation is required for pulmonary mycobacterial disease, resection of the diseased portion of the lung is the procedure of choice. Thoracoplasty and other procedures intended to collapse the infected portion of lung are rarely indicated and are of historic interest only. Guidelines for pulmonary resection in mycobacterial disease are listed below:

1. Persistently positive sputum cultures with cavitation following an adequate period of continuous chemotherapy with two or more drugs to which the organism has been proved sensitive requires surgical intervention.

2. Localized pulmonary disease caused by *M. avium–intracellulare* (or another mycobacterium broadly resistant to chemotherapy) is an indication for resection.

3. A mass lesion of the lung in an area of mycobacterial infection is an indication for resection for simultaneous diagnosis of the mass lesion and treatment of the mycobacterial disease.

4. Massive hemoptysis or recurrent severe hemoptysis is an indication for resection of the infected portion of the lung that is the source of the hemorrhage. Pulmonary hemorrhage is a rare but often fatal complication of pulmonary mycobacterial disease. Massive hemoptysis is defined as greater than 600 ml. per 24 hours; severe hemoptysis is defined as greater than 200 ml. per 24 hours. Asphyxiation rather than hypovolemia is the usual cause of death from hemoptysis. The site of bleeding is almost invariably a cavitary lesion. The

TABLE 2. Commonly Used Antimycobacterial Drugs

Drug	Daily Dosage		Comments
	Children	*Adults*	
Isoniazid (INH)	10–20 mg./kg. PO or IM	5 mg./kg. PO or IM	Bactericidal to both intracellular and extracellular organisms; pyridoxine 10–50 mg./day as prophylaxis for neuritis
Rifampin (RIF)	10–20 mg./kg. PO	10 mg./kg. PO	Bactericidal to both intracellular and extracellular organisms; colors urine orange; inhibits the effect of oral contraceptives, quinidine, digitalis, corticosteroids, and coumadin
Pyrazinamide (PZA)	15–20 mg./kg. PO	15–30 mg./kg. PO	Bactericidal to intracellular organisms; reduces total length of chemotherapy required
Streptomycin (SM)	20–40 mg./kg. IM	15 mg./kg. IM	Bactericidal to extracellular organisms within cavities; limit dose to 10 mg./kg. in elderly patients
Ethambutol (EMB)	15–25 mg./kg. PO	15–25 mg./kg. PO	Bacteriostatic for both intracellular and extracellular organisms

source of bleeding should be resected on an urgent basis following an episode of massive or recurrent severe hemoptysis, since mortality without resection is high. Tuberculosis remains the most common cause of severe hemoptysis.

5. A bronchopleural fistula secondary to mycobacterial infection that does not respond to tube thoracostomy may require surgical treatment.

Several special situations may rarely require surgical treatment of pulmonary mycobacterial disease. Patients severely symptomatic from a destroyed lobe or bronchiectatic area of the lung may benefit from resection. Patients with particularly thick-walled cavities who have reactivated or are clearly unreliable in complying with prolonged chemotherapy may require resection. A patient with a "trapped lung" following a tuberculous empyema may benefit from decortications with or without resection in order to allow full expansion of the underlying lung. Widespread pulmonary or endobronchial disease is generally a contraindication to resection. Children with mycobacterial disease rarely, if ever, require resection, since chemotherapy is usually curative in children, even in far-advanced disease.

OPERATIVE MANAGEMENT. Use of a double-lumen endotracheal tube can make resection for tuberculosis easier and safer. A double-lumen tube can protect the dependent lung from contamination by secretions from the infected upper lung while the patient is in a lateral position. In the setting of severe hemoptysis, a double-lumen tube protects the dependent lung from hemoptysis during resection of the bleeding portion of the upper lung. The extent of pulmonary resection is guided by the principle that all gross evidence of disease should be resected. Whereas conservation of pulmonary tissue is desirable, the dense pleural reaction that is characteristic in mycobacterial disease often makes separation of segments within a lobe difficult. For active mycobacterial disease, a lobectomy or pneumonectomy is usually required. A wedge resection can be used for a mass lesion that is being excised for exclusion of carcinoma or in a case of hemoptysis secondary to a localized peripheral cavity. Pneumonectomy is required only in the setting of a totally destroyed lung.

Patients requiring operation generally have associated problems that predispose them to complications. Administration of effective antimycobacterial drugs, judicious timing of operation, careful operative technique, and meticulous postoperative care are the critically important factors in avoiding complications from pulmonary resection for mycobacterial disease. Good pulmonary toilet and careful attention to the pleural drainage system are necessary to assure full reexpansion of the remaining lung in order to avoid apical space problems. The incidence of bronchopleural fistula after resection for mycobacterial disease is about 3 per cent. An apical space problem follows approximately 20 per cent of resections for mycobacterial disease, but only 10 to 15 per cent of these patients develop a bronchopleural fistula or empyema.

Resectional surgery for mycobacterial disease is now em-

ployed in a selected group of patients who have failed
chemotherapy or have a serious complication such as massive
hemoptysis or bronchopleural fistula. Mortality for pulmonary resection of mycobacterial disease varies from zero with
minimal morbidity when surgical intervention is elective, to
15 per cent or greater when resection is performed as an
emergency. Prognosis for long-term survival free of further
mycobacterial disease is excellent in operative survivors with
95 per cent of patients free of disease 5 to 8 years postoperatively.

X

Benign Tumors of the Trachea and Bronchi

James M. Douglas, Jr., M.D.

Benign tumors of the trachea and bronchi are rare neoplasms that present in a variety of histologic types. They are
found in patients at any age but are three times more common
in males than in females. The peak incidence is in the fifth
and sixth decades for the majority of these tumors; however,
the relative incidence of some of these tumors is age-related.

CLINICOPATHOLOGIC FEATURES. Although these lesions are occasionally asymptomatic, when symptoms occur,
they are most often the result of major airway obstruction or
overlying mucosal irritation. Typically, more than 75 per cent
of the airway must be obstructed before decreased airflow
symptoms develop. Dyspnea, hemoptysis, cough, wheezing,
stridor, atelectasis, and pneumonia are the most common
symptoms.

Although the malignant potential of a particular tumor of
the trachea or bronchus cannot be determined absolutely
without pathologic confirmation, several features suggest a
benign nature. Masses under 2 cm. in length within the
trachea are usually benign. Benign tumors are smoother and
more rounded than are malignant tumors. Although slow
growth suggests a benign nature, this does not guarantee
the absence of malignant potential. Moreover, the presence
of calcium does not distinguish a benign from a malignant
tumor of the trachea or bronchus. More than 90 per cent of
all tumors of the trachea and proximal bronchi in children
are benign. The most common of these are the squamous
papillomas, fibromas, and hemangiomas. In adults, benign

See the corresponding chapter or part in the *Textbook of Surgery*,
14th edition, pp. 1737–1742, for a more detailed discussion of this
topic, including a comprehensive list of references.

and malignant tumors appear with equal frequency. The most common adult benign tumors of the trachea and proximal bronchi are osteochondromas, papillomas, and fibromas.

The definitive diagnosis of these large airway tumors is most easily accomplished with bronchoscopy. They may be identified on routine radiographs or more sophisticated studies including plain tomograms, computed tomography, or magnetic resonance imaging. Cytologic evaluation is rarely helpful. Adjunctive studies before surgical intervention may include esophagoscopy or barium swallow for exclusion of esophageal invasion.

BENIGN TUMORS. The most common benign tumor of the airway is the *squamous papilloma*. These tumors are most commonly found in the larynx with only 2 to 3 per cent in the trachea or bronchi. In children, they present as multiple lesions with a cauliflower-like appearance. They have been associated with the human papilloma viruses types 6 and 11. Malignant degeneration has been identified in approximately 2 per cent of these lesions. The likelihood of malignant degeneration increases with a history of radiation therapy to the head or neck. In adults, these tumors may be isolated and composed of squamous epithelium with a core of connective tissue. The isolated form differs from typical squamous papillomatosis in that as many as 50 per cent of these solitary papillomas become squamous cell carcinomas. Multiple lesions typical of squamous papillomatosis is the usual appearance. The tracheal lesions are usually associated with laryngeal nodules. Laryngeal nodules may be symptomatic in the form of voice change. Numerous reports have documented the propensity for spontaneous regression of squamous papillomatosis. These nodules tend to regress usually by 16 years of age. Laser ablation of these lesions is the current treatment of choice; however, other direct surgical therapy has included excision and bronchoscopic fulguration. Several studies have suggested a role for interferon in the medical treatment of this disorder.

Benign cartilaginous tumors of the trachea and bronchi include chondromas and hamartomas. Each of these tumors has slow growth characteristics. *Chondromas* arise from the cartilaginous plates of the trachea and are usually multiple. Malignant degeneration may occur, and determination of malignancy is sometimes difficult on pathologic examination. Because of a tendency for local recurrence, these lesions are preferably treated with resection and end-to-end anastomosis. *Hamartomas* contain cartilage in addition to other components including fat, lymphoid tissue, or epithelial elements. When found within the lung parenchyma, they occasionally can be extruded without excision of surrounding tissue.

The most common benign vascular tumor of the trachea and bronchi is the *hemangioma*. This is the most common neoplasm in children and most often occurs in the subglottic region. They are rare in adults but, when present, are typically supraglottic or laryngeal. They are more frequently found in females. Ninety per cent of children with these lesions develop respiratory distress before 3 months of age.

In adults, hoarseness is a frequent presenting complaint. Spontaneous regression has been documented in these tumors; consequently, initial treatment should be observational. When respiratory distress develops, tracheostomy may be necessary; rarely, resection is required.

Fibromas usually occur in the cervical trachea. In 1767, Lieutaud first described at postmortem examination a tracheal tumor that was most likely a tracheal fibroma. These tumors are solitary and well defined.

Spindle cell tumors include *neurinomas* and *leiomyomas*. Malignant varieties of these tumors may be difficult to distinguish in the absence of metastases. The neural tumors have rarely been associated with the secretion of hormones. Leiomyomas are slow-growing intramural tumors commonly seen in the lower third of the trachea.

Granular cell myoblastoma is most commonly seen on the tongue but may be found in the larynx, major bronchi, or trachea. They are most often seen in black females 30 to 50 years of age. On histologic examination, they are characterized by large, foamy cells in syncytial masses. Malignant degeneration has been described.

Ectopic thyroid represents 7 per cent of all tracheal tumors. There is a female:male predominance of 3:1. These appear histologically as normal thyroid tissue. Malignancy has been found in 10 per cent of these tumors. They most frequently occur in the endemic areas of goiters including Germany and Switzerland. The majority of these tumors are associated with goiter and may connect through the tracheal wall with the thyroid.

Tracheobronchopathia osteoplastica is a very unusual appearing malady of the major airways that presents as multiple submucosal tumors extending the entire length of the trachea. These tumors are firm and composed of bone and cartilage. Peak incidence is in the sixth decade, and it has never been described in children. This entity is frequently asymptomatic, although occasionally it may be associated with cough, dyspnea, or hemoptysis. When symptomatic, bronchoscopic removal is adequate.

Direct surgical approaches to endotracheal or proximal endobronchial tumors are complicated by the need to provide air exchange to the nonoperated segments of the tracheobronchial tree. Special endobronchial or endotracheal intubation techniques may be required. Approximately 2 to 3 cm. of trachea may be resected and the trachea primarily reanastomosed without associated mobilization. However, as much as 6 cm. of trachea may be resected and primary anastomosis achieved if extensive mobilization is performed. This includes division of the inferior pulmonary ligament; mobilization of the right main stem bronchus from the pulmonary artery, pulmonary vein, and pericardium; and release of the larynx by separation of the thyrohyoid attachments. With most proximal airway tumors, local excision through tracheotomy or bronchotomy is the treatment of choice. The operative approach to tracheal tumors is determined by the level of involvement. Tumors in the upper third are approached transcervically. Middle-third tumors require a median sternotomy combined with a cervical incision. Distal-third tumors are most often approached via a right lateral thoracotomy. Intraoperative tumor localization is facilitated by bronchoscopy. The development of postoperative anastomotic granulomas is minimized by the use of absorbable polyglactin sutures.

Benign tumors of the trachea and bronchi are eminently treatable lesions. Disastrous results are avoidable if the clinician maintains a high level of suspicion and intervenes promptly with definitive therapy.

XI

Bronchial Adenoma
James M. Douglas, Jr., M.D.

Traditionally, carcinoid tumors of the lung, adenoid cystic carcinoma of the lung, and mucoepidermoid tumors of the lung have been classified together under the appellation *bronchial adenomas*. However, this has generally been recognized as a misnomer in that malignant activity has been demonstrated in each of these tumor types. Although each is pathologically distinct, these neoplasms are similar, since they typically present as slow-growing endobronchial tumors with symptoms related to bronchial obstruction or overlying mucosal irritation. Bronchial adenomas constitute approximately 5 per cent of all primary lung tumors.

BRONCHIAL CARCINOIDS

Carcinoid tumors represent 0.6 to 2 per cent of lung tumors. Additionally, they constitute 83 per cent of all bronchial adenomas. They have been identified in children and elderly adults and demonstrate no sexual or racial predilection. Carcinoid tumors are thought to arise from the Kulchitsky cells in the bronchial mucosa. They are included with the APUD tumors (amine precursor uptake and decarboxylation) and are characterized by the ability to produce numerous hormones, including serotonin, histamine, growth hormone, and many others. The pathologic correlate for this hormone production is the typical neurosecretory granule that can be identified in these tumors by argyrophilic staining or electron microscopy. Despite the recognized potential for hormone production in these tumors, the carcinoid syndrome is seen in only 3 per cent of patients.

See the corresponding chapter or part in the *Textbook of Surgery*, 14th edition, pp. 1742–1746, for a more detailed discussion of this topic, including a comprehensive list of references.

There is increasing evidence that the Kulchitsky cell is the parent cell for a tumor cell line of increasing malignant potential, beginning with the carcinoid tumor and progressing to the atypical carcinoid tumor and, finally, the small cell undifferentiated carcinoma of the lung. Whereas the typical carcinoid tumor presents as a central endobronchial lesion with rare evidence for metastases, the atypical carcinoid is more likely to be peripheral and associated with lymph node metastasis. Eleven per cent of all carcinoid tumors constitute this atypical group. On pathologic examination, they demonstrate increased mitotic activity and a less differentiated cellular appearance. Secretory granules are present, but fewer than are found in typical bronchial carcinoids.

With the exception of the occasional carcinoid syndrome, carcinoid tumors of the lung most often present with signs and symptoms of bronchial obstruction or irritation. The diagnosis may be suggested by the presence of atelectasis or hyperexpansion of lung parenchyma. Computed tomographic scanning of the lung may demonstrate the tumor mass. Frequently, a diagnosis can be made on bronchoscopic examination and accompanying biopsy.

Whenever possible, patients with carcinoid tumors should undergo surgical resection. Because of the low-grade malignant potential of the typical carcinoid tumor, conservative sleeve resections have been recommended for the treatment of these endobronchial tumors. For the atypical carcinoid tumor, a more radical surgical resection with the inclusion of lymph node dissection should be considered. The overall prognosis in patients with carcinoid tumors is good. Patients with typical carcinoid tumors may expect a 93 per cent 5-year survival rate following surgical resection. Those with atypical carcinoid may expect a 66 per cent 5-year survival following treatment.

ADENOID CYSTIC CARCINOMA

Adenoid cystic carcinomas of the lung constitute 12 per cent of all bronchial adenomas. They occur within a broad age range of patients but are most frequently identified in adults. There appears to be no sexual or racial predilection. On pathologic examination, these tumors resemble the tumors of the same name that originate in the salivary and lacrimal glands.

Adenoid cystic carcinomas of the lung are most often found in the distal trachea or proximal bronchus. They tend to be more centrally located than are carcinoid tumors. Three major pathologic subtypes have been identified. These include the tubular, cribriform, and solid cellular subtypes. The solid subtype appears to be the most undifferentiated form and is associated with more extensive extraluminal growth and a poorer prognosis. Approximately 75 per cent of adenoid cystic carcinomas are associated with lymph node involvement, and only 60 per cent of these tumors are completely resectable at the time of surgical intervention. Nonetheless, because of their slow-growing characteristics, the overall prognosis remains good.

MUCOEPIDERMOID TUMORS

Mucoepidermoid tumors constitute 1 to 5 per cent of all bronchial adenomas. They also occur throughout a wide age range with no sexual or racial predilection. These tumors arise within the conducting airways and produce symptoms of bronchial obstruction or irritation. Occasionally, these tumors may be associated with constitutional symptoms or be completely asymptomatic. Mucoepidermoid tumors are composed of a mixture of cell types and may be categorized as low- or high-grade tumors based on mitotic activity, cellular necrosis, or primary nuclear pleomorphism. The majority of tumors are low-grade cell type. Mucoepidermoid and adenosquamous carcinomas of the lung are probably directly related. The adenosquamous tumor occurs in the periphery of the lung and is usually of the high-grade cell type.

Mucoepidermoid tumors may be diagnosed definitively by means of bronchoscopy. Like other bronchial adenomas, occasionally the diagnosis is suggested on chest films. Computed tomography is useful for defining the extent of disease. Surgical resection remains the treatment of choice. Radiation therapy has not been shown to be of value. Patients with low-grade tumors have a good prognosis with approximately 100 per cent 5-year survival, whereas those with high-grade tumors have a poor prognosis with a 66 per cent 4-year survival.

XII

Carcinoma of the Lung
David C. Sabiston, Jr., M.D.

Primary carcinoma of the lung is the most common malignant neoplasm in males and the most common cause of death due to cancer in both sexes. Cigarette smoking is the usual etiologic agent. Surgical removal of the tumor, with or without chemotherapy and radiation, remains the treatment of choice for most patients except those with small cell ("oat cell") carcinoma. This form is usually best managed by chemotherapy and radiation, since metastases are generally present at the time of initial diagnosis.

PATHOLOGIC ASPECTS. Carcinoma of the lung is generally classified as follows: (1) squamous cell (epidermoid), (2) adenocarcinoma, (3) undifferentiated or anaplastic (includ-

---

See the corresponding chapter or part in the *Textbook of Surgery*, 14th edition, pp. 1746–1757, for a more detailed discussion of this topic, including a comprehensive list of references.

ing small and large cell carcinoma), and (4) bronchoalveolar carcinoma. *Squamous cell carcinoma* generally constitutes 40 to 70 per cent of lesions. These are usually centrally located in the larger bronchi and frequently metastasize to hilar, mediastinal, and supraclavicular lymph nodes. *Adenocarcinoma* represents 5 to 15 per cent of lesions, and this type tends to metastasize to the liver, brain, bone, and adrenals in addition to lymph nodes. *Undifferentiated carcinoma* including small (oat cell) and large cell lesions generally composes 20 to 30 per cent of the total and is highly malignant. *Alveolar carcinoma* is quite distinctive histologically and constitutes some 3 to 5 per cent of lesions. It is associated with the best prognosis and responds favorably to surgical excision.

CLINICAL MANIFESTATIONS. The clinical presentation ranges from patients who are totally *asymptomatic* to those with severe disease and *metastatic* lesions at the time of initial diagnosis. Cough, hemoptysis, anorexia, and weight loss are the most frequent clinical characteristics and are highly suggestive of carcinoma of the lung. If weight loss is considerable, there is a strong likelihood that metastases are present; metastases may present as a pleural effusion, often bloody. Less common signs include clubbing of the fingers and symptoms of bone pain and neuromyopathy (usually oat cell carcinomas). An interesting form of the disease involving the superior sulcus is the Pancoast tumor. This neoplasm generally infiltrates the mediastinum and involves the brachial plexus and cervical sympathetic nerves, with production of shoulder and arm pain as well as Horner's syndrome of the side involved.

DIAGNOSIS. The *chest film* is the primary assessment for carcinoma of the lung. A mass or lesion is usually located in the hilum or periphery of the lung and may be associated with lymph node metastases. Pleural effusion may follow pleural metastases, and paralysis of the diaphragm may be present following spread of the tumor to the phrenic nerve. Atelectasis may be caused by bronchial obstruction by tumor with collapse of a part or all of the lung. Computed tomography is useful in detecting local spread of the lesion as well as lymph node metastases. The computed tomographic scan is particularly important in assessing adrenal metastases, which are frequently present.

HISTOPATHOLOGY. A direct diagnosis by bronchoscopy or percutaneous needle aspiration is quite important in establishing a specific diagnosis. Sputum cytology and cell washings obtained at the time of bronchoscopy are equally helpful. More than 90 per cent of patients with carcinoma of the lung have a positive cytologic diagnosis before operation. In the presence of radiologic evidence of involvement of the bones, a bone marrow biopsy may be indicated. Signs of inoperability include a bloody pleural effusion, Horner's syndrome, diaphragmatic paralysis, recurrent laryngeal nerve paralysis, and the vena caval syndrome. Such metastases are usually considered contraindications to operation, but a positive response may be obtained by radiation and chemotherapy.

The *differential diagnosis* of carcinoma of the lung includes pneumonia, pulmonary abscess, tuberculosis, histoplasmosis, other fungal infections, and benign tumors. Metastatic lesions from tumors elsewhere occasionally cause radiologic changes suggestive of primary bronchogenic carcinoma. Lymphosarcoma may also simulate primary bronchogenic carcinoma.

SURGICAL MANAGEMENT. Approximately half the patients who initially present with carcinoma of the lung already have demonstrable metastases. The remaining half are generally candidates for surgical management, but half of these are found to have inoperable lesions. For localized pulmonary tumors, it is now recognized that many patients are appropriate candidates for local excision ("wedge"), generally with use of a stapling device. With more extensive neoplasms, a lobectomy and occasionally pneumonectomy are indicated. The patient should be carefully screened by use of the American Joint Committee System of Staging and End Results Reporting for estimation of long-term survival. Occasionally a palliative resection is indicated, especially when the tumor has caused severe bronchial obstruction with distal infection and an abscess in the management of severe hemoptysis.

RADIATION THERAPY. Irradiation has a useful palliative role in patients with lymph node metastases and in those with primary lesions that are not resectable. Although cure following radiation therapy is quite rare, it has nevertheless been reported.

CHEMOTHERAPY. Various chemotherapeutic agents including bleomycin, doxorubicin (Adriamycin), vincristine, and nitrosourea have been given with success. However, complications are frequent, and the long-term result is generally less than satisfactory. A combination of chemotherapy and radiation is preferred, since cerebral, hepatic, lymph node, and bone marrow metastases are common sites of initial metastatic spread. For small cell carcinoma of the lung (oat cell), chemotherapy consisting of two to four courses of cyclophosphamide, doxorubicin, and vincristine has been followed by successful results. In one series, 33 per cent were initially completely responsive and 54 per cent partially responsive with 13 per cent having stable disease. In selected patients, interleukin-2 lymphokine-activated killer (LAK) cells have been successful.

LASER THERAPY. In patients with inoperable carcinoma of the bronchus with either a massive hemorrhage or infection distal to the tumor, laser therapy has been useful in producing cessation of bleeding by destruction of the tumor and opening the bronchial airways in those with distal infection.

RESULTS. The natural history of bronchogenic carcinoma has been demonstrated in a series of more than 3800 patients. Those who were *untreated* had a 95 per cent mortality within 1 year. It is generally agreed that in a group of 100 patients with carcinoma of the lung, half are inoperable from the outset. Of the remaining 50 per cent on whom exploratory thoracotomy is performed, half or 25 per cent of the original group have such extensive disease that operation for cure cannot be done. The remaining patients are candidates for pulmonary resection, and of the 25 in this group, 25 to 35 per cent are alive at the end of 5 years. Therefore, in assessing the initial group of 100 patients, the 5-year survival is only 8 to 10 per cent.

SOLITARY PULMONARY NODULES ("COIN LESIONS"). A frequent clinical problem is the patient with a solitary pulmonary nodule. These should be thoroughly investigated so that a specific diagnosis can be established. Lesions with smoothly circumscribed margins or with concentric layers of calcification are more apt to be benign. The younger the patient, the more likely is the lesion to be benign. However, for patients over the age of 50 years, an isolated pulmonary nodule is probably carcinoma in half the group. The differential diagnosis of *coin lesions* includes tuberculoma, histoplasmosis, blastomycosis, coccidioidomycosis, primary carcinoma of the lung, metastatic carcinoma, and benign pulmonary neoplasms. Rarely, pulmonary arteriovenous fistulas or resolving pulmonary infarcts may present as isolated lesions.

XIII

Thoracic Outlet Syndrome
Alfred Harding, M.D. and Donald Silver, M.D.

The thoracic outlet syndrome is the preferred term for those disorders produced by compression of neurovascular structures in the thoracic outlet. The symptoms of the thoracic outlet syndrome vary depending on the nerves or vessels involved. Neurologic symptoms predominate in 90 to 95 per cent of cases. The syndrome occurs most often in the young to middle-aged female, although all age groups may be afflicted. Neurologic symptoms consist of pain, weakness, paresthesias, and numbness usually in the fingers and hands in an ulnar distribution but numbness may occur anywhere in the upper extremity, neck, or shoulder girdle. Late neurologic deficits include sensory loss, motor weakness, and atrophy.

Symptoms of arterial compression include ischemic pain, numbness, fatigue, paresthesias, coldness, and weakness in the arm or hand. These symptoms are accentuated by exercise and exposure to cold. Thrombosis may occur in the compressed or post-stenotic dilated areas of the subclavian artery. Distal embolization may be associated with vasomotor symptoms in the fingers consisting of episodic pain with pallor and/or cyanosis. Ulceration or gangrene of the fingertips may occur. Venous compression may produce arm swelling, pain,

See the corresponding chapter or part in the *Textbook of Surgery*, 14th edition, pp. 1757–1761, for a more detailed discussion of this topic, including a comprehensive list of references.

and cyanosis. The patient frequently complains of a sensation of heaviness or tightness in the arm. Distended superficial veins may be present.

The diagnosis is generally made by history and physical examination, although a number of ancillary tests are usually indicated. A careful neurologic examination may reveal motor or sensory deficits in the distribution of the brachial plexus, especially of the ulnar nerve. Occasionally symptoms may be reproduced by pressure or light percussion in the supraclavicular fossa. Signs of arterial involvement may include weakened distal pulses or a supraclavicular bruit. A chest film may reveal cervical ribs. Nerve conduction velocities should be obtained to exclude a carpal tunnel syndrome. The 3-minute elevated arm stress test is a useful diagnostic maneuver. The patient is asked to slowly open and close the hands while keeping both arms abducted, externally rotated, and flexed to 90 degrees at the elbow. Normal patients may experience fatigue but rarely have pain or paresthesias. The test may reproduce symptoms in patients with the thoracic outlet syndrome. The Adson, hyperabduction, and costoclavicular maneuvers are often positive in normal patients and are usually not helpful in establishing the diagnosis of a thoracic outlet syndrome.

For all patients, except those with symptomatic complete vascular occlusions, distal embolization, or a postcompression aneurysm, initial management should consist of a trial of weight reduction and an exercise program directed toward improving posture, strengthening the elevators of the shoulder girdle, and avoiding hyperabduction. These measures relieve symptoms in 50 to 70 per cent of patients. Nonoperative management appears to be most successful in the obese, young to middle-aged female with poor posture. When patients do not respond to a 4-month or longer trial of conservative treatment, surgical intervention should be considered. Currently, supraclavicular decompression of the thoracic outlet is favored. This operation consists of wide anterior scalenectomy, middle scalenectomy, removal of a cervical rib if present, and, on occasion, first rib resection. Resection of the first rib via a transaxillary approach is also popular and produces similar results. However, the transaxillary operation is associated with a higher incidence of serious complications. Vascular reconstruction may be required in those few cases with vascular thrombosis or arterial aneurysm.

XIV

Congenital Deformities of the Chest

David C. Sabiston, Jr., M.D.

The primary congenital chest wall deformities of surgical significance are pectus excavatum, pectus carinatum, and sternal fissure (bifid sternum).

PECTUS EXCAVATUM

The most common of these congenital malformations is *pectus excavatum*. In this condition, the abnormality primarily involves bilateral defects in the costal cartilages. It varies from a mild asymptomatic deformity to one that is quite severe and symptomatic. The anatomic problem primarily involves *costal cartilages*, which have developed in a concave position in a way that *depresses* the sternum posteriorly. A familial history is not uncommon.

CLINICAL MANIFESTATIONS. The majority of patients with pectus excavatum have few if any symptoms. However, when questioned carefully, older children and teenagers are apt to recognize that they do not have the same physical endurance as their peers do, especially in competitive sports. After correction of the defect, these patients spontaneously volunteer that they have additional respiratory reserve. With pectus excavatum, significant decreases have been demonstrated in the force of expiratory flow and in maximal voluntary ventilation. Cardiac catheterization at rest shows normal values; exercise under these circumstances has produced a subnormal response in some patients. Most patients with pectus excavatum are quite sensitive about the deformity and tend to be embarrassed when it is noted by others; they become withdrawn and are apt to have a poor self-image. Most patients with this defect are quite unlikely to remove clothing covering the chest, and few if any wish ever to be seen bare chested. These changes alter their social activities and may scar their personalities. For the majority of patients with pectus excavatum, surgical correction is performed to improve appearance and to increase the patient's self-image. In the more severe cases, respiratory insufficiency may manifest and constitute an additional reason for operation. In most circumstances, surgical correction should be performed between the ages of 2 and 3 and clearly before the age of 5 years. The psychological complications that occur in these patients should be reduced early in life so that the child is permitted to have a normal life-style.

TECHNIQUE. Surgical correction of pectus excavatum is straightforward, but it is nevertheless a major procedure.

See the corresponding chapter or part in the *Textbook of Surgery*, 14th edition, pp. 1761–1765, for a more detailed discussion of this topic, including a comprehensive list of references.

Primary features of the operation include the subperichondrial removal of all involved costal cartilages bilaterally and performance of a posterior wedge osteotomy of the sternum for elevation. In older children, the sternum may need support by a Steinmann pin placed beneath the sternum. A drain with multiple perforations is left in place and attached to sterile suction for removal of the serous fluid during the first several days. Mild temperature elevation may occur postoperatively primarily owing to atelectasis. The results are generally excellent with few if any complications.

PECTUS CARINATUM ("PIGEON BREAST")

Pectus carinatum is another malformation of the chest that should be corrected in most instances. A protrusion of the sternum caused by an upward curve in the lower costal cartilages, generally the fourth through the eighth, displaces the sternum superiorly. In most patients the condition is symmetrical, but it may primarily involve one side.

OPERATIVE CORRECTION. The majority of patients with this malformation should have surgical correction for prevention of psychological problems, primarily sensitivity to their physical appearance. The operative procedure is straightforward and consists of removal of all the deformed costal cartilages subperichondrially and removal of any bone prominences that may be present on the anterior sternum. The results are generally excellent with few if any complications.

STERNAL FISSURE

During embryologic development, the sternum originates from two lateral plates of mesoderm that also provide the pectoral muscles. By the tenth week of embryologic development, the two bands should be fused. However, in some instances fusion does not occur and may produce a defect of varying severity that allows herniation of the heart and pericardium through the defect so that they are covered only by the skin. In the *simple* sternal cleft, the two bands of the sternum are joined distally. The complete cleft of the sternum is a more serious deformity with a cleft in the distal sternum, a ventral omphalocele, a crescentic deficiency of the anterior diaphragm, a defect in the diaphragm and pericardium with free communication between the pericardium and peritoneal cavities, and congenital heart defects.

SURGICAL CORRECTION. Surgical correction of a simple sternal cleft is easily achieved by joining of the two bands with appropriate sutures. The complete defects present more technical problems, and each patient must be individualized.

XV

Extracorporeal Membrane Oxygenation
Robert H. Bartlett, M.D.

Extracorporeal circulation can be used for days or weeks to support the life of patients with severe cardiac or pulmonary failure. This procedure, referred to as extracorporeal membrane oxygenation (ECMO), involves cannulation of major vessels without thoracotomy, carefully titrated partial anticoagulation with heparin, and continuous high-flow extracorporeal circulation through a membrane lung. ECMO is not a therapy but a mechanical support system that allows time for the damaged heart or lungs to heal in a milieu of normal perfusion and gas exchange while the damaged organs are "resting" from the effects of mechanical ventilation. ECMO has been the most successful in neonatal respiratory failure and is considered standard therapy for this condition. It is also used for respiratory failure in children and adults and cardiac failure in children.

INDICATIONS. ECMO is indicated when conventional management of respiratory failure fails and mortality risk is high. In the neonate, the underlying pathophysiologic mechanism is pulmonary arterial vasospasm producing pulmonary hypertension and right-to-left shunting through the ductus arteriosus or foramen ovale. Shunting produces arterial hypoxemia measured by the alveolar-arterial oxygen gradient (A-aDO$_2$). ECMO should be considered when the A-aDO$_2$ is greater than 600 mm. Hg despite optimal therapy. ECMO is also indicated for barotrauma manifested by uncontrolled air leaks or poor compliance with mean airway pressure greater than 20 cm. H$_2$O.

For children and adults, ECMO is indicated when the A-aDO$_2$ is consistently greater than 600 mm. Hg (representing more than 30 per cent transpulmonary shunt) despite optimal therapy. Barotrauma with air leaks and compliance less than 0.05 ml/cm H$_2$O lag pressure are also indications.

ECMO is contraindicated in patients with severe brain injury, poor prognosis for a normal quality of life, active bleeding, and irreversible pulmonary injury (usually associated with mechanical ventilation longer than 10 days).

ECMO PROCEDURE

Because most of the clinical application of ECMO is currently in newborn infants, this description refers primarily to that group of patients. The basic principles of extracorporeal circulation, gas exchange, and systemic oxygen delivery apply to patients of all sizes and ages. The underlying patho-

---

See the corresponding chapter or part in the *Textbook of Surgery*, 14th edition, pp. 1765–1770, for a more detailed discussion of this topic, including a comprehensive list of references.

physiologic mechanism of respiratory failure in the newborn is pulmonary vasospasm with right-to-left shunting. The lung is intrinsically normal, and the recovery rate is excellent. The underlying pathophysiologic process in children and adults includes interstitial edema and inflammation, which cause necrosis and fibrosis, so patient recovery is related to the extent of irreversible pulmonary injury.

THE ECMO CIRCUIT AND MANAGEMENT. The circuit includes a servoregulated roller pump, membrane lung, heat exchanger, tubing, and connectors. Right atrial blood is drained via a right internal jugular catheter to the extracorporeal circuit. Blood is pumped by the servoregulated pump through the membrane lung and back into the patient. The size of catheters, tubing, and membrane lung are designed to be capable of total cardiopulmonary support, although partial support is adequate for most patients. Typical flow rates are 80 to 120 ml. per kg. per minute. In *venoarterial* circulation, the blood is perfused through a carotid, femoral, or axillary artery into the aortic arch, which provides both heart and lung support. In *venovenous* circulation, arterialized (oxygenated) blood is returned to the venous circulation, which supports gas exchange only and relies on cardiac function for perfusion. Cannulation is performed at the bedside in the intensive care unit. Supporting drugs are discontinued, and the ventilator is turned down to allow "lung rest." Extracorporeal circulation is continued at low ventilator settings until the lung recovers, typically 4 days for newborn infants. The adequacy of perfusion is monitored by the mixed venous saturation, which measures the adequacy of oxygen delivery in relation to metabolic needs. The patient is heparinized for maintenance of the whole blood activated clotting time between 200 and 240 seconds. The extracorporeal flow is gradually decreased as native lung function increases. When flow is approximately 20 ml. per kg. per minute, a trial off bypass at low ventilator settings is attempted. If pulmonary function is adequate, the cannulas are removed.

RESULTS. ECMO is used when the likelihood of survival is small, so that survival ranging from 40 to 90 per cent represents significant salvage from acute respiratory failure. When death occurs in newborn infants, it is caused by anoxic brain injury from the perinatal period or intracranial bleeding. When death occurs in children and adults, it is due to multiple organ failure and sepsis or diffuse pulmonary fibrosis.

Physiologic complications occur in approximately two thirds of patients, including intracranial bleeding (14 per cent), surgical site bleeding (14 per cent), seizures (20 per cent), hemolysis (7 per cent), and positive cultures (6 per cent). Mechanical complications occur in approximately one quarter of patients, including oxygenator change (7 per cent), tubing rupture (3 per cent), and cannula problems (7 per cent).

In follow-up examination, most of the survivors are normal. Abnormalities are related to neurologic and pulmonary systems and are generally caused by the primary disease rather than the ECMO procedure. Twenty per cent of newborn infants have detectable neurologic abnormality, and 10 per cent have bronchopulmonary dysplasia. Both of these problems improve with time. Follow-up in children and adults demonstrates the findings of pulmonary fibrosis and restrictive disease, which usually returns to normal within 1 year.

THE FUTURE OF EXTRACORPOREAL LIFE SUPPORT

In 1991, ECMO is the treatment of choice for infants with severe respiratory failure who fail to respond to conventional management. In the next decade, the use of heparin-coated circuits will decrease the risk of bleeding, and venovenous catheterization will simplify vascular access. Both of these improvements will permit earlier use of ECMO in respiratory failure, which will probably improve outcome results in children and adults. With these technical improvements, the use of ECMO for respiratory failure will become a standard adjunct to conventional mechanical ventilation, rather than a salvage procedure when mechanical ventilation fails or causes lung injury.

SUMMARY AND CONCLUSIONS

Extracorporeal life support has become standard treatment for term and near-term newborn infants with severe respiratory failure. The survival rate for 3094 cases in the Neonatal ECMO Registry was 82.6 per cent. The lesson learned from neonatal experience is that avoiding high-pressure, high-oxygen mechanical ventilation by means of extracorporeal life support will effect recovery of the lung and patient survival. In severe respiratory failure in children and adults, the use of ECMO effects survival in approximately 40 per cent of cases. The use of ECMO earlier in the course of disease will decrease the component of progressive lung injury related to mechanical ventilation. The use of heparin-coated circuits and simplified vascular access will expand the applications of all types of extracorporeal life support during the next decade.

54

THE MEDIASTINUM

R. Duane Davis, M.D.,
and David C. Sabiston, Jr., M.D.

The mediastinum is an important and complex anatomic division of the thorax defined by the following borders: the thoracic inlet superiorly, the diaphragm inferiorly, the sternum anteriorly, the vertebral column posteriorly, and the parietal pleura laterally. Because of the characteristic location of many tumors and cysts, the mediastinum has been artificially divided into three subdivisions: the anterosuperior, middle, and posterior. The anterosuperior mediastinum is anterior to the pericardium and the pericardial reflection extending over the great vessels. The posterior mediastinum is posterior to the pericardium and the pericardial reflection. The middle mediastinum is contained within the pericardial sac.

MEDIASTINAL EMPHYSEMA

Air within the mediastinum produces mediastinal emphysema or pneumomediastinum. The source of the air may be from the esophagus, trachea, bronchi, neck, or abdomen. Common causes of pneumomediastinum include penetrating wounds and perforations of these structures, blunt trauma that produces fractured ribs or vertebrae, and barotrauma caused by either blunt trauma or positive-pressure ventilation. Spontaneous pneumomediastinum occurs and usually is found in patients with exacerbation of bronchospastic disease. The clinical manifestations, initially described by Hamman, include substernal chest pain that may radiate into the back and crepitation in the region of the suprasternal notch, chest wall, and neck. With increasing pressure, the air can dissect into the neck, face, chest, arms, abdomen, and retroperitoneum. Rarely, sufficient pressure develops so that venous return is impaired, which produces venous distention in the head and upper extremities and impairment of cardiac output. Frequently, pneumomediastinum and pneumothorax occur simultaneously. The diagnosis of pneumomediastinum is confirmed by the presence of air in the mediastinum on the chest film. Treatment is directed toward correcting the inciting cause. Careful observation for the development of circulatory compromise is necessary. Surgical decompression is rarely required.

MEDIASTINITIS

Infection of the mediastinal space is a serious and potentially fatal process caused by perforation of the esophagus

---

See the corresponding chapter or part in the *Textbook of Surgery*, 14th edition, pp. 1771–1796, for a more detailed discussion of this topic, including a comprehensive list of references.

due to instrumentation, foreign body, and penetrating or, more rarely, blunt trauma; spontaneous esophageal disruption (Boerhaave's syndrome); leakage from an esophageal anastomosis; tracheobronchial perforation; and mediastinal extension from an infectious process originating in the pulmonary parenchyma, pleura, chest wall, vertebrae, great vessels, or neck. It also occurs following operations using median sternotomy. Wound infections after median sternotomy for cardiac operations occur in 2 per cent of patients; half of these involve the mediastinum. Mediastinitis is manifested clinically by fever, tachycardia, leukocytosis, and pain that may be localized to the chest, back, or neck. The lateral chest film and computed tomography (CT) may assist in the diagnosis by identifying air-fluid levels, abnormal soft tissue densities, and sternal dehiscence. Endoscopy, bronchoscopy, and contrast studies of the esophagus are useful in identifying esophageal and tracheobronchial etiologic factors. Treatment of mediastinitis requires correction of the inciting cause by débridement of necrotic tissue and surgical drainage and aggressive supportive therapy with appropriate antimicrobial coverage. A number of techniques for treating postoperative mediastinitis have been used, but the best results with the shortest hospitalization have occurred with use of tissue flaps (rectus or pectoralis muscle and omentum) for covering the mediastinum after surgical control of the wound infection has been obtained.

SUPERIOR VENA CAVAL OBSTRUCTION

A number of benign and malignant processes may cause obstruction of the superior vena cava with production of increased pressure in the venous system draining into the superior vena cava, which leads to the characteristic features of the superior vena caval syndrome including edema of the head, neck, and upper extremities, distended neck veins with dilated collateral veins over the upper extremities and torso, cyanosis, headache, and confusion. These findings are more pronounced when the patient is in a recumbent position. Sudden occlusion may cause rapid development of cerebral edema and intracranial thrombosis with resultant coma and death. Bronchogenic carcinoma of the right upper lobe is the most common etiologic factor, but a large number of malignant mediastinal tumors also commonly cause this syndrome. Less than 25 per cent of patients with superior vena caval obstruction have a benign etiologic factor. The syndrome occurs infrequently in children, with atrial level repairs for transposition of the great arteries being the most common cause. Malignant mediastinal neoplasms are the second most common cause. CT or magnetic resonance imaging (MRI) is usually sufficient for establishing the diagnosis of superior vena caval obstruction. A histologic diagnosis is attempted before therapy is initiated owing to the alteration in morphologic appearance of the tumor following treatment. Needle biopsy techniques and procedures performed under local anesthesia are utilized most frequently because of the hazards of cardiovascular compromise during general anesthesia. Radiation, corticosteroids, and chemotherapy are the usual modalities of treatment. When neurologic symptoms are present, urgent therapy is mandated. Surgical bypass with a variety of graft materials has been used with improving success.

PRIMARY NEOPLASMS AND CYSTS

A large number of neoplasms and cysts arise from multiple anatomic sites in the mediastinum and present with a myriad of clinical signs and symptoms. The most common mediastinal masses are neurogenic tumors (21 per cent), thymomas (19 per cent), primary cysts (18 per cent), lymphomas (13 per cent), and germ cell tumors (10 per cent). Many mediastinal masses occur in characteristic sites within the mediastinum. In the anterosuperior mediastinum, the most frequent neoplasms are thymoma (31 per cent), lymphoma (23 per cent), and germ cell tumor (17 per cent). Posterior mediastinal lesions are usually neurogenic tumors (52 per cent), bronchogenic cysts (22 per cent), and enteric cysts (7 per cent). Middle mediastinal masses are usually pericardial cysts (35 per cent), lymphomas (21 per cent), and bronchogenic cysts (15 per cent). Malignant neoplasms represent 25 to 42 per cent of mediastinal masses. Lymphomas, thymomas, germ cell tumors, primary carcinomas, and neurogenic tumors are the most common. The relative frequency of malignancy varies with the anatomic site in the mediastinum. Anterosuperior masses are most likely malignant (59 per cent), compared with middle mediastinal masses (29 per cent), and posterior mediastinal masses (16 per cent). Patients in the second through fourth decades have a greater proportion of malignant neoplasms; those in the first decade have a lower proportion. The incidence of various mediastinal masses varies in infants, children, and adults. In a series of 706 children with mediastinal masses, the most frequently occurring were neurogenic tumors (35 per cent), most commonly gangliomas, ganglioneuroblastomas, and neuroblastomas; lymphomas (25 per cent), usually non-Hodgkin's; germ cell tumors (11 per cent), predominantly benign teratomas; and primary cysts (16 per cent). Pericardial cysts and thymomas are uncommon in children.

SYMPTOMS. Among patients with a mediastinal mass, 56 to 65 per cent are symptomatic at presentation. Patients with a benign lesion are more often asymptomatic (54 per cent) than are patients with a malignant neoplasm (15 per cent). The absence of symptoms is associated with a benign histologic diagnosis in three quarters of patients. In contrast, almost two thirds of symptomatic patients have a malignant lesion. The most common symptoms were chest pain, cough, and fever. Although myasthenia gravis was present in only 7 per cent of patients from the overall series, in patients with thymoma, 43 per cent had myasthenia gravis. Infants most likely present with symptoms or findings (78 per cent) because of the relatively small space within the mediastinum.

Symptoms may be related to compression or invasion of mediastinal structures or production of hormones or antibodies causing systemic symptoms that characterize a specific syndrome. The pathophysiologic mechanism of some of the systemic syndromes is not well defined, although autoimmune mechanisms have been implicated.

DIAGNOSIS. The goal of the diagnostic evaluation is the precise histologic classification and staging of the lesion for determination of optimal therapy. Routine chest films demonstrate the location, size, relative density, and degree of calcification of the mediastinal mass, which greatly narrows the differential diagnosis. CT imaging increases the sensitivity and specificity of the diagnostic evaluation because of the improved spatial resolution, because of the ability to examine areas poorly visualized on chest films (aortopulmonary window and subcarinal region), and through the use of contrast for differentiating primary mediastinal lesions from a variety of cardiovascular abnormalities that mimic a mediastinal mass on chest film. CT imaging more accurately predicts resectability of a neoplasm than it indicates unresectability. MRI also differentiates primary masses from vascular lesions. CT and MRI are useful in determining the presence of spinal column involvement by posterior mediastinal tumors and airway compression by anterior and middle mediastinal masses.

Examples of useful nuclear scans include [131]I–*meta*-iodobenzylguanidine (MIBG), which identifies pheochromocytomas (particularly helpful when the tumor is located in the middle mediastinum), and radioisotopic iodine scans, which identify functioning ectopic thyroid tissue.

Monoclonal antibodies have been used to develop serologic markers for a variety of mediastinal tumors, the most important of which are those used to measure alpha-fetoprotein and beta-human chorionic gonadotropin. These tumor markers identify nonseminomatous germ cell tumors, and they should be obtained in all males in the second through fifth decades with a mediastinal mass.

Nonoperative methods of establishing a histologic diagnosis are available, including fine-needle biopsy (22-gauge needle) technique, which produces a cytologic specimen, and cutting-needle technique, which produces a histologic specimen. Significant complications include pneumothorax in 20 to 25 per cent of patients (only 5 per cent require tube thoracostomy), hemoptysis, and rare occurrence of significant hemorrhagic complications. A cytologic determination of malignancy can be made in 80 to 90 per cent of patients; however, a precise histologic diagnosis is determined less commonly. Because the precise diagnosis and, in particular, the subclassification of lymphomas require more tissue than can be obtained by use of needle techniques, more invasive procedures are often necessary. Mediastinoscopy and mediastinotomy provide access to the anterosuperior mediastinum for biopsy of lesions, whereas thoracotomy and median sternotomy provide greater exposure for biopsy or resection when indicated. The majority of patients can safely undergo these diagnostic procedures. However, patients with large anterior and middle mediastinal masses may be susceptible to cardiopulmonary collapse secondary to extrinsic compression of the trachea or bronchus or superior vena caval obstruction. CT, MRI, and pulmonary-flow mechanics are sensitive indicators of airway compromise and are useful in patients at high risk for general anesthesia. In these patients, diagnosis should be established by use of needle biopsy techniques or biopsy under local or regional anesthesia. Occasionally, a diagnosis cannot be established before initiation of empiric therapy.

Neurogenic Tumors

Neurogenic tumors are the most common neoplasm in the mediastinum, representing approximately 21 per cent of all primary tumors and cysts. These tumors are usually located in the posterior mediastinum and originate from the sympathetic ganglia (ganglioma, ganglioneuroblastoma, and neuroblastoma), the intercostal nerves (neurofibroma, neurilemoma, and neurosarcoma), and the paraganglia cells (paraganglioma). Although the peak incidence occurs in adults, neurogenic tumors comprise a proportionally greater percentage of mediastinal masses in children (35 per cent). Whereas the majority of neurogenic tumors in adults are benign, a greater percentage of neurogenic tumors are malignant in children.

The most common neurogenic tumor is the neurilemoma, which originates from the perineural Schwann cells. These tumors are well circumscribed and have a well-defined capsule. In contrast, neurofibromas are poorly encapsulated and originate as a proliferation of all the peripheral nerve elements. Both entities occur as a manifestation of neurofibromatosis. Surgical excision effects cure.

Ganglioneuromas, ganglioneuroblastomas, and neuroblastomas originate from the sympathetic chain and are composed of ganglion cells and nerve fibers; they are the most common neurogenic tumors of childhood. The degree of differentiation of the ganglion cells distinguishes these tumors: well-differentiated, ganglioneuroma; poorly differentiated, neuroblastoma; and mixture, ganglioneuroblastoma. Surgical excision is usually curative for ganglioneuromas, Stage I and Stage II ganglioneuroblastomas, and Stage I neuroblastomas. Radiation and multiagent chemotherapy are used in the treatment of higher stage malignant tumors. Children less than 1 year and those with less extensive disease have the best prognosis.

Mediastinal paragangliomas are rare tumors, representing less than 1 per cent of mediastinal masses and less than 2 per cent of all pheochromocytomas. The majority of these tumors occur in the paravertebral sulcus; however, a number occur in the middle mediastinum. Catecholamine production is less common than with adrenal paragangliomas, and when present, the product is usually norepinephrine. Catecholamine production causes the classic constellation of symptoms associated with pheochromocytomas, including periodic or sustained hypertension, often accompanied by orthostatic hypotension, hypermetabolism manifested by weight loss, hyperhidrosis, palpitations, and headaches. Measurement of elevated levels of urinary catecholamines or their metabolites, the metanephrines and vanillylmandelic acid, usually establishes the diagnosis. Tumor localization has improved remarkably through the use of CT and *meta*-iodobenzylguanidine (^{131}I-MIBG) scintigraphy, particularly when the tumors are hormonally active. When possible, resection is the appropriate therapy. Although many tumors appear morphologically malignant, only 3 per cent of patients develop metastatic disease. Multiple paragangliomas occur in 10 per cent of patients and more commonly in association with the multiple endocrine neoplasia syndrome, Carney's syndrome, or when a family history is present.

Thymoma

Thymoma is the most common neoplasm of the anterosuperior mediastinum and the second most common mediastinal mass (20 per cent). The peak incidence is in the third through fifth decades, and it is rare during childhood. Symptoms due to local mass effects such as chest pain, dyspnea, and cough are common. A number of systemic syndromes are associated with thymomas, most commonly myasthenia gravis and red cell aplasia. Myasthenia gravis occurs in 10 to 50 per cent of patients with a thymoma. In patients with myasthenia gravis, 10 to 42 per cent have a thymoma, with elderly and male patients having a higher incidence. The disease process is characterized by weakness and fatigue of the skeletal muscles associated with destruction of the postsynaptic nicotinic receptors. This process appears to be immune-related.

Whenever possible, the therapy for thymoma is surgical excision without removal of or injury to the vital structures. Even with well-encapsulated thymomas, extended thymectomy with eradication of all accessible mediastinal fatty-areolar tissue should be performed so that removal of all ectopic thymic tissue is ensured. This approach has been shown to lower the number of tumor recurrences. The best operative exposure is obtained with use of a median sternotomy. The differentiation between benign and malignant disease is determined by the presence of gross invasion of adjacent structures, metastasis, or microscopic evidence of capsular invasion. In patients with tumor invasion through the capsule or into surrounding structures, postoperative radiotherapy is recommended. Multiagent chemotherapy has been useful in patients with metastatic or recurrent disease.

Patients with thymoma and myasthenia gravis require careful perioperative management with use of plasmapheresis in the 72 hours before operation, discontinuation of anticholinesterase inhibitors, and good pulmonary therapy. Postoperatively, decisions regarding extubation are based on adequate respiratory mechanics.

Germ Cell Tumors

Germ cell tumors are benign and malignant neoplasms thought to originate from primordial germ cells that fail to complete the migration from the urogenital ridge and come to rest in the mediastinum. These tumors are classified as teratomas, teratocarcinomas, seminomas, embryonal cell carcinomas, choriocarcinoma, and endodermal cell (yolk sac) tumors and are identical histologically to those originating in the gonads. They occur most commonly in the anterosuperior mediastinum. Teratomas are neoplasms composed of multiple tissue elements derived from the three primitive embryonic layers foreign to the area in which they occur. The peak incidence is in the second and third decades of life. There is no sex predisposition. The teratodermoid is the simplest form, composed predominantly of derivatives of the epidermal layer (hair, sebaceous material, dermal and epidermal glands). Teratomas are histologically more complex. The solid component of the tumor contains well-differentiated elements of bone, cartilage, teeth, muscle, connective tissue, fibrous and lymphoid tissue, nerve, thymus, mucous and salivary glands, lung, liver, or pancreas. Malignant teratomas are differentiated by the presence of embryonic or primitive tissue. Surgical resection of benign teratomas, even partial, is the recommended therapy for prevention of complications.

Malignant Germ Cell Tumor

Malignant germ cell tumors occur predominantly in males with a peak incidence in the third and fourth decades. These tumors frequently cause symptoms due to local mass effects, including the superior vena caval syndrome. Serologic measurements of alpha-fetoprotein and beta-human chorionic gonadotropin are useful for the following tasks: differentiating seminomas from nonseminomas, quantitatively assessing response to therapy in hormonally active tumors (plasma half-life of alpha-fetoprotein and beta-human chorionic gonadotropin is 5 days and 12 to 24 hours, respectively), and diagnosing relapse or failure of therapy before changes that can be observed in gross disease. Seminomas rarely produce beta-human chorionic gonadotropin (7 per cent) and never produce alpha-fetoprotein; in contrast, over 90 per cent of nonseminomas secrete one or both of these hormones. The differentiation between seminomas and nonseminomatous germ cell tumors is important because of the radiosensitivity of seminomas and the contrasting insensitivity of the other germ cell tumors. Seminomas are also more likely to remain intrathoracic than are the other germ cell tumors. With seminomas, surgical therapy usually is limited to the establishment of the histologic diagnosis. Radiotherapy is the basis of therapy with the use of multiagent chemotherapy for patients with extrathoracic disease or tumor relapse. In contrast, the optimal treatment of nonseminomatous germ cell tumors is *cis*-platinum–based chemotherapy with subsequent resection of residual disease. Chemotherapy may be initiated based on the presence of an anterosuperior mediastinal mass in a male patient in the second through fifth decades with elevated beta-human chorionic gonadotropin or alpha-feto-protein, which emphasizes the importance of measuring these hormones. The presence of residual disease after surgical resection portends a grave prognosis.

Lymphomas

Although the mediastinum is frequently involved in patients with lymphoma sometime during the course of the disease (40 to 70 per cent), it is infrequently the sole site of disease at the time of presentation. These tumors frequently produce symptoms due to local mass effects, in addition to characteristic symptoms such a cyclic fevers (Pel-Ebstein) and chest pain associated with alcohol consumption. These tumors occur most commonly in the anterosuperior mediastinum or in the hilar region of the middle mediastinum. Mediastinal involvement with Hodgkin's disease is most common with nodular sclerosing and lymphocyte predominant subtypes. Patients with Stage IA and Stage IIA disease are treated with radiation therapy, whereas those with Stage IIB, Stage III, and Stage IV disease are treated with chemotherapy. Controversy exists regarding the use of chemotherapy for the treatment of patients with bulky mediastinal involvement owing to the higher relapse rate with radiation therapy. Non-Hodgkin's lymphomas are usually either of lymphoblastic morphologic type (60 per cent) or large cell morphologic type with a diffuse pattern of growth (40 per cent). Multiagent chemotherapy is the optimal treatment. Operative intervention is limited to providing adequate tissue for a precise histologic diagnosis. Because of the importance of precise immunotyping in the selection of the chemotherapeutic regimen, needle biopsy techniques are usually inadequate owing to the insufficient tissue sample obtained.

Primary Carcinoma

Primary carcinomas comprise between 3 and 11 per cent of mediastinal masses. Their origin is unknown, but it is important to differentiate these tumors from the neoplasms that may have a similar morphologic appearance such as thymoma, lymphoma, metastasis, and bronchogenic cancers by use of electron microscopy and immunohistochemistry. Primary carcinomas usually cause symptoms and are rarely resectable. Prognosis is poor with mean survival less than 1 year after diagnosis with minimal benefit from chemotherapy and radiation therapy.

Endocrine Tumors

Although substernal extension of a cervical goiter is common, totally intrathoracic thyroid tumors are rare and represent less than 1 per cent of mediastinal masses. Arising from ectopic thyroid tissue, these tumors occur most commonly in the anterosuperior mediastinum but also occur in the middle and posterior mediastinum. Symptoms are usually due to mass effect; however, hormone production can cause thyrotoxicosis. When functioning thyroid tissue is present, the radioactive iodine (^{131}I) scan is usually diagnostic. Significantly, the ^{131}I scan can determine if functioning cervical thyroid tissue is absent, which would contraindicate excision of an asymptomatic intrathoracic thyroid tumor. Because of thoracic derivation of the blood supply, intrathoracic thyroid tumors should be approached through a thoracic incision. Most tumors are adenomas, but carcinomas have been reported.

Mediastinal parathyroids occur in 10 per cent of patients; however, the majority are accessible through a cervical incision. Only 2 per cent of patients with hyperfunctioning parathyroid glands require a sternotomy for resection. These glands are usually adjacent or within the thymus. With use of CT, MRI, thallium and technetium scanning, venous angiography with selective sampling, and selective arteriography, preoperative localization of these tumors can be made in approximately 80 per cent of patients. Parathyroid carcinomas occur and tend to be more hormonally active.

Mediastinal carcinoid tumors arise from cells of Kulchitsky located in the thymus. Occurring more often in male patients, these tumors usually are located in the anterosuperior mediastinum. When hormonally active, these tumors usually produce adrenocorticotropic hormone, causing Cushing's syndrome. Hormonally inactive carcinoids tend to be larger and frequently are invasive locally. In addition, metastatic spread to mediastinal and cervical lymph nodes, liver, bone, skin, and lungs occurs in the majority of patients. Surgical removal when possible is the preferred treatment. Radiation and chemotherapy have not been demonstrated to be effective in the treatment of malignant disease.

Mesenchymal Tumors

Mediastinal mesenchymal tumors originate from the connective tissue, striated and smooth muscle, fat, lymphatic tissue, and blood vessels present within the mediastinum, which produces a diverse group of neoplasms. Relative to other sites in the body, these tumors occur less commonly within the mediastinum. Mesenchymal tumors comprised 7 per cent of the primary masses in the collected series. There is no apparent difference in incidence between sexes. The soft tissue mesenchymal tumors have a similar histologic appearance and generally follow the same clinical course as do the soft tissue tumors found elsewhere in the body. Fifty-five per cent of these tumors are malignant. The vascular tumors are poorly encapsulated, and even benign tumors may be locally invasive. Ten to 30 per cent are morphologically malignant, but only 3 per cent develop metastases. Surgical resection remains the primary therapy in the treatment of patients with mesenchymal tumors, since poor results have been obtained with use of radiation and chemotherapy.

Other uncommon mediastinal masses include giant lymph node hyperplasia, extramedullary hematopoiesis, and chondromas.

Primary Cysts

Primary cysts of the mediastinum comprise 20 per cent of the mediastinal masses in the collected series. These cysts can be bronchogenic, pericardial, enteric, or thymic or may be of an unspecified nature. More than 75 per cent of patients are asymptomatic, and these tumors rarely cause morbidity. However, due to the proximity of vital structures within the mediastinum, with increasing size even benign cysts may cause significant morbidity. In addition, these masses need to be differentiated from malignant tumors.

Bronchogenic cysts are the most common primary cyst. They originate as sequestrations from the ventral foregut, the antecedent of the tracheobronchial tree. The bronchogenic cyst may lie within the lung parenchyma or the mediastinum. The cyst wall is composed of cartilage, mucous glands, smooth muscle, and fibrous tissue with a pathognomonic inner layer of ciliated respiratory epithelium. When bronchogenic cysts occur in the mediastinum, they are usually located proximal to the trachea or bronchi and may be just posterior to the carina. Often these cysts will be poorly demonstrated by routine chest films but readily visualized by CT.

Pericardial cysts are the second most frequently encountered cysts within the mediastinum and comprise 6 per cent of all lesions and 33 per cent of primary cysts. These cysts classically occur in the pericardiophrenic angles, with 70 per cent in the right pericardiophrenic angle, 22 per cent in the left, and the remainder in other sites in the pericardium.

Enteric cysts (duplication cysts) arise from the posterior division of the primitive foregut, which develops into the upper division of the gastrointestinal tract. These cysts are found less frequently than are bronchogenic or pericardial cysts and comprise 3 per cent of the mediastinal masses in the collected series. Occurring most commonly in the posterior mediastinum and in children, these lesions are composed of smooth muscle with an inner epithelial lining of esophageal, gastric, or intestinal mucosa. When gastric mucosa is present, peptic ulceration with perforation into the esophageal or bronchial lumen may occur with production of hemoptysis or hematemesis. When enteric cysts are associated with anomalies of the vertebral column, they are referred to as neuroenteric cysts. Such cysts may be connected to the meninges, or, less frequently, a direct communication with the dural space may exist. In patients with neuroenteric cysts, preoperative evaluation for potential spinal cord involvement is mandatory, usually by use of CT or MRI.

Thymic cysts may be inflammatory, neoplastic, or congenital lesions. Congenital cysts are thought to originate from the third branchial arch and are not usually related to thymomas. These cysts are defined by the presence of thymic tissue within the cyst wall. An apparent increase in the incidence of thymic cysts following treatment of malignant anterior mediastinal neoplasms has been reported. Nonspecific cysts include those lesions in which a specific epithelial or mesothelial lining cannot be identified.

The optimal treatment of a mediastinal cyst is surgical excision primarily for diagnosis and for differentiation of these cysts from malignant lesions, although the bronchogenic and enteric cysts frequently can cause significant symptoms, particularly in children. Patients with characteristic lesions and classic CT findings for pericardial cysts have been managed with needle aspiration and serial follow-up with CT rather than surgical excision.

I

The Surgical Management of Suppurative Mediastinitis

Thomas J. Krizek, M.D., and John G. Lease, M.D.

Suppurative mediastinitis is largely a modern phenomenon occurring in most instances as a complication of surgical procedures utilizing median sternotomy, an approach introduced by Julien in 1957. Early reports of an incidence of 5 per cent with mortality in excess of 50 per cent greatly tempered initial enthusiasm for what has become the preferred access to the heart, great vessels, and mediastinum. Today this complication has been reduced to 1 to 2 per cent, and treatment with current techniques has reduced mortality to less than 5 per cent in most series. The incidence of nonoperative mediastinitis is only of historic note. Before the advent of antibiotics, mediastinitis occasionally occurred in conjunction with granulomatous infections, usually tuberculosis. It has also been described following closed chest cardiopulmonary resuscitation and in cases of sternal fracture as a result of trauma.

The chest wall serves the dual purpose of providing a rigid compartment for protecting the thoracic viscera from injury while allowing flexibility for accomplishing ventilation. Median sternotomy provides unparalleled access and produces minimal interference with these vital functions. Restoration of sternal integrity at the completion of operation has, in general, not utilized rigid fixation as might be applied to most other divided bones. The use of wire fixation may produce areas of avascularity and also provides poor immo-

---

See the corresponding chapter or part in the *Textbook of Surgery*, 14th edition, pp. 1796–1800, for a more detailed discussion of this topic, including a comprehensive list of references.

bilization. The stress of ventilation, therefore, effects constant motion at the fracture site, impedes healing, and increases the risk of hematoma formation, a known factor associated with wound infection.

Quantitative microbiology of wounds has demonstrated that it is not merely the presence of bacteria in a wound but rather a critical number of microorganisms per gram of tissue that determines clinical infection. Bacteria may invade a wound from external contamination or from "seeding" of the operative site by microorganisms found elsewhere in the body. When more than 10^5 microorganisms per gram of tissue become established, infection occurs; lower levels of inoculum can reach the critical level of 10^5 if either systemic or local defenses are lowered. The ecology of microorganisms tends to vary from institution to institution and may change in time, particularly with the changing use of antibacterials. *Staphylococcus epidermidis* and *Pseudomonas aeruginosa* are the most common microorganisms to cause infection, since they are the most indigenous to the patients. Other gram-negative species such as *Escherichia coli, Klebsiella, Serratia,* and *Proteus* have been implicated, and mixed infections represent 40 per cent of cases. *Candida* and pure anaerobic infections have also been identified, albeit rarely.

There are multiple factors, both nonspecific and specific, that predispose patients to mediastinitis. Nonspecific factors include obesity, diabetes, prolonged hospitalization, malnutrition, poor hemodynamics, and reoperation. More specifically, the type of operation influences infectious complications of median sternotomy. An incidence of less than 1 per cent is noted in cases of congenital heart defects, but a higher rate is found in cases of coronary artery bypass, particularly when the internal mammary artery is used. As techniques of sternotomy have improved with the use of high-speed mechanical saws, problems have been reduced. Long operative times also correlate with increased rates of infection, especially when pump bypass times exceed 3 hours.

The use of antibacterials as a preventive measure against mediastinitis requires an adequate dose combined with administration in a timely manner and by the proper route. In the surgical patient, this means establishing therapeutic tissue levels of antibacterials at the time of operation. Suppurative mediastinal wound infections usually present within 4 to 30 days postoperatively, usually within 2 weeks, but have been reported as late as 5 months. In 70 to 90 per cent of patients with mediastinitis, wound drainage is the first sign. Sternal instability is also a common finding, but this alone is not diagnostic and may indicate only failure of sternal fixation. Sternal tenderness that follows a progressive course may also be suggestive. Occult sepsis with fever and leukocytosis must be evaluated for a mediastinal source. Chest films may reveal a widened mediastinum, but this finding is not diagnostic. Mediastinal needle aspiration is a simple diagnostic test and is useful when positive.

The therapy of mediastinal wound infections follows the same principles of treatment applied to any infected wound. These include initial adequate drainage, débridement of all ischemic or necrotic tissues and closure with sufficient soft tissue to fill all dead space. This should be approached in a systematic and expeditious manner in order to achieve the best possible outcome. When the presence of infection within the mediastinal wound is confirmed, initial treatment should be to establish adequate drainage. This condition demands urgency because the often debilitated state of the patient is compromised further by the presence of a mediastinal abscess. Drainage procedures can be performed at the bedside or in an office setting in an emergency, but general anesthesia is usually required. The wound should be opened and all suture materials removed. If the infection is confined to the subcutaneous space, the deep margins of the wound can remain intact. If the abscess extends into the sternal and pericardial space, the entire extent of the wound should be opened. The pleural spaces, which are often in communication with the mediastinum following cardiac surgery, should also be inspected for the presence of loculated infection. If this is found, drainage should be accomplished through the mediastinum.

Débridement of all clearly necrotic or ischemic tissue should follow, either at the time drainage is accomplished or as a secondary procedure if the patient's clinical course precludes this initially. Excision of a narrow rim of skin and subcutaneous tissue usually suffices, and only rarely is extensive soft tissue resection required. Care should be taken to preserve, if possible, the medial blood supply of the pectoralis major muscle via the internal mammary artery perforators, since this may prove useful in the subsequent closure. Any remaining sternal wires or tapes should be removed. In many cases, the entire sternum must be excised, since it may be comminuted and nonviable. Costal cartilages are resected because their poor blood supply tends to create a site for chronic infection. Jet or pressure lavage of the wound with warm normal saline completes the débridement procedure. If all tissues with high bacterial counts have been débrided, closure can proceed. Quantitative wound bacteriology, by use of a rapid slide method, can serve as a guide to assessing the adequacy of the débridement. If closure is to be delayed, the wound is dressed with an appropriate topical antimicrobial.

Such factors as nutritional, hemodynamic, and pulmonary status should be improved in the interim between débridement and delayed closure. When the clinical condition is appropriate, definitive closure can proceed.

Although rigid fixation of the rib cage may be an issue for proper closure of acute sternal resections, it is rarely a concern in closure of this type of chronic wound. Scarring and tissue fibrosis serve to stabilize the chest wall. The main focus of closure should address proper soft tissue obliteration of dead space.

The pectoralis major muscle, either unilaterally or bilaterally, is useful for closure of the middle or superior aspects of the mediastinal wound. The muscle can be reliably rotated as a flap on its dominant vascular pedicle, the thoracoacromial vessels. Detachment of its medial costal origin and its humeral insertion allows a wide arc of rotation. The muscle can also be used as a turnover flap based on the medial perforators of the internal mammary artery when intact. Following the positioning of the flaps, direct skin closure is usually possible. Use of one or even both pectoralis major muscles produces little functional or esthetic deformity.

The rectus abdominis muscle provides the best coverage for the inferior aspect of a mediastinal wound. The muscle is transferred on the superior epigastric vessels or intercostal perforators at the superolateral border. The inferior epigastric vessels, which are the dominant blood supply to the muscle, can be used only through microvascular transfer techniques. As in the pectoralis major flap, use of either one or both rectus muscles creates little functional or esthetic deformity for the patient.

The omentum can provide adequate coverage for a portion or all of the mediastinal wound. The omental blood supply is based on either the left or right gastroepiploic vessels. Access to the flap is through a short upper midline incision. Although this technique can prove quite versatile, it does have the disadvantage of requiring an intra-abdominal procedure.

Other flaps such as latissimus dorsi or serratus anterior muscles may be considered. In unusual circumstances when flap closure is not possible, free tissue transfer is an option. All wounds should be closed over closed-suction drains, which are removed appropriately in the early postoperative period.

In summary, suppurative mediastinitis is an uncommon complication of cardiac surgical procedures. These patients are often ill preoperatively and often have a number of factors predisposing to wound infection. The principles of management include early and aggressive débridement, reduction of bacterial counts with topical antimicrobials, and closure often by the use of muscle flaps. These techniques have produced a reduction of mortality from 73 to 100 per cent with nonoperative management to less than 5 per cent with current techniques.

II

Surgical Management of Myasthenia Gravis

C. Warren Olanow, M.D.,
and Andrew S. Wechsler, M.D.

Myasthenia gravis is a disorder of neuromuscular transmission. It is characterized by weakness and fatigue of

See the corresponding chapter or part in the *Textbook of Surgery*, 14th edition, pp. 1801–1814, for a more detailed discussion of this topic, including a comprehensive list of references.

voluntary muscles. It is generally accepted that the disease is due to an autoimmune attack directed against postsynaptic nicotinic acetylcholine (ACh) receptors of voluntary muscles. The consequence is a reduced number of acetylcholine receptors (AChR) on the postsynaptic membrane of the neuromuscular junction. For any amount of ACh released, the likelihood of an interaction with the AChR is diminished.

CLINICAL FEATURES

Myasthenia gravis tends to occur in younger women and elderly men. Males have a higher incidence of thymoma. The hallmarks of myasthenia gravis are weakness and fatigue. Weakness increases as the day progresses or after exercise. The ocular muscles are affected most frequently and are the presenting feature in 50 to 60 per cent of patients, with ultimate involvement in 90 per cent of patients. This is manifest by ptosis and diplopia. Involvement of other cranial nerves may cause potentially fatal complications such as dysphagia and respiratory distress. In older patients, impaired chewing, dysarthria, and nasal speech are common.

In extremities, there is generally a symmetrical weakness involving proximal muscles more than distal groups and the arms more than the legs. The symptom onset may be insidious or sudden. Symptoms may initially be confined to the ocular muscles, but more than 80 per cent of patients develop generalized weakness within a year. The Osserman classification is used for clinical classification of the disease.

Myasthenia gravis may occur transiently in neonates of mothers with myasthenia gravis. A congenital variety is more common in males and is often familial and generally improves after 6 to 10 years of symptoms; it is unresponsive to drugs or thymectomy.

The Lambert-Eaton syndrome is a disorder of peripheral cholinergic transmission characterized by weakness and fatigability of proximal muscles, particularly in the lower extremities. Ocular bulbar involvement is minimal. There are abnormalities of deep tendon reflexes. The Lambert-Eaton syndrome is the consequence of deficient release of acetylcholine from nerve terminals. This is an autoimmune disorder, and unlike for myasthenia gravis, anticholinesterase agents are generally not effective. The Lambert-Eaton syndrome is often seen in association with underlying carcinoma, predominantly oat cell carcinoma of the lung, and may occasionally occur in association with chronic disease states.

THYMIC ABNORMALITIES

The thymus gland is abnormal in 75 to 80 per cent of patients with myasthenia gravis; 10 to 15 per cent of patients with myasthenia gravis have thymomas, generally benign. Two thirds of thymomas are not associated with myasthenia gravis. Malignancy is a rare occurrence and is generally defined by the biologic behavior of the tumor, rather than the histologic type. Almost all thymomas can be detected by computed tomographic scan of the mediastinum.

The most common finding in young patients with myasthenia gravis is lymphoid hyperplasia of the thymus gland. There are increased numbers of B cells in the thymus glands of patients with myasthenia. In late-onset myasthenia gravis (after 55 years of age), the thymus gland is most often atrophic and involuted. All patients with myasthenia gravis have a relative lymphopenia in their peripheral blood consisting primarily of a reduction in T lymphocytes and $3A1^+$ and OKT4 T cell subsets.

DIAGNOSTIC STUDIES

Myasthenia gravis is frequently diagnosed by the injection of edrophonium (Tensilon). This anticholinesterase agent improves the probability of ACh-AChR interaction, and injection of 2 to 10 mg. intravenously frequently improves symptoms.

Electrophysiologic studies may be helpful. The Jolly test utilizes supramaximal repetitive stimulation of a peripheral nerve and in myasthenia gravis is associated with a gradual decrease in the amplitude of the evoked action potential without a change in antidromic conduction. Unfortunately, the test is somewhat insensitive, and changes are not detected in more than 50 per cent of patients with myasthenia gravis, particularly in the early stages. Single-fiber electromyography is more sensitive. The test performed is known as the "jitter" test and is abnormal in 95 per cent of patients with myasthenia gravis if multiple muscle groups are studied.

In 85 to 90 per cent of patients with myasthenia gravis, it is possible to demonstrate antibodies directed against the acetylcholine receptor.

PATHOGENESIS

Important to theories of pathogenesis has been the demonstration of antibodies directed against the acetylcholine receptor. Mechanisms proposed by which the antibody may be causal in myasthenia gravis include (1) accelerated degradation of AChR on the postsynaptic membrane, (2) immunopharmacologic blockade in which the antibody hinders interaction between ACh and the AChR, (3) modulation or accelerated internalization with intracellular degradation of the AChR–AChR antibody complex, and (4) reduced synthesis of AChR.

Anti-AChR antibody may not be the sole factor responsible for clinical weakness. Studies at Duke University in which all patients underwent thymectomy demonstrated dramatic clinical improvement in most patients without reduction in the anti-AChR antibody titer. Moreover, there was no direct correlation between the serum-AChR antibody level and the clinical status of individual patients. These data suggest that the presence of a thymic factor is essential to the development of clinical weakness in myasthenia gravis.

ROLE OF THE THYMUS GLAND

Seventy-five to 85 per cent of patients with myasthenia have pathologic changes in the thymus gland. For 50 years, thymectomy has been known to influence the clinical course of myasthenia gravis. Nonetheless, the exact role of the thymus gland remains to be defined. The mechanism by which thymectomy provides clinical benefit has not yet been elucidated. Thymectomy influences cell-mediated immunity and peripheral T cell counts in patients with late onset myasthenia gravis. The clinical relevance of this finding has not been established. Thymectomy may remove a source of (1) AChR antigen that is a source of autosensitization against AChR antigenic determinants; (2) anti-AChR antibody production; (3) sensitized helper T cells that facilitate the production of anti-AChR antibody by peripheral lymphocytes; (4) sensitized killer T cells directed against the neuromuscular junction; and (5) a putative thymic factor that may act directly at the acetylcholine receptor or may activate complement-mediated lysis at antibody-labeled receptor cites. It is possible that thymectomy acts by multiple or unknown mechanisms and has different effects in individual patients.

Failure of thymectomy to induce clinical remission might be due to (1) incomplete thymectomy, (2) permanent irreparable damage to the neuromuscular junction, (3) immune complex from damaged end plates with perpetuation of the immune response and lymphocytes within the spleen and lymph nodes that are unaffected by the thymectomy, and (4) the influence of long-lived peripheral T cells.

TREATMENT

The authors favor thymectomy as early as possible after development of generalized weakness as preferred therapy, particularly for younger patients. This approach avoids side effects of anticholinesterase medications and may influence the disease to assume a more benign course. Nonetheless, it is important to be aware of medical treatments available.

Medical treatment includes the use of anticholinesterase agents, corticosteroids, plasma exchange, and immunosuppressant agents.

ANTICHOLINESTERASE AGENTS. Anticholinesterase agents have been a standard medical treatment for the past 60 years and act by inhibiting breakdown of acetylcholine. The likelihood of interactions between acetylcholine and the acetylcholine receptor is increased, thereby increasing the safety margin for neuromuscular transmission. Long-acting anticholinesterase agents most commonly used are neostigmine (Prostigmin) and pyridostigmine (Mestinon).

CORTICOSTEROIDS. Clinical response to corticosteroids may be dramatic, and unlike the effect of anticholinesterase agents, true remission may occur. Initiation of large-dose corticosteroid treatment in severely weakened patients may produce deterioration in the clinical condition 4 to 8 days after onset of therapy. When myasthenia is confined to ocular muscles, a much smaller dose (5 mg. compared with 60 mg.)

may be utilized on an every-other-day schedule, with increases as necessary. Although steroids may produce a dramatic clinical response, they are less desirable than is thymectomy and are best reserved for patients who have failed to respond to thymectomy. Complications of steroid therapy are significant.

PLASMA EXCHANGE. Plasma exchange permits selective removal of plasma or plasma components by centrifugal methods with return of the red cells to the patient. This procedure is easy to accomplish and produces rapid clinical improvement in patients with myasthenia gravis. It is an ideal method for preparing patients for operation rather than initiating complex medical treatment. Usually four to six treatments restore clinical strength.

IMMUNOSUPPRESSIVE AGENTS. Azathioprine (Imuran) has been widely used in doses of 1.5 to 3 mg. per kg. There is a latent period of 6 to 12 weeks before any effect is seen, and the maximal benefit may not be realized for a year or longer. The drug has been used more in Europe than in North America, and favorable responses have been reported in most patients. As is the case with corticosteroids, there are significant side effects associated with the use of azathioprine. Clinical trials are currently in progress utilizing cyclosporine. Experience with cyclosporine suggests that a better response is obtained when it is introduced early in the course of myasthenia gravis. The major side effect of cyclosporine is nephrotoxicity.

Ideal immunotherapy for myasthenia gravis would selectively delete the autoimmune reaction directed at the AChR in a permanent manner without toxicity. The strategies that might provide a "cure" for myasthenia gravis include (1) attempts to inhibit the accelerated degradation of the AChR by use of methylation inhibitors, (2) elimination of specific B cells that produce anti-AChR antibodies, (3) total body lymphoid irradiation if immunologic precursor cells could be protected, (4) selected proliferation of anti-idiotype antibodies directed against the anti-AChR antibody, and (5) generation of antigen-specific suppressor cells.

SURGICAL TREATMENT

Patients with myasthenia gravis are considered for thymectomy as soon as possible after the development of generalized weakness. Plasma exchange is used to optimize medical status before thymectomy, if patients have significant weakness. Patients on anticholinesterase medications have these agents slowly withdrawn during the course of plasma exchange. Patients receiving corticosteroids are maintained on them throughout the postoperative period for prevention of adrenal insufficiency; after this period, attempts are made to gradually lower the dosage as tolerated. Operative mortality should be less than 1 per cent and should occur only in high-risk patients with profound clinical weakness. Preoperative sedation should be given in smaller doses than is customary; atropine should be avoided.

SURGICAL ANATOMY OF THE THYMUS GLAND. The thymus gland overlies the pericardium and great vessels at the base of the heart and is in proximity to the left innominate vein. It generally has an H-shaped configuration with variable fusion of the right and left lobes at about the midportion of the gland. There are many variations in regional anatomy of the thymus gland, and thymic remnants may be left along its embryonic migratory route from the third and occasionally fourth branchial pouches. The thymus gland normally undergoes marked reduction in size from the time of puberty.

SURGICAL TECHNIQUE. Five approaches have been recommended for thymectomy. These include (1) transcervical, (2) median sternotomy, (3) partial median sternotomy, (4) median sternotomy plus cervical incision, and (5) upper median sternotomy combined with transcervical. The authors prefer median sternotomy and radical thymectomy. This procedure requires a slightly longer hospital stay and has slightly greater morbidity than does transcervical thymectomy but allows a more total removal of thymic tissue. The thymus gland is removed along with all perithymic and most mediastinal fat. The upper poles of the thymus gland are followed into the neck to their attenuation into the thymic ligaments. Safety is ensured by excellent visibility. Complete resection of thymic tumors is most likely with this approach. Since results of thymectomy from myasthenia must continually be evaluated and compared against other therapies, the most controlled data are obtained when complete thymectomy has been performed.

Cervical thymectomy, however, has proved extremely effective in treating myasthenia gravis, and recent reports suggest success rates comparable to those of median sternotomy. The learning curve for successful performance of the procedure is greater, and the ability to perform more radical thymectomy is distinctly limited.

With use of either technique, great care is taken for avoidance of inadvertent injury to the phrenic nerve with the electrocautery or by excessive traction. At the time of thymectomy, attempts are made to retain the thymus gland within its normal thin capsule. It is important to be aware of the multiple potential locations for thymic tissue.

THYMECTOMY FOR THYMOMA

The diagnosis of thymoma is usually made prior to thymectomy on the basis of a mediastinal computed tomographic scan. Unusual firmness of the thymus gland suggests thymoma at operation. Malignancy of the thymic tumor is determined by the surgeon at the time of operation based on its biologic rather than histologic behavior. Complete resection of the tumor is optimal and may be accompanied by removal of portions of pericardium, a single phrenic nerve, the left innominate vein, and pleural reflections or pulmonary tissue. Margins of the tumor should be marked with metallic clips for future identification of radiation ports.

POSTOPERATIVE CARE

Postoperative care should be provided jointly by the neurologist and the surgeon. Following thymectomy, patients are unusually sensitive to anticholinesterase agents, and cholinergic crises have been precipitated by injudicious use of these drugs after operation. Deterioration of ventilatory status may occur several days postoperatively, possibly related to the increased corticosteroid response associated with operation and its subsequent salutary effect on symptoms of myasthenia gravis. For most patients having median sternotomy, hospital discharge is possible a few days after operation; for minimally symptomatic patients having transcervical thymectomy, hospital discharge may be possible 1 or 2 days following operation.

RESULTS OF THYMECTOMY

Improvement after thymectomy had been reported in 57 to 86 per cent of patients with permanent remission in 20 to 36 per cent. There may be significant delay between the time of operation and remission. In general, patients with nonthymomatous myasthenia gravis have better remission rates and long-term survival than do those with thymomatous myasthenia gravis. Only 10 per cent of patients with noninvasive thymoma are reported to have remission. When the tumor is invasive, remission is even less likely, and more than 50 per cent of patients die within 5 years. Most of these deaths occur in the first year and are related to myasthenic complications.

There has not been a prospective randomized study comparing effects of thymectomy with other forms of management for myasthenia gravis. The authors initiated a prospective study in which all patients with generalized myasthenia were subjected to thymectomy as primary therapy. Plasmapheresis was used to improve the clinical state of any patients who were receiving cholinesterase inhibitors. Following operation, 46 of 47 patients were improved at a mean follow-up of 25.5 months, and myasthenic symptoms were confined mainly to the ocular muscles in patients who did not have complete response. An additional 55 patients received thymectomy as primary therapy by the authors, and none of the patients were receiving long-term medical management. The mean follow-up for this group of patients was 39 months, and at that time 64 per cent of the patients were asymptomatic with no functional neurologic deficit. Ten patients continued to have mild generalized weakness, but none had residual bulbar dysfunction. Ninety-two per cent of the patients were improved by at least one stage in the Osserman classification system compared with their prethymectomy status. Seventy-one per cent improved by two or more stages; 55 per cent of the patients required no further medication, and only 22 of the patients required chronic prednisone therapy for generalized myasthenic symptoms. An additional 24 per cent of the patients received low-dosage prednisone therapy every other day for management of ocular symptoms. Thus, by use of thymectomy as primary treatment for generalized myasthenia gravis, 92 per cent of patients enrolled in the series were improved and 80 per cent were free of generalized weakness at the time of latest medical follow-up.

ALGORITHMS FOR MANAGEMENT OF PATIENTS WITH MYASTHENIA GRAVIS

Critical in the evaluation phase is the determination of whether the patient has myasthenia gravis or weakness associated with another clinical condition. The response to Tensilon, the Jolly and jitter tests, and determination of the level of anti-AChR antibodies identify the disease correctly in more than 95 per cent of cases. Radiologic studies are used to determine if a thymoma is present.

Patients enter the therapeutic phase following the diagnosis of generalized myasthenia. In the authors' algorithm, the primary treatment mode for generalized myasthenia is thymectomy. Patients with major ocular symptoms are cautioned that thymectomy produces unpredictable ocular responses and there may be a need for continuation of medical management. By use of this overall treatment plan, the systemic complications of pharmacologic management of myasthenia gravis can be avoided or minimized. Thymectomy as the primary therapy for myasthenia gravis yields remission in most patients and allows reduced pharmacologic requirements in patients with residual symptoms after thymectomy.

55

SURGICAL DISORDERS OF THE PERICARDIUM

Thomas L. Spray, M.D.

ACUTE PERICARDITIS

Acute pericarditis caused by inflammation is characterized by chest pain, pericardial friction rub, and electrocardiographic abnormalities. The most common causes of the syndrome include idiopathic or viral pericarditis, uremia, bacterial pericarditis, acute myocardial infarction, tuberculosis, trauma, or neoplastic infiltration of the pericardium. Chest pain is the most frequent complaint of patients with acute pericarditis and is often exacerbated by lying supine, coughing, deep inspiration, or swallowing and is eased by sitting up and leaning forward.

The pathognomonic physical finding of acute pericarditis is the pericardial friction rub, which classically has three components related to cardiac motion during atrial systole, ventricular systole, and rapid ventricular filling in diastole. The rub may be variable and evanescent. Four stages of electrocardiographic changes occur in acute pericarditis; however, S-T segment elevation present in all leads except aVR and V_1 with upright T waves is most common and essentially diagnostic of pericarditis. Intermittent atrial fibrillation, supraventricular tachycardia, or atrial flutter occurs in approximately 20 per cent of patients. The chest film is of little diagnostic value unless the pericarditis is accompanied by a large pericardial effusion, which may enlarge the cardiac silhouette. The most sensitive test for evaluation of the magnitude of pericardial effusion is the echocardiogram. Most acute pericarditis is self-limiting with gradual improvement over 2 to 6 weeks. The pericardial inflammation may recur weeks or months after the initial episode with remissions and exacerbations lasting several months.

Treatment includes bed rest until the pain and fever subside, exclusion of any underlying etiologic factor that requires specific treatment, and control of pain with nonsteroidal anti-inflammatory agents. If pain fails to respond within 48 hours, corticosteroids (up to 60 mg. of prednisone daily) may be given. The steroids are then gradually tapered to the smallest dose that controls symptoms.

Development of life-threatening hemodynamic complications may occur as a result of cardiac compression by pericardial effusion, development of fibrosis causing constriction, or a combination of both effusive and constrictive processes.

See the corresponding chapter or part in the *Textbook of Surgery*, 14th edition, pp. 1815–1825, for a more detailed discussion of this topic, including a comprehensive list of references.

PERICARDIAL EFFUSION

The development of cardiac tamponade by effusion depends on the volume of the pericardial effusion, the rate of accumulation of fluid, and the relative thickness and elasticity of the pericardium. If the accumulation of fluid is gradual, few symptoms are noted. On physical examination, the heart sounds may be distant and rales may be heard over the lung fields. Chest film is often unrevealing unless a large effusion is present, and the cardiac silhouette then may have a water-bottle shape. The electrocardiogram may show nonspecific reduction in Q or S voltage and flattening of the T waves. The most accurate diagnostic test currently available for pericardial effusion is two-dimensional echocardiography, which may localize even small loculated effusions. Pericardial effusions do not require treatment unless there is hemodynamic compromise from increasing pericardial pressure or unless aspiration of fluid is necessary for diagnosis. Pericardiocentesis for acute effusions may be curative; however, chronic effusion with significant or recurrent symptoms may require total pericardiectomy for control.

CARDIAC TAMPONADE

Cardiac tamponade is characterized by an elevation of intrapericardial pressure, which may rise to the level of right atrial and right ventricular diastolic pressures. A decline in the transmural filling pressures results and, therefore, decreases cardiac output. Although initial reduction in stroke volume is compensated by increases in heart rate and adrenergic tone, as these compensatory mechanisms fail, evidence of severe circulatory compromise is noted.

The pathognomonic finding in cardiac tamponade is pulsus paradoxus, an inspiratory fall of aortic systolic pressure greater than 10 mm. Hg. Cardiac tamponade may occur in almost any type of pericarditis and is commonly associated with chest trauma or penetrating injury. Jugular venous pressure is usually markedly elevated, and precordial cardiac activity is faint. Heart sounds are distant or inaudible, and tachypnea and tachycardia may be apparent clinically. The electrocardiogram may show signs of electrical alternans, a phasic alteration of the amplitude of the R wave, which is highly suggestive of cardiac tamponade. In acute cardiac tamponade, the patient is clinically in shock. Venous distention is striking at a time when other signs of circulatory failure are similar to those observed in hemorrhagic shock, and measurement of elevated central venous pressure often confirms the diagnosis. Prompt *treatment* of acute tamponade is mandatory, and immediate pericardial aspiration may be life-saving. Aspiration of only a small amount of pericardial fluid may produce a striking reduction in pericardial pressure and improvement in cardiac output.

CONSTRICTIVE PERICARDITIS

Constrictive pericarditis occurs when fibrosed and adherent pericardium restrict diastolic filling of the cardiac chambers.

Most cases of constrictive pericarditis are of unknown etiology. In classic constrictive pericarditis, the pericardial scarring restricts diastolic filling of the heart, with resultant equilibration of diastolic pressures in all four cardiac chambers. In early diastole, filling is unimpeded owing to the elevated venous pressures. When intracardiac volume reaches the limit of the noncompliant pericardium, diastolic filling rapidly ceases, with creation of the characteristic early diastolic dip and plateau waveform in the right and left ventricular pressure tracings. Usually systolic contraction of the ventricles is normal, although in long-standing cases myocardial atrophy may occur.

Symptoms of constrictive pericarditis include weakness, easy fatigability, and shortness of breath with exertion. Unlike those with congestive heart failure, patients with constrictive pericarditis often develop ascites without peripheral edema. Syncope is occasionally seen. The primary physical finding is elevation of jugular venous pressure, occasionally with an increase on inspiration (Kussmaul's sign). The precordium is quiet, with no right ventricular lift. The liver may be enlarged and tender with prominent hepatojugular reflux. Arterial blood pressure is often low and pulse pressure narrow. Atrial arrhythmias are seen in approximately one third of patients, and on chest film the heart is usually normal or mildly enlarged, occasionally with calcium deposits in the pericardium.

The electrocardiogram often shows low-voltage Q or S complexes with flat or inverted T waves. Serum proteins may be low from a loss of protein through the gastrointestinal tract. Confirmation of the diagnosis of constrictive pericarditis may be difficult. Cardiac catheterization offers the most reliable technique for differentiating myocardial and pericardial diseases. Left ventricular end-diastolic pressure is usually normal with constrictive pericarditis, and restrictive cardiomyopathy is more likely when right ventricular systolic hypertension is present. In contrast to patients with constrictive pericarditis, patients with cardiac tamponade often show marked pulsus paradoxus.

Computed tomographic scans often show pericardial thickening but are not diagnostic of constrictive disease without hemodynamic confirmation. Nuclear magnetic resonance images can show both the thickened pericardium and the dilation of hepatic veins and right atrium and small right ventricle characteristic of constriction.

Patients with constrictive pericarditis often become progressively disabled by weakness, ascites, and cardiac cachexia. Optimal treatment for constrictive pericarditis is complete resection of the pericardium.

SURGICAL TECHNIQUES

PERICARDIOCENTESIS. Aspiration of the pericardial sac can be life-saving in the case of cardiac tamponade or a diagnostic procedure for determining the etiologic basis of pericardial effusion. Pericardiocentesis is performed by the left parasternal approach in the fourth or fifth intercostal space or preferably via the subxiphoid route, under local anesthesia. A long needle and catheter are attached to a stopcock and syringe and inserted just beneath and to the left of the xiphoid process. Although two-dimensional echocardiographic-guided aspiration is the preferred technique when the equipment is available, attachment of a precordial electrogram lead to the pericardiocentesis needle hub by a small clip may show contact with the epicardium by negative deflection of the Q or S complex. The aspirating needle is inserted at a 30- to 45-degree angle posteriorly toward a point midway between the scapulae. The needle is then advanced slowly until fluid is encountered or the echocardiogram shows contact with the surface of the heart. A catheter can then be advanced safely into the pericardial space over a guidewire.

Open drainage of the pericardium is often required in the presence of chronic pericardial effusion or purulent pericarditis. The subxiphoid approach is commonly used for drainage of large effusions: dependent drainage is effectively established, and catheters can be placed via this approach for irrigation. In addition, small portions of pericardium for biopsy can be obtained.

An alternative approach for pericardial biopsy is through a left anterior thoracotomy incision in the fourth intercostal space. The pleura may be opened for wide drainage of pericardial fluid. Excision of the maximal amount of pericardium possible through the left thoracotomy approach is the preferred treatment for large pericardial effusions, since recurrent effusion or constriction can develop.

PERICARDIECTOMY. Pericardiectomy for constrictive pericarditis has an operative mortality of 4 to 6 per cent with long-term improvement in approximately 75 per cent of the survivors. The preferred approach for complete excision of the pericardium is the left anterior thoracotomy through the left fourth interspace, with initial removal of the scar over the left ventricle, although a median sternotomy may also be used. Occasionally, cardiopulmonary bypass may be used to control bleeding from friable areas of the heart. In most patients, progressive hemodynamic and symptomatic improvement is apparent after operation, although low cardiac output syndrome in the immediate postoperative period is common.

SPECIFIC PERICARDIAL DISEASES

TUBERCULOUS PERICARDITIS. Tuberculous pericarditis probably is due to early dissemination following a primary infection. Symptoms are often nonspecific with malaise, fever, sweats, and cough. It is important to treat tuberculous pericarditis early because gradual fibrosis and scarring prevent effective delivery of antibiotics, and fibrosis and calcification with eventual constriction are common. Combination chemotherapy with two and usually three agents should be begun, and operative resection of the pericardium is warranted early when the patient is clinically well.

UREMIC PERICARDITIS. Uremic pericarditis is a frequent complication of chronic renal failure and may be detected in approximately 50 per cent of patients with untreated renal disease. No treatment is required for small effusions; however, large effusions may occasionally be improved by increasing the frequency of dialysis. Management of symptoms of fever and pain may include a nonsteroidal anti-inflammatory agent or administration of steroids. Pericardiectomy is generally reserved for patients with recurrent effusion, evidence of tamponade, or pericardial constriction. Echo-guided aspiration of fluid and placement of a drainage catheter may also be considered.

PURULENT PERICARDITIS. Purulent pericarditis occurs as a direct contamination of the pericardium following penetrating injury or pneumonia. Severe chest pain and fever are common. The most common infectious agents are *Staphylococcus* or gram-negative bacteria in adults and *Staphylococcus* or *Haemophilus influenzae* in children. Aspiration of the pericardium and treatment with antibiotics are indicated, with pericardiectomy and drainage deferred for resistant cases.

NEOPLASTIC PERICARDITIS. The heart is involved in about 10 per cent of patients with malignant neoplasms, 85 per cent of whom have pericardial tumor. Common neoplasms that develop pericardial metastases are tumors of the lung and breast, melanoma, leukemia, and lymphoma. Effusions are the most significant sign of pericardial involvement and may require drainage if hemodynamically significant.

56

THE HEART

I

Cardiac Catheterization

Christopher E. H. Buller, M.D.,
and Richard S. Stack, M.D.

Diagnostic cardiac catheterization combines high-resolution dynamic imaging of the cardiac chambers, great vessels, and coronary arteries with quantitative hemodynamic measurements. Findings at cardiac catheterization are often critical in patient management, guiding the selection of appropriate medical and surgical therapy in ischemic, valvular, myopathic, and congenital heart diseases.

INDICATIONS

Cardiac catheterization is indicated when clinically important information obtainable by the study is not otherwise reliably available by clinical and noninvasive evaluation. The inherent risks and discomfort of the procedure demand consideration of the risk:benefit ratio for each patient. Indications are shown in Table 1. Complications associated with cardiac catheterization are listed in Table 2.

TECHNIQUE

Proper preparation for cardiac catheterization should address the issues outlined in Table 3. Most diagnostic and interventional catheterizations are performed percutaneously via the right or left femoral artery and vein from a site 2 to 3 cm. below the inguinal ligament. In a sterile field, the femoral

TABLE 1. Indications for Cardiac Catheterization

Category	Example
Diagnosis of symptoms	Chest pain, equivocal noninvasive studies
Determine the severity of disease	Aortic stenosis, mitral stenosis
Plan a specific operative approach	Complex congenital heart disease
Evaluate therapy	Post-thrombolytic therapy
Therapeutic intervention	Percutaneous transluminal coronary angioplasty

See the corresponding chapter or part in the *Textbook of Surgery*, 14th edition, pp. 1826–1843, for a more detailed discussion of this topic, including a comprehensive list of references.

841

TABLE 2. Complications of Right Heart Catheterization

Insertion Complications
Local hematoma
Inadvertent arterial puncture
Pneumothorax
Hemothorax
Right bundle branch block
Dysrhythmias (atrial and ventricular)
Intracardiac catheter knotting*
Cardiac perforation*

Maintenance Complications
Dysrhythmias (especially ventricular)
Venous thrombosis
Pulmonary artery rupture*
Infection
Air embolism
Balloon rupture
Endocarditis*

Major Complications of Cardiac Catheterization

Complication	Percentage of Total Cases
Death	0.14
Nonfatal myocardial infarction	0.07
Stroke	0.07
Major arrhythmia	0.56
Vascular	0.57
Other	0.41
Total	1.82

*Rare.
Data from Kennedy, J. W.: Complications associated with cardiac catheterization and angiography. From the Registry Committee of the Society for Cardiac Angiography. Cathet. Cardiovasc. Diagn., 8:5, 1982.

artery or vein, as required, is cannulated by use of the Seldinger technique.

The brachial artery and vein provide alternative access for both diagnostic and interventional procedures (Sones technique). This approach is useful in patients with occlusive peripheral vascular disease involving the aorta, both iliac arteries, or both femoral arteries.

Access via the internal jugular or subclavian veins is re-

TABLE 3. Patient Preparation for Elective Cardiac Catheterization

Informed consent
NPO > 6 hours
Light sedation
Hydration of patients at risk for contrast nephropathy (diabetes, pre-existing renal dysfunction)
Prophylaxis against contrast allergy when known or suspected (H_1- and H_2-blockade plus corticosteroids for 24 hours)
Reversal of chronic anticoagulation (prothrombin time < 1.5 times control)

served for bedside insertion of flow-directed pulmonary artery catheters. Their corresponding arteries cannot be safely cannulated.

Left heart catheterization by the retrograde arterial approach is sometimes undesirable, and the procedure may then be performed by a transseptal approach employing a Brockenbrough catheter (Table 4). This device consists of a tapered end-hole catheter snugly fitted over a removable steel needle. The catheter tip is positioned in the right atrium against the fossa ovalis, and the needle is then abruptly advanced into the left atrium by puncturing the atrial septum. When correct positioning is confirmed, the catheter is advanced over the needle to the left atrium, and the needle is removed. The Brockenbrough technique is contraindicated if a patient has received anticoagulants, since inadvertent perforation of the atrium occasionally occurs. Suspicion of left atrial thrombus or tumor contraindicates left atrial catheterization because of the risk of systemic embolism.

HEMODYNAMICS

Cardiac catheterization allows multiple hemodynamic measurements to be recorded simultaneously. The known relationships between these measurements may then be used to infer or calculate parameters of ventricular function, valvular stenosis or regurgitation, vascular resistance, shunts, and pericardial effects. Interpretation of hemodynamic data first requires familiarity with normal measurements. The range of normal measured and derived hemodynamic variables is given in Table 5.

Accuracy requires careful calibration of the hydraulic and electronic portions of the system. When the transducer diaphragm is exposed to ambient atmospheric pressure at the level of the patient's mid right atrium (5 cm. below the sternal angle), the system should be calibrated to record zero pressure. Calibration of amplifier gain is performed with use of a mercury manometer or the internal calibration circuits provided in most equipment.

Measurement of Cardiac Output

There are three main ways to measure cardiac output during cardiac catheterization: the Fick method, the indicator-dilution methods, and the angiographic method.

The Fick method of cardiac output measurement is based

TABLE 4. Indications for Transseptal Left Heart Catheterization

Tilting disc or bileaflet mechanical aortic valve prosthesis
Severe aortic stenosis with inability to cross retrograde
Direct measurement of left atrial pressure of transmitral pressures is required
Mitral valvuloplasty

**TABLE 5. Normal Hemodynamic Values
(Recumbent Adults)**

Pressure Site	Systolic (mm. Hg)	Diastolic (mm. Hg)	Mean (mm. Hg)
Right atrium	—	—	0–8
Right ventricle	5–30	0–8	—
Pulmonary artery	15–30	5–15	10–18
Pulmonary artery wedge	—	—	1–12
Left ventricle	90–140	2–12	—
Aorta	90–140	60–90	70–105

Fick Cardiac Output Parameter	Normal Range
AV O_2 difference	30–50 ml./L.
O_2 consumption	140–390 ml./min.
O_2 consumption index	110–150 ml./min./m.^{2}
Cardiac output	3.5–8.5 L./min.
Cardiac index	2.5–4.5 L./min./m.^{2}

Vascular Resistances	Normal Range
Systemic vascular resistance	8–15 units*
Pulmonary vascular resistance	≤2.0 units*

Valve Gradients	
Aortic valve	<10 mm. Hg
Mitral valve	Negligible

Valve Areas	
Aortic valve	2.0–3.0 sq. cm.
Mitral valve	4.0–6.0 sq. cm.

AV, arteriovenous.
*To convert Wood units to dyne-sec.-cm.$^{-5}$, multiply by 80.

on the principle that the amount of oxygen extracted by the lungs from air is equal to the amount taken up by blood in its passage through the lungs. By measuring the rate of lung oxygen extraction and the oxygen content of pulmonary arterial and pulmonary venous blood, the rate of pulmonary blood flow can be calculated. Traditionally, the rate of lung oxygen extraction (oxygen consumption), is measured by collecting expired gas over a known period of time. More recently, methods of measuring oxygen consumption by continuous sampling of exhaled gas have become available. If oxygen consumption cannot be measured, assumed oxygen consumptions calculated from body surface area may be substituted but are prone to error introduced by age, sex, disease, and nonbasal conditions.

Calculation of blood oxygen content (where K = 1.36 ml. O_2/gm. hemoglobin):

$$O_2 \text{ content(ml. } O_2 \text{/liter)} = \text{(saturation)} \times \text{([hemoglobin, gm./liter]} \times K)$$

Calculation of arteriovenous oxygen difference:

$$AV\ O_2\ \text{diff. (ml. } O_2\ \text{/liter)}$$
$$= (O_2\ \text{content PV}) - (O_2\ \text{content PA})$$

Calculation of cardiac output (CO) follows:

$$CO\ \text{(liter/min.)} = \frac{O_2\ \text{consumption (ml./min.)}}{AV\ O_2\ \text{diff. (ml./liter)}}$$

In practice, systemic arterial or left ventricular samples are substituted for pulmonary venous samples.

The indicator-dilution technique is based on the principle that the dilution of an indicator is proportional to the volume of fluid to which it is added. Thus, if the amount and concentration of indicator is known, the volume of fluid in which it is diluted can be calculated. This relationship is easily modified for circulating fluids. When a known bolus of indicator is added, the time-concentration curve generated at a point downstream is related to flow as follows:

$$\text{Flow} = \frac{\text{Amount of indicator}}{C \times T}$$

where C is the mean concentration of indicator and T the time for first pass.

Whereas several specific indicator methods have been proposed, only two are used clinically: thermodilution and indocyanine green. Thermodilution is now widely used in both the catheterization laboratory and intensive care unit. A known amount (usually 10 ml.) of iced 5 per cent dextrose (approximately 0° C.) is injected rapidly through the right atrial port of a thermistor-tipped pulmonary artery catheter. The temperature of blood passing the catheter tip is then used to generate a time-concentration curve from which cardiac output is calculated. The popularity of this method can be attributed to the thermal indicator, which is nontoxic, has no significant recirculation, and does not accumulate. These properties permit frequent measurements to be performed. Indocyanine green dye is now used infrequently.

Comparisons of Fick, indocyanine green, and thermodilution methods have shown good agreement. The Fick method, however, is the most *accurate* method in patients with reduced cardiac output. For purposes of measuring cardiac output, the presence of a shunt or regurgitant lesion between the indicator injection site and the sampling site invalidates the time-concentration curve. Therefore, tricuspid or pulmonary regurgitation invalidates thermodilution measurements, and mitral or aortic regurgitation invalidates green dye measurements. The Fick method provides direct measurement of pulmonary (but not systemic) blood flow despite intracardiac shunts.

Cardiac output may also be measured angiographically by multiplying the angiographic left ventricular stroke volume by the heart rate (see Left Ventriculography).

Vascular Resistance

The opposition to blood flow created by frictional and other losses within a vascular bed is termed *vascular resistance*. It is defined by analogy to Ohm's law for electrical currents:

$$\text{Resistance} = \frac{\text{Driving Pressure (volts)}}{\text{Flow (current)}}$$

Systemic (peripheral) vascular resistance (SVR) is calculated as follows:

$$\text{SVR} = \frac{P_{Ao} - P_{Ra}}{Q_s}$$

where P_{Ao} is mean aortic pressure (mm. Hg), P_{Ra} is mean right atrial pressure, and Q_s is systemic blood flow (liters per minute). Measurement of systemic vascular resistance is most useful in the management of critically ill patients with shock. In this setting, the profile of systemic vascular resistance, cardiac output, and ventricular filling pressures obtained with a pulmonary artery catheter can help distinguish cardiogenic, hypovolemic, and vasodilatory causes. Sequential measurements allow objective assessment of specific therapeutic interventions.

Pulmonary vascular resistance (PVR) is calculated similarly:

$$\text{PVR} = \frac{P_{Pa} - P_{La}}{Q_p}$$

where P_{Pa} is mean pulmonary artery pressure (mm. Hg), P_{La} is mean left atrial or pulmonary artery wedge pressure, and Q_p is pulmonary blood flow (liters per minute).

Calculation of Stenotic Orifice Area

The pressure gradient produced by a stenotic valve is inversely proportional to valve area and directly proportional to the *square* of blood flow across the valve. Cardiac valve areas are calculated with formulas developed by Gorlin. The general form of this equation is

$$A = \frac{Q}{C \, (P^{1/2})}$$

where A is valve orifice area (sq. cm.), Q is flow rate across valve (ml. per minute), P is mean pressure gradient across valve (mm. Hg), and C is an empiric constant (C = 37.7 for mitral valve; C = 44.5 for aortic valve). Cardiac valves open for only a portion of the cardiac cycle. Valve flow rates (Q) are therefore calculated by dividing the cardiac output (ml. per minute) by the fraction of time the valve is open (seconds per minute).

$$Q = \frac{CO}{\text{DFP or SEP}}$$

where CO is cardiac output (ml. per minute), DFP is diastolic filling period (seconds per minute), and SEP is systolic ejection period (seconds per minute). Diastolic filling periods (for atrioventricular valves) and systolic ejection periods (for semilunar valves) are derived by multiplying the appropriate systolic or diastolic interval measured from pressure tracings (seconds per beat) by the heart rate (HR, beats per minute). Thus, the final equations are as follows:

$$\text{Mitral valve A} = \frac{CO[\text{ml./min.}]/(HR[\text{beats/min.}])(DFP[\text{sec./beat}])}{37.7(P^{1/2})}$$

$$\text{Aortic valve A} = \frac{CO[\text{ml./min.}]/(HR[\text{beats/min.}])(SEP[\text{sec./beat}])}{45.5(P^{1/2})}$$

It is important to realize that cardiac output as used in the formula must represent the flow across the valve in question. In mixed stenotic and regurgitant mitral valve disease, for example, diastolic mitral flow is equal to the sum of forward cardiac output plus regurgitant output.

Shunts

Evaluation of shunts requires their detection, classification (Table 6), localization, and quantitation. Analysis of oxygen saturation data (oximetry) is the principal means for detecting and localizing shunts. Sampling of blood oxygen saturation is performed proximal and distal to a suspected shunt. An abnormal increase (step-up) or decrease (step-down) is detected immediately distal to the shunt, with the magnitude of the change being proportional to the size of the shunt.

Left-to-right shunts are characterized by a right heart oxygen saturation step-up as arterial or pulmonary venous blood is added to desaturated systemic venous or pulmonary arterial blood, and an increase in pulmonary blood flow relative

TABLE 6. Common Cardiac Shunts

Left to Right
Atrial septal defect (ASD)
Ventricular septal defect (VSD)
Persistent ductus arteriosus (PDA)
Anomalous pulmonary venous return
Aortopulmonary window
Coronary fistula
Surgical shunts

Right to Left
Tetralogy of Fallot
Pulmonary atresia
ASD or VSD with severe pulmonary hypertension

Bidirectional
ASD, VSD, or PDA with moderate pulmonary hypertension
Atrioventricular canal defects
Complex congenital heart disease

to systemic blood flow (Table 7). Step-ups of less than 5 to 7 per cent may reflect normal physiology and cannot be relied upon as evidence for a shunt (Table 2, Chapter 6-I). Right-to-left shunts result in mixing of desaturated (systemic venous or pulmonary arterial) with saturated (systemic arterial or pulmonary venous) blood on the left side of the circulation, creating an oxygen step-down and a decrease in pulmonary blood flow relative to systemic blood flow. Right-to-left shunting is implied by the presence of systemic arterial desaturation (arterial oxygen saturation below 95 per cent) without significant pulmonary disease. Administration of supplemental oxygen fails to correct desaturation due to shunting.

Complex congenital heart disease may result in bidirectional shunting characterized by an oxygen step-up between systemic venous and pulmonary arterial saturation, and a step-down between pulmonary venous and systemic arterial saturation.

CARDIAC ANGIOGRAPHY

Left Ventriculography

A contrast cineangiogram of the left ventricle is a routine part of most left heart catheterization studies (Table 8). The standard view for left ventriculography is 30-degree right anterior oblique (RAO), which projects the ventricle close to

TABLE 7. Calculation of Shunts

Left to right shunts:

$$Q_s = Q_p - Q_{sys}$$

$$\text{where } Q_p = \frac{O_2 \text{ consumption}}{(O_2 \text{ content Ao}) - (O_2 \text{ content PA})}$$

$$\text{and } Q_{sys} = \frac{O_2 \text{ consumption}}{(O_2 \text{ content Ao}) - (O_2 \text{ content MV})}$$

Mixed venous O_2 content is estimated from superior (SVC) and inferior vena caval (IVC) saturations as follows:

$$O_2 \text{ content MV} = \frac{1(O_2 \text{ content SVC}) + 2(O_2 \text{ content IVC})}{3}$$

Right to left shunts:

$$Q_s = Q_{sys} - Q_p$$

$$\text{where } Q_p = \frac{O_2 \text{ consumption}}{(O_2 \text{ content PV}) - (O_2 \text{ content PA})}$$

$$\text{and } Q_{sys} = \frac{O_2 \text{ consumption}}{(O_2 \text{ content Ao}) - (O_2 \text{ content PA})}$$

Ao, aorta; MV, mixed venous; PA, pulmonary artery; PV, pulmonary vein.

TABLE 8. Interpretation of the Left Ventriculogram

Chamber dimensions
Global systolic function (ejection fraction)
Segmental wall motion
Ventricular aneurysms and pseudoaneurysms
Mitral calcification, prolapse, or regurgitation
Aortic valve calcification and mobility
Ventricular septal defects
Mural thrombi

its long axis with the beam passing at right angles to the trabeculated muscular interventricular septum. The anterior, apical, and inferoposterior wall segments as well as the mitral anulus are therefore viewed tangentially. For assessment of septal and posterolateral wall motion, however, a 60-degree left anterior oblique (LAO) view, which projects the ventricle close to its short axis, is required. In order to fully define the anatomy of the ventricular septum and outflow tract, compound angulations are required.

Calculation of left ventricular volume is based on the modeling of left ventricular geometry as half a prolate ellipsoid (the shape produced by an ellipse rotated in space about its long axis). By planimetering the area (A, sq. cm.) of left ventricular images in RAO and LAO projections, left ventricular volume (V, ml.) can be calculated as follows:

$$V = \frac{8}{3\pi} \cdot \frac{A_{RAO}A_{LAO}}{L}$$

where L is the long axis of the ventricle (cm.).

By calculating left ventricular volume at end diastole (EDV) and end systole (ESV), the stroke volume and ejection fraction (EF) may be calculated.

$$EF = \frac{EDV - ESV}{EDV}$$

Left ventricular ejection fraction is a powerful predictor of prognosis in many cardiac diseases. Its limitations, however, should be recognized. The ejection fraction varies inversely with afterload and directly with preload. Thus, conditions that decrease afterload (i.e., mitral regurgitation, vasodilator therapy) or increase preload (i.e., aortic regurgitation, mitral regurgitation) may misleadingly normalize the ejection fraction despite important deterioration of ventricular function.

Valvular Regurgitation

Angiographic assessment of the severity of valvular regurgitation is an important factor in determining the need for surgical correction. Mitral regurgitation is assessed during left ventriculography. Aortic regurgitation is evaluated during aortography. Subjective grading of both mitral and aortic regurgitation is done on a 1+ to 4+ scale (Table 9).

TABLE 9. Grading of Valvular Regurgitation

Grade	Aortic Regurgitation*	Mitral Regurgitation†
1+	Small jet of contrast into LV that clears with each beat	Small jet of contrast into LA that clears with each beat
2+	Moderate opacification of LV but less than Ao; incomplete clearing with each beat	Moderate opacification of LA but less than LV; incomplete clearing with each beat
3+	Persistent marked opacification of LV, equal to Ao *after* 3 beats	Persistent marked opacification of LA, equal to LV after 3 beats
4+	Persistent marked opacification of LV, equal to Ao *within* 3 beats	Persistent marked opacification of LA, equal to LV within 3 beats; systolic reflux into pulmonary veins may be observed

LV, left ventricle; LA, left atrium; Ao, aorta.
*Assessed by aortography.
†Assessed by left ventriculography.

Coronary Angiography

An appreciation of three-dimensional coronary anatomy is helpful for performing or interpreting coronary angiograms. In approximately 85 per cent of individuals, the right coronary artery is said to be dominant. Dominance is assigned to the vessel traversing the posterior crux of the heart, thus giving rise to the posterior descending and atrioventricular nodal arteries. In about 10 per cent of individuals, these branches arise from the distal left circumflex artery, and the left coronary is therefore dominant. In the remaining 5 per cent, a codominant pattern exists in which one or two posterior descending arteries are supplied by both the right coronary and left circumflex arteries.

The purpose of coronary angiography is to demonstrate the severity and distribution of coronary stenoses. In order to accomplish this, each segment of the coronary tree should be demonstrated in at least two views. A simple and widely used convention for grading the severity of discrete coronary lesions compares the minimal luminal diameter of the lesion with that in an adjacent normal vessel. The degree of stenosis is expressed as percentage reduction of luminal diameter or cross-sectional area. This method provides a valuable although imperfect clinical guide to lesion severity.

Lesions characterized by multiple irregularities, overhanging edges, intraluminal filling defects, or persistent staining with contrast are more likely to be seen in the setting of unstable angina or after myocardial infarction. These changes are thought to represent plaque rupture or ulceration, and intraluminal thrombus.

The most common convention for describing the extent of coronary disease is to categorize patients according to the number of major coronary vessels (left anterior descending, left circumflex, right coronary, or their large branches) containing a stenosis of greater than 50 per cent. In a large study of coronary bypass surgery, 5-year mortality of medically treated patients ranged nearly threefold, depending on the presence of single-, double-, or triple-vessel disease at the time of index angiography. Patients with left main coronary stenosis are at highest risk.

Categorizing the distribution of coronary disease is central to predicting whether bypass surgery will improve prognosis. Patients with left main coronary obstruction enjoy longer survival regardless of symptoms. The benefit is greatest in those with severe left main coronary artery stenosis and those with coincident ventricular dysfunction. Patients with triple-vessel disease and moderate left ventricular dysfunction or severe ischemia also live longer after bypass surgery.

When surgical revascularization is being considered, interpretation of the coronary angiogram must include an assessment of the distal coronary bed. Grafting to small (less than 1.5 mm.) or diffusely diseased distal vessels is less likely to result in long-term graft patency.

II

Cardiac Arrest
Louis A. Brunsting, M.D.

Sudden cardiac death represents an unexpected circulatory arrest from cardiac causes with no antecedent symptoms or with symptoms of less than 1 hour in duration. In the United States, approximately 400,000 people die of cardiac arrest each year. Sudden death is the initial clinical manifestation of symptomatic coronary atherosclerosis in 20 to 25 per cent of patients. It has been demonstrated that immediate institution of cardiopulmonary resuscitation (CPR) and defibrillation at the scene of the arrest successfully resuscitates over 40 per cent of out-of-hospital arrest victims with ventricular fibrillation, potentially saving 100,000 lives annually.

HISTORICAL DEVELOPMENT

Early reports of CPR include Sherwin's suggestion in 1786 that "the surgeon should go on inflating the lungs and alternately compressing the sternum." Ingelsrud introduced open-chest cardiac massage in 1901, which became the stan-

See the corresponding chapter or part in the *Textbook of Surgery*, 14th edition, pp. 1844–1850, for a more detailed discussion of this topic, including a comprehensive list of references.

dard of practice during the next 60 years. Wiggers investigated the physiology of ventricular fibrillation in dogs in the 1930s and 1940s. His student Claude Beck first successfully applied internal cardioversion in man in 1947. In 1956, Zoll demonstrated the possibility of external cardioversion. The American Heart Association formed the Committee on Cardiopulmonary Resuscitation in 1963, which has provided continuing leadership in standardization and education.

ETIOLOGY

The etiologic factor of cardiac arrest may be cardiac, pulmonary, or metabolic. The most common cause is ventricular fibrillation from acute myocardial ischemia or infarction. Other cardiac causes include asystole, bradycardia, and recurrent ventricular tachycardia. Inadequate ventilation and gas exchange cause hypoxia, hypercarbia, and acidosis, which cause circulatory decompensation and ventricular fibrillation. Causes of acute pulmonary insufficiency are suffocation, drowning, drug overdose, foreign body aspiration, electrocution, and stroke. Metabolic causes of cardiac arrest include hyperkalemia, hypocalcemia, hypoglycemia, and metabolic acidosis.

BASIC LIFE SUPPORT

When cardiac arrest is diagnosed, a call for help is made and basic life support is initiated. First, patency of the airway is assessed. If obstruction exists, back blows and abdominal thrusts are applied in combination and the oropharynx is swept with a finger for clearance of any foreign object. Initial ventilation should be performed with a mask or mouth-to-mouth. Endotracheal intubation should be performed only when satisfactory mask ventilation has been established and trained personnel with appropriate equipment are present. With either mask or endotracheal ventilation, 100 per cent oxygen should be delivered at 12 breaths per minute.

Before chest compression is begun, especially in a witnessed arrest, a precordial thump is delivered in an attempt to restore cardiac rhythm. If it is not successful, external massage is initiated. The patient is placed supine in the horizontal position with a board or other rigid surface under the back to provide support. The heel of one hand is placed over the other, and force is applied rhythmically over the lower half of the sternum. The resuscitator's arms are locked at the elbows for transmission of the full momentum of the upper body to the patient's chest. The mechanism of effective external cardiac massage is transmission of energy to the circulatory system by direct cardiac compression. Compression of the ventricular chambers closes the mitral valve, opens the aortic valve, and produces unidirectional arterial flow and pressure. Cardiac stroke volume is optimized by compressions of high velocity, moderate force, and brief duration (high-impulse CPR). High-impulse CPR at a rate of 100 to 120 compressions per minute has been demonstrated to maximize cardiac output, brachiocephalic blood flow, coronary blood flow, and arterial pressure. The American Heart Association has changed its recommendation for adult chest compression from 60 to 100 compressions per minute.

In hospitalized arrest victims, external chest compression is occasionally unsuccessful. In this case, or if a diagnosis of pericardial tamponade is entertained, open-chest cardiac massage should be initiated through a left anterior thoracotomy. Cardiac output and diastolic coronary perfusion pressure are better with open chest massage. A compression rate of 60 to 80 per minute is recommended to allow adequate diastolic filling, as ventricular emptying is more efficient with open massage. Internal defibrillation, which is more effective than external, is also possible. If resuscitation is successful, chest closure is performed in the operating room.

ADVANCED LIFE SUPPORT

Cardiac arrest occurring in a hospital setting is treated with the techniques of advanced life support. While basic life support is initiated, an electrocardiographic tracing is obtained, often directly with the defibrillator paddles. If ventricular tachycardia or fibrillation is present, immediate cardioversion or defibrillation is performed with maximal energy (360 to 400 joules). Venous access, preferably via a central vein, is established for administration of sodium bicarbonate to reverse acidosis, cardiotonic agents such as epinephrine and calcium, and antiarrhythmic drugs such as lidocaine, procainamide, and bretylium. Arterial blood gas analysis allows accurate treatment of hypoxia, hypercapnia, and acidosis.

Cardiac arrest upon induction of anesthesia for noncardiac procedures is treated by resuscitation, termination of the procedure, and monitoring of the patient in an intensive care unit. For arrest during induction for cardiac procedures, the operation is initiated immediately and the patient placed on cardiopulmonary bypass as rapidly as possible. The cardiopulmonary bypass apparatus may be viewed as the ultimate in cardiopulmonary resuscitation.

MANAGEMENT AFTER RESUSCITATION

The two most critical factors determining the success of resuscitation are (1) the severity and reversibility of the patient's underlying disease and (2) the time from arrest to defibrillation. The likelihood of successful resuscitation diminishes with time, in part because CPR maintains only 25 to 40 per cent of the normal cardiac output. Therefore, the goal of every resuscitation should be to restore the patient's own cardiac function as quickly as possible. After successful resuscitation in any setting, appropriate evaluation and therapy of the underlying cause is essential. Patients with acute coronary syndromes should be stabilized, catheterized, and revascularized if possible for improving their survival and reducing the incidence of subsequent sudden death.

III

Penetrating Cardiac Injuries
Fred A. Crawford, Jr., M.D.

Although cardiac injuries have been described for thousands of years, the first successful repair was accomplished less than 100 years ago when Rehn (1896) successfully sutured a stab wound of the right ventricle. Subsequently, numerous series have documented the ability to successfully repair penetrating cardiac injuries. This is fortunate, since the incidence of such injuries has increased dramatically during the past several decades. Most penetrating cardiac injuries formerly were caused by stab wounds, but more recently there has been an increase in the frequency of injuries due to gunshot wounds. Penetrating cardiac injuries occur most often in the home (70 per cent) by a known assailant (83 per cent) and are due to domestic or social disputes (73 per cent). Victims are commonly male (83 per cent). Approximately 60 to 80 per cent of individuals with penetrating cardiac injuries die at the scene or before arrival at a trauma facility. Factors that influence mortality include, in order of decreasing significance, (1) coronary artery injury, (2) multiple chamber injury or isolated left atrial or left ventricular injury, (3) comminuted tear of a single chamber, (4) single right-sided chamber injury, and (5) tangential injuries that do not penetrate the endocardium.

DIAGNOSIS. Any patient with a penetrating injury to the chest, neck, upper abdomen, or back should be suspected of having a cardiac injury. The right ventricle is the most common chamber injured, followed by the left ventricle, right atrium, left atrium, and great vessels.

Patients with penetrating cardiac injuries present with cardiac tamponade or in hemorrhagic shock. Stab wounds to the heart may bleed a small amount and seal spontaneously, but if bleeding is significant, cardiac tamponade may develop. A relatively small amount of blood in the pericardium can produce acute cardiac tamponade because of the nondistensibility of the intact pericardium. These patients may present with classic findings of tamponade including hypotension, elevated venous pressure (distended neck veins), and decreased heart sounds. If the blood loss from the cardiac injury or from other injuries is significant, the neck veins may not be distended, and the findings of tamponade are not so apparent. When hypotension and distended neck veins are present in a cooperative patient with a penetrating chest wound, some degree of cardiac injury must be assumed, but the absence of classic findings of tamponade does not exclude a cardiac injury.

The chest film is generally of little help in making the diagnosis. Likewise, an electrocardiogram is rarely useful

---

See the corresponding chapter or part in the *Textbook of Surgery*, 14th edition, pp. 1851–1855, for a more detailed discussion of this topic, including a comprehensive list of references.

unless obvious ischemic changes suggest a coronary artery injury. Echocardiography may be helpful, particularly in detecting an intracardiac shunt, but may not be available at the time these patients present, and this study may be difficult to perform in uncooperative patients. Pericardiocentesis is a somewhat difficult technical procedure, especially in an uncooperative patient, and both false-negative and false-positive diagnoses are reported. However, the removal of a small amount of blood from the pericardial space in a patient with acute pericardial tamponade can provide significant hemodynamic improvement, but this is most often transient in nature. Some have advocated a subxyphoid pericardial window, and if this is performed, the surgeon must be ready to proceed immediately to a thoracotomy should a cardiac injury exist.

If the cardiac injury is large, either secondary to a stab wound or more commonly from a gunshot wound, cardiac tamponade is uncommon and the mode of presentation is most frequently that of hemorrhagic shock. Thus, the diagnosis of significant cardiac injury should be suspected in any patient with evidence of penetrating injury to the chest, obvious bleeding, and profound hypotension.

TREATMENT. Patients with penetrating chest trauma should undergo standard initial resuscitative measures including airway control, insertion of large intravenous lines, and fluid replacement. When the patient is stable and the diagnosis of cardiac injury is strongly suspected, thoracotomy with prompt repair of the injury is indicated. Although conservative management (pericardiocentesis and observation) has been advocated by some, most agree now that all such patients should undergo prompt operative intervention. Emergency room thoracotomy has been advocated for those patients who present in extremis or who deteriorate rapidly following arrival in the emergency room. A significant number of these individuals may be salvaged by prompt thoracotomy, and complications are relatively uncommon.

Penetrating cardiac injuries may be approached through either a left anterior thoracotomy or a median sternotomy incision. The left anterior thoracotomy requires no special equipment and is more easily performed in the emergency room than is a sternotomy. However, most current operative procedures on the heart employ a median sternotomy incision, and this is the author's preferred approach when time permits. Cardiopulmonary bypass is rarely necessary but should be available if needed.

When the pericardium is opened and blood evacuated, the point of injury can usually be controlled with digital pressure and the laceration or defect closed with several interrupted sutures. Injuries to the atrium or great vessels may be similarly repaired or may be repaired after a tangential side-binding clamp has been applied. Injuries adjacent to coronary arteries can usually be repaired by placing the sutures such that flow through the arteries is not compromised. Injuries to distal small branches of the coronary artery can be repaired by ligating the coronary artery, but proximal coronary artery injuries should be repaired or the vessel should be bypassed with a saphenous vein or internal mammary artery.

Penetrating cardiac wounds may also cause injury to valves and the development of intracardiac or extracardiac shunts in as many as 5 per cent of patients. Most commonly the shunt occurs between the left and right ventricles (ventricular septal defect), but it may also occur between the atria, or between other great vessels or cardiac chambers. Such fistulas are usually small and rarely appreciated on initial examination in the emergency facility. When they are suspected, intraoperative echocardiography may be useful in making the definitive diagnosis, but rarely is it necessary to repair them at the time of initial operation. Careful repeated physical examinations are required following operation in order to detect any residual defects, and these examinations should be supplemented with thorough echocardiographic studies if a residual defect is suspected. Tiny residual defects or insignificant shunts may be left alone and may close spontaneously, but larger shunts (greater than 1.5:1 left-to-right) may require reoperation for closure of the shunt.

In gunshot wounds to the heart, foreign bodies may be retained in the pericardium, in the wall of the heart, or in a cardiac chamber. Indications for operative removal of such retained fragments include (1) large vessels, (2) symptomatic patients, and (3) intracardiac location, especially left side. It is clear that not all retained missiles in or around the heart require removal, and thus these patients must be individualized.

Although the majority of the patients who sustain penetrating cardiac injuries die at the scene or before arrival at a treatment facility, some who arrive in extremis and without vital signs survive, and for those in whom vital signs are present on arrival in the emergency room, survival of 60 to 70 per cent can be expected.

IV

Patent Ductus Arteriosus, Coarctation of the Aorta, and Anomalies of the Aortic Arch

J. William Gaynor, M.D.

PATENT DUCTUS ARTERIOSUS

The ductus arteriosus is a fetal structure derived from the left sixth aortic arch. The ductus extends from the main or

See the corresponding chapter or part in the *Textbook of Surgery*, 14th edition, pp. 1855–1872, for a more detailed discussion of this topic, including a comprehensive list of references.

left pulmonary artery to the descending aorta, inserting just distal to the origin of the left subclavian artery. The size of the ductus is variable, and the aortic orifice is generally larger than the pulmonary orifice. *In utero,* most of the blood ejected by the right ventricle bypasses the high-resistance pulmonary circuit and flows almost exclusively through the ductus to the lower extremities and the placenta. At birth, during the transition from the fetal to adult circulation, the lungs expand with the first breath, which decreases the pulmonary vascular resistance resulting in increased pulmonary blood flow and increasing arterial oxygen concentration. In normal, full-term neonates, functional closure of the ductus occurs in the first 10 to 15 hours of life as rising arterial oxygen tension causes constriction of muscle fibers in the wall. The ductal smooth muscle in premature infants is less sensitive to oxygen-induced constriction. Anatomic closure by fibrosis produces the ligamentum arteriosum, and closure is complete in 88 per cent of full-term newborns by the age of 8 weeks.

Prolonged patency of the ductus produces a left-to-right shunt with pulmonary congestion and left ventricular volume overload. The magnitude of the shunt depends on the size of the ductus. With a large, nonrestrictive ductus, the level of the pulmonary vascular resistance is important in determining the severity of shunting. Shunting occurs throughout systole and diastole, with production of diastolic hypotension and possibly impaired systemic perfusion. Isolated patent ductus arteriosus (PDA) occurs approximately once in every 2500 to 5000 live births. The incidence increases greatly with prematurity and with decreasing birth weight. The incidence may be greater than 80 per cent in infants weighing less than 1000 gm. at birth.

PDA is not a benign entity, although prolonged survival has been reported. In the preantibiotic era, 40 per cent of patients with PDA died of bacterial endocarditis, and most of the remainder died of congestive heart failure. Premature infants with PDA often have associated problems of prematurity that are aggravated by the left-to-right shunting and abnormal hemodynamics. In patients surviving to adulthood, severe pulmonary hypertension with reverse shunting through the ductus may develop.

The signs and symptoms of PDA depend on the size of the ductus, the pulmonary vascular resistance, the age at presentation, and associated anomalies. Full-term infants usually do not become symptomatic until the pulmonary vascular resistance decreases at 6 to 8 weeks of life, allowing a significant left-to-right shunt. Because premature infants have less smooth muscle in the pulmonary arterioles, vascular resistance decreases earlier, and symptoms may develop in the first week of life. A large, hemodynamically significant PDA usually presents in infancy with congestive heart failure. Afflicted infants are irritable, tachycardic, and tachypneic and take feedings poorly. The physical examination is almost diagnostic and reveals evidence of a hyperdynamic circulation with a hyperactive precordium and bounding peripheral pulses. The systolic blood pressure is usually normal, but diastolic hypotension may be present. Auscultation reveals a systolic or continuous murmur termed a machinery murmur, which is best heard in the pulmonic area and radiates toward the middle third of the clavicle. Absence of the characteristic murmur does not exclude the presence of a PDA, especially in premature infants. The chest roentgenogram may show cardiomegaly and pulmonary congestion. Two-dimensional and Doppler echocardiography can be used to demonstrate abnormal aortic flow patterns and can provide an estimate of the shunt magnitude. Formal cardiac catheterization is not required in children and young adults with classic findings and should be reserved for older patients or those with atypical findings, suspicion of associated anomalies, or pulmonary hypertension.

The presence of a persistent PDA in a child or adult is sufficient indication for surgical closure because of the increased mortality and risk of endocarditis. In symptomatic patients, closure should be performed when diagnosis is made. In asymptomatic children, intervention can be postponed if desired but should be done in the preschool years. Older patients should have the ductus closed when the diagnosis is made. If severe pulmonary hypertension has occurred with reversal of the ductal shunting, closure is associated with a higher mortality and may not improve symptoms.

When surgical therapy is indicated, either division or multiple suture ligation of the ductus via a left anterior or a posterior thoracotomy may be performed. In neonates, single or double ligation of the ductus is usually the procedure of choice. The calcified ductus in older patients presents a difficult surgical problem and may require the use of cardiopulmonary bypass. Recently there has been increasing interest in the nonoperative closure of PDA, and successful transcatheter techniques have been developed. However, these techniques are still investigational, and their role in the management of PDA has not been determined.

Management of PDA in premature infants is controversial. In infants with severe pulmonary disease, little or no improvement may follow closure of a PDA. A child with evidence of PDA and persistent congestive heart failure, continuing need for mechanical ventilation, or inability to receive adequate nutrition secondary to fluid restriction requires further intervention. Two therapeutic options for closure of PDA are available. Pharmacologic closure can be attempted with prostaglandin inhibitors such as indomethacin, which may be successful in more than 70 per cent of infants. Surgical closure of an isolated PDA is also an option. A recent study reported a 42 per cent failure rate with indomethacin in infants of very low birth weights and suggested that primary surgical closure remains more predictable with minimal morbidity.

Surgical closure of PDA has become a very safe procedure. Operative mortality approaches zero even in critically ill neonates. In premature infants, hospital mortality and long-term results depend primarily on associated pulmonary disease, coexistent anomalies, and the degree of prematurity. Mortality of PDA closure is increased and long-term results are poor in older patients with a calcified ductus and are poorest in those patients with severe pulmonary hypertension and reverse shunting. Most patients with PDA become functionally normal and have a normal life expectancy after closure.

COARCTATION OF THE AORTA

Coarctation of the aorta is a narrowing that diminishes the lumen and produces an obstruction to the flow of blood. The lesion may be a localized obstruction or a diffusely narrowed segment, which is termed *tubular hypoplasia*. Coarctation may occur at any site in the aorta, but the most common site is at the insertion of the ligamentum arteriosum. Externally there appears to be an obstructing indentation on the posterior wall of the aorta, whereas internally there is an infolding of the aortic media with a ridge of intimal hyperplasia.

Coarctation of the aorta represents 5 to 10 per cent of congenital heart disease, and the autopsy incidence is 1 per 3000 to 4000 autopsies. With isolated coarctation, males predominate, but there is no sex difference in patients with more complex lesions. Several anomalies occur commonly in patients with coarctation of the aorta: bicuspid aortic valve, ventricular septal defect, PDA, and various mitral valve disorders. The age of presentation and the mode of presentation depend on the location of the coarctation and the associated anomalies. When the obstruction is preductal, there is an increased incidence of other cardiac defects, and the patients usually present in infancy with congestive heart failure.

Preductal coarctation may not seriously alter the normal fetal circulation and therefore does not provide a stimulus to the development of collateral circulation *in utero*. Infants with severe narrowing may appear normal at birth and have palpable femoral pulses, if a PDA allows blood flow around the obstructing shelf. Significant aortic obstruction develops as the PDA closes. The infants are irritable, tachypneic, and uninterested in feeding. A systolic murmur may be present over the left precordium and posteriorly between the scapulae. Moderate upper extremity hypertension and an arm-leg pressure gradient are usually present even in neonates. These findings may be absent in critically ill infants with a low cardiac output. Hypotension, oliguria, and severe metabolic acidosis may be present in severely ill infants.

Older children and adults often present with unexplained headache, epistaxis, visual disturbances, hypertension, and exertional dyspnea. Some patients present with a cerebrovascular accident, aortic rupture, dissecting aneurysm, or bacterial endocarditis. Many cases are discovered during evaluation of hypertension or unexplained murmur heard on routine examination. Findings on physical examination include hypertension, a systolic pressure gradient between the arms and legs, a systolic murmur heard over the left precordium and posteriorly between the scapulae, and diminished or absent femoral pulses. An anterior diastolic murmur may indicate aortic regurgitation secondary to a bicuspid aortic valve. There may be evidence of collateral circulation in older children and adults involving branches of the subclavian arteries that are proximal to the obstruction.

The electrocardiogram in infancy may show right, left, or biventricular hypertrophy. In older children and adults, it may be normal or show evidence of left ventricular hypertrophy. A chest film may reveal rib notching secondary to the enlarged, tortuous intercostal vessels that are part of the collateral circulation. This finding is almost pathognomonic. Angiocardiography remains the most objective method of showing the coarctation and provides evidence of the location and extent of narrowing, the involvement of the great vessels, and associated anomalies. The pressure gradient can be measured, and associated cardiac defects can be evaluated. Two-dimensional echocardiography with spectral and color-flow Doppler echocardiography may show the site of obstruction, suggest or exclude associated anomalies, and provide an estimate of the arterial pressure gradient.

The natural history of untreated coarctation of the aorta depends on the age at presentation and associated anomalies. Symptomatic infants have a high mortality, depending on the severity of the coarctation and the presence of associated defects. Patients surviving until adulthood have a greatly diminished life expectancy. The most common causes of death in untreated coarctation are spontaneous rupture of the aorta, bacterial endocarditis, cerebral hemorrhage, and congestive heart failure.

The pathogenesis of hypertension in coarctation is multi-factorial, and the most prominent causes appear to be mechanical and renal factors. Scott and Bahnson were the first to definitively demonstrate the role of the kidneys in the pathogenesis of coarctation hypertension. In experimental coarctation, they found that hypertension could be eliminated by transplanting one kidney to the neck (proximal to the obstruction) with contralateral nephrectomy. It is thought that coarctation hypertension is a variant of the single-clip, single-kidney Goldblatt model, although other factors including abnormal rigidity of the prestenotic aortic wall and abnormal baroreceptor function have been demonstrated.

The presence of coarctation is generally sufficient indication for surgical correction. The major decisions are the timing and method of repair. Symptomatic infants usually require surgical intervention, although a few improve with conservative medical management. A major advance in the treatment of the critically ill neonates with coarctation has been the introduction of prostaglandin E_1 therapy. Infusion of prostaglandin E_1 can reopen and maintain patency of the ductus arteriosus in many neonates and allows perfusion of the lower body with correction of the metabolic acidosis and oliguria. Stabilization of these severely ill infants allows surgical correction to be accomplished under more optimal conditions.

The timing of elective repair of coarctation of the aorta is an important determinant of surgical outcome. Repair in late childhood or adulthood, although providing relief of some symptoms, has an increased incidence of persistent hypertension. Repair in infancy may cause a high incidence of residual or recurrent stenosis. The current trend is for elective repair at an early age, and many authors believe that repair should be undertaken at the time of diagnosis in symptomatic and asymptomatic infants to prevent the development of complications. Others prefer elective repair in asymptomatic children at the age of 1 to 6 years to decrease the recoarctation rate.

Three surgical techniques have been developed for repair of coarctation of the aorta. The classic method of repair used by Crafoord and by Gross is resection of the area of obstruction with primary end-to-end anastomosis. Advantages of the classic repair include complete resection of the abnormal tissue, preservation of normal vascular anatomy, and no requirement for prosthetic material.

Because of early unsatisfactory results with resection with primary anastomosis, other techniques of repair were developed. In the prosthetic patch aortoplasty, the area of constriction is incised, and a prosthetic patch is used to enlarge the lumen. Advantages of this technique include decreased operative time, decreased dissection, maximal augmentation of the area of stenosis, preservation of the collateral vessels, and no need for sacrifice of normal vascular structures. However, the use of prosthetic material may predispose to infection, and there are increasingly frequent reports of the formation of aneurysms and pseudoaneurysms. The subclavian flap aortoplasty was introduced by Waldhausen and Nahrwold in 1966. The subclavian artery is ligated, incised, and turned down as a flap for enlarging the area of constriction. Advantages include avoidance of prosthetic material, decreased dissection, decreased aortic cross-clamp time, and increased anastomotic growth since there is no circumferential suture line.

Correction of coarctation may be complicated by hemorrhage, chylothorax, recurrent nerve paralysis, infection, and suture line thrombosis. Postoperative paradoxical elevation of the blood pressure to greater than preoperative levels may occur. This paradoxical hypertension may be associated with the postcoarctectomy syndrome of abdominal pain and distention. The most dreaded complication of coarctation repair is paraplegia, which occurs in 0.3 to 1 per cent of patients. Variations in the blood supply to the anterior spinal cord, poor collateral formation, anomalous origin of the right subclavian artery, distal hypotension during the period of aortic cross-clamping, and reoperation all may predispose to paraplegia. Outcome after surgical correction depends on the age at the time of operation, the method of operation chosen, and, especially, the presence of associated anomalies. The optimal management of associated anomalies remains controversial. PDA is frequently present and should be divided or ligated. Appropriate management of an associated ventricular septal defect is unclear, since many are of a type with a high incidence of spontaneous closure. Many infants improve sufficiently after repair of the coarctation to allow elective repair at a later date if the ventricular septal defect fails to close. Other options include pulmonary artery banding or primary repair of the ventricular septal defect at the time of coarctation repair.

Recoarctation usually manifests itself as a persistent hypertension or arm-leg pressure gradient. Some patients are normotensive at rest and develop severe hypertension with an arm-leg pressure gradient following exercise. Reoperation is indicated if significant hypertension or other symptoms occur and a pressure gradient can be demonstrated. Reoperation is more difficult secondary to scarring and is associated with a higher morbidity and mortality.

Percutaneous transluminal angioplasty has been introduced as an alternative therapy for native and recurrent coarctation. The initial results were encouraging; however, aneurysmal dilation following balloon angioplasty of native coarctation has been reported. Balloon dilation of recurrent coarctation has been successful, and there have been fewer reports of aneurysm formation. The long-term results of balloon angioplasty of coarctation in terms of restenosis and aneurysm formation are unknown, and the technique must be considered investigational.

Some patients who have had a technically excellent repair may not have complete resolution of the hypertension. The cause of this persistent hypertension is unclear, but it is related to the age at repair and the duration of the preoperative hypertension. Follow-up of surgical patients indicates that they are not rendered entirely normal. There is an increase in premature death rates, which is related to cardiovascular disease. Aortic stenosis or regurgitation secondary to a bicuspid aortic valve may develop and necessitate valve replacement. As has been emphasized, the long-term prognosis of many patients is determined primarily by the presence or absence of associated anomalies.

ANOMALIES OF THE AORTIC ARCH

Vascular rings are developmental anomalies of the aorta and great vessels that encircle and may constrict the esophagus and trachea. The natural history of vascular rings is obscured by the wide spectrum of anomalies and range of symptoms. Vascular rings should be suspected in any infant with stridor, dysphagia, recurrent respiratory tract infections, difficulty in feeding, or failure to thrive. Vascular rings are not necessarily inconsistent with prolonged survival. Infants with symptomatic rings most commonly present with respiratory difficulties, tachypnea, stridor exacerbated by feeding, and recurrent respiratory infection. The physical examination is usually nondiagnostic. The chest roentgenogram may be normal or show pneumonia or, occasionally, compression of the air-filled trachea. A right aortic arch is seen in some anomalies. The barium esophagogram is the most valuable study for evaluation of patients with a suspected vascular ring. The combination of posterior compression of the esophagus with anterior tracheal compression is diagnostic of a vascular ring.

Although a few patients with symptomatic constricting vascular rings improve as they grow, the long-term prognosis of the medical therapy is poor. Despite the wide spectrum of anomalies, the principles of surgical therapy are simple. Surgical intervention should be undertaken at the time of diagnosis and is designed to divide the vascular ring, relieve the constriction, and preserve circulation to the aortic branches.

The most common anomaly producing a true vascular ring is persistence of the right and left fourth aortic arches with formation of a *double aortic arch.* The right or posterior arch is usually larger, and there is usually a left descending aorta and a left ductus arteriosus. The right carotid and subclavian arteries arise from the right arch, and the left carotid and subclavian arteries arise from the left arch. Patients with double aortic arch are usually symptomatic in early infancy. The diagnosis of double aortic arch can easily be made from the barium esophagogram. Surgical intervention is indicated at the time of diagnosis. In the usual situation, a left thoracotomy is done, and the smaller anterior arch is divided at its junction with the descending aorta so that the left carotid and subclavian arteries arise from the ascending aorta.

Aberrant origin of the right subclavian artery is a very common anomaly but rarely causes symptoms. This defect is due to regression of the right fourth aortic arch between the carotid and subclavian arteries rather than distal to the subclavian. The anomalous artery most often courses posterior to the esophagus but may pass between the trachea and esophagus or anterior to the trachea. Anomalous origin of the right subclavian artery is not a true vascular ring. However, the aberrant artery may compress the esophagus, causing dysphagia (dysphagia lusoria). The diagnosis of aberrant origin of the right subclavian artery can be made by a barium esophagogram. In children, the artery may be simply ligated and divided without sequelae. In adults, division with anastomosis to the ascending aorta is usually necessary.

Pulmonary artery sling is a rare cardiac anomaly occurring when the left pulmonary artery arises from the right pulmonary artery and courses between the trachea and esophagus, but it is not a true vascular ring. Compression of the distal trachea and main stem bronchi may occur. Tracheal stenosis with complete cartilaginous rings and absence of the membranous portion of the trachea is frequently associated with pulmonary artery sling. Infants with pulmonary artery sling often present with respiratory symptoms at birth, and most are symptomatic by 1 month of age. The physical examination is not helpful in the diagnosis. A barium esophagogram may show anterior pulsatile compression of the esophagus. Bronchoscopy is particularly useful in these patients for evaluation of associated tracheobronchial anomalies. Surgical intervention is indicated in any patient with pulmonary artery sling and symptoms of significant respiratory obstruction. The recommended procedure is division of the anomalous artery with anastomosis to the main pulmonary artery anterior to the trachea. Mortality is usually related to the severity of the tracheobronchial stenosis and associated defects. Survivors generally have a benign course, although occlusion of the left pulmonary artery may occur.

The results of surgical therapy in infants with vascular rings are good in terms of both survival and relief of symptoms. Operative mortality is low but not zero. Postoperative morbidity is often related to tracheomalacia following vascular compression and to associated anomalies.

V

Atrial Septal Defects, Ostium Primum Defects, and Atrioventricular Canals

Ross M. Ungerleider, M.D.

An atrial septal defect (ASD) is a defect in the atrial septum that enables mixing of blood from the systemic and pulmonary venous circulations. These defects may develop in a number of locations that relate to the formation of the intra-atrial septation, and the embryology of this region should be carefully reviewed. The most common ASDs are (1) *secundum*, (2) *sinus venosus*, and (3) *ostium primum*. ASDs can occur in other locations, such as around the coronary sinus, but are quite unusual and are not discussed in this chapter.

Secundum ASDs occur in the fossa ovalis and develop owing to a deficiency of septum primum tissue or lack of fusion between the septum primum and the limbus of the septum secundum. These defects are clearly in the wall between the two atria and can range in size from a small patent foramen to a large defect that has the appearance of a common atrium. The lower boundary can extend inferiorly toward the eustachian valve of the inferior vena cava and superiorly to the superior limbus of the septum secundum. These are the most common ASDs and can be observed in association with almost any other type of cardiac anomaly. Approximately 30 per cent of secundum ASDs occur with other cardiac defects. Moreover, intra-atrial communication at the level of the foramen ovale is essential for survival in certain forms of congenital heart disease, such as tricuspid atresia or total anomalous pulmonary venous return. In addition, enlargement of a defect at this location is a common palliative maneuver for patients with transposition of the great arteries (Rashkind balloon septostomy) to allow mixing of blood at the atrial level. Secundum ASDs occur more

---

See the corresponding chapter or part in the *Textbook of Surgery,* 14th edition, pp. 1873–1892, for a more detailed discussion of this topic, including a comprehensive list of references.

frequently in females than in males with a ratio of 3:1. Familial inheritance on the basis of a dominant autosomal gene with incomplete penetrance has been reported and may help to explain the appearance of ASDs of the secundum type within a family lineage. Nevertheless, most secundum ASDs are caused by unknown and random disturbances in development.

Sinus venosus defects are less common than are secundum defects and represent about 10 per cent of ASDs. Sinus venosus ASDs are commonly associated with partial anomalous pulmonary venous return, especially of the right superior pulmonary veins draining into the lateral aspect of the superior vena cava. These defects occur high in the atrial septum and actually represent a deficiency between the posterior wall of the superior vena cava and the anterior wall of the left atrium. In part because of the commonly associated anomalous pulmonary venous return, the left-to-right shunt across these defects can be quite large.

Ostium primum ASDs are located at the anulus of the tricuspid and mitral valves and represent a defect in endocardial cushion formation. This region of the atrium, referred to as the triangle of Koch, marks the location of the atrioventricular (AV) node and corresponds to the septation between the left ventricle and the right atrium. In this respect, this small region is referred to as the atrioventricular septum, and defects in this location are referred to as atrioventricular septal defects. An ostium primum ASD is a defect of the atrioventricular septum of the "partial" type so that an intracardiac communication exists only at the intra-atrial level. This is an ostium primum ASD, and because the endocardial cushions are involved in the formation of the mitral and tricuspid valves, these defects are often associated with a "cleft" in these valves, especially of the anterior leaflet of the mitral valve. When deficiency also occurs in the ventricular septum, the resulting defect is a "complete" atrioventricular septal defect or complete AV canal, which causes both an intra-atrial and intraventricular communication with a common AV valve that bridges the defect. Both partial and complete AV canal defects are sometimes found in association with more complex and severe forms of congenital heart disease. It is not uncommon for these patients to also have a small secundum type ASD as well as a patent ductus arteriosus. Some form of this defect may be present in as many as 30 per cent of children with Down's syndrome.

NATURAL HISTORY. The natural history of an ASD is related to the type of defect and any other associated anomalies. Most secundum ASDs can exist for years without recognition and constitute one of the more common congenital heart defects that present initially in adulthood. Similarly, sinus venosus defects with partial anomalous pulmonary venous return are also frequently first recognized in late childhood or early adulthood. AV canal defects, because of the degree of physiologic shunting involved, are usually detected at an earlier age. Despite the relatively benign nature of most of these defects, long-term survival of patients with an ASD compared with age-matched controls is diminished, becoming significant by the time these patients reach the third and fourth decades of life. Long-term complications attributable to ASDs include the development of progressive congestive heart failure and atrial arrhythmias. In addition, the potential for paradoxical embolization is always present in patients with these defects. Pulmonary hypertension is reported but unusual as a late development in these patients. The functional status of patients with ASDs deteriorates with age so that concomitant with the decline of life expectancy, patients experience increasing symptoms of easy fatigability, exercise intolerance, and palpitations. Patients with complete AV canal defects have a much more malignant natural history with 80 per cent of unoperated patients dying by age 2 years. Those patients who survive often do so because of the development of pulmonary hypertension with progression to inoperability at an early age.

PHYSIOLOGY. The direction of an intracardiac shunt is toward the most compliant downstream chamber. When the defect occurs at the level of the atrial septum, the compliance of the right and left ventricles dictates the amount and direction of shunt flow. The size of the ASD itself is not a factor as long as the defect is large enough to be unrestrictive to flow. Most atrial level shunts are in the left-to-right direction, since the right ventricle is more compliant (distensible) and offers less resistance to being filled with increasing volume during diastole. Shunt flow across an ASD can be in a right-to-left direction, especially as right ventricular compliance diminishes, such as is common if the ventricle hypertrophies in response to pulmonary stenosis. The impact of left-to-right shunting is increased flow through the lungs and a tendency for these patients to have frequent pulmonary infections. Patients who have right-to-left shunting present with cyanosis. If the cyanosis is a reflection of right-to-left shunting due to pulmonary hypertension, it may be a sign that the patient's defect is no longer surgically correctable. Patients with partial (ostium primum) and complete AV canal defects may also have mitral regurgitation that impacts on the physiology of their lesion.

PHYSICAL FINDINGS AND DIAGNOSIS. Patients with ASDs may have few physical findings. If the left-to-right shunt is greater than 1.8:1, there may be a visible left parasternal heave with a palpable right ventricular lift. Auscultation reveals prominence of the first heart sound with fixed splitting of the second heart sound. A soft systolic ejection murmur is present in the second or third left intercostal space, and a mid-diastolic tricuspid flow rumble may also be audible in the fourth or fifth left intercostal space. A chest film shows mild to moderate cardiomegaly and prominence of a pulmonary artery shadow. In addition, there are increased pulmonary vascular markings. Patients with partial and complete AV canal defects may have cardiomegaly of a more pronounced degree due to the mitral insufficiency. An electrocardiogram usually shows an incomplete right bundle branch block in lead V_1 for patients with secundum level defects, whereas patients with ostium primum defects show left axis deviation. Diagnosis is usually confirmed by two-dimensional echocardiography with color-flow mapping. This technology can also provide excellent information about the AV valves. Cardiac catheterization is rarely necessary for patients with secundum or sinus venosus defects and is usually necessary in complete AV canal defects when there is a concern about pulmonary artery hypertension. Patients with pulmonary vascular resistance greater than 12 units per sq. m. are considered to be inoperable. If the pulmonary vascular resistance is less than 6 units, the patient can usually be safely corrected.

TREATMENT. Spontaneous closure of ASDs may occur early in life but is unusual after the first year of life. It is also unlikely to occur in patients with hemodynamically significant shunts that produce right ventricular enlargement and symptoms. The safety of modern cardiopulmonary bypass techniques has enabled most ASDs to be approached and repaired with a low mortality and morbidity. Secundum defects can be closed primarily or with a patch of pericardial or prosthetic material. Sinus venosus defects are usually closed with use of a patch for redirection of the anomalous pulmonary venous return toward the left atrium. Ostium primum defects also require a patch as well as repair of the involved AV valves. This usually entails repair of a "cleft" in the mitral valve. The adequacy of the surgical repair can be evaluated by use of intraoperative color-flow Doppler. Operative mortality for closure of uncomplicated secundum and sinus venosus ASDs approaches zero and should be no greater than 1 to 2 per cent even in older patients. Long-term results are very good with survival statistics comparing with those of normal age-matched controls, especially if the repair is undertaken before age 5 years. Outcome is less predictable if the repair is delayed past 60 years of age. Repair of AV canal defects has a somewhat higher risk, but uncomplicated partial AV canal defects should have a mortality near zero. Mortality for repair of complete AV canal defects is highly inconsistent because of the wide variation and anatomic patterns with this anomaly but should be 5 to 13 per cent. This risk is influenced by the nature of the common AV valve and the adequacy of the right and left ventricles. The long-term outcome for patients after repair of AV canal defects is also related to the degree of defect as well as to other anomalies but in appropriately selected cases can be very good.

VI

Disorders of Pulmonary Venous Return

Richard A. Jonas, M.D., and Aldo R. Castaneda, M.D.

Abnormalities of pulmonary venous return are most commonly due to anomalous connection of the pulmonary veins, which can involve all pulmonary veins (i.e., total anomalous pulmonary venous connection) or fewer pulmonary veins (partial anomalous pulmonary venous connection). A critical determinant of the hemodynamic consequences of anomalous pulmonary venous connection is the presence of obstruction within the pulmonary venous pathway. Rarely, pulmonary venous obstruction can occur despite normal connection of the pulmonary veins to the left atrium, in the form of individual pulmonary vein stenosis or owing to an obstructive membrane within the left atrium, *cor triatriatum.*

TOTAL ANOMALOUS PULMONARY VENOUS CONNECTION

Total anomalous pulmonary venous connection (TAPVC) is relatively rare, representing 2.5 per cent of all cases of congenital heart disease. The anomaly is due to failure of the pulmonary vein evagination from the posterior surface of the left atrium to fuse with the pulmonary plexus of veins surrounding the lung buds. A connection persists between the pulmonary plexus and the primitive systemic venous plexus. A common classification of TAPVC is as follows: supracardiac: 45 per cent of cases connect to a left ascending vertical vein to the innominate vein (occasionally to the right superior vena cava); cardiac: 25 per cent of cases connect to the coronary sinus (occasionally directly to the right atrium); infracardiac: 25 per cent of cases connect to the intra-abdominal vein; mixed: 5 per cent of cases.

Severe obstruction to pulmonary venous return is very common with infracardiac TAPVC but is rare with other forms. Patients with obstruction present in early infancy with failure to thrive and respiratory distress; if obstruction is particularly severe, neonates may present with severe hypoxia, acidosis, and circulatory collapse. *Diagnosis* is established by a pattern of desaturation on arterial blood gas analysis with the chest film revealing a normal cardiac silhouette and pulmonary edema. Two-dimensional echocardiography accurately defines the anomalous connection and provides an estimate of right ventricular pressure. Cardiac catheterization is best avoided, since the osmotic load of angiographic dye as well as the invasive intracardiac manipulations can further compromise the seriously ill child. The

---

See the corresponding chapter or part in the *Textbook of Surgery,* 14th edition, pp. 1892–1898, for a more detailed discussion of this topic, including a comprehensive list of references.

child with no pulmonary venous obstruction may be asymptomatic for many years.

MANAGEMENT OF TAPVC

Obstructed TAPVC. There is no medical palliation; therefore, urgent surgical correction should be undertaken. Deep hypothermic circulatory arrest provides optimal exposure as well as cerebral and myocardial protection. The descending vertical vein is ligated and divided at the diaphragm. It is filleted open and anastomosed to a parallel vertical incision in the posterior wall of the left atrium.

Intensive Care Management. Careful monitoring of pulmonary artery pressure in the early postoperative period is essential. Pulmonary vasoreactivity can be minimized with use of a fentanyl infusion with pancuronium boluses, thereby avoiding pulmonary hypertensive crises in response to stress such as endotracheal tube suctioning. Pulmonary resistance should be minimized by appropriate ventilatory management.

Nonobstructed TAPVC. This is generally best repaired during infancy at a convenient elective time. For supracardiac TAPVC, the anomalous vertical vein is ligated and a direct anastomosis made between the horizontal pulmonary venous confluence and the posterior wall of the left atrium. For cardiac TAPVC to the coronary sinus, the coronary sinus is unroofed into the left atrium. The resultant atrial septal defect is closed with a pericardial patch.

RESULTS. Surgical results even for very ill neonates with severe obstruction have dramatically improved over the last 3 decades. Currently, the overall risk for surgical repair is less than 10 per cent. For patients repaired electively, the risk of mortality is low, being less than 2 per cent. Late pulmonary vein stenosis is a process of fibrous intimal hyperplasia that can cause progressive pulmonary vein stenosis following repair of TAPVC, usually obstructed infradiaphragmatic TAPVC. Management, either surgically or by balloon dilation, is rarely successful.

PARTIAL ANOMALOUS PULMONARY VENOUS CONNECTION

The right pulmonary veins are most commonly involved, either in association with a sinus venosus atrial septal defect (usually right upper and right middle lobe pulmonary veins draining to the superior vena cava) or as part of the scimitar syndrome in which the right pulmonary veins drain through a curved descending vertical vein to the inferior vena cava–right atrium junction.

The hemodynamic impact of partial anomalous pulmonary venous connection is generally no more than that of a left-to-right shunt at atrial level. Thus, most children can remain asymptomatic for many years. Repair can be undertaken electively during the preschool years.

MANAGEMENT. The pulmonary venous blood from the anomalously connected veins is baffled through the associated atrial septal defect to the left atrium by use of a pericardial patch baffle. Care must be taken to avoid caval obstruction by the baffle. Where the anomalous veins enter very high in the superior vena cava, an alternative procedure involving division of the superior vena cava can be employed.

COR TRIATRIATUM

Cor triatriatum is a very rare anomaly related to TAPVC. Although pulmonary venous blood drains appropriately to the left atrium, there is obstruction at the point of connection. There is an upper common pulmonary vein chamber that receives the pulmonary veins and a lower left atrial chamber including the left atrial appendage. The foramen ovale is generally present between the right atrium and common pulmonary vein chamber. The diameter of the orifice in the fibrous membrane that separates the upper and lower chambers determines the degree of pulmonary venous obstruction and thus the timing and mode of presentation.

MANAGEMENT. Cor triatriatum is amenable to surgical correction. Under conditions of either deep hypothermic circulatory arrest in the infant or cardiopulmonary bypass in the older child, the obstructive membrane is completely excised. Early and late mortality approach zero.

PULMONARY VEIN STENOSIS

Pulmonary vein stenosis is also an extremely rare anomaly that has a dismal prognosis, with or without surgical management. The anomaly is generally fibrous intimal hyperplasia, which most commonly affects the point of junction between the pulmonary veins and left atrium but can progress to complete obliteration of the veins. Diagnosis is generally made in infancy when the child presents with respiratory distress and failure to thrive.

MANAGEMENT. Numerous surgical procedures have been attempted, but success has been rare. Although early survival can be achieved, there is often inexorable progression of the disease process.

VII

Ventricular Septal Defects
Albert D. Pacifico, M.D., John W. Kirklin, M.D., and James K. Kirklin, M.D.

Ventricular septal defect (VSD), in its isolated form, is the most common congenital cardiac lesion and represents 30 to

See the corresponding chapter or part in the *Textbook of Surgery*, 14th edition, pp. 1898–1909, for a more detailed discussion of this topic, including a comprehensive list of references.

40 per cent of all congenital heart disease at birth. Initially, it was surgically managed by banding the pulmonary artery; subsequently it was repaired in 1954 by use of controlled cross-circulation with an adult human being as the oxygenator, and in 1955 by use of a pump oxygenator for cardiopulmonary support.

ANATOMIC ASPECTS. The interventricular septum can be divided into a fibrous component, termed the membranous septum, and three muscular components, the inlet septum, the apical trabecular septum, and the outlet (or infundibular) septum. The tricuspid and mitral valves in the normal heart are attached to the ventricular septum at different levels so that the tricuspid valve attachment is apically displaced compared with that of the mitral valve. The intervening portion of the ventricular septum separating the left ventricle from the right atrium is termed the atrioventricular septum. It has a fibrous component anteriorly and a muscular component posteriorly. VSDs can have a partially fibrous rim or be completely surrounded by muscle. Defects with a partly fibrous rim are termed perimembranous when they are in the general area of the membranous septum, or subarterial infundibular defects when either the aortic or pulmonary valve forms part of the rim of the defect within the infundibular or outlet septum. The atrioventricular canal type of VSD is a perimembranous defect that extends into the inlet septum with the septal leaflet of the tricuspid valve forming its rightward border. Perimembranous defects are related to the anteroseptal commissure of the tricuspid valve and also to the aortic valve. The anulus of these valves often forms part of the rim of the defect but sometimes is separated from the VSD by a thin rim of muscular tissue.

Muscular defects are completely surrounded by muscular tissue and may be located in the infundibular, trabecular, or inlet portions of the ventricular septum. Most are located in the trabecular portion of the ventricular septum where they may be single or multiple. Most multiple defects are located in the anterior portion of the trabecular septum.

About 10 per cent of VSDs are located in the infundibulum or outlet septum. When the aortic and/or pulmonary valve anuli form part of the rim of the defect, they are termed subarterial and form the majority of defects in this location. Less commonly, defects in the infundibular septum may be completely surrounded by muscle and are infundibular muscular defects. Classification of VSDs according to size is arbitrary, but a large VSD is approximately the size of the aortic orifice or larger and is nonrestrictive, causing systemic–right ventricular pressure. Small defects have insufficient size to raise right ventricular systolic pressure, and the pulmonary:systemic flow ratio ($Q_p:Q_s$) does not increase above 1.75. Moderate-sized VSDs are "restrictive" but have sufficient size to raise the right ventricular systolic pressure to approximately half of the left ventricular pressure and may produce a $Q_p:Q_s$ of 2:3.5. Coexistent associated cardiac defects are present in about 50 per cent of patients undergoing surgical treatment for primary VSD. These include patent ductus arteriosus, coarctation of the aorta, valvular or subvalvular aortic or pulmonary stenosis, and congenital mitral valve disease.

PATHOPHYSIOLOGY. The direction and size of the shunt in patients with VSD depend on the size of the defect and the differences in pressure between the ventricles during systole and diastole as well as the relative compliance of each ventricle and the relative resistance to ejection offered by the systemic and pulmonary vasculature. Large defects offer little resistance to flow, and similar peak pressures are present in both the left and right ventricles. Small defects are restrictive, producing higher pressure in the left ventricle than in the right ventricle. When a left-to-right shunt is present at the ventricular level, pulmonary blood flow is increased above normal and above systemic blood flow. Flow through the left atrium and mitral valve orifice is increased, and more work is done by both the left and right ventricles. In the absence of a large atrial septal defect, the left atrium becomes enlarged to a degree corresponding to the magnitude of increased pulmonary blood flow.

Patients with a small VSD usually have normal right ventricular and pulmonary arterial pressure and slightly elevated pulmonary blood flow relative to systemic blood flow. When the defect is large, the hemodynamic state is determined by the pulmonary vascular resistance, which in these patients may be mildly, moderately, or severely elevated because of varying degrees of hypertensive pulmonary vascular disease. Pulmonary vascular resistance (R_p) is numerically expressed in resistance units normalized to body surface area (units per sq. m.) and is equal to the mean pulmonary artery pressure minus the mean left atrial pressure divided by the cardiac index. Significant pulmonary vascular disease is present when the pulmonary resistance is greater than 8 units per sq. m. When the resistance is greater than about 10 units per sq. m., the flow across the defect is usually bidirectional or right to left, and the pulmonary blood flow is similar to or less than systemic blood flow. Severe elevation of pulmonary vascular resistance contraindicates closure of a VSD. When such patients exercise, systemic blood flow is augmented by right-to-left shunting, since the pulmonary vascular resistance is "fixed." Closure of the defect in this circumstance is hazardous, since the fixed pulmonary vascular resistance prevents an increase in systemic blood flow during exercise postoperatively.

NATURAL HISTORY. Spontaneous closure of a VSD has been estimated to occur in 25 to 50 per cent of patients during childhood. The probability of eventual spontaneous closure is inversely related to the age at which the patient is observed. The mechanism of closure is usually related to ingrowth of fibrous tissue from the margins of the defect or adherence of the septal leaflet of the tricuspid valve to the margins of the defect. Infants with large defects usually do not have symptoms until they reach the age of 6 weeks to 3 months. At this time, the pulmonary vascular resistance has fallen from elevated levels present at birth, and maximal left-to-right shunting across the defect occurs. The increase in pulmonary blood flow is manifest by tachypnea, poor feeding, growth failure, pneumonia, and severe cardiac failure. Those with small defects are usually asymptomatic. Patients with marked elevation of pulmonary vascular resistance and predominant right-to-left shunting across the defect (Eisenmenger's complex) are cyanosed, polycythemic, and severely limited in their activities. The diagnosis can be made noninvasively by Doppler echocardiography with color-flow mapping, and cardiac catheterization studies are useful to confirm the diagnosis, to define the hemodynamic state, and to search for additional defects.

INDICATIONS FOR OPERATION. Prompt intracardiac repair is indicated for infants with large defects, large shunts, and pulmonary hypertension who present with left ventricular failure, recurrent pulmonary infections, severe growth failure, or evidence of increasing pulmonary vascular disease. The authors do not believe that pulmonary arterial banding has a place in the management of these patients unless a true "Swiss-cheese" septum is present. Operation at any age is contraindicated when severe pulmonary vascular disease is present and a pulmonary vascular resistance of greater than 10 to 12 units per sq. m. is measured. The presence of severe pulmonary hypertension is not a contraindication to operation if the pulmonary vascular resistance is greater than 10 units per sq. m. If the defect is small or moderate in size, the possibility of spontaneous closure and the general well-being of the patient support the decision to defer operation. If such defects remain patent in patients who reach the age of 10 to 12 years, surgical repair is usually recommended when the $Q_p:Q_s$ is 1.5 or greater. The development of aortic valve incompetence in a child with a VSD is an indication for prompt closure of the defect for prevention of further prolapse of the aortic cusps and progression of the aortic incompetence.

SURGICAL TREATMENT

Intracardiac Repair. Closure of the VSD is performed through a median sternotomy incision usually with employment of standard cardiopulmonary bypass methods cannulating each vena cava directly for venous return and the ascending aorta for arterial return from the pump oxygenator. In some small infants, some surgical groups prefer the use of profound hypothermia induced with a pump oxygenator and repair of the defect during a period of circulatory arrest. The right atrial approach is preferred for most perimembranous and mid-muscular VSDs and for some apical and subarterial defects. The right ventricular approach provides good exposure through a transverse infundibular incision for subarterial and infundibular defects, through an apical ventriculotomy for apical muscular defects, and through a longitudinal right ventriculotomy for some multiple muscular VSDs. Rarely, a left ventriculotomy is employed for multiple muscular defects in the trabecular septum. It is essential to have knowledge of the location of the atrioventricular node and penetrating portion of the bundle of His relative to the margins of the defect in order to avoid injuring this tissue, which produces surgically induced complete heart block. This tissue is on the inferior margin of perimembranous and atrioventricular canal type VSDs. It is not related to muscular VSDs located in the trabecular or infundibular septum.

Postoperative Care. Most infants convalesce normally after repair of VSD and do not require special supportive treatment. Small sick infants may be at risk for postoperative pulmonary hypertensive crises, which are episodes characterized by sudden marked increases in pulmonary vascular resistance that may produce suprasystemic pulmonary artery pressure and severe acute cardiac failure. Management may be difficult but is aided by leaving a monitoring catheter within the pulmonary artery for continuous postoperative measurement of pulmonary artery pressure and by maintenance of alkalosis, hyperventilation, and the use of narcotic analgesia, prostaglandins, and tolazoline.

Whenever low cardiac output is present after operation, consideration should be given to the possibility of an overlooked or incompletely closed VSD, and Doppler echocardiography with color-flow mapping should be performed.

Results of Surgical Treatment. Hospital mortality after closure of a VSD now approaches zero. Younger age in earlier years was an incremental risk factor in some surgical experiences, but this effect has been neutralized during the past decade. Multiple VSDs also represented an important incremental risk factor for hospital mortality, but currently it is only a weak one. In contrast to earlier years, pulmonary artery pressure and pulmonary vascular resistance are no longer determinants of hospital mortality. In contrast, the presence of major associated lesions, particularly when present in symptomatic infants with large VSDs, does have an incremental risk effect on hospital mortality.

Permanent surgically induced heart block has occurred in the very early years of cardiac surgery after repair of VSD, but currently this complication is quite unusual and its incidence approaches zero. Postoperatively, tiny residual defects may sometimes be demonstrated by color Doppler echocardiographic studies. However, residual shunts of sufficient magnitude to indicate reoperation are uncommon and in the authors' series occurred in only 1 (0.7 per cent) of 138 patients undergoing repair of a large VSD.

Premature late death after repair of VSD rarely occurs when pulmonary vascular resistance is low preoperatively. Such deaths presumably are due to arrhythmias, either ventricular fibrillation or the sudden late development of heart block. Patients with high pulmonary vascular resistance preoperatively have a tendency for this to progress and cause premature death, and about 25 per cent die within 5 years of operation when the pulmonary vascular resistance is more than 10 units per sq. m. In the presence of normal or mild elevation of pulmonary vascular resistance preoperatively, late functional results are excellent and cardiac function is essentially normal when repair is done within the first 2 years of life by current techniques.

VIII

The Tetralogy of Fallot

Ross M. Ungerleider, M.D.,
and David C. Sabiston, Jr., M.D.

Tetralogy of Fallot (TOF) is one of the most common congenital heart malformations and can be present in 3 to 6 infants for every 10,000 births. The anomaly was originally described by Fallot in 1888 and was thought to consist of (1) pulmonary stenosis, (2) an intraventricular communication (ventricular septal defect), (3) dextroposition of the aorta, and (4) hypertrophy of the right ventricle. In 1944, Alfred Blalock performed a subclavian artery to pulmonary artery anastomosis, and the creation of this *shunt,* which provided increased pulmonary blood flow for a severely cyanotic 4.5-kg. child, has been considered by many to be the beginning of modern congenital heart surgery. Several patients treated with shunts in the era prior to the introduction of cardiopulmonary bypass (in the early 1950s) later received total correction with the technology of extracorporeal circulation.

ANATOMY. As is true for most congenital heart lesions, there is wide variability in the anatomic spectrum of TOF. This can encompass the size of the right ventricle, the size and distribution of the pulmonary arteries, and the location of the pulmonary stenosis as well as additional sources of pulmonary blood flow. The most common variability involves the degree of pulmonary stenosis and the size of the pulmonary arteries. Patients with high-grade obstruction of the right ventricular infundibulum or pulmonary valve present with cyanosis immediately after birth as the ductus arteriosus begins to close. Patients with less severe pulmonary outflow obstruction may receive enough antegrade pulmonary flow from the right ventricle to appear only mildly cyanotic in infancy. Similarly, patients with hypoplastic pulmonary arteries present with more obstruction to pulmonary blood flow and increased cyanosis at an earlier age. Occasionally, one of the pulmonary arteries may be absent. TOF also encompasses the spectrum of defects with atresia of the main pulmonary artery. Complete obstruction between the right ventricle and pulmonary arteries forces all right ventricular blood flow to exit the heart through the aorta by way of the ventricular septal defect. Patients with TOF may also have abnormalities of the coronary arteries (5 per cent) with the most frequent anomaly being the left anterior descending coronary artery arising from the right coronary artery and crossing the right ventricular outflow tract just below the pulmonary valve anulus. A right aortic arch (25 per cent of patients) or a retroesophageal subclavian artery (5 to 10 per cent) may also be present. The degree of the pulmonary blood flow is dependent on the size of the pulmonary arteries

---

See the corresponding chapter or part in the *Textbook of Surgery,* 14th edition, pp. 1909–1923, for a more detailed discussion of this topic, including a comprehensive list of references.

and the degree of right ventricular outflow tract obstruction. Moreover, additional sources of pulmonary blood flow (a ductus arteriosus or bronchial collaterals) can also influence the amount of pulmonary blood flow present in individual patients. The predominant physiology is right-to-left shunting across the ventricular septal defect. This shunt flow is increased by a fall in systemic vascular resistance, which further diminishes pulmonary blood flow and increases cyanosis. Pulmonary blood flow in these patients can be enhanced by increasing systemic vascular resistance (e.g., squatting) or by raising the systemic arterial pressure. Since the ventricular septal defect is nonrestrictive, it is not a limiting factor in the amount of shunt flow. The shunt is more affected by the degree of pulmonary stenosis, with greater right-to-left shunt occurring in patients with the most significant degrees of pulmonary outflow obstruction.

NATURAL HISTORY AND DIAGNOSIS. If untreated, TOF is associated with a 30 per cent mortality by age 6 months that increases to 50 per cent by 2 years. Only 20 per cent of patients can be expected to reach 10 years of age, and not more than 5 to 10 per cent live to reach 21 years. The greatest risk is paradoxical emboli, cerebral or pulmonary thrombosis, or subacute bacterial endocarditis. Patients may appear smaller than expected for age and usually have cyanosis of some degree. Almost all present with a systolic ejection murmur, and the second heart sound is usually single and rarely increased in intensity. This is because pulmonary hypertension is distinctly unusual in these patients. Those who have been cyanotic for several years may have an increase in their hemoglobin, and the platelet count and total blood fibrinogen are frequently slightly diminished. In early infancy, the chest film may appear normal. The pulmonary vascular markings may be somewhat decreased depending on the amount of pulmonary blood flow. With time, a classic boot-shaped heart (*coeur en sabot*) may develop and is the recognized hallmark of tetralogy of Fallot. The chest film may also show evidence of a right aortic arch. This finding in the presence of cyanosis is very suggestive of TOF. Recent advances in two-dimensional echocardiography and color-flow Doppler have elevated the diagnostic capabilities, and almost all infants with TOF can be diagnosed with this procedure. Classically, these images demonstrate a large perimembranous ventricular septal defect with an overriding aorta and bidirectional shunting across the ventricular septal defect. The pulmonary outflow tract appears narrowed or even atretic. Angiography with cardiac catheterization is necessary for demonstration of the pulmonary artery anatomy and sources of pulmonary blood flow. Typical findings at catheterization include equal right ventricular and left ventricular pressures (due to the unrestrictive ventricular septal defect) and mild to moderate systemic arterial desaturation from right-to-left shunting.

SURGICAL CORRECTION. As suggested by the natural history of this lesion, most patients require surgical intervention. Current trends are to provide surgical correction as soon as possible (often electively before the first year of life) and generally by the time the patient has reached the age of 2 years. The urgency with which surgical therapy is performed is affected by numerous variables, which include the symptoms at presentation, age at presentation, and associated lesions. The use of prostaglandins (PGE_1) for stabilizing patients with diminished pulmonary blood flow has greatly influenced the emergent care of these patients. Prostaglandins reopen the ductus arteriosus and help to maintain patency, thus providing pulmonary blood flow to these critically ill infants. This enables transport of these infants to institutions with tertiary facilities for appropriate treatment. Prior to the recognition of the value of prostaglandins in these patients, infants were transported with critical cyanosis and marginal pulmonary blood flow and often reached the referral institution in a condition beyond salvage.

Surgical management can be varied and ranges from total correction of the entire defect in early infancy to palliation in infancy followed by total correction at a later time. Total operative correction during infancy is accomplished with the utilization of cardiopulmonary bypass. It includes patch closure of the ventricular septal defect and enlargement of the right ventricular outflow tract for providing unobstructed flow into the pulmonary bed. This often requires placement of a patch from the right ventricle across the pulmonary valve anulus extending out the main pulmonary artery to the bifurcation of the right and left branches. Patients with small pulmonary arteries or with anomalies that require placement of a conduit for establishing right ventricle to pulmonary artery continuity (such as patients with pulmonary atresia or anomalous coronary arteries) may be safely palliated with the creation of a shunt to provide pulmonary blood flow until they attain ample growth that enables total correction. Some surgeons prefer placement of a shunt as an initial procedure for patients with TOF, since this can often be done without the use of cardiopulmonary bypass and, in their experience, enables staged correction at a later date with results similar to early total correction. Surgeons who favor shunts choose the Blalock-Taussig shunt (subclavian artery to pulmonary artery), the modified Blalock-Taussig shunt (a prosthetic tube placed between the subclavian artery and pulmonary artery), or a central shunt (a prosthetic tube placed between the aorta and main pulmonary artery). Each of these shunts provides an increase in pulmonary blood flow and alleviates the cyanosis while enabling deferment of total surgical correction until a later date.

Tetralogy of Fallot is now being corrected with an ever-diminishing mortality. Overall, survival with operative repair should be greater than 95 per cent when the repair is done primarily or after a single systemic to pulmonary artery shunt. Improved techniques of myocardial protection with hypothermia, cold cardioplegia, or total circulatory arrest are enabling more precise anatomic repairs in younger infants with excellent results. Early postoperative risks include the creation of heart block, which should occur in less than 1 per cent of patients of all ages, and residual ventricular septal defects, which should occur in less than 4 per cent of patients.

PULMONARY STENOSIS WITH INTACT VENTRICULAR SEPTUM

Stenosis of a pulmonary valve with an intact ventricular septum can range from a highly favorable to a highly lethal lesion. The most important prognostic factor is the size of the right ventricular chamber. Patients who present at an older age often are in a more favorable category with respect to long-term outcome. This is not necessarily true if a patient with a hypoplastic right ventricle presents at a later age because pulmonary blood flow has been adequately maintained through a patent ductus arteriosus during the interim period. Patients with severe hypoplasia of the right ventricle may never be candidates for a biventricular repair and may instead need to be staged toward a Fontan type operation. A Fontan operation corrects the systemic venous return directly into the pulmonary bed and utilizes the single adequate ventricle as the systemic pumping chamber. These patients are usually managed with the placement of a systemic to pulmonary artery shunt at the time of initial presentation in infancy. This enables the pulmonary artery to grow so that conversion to Fontan physiology can be accomplished by the time the patient reaches the age of 5 years. Twenty per cent may also have severe coronary artery anomalies producing coronary ischemia with myocardial infarction. These patients, especially if they need to be staged toward a Fontan operation, may be more suitable candidates for cardiac transplantation. Those with right ventricles that approximate a more normal size may be adequately treated with enlargement of the pulmonary outflow tract alone, and the long-term outcome in this group can be quite satisfying.

IX

Double Outlet Right Ventricle

Albert D. Pacifico, M.D., John W. Kirklin, M.D., and James K. Kirklin, M.D.

DEFINITION AND MORPHOLOGY. Double outlet right ventricle (DORV) is present when more than 50 per cent of each great artery arises from the morphologic right ventricle. A ventricular septal defect (VSD) is the only outlet from the left ventricle. In general, when one great artery overlies the ventricular septum, it is assigned to the ventricle connected to its greater part. The malformation is usually present in

---

See the corresponding chapter or part in the *Textbook of Surgery*, 14th edition, pp. 1923–1928, for a more detailed discussion of this topic, including a comprehensive list of references.

hearts with atrioventricular concordant connections but can also exist in hearts with atrioventricular discordant connections.

A VSD is almost uniformly present but may vary in size and location. The hemodynamics, clinical course, and specific type of operation employed depend on the relation of the VSD to either great artery and the relation of the great arteries to each other. Lev and colleagues have described the commitment of the VSD to either or both great arteries and classified them as subaortic, doubly committed, or noncommitted. The precise location of the VSD within the ventricular septum does not uniformly predict its commitment to either great artery. Thus, a perimembranous VSD can have any type of commitment or be noncommitted. When the defect is subpulmonary, it is related to the pulmonary artery, and the heart is generally categorized as the Taussig-Bing type of DORV.

PHYSIOLOGY, CLINICAL COURSE, AND DIAGNOSIS. Patients with DORV and a subaortic VSD are acyanotic because of streaming of oxygenated left ventricular blood into the aorta. The clinical course is similar to patients with an isolated large VSD, and they may develop congestive heart failure early in life as well as severe pulmonary vascular disease. Pulmonary stenosis, however, is usually present in those with a subaortic VSD (and usually absent in those with a subpulmonary VSD). It protects the lungs from pulmonary vascular disease; a clinical course similar to that of patients with tetralogy of Fallot also results. Patients with a subpulmonary VSD and no pulmonary stenosis have a clinical course similar to that of patients with transposition of the great arteries with VSD. Cyanosis is present from birth, since desaturated systemic venous blood streams toward the aorta and oxygenated left ventricular blood toward the pulmonary artery. They develop early congestive heart failure or severe pulmonary vascular disease and usually present with symptoms in the first few months of life. Diagnosis can be made by two-dimensional echocardiography and is enhanced by color-flow mapping. Angiocardiograms with axial projections after separate injection of contrast media into the left and right ventricle offer the greatest diagnostic reliability.

SURGICAL METHODS AND RESULTS. The goals of corrective surgery are to relieve pulmonary stenosis when it is present, to provide separate unobstructed outflow pathways from each ventricle to a great artery, and to separate the pulmonary and systemic circulations. This is usually accomplished by a tunnel-type repair connecting the committed VSD with its respective great artery. When the VSD is subaortic or doubly committed, the tunnel-type repair connects the left ventricle via the VSD and tunnel to the aorta, leaving a "venoarterial" concordant arrangement.

However, when the VSD is subpulmonary in commitment, the tunnel repair connecting the VSD with the pulmonary artery leaves a "venoarterial" discordant arrangement similar to that found in patients with transposition of the great arteries. Venous switching, or more preferably arterial switching, must be concomitantly performed for complete repair to be accomplished. In the most common anatomic circumstance, the aorta is more or less anterior to the pulmonary artery, and pulmonary stenosis is absent. When the great arteries are more or less side-by-side and chordae tendineae from the tricuspid valve do not insert upon the infundibular septum (which separates the aortic and pulmonary outlet), resection of the infundibular septum and construction of a straight tunnel connecting the VSD with the aorta and leaving an unobstructed outlet from the right ventricle to the pulmonary artery is sometimes possible.

When a noncommitted VSD is present, repair can sometimes be accomplished by constructing an intraventricular tunnel connecting the VSD with both the aorta and pulmonary artery. The pulmonary artery is then closed, and a valved extracardiac conduit is placed from the right ventricle to the pulmonary artery. Other alternatives include closure of the VSD, closure of the pulmonary artery, and placing a valved extracardiac conduit from the left ventricle to the pulmonary artery coupled with venous switching by the Senning or Mustard technique. Repair including an arterial switch operation has also been successfully accomplished as well as repair by a modification of the operation described by Fontan. Complete anatomic repair has also been achieved when a complete atrioventricular canal defect is associated with DORV.

Hospital mortality is less than 5 per cent when a subaortic VSD is present, and late reoperation for tunnel obstruction is uncommonly required. When the VSD is subpulmonary in location, results are less favorable and are better with concomitant arterial switching compared with venous switching. Repair of more complex forms is less favorable, but encouraging success has recently been achieved.

SURGICAL INDICATIONS AND TIMING. Patients with DORV and a subaortic VSD without pulmonary stenosis have a natural history similar to those with isolated large VSD. They are prone to develop congestive heart failure early in life and early pulmonary vascular disease. Operation is advised at any age to control symptoms of congestive heart failure or electively at about 6 months of age to prevent the development of severe pulmonary vascular disease.

When pulmonary stenosis is absent, elective repair is advised by the age of 2 years or sooner if significant cyanosis or cyanotic episodes are present. In some circumstances, it is best to advise an initial systemic–pulmonary artery shunt with later repair.

When a subpulmonary VSD is present in patients with DORV, pulmonary stenosis is usually absent, and patients tend to develop early congestive heart failure or severe pulmonary vascular disease. Elective operation is advised within the first 3 months of life by methods that will leave the left ventricle as the systemic ventricle. When pulmonary stenosis is present, a balloon atrial septostomy is initially recommended within the first few weeks of life to improve mixing of systemic and pulmonary venous blood. The usual elective repair employing a cryopreserved homograft valved extracardiac conduit (Rastelli-type procedure) is advised between ages 2 and 5 years. Some patients will require a systemic–pulmonary artery shunt in the interim.

Patients with DORV, noncommitted VSD, and absent pulmonary stenosis should have pulmonary artery banding at about 6 months of age or sooner for control of heart failure and for preventing the development of advanced pulmonary vascular disease. When pulmonary stenosis is present, an initial systemic–pulmonary artery shunt is performed to relieve cyanosis when required in patients less than about 2 years of age. Repair usually includes a valved extracardiac conduit or a modification of the Fontan operation and ideally should be delayed until about 3 to 5 years of age.

When DORV is associated with a complete atrioventricular canal defect, repair is advised by 6 months of age if pulmonary stenosis is absent and repair by use of an intraventricular tunnel connecting the left ventricle with the aorta can be accomplished. When pulmonary stenosis is present, management is similar to that of patients with tetralogy of Fallot. When the interventricular communication is not related to the aorta, a valved extracardiac conduit is necessary as part of the repair. If pulmonary stenosis is absent, early pulmonary artery banding for control of congestive heart failure and protection of the pulmonary vasculature is advised. When pulmonary stenosis is present, an initial systemic–pulmonary artery shunt is constructed when needed, and later repair at about 3 years employing an extracardiac conduit or by Fontan methods is accomplished.

X

Tricuspid Atresia
Harvey W. Bender, Jr., M.D.

The primary malformation in tricuspid atresia is the failure of development of the right atrioventricular valve. Associated with this are varying degrees of hypoplasia of the right ventricle and infundibulum and, in most patients, an atrial septal defect. This malformation may occur in patients with normally related great arteries or in patients with transposition of the great arteries. Ventricular septal defect can also occur with or without stenosis of the pulmonary outflow tract.

A clinical anatomic classification has been proposed by Rudolph. Each of Rudolph's three classes has a characteristic clinical presentation. In Group I, tricuspid atresia with intact

See the corresponding chapter or part in the *Textbook of Surgery*, 14th edition, pp. 1928–1929, for a more detailed discussion of this topic, including a comprehensive list of references.

ventricular septum and hypoplastic right ventricle, infants present with hypoxemia and acidemia. Pulmonary blood flow is dependent on the presence of a patent ductus arteriosus. All systemic and pulmonary venous return mixes in the atria. The degree of cyanosis in these infants depends primarily on the size and patency of the ductus and the ratio of systemic to pulmonary vascular resistance. In Group II, tricuspid atresia with ventricular septal defect and normally related great arteries, cyanosis occurs during the first few days of life and is then accompanied by left ventricular failure and pulmonary edema as pulmonary vascular resistance falls. Congestive heart failure develops in this group of infants within the first 2 to 3 weeks of life and increases as pulmonary vascular resistance decreases. In Group III, tricuspid atresia with ventricular septal defect and transposed great arteries, the infant may present with only mild cyanosis; however, the hypoplastic right (or systemic) ventricle will be unable to sustain an adequate cardiac output in the absence of pulmonary stenosis and a ventricular septal defect.

All current treatment for infants with tricuspid atresia should be considered palliative. In the cyanotic infant, augmentation of pulmonary blood flow is required. This is accomplished by a shunt for increasing pulmonary blood flow. This may be in the form of an aortopulmonary shunt, subclavian to pulmonary artery shunt, or superior vena cava to pulmonary artery shunt. Few infants in Rudolph's Group I survive the first 6 months without treatment.

The various types of systemic pulmonary artery shunts are associated with their certain complications and results. With the improvement of operative techniques, particularly the use of magnification and fine monofilament suture, the subclavian to pulmonary artery anastomosis is now performed in newborns with increasing success. This appears to be the procedure of choice in patients who require a shunt in the first few weeks of life. In older children, the superior vena cava to right pulmonary artery shunt is quite satisfactory with good relief of symptoms for several years.

In infants in Rudolph's Group II and Group III with increased pulmonary blood flow, medical management with digitalis and diuretics should be undertaken. If this treatment regimen fails, banding of the pulmonary artery may be necessary. In all groups, a satisfactory interatrial communication is necessary.

In 1971, Fontan and Baudet reported an operative procedure for "correction" of tricuspid atresia. This consisted of diverting all systemic venous return through a valve-containing conduit to the lungs with closure of the interatrial septal defect. Originally they incorporated an aortic valve homograft into the inferior vena cava–right atrial junction for prevention of reflux into the inferior vena cava. This is no longer used, and the procedure has been modified in the last 2 decades with steadily improving results. Predictable good results can be obtained with this procedure in patients with low pulmonary vascular resistance, good left ventricular function, no mitral valve incompetence, and no obstruction in the pulmonary arterial tree. The essential feature of the procedure, however it is modified, is to provide a wide-open, unimpeded connection between the right atria or venae cavae and the pulmonary artery with subsequent closure of the atrial communication.

Whereas results of the intracardiac procedures for tricuspid atresia are encouraging, it must be recognized that they are palliative procedures and that careful selection is essential to identify patients who might be candidates for intracardiac repair. Although it has been shown that good results can be achieved in patients who do not meet Fontan's original criteria, these standards remain important in patient selection.

XI

Hypoplastic Left Heart Syndrome
William I. Norwood, M.D.

Hypoplastic left heart syndrome is the fourth most common congenital cardiac anomaly presenting in the first year of life. It is the most common malformation in which there is only one ventricle and as such is amenable to application of Fontan's procedure. However, development of operative therapy for hypoplasia of left heart structures during the first 2 decades of open heart procedures appeared remote. Lev first described the pathologic process of "hypoplasia of the aortic tract complexes." This category included (1) isolated hypoplasia of the aorta, (2) hypoplasia of the aorta with ventricular septal defect, and (3) hypoplasia of the aorta with aortic stenosis or atresia with or without mitral stenosis or atresia. Noonan and Nadas referred to these lesions as hypoplastic left heart syndrome. Although the anatomic factors that comprise the hypoplastic left heart syndrome are varied, the physiologic similarities among this collection of lesions have resulted in acceptance of this term.

DEFINITION AND ANATOMY

Hypoplastic left heart syndrome consists of a group of cardiac malformations in which there is aortic valve hypoplasia, stenosis, or atresia with hypoplasia or absence of the left ventricle and, as a consequence, hypoplasia of the ascending aorta. This syndrome coexists most frequently with severe mitral hypoplasia or mitral atresia. A less common variation includes malalignment of the common atrioventricular canal

See the corresponding chapter or part in the *Textbook of Surgery*, 14th edition, pp. 1930–1935, for a more detailed discussion of this topic, including a comprehensive list of references.

with regard to the muscular ventricular septum over the right ventricle.

In a study by Bharati and Lev, 87 per cent of the patients had aortic atresia and 13 per cent had aortic stenosis. The coronary arteries originate normally from the aortic root and have a normal distribution. The ascending and transverse portions of the aorta are hypoplastic. With aortic atresia, the size of the ascending aorta is usually 1 to 3 mm. In rare cases, with aortic stenosis, the mean size of the ascending aorta has been reported to be as large as 5 to 6 mm. True coarctation of the aorta is not a common finding. There is, however, a posterolateral intimal ridge at the junction of the aortic isthmus, ductus arteriosus, and thoracic aorta in most patients.

EPIDEMIOLOGY

Hypoplastic left heart syndrome has been reported to occur in at least 0.016 to 0.036 per cent of live births, making it the most common defect in which there is only one ventricle. In pathologic series, it represents 1.4 to 3.8 per cent of congenital heart disease and has been reported to cause 23 per cent of the deaths due to congenital heart disease in the newborn period.

PHYSIOLOGY

The physiology of hypoplastic left heart syndrome is complex. The left ventricle is essentially a nonfunctional structure. Pulmonary venous return must therefore be to the right atrium through an atrial septal defect, through a stretched foramen ovale, or, rarely, by a total anomalous pulmonary venous connection. In the right atrium, systemic and pulmonary venous return mix. The right ventricle must maintain both the pulmonary and systemic output, and the ductus arteriosus must remain patent for systemic perfusion.

Systemic blood flow is maintained as long as the ductus arteriosus remains patent. Perfusion is retrograde through the transverse arch and ascending aorta to the carotid and coronary arteries. With the left and right pulmonary arteries connected parallel with the ductus arteriosus and descending aorta, the relative ratio of pulmonary to systemic blood flow depends on a delicate balance between pulmonary and systemic vascular resistances.

NATURAL HISTORY

Untreated, more than 95 per cent of infants with hypoplastic left heart syndrome die within the first month of life. This syndrome is responsible for approximately 25 per cent of cardiac deaths during the first week and 15 per cent of cardiac deaths during the first month of life.

PREOPERATIVE CARE

Two approaches to the surgical management of hypoplastic left heart syndrome have been advanced: reconstructive procedure and cardiac replacement. The basis for reconstructive procedures is the fact that the lungs, coronary anatomy, and myocardial biochemistry are inherently normal in this condition. Thus, if hypoplastic left heart syndrome is considered to be one of several cardiac malformations in which only one ventricle is effective, a surgical approach may be devised, with use of a modification of Fontan's procedure. A good functional result after Fontan's procedure can be expected when the pulmonary artery architecture is almost normal, the pulmonary vascular resistance is that of the normal mature lung, and ventricular function has been preserved (low end-diastolic pressure). However, because the systemic circulation in neonates with hypoplastic left heart syndrome depends on the patency of the ductus arteriosus, which characteristically closes in the first days of life, an urgent operative procedure is necessary. The pulmonary vascular resistance of the neonate is prohibitively high for Fontan's procedure; therefore, staged surgical therapy is necessary. The general goals of the initial stage are to establish unobstructed systemic output from the right ventricle, to ensure normal maturation of the pulmonary vasculature by regulating pulmonary arterial blood flow and pressure, and to ensure a widely patent interatrial communication, thus avoiding pulmonary venous hypertension. Although several approaches to these goals have been conceived, the surgical techniques outlined here are designed additionally to incorporate as much as possible of the patient's own tissues and to avoid conduits or circumferential suture lines, thus minimizing the number of surgical interventions.

PALLIATION (STAGE I)

After removal of the arterial and venous cannulas, the atrial septum is excised to allow unimpeded pulmonary venous return to the right atrium. The main pulmonary artery, which has been separated from the diminutive ascending aorta during the cooling phase of cardiopulmonary bypass, is transected adjacent to the takeoff of the right pulmonary artery, and the distal stump of the main pulmonary artery is closed with a patch. Patch closure is recommended in order to ensure continuity between the right and left pulmonary artery branches. The ductus arteriosus is then exposed, ligated, and transected at its entrance to the thoracic aorta. An incision in the aorta is extended distally 1 to 2 cm. into the thoracic aorta and also proximally into the aortic arch and ascending aorta to the level of the rim of the transected proximal main pulmonary artery. Because the isthmus of the aorta and the aortic arch actually function as a branch of the main pulmonary artery–ductus–thoracic aorta continuum, the junction of the isthmus and thoracic aorta is gusseted with a patch in order to avoid subsequent development of distal aortic arch obstruction. A pulmonary homograft is used for this patch because it is thin, pliable, and hemostatic.

At this point, the author favors the construction of a short central shunt of 4 mm. tube graft between the inferior aspect of the augmented aortic arch and the confluence of branch pulmonary arteries. The rationale for a central shunt is to obtain more even distribution of flow and thus uniform growth of the right and left pulmonary arteries. The remaining pulmonary homograft gusset is then extended to 5 mm. above the end of the most proximal incision in the ascending aorta. The proximal transected main pulmonary artery is then anastomosed to the ascending aorta and homograft gusset, thus creating outflow from the right ventricle to the augmented aorta through the pulmonary valve.

FONTAN'S PROCEDURE (STAGE II)

During a period of circulatory arrest, the pulmonary arteries are opened and an incision in the right atrium is made from the sulcus terminalis superiorly to the right lateral insertion of the eustachian valve inferiorly. The interatrial communication is inspected and enlarged if possible. A final incision is then made in the superior right atrium adjacent to the right pulmonary artery and carried into the posterior aspect of the right superior vena cava immediately adjacent to the most rightward aspect of the incision in the right pulmonary artery. A suture line is begun between the inferior lip of the incised right pulmonary artery and the posterior lip of the right superior vena caval–right atrial incision. This provides the floor for the anastomosis of the systemic venous return to the pulmonary arterial tree.

A tube graft 10 mm. in diameter, of sufficient length to extend from the inferior vena caval–right atrial junction to the right superior vena caval–right atrial junction, is cut in half lengthwise. This is used as a baffle to channel inferior vena caval flow along the right lateral aspect of the right atrium to the anastomosis between the right atrium and the pulmonary arterial tree superiorly. The baffle is sutured around the orifice of the inferior vena cava along the right lateral floor and free wall of the right atrium and around the patulous orifice in the superior dome of the right atrium. This particular baffling technique was introduced to minimize problems associated with tricuspid prolapse or regurgitation, or obstruction of pulmonary venous return to the right ventricle, which was experienced early in this series with an alternative baffling technique.

The construction of the systemic venous pulmonary arterial system is completed by gusseting the pulmonary arterial incision with an elongated triangular patch, beginning on the left pulmonary artery. As the right pulmonary artery and adjacent right superior vena cava are approached, the base of the triangular patch is sutured onto the anterior lip of the right superior vena caval–right atrial incision, providing a roof for the anastomosis. The patient is placed back on cardiopulmonary bypass after closure of the initial right atriotomy and rewarmed to 37°C.

CONCLUSION

From October 1984 through June 1988 at the Children's Hospital of Philadelphia, 198 newborns had palliative operative procedures similar to those described for hypoplastic left heart syndrome. The hospital mortality among those patients was 28 per cent. The 18-month actuarial survival was 61 per cent. To date, 52 patients have undergone application of Fontan's procedure for the treatment of hypoplastic left heart syndrome. Of these 52 patients, there were 16 early and 2 late deaths, with 2 deaths in the last 15 patients. The results continue to improve for both initial palliation and later reconstructive procedures as an increasing knowledge of the anatomy and physiology of this complex group of patients is gained. The approach outlined for reconstructive therapy for this malformation will continue to evolve. The challenge for the future is to better characterize this group of lesions so that the preoperative, operative, and postoperative management may be further improved.

XII

Truncus Arteriosus
Robert B. Wallace, M.D., and Richard A. Hopkins, M.D.

ANATOMY AND CLASSIFICATION. Truncus arteriosus is a rare congenital cardiac malformation characterized by a single arterial vessel arising from the heart, receiving blood from both ventricles, and supplying blood to the aorta, lungs, and coronary arteries. Truncus arteriosus is due to a lack of partitioning of the embryonic conus during the first few weeks of fetal development and is usually associated with a ventricular septal defect. Collett and Edwards classified truncus arteriosus into four types, based on the origin of the pulmonary arteries. In Type I, a single arterial trunk gives rise to the aorta and main pulmonary artery. In Type II, the right and left pulmonary arteries arise immediately adjacent to one another from the dorsal wall of the truncus. In Type III, the right and left pulmonary arteries arise from either side of the truncus. In Type IV, the proximal pulmonary arteries are absent, and pulmonary blood flow is by way of bronchial arteries. Type I and Type II composed 76 per cent of Collett and Edwards' series, and Type III, 13 per cent. From a surgical perspective, Type II and Type III are grouped

See the corresponding chapter or part in the *Textbook of Surgery*, 14th edition, pp. 1935–1940, for a more detailed discussion of this topic, including a comprehensive list of references.

together. Type IV, in which there are no pulmonary artery trunks, more appropriately should be considered a severe form of tetralogy of Fallot with complete pulmonary atresia.

HEMODYNAMICS. All of the blood from both the left and the right ventricles is ejected into the truncus arteriosus. The systemic and pulmonary venous blood mixes, and the degree of arterial oxygen unsaturation is dependent on the amount of pulmonary blood flow. Pulmonary blood flow may be limited by stenosis of the pulmonary arteries, but this is uncommon. In most instances, pulmonary blood flow (and thus arterial oxygen saturation) is determined by the resistance to flow in the pulmonary vascular bed. As with isolated ventricular septal defect, the pulmonary vascular bed in truncus arteriosus is exposed to high flow at systemic pressure, a condition that may produce progressive pulmonary vascular obstructive disease.

PROGNOSIS, SYMPTOMS, AND DIAGNOSIS. Most patients with persistent truncus arteriosus die in early infancy from congestive heart failure. Death for those who survive the first 2 years of life is generally related to pulmonary vascular obstructive disease. During the first few weeks of life, when pulmonary vascular resistance is normally increased, symptoms are usually absent, unless there is associated significant truncal valve incompetence. With maturation of the fetal pulmonary vascular bed associated with a decrease in pulmonary vascular resistance and an increase in pulmonary blood flow, symptoms of congestive heart failure develop. These include dyspnea, excessive perspiration, and failure to thrive. Cyanosis is not usually apparent because the arterial oxygen saturation is generally greater than 85 per cent.

Physical examination usually reveals a systolic thrill and murmur over the left third and fourth intercostal spaces parasternally. When truncal valve incompetence is present, a diastolic murmur follows the second heart sound. Chest roentgenography shows cardiomegaly with biventricular enlargement. The peripheral pulmonary vasculature is increased unless there is advanced pulmonary vascular obstructive disease. The electrocardiogram is nonspecific.

Right and left heart catheterization and angiocardiographic studies are indicated in all patients suspected of having truncus arteriosus. Ventricular pressures are equal, and in the absence of pulmonary artery stenosis, there are equal pressures in the ventricles, truncus, and pulmonary arteries. Oxygen saturation studies indicate bidirectional shunting at the ventricular level, the predominant shunt being left-to-right. Pulmonary flow and resistance should be determined by measurement of pressures and oxygen saturations in both pulmonary arteries.

TREATMENT. Definitive treatment for truncus arteriosus is complete repair. Ideally, operation should be performed in the first 3 months of life, during which time approximately 80 per cent of patients die without correction. Operation at this age also protects against the development of pulmonary vascular obstructive disease. Although conduit replacement is required when operation is performed in infancy, it has been shown that this can be accomplished at a low risk. The high mortality in infants with unrepaired truncus arteriosus attests to the ineffectiveness of medical management in most patients.

Complete Surgical Repair. The operation is performed through a median sternotomy with utilization of total cardiopulmonary bypass and deep hypothermia, either with total circulatory arrest or low flow. Myocardial protection is provided by cold cardioplegic arrest during aortic cross-clamping. The pulmonary arteries can usually be excised from the truncus as a single segment, even in Type II truncus. In smaller infants, the posterior defect is usually closed with a patch for avoidance of distortion of the truncal valve pillars. The incision in the right ventricle is made high in the ventricle in the planned direction of the conduit. If truncal regurgitation is severe, valve replacement must be considered. A patch is used to close the ventricular septal defect. An appropriate-sized valved Dacron or homograft conduit is cut to proper length and used to establish continuity between the right ventricle and the pulmonary arteries.

RESULTS. The Mayo Clinic experience with 167 patients with Type I and Type II truncus arteriosus who underwent surgical repair between 1965 and 1982 has been reported. There were 48 hospital deaths (28.7 per cent). The most significant risk factors in this early series were age at operation of less than 2 years and a postrepair right ventricle to left ventricle pressure ratio greater than 0.8. During this era, children under 2 years were repaired only when medical management failed. Recent experiences from institutions in which elective repair in infancy has been performed indicate that this can be accomplished at an acceptable mortality. Bove and colleagues have reported neonatal repairs in 11 patients with a 9 per cent mortality. Ebert reported an 11 per cent hospital mortality in 100 consecutive patients operated on under 6 months of age. Eighty-six patients were alive at 16 months to 8 years postoperatively and 55 of the survivors required conduit replacement (accomplished without mortality). Early complete repair is currently the procedure of choice.

XIII

Transposition of the Great Arteries

Gary K. Lofland, M.D.

Transposition of the great arteries is a congenital cardiac anomaly that in its anatomically simplest form is pathophysiologically the most severe. It is a lesion that may coexist with essentially any cardiac lesion. This section is confined to *complete transposition, complete transposition with a ventricular septal defect,* and *complete transposition with left ventricular outflow tract obstruction.* Data from the New England regional infant cardiac program indicate that complete transposition of the great arteries is the second most frequently encountered disorder in their registry. It was found in 9.9 per cent of infants with congenital heart disease and occurred with a frequency of 0.206 per 1000 live births. There is a distinct male preponderance. Transposition of the great arteries represents approximately 15 per cent of congenital cardiac anomalies seen at autopsy in infants less than 1 month of age.

CLINICAL MANIFESTATIONS. The greater the size or larger the number of shunts, the less the degree of cyanosis. Infants with smaller degrees of intracirculatory shunting are thus more cyanotic. When the anatomic diagnosis of transposition of the great arteries is established, subsequent management before the time of definitive correction is based on the adequacy of the intracirculatory shunting. The most common clinical findings in infants with complete transposition of the great arteries are cyanosis and congestive heart failure. Cyanosis is usually striking and present at birth.

DIAGNOSIS. With *echocardiography* and antenatal screening, the diagnosis is usually made within the first few days of life. Infants with simple complete transposition usually have a normal birth weight, but subsequent physical development is impaired because of cyanosis. Symptoms of heart failure are present within the first week of life in approximately 10 per cent of patients but usually appear by 1 month and are associated with the decline in pulmonary vascular resistance normally expected. Most patients have a systolic murmur with an accentuated second heart sound, and diastolic gallops are common. Children with left ventricular outflow tract obstruction have a murmur that is characterized by a long crescendo-decrescendo systolic component. *Electrocardiographic* findings include right atrial hypertrophy, right or combined ventricular hypertrophy, and right axis deviation. These findings obviously vary depending on the presence or absence of ventricular septal defect and the degree of pulmonary vascular resistance. The *chest film* is frequently diagnostic with demonstration of cardiomegaly, an oval or

See the corresponding chapter or part in the *Textbook of Surgery*, 14th edition, pp. 1940–1950, for a more detailed discussion of this topic, including a comprehensive list of references.

egg-shaped cardiac configuration, and a narrow superior mediastinum. Pulmonary markings are usually increased even in the absence of overt congestive heart failure.

Echocardiography has become the mainstay of anatomic diagnosis and demonstrates an aorta that is located anterior to the pulmonary artery. Although the aorta–pulmonary arterial relationship may approach side-by-side, *the aorta is located anterior to the pulmonary artery*. Intracardiac structures can also be defined by echocardiography, which demonstrates the relative size of the left atrium, the size of the interatrial communication, the presence or absence of a ventricular septal defect, and the relationship of the atrioventricular valves to the ventricles and great arteries. Echocardiography also demonstrates the presence or absence of a ductus arteriosus, the presence or absence of arch anomalies, and the location of pulmonary venous drainage. In addition, echocardiography can be used to assess the adequacy of left ventricular volume, wall thickness, and function.

Cardiac catheterization is performed if there is a question about intra- or extracardiac diagnosis or adequacy of intracirculatory shunting as manifested by oxygen saturations and degree of cyanosis. Cardiac catheterization demonstrates a left atrial pressure that is usually greater than the right atrial pressure and some elevation of pulmonary vascular resistance. Catheterization might also be used to better define the relationship of a ventricular septal defect to the great arteries and the presence or absence of gradients across the left ventricular outflow tract. Catheterization must be performed expediently in a warm room and with minimal stress.

When the diagnosis is confirmed in the newborn, decisions must be made concerning the subsequent long-term management of the patient. Definitive surgical correction must consider all of the anatomic data, including most significantly the presence of a ventricular septal defect, left ventricular outflow tract obstruction, and the propensity for subsequent development of left ventricular outflow tract obstruction if a ventricular septal defect is malaligned posteriorly. If ultimately an atrial correction is planned, effective palliation must be accomplished by optimizing intracirculatory shunting until such time as the definitive correction can be performed. If ultimately an arterial switch procedure is planned, it is best accomplished early in the newborn period, and an interval palliative procedure may not be necessary. If an arterial switch procedure is planned, cardiac catheterization may not be necessary. Palliation of these infants consists of optimizing intracirculatory shunting. This is best accomplished by increasing the size of the interatrial communication, thus allowing better admixture of the systemic and pulmonary venous blood. The technique for this involves passing a balloon-tipped catheter through a systemic vein into the right atrium and through the foramen ovale into the left atrium. If the atrial septum is somewhat thickened and the patent foramen ovale small because of concomitant congenital anomalies, a blade can be used to first enlarge the foramen ovale and allow the subsequent passage of the balloon-tipped catheter. The balloon is then inflated with

1 to 3 ml. of contrast material so that it can be visualized on an image intensifier, and it is then pulled vigorously across the atrial septum to enlarge or tear the foramen ovale. This septostomy can be repeated at subsequent intervals as cyanosis becomes unmanageable. If it is determined that the patient is a good candidate anatomically for an arterial switch procedure, enlargement of the atrial septum has been found at times to be a disadvantage, since it can decompress the left ventricle, producing a ventricle that is poorly prepared to accommodate systemic circulation at the conclusion of the operation.

CORRECTIVE SURGERY. Definitive surgical correction of transposition of the great arteries involves rerouting of systemic venous blood into the pulmonary circulation and pulmonary venous blood into the systemic circulation. This can be accomplished at either an atrial or a great arterial level. If it is accomplished at an atrial level, the systemic ventricle remains the morphologic right ventricle. If it is accomplished at an arterial level, the systemic ventricle becomes the morphologic left ventricle. Each of these definitive corrective approaches has inherent advantages and disadvantages. All definitive surgical corrections are accomplished through a median sternotomy incision and utilize cardiopulmonary bypass and hypothermia. Some institutions also prefer the use of profound hypothermia and complete circulatory arrest in younger infants.

The first diversion of venous inflow successfully accomplished at the atrial level was by *Senning* in 1959, and this procedure has continued to bear his name. It is an ingenious operation that utilizes autologous atrial tissue and ultimately creates two large channels crossing the systemic and pulmonary venous circulations. This proved to be conceptually difficult, and these difficulties were translated into poor results in the early experience. Consequently, when *Mustard* described his operation in 1964, it generated considerable enthusiasm because the operation was conceptually and technically simpler. The Mustard operation utilizes an intra-atrial baffle for diversion of the systemic venous return to the posterior ventricle and allows the pulmonary venous return to enter the more anteriorly located systemic ventricle (morphologic right ventricle). The intra-atrial baffle is usually constructed from pericardium, but synthetic materials may be used. Problems with the operation have concerned baffle obstruction, which physiologically translates into vena caval or pulmonary venous obstruction. Other problems have included a high incidence of atrial arrhythmias. Despite these problems, early success with both the Mustard and Senning procedures has been excellent. Both the Mustard and Senning operations, in accomplishing definitive correction at an atrial level, have the disadvantage of leaving residual ventriculoarterial discordance. Thus, the morphologic right ventricle remains the systemic ventricle.

Because of the concerns about the right ventricle being able to function as a high-pressure, systemic ventricle over a long period, plus the incidence of intractable atrial arrhythmias and systemic (morphologic right ventricular) failure, there has long been interest in achieving a definitive anatomic and physiologic correction. In 1975, *Jatene* described anatomic correction of transposition of the great arteries in infants by dividing both the aorta and the pulmonary artery with removal of a "button" of aorta around the origin of the coronary arteries for repositioning and anastomosis of the coronary arteries into the pulmonary artery. Yacoub also reported initial success with this technique, but initial application of the arterial switch procedure worldwide was accompanied by high mortality. Consequently, the arterial switch procedure was less frequently performed during the decade of the 1970s and early 1980s than was the Senning procedure. Quaegebure in 1986 reported a large series of patients undergoing an arterial switch procedure for both transposition and transposition with ventricular septal defect. Mortality in this series was very acceptable, and interest in the arterial switch procedure was rekindled. The technique of the arterial switch procedure involves mobilization and transection of both the aorta and the pulmonary artery, detachment of the coronary arteries from the aorta, and reattachment of the coronary arteries to the pulmonary artery, which becomes the neo-aorta. The neo–pulmonary artery is then reconstructed, and the great vessels are reanastomosed. This is a technically demanding procedure, and operative results are directly influenced by surgical technique. In addition, operative results are directly influenced by the events occurring immediately postoperatively, and there has been a trend to perform this operation as early in the neonatal period as possible. Ventricular septal defects are managed at the time of definitive correction, are usually perimembranous in location, and are usually closed through a standard transatrial approach. Since the great vessels have been transected, additional exposure can be achieved through the pulmonary valve. A large ventricular septal defect may allow delay in timing of operation, since the degree of intracirculatory shunting is more than adequate. Operations should not be delayed until pulmonary vascular resistance changes occur, however. Patients with simple complete transposition and intact ventricular septum are best corrected as early as possible in the neonatal period if an arterial switch procedure is chosen.

The presence of pulmonary stenosis has been a more difficult problem to manage in the child with transposition of the great arteries. If pulmonary stenosis is present along with a ventricular septal defect, the technique described by Rastelli can be utilized. This consists of construction of an intraventricular conduit so that left ventricular drainage is diverted across the ventricular septal defect and into the aorta, followed by construction of a right ventricular to pulmonary arterial conduit placed in an extracardiac position. This has proved to be most effective but is best accomplished in a somewhat older child to allow placement of a larger conduit and a reduction in frequency of conduit changes necessitated by growth of the child. Timing of a Rastelli-type repair is a judgmental decision made by the cardiologist and cardiac surgeon. The presence of pulmonary stenosis with a restrictive or absent ventricular septal defect is an extremely difficult problem because repeated resections of fibrous tissue may be necessary, with culmination in an extracardiac conduit from the left ventricle to the pulmonary arteries. Fortunately, this is the most rare of the subsets composing transposition of the great arteries.

Additional operative and postoperative management consists of careful hemostasis, since infants and children are extremely sensitive to any degree of fluid accumulation and resultant tamponade. The slightest compression of the right anterior atrial wall may impair filling of the systemic ventricle and cause low cardiac output and elevated pulmonary venous pressure. Baffle obstruction may also occur with either of the atrial repairs. Rhythm disturbances in the immediate postoperative period have been quite common and have consisted primarily of nodal rhythms and occasional junctional ectopic tachycardia. A nodal rhythm is generally well tolerated, but junctional ectopic tachycardia might continue to accelerate and must be managed very aggressively. Currently in this country, digoxin is the drug of choice for the management of junctional ectopic tachycardia, and complete loading must be accomplished rapidly. In Europe, intravenous amiodarone has proved very effective in the management of junctional ectopic tachycardia. Some degree of cardiac failure may be present in the immediate postoperative period and is managed with judicious fluid administration, inotropic support, and afterload reduction. In addition, it is very important in the neonate to control pulmonary vascular resistance, which can change instantaneously and dramatically.

RESULTS. Early results with both the Mustard and Senning procedures have been excellent, and worldwide there has been considerable accumulation of experience with both of these procedures. A distressing note, however, is that the incidence of atrial arrhythmias is quite common, and decreased contractility of the right or systemic ventricle has been observed in a number of children. Excellent results have also been obtained in the recent past with the arterial switch procedure, although longer follow-up is obviously needed. Late functional results of the left ventricle have been excellent, and the incidence of rhythm disturbances has been as low as 5 per cent.

In conclusion, the management of patients with transposition of the great arteries has undergone considerable evolution over the past 30 years and continues to evolve. Several treatment options are available that are quite satisfactory, and a satisfactory result can be expected with definitive correction of this lesion.

XIV

Congenital Aortic Stenosis

James D. Sink, M.D.

Congenital obstruction of the left ventricular outflow tract is not uncommon, occurring in approximately 7 per cent of patients with congenital heart disease. Sites of obstruction, in decreasing order of frequency, are (1) valvular, (2) subvalvular, and (3) supravalvular. Whereas there are no known genetic or etiologic factors associated with valvular or discrete subvalvular aortic stenosis, diffuse subaortic stenosis can be associated with Turner's syndrome, Norman's syndrome, and congenital rubella. Supravalvular aortic stenosis may occur with infantile hypercalcemia and derangements in vitamin B metabolism.

Eighty per cent of patients with congenital aortic stenosis have valvular aortic stenosis. Frequently, the aortic valve is bicuspid with two commissures that are fused to a varying degree with a slitlike opening. The valve can be tricuspid, and rarely a unicuspid valve is found. Subaortic stenosis is the second most common type of congenital aortic stenosis. Subaortic stenosis may be a localized fibrous shelf located below the aortic valve, or a fibromuscular type of obstruction that has a longer stenotic area including both a muscular and fibrous component; or, in its most severe form, the obstruction can extend for several centimeters and be associated with a small aortic anulus. Supravalvular aortic stenosis is the least common and may be either localized or diffuse.

CLINICAL FEATURES. The clinical presentation is essentially identical in each type of congenital aortic stenosis. Symptoms appear as the left ventricle is no longer able to compensate for pressure overload at rest or at exercise. As cardiac output decreases below demand, patients develop symptoms of exertional syncope, angina pectoris, or congestive heart failure. Neonates with severe aortic stenosis may present at birth or shortly thereafter with pallor, perspiration, inability to feed, shortness of breath, and cyanosis. Infants presenting with congestive heart failure in the first 2 weeks of life are usually critically ill and represent true emergencies. Most young patients are asymptomatic, and the detection of a systolic murmur substantiates the diagnosis of aortic stenosis.

DIAGNOSIS. The chest film is similar in all three types of congenital left ventricular outflow tract obstruction. The overall heart size is usually normal, but cardiomegaly can be present if congestive heart failure exists. Post-stenotic dilatation of the aorta is evident in about one half the cases of valvular aortic stenosis. The electrocardiogram may be normal, but in most patients it demonstrates left ventricular hypertrophy. Characteristic M-mode and two-dimensional echocardiogra-

---

See the corresponding chapter or part in the *Textbook of Surgery*, 14th edition, pp. 1950–1956, for a more detailed discussion of this topic, including a comprehensive list of references.

phy patterns distinguish valvular, subvalvular, and supravalvular aortic stenosis. Continuous-wave Doppler echocardiography enables determination of the velocity of flow across
the aortic valve. From this information, the transvalvular
gradient can be calculated. Echocardiographic diagnosis is
sufficiently accurate that catheterization and angiography are
unnecessary prior to surgical therapy. Definitive diagnosis is
provided by demonstration of a systolic gradient across the
stenotic area at catheterization. Angiography demonstrates
this site of obstruction in all types of congenital aortic stenosis.

TREATMENT

Valvular Aortic Stenosis. Valvular aortic stenosis presenting in infancy is usually severe and may rapidly progress to
congestive heart failure and death. Symptomatic infants require emergency surgical intervention as soon as the diagnosis is made. If the patient is moribund or has metabolic
acidosis, administration of prostaglandin E often opens the
ductus arteriosus and improves systemic circulation, thereby
relieving the acidosis. In older infants or children, a gradual
progression in severity of the pressure gradient across the
outflow tract obstruction has been documented in many.
Surgical therapy is indicated for left ventricular to aortic
pressure gradient in excess of 75 mm. Hg and for calculated
aortic valve index less than 0.5 sq. cm. per sq. m. Angina
and syncope are also indications for surgical therapy, as are
progressive symptoms, severe hypertrophy on the electrocardiogram, or increasing cardiac enlargement even if the
measured gradient is less than 50 mm. Hg.

Operation is performed with use of cardiopulmonary bypass, moderate hypothermia, and cold cardioplegic solution.
After the aorta is cross-clamped, a scalpel is used to divide
fused commissures to within 1 mm. of the aortic wall. Care
must be taken to divide only true commissures with adequate
leaflet attachment to the aortic wall, since division of incomplete or false commissures can cause aortic insufficiency. The
subvalvular area must be examined for associated pathologic
conditions before closure of the aorta. Some groups have
recommended inflow occlusion without cardiopulmonary bypass for valvotomy in the infant with critical aortic stenosis.
Operative mortality and morbidity in the older infant or child
is quite low, and relief of left ventricular outflow tract obstruction is good. Aortic valvotomy must be considered palliative,
however, since recurrent aortic stenosis or progressive insufficiency is the usual late sequela. A repeat valvotomy or aortic
valve replacement often becomes necessary in the future.
Mortality following aortic valvotomy in the critically ill infant
remains high, with mortality of 50 to 100 per cent recorded.

Subvalvular Aortic Stenosis. Unlike valvular aortic stenosis, subvalvular aortic stenosis rarely causes symptoms in
infancy. In most patients, the obstruction becomes evident
in early childhood or young adulthood. Obstruction is progressive and can be rapid. Associated aortic regurgitation is
often seen and is also progressive. Operation is recommended when a left ventricular to aortic gradient is greater
than 50 mm. Hg. Surgical treatment of the membranous type

of subvalvular stenosis consists of excision of the membrane during cardiopulmonary bypass, after the aorta has been cross-clamped and the heart has been arrested with cold cardioplegia. In addition to removal of the obstructing membrane, the ventricular septum is always hypertrophied, and a myotomy or myectomy is usually indicated. Tunnel subaortic obstruction is much more difficult to treat surgically. Surgical options include an aortoventriculoplasty as first proposed by Konno and Rastan. Other authors have suggested homograft replacement of the entire aortic root with reimplantation of the coronary arteries, whereas others report excellent results with left ventricular apex to aortic conduits.

The surgical mortality for localized subvalvular aortic stenosis is between 2 and 4 per cent. Mortality for the more extensive Konno procedure has been reported between 6 and 12 per cent. The best operation for tunnel aortic stenosis remains unclear, with some groups preferring the Konno procedure, whereas others prefer the apicoaortic conduit.

Supravalvular Aortic Stenosis. Progressive stenosis with the appearance of symptoms and electrocardiographic changes has been demonstrated in patients with supravalvular stenosis. Operation is indicated at any age when the pressure gradient across the aorta is 50 mm. Hg or more. Patients may have coexisting pulmonary artery stenosis, which may be uncorrectable. Operation is performed with use of cardiopulmonary bypass and cold cardioplegia. After the aorta is cross-clamped, an incision is made across the aortic root, crossing the stenotic area and extending down into the noncoronary sinus of Valsalva. The stricture, which often consists of a ridge protruding into the lumen of the aorta, is excised; a patch graft is used to close the aortotomy, with enlargement of the stenotic area. Doty has recommended a more extensive aortoplasty in which the supravalvular ring is divided by extending the aortic incision into the noncoronary and right coronary sinuses of Valsalva and closing the incision with an inverted Y-patch. This method is designed to provide a more symmetric reconstruction of the aorta. Diffuse supravalvular aortic stenosis requires a more complex repair. If the stenosis extends into the transverse arch, circulatory arrest under deep hypothermia may be necessary. A left ventricular apex to aorta conduit has also been suggested for patients with diffuse supravalvular stenosis. Mortality in patients with isolated supravalvular aortic stenosis is minimal. Mortality is considerably greater, however, in patients with diffuse stenosis.

XV

The Coronary Circulation
David C. Sabiston, Jr., M.D.

Coronary atherosclerotic heart disease continues as the leading cause of death in the United States. Approximately 1,500,000 Americans have a myocardial infarction each year, and of these, over 500,000 die from complications. The surgical management of myocardial ischemia has become a frequent procedure that relieves the pain of angina pectoris and also extends the length of life. Because the population is gaining in longevity each year, it is expected that the incidence of this disease will continue to increase. In the original description of angina pectoris in 1759, Heberden poignantly said, "The termination of angina pectoris is remarkable. For if no accident intervene, but the disease go on to its height, the patients all suddenly fall down and perish almost immediately."

PATHOLOGY

The coronary arteries are especially susceptible to development of atherosclerosis, which is a progressive disease. The surprising presence of extensive coronary atherosclerosis in healthy young males was emphasized among autopsies on Korean military casualties. In a carefully conducted study, it was shown that 77 per cent of these otherwise healthy young men had *gross* evidence of coronary atherosclerosis, and 10 per cent showed advanced disease with a 70 per cent or greater occlusion of one of the major coronary arteries. The anterior descending coronary artery is most frequently involved, followed by the right coronary, the left circumflex, and the left main coronary artery. The most severe changes occur in the proximal one third or half of these vessels, and most of the stenoses or occlusions are short, usually less than 5 mm. in length. When an atherosclerotic lesion decreases the cross-sectional area 75 per cent or more, the resistance becomes significant, and blood flow is decreased. Whereas coronary flow may be adequate at rest, exercise or other factors that increase myocardial oxygen consumption cause a decrease in the coronary pressure distal to the stenosis and blood flow is redistributed away from the subendocardium, making it ischemic.

In many arterial beds, stenosis or occlusion of a major vessel is followed by development of extensive arterial collateral vessels. However, the human heart has few natural collaterals that are of sufficient diameter to deliver a significant quantity of blood in the event of a major coronary occlusion. Even with prolonged stenosis and occlusion, the

---

See the corresponding chapter or part in the *Textbook of Surgery,* 14th edition, pp. 1957–1972, for a more detailed discussion of this topic, including a comprehensive list of references.

development of collaterals is usually inadequate for preventing myocardial ischemia.

PERCUTANEOUS TRANSLUMINAL CORONARY ANGIOPLASTY VERSUS CORONARY ARTERY BYPASS GRAFTS

The first percutaneous transluminal coronary angioplasty was performed by Grüntzig in 1977 and has since become quite popular. Current results indicate that successful dilation rates are achieved in about 90 per cent of patients. Major complications of angioplasty have decreased to approximately 5 per cent, and myocardial infarction and death following dilation are uncommon. However, repeat dilation is frequently necessary, and many patients initially treated by this approach ultimately require coronary artery bypass graft (CABG).

CLINICAL DIAGNOSIS

The most common clinical manifestations of myocardial ischemia are substernal pain, a choking sensation, and tightness in the chest with augmentation of pain during exercise, exposure to cold, or emotional distress. The pain frequently radiates into the left arm, sometimes into the left neck, and less often down the right arm. In the later stages, ischemia occurs at rest. When the pain becomes continuous and refractory, the condition is termed *unstable angina.* Many patients do not have significant symptoms, and the initial presentation may be acute myocardial infarction frequently associated with sudden death.

The physical examination is usually unremarkable. The chest film may show evidence of cardiac enlargement in patients with advanced disease. In many, the electrocardiogram is normal; but in an appreciable number, abnormal findings including myocardial ischemia are evident by inverted T waves on the resting electrocardiogram or alternatively by transient ST segment and T wave changes during the course of angina. ST segment elevation or depression is an especially reliable sign; if it is not present at rest, it may be stimulated by an exercise stress test. Exercise treadmill testing is most useful as a screening test for identifying the need for coronary angiography.

Cardiac catheterization and coronary arteriography are now considered essential in defining the presence and extent of coronary atherosclerotic lesions. This is particularly important because there has been a definite trend toward early surgical therapy since CABG not only relieves the pain of angina but also significantly extends life expectancy. The cardiac output and ejection fraction can be determined at the time of cardiac catheterization. Cardiac catheterization is especially important because the ejection fraction of the left ventricle may be considerably depressed in severe coronary heart disease. The extent can be carefully assessed by the number of vessels involved and the anatomic site and characteristics of the lesions. Physiologic assessment with radionuclide exercise angiography can be quite useful in selecting patients for operation and in particular shows the effect of exercise on the ejection fraction. If the ejection fraction falls significantly during exercise, it increases the need for bypass surgery.

MEDICAL MANAGEMENT

Careful attention should be paid to the risk factors associated with coronary artery disease including hypertension and smoking. Hypertensive patients should be placed on an appropriate medical regimen; the patient should be urged to cease smoking, by use of psychological therapy if necessary. Hyperlipidemia should also be controlled. For patients with low-risk coronary lesions, medical management may be indicated. Coronary vasodilators as well as beta-blocking agents such as propranolol and atenolol are often effective. Antiplatelet agents, primarily such as aspirin, have a definite prophylactic and therapeutic role and have been shown to decrease coronary events.

SURGICAL MANAGEMENT

In addition to standard preoperative preparation, special attention should be given to examination of the carotid system for the presence of bruits. Anesthesia in these patients is of extreme importance and should be undertaken by those especially trained in the field. Prophylactic broad-spectrum antibiotics are administered intravenously immediately before induction of anesthesia and for 24 to 48 hours postoperatively. The blood should be assessed for possible defects of coagulation.

The surgical procedure consists of the placement of coronary artery bypass grafts. In the majority of patients, the left internal mammary artery is used to bypass the left anterior descending coronary artery, and saphenous vein grafts are generally used for the other anastomoses. The procedure is usually performed with use of extracorporeal circulation with general body hypothermia (28 to 30° C.). Since the blood flow passing through the heart is great, its temperature rapidly falls and it reaches 28° C. The ascending aorta is occluded, and potassium-containing cardioplegic solution is infused into the coronary circulation. The potassium places the heart in diastolic arrest and provides a motionless and dry field for performance of the anastomoses; oxygen usage can be reduced even further by local cooling of the heart with cold saline on ice slush. In general, all coronary arteries 1.5 mm. or more in diameter with stenoses greater than 50 per cent are chosen for bypass. In recent years, nearly all significant vessels are bypassed. In most patients, three to four bypass grafts are inserted. It is quite important to utilize the internal mammary artery, which is now anastomosed in 95 per cent of patients. The technique of coronary anastomosis is very significant; emphasis should be placed on this aspect of the procedure because it is crucial in the immediate as well as long-term results. After completion of all bypass grafts, the body temperature is raised, the heart generally resumes its beat, and appropriate pharmacologic agents for stabilizing the circulation are administered.

POSTOPERATIVE MANAGEMENT

Postoperatively, patients undergoing CABG require careful observation with continuous registration of arterial blood pressure, venous pressure, urinary output, and the electrocardiogram with periodic determinations of arterial blood gases (PO_2, PCO_2, and pH) and cardiac output. Cardiac output can be determined by a pulmonary arterial catheter with a thermodilution device for indicating cardiac output and pulmonary wedge capilliary pressure. Body weight should be recorded daily for assessment of potential fluid retention.

POSTOPERATIVE COMPLICATIONS

In many patients, few if any complications follow CABG. However, strict attention should be given the possible development of hypovolemia, cardiac tamponade, concealed bleeding, dysrhythmias, myocardial insufficiency, and occlusion of coronary anastomoses in the postoperative period. Fortunately, the long-term results are excellent.

Cardiac *tamponade* due to collection of blood and clots around the heart that interfere with cardiac filling is a serious postoperative complication. It causes a low cardiac output and hypotension with equalization of central venous and pulmonary arterial wedge pressures. A chest film may demonstrate mediastinal widening from the collection of blood or clots. However, it should be remembered that a *significant* amount of tamponade may occur with minimal evidence on the chest film. Tests for blood clotting defects should be performed; if blood clotting defects are present, they should be managed by blood component therapy. Reoperation should be undertaken without delay and is necessary in 2 to 3 per cent of patients undergoing CABG.

ATRIAL DYSRHYTHMIAS

Premature atrial contractions, atrial fibrillation, or atrial flutter occurs in 10 to 30 per cent of CABG patients postoperatively. Atrial tachycardia can be controlled by intravenous digoxin followed by an attempt at pharmacologic cardioversion with atenolol, procainamide, or calcium channel-blocking agents. Atrial pacing or direct cardioversion can be effective in managing atrial flutter after initial drug therapy. The important feature is conversion of the dysrhythmia for prevention of prolonged hypotension and low cardiac output. Ventricular arrhythmias may also occur, including frequent or multifocal premature ventricular contractions, ventricular tachycardia, or ventricular fibrillation. These are best managed by intravenous lidocaine and/or procainamide together with direct current cardioversion when necessary. Serious and repetitive ventricular dysrhythmias are usually a manifestation of significant myocardial ischemia, and attention should be focused on whether the grafts are occluded or if a myocardial infarction has occurred. Beta-blocking agents and oral procainamide are used for long-term management of persistent ventricular ectopy.

Ventilatory support is usually provided immediately after operation, and most patients can be extubated the same day or following morning. Those with preoperative respiratory insufficiency usually require longer periods of ventilatory support with endotracheal intubation. If the patient requires ventilatory support after 10 days, consideration should be given to the placement of a tracheostomy for prevention of permanent damage from the endotracheal tube.

Postoperative renal dysfunction may become manifest by low output and elevations of the blood urea nitrogen and creatinine. Most often it is due to a low cardiac output or presence of renal insufficiency preoperatively. Management consists of correcting the primary cause, usually hypotension, with low-dose intravenous dopamine, adequate hydration, and general support of cardiac output. Care must be taken to prevent overhydration or hyperkalemia. Should dialysis be required, peritoneal dialysis is preferable to hemodialysis.

Superficial wound infections may occur in the median sternotomy incision postoperatively but are usually inconsequential. The combination of diabetes and bilateral internal mammary grafts may predispose some patients to a higher incidence of sternal infection. Severe sternal wound infection with mediastinitis is quite serious and occurs in 1 to 2 per cent of patients following CABG. Fever often precedes local evidence of the infection. Separation of the sternum with instability is often present. With a definite sternal infection, open drainage and antibiotics with concomitant or subsequent placement of muscle or omental flaps should be performed to speed healing. Although the mortality of this complication was formerly high, with appropriate therapy it is now generally less than 10 per cent. Perioperative myocardial infarction occurs in about 1 to 2 per cent of patients after CABG.

Currently the overall postoperative mortality ranges between 1 and 2 per cent for most patients with a 4-year survival greater than 90 per cent. Good-risk patients, less than age 65 years or who have an ejection fraction greater than 0.40, have a lower operative mortality and survive longer.

Postoperative studies indicate that the primary physiologic effect of CABG is augmentation of left ventricular function with definite improvement in cardiac hemodynamics including an increased ejection fraction, higher cardiac output, decreased diastolic volume, and improved left ventricular wall motion. These can be demonstrated in a significant proportion of patients after CABG. Exercise function is also definitely increased in the majority of patients.

1. SURGICAL MANAGEMENT OF FAILED ANGIOPLASTY

Peter Van Trigt, M.D.

As percutaneous transluminal coronary angioplasty (PTCA) has gained increasing popularity as a primary treatment for coronary atherosclerotic heart disease (more than 450,000 PTCA procedures will be performed in 1991), surgeons have encountered a concomitant rise in the need for emergency surgical myocardial revascularization for acute coronary angioplasty failure. Emergency coronary artery bypass grafting for acute myocardial ischemia secondary to vessel dissection, thrombosis, or spasm has significant morbidity and definite mortality. Currently, a PTCA failure rate of 4 to 5 per cent is reported by most centers performing a large number of coronary angioplasties, and these patients require expeditious surgical revascularization. Rapid surgical revascularization with careful management of the patient during the period of vessel closure for minimization of ischemia is required for optimizing the clinical outcome of these compromised patients.

Percutaneous transluminal coronary angioplasty utilizes intracoronary balloon inflation to approximately four atmospheres of pressure for production of localized trauma to the coronary artery wall; the intended result is atheroma fracture and arterial expansion that produce an increase in luminal area. Unfortunately, balloon inflation or guidewire and catheter manipulation can cause more extensive arterial wall damage with medial dissection and creation of an occlusive intimal flap. Thrombosis or spasm may also occur at the dilation site. In the absence of a well-developed collateral circulation, acute coronary occlusion produces severe myocardial ischemia and evolving myocardial infarction. The intracoronary reperfusion catheter has been used clinically to sustain coronary flow beyond an occlusion following failed angioplasty and can reverse myocardial ischemia and allow stabilization of the patient during the transport to the operating room. Re-establishment of coronary flow through the reperfusion catheter before operation can have a direct influence on reducing the extent of myocardial infarction, which occurs in 30 to 40 per cent of angioplasty failures despite successful later surgical revascularization. Reversal of acute ischemia also allows the surgeon time to harvest the internal mammary artery for use in surgical revascularization as the optimal bypass conduit. The intra-aortic balloon pump has also been used to stabilize patients following failed PTCA. However, intra-aortic balloon pumping has generally been reserved for those patients with hemodynamic instability following vessel closure after PTCA failure. Diastolic augmentation from the intra-aortic balloon pump does not greatly

---

See the corresponding chapter or part in the *Textbook of Surgery*, 14th edition, pp. 1972–1977, for a more detailed discussion of this topic, including a comprehensive list of references.

alter blood flow through the occluded vessel but can assist in maintaining viability of marginal myocardium that is supplied by collateral vessels at the border of the infarct zone. It should be emphasized that rapid transport of the patient to the operating room and placement on cardiopulmonary bypass is the *major objective* during the period of vessel closure, since this has been shown to be the only effective means of reducing a significant perioperative myocardial infarction rate.

Most recent series of emergent coronary surgical revascularization following angioplasty failure cite an operative mortality of approximately 5 per cent with a perioperative infarction incidence of approximately 30 per cent. If active ischemia is present on the presurgical electrocardiogram following failed PTCA, the postoperative myocardial infarction rate approaches 50 per cent despite successful surgical revascularization. This is the result of a necessary period for transportation of the patient from the catheterization laboratory to the operating room, placement of the patient on cardiopulmonary bypass, and establishment of surgical revascularization. The predictors of operative mortality in patients undergoing emergency coronary artery bypass grafting for failed PTCA include cardiogenic shock, previous coronary artery bypass surgery, and the presence of multiple vessel disease. A large series of 316 patients undergoing emergency or elective coronary artery bypass grafting following angioplasty failure at Emory University found that patients undergoing emergency surgical revascularization sustained a 2.5 per cent operative mortality and a 27 per cent incidence of perioperative myocardial infarction. In contrast, those patients undergoing elective coronary bypass grafting following failed PTCA, in the absence of active ischemia, sustained a perioperative myocardial infarction rate of only 4 per cent. Patients undergoing emergency surgical revascularization for failed PTCA also encounter a higher incidence of postoperative complications other than myocardial infarction, including hemorrhagic complications and respiratory failure.

Management of the patient who has sustained a failed coronary angioplasty and requires emergent coronary artery

TABLE 1. Techniques to Minimize Ischemic Injury After Failed PTCA

Within Catheterization Laboratory
 Coronary vasodilators
 Intracoronary thrombolytic therapy
 Repeat balloon inflations
 Prolonged balloon inflation with perfusion balloon catheter
 Reperfusion catheter placed across lesion
 Insertion of intra-aortic balloon pump

Within Operating Room
 Expeditious placement on cardiopulmonary bypass
 Systemic hypothermia
 Hyperkalemic hypothermic cardioplegic arrest
 Internal thoracic artery or saphenous vein bypass grafts
 Rapid revascularization

bypass grafting requires careful attention to strategies for minimizing myocardial ischemia incurred following vessel closure and before surgical revascularization can be accomplished (Table 1). Paramount importance is rapid surgical revascularization, which requires cardiac anesthesia and cardiac surgery well-coordinated with the cardiac catheterization laboratory. Current experience has shown that operative mortality can be reduced to a low level (although not equivalent to elective surgical coronary mortality). However, the in-hospital morbidity remains quite high, especially perioperative myocardial infarction of approximately 30 per cent. Attempts to reduce this rate of perioperative infarction must involve intervention techniques for restoration of perfusion to the ischemic region preoperatively.

2. RADIONUCLIDE EVALUATION OF CORONARY ARTERY DISEASE

Robert H. Jones, M.D.

The first use of radioactive tracers for assessment of any biologic process in man was for evaluation of blood flow. Modern radionuclide cardiac procedures permit assessment of cardiac function, myocardial perfusion, and metabolism. Characterization of these physiologic processes adds important information to depiction of coronary arterial anatomy on the coronary arteriogram and aids the management of patients with coronary artery disease.

MEASUREMENT OF CARDIAC FUNCTION. The two radionuclide techniques that can be used to measure left ventricular function noninvasively in patients are initial-transit radionuclide angiocardiography and gated equilibrium ventriculography. Data are acquired for the gated equilibrium technique during 100 to 300 heart beats after an intravenously injected blood pool tracer reaches equilibrium. Counts are synchronized to the cardiac cycle by the electrocardiogram and compressed into a single averaged heart beat. This then permits assessment of wall motion on dynamic images and calculation of left ventricular ejection fraction from left ventricular count changes. Initial-transit radionuclide angiocardiography uses a high-sensitivity gamma camera to dynamically record a single transit of a discrete tracer bolus through the heart. Assessment of the left ventricular function requires data from less than 10 heart beats. The short imaging time makes initial-transit radionuclide angiocardiography especially useful for obtaining hemodynamic measurements during the stress of exercise.

MYOCARDIAL PERFUSION AND METABOLISM. Radionuclides that have a high extraction during initial myocardial transit can be used to assess regional blood flow.

See the corresponding chapter or part in the *Textbook of Surgery*, 14th edition, pp. 1981–1986, for a more detailed discussion of this topic, including a comprehensive list of references.

[201]Thallium is a potassium analog that has been used extensively to assess the distribution of regional myocardial blood flow. Tracer injected during the peak of exercise stress, and imaged soon thereafter, depicts the distribution of myocardial blood flow during exercise. Perfusion defects on exercise [201]thallium images correspond to myocardium beyond a stenosis that fails to augment blood flow normally during exercise. During the initial few hours after injection, [201]thallium gradually redistributes in the myocardium proportional to tissue potassium content. Therefore, redistribution images are influenced more by myocardial mass than by differences in regional myocardial blood flow. Ischemic myocardial regions typically show defects during exercise that normalize on redistribution images. In contrast, regions of prior myocardial infarction and scar cause defects on exercise images that persist on redistribution images. The three-dimensional distribution of gamma-emitting tracers, such as [201]thallium, is commonly quantitated by use of single photon emission computed tomography.

A number of specific radiopharmaceuticals have been designed to reflect myocardial metabolism and integrity. [99m]Technetium pyrophosphate and labeled antimyosin accumulate in infarcted myocardium. Positron-emitting radiopharmaceuticals have been developed that permit assessment of regional accumulation and utilization of glucose, fatty acids, and amino acids. Use of positron-labeled radiopharmaceuticals requires special instrumentation comprised of a number of detectors encircling the patient. Further development of this promising technology, which measures regional metabolism in the myocardium, may greatly enhance understanding of ischemic processes in patients.

APPLICATION OF RADIONUCLIDE TECHNIQUES IN PATIENTS WITH CORONARY ARTERY DISEASE. Radionuclide techniques are most useful for risk stratification of patients with known or suspected coronary artery disease. Global and regional function and perfusion abnormalities are highly sensitive indicators of myocardial ischemia that usually appear at a lower ischemia threshold than evokes chest pain or electrocardiographic change. Radionuclide techniques measuring ventricular function and myocardial perfusion reflect similar biologic processes because of the close link between myocardial integrity and blood flow.

The three variables on [201]thallium studies that relate most closely to the risk of death from coronary artery disease are the number of reversible thallium defects, the magnitude of initial reversible defect, and the maximal heart rate achieved during exercise. The variable on radionuclide angiocardiography that relates most to subsequent cardiac death or myocardial infarction is the exercise ejection fraction. A lesser amount of prognostic information is contributed by the exercise increase in heart rate and the resting end-diastolic volume. Measurement of the magnitude of myocardial ischemia by these radionuclide tests provides prognostic information not available from cardiac catheterization or routine clinical assessment. The accuracy of physiologic assessment obtained simply and at a relatively low cost makes radionuclide measurements ideally suited for initial evaluation of patients with coronary artery disease. Patients recognized by radionuclide testing to have a high risk of subsequent cardiac event should undergo cardiac catheterization and evaluation for possible interventional therapy.

Patients with good anatomic results after interventional therapy commonly normalize cardiac function and myocardial perfusion during exercise. The amount of improvement in individual patients objectively documents the effectiveness of interventional therapy and relates to subsequent freedom from untoward cardiac events. Radionuclide studies are also useful for evaluating the magnitude of recurrent ischemia in patients who subsequently become symptomatic for identification of those who might benefit from repeat interventional procedures.

3. VENTRICULAR ANEURYSM

William A. Gay, Jr., M.D.

Although true aneurysms of the left ventricle may be caused by trauma or congenital cardiac malformations, the majority follow acute transmural myocardial infarction. The typical ventricular aneurysm has been described as "a thinned-out transmural scar that has completely lost its trabecular pattern." It is estimated that approximately 10 per cent of patients sustaining an acute transmural myocardial infarction will develop a left ventricular aneurysm. However, it is likely that this incidence will decrease with recent advances in the care of patients with acute infarcts including careful hemodynamic control and aggressive reperfusion efforts.

Although the relationship between coronary occlusion and aneurysm formation has been well established, until recently it was poorly understood why some infarctions produced aneurysms whereas others did not. Recent studies indicate that the absence of significant collateral circulation in the distribution of the left anterior descending coronary artery is a major determining factor in the formation of ventricular aneurysm following anterior infarction.

Whereas some patients with ventricular aneurysm may be asymptomatic, most have some combination of dyspnea, angina, and palpitations. Peripheral arterial embolization from mural thrombi within the aneurysm is rare. Those patients whose aneurysms produce symptoms should be considered candidates for surgical resection. Moreover, if coronary bypass surgery is being planned for a patient with a ventricular aneurysm, the aneurysm should be resected concomitantly. Although ventricular aneurysm may be accurately diagnosed by use of noninvasive means, ventricu-

---

See the corresponding chapter or part in the *Textbook of Surgery*, 14th edition, pp. 1986–1989, for a more detailed discussion of this topic, including a comprehensive list of references.

lography and selective coronary arteriography should be done in all patients being considered for operation. Visualization of the coronary arteries allows bypass of all significant occlusive lesions at the time of aneurysmectomy.

Aneurysmectomy is performed via a midline sternotomy incision with use of cardiopulmonary bypass. The aneurysm is opened and its "neck" identified and closed with a patch trimmed to cover the defect. The aneurysm sac is then trimmed and closed over the patch, usually without buttresses or pledgets. This surgical approach best reconstructs left ventricular geometry and appears most likely to optimize cardiac function. Early operative mortality is 5 to 10 per cent. Moreover, it has been found that 80 per cent of survivors are living 4 years later. These figures are in dramatic contrast with a nearly 90 per cent 5-year mortality among patients whose aneurysms were not resected. Factors that increase operative risk include advanced age (more than 65 years), left main coronary artery disease, renal failure, and NYHA Class IV status. Late survival is negatively affected by severe right coronary artery disease and/or posterobasal left ventricular dysfunction. Whereas there is little question that there is both subjective improvement and better survival among patients having aneurysmectomy, data documenting objective improvement in ventricular function are sparse. However, with such modalities as intraoperative echocardiography and radionuclide ventriculography, data are being accumulated to suggest that objective as well as subjective improvement occurs.

4. KAWASAKI'S DISEASE

Thomas A. D'Amico, M.D.

Kawasaki's disease is a multisystemic disorder of undetermined etiology that is now the leading cause of acquired cardiac disease in children in both Japan and the United States. Described in Japan by Kawasaki in 1967, the disorder was first presented in English in 1974. This acute illness presents with fever, sterile conjunctivitis, cervical lymphadenopathy, mucocutaneous changes, and prominent vasculitic features. Although usually indolent and self-limiting, in its advanced stage the syndrome is characterized by coronary and peripheral artery aneurysms, coronary stenoses, mitral valve insufficiency, and left ventricular dysfunction. In Kawasaki's original description, the syndrome was thought to be limited to Japanese children. The syndrome was recognized in the United States in 1973, and to date, more than 2200 cases have been reported nationally. Kawasaki's disease has been described throughout North America, Europe, and

See the corresponding chapter or part in the *Textbook of Surgery*, 14th edition, pp. 1989–1995, for a more detailed discussion of this topic, including a comprehensive list of references.

the Pacific, in addition to approximately 80,000 cases in Japan alone.

Kawasaki's disease predominantly affects infants and children, the highest incidence being at 12 to 16 months, and has been found to be more common in males than in females (3:2), in Asians and blacks, and in siblings. Various causative agents have been proposed, but the etiologic agent of Kawasaki's syndrome remains unclear. The pathophysiologic mechanism has been well described, but the infrequent progression to severe cardiovascular manifestations is not well understood. Current management consists of aspirin and gamma globulin as well as surgical intervention in patients with advanced disease. An ideal treatment that ameliorates the early inflammatory symptoms, arrests the vasculitic progression, and prevents the formation of coronary aneurysms has not yet been discovered.

CLINICAL MANIFESTATIONS

Symptoms. The diagnosis of Kawasaki's disease is secured by the presence of five of the six major criteria: fever, conjunctivitis, mucocutaneous changes, vasculitic changes in the extremities, truncal rash, and cervical adenopathy. The presentation of this syndrome is acute, and the symptoms evolve during a period of a few days, a stereotypical clinical pattern that usually is diagnostic. The principal presenting symptom is fever, which usually has an abrupt onset, may be prolonged or intermittent, and does not respond to antibiotics. The fever lasts from 7 to 14 days but may persist in more severe cases. The appearance of fever is often accompanied by the presence of congested ocular conjunctivae. After the appearance of conjunctivitis, several changes in the lips and oral cavity occur: there is a reddening of the lips, the tongue may appear prominently, with protuberant papillae ("strawberry tongue"), or there may be only diffuse reddening of the oropharyngeal mucosa.

By the third day of the illness, a polymorphous macular erythematous rash appears. The rash begins with reddening of the palms and soles; individual lesions may coalesce as the rash progresses proximally to spread over the trunk, usually over 48 hours. In less than 50 per cent of patients, nonpurulent cervical lymphadenopathy develops.

Physical Examination. The principal physical findings are easily recognized. Elicitation of the more subtle physical findings early in the course of Kawasaki's disease may facilitate the prompt diagnosis of its numerous complications. Examination of the heart may reveal tachycardia, distant heart sounds, or a gallop, suggestive of myocarditis or congestive failure. A holosystolic apical murmur signifies mitral valve insufficiency, which may be secondary to cardiomegaly, endocarditis, or papillary muscle dysfunction. Palpation of the peripheral arteries, especially in the axillary and inguinal regions, may reveal an aneurysm. Palpation of the abdomen may show hepatomegaly secondary to congestive heart failure, or right upper quadrant tenderness secondary to hydrops of the gallbladder. Auscultation of the abdomen may reveal the bruit of an aneurysm of the renal, celiac, mesenteric, or iliac arteries. Neurologic examination may reveal meningeal signs as well as emotional lability, irritability, stupor, or coma secondary to aseptic meningitis.

Laboratory Studies. Leukocytosis is invariably present and is often accompanied by a shift to the left. Anemia and thrombocytosis may be present. Other findings include an increase in the red blood cell sedimentation rate, C-reactive protein, factor VII concentration, and fibrinogen level as well as low antithrombin III concentration.

The electrocardiogram is abnormal in 70 per cent of patients, the most common findings being sinus tachycardia, prolonged PQ and QR intervals, second-degree atrioventricular block, decreased voltage, ST segment changes, and T wave changes.

Admission radiologic studies are often abnormal. Chest roentgenograms may reveal cardiomegaly or pleural effusions. Echocardiograms are positive in 45 per cent, providing early objective evidence of cardiovascular dysfunction.

Natural History. There are three clinical stages of Kawasaki's disease. The acute phase lasts approximately 10 days, during which time fever and the development of the characteristic rash predominate. The subacute phase ensues, during which time the cardiac complications commonly occur. The convalescent phase is defined as the period during which the red blood cell sedimentation rate remains elevated. Although the course of Kawasaki's disease is typically acute with resolution of symptoms and complications, it may recur, presenting with vasculitic symptoms or with sudden death.

A spectrum of cardiovascular manifestations may occur in Kawasaki's disease, although they are usually self-limited and benign. Myocarditis, diagnosed clinically and by electrocardiographic criteria, is present in as many as 50 per cent of patients. Mitral regurgitation occurs in only 5 per cent of patients with Kawasaki's disease; however, in patients with coronary aneurysms, the incidence is 25 per cent. Myocardial infarction, a rare complication of Kawasaki's disease, may occur after diffuse ischemia or a thromboembolic event.

The most serious complication of Kawasaki's disease is the formation of coronary artery aneurysms, which has an incidence of 20 to 40 per cent in the subacute phase. Coronary aneurysms are responsible for at least 85 per cent of the mortality associated with Kawasaki's disease. The aneurysms may be asymptomatic or may not present symptoms until years later; others may initially present with myocardial infarction, cardiogenic shock, or sudden death.

The diagnosis of Kawasaki's disease should be accompanied routinely by echocardiography, which has demonstrated a sensitivity of greater than 90 per cent in detecting coronary aneurysms. Selective coronary angiography is reserved for patients with complications of known coronary aneurysms.

PATHOLOGY. The pathologic basis of Kawasaki's disease is the progression of a nonspecific vasculitis that involves the microvasculature of the aorta and its major branches and is manifested by endarteritis of the vasa vasorum of the coronary, brachiocephalic, celiac, renal, and iliofemoral systems. As the inflammatory process of the intima and adventitia progresses, aneurysms form in these vessels and produce stenosis, thromboembolism, ischemia, rupture, or asymptomatic healing. Kawasaki's disease can be described in four pathologic phases: acute, subacute, convalescent, and chronic.

The acute phase, characterized by perivasculitis, corresponds to the febrile period and usually involves the first 10 days of the illness. During this period, the oral changes, skin changes, and conjunctivitis also develop. Death in the acute phase is usually secondary to advanced myocarditis but is rare.

During the subacute phase, typically the second 10 days of the illness, most of the clinical findings may resolve, although fever and irritability often persist. Coronary artery aneurysms develop during this phase, and thrombotic occlusion may ensue with subsequent myocardial infarction. Death in the subacute phase is often caused by a ruptured coronary artery aneurysm.

The convalescent phase, which extends into the second month, is characterized by decreased arterial inflammation. Granulation changes are seen in this phase, since internal proliferation within the aneurysm may ameliorate luminal defects. Aneurysmal dilatation may persist and produce progressive stenosis and further risk of thromboembolism. Death in this phase is usually secondary to diffuse myocardial ischemia. The disease rarely enters a chronic phase during which scarring continues, as does myocardial ischemia secondary to coronary stenoses.

ETIOLOGY. Kawasaki's disease is the main cause of acquired heart disease in children in the United States and Japan. Despite the prevalence of the disorder, investigations of the etiologic origin have been unsuccessful. Possibilities include mite-associated antigens, rickettsiae, spirochetes, *Propionibacterium, Borrelia, Pseudomonas,* and Epstein-Barr virus, all without confirmation. The lack of evidence for person-to-person transmissibility has made it difficult to isolate a single etiologic factor.

Analysis of blood from patients in the acute stage of Kawasaki's disease showed increased helper T lymphocyte activity, decreased suppressor T lymphocyte activity, and elevated reverse transcriptase activity, which suggest a retroviral component in the causation of Kawasaki's disease. However, there is no conclusive evidence of a specific viral agent, since cell lines and culture conditions have not been discovered, and there is no serologic evidence of a specific antiviral antibody.

TREATMENT. The mortality of Kawasaki's disease before 1976 was 1 to 2 per cent. Since 1976, the mortality has decreased to approximately 0.5 per cent because of earlier diagnosis and the evolution of effective treatment modalities, including surgical intervention. Optimal therapy depends ultimately on the discovery of the etiologic agent of Kawasaki's disease.

When Kawasaki's disease is diagnosed, children are given a regimen of aspirin, 100 mg. per kg. per day, which is continued until defervescence. Thereafter, they are maintained on aspirin, 10 mg. per kg. per day, for 8 weeks or until the red blood cell sedimentation rate is normal. The goal of aspirin therapy is the amelioration of symptoms and the prevention of the thrombotic and embolic complications of Kawasaki's disease. Aspirin does *not* decrease the risk of the development of coronary aneurysms. Treatment with intravenous gamma globulin has been shown to decrease the duration of fever, to decrease the prevalence of coronary abnormalities, and to prevent the progression to giant coronary aneurysms. Moreover, gamma globulin therapy improves cardiac function in patients with wall motion abnormalities secondary to diffuse myocarditis.

Advanced cardiovascular complications require surgical intervention. The first use of coronary artery bypass grafting for obstructive coronary aneurysms in Kawasaki's disease was reported in 1976 by Kitamura. General problems with coronary artery bypass grafting became apparent: the use of saphenous vein grafts showed frequent early occlusion of the grafts. Kitamura also described the first successful use of an internal mammary artery graft for treatment of coronary aneurysms in Kawasaki's disease. Before the use of arterial bypass grafts, venous graft closure at 1 year was greater than 50 per cent. With the use of internal mammary artery grafting, patency is now 85 per cent at 1 year, and late patency is nearly 60 per cent.

Mitral valve insufficiency in Kawasaki's disease is due to papillary muscle dysfunction secondary to ischemia. Mitral regurgitation is associated with high mortality when accompanied by poor left ventricular function. Surgical correction, in the presence of myocarditis and compromised left ventricular function, presents a more difficult problem than is usually encountered with valve replacement for rheumatic disease. Experience with ineffective valve repair has shown that mitral valve replacement is the most certain means of ensuring the management of severe mitral insufficiency, despite the absence of valvulitis.

CONCLUSION. Kawasaki's disease is a fascinating disorder with many cardiovascular manifestations. Aspects of this disease yet to be explained include its etiology, selectivity for children, and ability to progress to severe stages in view of its usually benign and self-limited nature.

5. CHANGES IN VENOUS AUTOGRAFTS USED AS AORTOCORONARY CONDUITS

William C. Roberts, M.D.

FINDINGS IN REMNANT SAPHENOUS VEINS EXCISED FOR AORTOCORONARY CONDUITS BUT NEVER USED. Some degree of intimal fibrous thickening occurs

See the corresponding chapter or part in the *Textbook of Surgery,* 14th edition, pp. 1995–2001, for a more detailed discussion of this topic, including a comprehensive list of references.

commonly in saphenous veins excised for aortocoronary bypass but never utilized. Approximately 1 per cent of saphenous veins excised for coronary bypass are narrowed more than 50 per cent in cross-sectional area by fibrous tissue before they are used as aortocoronary conduits.

EARLY CHANGES IN SAPHENOUS VEINS USED AS AORTOCORONARY CONDUITS. In 1906, Carrel and Guthrie described intimal thickening of veins implanted into the arterial system in dogs and concluded that veins placed in the arterial circulation had a strong tendency to assume the character of an artery. Carrel described four characteristic changes in veins used as arteries in the peripheral circulation: (1) intimal thickening, (2) adventitial thickening (from fibrosis), (3) loss of the inner third of the media, and (4) loss of elastic fibers with production of a fibrous tube.

Spray and Roberts studied a large number of saphenous vein grafts from patients dying within a year after aortocoronary bypass. By 2 weeks postoperatively, mural edema was pronounced, some medial smooth muscle cells were necrotic, and inflammatory infiltrates were present. The endothelium often was disrupted, and the intimal surface usually was covered, either partially or completely, by fibrin. By 3 weeks, cells with characteristics of smooth muscle appeared in the subendothelial portion of the intima. Thereafter, the subendothelial intimal lesions became more generalized and less cellular, ground substance appeared in abundance, and short elastic fibers and vascular channels occasionally were present. The smooth muscle fibers of the media gradually diminished in number and were replaced, in part or in whole, by fibrous tissue. Fibrous tissue also increased in the adventitia. Thus, the saphenous vein used as an artery becomes a stiff, fibrous-tissue conduit.

LATE CHANGES IN SAPHENOUS VEINS USED AS AORTOCORONARY CONDUITS. Kalan and Roberts described at necropsy findings in saphenous vein grafts in the aortocoronary position from 13 to 185 months (mean 58 months). Of the 53 patients, 31 (58 per cent) had at least one bypass graft maximally narrowed greater than 75 per cent in cross-sectional area at some point by fibromuscular tissue with or without lipid; 12 patients (23 per cent) had maximal graft narrowing of 51 to 75 per cent; 8 patients (15 per cent), 26 to 50 per cent; and 2 patients (4 per cent), 0 to 25 per cent. The percentage of patients with a graft narrowed over 75 per cent at necropsy did not increase as the interval from bypass surgery to death increased. Of the 123 saphenous vein grafts, 47 (38 per cent) were maximally narrowed greater than 75 per cent in cross-sectional area; 44 (36 per cent), 51 to 75 per cent; 22 (18 per cent), 26 to 50 per cent; and 10 (8 per cent), 0 to 25 per cent. The degree of narrowing of the saphenous vein graft was related to the degree of luminal narrowing of the native coronary artery at or within 2 cm. distal to the saphenous vein–coronary artery anastomosis. Analysis of the 1865 5-mm. long saphenous vein segments disclosed that 209 segments (11 per cent) were narrowed 96 to 100 per cent in cross-sectional area; 172 (9 per cent), 76 to 95 per cent; 407

(22 per cent), 51 to 75 per cent; 685 (37 per cent), 26 to 50 per cent; and 392 (21 per cent), 0 to 25 per cent.

Essentially all saphenous veins used as aortocoronary conduits for longer than a year develop atherosclerotic plaques in each 5-mm. segment of their entire lengths. Thus, the atherosclerotic plaquing late in saphenous veins used as aortocoronary conduits is diffuse, just as it is in native coronary arteries in patients with fatal myocardial ischemia. The amount of luminal narrowing in the saphenous veins used as aortocoronary conduits is significantly greater in those patients who die from a cardiac cause compared with those who die from a noncardiac cause. The interval from coronary bypass to death does not correlate with either the percentage of vein conduits or the percentage of 5-mm. segments of vein conduit narrowed over 75 per cent in cross-sectional area by plaque.

COMPOSITION OF TISSUE CAUSING LUMINAL NARROWING IN SAPHENOUS VEINS USED AS AORTOCORONARY CONDUITS. The composition of the plaques in the saphenous venous conduits is similar to that in the native coronary arteries. Fibrous tissue or fibromuscular tissue is the dominant component of the plaques in saphenous vein conduits just as it is the dominant component of plaques in the native coronary arteries in patients with fatal coronary artery disease without coronary bypass.

COMPARISON OF MORPHOLOGIC CHANGES IN SAPHENOUS VEINS WITH THOSE IN INTERNAL MAMMARY ARTERIES USED AS AORTOCORONARY CONDUITS. None of the aforedescribed changes in saphenous veins used as aortocoronary conduits is found in internal mammary arteries used in the coronary position. The internal mammary artery late after bypass remains much smaller than does the saphenous vein when each is utilized in the same patient.

XVI

Congenital Lesions of the Coronary Circulation

James E. Lowe, M.D., and David C. Sabiston, Jr., M.D.

Congenital coronary arterial malformations have long been recognized, but the number of reported patients has increased markedly since the introduction of selective coronary arteriography in 1959.

See the corresponding chapter or part in the *Textbook of Surgery*, 14th edition, pp. 2001–2011, for a more detailed discussion of this topic, including a comprehensive list of references.

CORONARY ARTERY FISTULAS

Congenital coronary fistulas are the most common of the congenital coronary malformations. They are characterized by normal origin of the involved coronary artery from the aorta with a fistulous communication with the atria or ventricles or with the pulmonary artery, coronary sinus, or superior vena cava.

CLINICAL MANIFESTATIONS. Formerly, it was believed that most patients with coronary artery fistulas were asymptomatic. However, based on the authors' experience with 30 patients and supported by a review of 258 others reported in the literature, 55 per cent are symptomatic at the time of presentation. Because the underlying pathophysiologic process is essentially that of a left-to-right cardiac shunt, the most common manifestation is congestive heart failure. Other symptoms are angina pectoris, secondary to a steal of coronary arterial flow through the fistulous communication, and subacute bacterial endocarditis. The major clinical finding secondary to a coronary artery fistula is a continuous murmur over the site of the abnormal communication. This murmur may closely resemble that of a patent ductus arteriosus.

The right coronary artery is most often involved in the development of the congenital coronary fistula (56 per cent) and usually communicates with a chamber of the right side of the heart. The fistula usually involves the right ventricle (39 per cent), followed closely in incidence by drainage into the right atrium (33 per cent), including the coronary sinus and superior vena cava, or the pulmonary artery (20 per cent). Left coronary artery fistulas are less common but usually drain into the right ventricle or right atrium. Rarely, coronary artery fistulas may drain into the left atrium or left ventricle.

EVALUATION. The precise diagnosis of coronary artery fistulas requires arteriographic demonstration of the involved coronary artery, the recipient cardiac chamber, and the exact site of communication. In patients with a large fistula, injection of contrast medium into the aortic root may clearly delineate the lesion. In patients with a smaller fistula or fistulous communications from both coronary arteries, selective coronary arteriography is essential for establishing the diagnosis.

SURGICAL MANAGEMENT. Patients with a single coronary fistula that is easily dissected usually do not require cardiopulmonary bypass for suture obliteration. However, in patients with multiple communications or large, tortuous, draining channels, the fistula is best obliterated by opening the recipient cardiac chamber with the patient on cardiopulmonary bypass in order to completely close all fistulous tracts.

RESULTS. Thirty patients with congenital coronary artery fistulas have been evaluated by the authors, and 23 patients have undergone surgical repair. The mean time of follow-up for these patients has been 10 years. There were no operative deaths, and all patients are well and do not have evidence of recurrent fistula formation, although one patient with a complex fistula of the circumflex coronary artery to the right ventricle has a small residual shunt.

ORIGIN OF THE LEFT CORONARY ARTERY FROM THE PULMONARY ARTERY

It is generally recognized that the prognosis for most patients with origin of the left coronary artery from the pulmonary artery is poor. It has been estimated that 95 per cent of patients with this anomaly die within the first year of life unless surgical therapy is undertaken.

CLINICAL MANIFESTATIONS. The pathophysiologic mechanism of this malformation is that blood from the right coronary artery flows, via collaterals, into the left coronary artery and then into the pulmonary artery. The resultant symptoms and clinical manifestations are secondary to left ventricular myocardial ischemia, which results either from inadequate collateral flow from the right coronary artery to the left coronary artery or from a steal of adequate collateral flow into the low-pressure pulmonary arterial system. Clinical manifestations become apparent in infancy in most patients. When symptoms appear, the course is one of progressive deterioration. Unless operative therapy is undertaken, progressively worsening left ventricular dysfunction occurs, usually leading to death in infancy.

The characteristic findings on physical examination include rapid respiratory rate, tachycardia, and cardiac enlargement. A murmur is not usually present early in life, and congenital origin of the left coronary artery from the pulmonary artery is one of the few malformations in infancy that can cause congestive heart failure without a murmur. The liver is characteristically enlarged, and the spleen is palpable in a smaller number of patients. Occasionally, patients first present with signs of cardiovascular collapse and shock similar to those shown by adults with sudden coronary artery occlusion.

EVALUATION. Considerable emphasis has been placed on the changes that occur on the electrocardiogram in establishing a diagnosis. Bland and associates in 1933 first described myocardial ischemia on the electrocardiogram of an infant with this condition. Based on this work, congenital origin of the left coronary artery from the pulmonary artery has also been referred to as the Bland-White-Garland syndrome. Cardiac catheterization usually reveals the right side of the heart to be normal. The pulmonary vasculature may show slight engorgement and enlargement. The most striking feature is enlargement of the left atrium and particularly of the left ventricle. The wall of the left ventricle may be quite thin, especially the anterolateral aspect near the apex. A true ventricular aneurysm with paradoxical pulsations may be present, and mitral insufficiency is relatively common. The passage of contrast medium into the aorta demonstrates a single right coronary artery, although selective coronary arteriography is more reliable for precise demonstration of this feature. The right ventricular and pulmonary artery pressures may be elevated. It is usually possible to show a left-to-right shunt at the pulmonary artery level by injection of contrast material. Although the oxygen saturation may sometimes show a significant increase from the right ventricle to the pulmonary artery, this increase is not always present, even when it can be shown that the left coronary artery arises from the pulmonary artery.

SURGICAL MANAGEMENT. Two basic approaches are available for the surgical treatment of origin of the left coronary artery from the pulmonary artery. Simple ligation at the site of origin from the pulmonary artery is effective treatment if there are enough collaterals from the right coronary artery to adequately supply the left coronary arterial system. This approach is usually reserved for small infants, in whom the left coronary artery is too small for a direct anastomosis. Ligation prevents the steal of right coronary collateral flow into the low-pressure pulmonary artery system. If collateral flow from the right coronary artery is inadequate or if the patient is an older infant, the initial repair can be designed to reconstruct a two–coronary artery system. At present, this is best accomplished by either ligation and saphenous vein bypass grafting or ligation and left or right subclavian artery–left coronary artery anastomosis. In younger children and infants, the latter form of therapy has technical advantages, because in this group, the subclavian artery is usually larger than is the autologous saphenous vein. Direct reimplantation of the left coronary artery to the aorta has also been reported. In addition, a two–coronary artery system can also be created by intrapulmonary conduits from the left coronary ostia to the aorta. Segments of saphenous vein, free subclavian arterial grafts, flaps of pulmonary artery, pericardial tubes, and prosthetic conduits have all been successfully used, but their long-term patency rates are unknown. Because of the 95 to 100 per cent mortality in those treated nonoperatively, surgical therapy is always indicated following diagnosis.

ORIGIN OF THE RIGHT CORONARY ARTERY FROM THE PULMONARY ARTERY

St. John Brooks in 1886 originally described this rare malformation in two cadavers. Both lesions occurred in adults, neither of whom had evidence of heart disease. Brooks noted dilated collaterals from the left coronary artery feeding the right coronary artery and correctly postulated, based on this observation, that flow in the right coronary artery might actually be retrograde into the pulmonary artery.

CLINICAL MANIFESTATIONS. The clinical manifestations of this condition are usually minimal or absent. In the 17 cases collected from the literature, the abnormal artery was discovered in individuals whose ages ranged from 17 to 90 years. The malformation was thought to have been associated with death in only two cases. Even though origin of the right coronary artery from the pulmonary artery is a rare anomaly with a benign natural history in most patients, it can cause myocardial ischemia, infarction, congestive heart failure, and myocardial fibrosis. Because it can be safely corrected when diagnosed, operative correction is indicated.

EVALUATION. In the rare patient with this condition who comes to medical attention, the diagnosis is established by aortography and selective coronary arteriography. The left coronary artery is found to be dilated, and large intercoronary collaterals feed the right coronary artery. Flow in the right coronary artery is retrograde, emptying into the pulmonary artery. In contrast to patients who have the more frequently occurring malformation or origin of the left coronary artery from the pulmonary, there are usually no electrocardiographic or radiographic abnormalities.

SURGICAL MANAGEMENT AND RESULTS. At operation, a narrow rim of tissue from the pulmonary artery is removed with the origin of the right coronary artery, and this is then reimplanted into the ascending aorta. This represents the ideal form of surgical management and has been performed by several groups with no operative or late mortality. Other alternatives include simple ligation at the site of anomalous origin with or without saphenous vein bypass grafting.

ORIGIN OF BOTH CORONARY ARTERIES FROM THE PULMONARY ARTERY

Twenty-five infants in whom both coronary arteries arose from the pulmonary artery have been reported. The malformation has been diagnosed by cardiac catheterization, and surgical repair has been attempted but to date has not been successful.

ANEURYSMS OF THE CORONARY ARTERIES

Congenital aneurysms of the coronary arteries are most often asymptomatic until complications occur. Complications include thrombosis or embolization with subsequent myocardial ischemia or infarction or actual rupture of the aneurysm. Surgical management of a coronary artery aneurysm is indicated if the aneurysm is symptomatic, especially if there is evidence of emboli arising from the aneurysm with production of myocardial ischemia in the distal coronary bed.

XVII

Acquired Disorders of the Aortic Valve

Glenn J. R. Whitman, M.D.,
and Alden H. Harken, M.D.

AORTIC STENOSIS

PATHOPHYSIOLOGY. Left ventricular outflow tract obstruction becomes severe when normal flow generates a transvalvular gradient of 60 mm. Hg or produces a calculated valve area of less than 0.7 sq. cm. The accompanying left ventricular hypertrophy, when severe, is associated with a decrease in compliance. In this situation, atrial contraction has a crucial role in diastolic loading, and loss of a normal sinus mechanism may cause acute cardiac decompensation. Moreover, with prolongation of the ejection period and elevation of the end-diastolic pressure, diastolic coronary blood flow diminishes, and ischemic subendocardial fibrosis may occur.

CLINICAL COURSE. Initially, patients may present with angina (medical survival 5 years) due to an imbalance of oxygen delivery and consumption. Exercise-induced syncope, the result of baroreceptor dysfunction in the presence of a fixed cardiac output, may then follow (medical survival 3 years), after which left ventricular dysfunction occurs with resultant dyspnea and failure (medical survival 2 years).

DIAGNOSIS. Auscultation reveals a crescendo-decrescendo murmur. The carotid pulse is characterized by a prolonged slow rise. Doppler echo can evaluate the peak valvular gradient, such that

$$\text{Predicted peak transvalvular gradient} = 4 \cdot v^2$$

where v equals blood velocity (liters per minute). However, the most accurate measure of obstruction is with cardiac catheterization; a simplified Gorlin formula demonstrates.

$$\text{AVA} = \frac{\text{CO}}{\sqrt{\Delta}}$$

where AVA is the aortic valve area, CO is the cardiac output, and Δ is the transvalvular gradient.

TREATMENT. The onset of symptoms is an indication for valve replacement, the only effective therapy for aortic stenosis, which is performed electively for angina and syncope and more urgently for symptoms of left ventricular failure. Asymptomatic patients should be recommended for aortic valve replacement when they exhibit left ventricular chamber

---

See the corresponding chapter or part in the *Textbook of Surgery*, 14th edition, pp. 2011–2018, for a more detailed discussion of this topic, including a comprehensive list of references.

enlargement. In general, there are no contraindications to surgical therapy for aortic stenosis. A small group of patients present with end-stage myocardial dysfunction disproportionate to their degree of stenosis. This may be the only group who derive little benefit from surgical therapy.

Surgical mortality for aortic valve replacement is 2 to 8 per cent. Risk factors include age, left ventricular function, NYHA class, and pulmonary function. In patients with aortic stenosis and coronary artery disease, valve replacement and revascularization should be performed simultaneously.

Percutaneous aortic balloon valvuloplasty is an option in the treatment of aortic stenosis. The immediate results show an increase in the aortic valve area of only 50 per cent with a 3 to 10 per cent mortality. Recurrence of symptoms, hemodynamic evidence of restenosis, or a combination of these or death may occur in over 50 per cent of patients at 6 months. Consequently, if balloon valvuloplasty is employed, it should be limited to patients with a poor prognosis due to other organ system failure.

AORTIC INSUFFICIENCY

PATHOPHYSIOLOGY. The primary pathophysiologic result of aortic insufficiency is an increase in preload. For sustaining a normal effective cardiac output, left ventricular dilation and wall thickening occur for maintenance of a normal ejection fraction. However, in time, wall thickness does not keep pace with increasing end-diastolic volumes, wall tension increases, and systolic dysfunction occurs. At this point, end-diastolic pressure rises, and patients often become symptomatic. Frequently, however, significant cardiac dysfunction can occur without symptoms. Acute aortic insufficiency produces high left ventricular end-diastolic pressures as the regurgitant fraction encounters an unconditioned ventricle. Symptoms develop immediately.

CLINICAL COURSE. Chronic aortic insufficiency is surprisingly well tolerated. Patients may have essentially no cardiorespiratory symptoms until symptoms of left ventricular failure occur. Angina may also occur and is the result of low aortic diastolic pressure with resultant poor coronary blood flow.

TREATMENT. Survival of a population of medically treated patients with moderate to severe aortic insufficiency is 75 per cent at 5 years and 50 per cent at 10 years. When symptomatic, these patients should be referred for surgical therapy; however, treatment of the asymptomatic patient is more controversial. Survival, either medical or surgical, is dependent on left ventricular function. Elevation of end-systolic volumes can be used as an indicator for surgical intervention. Preoperative resting left ventricular ejection fraction, fractional shortening, and end-systolic dimension are strong predictors of long-term survival despite surgical intervention. Persistent medical management of dysfunction for more than 1 year can severely jeopardize survival. Early and late results are improved by early surgical intervention.

CHOICE OF VALVE PROSTHESIS

Three broad categories of valves are available: mechanical valves, xenograft (porcine) prostheses, and free-sewn homograft valves. At the University of Colorado Health Science Center, the authors currently use a tilting disc valve (St. Jude). The tilting disc prosthesis functions hemodynamically better in small sizes when compared with the high-profile ball and cage prosthesis. It has a much smaller profile compared with the Medtronic-Hall valve. A 21-mm. St. Jude valve has an effective orifice area of approximately 1.5 sq. cm. Thromboembolic complication rates for these prostheses are 1 to 1.7 events per patient year. These valves require anticoagulation with an associated complication rate of 5 per cent per year and a 1 per cent yearly anticoagulation-related mortality.

The porcine bioprostheses (Hancock and Carpentier-Edwards) utilize the aortic valve of the pig fixed in glutaraldehyde. The main appeal of these valves is that they do not require anticoagulation. In a prospective study, freedom from all aortic valve–related complications at 5 to 8 years, fatal or nonfatal, was 63 per cent for the bioprosthetic valve versus 53 per cent for a mechanical valve. The bioprosthetic advantage was due entirely to fewer bleeding complications because of the lack of anticoagulation. The bioprosthetic valve, however, exhibits poor long-term durability. Although valve performance is excellent up to 60 months, it then falls precipitously. In patients less than 30 years old, 75 per cent require reoperation for valve replacement at 10 years. Moreover, the hemodynamic profile of the bioprostheses is not as good as that of the mechanical prostheses. Consequently, bioprostheses should be used cautiously in sizes smaller than 23 mm.

Unlike the bioprostheses, the free-sewn homograft valve is not stented and is sewn into the native annulus freehand. This is a significantly more difficult and time-consuming operation than is a prosthetic aortic valve replacement. As with the bioprostheses, these valves require no anticoagulation. Long-term morbidity relates exclusively to valve degeneration and progressive aortic regurgitation. With the antibiotic-preserved valve, the best reports show a freedom from incompetence of approximately 94 per cent at 9 years, which falls to only 62 per cent at 13 years. The cryopreserved homograft valve may have an entirely different natural history. With this valve, freedom from *all* valve-related complications has been shown to be over 90 per cent at 10 years. Follow-up data significantly longer than 10 years are not yet available.

1. SURGICAL TREATMENT OF HYPERTROPHIC CARDIOMYOPATHY

H. Newland Oldham, Jr., M.D.

Cardiomyopathy is a primary disorder of cardiac muscle that is subclassified into hypertrophic cardiomyopathy (HCM) and dilated cardiomyopathy. This terminology has replaced the earlier title of idiopathic hypertrophic subaortic stenosis. Cardiomyopathy of all types is responsible for less than 1 per cent of cardiac deaths in the United States. Symptoms are related to dynamic systolic obstruction of left ventricular outflow, abnormalities of diastolic function, alterations in coronary blood flow, and cardiac arrhythmias. Most patients respond to medical therapy, and surgical therapy has been reserved for those with significant obstruction whose symptoms are unresponsive to medical treatment.

PATHOLOGIC ANATOMY. The two major pathologic features are asymmetric septal hypertrophy and microscopic evidence of disorganized muscle bundles. Septal hypertrophy begins several centimeters below the aortic valve and primarily involves the upper septum in 90 per cent of patients. Septal thickness is greatest at the level of the mitral valve, and the valve may be abnormally positioned. Disagreement persists concerning the specificity of the microscopic disorganization, but it probably is not unique to HCM. Additional histologic features include myocardial scarring and abnormalities of the intramural coronary arteries.

PHYSIOLOGY. The three basic pathophysiologic processes in HCM are dynamic systolic subaortic obstruction, diastolic dysfunction, and myocardial ischemia. Systolic obstruction is caused by contact between the mitral valve and the septum. This obstruction is dynamic and may change spontaneously or after physiologic or pharmacologic provocation. A reduction in the gradient is caused by decreased myocardial contractility, increased ventricular volume, or increased arterial pressure, and the gradient is increased by the opposite influences. Rapid ejection through a narrow outflow tract creates Venturi forces that draw the anterior mitral leaflet toward the septum. Abnormal papillary muscle support may contribute to systolic anterior motion of the mitral valve. Diastolic dysfunction of HCM is less well understood. Abnormalities in relaxation, compliance, and filling have been identified in the majority of patients. Atrial fibrillation causes loss of atrial contribution to systolic filling and shortened diastole, and it may cause further clinical deterioration. Myocardial ischemia is an important cause of chest pain and progression of the disease. Elevated left ventricular pressure increases myocardial oxygen demand, contributing to ischemia. Ischemia may additionally be caused by abnormalities

---

See the corresponding chapter or part in the *Textbook of Surgery,* 14th edition, pp. 2018–2026, for a more detailed discussion of this topic, including a comprehensive list of references.

in capillary density, small vessel vasodilator reserve, and wall thickness of intramural myocardial arteries.

CLINICAL FEATURES. HCM may present between infancy and old age. When symptoms occur in the first year, death is common and usually from congestive failure. In elderly patients, HCM is associated with distorted ventricular geometry and mitral annular calcification. The calcified annulus contributes to obstruction and occasionally necessitates mitral valve replacement. More typical patients demonstrate morphologic abnormalities by 20 years of age and symptoms by the age of 40 years. The disease is more common in males and is familial in approximately 60 per cent of patients. The classic symptoms of HCM are dyspnea, chest pain, and presyncope or syncope. There is poor correlation between symptoms and underlying pathophysiologic mechanisms. Symptoms may be caused by dynamic ventricular obstruction, alteration in diastolic function, myocardial ischemia, mitral regurgitation, or cardiac arrhythmias. Identical symptoms may be caused by several mechanisms, and their severity does not correlate with the magnitude of the pathophysiologic abnormality.

Sudden death is the most ominous clinical feature of HCM. There is no clear relationship between the incidence of sudden death and extent of hypertrophy, severity of symptoms, functional limitations, hemodynamic abnormalities, or degree of outflow tract obstruction. The annual mortality for sudden death is 2 to 3 per cent with a slightly higher incidence in younger patients. Sudden death is due to arrhythmia, and the most common is probably ventricular tachycardia. The mechanism is unknown but may be related to disorganized myocardial cells, elevated ventricular pressure, or ischemia and fibrosis. The most useful marker has been nonsustained ventricular tachycardia during 48-hour electrocardiographic monitoring.

DIAGNOSTIC EVALUATION. Echocardiography has been helpful in understanding and evaluating HCM. The characteristic findings of asymmetric septal hypertrophy and systolic anterior motion of the mitral valve are recognized and may be followed serially. Mitral valve systolic anterior motion occasionally occurs with other abnormalities, and asymmetric septal hypertrophy may rarely be associated with valvular aortic stenosis. Two-dimensional echo has been beneficial in identifying the mechanism by which systolic anterior motion of the mitral valve contributes to the subaortic gradient. Echo Doppler has demonstrated diastolic dysfunction in the majority of patients even in the absence of symptoms or subaortic gradients. Intraoperative echocardiography has been used to identify atypical patterns of septal hypertrophy in order to modify the operation to match the specific type and location of obstruction. Complete cardiac catheterization is rarely necessary, but coronary angiography is recommended before surgical intervention.

NATURAL HISTORY AND OPERATIVE INDICATIONS. Typical patients develop symptoms in mid life, although increasing numbers of elderly patients are being recognized. Treatment is designed to alleviate symptoms but does not reverse the basic hypertrophic process or eliminate sudden death. Most patients respond to beta-blockers with reduction in heart rate, contractility, systolic wall stress, and myocardial oxygen consumption and have improvement in angina, congestive failure, and presyncope. Calcium channel blockers have been beneficial in patients with alterations in diastolic relaxation and filling. Amiodarone improves survival of patients with nonsustained ventricular tachycardia but has serious side effects and does not benefit all patients. Failure of drugs to relieve symptoms in the presence of a significant resting gradient indicates the advisability of surgical treatment. Treatment of asymptomatic patients and treatment of patients with gradients that can be demonstrated only by provocative measures remain controversial.

SURGICAL TREATMENT. Two thirds of patients with HCM respond well to medical treatment. Those who remain symptomatic usually have dynamic outflow tract obstruction, diastolic dysfunction, or severe mitral regurgitation. The goals of surgical therapy are relief of symptoms and improvement in the quality of life and are attainable in 70 per cent of patients. The two main treatments are septal myotomy-myectomy (M-M) and mitral valve replacement (MVR). Septal M-M is performed through a transaortic approach and two parallel incisions are made into the septal muscle away from the conduction tissue, and a strip of septum extending to below the site of mitral valve–septal contact is excised. Removal of this rectangle of muscle enlarges the left ventricular outflow tract, reduces the velocity of blood flow, and decreases Venturi forces on the mitral valve and septum. Subaortic obstruction may also effectively be eliminated by MVR. Advantages of this operation include elimination of ventricular septal perforation and decreased injury to the conduction system. Recent reports indicate that MVR is utilized in up to one third of patients. Indications for MVR include severe mitral disease other than systolic anterior motion and reoperation following a previous septal M-M. Relative indications include older patients with severe mitral regurgitation or very large gradient. The best method of choosing between these two procedures currently is not established. Most surgeons have based their decision on preoperative criteria, but the NIH group has depended on the use of intraoperative echocardiography. Their primary indications for MVR are inaccessible septal hypertrophy and relative thinness of the basal septum.

RESULTS OF SURGICAL TREATMENT. Operative mortality is 5 to 8 per cent with no clear difference between septal M-M and MVR. Ventricular septal defect, complete heart block, and aortic or mitral valve damage may occur with an incidence less than 5 per cent. These complications do not follow MVR, but it is accompanied by the well-known sequelae of prosthetic valves, which include endocarditis, thromboembolism, anticoagulant-related bleeding, and deterioration of the prosthesis. Seventy per cent of 240 patients having septal M-M performed by Morrow between 1960 and 1982 achieved long-lasting symptomatic relief. The resting gradient was effectively eliminated, but it was usually possible to provoke a postoperative gradient. Mitral regurgitation was usually improved by operation.

There are no randomized comparisons of surgical and medical treatment, nor are there randomized studies comparing MVR with septal M-M. McKenna reported the incidence of sudden death of 2 to 3 per cent per year. The longest available surgical results report a 2.2 per cent annual mortality over an 11.5-year period. Recent reports describe an annual mortality of 1 per cent in patients less than 65 year of age. The operation of choice continues to be septal M-M, based on current excellent results. Some centers, however, are presently treating up to one third of patients with MVR. There are, therefore, two acceptable operations for HCM that provide comparable immediate and late results. The exact indications for each of these procedures await further studies including additional experience with intraoperative echocardiography.

XVIII

Mitral and Tricuspid Valve Disease

J. Scott Rankin, M.D., and Donald D. Glower, M.D.

NORMAL ANATOMY AND PHYSIOLOGY

Although the mitral valve is initially quadricuspid in the fetus, most adults have only two leaflets, the anterior leaflet and the posterior leaflet. Both leaflets are attached by fibrous chordae tendineae to both the anterior and posterior papillary muscles. Although the anterior and posterior leaflets have similar surface areas, the anular circumference of the posterior leaflet is twice as great as that of the anterior leaflet. The anterolateral papillary muscle is supplied by high lateral branches of the left anterior descending or circumflex system, and the posteromedial papillary muscle usually receives blood from the posterolateral branches of the right coronary artery.

The anatomy of the tricuspid valve apparatus is similar except that three valve leaflets are usually evident: anterior, posterior, and septal. The anterior leaflet is usually the largest of the three and the posterior the smallest, although multiple variations occur. The papillary muscles tend to be multiple but can be grouped into three complements: anterior, inferior, and septal.

See the corresponding chapter or part in the *Textbook of Surgery*, 14th edition, pp. 2026–2043, for a more detailed discussion of this topic, including a comprehensive list of references.

The function of the atrioventricular valves is to permit uninhibited blood flow from the atria to the ventricles during ventricular diastole and to prevent reflux of blood into the atria during ventricular systole. With isovolumic relaxation, left ventricular pressure falls; and when ventricular pressure becomes lower than that of the full atrium, the valve opens and initiates rapid filling of the ventricle. Mitral valve closure is produced by a combination of events. Deceleration of blood flow across the valve produces positive pressure gradients from the ventricle to the atrium with ring vortices around the incoming jet of blood. Additionally, left ventricular pressure is increased during early ventricular systole.

MITRAL STENOSIS

PATHOPHYSIOLOGY. Rheumatic fever remains a common etiologic factor of mitral stenosis, and a strong relationship exists between rheumatic fever and an antecedent episode of group A streptococcal pharyngitis. Rheumatic fever is characterized by exudative and proliferative inflammatory reactions in the heart, joints, and skin with residual myocardial Aschoff nodules and interstitial fibrous scars. The leaflets become thickened with fusion of the commissures, and the chordae also become thickened, shortened, and fused, often with calcification of the mitral valve and anulus. Other causes of mitral stenoses include malignant carcinoid, systemic lupus erythematosus, rheumatoid arthritis, endomyocardial fibrosis, and congenital "parachute" deformity of the mitral valve. The result of long-standing obstruction to mitral flow can be left atrial dilation and hypertrophy, atrial fibrillation, left atrial thrombi with or without embolization, and ultimately pulmonary hypertension.

CLINICAL DIAGNOSIS. Clinical symptoms of mitral stenosis may include exertional dyspnea, orthopnea, easy fatigability, and occasional hoarseness or dysphagia from left atrial enlargement. Physical examination may be remarkable for cachexia and "mitral facies" with ruddiness of cheeks and peripheral cyanosis. Right-sided heart failure may be evident with peripheral edema, hepatojugular reflux, and a sternal heave. Auscultation of the heart may reveal either accentuation or diminution of the first heart sound, depending on the pliability of the mitral valve; an accentuated pulmonary component of the second heart sound if pulmonary hypertension is present; an opening snap shortly after the second heart sound; and a mid-diastolic rumbling murmur.

In mitral stenosis, the electrocardiogram may reveal a broad, notched P wave in lead II, atrial fibrillation, right ventricular hypertrophy, and right axis deviation. Chest radiograph may show left atrial enlargement with prominence of the left atrial appendage, elevation of the left main stem bronchus, an ovoid double density through the central heart shadow, and posterior displacement of the left atrium on the lateral projection. Pulmonary venous hypertension may be accompanied by engorged superior pulmonary veins termed "cephalization of pulmonary blood flow," right ventricular enlargement, and Kerley B-lines corresponding to hypertrophy of pulmonary lymphatics. Cardiac catheterization will demonstrate an elevated diastolic pressure gradient across the mitral valve. Mitral valve orifice area can be derived from measurements of mean diastolic mitral gradient (ΔP) in millimeters of mercury and average diastolic mitral flow (F) in milliliters per second:

$$\text{Mitral valve area (cm}^2\text{)} = F/[38\sqrt{(\Delta P)}]$$

The normal mitral orifice area is 3 sq. cm. per sq. M., and significant mitral stenosis is suggested when the calculated area approaches 1 sq. cm. per sq. M.

OPERATIVE INDICATIONS. The natural history of medically treated mitral stenosis includes an average latent period of 19 years from an episode of rheumatic fever to onset of symptoms with progression of symptoms to total incapacity over the next 7 years. Overall medical survival at 10 years is 34 per cent with causes of death being congestive heart failure, thromboembolism, and infectious endocarditis.

In the presence of clinically or hemodynamically significant valvular obstruction, firm indications for operation include NYHA Class III or Class IV symptoms, the onset of atrial fibrillation independent of symptoms, worsening of pulmonary hypertension, an episode of systemic embolization, and infective endocarditis. Class II patients who are over the age of 40 years, have severe reduction in valve area, or experience limitations in life-style should also be recommended surgical therapy. Recently, percutaneous balloon mitral valvuloplasty has been introduced as an alternative approach to surgical therapy, but the exact role of balloon valvulopasty remains to be defined.

SURGICAL RESULTS. Operations for mitral stenosis include closed commissurotomy, open commissurotomy, and mitral valve replacement with operative mortality ranges from 1 to 5 per cent depending on the severity of preoperative symptoms, the presence of hypertension or right ventricular failure, and the need for mitral valve replacement. After mitral commissurotomy, most patients experience significant improvement in symptoms followed by clinical deterioration over 8 to 10 years, although 10-year survival exceeds 90 per cent. Mitral valve replacement generally is required as a second procedure.

MITRAL REGURGITATION

PATHOPHYSIOLOGY. Mitral regurgitation can be caused by abnormalities of the mitral anulus, the valve leaflets, the chordae tendineae, the papillary muscles, or the ventricular wall. Rheumatic heart disease with shortening and fibrosis of the cusps and chordae produces 35 to 45 per cent of mitral regurgitation cases. Idiopathic mitral calcification may cause regurgitation in association with aging, hypertension, aortic stenosis, diabetes, or chronic renal failure. Mitral valve prolapse may produce mitral regurgitation through myxomatous degeneration of the leaflets and chordae, often with ruptured chordae. Chordal rupture and regurgitation can also result from chest trauma, infective endocarditis, and ischemic papillary muscle rupture. Hypertrophic obstructive cardiomyopathy may produce mitral regurgitation by anterior displacement of the anterior mitral leaflet into the outflow tract during systole. Coronary artery disease may cause ischemic mitral regurgitation by papillary muscle rupture, generalized anular dilation, and papillary-anular dysfunction.

Physiologic derangements caused by mitral regurgitation are similar to mitral stenosis, with left atrial hypertension, pulmonary arterial hypertension, right ventricular failure, and functional tricuspid regurgitation all possible. Chronic augmentation of diastolic filling pressure and cardiac dilation in untreated patients may ultimately cause death from biventricular cardiac failure, low cardiac output, and pulmonary edema.

CLINICAL DIAGNOSIS. Symptoms of mitral regurgitation include exertional dyspnea, orthopnea, easy fatigability, cardiac cachexia, rare hemoptysis, atrial fibrillation, systemic emboli, bacterial endocarditis, and rare angina. Physical findings are similar to those of mitral stenosis with a sternal heave, an accentuated third heart sound, an increased second heart sound with pulmonary hypertension, and an apical, high-pitched, holosystolic murmur radiating to the axilla and back. The electrocardiogram may show left ventricular or biventricular hypertrophy, atrial fibrillation, or "P mitrale." On chest radiograph, left atrial enlargement, right ventricular enlargement, left ventricular dilation, pulmonary cephalization, and Kerley B-lines may be observed. Cardiac catheterization will commonly demonstrate left atrial V waves, elevated left ventricular end-diastolic pressure and volume, and mitral regurgitation on left ventriculogram.

OPERATIVE INDICATIONS. The natural history of mitral regurgitation is more variable than that of mitral stenosis but is affected primarily by the degree of regurgitation, the status of left ventricular function, and the cause of valve disease. Surgical intervention is recommended in chronic mitral regurgitation if symptoms significantly limit life-style or for NYHA Class III or Class IV congestive heart failure. Because symptoms may not correlate well with outcome after medical therapy, surgical therapy should be considered in Class I or Class II patients if pulmonary hypertension is progressing, if atrial fibrillation occurs, or if the left ventricle is dilating. In mitral regurgitation due to infective endocarditis, trauma, or ruptured chordae tendineae, emergency operative therapy may be indicated with failure to respond to antibiotics, pulmonary or systemic emboli, evidence of an abscess involving the valvular ring, fungal endocarditis, or hemodynamic deterioration.

SURGICAL RESULTS. Using a Cox multivariate regression model, Hammermeister demonstrated a surgical survival benefit in all types of mitral valve disease, and the improved longevity was especially significant in patients with moderate left ventricular dysfunction. The overall operative mortality for elective isolated mitral valve procedures averages 3 to 10 per cent in most centers and is influenced by preoperative symptomatic status, age, and the cause of mitral regurgitation.

TRICUSPID VALVE DISEASE

PATHOPHYSIOLOGY. Tricuspid regurgitation is usually a functional derangement that is secondary to right ventricular dilation and enlargement of the free wall tricuspid anulus due to mitral valve disease, cor pulmonale, primary pulmonary hypertension, right ventricular infarction, or congenital heart disease. Organic causes of tricuspid regurgitation affect the valve apparatus directly and include rheumatic fever, congenital malformations, papillary muscle rupture, trauma, Marfan's syndrome, infective endocarditis, carcinoid syndrome, and cardiac tumors. Tricuspid stenosis is generally rheumatic in origin with thickening and fusion of the leaflets and chordae, but it may also result from carcinoid syndrome, congenital defects, and cardiac tumors. Both tricuspid stenosis and regurgitation may produce right atrial hypertension, systemic venous engorgement, and hepatic congestion ultimately with severe fluid retention, edema, hepatic failure, cardiac cirrhosis, anasarca, and renal failure.

CLINICAL DIAGNOSIS. Symptoms of tricuspid stenosis or regurgitation include weakness and fatigue. Physical examination may demonstrate an enlarged and pulsatile liver, ascites, edema, a tricuspid opening snap, and either holosystolic or mid-diastolic murmurs augmented by inspiration. At cardiac catheterization, tricuspid stenosis is demonstrated by a mean diastolic gradient across the tricuspid valve of greater than 3 to 5 mm. Hg, and tricuspid regurgitation is characterized by a prominent V wave in the right atrial pressure tracing and tricuspid regurgitation on right ventriculography.

SURGICAL MANAGEMENT. Although rheumatic tricuspid stenosis may occasionally be treated by commissurotomy, a significantly diseased tricuspid valve generally requires tricuspid valve replacement with a tissue valve. Tricuspid endocarditis in drug addicts with active infection may require total excision of the valve with possible valve replacement at a later date. Functional tricuspid regurgitation can usually be managed by tricuspid anuloplasty.

OPERATIVE TECHNIQUE

OPEN MITRAL COMMISSUROTOMY. Open commissurotomy is usually performed for mitral stenosis with good leaflet pliability, minimal or no leaflet calcification, and insignificant regurgitation. The operation is performed through a median sternotomy with the support of cardiopulmonary bypass and cardioplegia. The left atrium is opened, any thrombotic material is removed, the commissures are opened with sharp and blunt dissection, and the fused chordae are mobilized.

TRANSATRIAL CARPENTIER VALVE REPAIR. Valve repair is most commonly performed by the methods devised by Carpentier for the complications of myxomatous degeneration including anular dilation, leaflet prolapse, or chordal rupture. Median sternotomy, cardiopulmonary bypass, and cardioplegia are generally employed. Anular dilation is treated with a prosthetic ring anuloplasty that reduces posterior anular circumference. Redundancy of the posterior leaflet or rupture of the posterior chordae is treated by resection of the central posterior leaflet. Elongated chordae are shortened, and a ruptured papillary head may occasionally be reimplanted into the ventricular wall with pledgeted mattress sutures.

TRANSATRIAL KAY ANULOPLASTY. A valve with a dilated anulus but little prolapse may be repaired with a Kay anuloplasty with use of pledgeted mattress sutures at each commissure for reduction of the posterior anular circumference.

TRANSVENTRICULAR MITRAL VALVE REPAIR. In the presence of a thinned out transmural infarct or aneurysm, the mitral valve may be repaired through a longitudinal posterior ventriculotomy. Pledgeted mattress sutures are placed at the commissures for reduction of the posterior anular circumference, and elongated chordae may be shortened.

In all types of mitral valve repair, intraoperative and postoperative Doppler echocardiography has been useful in assessing the quality of the repair and in long-term follow-up of patients.

MITRAL VALVE REPLACEMENT. Mitral valve replacement may be necessary for severely deformed rheumatic valves, valves with significant leaflet or submitral calcification, or valves with prolapse or chordal rupture compromising integrity of the anterior leaflet. Mitral valve replacement is generally performed through a median sternotomy with cardiopulmonary bypass and cardioplegia. The left atrium is opened, the thrombotic material removed, the mitral valve excised, and the prosthetic valve secured with pledgeted horizontal mattress sutures.

TRICUSPID VALVE ANULOPLASTY OR REPLACEMENT. Tricuspid valve anuloplasty is usually performed during the reperfusion period of cardiopulmonary bypass after a mitral valve procedure if Doppler evidence of significant tricuspid incompetence exists before or after cardiopulmonary bypass. The circumference of the dilated right ventricular free wall segment of the anulus is reduced by use of a Carpentier tricuspid ring, bicuspidization anuloplasty, or a DeVega anuloplasty. If organic disease of the tricuspid valve is encountered, the tricuspid valve is excised and replaced with a bioprosthesis.

POSTOPERATIVE CARE. Depending on the patient's valve disease, marginal cardiac output may be encountered postoperatively and may require inotropic agents and the intra-aortic balloon pump. Patients with tissue valves generally are anticoagulated with aspirin and dipyridamole; patients with mechanical valves are anticoagulated with warfarin (Coumadin) initiated on the fourth or fifth postoperative day with maintenance of a prothrombin time ratio of approximately 1.5. Because of the high incidence of long-term valve-related complications, patients with prosthetic valves should be examined at least once yearly by a physician who is familiar with the associated problems.

VALVE SELECTION

BIOPROSTHETIC VALVES. Bioprosthetic valves rarely induce hemolysis and are inaudible. The incidence of thromboembolism is low (0.1 to 2 per cent per patient year) so that warfarin (Coumadin) anticoagulation is not required. The incidence of postoperative prosthetic valve endocarditis is approximately the same as with mechanical valves (5 to 10 per cent over the valve's lifetime). The major concern with all tissue valves is durability with degeneration of leaflet tissue, calcification, and structural failure causing prosthetic valve dysfunction after an average of 7 to 10 years in porcine heterografts. The rate of valve failure is higher in the mitral than in the aortic position.

MECHANICAL VALVES. Current mechanical heart valves offer better predictability of performance and durability than do tissue valves. However, all patients require warfarin therapy, and valve thrombosis or thromboembolism can occur despite adequate anticoagulation. The thromboembolic rate for most mechanical valves with adequate anticoagulation is approximately 2 to 5 per cent per patient year, and the mortality attributable to warfarin therapy approaches 1 per cent per year.

SPECIFIC INDICATIONS. In all tissue valves, the rate of leaflet calcification and degeneration is unacceptable in patients less than 20 to 30 years of age or in patients with chronic renal failure. In children, the St. Jude valve is employed because of good flow characteristics in small sizes, but it requires warfarin anticoagulation. Young females desiring children and patients with specific contraindications to anticoagulation are candidates for tissue valves. Elderly patients and patients undergoing complicated valve procedures may receive mechanical valves because of higher mortality associated with reoperation in these groups. Tricuspid valve replacement is performed exclusively with tissue valves. In the final analysis, the thromboembolic and anticoagulation complications of mechanical valves are approximately equivalent to the durability problems of bioprostheses. As a result, application of techniques for valve reconstruction has increased in recent years but still needs more detailed analysis of long-term survival and complications.

XIX

Ebstein's Anomaly

James A. Alexander, M.D., and Daniel J. O'Brien, Ph.D.

Ebstein's anomaly is an extremely rare and variable defect of the tricuspid valve that represents less than 1 per cent of all congenital cardiac disorders. Approximately one third of patients with Ebstein's anomaly die before the age of 10 years, most in early infancy. The mean age of death is near the second decade of life, although a number of patients have survived into the sixth decade.

ANATOMY AND PATHOPHYSIOLOGY. It is speculated that during embryologic development, the tricuspid valve is almost exclusively derived from the interior of the embryonic right ventricular myocardium and involves a process of undermining the right ventricular wall. It is reasoned that the undermining process of the right ventricular wall does not reach the anulus of the tricuspid valve and that the degree of undermining determines the marked variations in appearance of the tricuspid valve. These variations range from lack of undermining of all three valve cusps with only a small free valve edge at the apex of the right ventricle to an almost normal-appearing tricuspid valve with a small septal leaflet adherent to the ventricular septal surface.

In Ebstein's malformation, the right atrium is dilated and, in advanced cases, may be enormous. Atrial septal defects are common. The anulus of the tricuspid valve is generally dilated. The septal leaflet is small and firmly attached to the ventricular septum with cords that appear to directly enter the myocardium. The posterior leaflet may be firmly attached to the right ventricular myocardium or, in some cases, may be absent. If undermining has occurred, the anterior leaflet of the tricuspid valve is generally redundant and has the appearance of a sail. The papillary muscles of the tricuspid valve are anomalous and may be malpositioned. The valve is generally incompetent. When the valve leaflets are displaced to the apex of the right ventricle, the atrialized portion of the right ventricle may be markedly thinned and dilated. In more severe cases, this atrialized portion appears as a parchment right ventricle. In other cases, the tricuspid valve leaflets may be attached at the apical portion of the right ventricle with only a perforation in the leaflet for an exit of blood flow to the infundibulum. In the presence of an atrial septal defect, cyanosis develops owing to increased right-to-left shunting of blood flow. Several mechanisms that enhance cyanosis include aneurysmal formation in the atrialized portion of the right ventricle, increased pulmonary vascular resistance due to pulmonary embolism, and atrial dysrhythmias.

CLINICAL MANIFESTATIONS. The clinical manifesta-

See the corresponding chapter or part in the *Textbook of Surgery*, 14th edition, pp. 2043–2048, for a more detailed discussion of this topic, including a comprehensive list of references.

tions of Ebstein's anomaly are principally caused by the combination of right ventricular dysfunction and tricuspid insufficiency and/or stenosis, especially with the presence of an atrial septal defect. Patients are generally symptomatic during the newborn period and demonstrate signs of cyanosis and rapid respirations. However, these signs may disappear as pulmonary vascular resistance decreases, only to return in childhood or early adult life. Other signs that may be prominent are fatigue, cardiomegaly, hepatomegaly, and peripheral edema. Palpitations are frequent, and some patients may complain of dizziness and transient visual loss. In addition, patients may exhibit signs and symptoms of pulmonary or systemic embolization. In patients with long-standing cyanosis, clubbing is usually present. On auscultation, the first and second heart sounds are usually normal. In the majority of patients, a systolic murmur is heard.

DIAGNOSIS. The electrocardiogram is always abnormal. Usually present is a right ventricular bundle branch block with a characteristically prolonged P-R interval. Generally, the P wave has an increased duration and increased amplitude owing to the size of the right atrium. Dysrhythmias, especially atrial flutter, atrial fibrillation, and ventricular ectopy, occur in more than one half of patients with Ebstein's disease. Approximately 5 to 20 per cent of these patients have Wolff-Parkinson-White syndrome, usually of the Type B pattern resembling left bundle branch block. Multiple accessory pathways may be present. Roentgenographic evaluation of the cardiac silhouette may vary from essentially normal to the classic globular heart. Cardiomegaly may be striking, and the pulmonary vasculature is either normal or decreased.

At cardiac catheterization, there may be a dominant v wave owing to tricuspid insufficiency. A right ventriculogram usually demonstrates abnormal attachments of the valve leaflets. The *sine qua non* of Ebstein's anomaly is a pullback of an electrode catheter from the right ventricular outflow tract/apex with a ventricular complex associated with a ventricular pressure tracing. Withdrawal of the catheter back into the atrialized portion of the ventricle yields a ventricular complex with an atrial pressure tracing.

Two-dimensional echocardiography is useful in assessing tricuspid valve mobility and valve attachments. The degree of right ventricular wall thickness and paradoxical motion of the atrialized posterior right ventricular wall can also be visualized. Color-flow Doppler studies demonstrate stenosis of the displaced tricuspid valve as well as blood flow through the atrial septum. During pregnancy, fetal echocardiography is useful in diagnosing Ebstein's anomaly and accompanying cardiac defects. Magnetic resonance imaging is useful in providing additional information about the relationship of the tricuspid valve to the right ventricular outflow tract.

PATIENT MANAGEMENT. Children with Ebstein's anomaly should not be placed in competitive athletics, and all these patients should receive antibiotics before dental or endoscopic procedures as prophylaxis against subacute bacterial endocarditis. Patients, children and adults, with Ebstein's anomaly who are judged Class I or Class II according to the New York Heart Association (NYHA) Functional Classification System are generally followed and treated medically. Exceptions to following Class I and Class II patients include paradoxical emboli, right ventricular outflow tract obstruction, moderate-to-severe cyanosis, and tachydysrhythmias refractory to drug therapy. Paroxysmal tachydysrhythmias should be treated aggressively. In asymptomatic patients with Wolff-Parkinson-White syndrome, surgical ablation of accessory tracts with or without valve reconstruction or replacement should be considered. Palliative surgical procedures for symptomatic patients with Ebstein's anomaly have generally produced poor results. The superior vena cava to right pulmonary artery anastomosis (Glenn shunt) has some limited benefit to severely cyanotic patients.

Patients with NYHA Class III or Class IV require surgical intervention for either repair or replacement of the tricuspid valve and closure of the atrial septum. In the past decade, tricuspid valvuloplasty with reconstruction has become a significant part of the surgical armamentarium for Ebstein's anomaly. Danielson and associates have employed plastic procedures in approximately 72 per cent of 134 consecutive patients undergoing surgical repair. In this series, the majority of patients had tricuspid valve reconstruction by creation of a monocusp tricuspid valve. This technique entails plication of the atrialized ventricular portion, reduction of the giant right atrium, closure of the atrial septal defect, and narrowing of the true tricuspid anulus.

Recently, Carpentier and associates introduced a slightly different approach to tricuspid valve reconstruction in which the atrialized ventricular portion is plicated on the long axis of the right ventricle in a vertical direction. This procedure differs from the approach by Danielson in which the atrialized portion of the right ventricle is plicated in a horizontal or apex-to-base position, which shortens the long axis of the ventricle. Carpentier also recommends detaching the anterior leaflet and a portion of the posterior leaflet from the annulus as well as detaching secondary cords. The leaflets are then resutured to the anulus after the appropriate vertical plication is performed. A tricuspid valvuloplasty ring is then inserted below the coronary sinus. Atrial plication is also performed. Despite the trend toward repair rather than replacement of abnormal cardiac valves, some variations of Ebstein's anomaly require prosthetic valve replacement, which usually requires placement of the sewing ring above the coronary sinus for prevention of heart block. When valve replacement is necessary, the risk to benefit ratio of using bioprosthetic valves versus mechanical valves must be evaluated carefully, particularly in children.

General postoperative concerns include maintaining adequate cardiac performance, reducing pulmonary vascular resistance, and optimizing the heart rate and rhythm. However, the need for catecholamine support must be carefully balanced against the dysrhythmogenic effects of inotropic agents. Conversely, the benefits of antidysrhythmic medications must be balanced against the myocardial depressant properties of these agents. Mortality following surgical repair of Ebstein's anomaly has been reported to be as high as 50 per cent. Danielson reported an overall operative mortality of 4.9 per cent for 134 patients undergoing either valve repair or replacement. In that series, the late mortality was an additional 3 per cent.

XX

Surgical Treatment of Cardiac Arrhythmias

James L. Cox, M.D.

During the past 2 decades, surgical intervention has become an important part of the treatment of cardiac arrhythmias. Although the main indication for cardiac arrhythmia surgery is medical refractoriness, surgical therapy is considered the conservative alternative to a lifetime of medical therapy for a number of arrhythmias that occur in young, otherwise healthy patients.

SUPRAVENTRICULAR TACHYARRHYTHMIAS

Wolff-Parkinson-White Syndrome

ANATOMIC-ELECTROPHYSIOLOGIC BASIS. The Wolff-Parkinson-White (WPW) syndrome is an electrophysiologic abnormality that occurs secondary to an anatomic congenital cardiac abnormality. Normally, the only electrical connection between the atria and ventricles is the atrioventricular (AV) node–His bundle complex. In patients with the WPW syndrome, there is an accessory anatomic atrioventricular connection that is capable of conducting electrical impulses. During sinus rhythm or atrial pacing, electrical activity is conducted in an antegrade manner (atrium to ventricle) across the accessory pathway, with production of early excitation of the ventricles (ventricular pre-excitation) and an abnormal electrocardiogram that includes a short P-R interval, a wide QRS complex, and a delta wave. If antegrade conduction block occurs in the accessory pathway, retrograde conduction from the ventricle across the accessory pathway can occur with resultant pre-excitation of the atrium. The retrograde atrial impulse can then re-enter the AV node–His bundle

---

See the corresponding chapter or part in the *Textbook of Surgery*, 14th edition, pp. 2048–2069, for a more detailed discussion of this topic, including a comprehensive list of references.

complex to establish a closed re-entrant circuit. The resultant reciprocating tachycardia is then perpetuated by electrical activity traveling antegrade through the AV node–His bundle complex to activate the ventricles, and retrograde across the accessory pathway to activate the atria. The accessory pathways responsible for the WPW syndrome may occur in the AV groove anywhere around the base of the heart. Their location has traditionally been classified into four categories: left free wall, posterior septal, right free wall, and anterior septal, in decreasing order of frequency.

SURGICAL INDICATIONS AND PREOPERATIVE EVALUATION. The major indication for surgical intervention in the WPW syndrome is medical refractoriness. Other common surgical indications include patient intolerance to drug therapy, detrimental side effects of anti-arrhythmic agents, and poor patient compliance. Recently, young, otherwise healthy patients with recurrent supraventricular tachycardia have been offered surgical therapy if they prefer it to medical therapy. Spontaneous atrial fibrillation occurring in the presence of the WPW syndrome may cause conduction of the atrial fibrillation across the accessory pathway to the ventricles, with resultant ventricular fibrillation and sudden death. Therefore, the combination of atrial fibrillation and WPW syndrome is considered an absolute indication for surgical intervention. Patients who are to be subjected to surgical therapy undergo a preoperative endocardial catheter electrophysiology study. The objectives of this study are to document the presence of the WPW syndrome, to determine the location of the accessory pathway, and to exclude other associated electrophysiologic abnormalities.

SURGICAL THERAPY AND RESULTS. The objective of surgical therapy for the WPW syndrome is to localize the accessory pathway and divide or ablate it. Although most of the accessory pathways can be adequately localized preoperatively, intraoperative mapping is performed for confirming the location of the pathway and for determining whether other accessory pathways exist that might have been overlooked during the preoperative study. The intraoperative study is particularly useful in identifying the presence of multiple accessory pathways, which may occur in 20 per cent of the patients.

There are two surgical techniques that are used to divide or ablate accessory pathways in patients with the WPW syndrome: the endocardial approach and the epicardial approach. The endocardial approach is performed from inside the appropriate atrium, where a supra-annular incision is placed just above the valve annulus for exposing the AV groove fat pad harboring the accessory pathway. A plane of dissection is established between the underlying AV groove fat pad and the top of the ventricle throughout the length of the supra-annular incision. There are basically four separate endocardial operations for the WPW syndrome, one for each of the four anatomic spaces where the accessory pathways may reside. The endocardial approach is directed toward dividing the ventricular end of the accessory pathway.

The epicardial technique involves dissection of the AV

groove fat pad away from the outside of the appropriate atrium in an effort to divide the atrial end of the accessory pathway. When the AV groove fat pad has been dissected away from the external surface of the atrium, cryolesions are placed at the level of the valve anulus at the suspected site of the accessory pathway. Cryosurgery is an adjunctive procedure that may be necessary in only a small percentage of patients, but with utilization of the epicardial technique, it is not possible to determine which patients require cryosurgery. As a result, it is routinely applied as an adjunctive procedure to the epicardial technique in all patients.

The surgical results with both the endocardial approach and the epicardial approach are excellent. The operative mortality is 0 to 0.5 per cent, with an overall cure rate that approaches 100 per cent. Because of these excellent results, surgical therapy has been liberalized during the past decade.

AV Node Re-entry Tachycardia

ANATOMIC-ELECTROPHYSIOLOGIC BASIS. The basis of AV node re-entry tachycardia is the presence of two functional conduction pathways through the AV node, one slow pathway and one fast pathway. During sinus rhythm, antegrade conduction through the AV node–His bundle complex occurs preferentially through the fast conduction pathway. However, if antegrade conduction block occurs in the fast pathway, electrical conduction may occur in an antegrade direction down the slow pathway and in a retrograde direction up the fast pathway, establishing a re-entrant circuit and immediate supraventricular tachycardia. Whether there is an anatomic correlate for the physiologic process of dual AV node conduction pathways is unknown. In addition, considerable controversy exists regarding whether the perinodal tissues form an active limb of the re-entrant circuit or the circuit is confined to the anatomic AV node. Recent experimental and clinical data, however, strongly suggest that the perinodal tissues are involved in the re-entrant circuit.

SURGICAL INDICATIONS AND PREOPERATIVE EVALUATION. The present indications for surgical intervention in patients with AV node re-entry tachycardia are similar to those applied to patients with the WPW syndrome and include medical refractoriness, drug intolerance, poor patient compliance, and patient preference for surgical over medical treatment. All patients who are to be subjected to surgical intervention for AV node re-entry tachycardia undergo a preoperative endocardial catheter electrophysiology study. The objectives of this study are to document the presence of dual AV node pathways and AV node re-entry tachycardia and to identify other associated electrophysiologic abnormalities.

SURGICAL THERAPY AND RESULTS. Prior to 1982, the only surgical therapy available for patients with refractory AV node re-entry tachycardia was elective ablation of the His bundle by surgical dissection or by cryosurgery, both of which require an open heart procedure. In 1982, a technique was described in which a catheter could be placed along the His bundle and an electric shock could be delivered through the catheter for ablation of the His bundle and permanent interruption of all AV conduction. This procedure rapidly replaced surgical division or ablation of the His bundle, since it was a closed chest procedure. However, ablation of the His bundle, whether by surgical means or via a transvenous catheter, required the implantation of a permanent pacemaker system. As a result, the author and associates developed a discrete perinodal cryosurgical technique that is capable of interrupting only one of the two pathways of conduction through the AV node, leaving the other intact. This cryosurgical technique is thus capable of curing the AV node re-entry tachycardia while leaving normal AV conduction intact, thereby precluding the necessity for a pacemaker. Others subsequently developed a surgical dissection technique that accomplishes the same result as the cryosurgical procedure, albeit with a slightly higher incidence of complete heart block, a lower cure rate, and a higher recurrence rate of the tachycardia.

Both the cryosurgical procedure and the surgical dissection procedure require cardiopulmonary bypass and a right atriotomy. Several 3-mm. cryolesions are placed around the borders of the AV node for interrupting one of the two dual AV node conduction pathways. AV conduction is monitored on a beat to beat basis so that the possibility of development of complete heart block is precluded. This is the major advantage of the cryosurgical technique over surgical dissection, since if heart block occurs with the latter, it is not reversible. Since the majority of these patients can be cured with either of these surgical approaches, they are now performed in preference to catheter ablation of the His bundle.

Automatic Atrial Tachycardia

ANATOMIC-ELECTROPHYSIOLOGIC BASIS. Automatic atrial tachycardia is caused by an automatic focus of arrhythmogenic tissue lying outside the region of the normal anatomic sinus node. Histologic examination of the atrial tissue excised at the site of origin of automatic atrial tachycardia has not revealed a specific finding common to all patients. Although the precise electrophysiologic differences between automatic and re-entrant tachycardias have not been documented, clinical arrhythmias are classified into one of these categories on the basis of their response to programmed electrical stimulation techniques. Automatic atrial tachycardias are those that do not respond to programmed stimulation, and re-entrant arrhythmias are those that can be induced and terminated by these stimulation techniques. Automatic atrial tachycardias are uncommon, with only 125 patients having been reported in the literature. Sixty-eight per cent are located in the right atrial free wall, 6 per cent in the atrial septum, and 26 per cent in the left atrium.

SURGICAL INDICATIONS AND PREOPERATIVE EVALUATION. Automatic atrial tachycardias frequently occur in pediatric patients in whom the tachycardia may be asymptomatic or may present with vomiting and epigastric pain.

Adult patients more commonly present with palpitations, presyncope, syncope, or symptoms of congestive failure. One of the most common manifestations of automatic atrial tachycardia is cardiomegaly and congestive heart failure, with the overall incidence being slightly above 50 per cent. Thus, the indications for surgical intervention in patients with automatic atrial tachycardias include medical refractoriness, intolerable side effects of anti-arrhythmic drugs, poor patient compliance, patient preference to medical therapy, tachycardia-induced ventricular dysfunction, and congestive heart failure.

The standard electrocardiogram during an automatic atrial tachycardia demonstrates a P wave morphologic pattern that is different from that seen in sinus rhythm, which suggests the presence of an ectopic focus remote from the sinus node. The preoperative electrophysiology study documents failure to initiate or terminate the tachycardia by programmed electrical stimulation techniques. However, these tachycardias are frequently incessant, and as a result, it is commonly possible to localize their site of origin with a reasonable degree of accuracy during the preoperative electrophysiology study.

SURGICAL THERAPY AND RESULTS. Intraoperative mapping is extremely important in patients with automatic atrial tachycardias, but unfortunately, general anesthetic agents frequently suppress these arrhythmias. As a result, it may be impossible to localize the site of origin of the tachycardia by intraoperative mapping. The development of computerized intraoperative mapping systems has greatly enhanced the ability of the surgeon to identify the precise location of automatic tachycardias during the past several years. If the site of origin of an automatic atrial tachycardia can be localized precisely by intraoperative mapping, the arrhythmogenic focus may be either excised or cryoablated. Automatic foci located in the free wall of the left atrium or in either of the atrial appendages are ideal for excision or cryoablation. Automatic atrial tachycardias arising near the orifices of the pulmonary veins are best treated either by pulmonary vein isolation or by left atrial isolation. Because automatic tachycardias arising in the free wall of the body of the right atrium are frequently multifocal in origin, they are best treated by isolation of the body of the right atrium, even though the site of origin of the tachycardia may be well defined by intraoperative computerized mapping. Lowe reports that electrophysiologically guided operative procedures have been performed in 63 of the 125 patients available for review. Fifty-six (89 per cent) have been completely cured without the need for permanent pacemaker implantation or postoperative anti-arrhythmic therapy; there has been one operative death.

Atrial Flutter and Fibrillation

ANATOMIC-ELECTROPHYSIOLOGIC BASIS. Experimental and clinical studies during the past decade have documented that atrial flutter and atrial fibrillation occur on the basis of re-entry. The re-entrant circuits in the atria may propagate through the septum around the pulmonary veins, inferior vena cava, or superior vena cava. More complex patterns of activation frequently exist in which re-entrant loops cannot be documented. Although anatomic obstacles such as the pulmonary veins, inferior vena cava, and superior vena cava are frequently involved in the re-entrant loops, complete re-entrant circuits may occur in the absence of these anatomic obstacles. These re-entrant loops rotate around areas of functional conduction block, the most common site being along the sulcus terminalis. As the atrial size increases, the number of wavefronts during atrial fibrillation and the duration of atrial fibrillation increase.

SURGICAL INDICATIONS AND PREOPERATIVE EVALUATION. The present indications for surgical intervention in patients with atrial fibrillation are extremely limited. However, the potentially life-threatening complications of atrial fibrillation and the number of patients suffering from this arrhythmia (a minimum of one million people in the United States alone) dictate that should a safe and effective surgical procedure be developed to cure atrial fibrillation, the surgical indications would expand dramatically. Should such an effective surgical therapy for atrial fibrillation become available, surgical indications would include medical refractoriness, intolerable drug side effects, poor patient compliance, preference to medical therapy, congestive heart failure due to atrial fibrillation, and thromboembolic episodes due to atrial fibrillation.

The preoperative catheter electrophysiology study is of limited value in patients with atrial fibrillation. Nevertheless, those patients who are to be subjected to some of the newer techniques designed to cure atrial fibrillation undergo a preoperative electrophysiology study primarily for exclusion of other associated electrophysiologic abnormalities, especially the WPW syndrome. Because the surgical techniques employed to treat atrial fibrillation are still in their developmental stages, they have thus far been applied only to patients who have normal ventricular and valvular function as determined by two-dimensional echocardiography, radionuclide ventriculography, and cardiac catheterization.

SURGICAL THERAPY AND RESULTS. Intraoperative electrophysiologic mapping is not absolutely essential before the surgical procedures that are currently available for the treatment of atrial fibrillation are employed. However, the author routinely performs computerized intraoperative mapping in these patients because of the possibility that a single, dominant re-entrant circuit might be identified and treated by a less complex surgical procedure. Prior to 1980, the only surgical procedure capable of alleviating some of the detrimental effects of atrial fibrillation was elective His bundle ablation. In 1980, the author and associates introduced the left atrial isolation procedure, which is capable of confining atrial fibrillation to the left atrium. By confinement of the arrhythmia to the left atrium, the sinoatrial node is allowed to drive the remainder of the heart in a normal sinus rhythm. This procedure alleviates the arrhythmia and restores normal hemodynamics, but it does not decrease the vulnerability to thromboembolism, since the left atrium may still fibrillate. In 1985, the corridor procedure was introduced in which a strip of atrial septum connecting the sinoatrial node to the AV node is isolated from the remainder of the atrial myocardium, allowing the sinoatrial node to drive the ventricles in a regular manner. This procedure alleviates the arrhythmia, but it does not restore normal hemodynamics because of loss of both right and left AV synchrony, and it does not decrease the vulnerability to thromboembolism, since the atria may continue to fibrillate.

The author's group has recently introduced the maze procedure, which is specifically designed to interrupt the re-entrant circuits responsible for atrial fibrillation. The incisions that interrupt the re-entrant circuits also direct the sinus impulse across both atria in such a way that atrial transport function is preserved bilaterally. Normal AV conduction also produces bilateral AV synchrony. Thus, the maze procedure is designed to ablate atrial fibrillation and restore normal sinus rhythm, which then restores normal hemodynamics and abolishes the vulnerability to thromboembolism. This procedure has now been performed in 22 patients successfully.

VENTRICULAR TACHYARRHYTHMIAS

Nonischemic Ventricular Tachyarrhythmias

ANATOMIC-ELECTROPHYSIOLOGIC BASIS. Ventricular tachyarrhythmias may be conveniently divided into two types, the more common type being associated with ischemic heart disease and the less common type being unrelated to myocardial ischemia. Most nonischemic ventricular tachyarrhythmias arise in the right ventricle, and most ischemic tachyarrhythmias arise in the left ventricle. Nonischemic ventricular arrhythmias may be due to cardiomyopathy, arrhythmogenic right ventricular dysplasia, or the long Q-T interval syndrome, or they may be idiopathic. Arrhythmogenic right ventricular dysplasia is the most common cause of nonischemic ventricular tachycardia. This is a congenital myopathy in which there is transmural infiltration of adipose tissue in the right ventricular free wall, with aneurysm formation in the infundibulum, apex, and/or posterior basilar region. Any or all of these regions may produce refractory ventricular tachycardia. Life-threatening ventricular tachyarrhythmias may occur as a result of familial or idiopathic prolonged Q-T interval syndrome. The ventricular tachycardia that occurs in this setting is frequently of a distinct type termed "torsades de pointes," which is characterized by inconsistent polarity of the tachycardia on standard electrocardiogram. This tachycardia is believed to be an abnormality of myocardial repolarization in contradistinction to other types of ventricular tachycardias that are thought to be abnormalities of myocardial depolarization.

SURGICAL INDICATIONS AND PREOPERATIVE EVALUATION. Nonischemic ventricular tachycardias are notoriously resistant to medical therapy. Therefore, essentially all patients with nonischemic ventricular tachyarrhythmias who require surgical therapy do so because of medical refractoriness. Since most of these arrhythmias arise in the right ventricle, the single distinguishing characteristic of these arrhythmias is the presence of a left bundle branch block pattern during the tachycardia. A preoperative right ventricular angiogram in patients with arrhythmogenic right ventricular dysplasia usually shows aneurysmal bulging in one of the areas of the right ventricular free wall mentioned previously. Catheter mapping during the preoperative electrophysiology study usually localizes the site of origin of the tachycardia in these patients. Generally, patients who are to undergo surgical intervention for the long Q-T syndrome do not require a formal preoperative electrophysiology study.

SURGICAL THERAPY AND RESULTS. The materials and methods used for intraoperative mapping of nonischemic ventricular tachyarrhythmias are identical to those employed for ischemic ventricular tachyarrhythmias. The objective of the intraoperative mapping procedure is to localize as precisely as possible the site of origin of the nonischemic ventricular tachycardia and to determine if more than one site of origin exists. Left cervical thoracic sympathectomy with removal of the left stellate ganglion and the first three to four left thoracic sympathetic ganglia has been advocated for patients requiring surgical intervention for the long Q-T syndrome. However, because of equivocal results with this approach, the author presently recommends implantation of an automatic internal cardioverter-defibrillator as an adjunct to the sympathectomy in these patients. If nonischemic ventricular tachycardia can be shown to originate from a single site in the right ventricular free wall, it may be treated by surgical excision, cryoablation, or isolation. Localized surgical isolation procedures are preferred for all right free wall nonischemic ventricular tachycardias. If the site of origin can be localized, a localized isolation procedure is performed. If the tachycardia cannot be mapped precisely, but is known to arise in the right ventricular free wall, a right ventricular disconnection procedure can be performed in which the entire free wall of the right ventricle is surgically isolated from the rest of the heart.

Ischemic Ventricular Tachyarrhythmias

ANATOMIC-ELECTROPHYSIOLOGIC BASIS. Ventricular tachycardia associated with ischemic heart disease occurs on the basis of re-entrant circuits that are located primarily in the endocardial and subendocardial layers of the heart, especially at the periphery of myocardial infarcts or ventricular aneurysms. The re-entrant ischemic ventricular arrhythmias are due to a complex interplay of (1) a nonuniform (heterogeneous) state of repolarization, (2) slow desynchronized conduction over abnormal myocardial pathways created by fibrotic or ischemic discontinuity, and (3) ventricular ectopy. Since fibrosis is nonuniform at the borders of infarcts, it produces complex interdigitations between normal myocardium and scar. A synchronous wavefront, upon approaching such an area, may become desynchronized, fragmenting into many individual wavelets. A slowing of conduction time accompanies the desynchronization.

SURGICAL INDICATIONS AND PREOPERATIVE EVALUATION. During the preoperative electrophysiology study, electrical activity is thought to be identifiable as part of the re-entrant tachycardia circuit if it precedes the onset of ventricular depolarization evident on the surface electrocardiogram and is required for the initiation and perpetuation of the tachycardia. The site of origin of the tachycardia is thought to be the area exhibiting the earliest presystolic electrical activity in the latter half of diastole and represents the region of myocardium that must be identified and removed at the time of operation in order to prevent the arrhythmias. The decision regarding surgical therapy for ischemic ventricular tachycardia is based on a number of preoperative clinical factors. The primary indication is refractoriness to medical therapy. The only absolute contraindication to surgical therapy for ischemic ventricular tachycardia is left ventricular dysfunction so severe that the preoperative risk is judged to be prohibitive.

SURGICAL THERAPY AND RESULTS. A computerized multipoint mapping system is used to map the heart intraoperatively in patients with ventricular tachycardia. A sock electrode with 96 bipolar contact points is first used to determine the epicardial activation sequence in sinus rhythm and during induced ventricular tachycardia. The sock electrode is then removed, and multiple plunge needle electrodes with four bipolar contact points along each needle shaft are inserted into the left ventricle to record up to 156 simultaneous transmural electrograms during normal sinus rhythm and during induced ventricular tachycardia. When the site of origin of the ventricular tachycardia has been localized, any one of several surgical approaches may be taken.

Following the intraoperative mapping procedure, the author prefers to resect all of the endocardial scar associated with the infarct or aneurysm, regardless of the site of origin of the tachycardia. Following removal of all of the endocardial scar, endocardial cryolesions are placed at the site of origin of the tachycardia in order to ablate tissue at the arrhythmogenic sites deeper than the endocardial fibrosis. If the endocardial fibrosis involves the base of the papillary muscles, it is not resected but is cryoablated. This has avoided the necessity of resecting the papillary muscles and replacing the mitral valve.

Other successful surgical techniques have included resection of the endocardial fibrosis at the site of origin of the tachycardia with no adjunctive cryosurgery, resection of all endocardial fibrosis without adjunctive cryosurgery, place-

ment of a deep endocardial incision at the junction of endocardial fibrosis and normal myocardium near the site of origin
of the tachycardia (the "partial encircling endocardial ventriculotomy"), and laser photoablation of the site of origin of the
tachycardia without endocardial scar resection or other adjunctive measures. All of these surgical approaches have
been characterized in large series by a high operative mortality (average 12.4 per cent) and a low incidence of sudden
death on long-term follow-up (approximately 0.5 per cent
per year).

Because of the excessive operative mortality that has been
reported following ventricular tachycardia surgery during the
past decade, some authors have proposed that it be abandoned. They have advocated routine coronary artery bypass
grafting, plus the implantation of an automatic internal cardioverter-defibrillator (AICD). The major reason for recommending this approach is the excessive operative mortality
associated with ventricular tachycardia surgery. However, it
should be remembered that the AICD was not routinely
available to most surgeons performing ventricular tachycardia
surgery during the first 5 to 8 years following the introduction
of the direct surgical procedures in the late 1970s. As a result,
patients who were medically refractory had to be subjected
to ventricular tachycardia surgery regardless of the degree of
ventricular dysfunction present. Those essentially inoperable
patients who had failed all forms of medical therapy and
persisted in having intractable ventricular tachycardia comprised the majority of operative deaths associated with the
direct surgical procedures. The AICD represents the previously missing therapeutic option that can now be applied to
patients with intractable, medically refractory ventricular
tachycardia who are inoperable because of severe left ventricular dysfunction. Since the long-term results of ventricular
tachycardia surgery are superior to the long-term results of
AICD implantation in terms of the prevention of sudden
death (0.5 per cent per year for surgical therapy versus 1.5
to 2.0 per cent per year for the AICD), ventricular tachycardia
surgery should be applied to any patient who is considered
to be an operable candidate. If the patient is considered too
high a risk for undergoing operation, an AICD should be
implanted. Thus, the two therapeutic modalities, ventricular
tachycardia and AICD implantation, should be viewed as
complementary procedures for the treatment of medically
refractory ischemic ventricular tachycardia.

XXI

Cardiac Neoplasms

Norman A. Silverman, M.D.,
and David C. Sabiston, Jr., M.D.

Cardiac tumors have evolved from pathologic curiosities to a surgically curable form of heart disease. Whereas prior to 1960 over 60 per cent of these lesions were found at postmortem examinations, cardiac tumors are now recognized during life.

INCIDENCE AND CLINICAL PRESENTATION. The rarity of primary cardiac tumors is evidenced by an autopsy incidence of 0.002 to 0.33 per cent. Eighty per cent of primary cardiac tumors are benign, with myxoma being by far the most common. Malignant neoplasms are relatively more common in adults but represent less than 10 per cent of primary cardiac tumors in children. Malignant tumors are predominantly various forms of sarcoma. In patients having known cancers, nearly 10 per cent have secondary cardiac involvement at necropsy. Cardiac tumors produce symptoms by their mass effect, local invasion, embolization, or systemic constitutional signs. Cardiac performance is compromised when an intracavitary tumor obstructs blood flow or prevents normal valvular function and when an intramural tumor infiltrates and destroys ventricular myocardium. Systemic emboli occur frequently with left atrial myxoma, but right heart tumors also can embolize to the pulmonary arteries. Particularly in the pediatric age group, these lesions cause recurrent dysrhythmias or injure the conduction system. Most intriguing are the systemic constitutional symptoms of fever, malaise, weight loss, polymyositis, hepatic dysfunction, Raynaud's phenomenon, hyperglobulinemia, and elevated erythrocyte sedimentation rate that are associated with left atrial myxomas.

DIAGNOSIS. Echocardiography is the technique of choice in the initial evaluation of intracardiac tumors. The M-mode technique was introduced first, but improved accuracy for real-time imaging of all cardiac chambers and more precise quantitation of tumor size, shape, location, consistency, and mobility are afforded by two-dimensional echocardiography. Findings suggestive of myxoma occur in 95 per cent of patients examined by echocardiography. In selected patients, computed tomography is a valuable alternative for imaging primary and metastatic cardiac tumors. Computed tomographic scanning is best utilized for demonstrating the myocardial and intrapericardial extension of tumor. Magnetic resonance imaging is a newer technique that also enables high-resolution tomography in three dimensions. The plain chest film and electrocardiogram show only indirect evidence of cardiac neoplasm by demonstrating chamber enlargement

See the corresponding chapter or part in the *Textbook of Surgery*, 14th edition, pp. 2069–2074, for a more detailed discussion of this topic, including a comprehensive list of references.

or rhythm disturbances. In addition, cardiac catheterization and angiography visualize intracavitary defects and document the hemodynamic sequelae of valvular dysfunction. However, echocardiography has supplanted this invasive procedure as the diagnostic modality of choice.

BENIGN NEOPLASMS

Myxomas constitute 50 per cent of benign primary cardiac tumors. Seventy-five per cent originate in the left atrium, and 20 per cent occur in the right atrium. Ventricular myxomas are rare. The majority of myxomas are solitary lesions. A familial incidence and associated skin tumors predispose to synchronous tumors. Although a "benign" tumor, myxomas can rarely undergo malignant degeneration and metastasize. Because they often obstruct the mitral orifice and produce systemic emboli, left atrial myxomas frequently masquerade as rheumatic mitral stenosis. When constitutional symptoms predominate, infective endocarditis, collagen vascular disease, and occult malignancy or infection enter the differential diagnosis. Right atrial myxomas produce signs and symptoms of right-sided heart failure by obstructing vena caval return or the tricuspid valve orifice. The rare ventricular myxomas arise from the outflow tract or interventricular septum and may induce syncope owing to transient obstruction of ventricular ejection.

Rhabdomyoma is a congenital, glycogen-rich hamartoma that is the most common cardiac tumor of childhood. These lesions are most often multicentric, ventricular masses that cause recurrent tachyarrhythmias and have a poor prognosis. In contrast, the rare cardiac *fibromas* are well circumscribed, solitary ventricular tumors of childhood that are more amenable to surgical cure. Lipoma, hemangioma, lymphangioma, teratoma, chemodectoma, neurilemoma, ganglioneuroma, and granular cell myoblastoma have also been reported to arise from the heart.

MANAGEMENT. The diagnosis of primary cardiac tumor mandates prompt operative intervention. All resections should be complete, but zealous removal of normal myocardium or trauma to intrinsically normal valvular apparatus should be avoided. After complete tumor resection, the prognosis is excellent with complete symptomatic relief and less than 1 per cent recurrence.

MALIGNANT NEOPLASMS

Malignant tumors are usually some variant of a sarcoma. Most often they originate from the right side of the heart to invade adjacent mediastinal structures and metastasize widely. The characteristic clinical presentation is progressive, unrelenting congestive heart failure, cardiomegaly, chest pain, fever, hemopericardium, and arrhythmia. When the diagnosis is made at exploratory surgery, the growth pattern of these lesions most often makes them unresectable. Mediastinal irradiation and systemic chemotherapy have also been ineffective in controlling primary malignant tumors.

METASTASES

Tumors that most frequently metastasize to the heart include lung and breast carcinoma as well as leukemia, lymphoma, and melanoma. The pericardium can also be invaded by direct extension of adjacent intrathoracic malignancies, in particular, bronchogenic carcinoma. Pericardial metastases cause tamponade or constriction. Myocardial metastases often cause rhythm disturbances or congestive heart failure. Treatment for cardiac metastases is generally palliative. Limited benefit has accrued from systemic chemotherapy and radiation therapy. Surgical intervention is indicated to establish a tissue diagnosis, to effect electrical pacing, or to decompress symptomatic pericardial effusion.

XXII

Cardiac Pacemakers
James E. Lowe, M.D.

The current artificial cardiac pacemaker is the result of technologic advances during the past two decades from aerospace and computer industries. The implantable pacemaker is one of medicine's greatest contributions to prolonging and improving human life.

INDICATIONS FOR PACEMAKER THERAPY

Indications for permanent pacing have been outlined in detail by a joint task force of the American College of Cardiology and the American Heart Association in 1984 and are shown in Table 1. In the early 1960s, after the introduction of the completely implantable pacing system, the major indication for permanent pacemaker therapy was complete atrioventricular (AV) block associated with presyncope or syncope. During the past several years, however, indications for implantation of permanent pacemakers have changed. Although complete AV block remains a definite indication for permanent pacing, most permanent pacemakers implanted are in patients with the sick sinus syndrome.

See the corresponding chapter or part in the *Textbook of Surgery*, 14th edition, pp. 2074–2095, for a more detailed discussion of this topic, including a comprehensive list of references.

TABLE 1. Indications for Permanent Pacing

Complete AV block with:
  Syncope or presyncope
  Congestive heart failure
  Ventricular tachycardia
  Heart rate less than 40 or asystole greater than 3 seconds
  Cerebral hypoperfusion
Second-degree AV block with symptoms
Acute myocardial infarction with persistent second-degree AV block
  or complete AV block
Chronic bifascicular or trifascicular block with symptomatic
  intermittent complete or second-degree AV block
Sinus bradycardia or sinus pauses with symptoms
Hypersensitive carotid sinus syndrome with recurrent syncope
Atrial fibrillation with slow ventricular rate and symptoms

Sick Sinus Syndrome and Bradycardia-Tachycardia Syndrome

Pharmacologic therapy alone is often ineffective in patients with the sick sinus syndrome, and permanent pacing is indicated in those who remain symptomatic because of bradycardia. The most common manifestation of the sick sinus syndrome is marked sinus bradycardia associated with intermittent sinus arrest or sinoatrial node block and episodes of A1V junctional escape rhythm. In more advanced forms of the sick sinus syndrome, chronic atrial fibrillation may develop and be associated with a slow ventricular rate secondary to advanced AV block. An additional group of patients develop various atrial tachyarrhythmias, which are a common result of advanced sick sinus syndrome.

In many patients, a ventricular inhibited-demand pacemaker is adequate therapy. However, in patients in whom the atrial contribution to cardiac output is essential, dual-chamber pacing should be used. Atrial arrhythmias can be suppressed occasionally by atrial pacing. In patients with the bradyarrhythmia-tachyarrhythmia syndrome, one or more antiarrhythmic agents are frequently required in addition to permanent pacemaker therapy.

Mobitz Type II AV Block

It is generally believed that permanent pacing is indicated for patients with Mobitz Type II AV block associated with a wide QRS complex, regardless of whether the patient is symptomatic. It has been documented that Mobitz Type II AV block frequently produces advanced AV block.

Complete AV Block

Before pacemaker therapy became clinically available, 50 per cent of patients with complete heart block died within 1 year. Complete heart block is frequently caused by sclerodegenerative disease of the cardiac skeleton or of the conduction system itself and is often preceded by the development of bifascicular blocks such as right bundle branch block with left- or right-axis deviation and left bundle branch block. Therefore, most surgeons agree that complete AV block represents a definite indication for permanent cardiac pacing. In addition to sclerodegenerative diseases, other causes of acquired complete AV block include ischemic myocardial injury, infiltrative cardiomyopathies, Chagas' disease, traumatic injuries, and cardiac procedures. Permanent pacing is usually recommended for surgically induced complete heart block continuing more than 1 week after operation. Complete AV block associated with acute anterior wall myocardial infarction is often irreversible and requires permanent pacemaker implantation. Conversely, complete AV block after a diaphragmatic myocardial infarction can usually be reversed and may require only temporary pacing. Permanent pacing is generally recommended in all patients with myocardial infarction when complete AV block continues for more than 10 to 14 days.

Symptomatic Bifascicular and Trifascicular Block

Bifascicular or trifascicular block usually signifies extensive conduction system disease. Symptoms in patients with bundle branch block may be due to intermittent episodes of advanced or complete AV block or to ventricular tachycardia. Permanent pacing should be considered in symptomatic patients with bifascicular or trifascicular block and prolonged H-V intervals of 100 msec. or longer. In patients with documented episodes of complete AV block associated with bundle branch block, implantation of a permanent pacemaker should be an urgent consideration. Dual-chamber pacing is generally preferred in patients in whom progression to permanent complete AV block is likely.

Bifascicular or Trifascicular Block with Intermittent Complete AV Block After Acute Myocardial Infarction

Clinical studies have shown that the potential risk of sudden death within 6 months after acute myocardial infarction increases in patients with bifascicular or incomplete trifascicular block associated with intermittent complete AV block during the peri-infarction period. Therefore, it is now recommended that this group of patients be considered candidates for permanent pacemaker implantation after their infarction before discharge from the hospital.

Carotid Sinus Syncope

A permanent pacemaker may be indicated in patients with carotid sinus syncope or near-syncope when a significant cardioinhibitory component can be implicated.

Recurrent Drug-Resistant Tachyarrhythmias Improved by Temporary Pacing

Some patients with tachyarrhythmias, particularly paroxysmal ventricular tachycardia, can be managed successfully by temporary pacing. In patients who respond, permanent pacing techniques can be considered to be part of their therapy. Because of the excellent surgical results obtained in patients with the Wolff-Parkinson-White syndrome and ventricular tachycardia associated with left ventricular aneurysms and micro–re-entry, operation should be considered to be primary therapy. However, in patients who are not surgical candidates, various antitachycardia pacing techniques are useful. Torsades de pointes due to a long Q-T interval as encountered with drug toxicity or electrolyte imbalance can be managed successfully with temporary overdrive pacing.

Intractable Congestive Heart Failure and Cerebral or Renal Insufficiency Benefited by Temporary Pacing

Patients with refractory congestive heart failure and decreased perfusion causing cerebral or renal insufficiency may be improved occasionally by increasing heart rate with temporary pacing. If temporary pacing has proved to be effective under these conditions and long-term therapy is indicated, permanent pacing should be considered. Most of these patients require atrial contraction for improvement of cardiac output. Therefore, dual-chamber atrial synchronous pacing is usually indicated in this subgroup. In patients with sinus bradycardia or atrial arrhythmias, single-chamber rate-modulated pacing should be considered. These examples indicate that choice of the exact mode of pacing depends on a thorough knowledge of the underlying conduction disturbance.

PHYSIOLOGY OF PACING

Pacing Modes

In order to meet the need for a uniform method of describing pacemaker function, the Intersociety Commission for Heart Disease Resources (ICHD) recommended a five-letter code that succinctly and accurately describes various pacing modes. This code was updated in 1987 to accommodate newer pacemakers.

The ICHD code uses the letters A and V for atrium and ventricle. The letter D stands for *dual,* which signifies both chambers or, when indicating a mode of response, more than one mode. The two traditional response modes to sensed activity, either inhibition or triggering, are indicated by I and T. When no function or response is possible, the letter O is used. In the three-letter code system, the first letter designates the chamber(s) paced, the second letter the chamber(s) sensed, and the third letter the mode of response of the pacemaker to sensed activity. Thus, a pacemaker that paces only the ventricle, senses ventricular activity when intrinsic beats are present, and responds to the sensed activity by inhibiting its output (the well-known ventricular-demand pacemaker) is designated VVI in the ICHD code. An asynchronous ventricular pacemaker that does not sense but paces at a constant rate regardless of intrinsic cardiac rhythm would be designated VOO (the ventricle is paced, neither chamber is sensed, and there is therefore no response mode to sensed events). In the case of the standard AV sequential pacemaker in which both the atrium and ventricle are paced but only ventricular activity is sensed, the designation is DVI.

The five-letter code has a tremendous advantage in describing not only a certain pacemaker but also various possible modes of function incorporated into a single programmable pacemaker. The magnet mode of a pacemaker may also be described. This is the test mode in which a pacemaker functions when the internal reed switch is closed by the external application of a strong magnet. Thus, a VVI pacemaker generally functions in the VOO (asynchronous) mode when an external magnet is applied. Similarly, a sophisticated DDD pacemaker, discussed later, may be programmed to function in one of many modes, including DVI, VVI, AAI, AOO, VDD, and many more.

Fourth and fifth letters are used to denote programmability and antitachycardia capabilities, respectively. In this system, the letter P in the fourth position indicates the ability to program one or two parameters, and the letter M represents multiprogrammability. The letter R in the fourth position is used to designate a rate-modulated pacemaker (e.g., VVI-R); an O in the fourth position indicates a nonprogrammable pacemaker. In the fifth position, various antitachycardia functions may be indicated, including P for pacing, S for shock, and D (for both pacing and shock). These modes are discussed later in detail.

Multiple pacing modes are potentially feasible, although only seven modes have real significance in clinical practice. Of these, until recently, two (VVI and DVI) have comprised the majority of pacing applications.

VVI PACING. Single-chamber ventricular pacing has been the main type of cardiac pacing but is being replaced by more physiologic pacing modes. This mode, often referred to as ventricular-demand pacing, is the simplest of the pacing modes routinely used. As the ICHD code states, the pacemaker senses intrinsic ventricular activity and is inhibited when this activity exceeds the standby or escape rate of the pacemaker. When the intrinsic ventricular rate falls below the escape rate of the pulse generator, the pacemaker begins to function at its programmed rate. The escape rate and the automatic rate (pacing rate) may be identical or may be different if hysteresis is programmed into the pacemaker.

Potential disadvantages of VVI pacing are the lack of AV synchrony and the inability to increase heart rate with physiologic stress. Loss of coordinated contraction of the atria and ventricles may cause unpleasant symptoms due to atrial contraction against a closed tricuspid valve and may produce symptoms of low cardiac output referred to as the pacemaker syndrome. The magnet code for VVI pacemakers (VOO) allows the function of the pacemaker to be observed even when an intrinsic rhythm is present that would otherwise inhibit pacemaker function.

Asynchronous ventricular pacing was used clinically before units capable of inhibition were available. Because of the potential dangers of asynchronous pacemaker function, with paced beats falling in the T wave of preceding spontaneous beats and inducing ventricular arrhythmias, VOO pacing is now relegated to the rare situation in which oversensing produces inappropriate inhibition that cannot be corrected by programming.

AAI PACING. Atrial pacing is potentially of great benefit in patients with intact AV conduction and sinus bradycardia as in the sick sinus syndrome. Until recently, atrial pacing was not used extensively because of technical problems related to stability of endocardial atrial leads. In addition to achieving stable pacing, the atrial electrode must be able to sense an adequate atrial electrogram for avoidance of asynchronous atrial pacing, although this is not fraught with the potential hazards of asynchronous ventricular pacing. Advances in electrode technology have produced preformed J-shaped atrial tined leads that may be placed in position in the atrial appendage and active fixation leads that can be screwed into the atrial endocardium in other locations. These leads are capable of providing reliable atrial pacing in most patients.

SINGLE-CHAMBER RATE-MODULATED PACING. Single-chamber rate-modulated pacing (VVI-R or AAI-R) has become an important and frequently used pacing mode with the commercial availability of pacemakers using various sensors to regulate the pacing rate. In rate-modulated pacing, the pacing rate is determined by a physiologic parameter, other than atrial rate, that is measured by a special sensor in the pacemaker or pacing lead. Examples of physiologic parameters that are currently used in rate-modulated pacing include body motion, venous blood temperature, the Q-T interval, and respiratory rate. Other parameters that are being developed include mixed venous oxygen saturation, contractility, and stroke volume. Although these pacing systems can theoretically respond to various physiologic stimuli with an increase in heart rate, their primary use is to provide an increase in cardiac output with exercise.

Patients who have chronic or intermittent atrial fibrillation and in whom atrial synchronous pacing is impossible may be able to maintain normal heart rate responses to exercise through the use of ventricular rate-modulated pacing. In patients with normal AV conduction and sinus bradycardia that does not respond to exercise, rate-modulated atrial pacing may be indicated.

DVI PACING. Dual-chamber pacing has provided an important improvement over simple ventricular pacing in approximately 40 per cent of patients in whom optimal cardiac function depends on the atrial contribution to cardiac output.

Before the development of atrial synchronous pacing, *bifocal* or AV sequential pacing was the only modality available.

In this mode, both the atrium and the ventricle are paced with an artificial AV delay programmed between the atrial and ventricular impulses. In other respects, these devices function in a manner similar to VVI pacemakers. Only ventricular activity is sensed; thus, atrial stimulation is asynchronous if the spontaneous atrial rate exceeds the paced rate. DVI pacemakers may be of two types: committed or noncommitted. Committed systems are those in which the ventricular output must be delivered when the atrial pulse has occurred. In these systems, a QRS appearing in the AV interval will not inhibit ventricular output, and the ventricular pulse will fall in the QRS or ST segment. The advantage of the committed system is that false inhibition of the ventricular output due to cross-talk from the atrial channel cannot cause inappropriate failure to pace. In noncommitted systems, ventricular activity occurring in the AV interval inhibits the ventricular output. Cross-talk from the atrial channel is prevented by means of a blanking period of approximately 20 to 30 msec. after atrial output during which the ventricular sensing circuits are closed. Some systems have used a compromise between these two modes in which sensed ventricular activity after the atrial output causes a paced beat with a shortened AV interval, thus providing protection from failure to pace and diminishing the likelihood that the paced beat will fall in the vulnerable period, causing an arrhythmia.

VDD PACING. One of the primary limitations of DVI pacing is its fixed rate and the need for pacing at a rate faster than the patient's intrinsic sinus rate if the benefits of AV synchrony are to be maintained. Atrial synchronous pacing allows the ventricle to be paced after sensed atrial activity. This method has the advantage of preserving AV synchrony and allowing the ventricular rate to vary with the sinus rate. VDD pacing is differentiated from an earlier form of atrial synchronous pacing (VAT) in which the ventricle was paced synchronously with atrial activity, but without sensing in the ventricle.

Advanced forms of dual-chamber pacing (VDD or DDD) have no fixed rate, but rather are programmed to lower and upper rate limits. The way in which the pacemaker functions when the atrial rate exceeds the upper rate limits is also an important feature of these devices.

The upper rate limit is the rate beyond that which the pacemaker does not continue to track atrial activity. This is a programmable function that can be set according to the patient's needs. When the atrial rate reaches the upper rate limit, the pacemaker continues to pace at a constant rate (the upper rate), and an apparent Wenckebach's sequence appears.

When atrial activity decreases to the rate programmed as the lower rate limit of the pacemaker, the pacemaker responds in much the same manner as a VVI pacemaker at its escape interval. Because the VDD pacemaker cannot pace the atrium, VVI pacing occurs at the pacemaker's lower rate limit. Failure to sense in the atrium causes pacemaker function at lower rate limits despite the presence of faster atrial activity. A VDD pacemaker has no technologic advantage over present DDD units because both require atrial and ventricular leads, and devices capable only of VDD pacing are now obsolete.

DDD PACING. "Universal" or "automatic" pacing represents the height of pacing technology at present although, as discussed in the section on physiologic pacing, not necessarily the optimal form of pacing for every patient. The primary difference between early DDD pacemakers and VDD pacemakers was the ability to pace the atrium at the lower rate limit. Thus, instead of VVI pacing at the low rate, AV synchrony was maintained by DVI pacing. Newer and more sophisticated DDD pacemakers can now be programmed to almost every pacing mode conceivable in addition to DDD, including AAI, VVI, DVI, VVT, and VOO.

With atrial rates above the lower rate limit of the pacemaker, the atrial output is inhibited and the pacemaker tracks atrial activity and responds with ventricular pacing after the programmed AV delay. This method provides a range of rate variation between the lower and the upper rate limits. An upper rate limit is programmed to avoid excessive paced rates in the event of rapid atrial rhythms. When the patient's atrial rate exceeds the upper rate limit of the pacemaker, the pacemaker maintains a fixed ventricular rate, producing an apparent Wenckebach's sequence with gradually lengthening AV intervals.

The fastest atrial rate the pacemaker can follow is also governed by the duration of total atrial refractoriness, composed of the AV interval and the postventricular atrial refractory period. If the atrial rate becomes so rapid that alternating P waves fall during the pacemaker's period of atrial refractoriness, they will not be sensed, and the pacemaker will track only every other P wave. Injudicious programming of the atrial refractory period of the pacemaker may therefore cause abrupt reversion to 2:1 conduction by the pacemaker at or near the upper rate limit, and the patient has an abrupt decrease in heart rate.

Programmability

Programming features that are desirable include the ability of the programmer to interrogate the pacemaker for retrieval of two types of information: (1) the programmed settings of the pacemaker, that is, what the pacemaker is supposed to be doing; and (2) measured data from the pacemaker that indicate what the pacemaker is actually doing, what kind of sensed electrograms the pacemaker is receiving, and the state of the electrode and battery.

Most pacemakers now use radiofrequency signals for transmitting coded information to and from the pacemaker. The functions that can be programmed in a specific pacemaker vary considerably depending on the manufacturer and model. Obviously, the functions subject to programmability depend largely on the type of pacemaker (e.g., VVI, DVI,

DDD). The most important functions for programmability are generally considered to be rate, pulse width, and sensitivity. Most of the potentially correctable problems encountered with implanted pacemakers can be managed by use of these functions.

Physiologic Pacing

Physiologic pacing is a term used to describe pacing modes that attempt to duplicate normally conducted sinus rhythm. This concept assumes an understanding of the physiologic relationships between the conduction of the cardiac impulse and the hemodynamic events it initiates and implies that duplication of this physiology can be achieved with an artificial pacemaker. At best, current artificial pacemakers are only crude substitutes for normal sinus rhythm; therefore, the term physiologic pacing must be considered to be an oversimplification. Physiologic pacing has also been recognized as synonymous with dual-chamber pacing, although this is not necessarily true.

It has been well established that AV synchrony—that is, the contraction of the atria and the ventricles with normal sequence and timing—provides some margin of improved cardiac output when compared with ventricular pacing alone at comparable rates. Appropriately timed atrial contraction has been shown to increase cardiac output by as much as 25 per cent. This difference may be even greater during exercise or in certain pathologic states. The deleterious effects of AV dissociation due to ventricular pacing vary greatly among individual patients and depend on the heart's ability to compensate for a fixed rate, the presence of retrograde AV conduction, and the patient's overall level of activity.

The ability to increase heart rate for meeting increased metabolic demand is an important feature of normal cardiac conduction. Cardiac output is related directly to heart rate and stroke volume, and when cardiac disease impairs the ability to increase stroke volume, increased heart rate is the only mechanism remaining to increase cardiac output. Therefore, a physiologic pacing system has two aspects: the maintenance of AV synchrony and the preservation of rate variation. Obviously, these two features can be separated and may not be found in the same pacemaker. The familiar DVI pacemaker, for example, preserves AV synchrony without being able to vary rate in response to physiologic demands. Rate-modulated pacemakers can respond to physiologic stimuli including respiratory rate, Q-T interval, body motion during exercise, mixed venous oxygen saturation, and temperature. These devices are particularly suited for patients with chronic atrial fibrillation. Thus, physiologic pacing should be thought of not only as dual-chamber pacing, but rather as a pacing system that meets the physiologic needs of the patient.

The pacing modes that offer some preservation of normal physiologic relationships include AAI-R, DVI, VVI-R, and DDD. AAI-R pacing has the advantages of maintaining normal AV conduction, requiring only one electrode, and offering rate variation and is used in patients with chronic sinus bradycardia with intact AV conduction. DVI pacing obviates the concern for AV conduction but has the limitation of fixed rate. DDD pacing offers both rate variation and AV synchrony and is the optimal pacing mode when normal sinus node function is present.

The acute benefits of AV sequential or atrial synchronous pacing compared with ventricular pacing have been well documented. Numerous studies have also substantiated a sustained hemodynamic benefit of physiologic pacing modalities compared with fixed-rate ventricular pacing. Improvement in acute and chronic exercise capacity, symptoms (dyspnea and fatigue), and even survival has been attributed to rate-modulated and dual-chamber atrial synchronous pacing when compared with simple ventricular pacing.

Indications for Pacing Modes

AAI PACING. Atrial fixed-rate pacing may be indicated in patients with resting sinus bradycardia and intact AV conduction. Patients with the sick sinus syndrome may be included in this category; however, the potential effects of antiarrhythmic drugs on AV conduction must be considered before an atrial pacing system is implanted. Similarly, the intermittent occurrence of atrial fibrillation would render this pacing mode ineffective. AAI-R (rate-modulated) pacing is indicated when a normal increase in sinus rate with exercise is absent.

VVI PACING. VVI pacing is indicated in patients who are receiving a pacemaker for the prevention of intermittent symptoms and who have normal sinus rhythm most of the time. VVI pacing systems should not be implanted in patients who would benefit from dual-chamber pacemakers because of unfamiliarity with these systems. The development and ready availability of more sophisticated pacing modalities compel the physician to decline to implant a VVI unit in favor of a dual-chamber or rate-modulated system.

VVI-R pacing is indicated when dual-chamber pacing is not possible because of atrial arrhythmias and when a normal chronotropic response of heart rate to exercise is not present.

VVT PACING. Ventricular-triggered pacing is rarely indicated. Inappropriate inhibition causing failure to pace may be managed by use of the VVT mode when reprogramming the sensing threshold is not successful. Another potential application of VVT pacing is in the treatment of re-entrant tachycardias. An external stimulator is used to trigger the pacemaker, which causes interruption of the arrhythmia. In order to prevent sensing of T waves and pacing in the vulnerable period, the sensing refractory period should be extended in pacemakers programmed to the VVT mode.

DVI PACING. Fixed-rate AV sequential pacing devices are rapidly replacing pulse generators capable of atrial synchronous pacing. The indications for the use of these systems now are essentially limited to patients with chronic stable sinus bradycardia with unstable AV conduction. As a pacing mode within the capabilities of a DDD system, DVI may be useful when atrial sensing is unreliable or concomitant antiarrhythmic therapy produces sinus bradycardia.

DDD PACING. Atrial synchronous pacing systems are indicated in patients with chronic AV block (second-degree or third-degree) with stable sinus rhythm. Patients with exercise-induced second-degree AV block are also good candidates for a DDD pacemaker.

COMPLICATIONS

Pacemaker complications can be divided into four categories: immediate surgical complications, wound problems, delayed complications, and pacemaker malfunctions. Fortunately, all are relatively uncommon, which makes pacemaker insertion an exceptionally safe procedure when it is done by experienced surgeons.

XXIII

The Use of Cardiovascular Pharmacologic Agents in Surgical Patients

Robert W. Anderson, M.D.

Many patients currently presenting for surgical therapy are elderly and have associated cardiovascular diseases that add significantly to their surgical risk. A careful clinical history and physical examination are the most important components of the preoperative assessment of the cardiac patient who is to undergo a noncardiac surgical procedure. From these factors and the nature of the surgical procedure planned, a reasonable estimate of potential cardiac risk can be formulated to guide judicious preoperative testing for further definition of potentially high-risk patients. The potential risks that may be associated with an invasive cardiac procedure or surgical intervention must always be considered, along with the potential benefits of such a procedure, in an attempt to reduce the cardiac risk of noncardiac operations. Another important aspect in planning the overall surgical management is the evaluation of how any cardiovascular pharmacologic agent may influence operative management.

See the corresponding chapter or part in the *Textbook of Surgery,* 14th edition, pp. 2095–2105, for a more detailed discussion of this topic, including a comprehensive list of references.

The drugs that are employed in the management of cardio-vascular diseases form five general categories: (1) antihypertensives and diuretics; (2) agents for the management of chronic congestive heart failure; (3) antianginal drugs; (4) inotropic drugs; and (5) antiarrhythmics.

ANTIHYPERTENSIVES AND DIURETICS

Antihypertensive drugs have an important role in current medical therapy, and all are potentially toxic and work by inhibiting or modifying normal physiologic regulatory mechanisms. They may be troublesome and potentially dangerous in surgical patients in whom the stress of disease and the use of anesthetic agents may unmask potentially hazardous reactions and responses.

The diuretic agents, such as the thiazides and furosemide, increase urinary excretion of salt and water. Their chronic use may produce volume depletion and a predisposition to hypotension when anesthetics are administered that interfere with sympathetic function and, therefore, block the reflex increase in cardiac output and peripheral vascular resistance that are normal homeostatic responses to decreasing blood pressure. In addition, hypokalemia may occur following the chronic administration of diuretics, and this condition predisposes to arrhythmias. Repletion of diminished volume and total body potassium stores before major surgical procedures is essential in order to prevent sudden episodes of hypotension or cardiac rhythm disturbances.

The peripherally acting adrenergic antihypertensive drugs that inhibit function of the sympathetic nervous system may depress cardiac output and produce hypotension secondary to blunted sympathetic responses in the presence of volume depletion or exposure to anesthetic agents. Abrupt withdrawal of the peripheral adrenergic inhibitors may cause hypertensive crisis or other evidence of profound sympathetic overactivity in the perioperative period. The same problem is not observed with the centrally acting adrenergic blockers such as clonidine, which is well tolerated.

Beta-blockers appear to be well tolerated in surgical patients and offer a significant degree of protection from postoperative rhythm disturbances and sudden episodes of hypertension. It is considered safer to continue the agents throughout the surgical period and to utilize specific beta-agonists if hypotension or bradycardia develops.

The peripheral vasodilators are rarely used for the chronic management of hypertension, but nitroprusside may be administered intravenously under carefully monitored circumstances and is the agent of choice for the control of acute hypertension in the operating room or during the postoperative period.

The angiotensin-converting enzyme inhibitors are particularly effective in patients with hypertension due to elevated renin levels. They are generally well tolerated and do not appear to interfere with normal cardiovascular homeostatic responses and should be used throughout the perioperative period. The calcium antagonists are currently being more widely employed for the treatment of hypertension. Nifedipine, in particular, is a profound peripheral vasodilator that is frequently employed in patients with both ischemic heart disease and hypertension. All of the calcium antagonists may unmask latent hypovolemia and cause profound hypotension after relatively minor amounts of volume loss in surgical patients, and this is a particularly troublesome side effect. Careful hemodynamic monitoring with attention to volume status is necessary in surgical patients who are taking these agents.

AGENTS FOR THE MANAGEMENT OF CONGESTIVE HEART FAILURE

During the past decade, it has been recognized that management of chronic congestive heart failure is best achieved by reduction of cardiac work by the use of vasodilators rather than vigorous stimulation of the failing heart with inotropic agents. Drugs that produce vasodilation of vascular smooth muscle favorably affect the performance of the heart by decreasing peripheral vascular resistance through the mechanism of arterial relaxation and also by relaxing venous smooth muscle, thereby shifting blood from the central circulation into the peripheral venous capacitance bed, which causes a decreased preload or end-diastolic volume in the heart. These effects facilitate ventricular emptying and enhance stroke volume, which is the fundamental objective of any form of therapy for congestive heart failure secondary to cardiac dysfunction.

The surgical management of patients with evidence of congestive heart failure has been greatly improved with the addition of vasodilator drugs. Any patient with cardiac disease sufficiently severe to produce symptoms or findings of congestive heart failure represents a substantial risk for any major surgical operation. A comprehensive evaluation of a patient's cardiac disease, the institution or continuation of appropriate therapy, and the judicious use of intraoperative monitoring of cardiac function are mandatory if surgical risk is to be reduced to an acceptable level. Drugs that have successfully controlled symptoms of cardiac failure before operation should be continued or more appropriate agents utilized throughout the preoperative, operative, and postoperative periods.

ANTIANGINAL DRUGS

Patients undergoing major surgical procedures who have any history of ischemic heart disease must be optimally managed from a cardiac standpoint. Many take drugs for control of symptoms of angina pectoris, but others may have equally severe coronary disease despite minimal clinical symptoms. Careful assessment through history and physical examination, noninvasive stress testing, and, possibly, cardiac catheterization is mandatory in order to appropriately lower the risk in these patients.

Three general classes of pharmacologic agents are specifically used for the treatment of angina pectoris. These include the nitrates, beta-blocking agents, and calcium antagonists. In general, cardiovascular medications for the control of angina should be continued up to the time of operation and resumed as soon as possible postoperatively, even by use of nasogastric tube administration. Initial concerns about precipitation of hypotension and bradyarrhythmias during general anesthesia because of the use of antianginal drugs are generally unfounded. Such therapy should be uninterrupted insofar as possible, especially in patients with ischemic heart disease in whom acute withdrawal may precipitate rebound myocardial ischemia.

INOTROPIC DRUGS

Inotropic drugs have an important role in the management of heart failure and are particularly important in the management of surgical patients with cardiac instability on the basis of either primary cardiac dysfunction or peripheral vascular instability. Certain problems may arise that predispose surgical patients to the toxic manifestations of digitalis compounds. Both acute hypoxemia and hypokalemia increase susceptibility to digitalis-induced ventricular arrhythmias, and these disturbances require prompt and specific correction. It is generally best to withhold digitalis compounds for a period of time before any surgical procedure and utilize safer pharmacologic inotropic agents throughout the operative and postoperative period for the management of cardiac failure or rhythm disturbances. Support of the poorly functioning myocardium in the surgical patient may require the use of an inotropic agent that improves cardiac contractility without producing an increase in cardiac rate or significant increases in peripheral vascular resistance. The inotropic agents that appear to best achieve these goals are dopamine, dobutamine, and amrinone, used either alone or in combination.

ANTIARRHYTHMIC AGENTS

The perioperative management of patients with cardiac arrhythmias and conduction disturbances is an important part of the care of surgical patients. The knowledge of the preoperative drug ingestion history, electrocardiographic status, and cardiovascular history is mandatory for the proper management of these patients. The surgical patient is particularly predisposed to the development of arrhythmias because of the frequency of ventilatory problems that produce hypoxia or respiratory alkalosis, the development of hypokalemia and other electrolyte abnormalities, the toxic effects of cardioactive anesthetics, episodes of hypotension or hypertension, reduced cardiac output, anemia, perioperative myocardial infarction, and the cardiac trauma and pericarditis that are invariably associated with open cardiac surgical procedures. These factors must always be considered in the evaluation of a surgical patient with cardiac rhythm disturbance, and initial treatment should always be directed toward correction of these abnormalities. In the case of arrhythmias that are life-threatening or produce hemodynamic compromise, appropriate pharmacologic therapy may be required for the nature of the rhythm disturbance.

During the postoperative period, premature ventricular contractions are considered significant if they occur more than ten times per minute from a single focus, are multifocal, occur two or more times consecutively (couplets), or fall close to the T wave. Such ectopic beats can produce ventricular tachycardia or ventricular fibrillation and should be suppressed by the use of intravenous lidocaine. When lidocaine is ineffective, procainamide is added or substituted. Atrial dysrhythmias are also common during the postoperative period, and atrial fibrillation and flutter are the most common abnormalities noted. Therapy should be directed to slowing ventricular response, and the drug of choice is usually digoxin. If there is hemodynamic compromise, cardioversion may be required, and intravenous verapamil has proved to be effective in slowing ventricular response rates in both atrial fibrillation and flutter.

XXIV

Cardiopulmonary Bypass for Cardiac Surgery

William L. Holman, M.D., and James K. Kirklin, M.D.

The development of methods for maintaining perfusion of the body while bypassing the patient's own heart and lungs was a singularly important event in the development of cardiac surgery. A *controlled cross-circulation* method for cardiopulmonary bypass was used clinically by Lillehei in 1954; however, this method was later abandoned in favor of the mechanical pump oxygenator device developed and used by Gibbon to support a patient during closure of an atrial septal defect in 1953. By 1955, Kirklin and colleagues at the Mayo Clinic had embarked on the world's first series of intracardiac operations using a pump oxygenator.

See the corresponding chapter or part in the *Textbook of Surgery*, 14th edition, pp. 2105–2115, for a more detailed discussion of this topic, including a comprehensive list of references.

PUMP OXYGENATOR APPARATUS

The precise apparatus available for cardiopulmonary bypass (CPB) changes frequently, but the basic components remain constant. *A venous reservoir* stores excess volume and allows escape of air bubbles returning with venous blood. The *oxygenator* provides oxygen to the blood and eliminates carbon dioxide. Currently, bubble oxygenators, membrane oxygenators, and microporous hollow-fiber oxygenators are available for clinical use. An efficient *heat exchanger* is necessary for control of the perfusate temperature in order to achieve systemic cooling and rewarming during CPB. The *arterial pump* is usually a roller pump, which should be adjusted to be slightly nonocclusive. Vortex pumps are also available; however, their use is generally restricted to extracorporeal membrane oxygenator or ventricular assist device circuits.

PHYSIOLOGIC RESPONSE TO CARDIOPULMONARY BYPASS

Many complex physiologic changes occur when a patient is temporarily supported by means of an oxygenator system. The term *total cardiopulmonary bypass* indicates that nearly all the systemic venous blood is returned to the oxygenator. *Partial CPB* implies that some of the systemic venous blood returns to the heart and is ejected into the aorta. Two main types of physiologic variables exist during CPB, that is, *externally controlled variables*, which are controlled by the surgeon and the perfusionist, and *patient variables*, which are less easily regulated.

Externally Controlled Variables

The *perfusion flow rate and temperature of the perfusate* are variables controlled by the perfusionist under the direct guidance of the operating surgeon. The authors and most other cardiac surgeons utilize some degree of hypothermia for nearly all cardiac operations and regard the decision concerning perfusion temperature as one of the most important decisions to be made during CPB. Although no absolute criteria exist for safe flow rates at a specific temperature, organ damage appears least likely to occur when the microvasculature is perfused at flows that maintain nearly normal tissue oxygen levels and maximal oxygen consumption. During CPB, maximal perfusion of the microcirculation probably occurs near the asymptote of the temperature-specific curve relating flow to oxygen consumption. Experimental and clinical data indicate that normothermic perfusion flow rates of 1.7 liters per minute per square meter or greater are usually acceptable, but flow rates of 2 to 2.5 liters per minute per square meter provide a more secure margin of safety for organ perfusion.

During CPB, the *systemic venous pressure* and *pulmonary venous pressure* (left atrial pressure) should be maintained near

0 on total cardiopulmonary bypass, and the *hematocrit* of the patient-oxygenator system should be maintained between 25 and 30 per cent. A low hematocrit during hypothermic perfusion theoretically provides optimal perfusion of the microcirculation by lowering blood viscosity; however, this advantage of hemodilution is balanced by an increase in extravasation of fluid as intravascular osmotic pressure decreases.

If the projected patient-oxygenator hematocrit is adequate, an *asanguineous priming solution* is used. The *glucose concentration* of the priming solution is increased to provide an energy source and promote an osmotic diuresis. *Arterial oxygen levels* are maintained between 100 and 250 mm. Hg while the *arterial carbon dioxide pressure* is maintained between 30 and 40 mm. Hg (measured at 37° C.).

Patient Variables

The body's physiologic response to CPB is extremely complex and only partially understood. The *systemic vascular resistance* falls abruptly with the onset of CPB. Thereafter it gradually increases throughout the period of bypass, although there is considerable variation among patients. The importance of maintaining a certain mean arterial perfusion pressure during bypass is controversial. The patient's oxygen consumption and venous oxygen saturation are both partially controlled by the perfusion flow rate and the patient's temperature. It is generally assumed that the microcirculation is being effectively perfused if the mixed venous oxygen pressure during CPB is 30 to 40 mm. Hg.

Metabolic acidosis is usually present during bypass, but lactate levels should not exceed 5 mEq. per liter if adequate perfusion rates are maintained. Extracellular fluid is increased after CPB. The magnitude of this increase is directly related to the duration of CPB and the degree of hemodilution.

DAMAGING EFFECTS OF CARDIOPULMONARY BYPASS

The majority of patients suffer no clinically apparent ill effects of CPB; however, an occasional patient develops severe multiorgan dysfunction despite an otherwise accurate intracardiac repair. In its most severe form, the post-perfusion syndrome is characterized by a diffuse whole-body inflammatory reaction with elements of increased capillary permeability, extravasation of plasma, increased interstitial fluid, leukocytosis, fever, peripheral vasoconstriction, breakdown of red blood cells, and a diffuse bleeding diathesis. Two risk factors for an adverse clinical response to CPB include *age* (very young and very old) and *duration of bypass* (sharply increased risk after 4 hours of CPB).

The *exposure of blood to abnormal events* is probably the most powerful determinant of post-perfusion injury and includes exposure to shear stresses, incorporation of abnormal substances, and exposure to unphysiologic (nonendothelial) surfaces. *Shear stresses* are generated by blood pumps, by suction devices, and by cavitation around the end of the arterial cannula. Shear stresses injure leukocytes and cause erythrocyte destruction.

The *incorporation of abnormal substances* during cardiopulmonary bypass includes air bubbles, fibrin, tissue debris, and platelet thrombi as well as defoaming agents. However, it is the *exposure to unphysiologic surfaces* that produces the greatest damage during CPB. The most critical surfaces are probably those of the oxygenating device. Exposure to the pump oxygenator promotes platelet aggregation, causing decreased platelet numbers and function after cardiopulmonary bypass. Platelet activation is probably mediated by fibrinogen adsorption to the surfaces of the oxygenator and tubing. Methods for attenuating postoperative bleeding by improving postbypass platelet function are being actively investigated.

The *humoral amplification system* is a complex system of plasma proteins that responds to a local stimulus with a self-perpetuating and expanding series of reactions. These normally involve an inflammatory reaction in a localized area of the body. The components of the humoral amplification system include the *coagulation cascade*, the *fibrinolytic cascade*, the *kallikrein system*, and the *complement system*. The authors believe that the damaging effects of CPB are related largely to the humoral amplification system that initiates a whole-body "inflammatory response" during CPB.

The complement system is integral to the body's inflammatory response following CPB. Two pathways exist for activation of the complement sequence. The classic pathway is usually initiated via interaction with antigen-antibody complexes. The alternative or properdin pathway is activated by exposure of blood to foreign surfaces, and it is this pathway that is initially activated during CPB with later activation of the classic pathway during protamine administration following CPB.

Activation of complement produces the anaphylatoxins C5a and C3a. C3a and C5a have physiologic effects similar to those observed in many patients after CPB, including vasoconstriction and increased capillary permeability. Complement activation is probably important in neutrophil activation and degranulation during CPB and is responsible for a portion of the hemolysis noted during CPB. Studies at the University of Alabama in Birmingham have correlated cardiac, pulmonary, renal, and hematologic dysfunction after CPB with higher levels of C3a after bypass, longer elapsed times of bypass, and younger age at operation.

An increased understanding of complement activation during CPB will allow the development of methods for attenuating complement activation and diminishing the deleterious effects of CPB. This may be achieved by designing oxygenator systems that produce less complement activation or developing pharmacologic methods for the inhibition of complement activation during CPB.

Low-Flow Perfusion

Particularly during infant intracardiac surgery, a nearly bloodless field can usually be achieved with hypothermic low-flow perfusion for a portion of the repair. At a nasopharyngeal temperature of 20° C., a flow rate of 1.2 to 1.6 liters per minute per square meter is well tolerated. At this temperature, the perfusion flow rate can be reduced to 0.5 liter per minute per square meter for 30 to 45 minutes.

Oxygen consumption is an important indicator of the adequacy of perfusion to the microcirculation. The relationship between oxygen consumption and the perfusion flow rate during hypothermic CPB (20° C.) is such that oxygen consumption decreases rapidly only after flow is reduced below 1 liter per minute per square meter. The adequacy of cerebral perfusion during low-flow hypothermic perfusion has been examined in animal experiments. Cerebral oxygen perfusion and calculated vascular resistance is maintained as flow is reduced from 1.5 to 0.5 liter per minute per square meter on CPB at 20° C. (Tables 1 and 2). The contribution of autoregulation to the maintenance of cerebral perfusion during hypothermic low-flow perfusion has been confirmed in human studies.

Blood Conservation

During the past decade, efforts have been directed toward conservation of blood and avoidance of nonautologous transfusions in patients undergoing CPB. Autotransfusion of shed mediastinal blood after cardiac operations has been shown to be a safe and effective method for minimizing postoperative transfusion requirements. Erythrocytes aspirated from the operative field can be separated by centrifugation and washing before reinfusion. Intraoperative ultrafiltration of blood by means of hollow-fiber hemofilters may also be used to conserve blood. Studies by Boldt and associates and Solem and associates have demonstrated that hemofiltration conserves the plasma fraction as well as erythrocytes. Hemofiltration or cell separation techniques can be used to conserve the blood that remains in the oxygenator after the termination of CPB.

Autologous blood donated before cardiac operations has been shown to reduce the need for homologous transfusion, and the preoperative administration of human recombinant erythropoietin is currently under investigation as a means of diminishing postoperative transfusion requirements. Ultimately, a much greater impact on postoperative hemostasis and transfusion requirements will result from the development of improved methods for platelet preservation during CPB.

Conduct of Cardiopulmonary Bypass

After the patient is heparinized, cannulation of the venous and arterial circulation is achieved and CPB is initiated. The

TABLE 1. Oxygen Consumption During Profoundly Hypothermic, Nonpulsatile, Hemodiluted Cardiopulmonary Bypass in Monkeys

Organ	Oxygen Consumption (ml./min./100 gm.)			p Value
	1.5*	1.0*	0.5*	
Whole body	0.119 ± 0.0077	0.086 ± 0.0045	0.056 ± 0.0029	<0.0001
	(17.3 ± 1.16)†	(12.5 ± 0.65)	(8.3 ± 0.44)	
Brain	0.51 ± 0.095	0.47 ± 0.076	0.45 ± 0.113	0.5
Whole body minus brain	0.114 ± 0.0074	0.081 ± 0.0085	0.0518 ± 0.00176	<0.0001

*Perfusion flow rate (L/min/m²)

†The numbers in parentheses are the whole-body oxygen consumption expressed as ml./min./sq. m.

From Fox, L. S., et al.: J. Thorac. Cardiovasc. Surg., 87:658, 1984.

TABLE 2. Resistance to Blood Flow in the Brain and Remainder of the Body at Various Perfusion Rates During CPB in Monkeys

| | Resistance (units/100 gm.) | | | | | | |
Organ	1.75*	1.5*	1.25*	1.0*	0.5*	0.25*	p Value
Brain	1.2 ± 0.51	0.80 ± 0.080	0.8 ± 0.22	0.78 ± 0.126	0.80 ± 0.117	1.02 ± 0.173	0.4
Whole body minus brain	2.8 ± 0.157	3.3 ± 0.22	3.3 ± 1.21	3.9 ± 0.24	5.1 ± 0.49	9.5 ± 0.70	<0.0001

*Perfusion flow rate (L/min/m²).
From Fox, L. S., et al.: J. Thorac. Cardiovasc. Surg., 87:658, 1984.

initial perfusate temperature is usually 30° C. After full CPB is established, the perfusion temperature is diminished. The intracardiac portion of the operation is generally performed with the aorta cross-clamped and with cardioplegia-induced cardiac arrest. The precise perfusate temperature selected during cardioplegic arrest depends on the expected duration of the ischemic period as well as the anticipated needs for low perfusion rates or total circulatory arrest.

Approximately 5 minutes before the aortic cross-clamp is removed, rewarming is initiated and the flow rate is increased to 2 to 2.5 liters per minute per square meter. The arterial line blood temperature should not exceed 39° C. so that heat damage to the blood elements is prevented. Air is evacuated from the cardiac chambers before the cross-clamp is removed. Suction is continued on the aortic needle vent until cardiopulmonary bypass is discontinued. When the cardiac action is vigorous, the venous line is partially occluded. This will elevate the left atrial pressure and promote effective cardiac action for debubbling the heart. Cardiopulmonary bypass is then gradually discontinued. Polyvinyl catheters are placed in the left and right atria for facilitation of postoperative hemodynamic management, and atrial and ventricular temporary pacing wires are placed for postoperative pacing and arrhythmia management.

XXV

Intra-aortic Balloon Counterpulsation: Physiology, Indications, and Techniques

W. Randolph Chitwood, Jr., M.D.

The intra-aortic balloon pump (IABP) is the circulatory assist device used most frequently. Balloon pumping provides concurrent diastolic coronary flow augmentation and systolic ventricular afterload reduction with mild preload reduction. These advantages often enable jeopardized myocardium to function more efficiently.

PHYSIOLOGIC EFFECTS OF INTRA-AORTIC BALLOON PUMPING

Major determinants of myocardial oxygen consumption include pulse rate, transmural wall stress, and intrinsic con-

See the corresponding chapter or part in the *Textbook of Surgery*, 14th edition, pp. 2116–2126, for a more detailed discussion of this topic, including a comprehensive list of references.

tractile properties. The IABP has been shown to modify left ventricular ejection pressure by altering afterload. During periods of cardiac failure, increased ventricular dilation and afterload cause augmented wall tension (stress). Maximal wall stress and oxygen requirements occur during isovolumic systole. Rapid collapse of the balloon reduces impedance to aortic flow. The additive effects from this singular event usually decrease ventricular end-diastolic pressure and ischemia. Secondary benefits are decreased heart rate and diminished peripheral vascular resistance.

In damaged hearts, most IABP benefits probably follow coronary flow augmentation. With ischemic myocardium, autoregulatory reserves generally are expended with transmural flow becoming more pressure dependent. Under these conditions, the IABP reduces the ventricular end-diastolic pressure, augmenting the endocardial perfusion pressure. Clinically, the diastolic pressure may be increased up to 90 per cent by counterpulsation.

INDICATIONS FOR INTRA-AORTIC BALLOON PUMPING

CARDIAC FAILURE FOLLOWING SURGERY. The IABP is very efficacious for weaning patients from cardiopulmonary bypass with ventricular failure following cardiotomy (3 to 6 per cent). These patients either had a severely damaged ventricle preoperatively and incurred additional ischemic injury or had good ventricular function but experienced profound intraoperative myocardial depression. Some patients with right ventricular failure may benefit from a pulmonary artery IABP. Also, satisfactory afterload reduction and diastolic augmentation have been effected in pediatric patients.

Of patients requiring IABP insertion during cardiopulmonary bypass, 75 to 85 per cent can be weaned effectively, and of these, 50 to 80 per cent leave the hospital with long-term survival. Specific guidelines have been established to aid in instituting balloon pumping following cardiac surgical operative procedures. When needed, balloon pumping should be compounded with vasodilator and inotropic drug therapy; however, for optimization of myocardial energetics, many institute the IABP before infusing large doses of inotropic agents.

MEDICALLY REFRACTORY ANGINA. The intra-aortic balloon pump is effective in treating pharmacologically refractory angina and enables angiography and angioplasty to be done more safely. At least 80 per cent of patients obtain pain relief from balloon pumping. Survival in patients with medically refractory angina has been excellent with use of IABP support followed by surgical revascularization.

MYOCARDIAL INFARCTION: COMPLICATIONS. Following myocardial infarction, severe acute mitral insufficiency, an acute ventricular septal defect, or intractable arrhythmias (with or without an aneurysm) often cause circulatory failure. These patients usually benefit from early

IABP support; however, the salutary effects may be short-lived, and emergent surgical intervention is required.

Most commonly, papillary muscle rupture or dysfunction follows an inferior myocardial infarction. Mitral regurgitation may cause cardiogenic shock even with minimal impairment of ventricular function. Inotropes may help but also enhance afterload, increasing regurgitation into the low-resistance left atrium. The IABP decreases afterload and atrial shunting, augmenting left ventricular ejection.

In approximately 60 per cent of those with acute ventricular septal defects, rapid hemodynamic deterioration occurs. The combination of IABP support and early repair has decreased the operative mortality to as low as 30 per cent. Long-term survival has been about 70 per cent when left ventricular function was preserved. IABP stabilization reduces left-to-right shunting (seen best by transesophageal color-flow echocardiography), right ventricular failure, and pulmonary wedge pressure, effecting an increase in cardiac output and systemic pressure. As with acute septal defects, these improvements follow afterload reduction by providing less resistance to systemic ejection.

Significant ventricular arrhythmias occur in 10 to 50 per cent of patients following acute myocardial infarctions. Up to 55 per cent may resolve following IABP institution. In 90 per cent, angina resolves and survival is increased, if IABP is followed by coronary grafting. When ischemia is the etiologic factor, placement of an IABP usually controls ventricular irritability. In contrast, when myocardial fibrosis or an aneurysm is the inciting arrhythmogenic focus, IABP is less effective. Ventricular aneurysms develop in up to 20 per cent of patients following myocardial infarctions. Significant irritability may occur with acute aneurysms; however, only 7 to 11 per cent require surgical intervention for treatment of arrhythmias. Those having congestive failure or residual ischemia usually improve hemodynamically with IABP therapy.

CORONARY ANGIOPLASTY FAILURE. For patients requiring emergent surgical therapy because of a failed angioplasty, balloon counterpulsation provides optimal stabilization. This is especially important with multivessel coronary disease or markedly impaired ventricular function. Current reperfusion catheters allow the counterpulsed IABP waveform to reach the coronary segment distal to the occlusion. Because of IABP stabilization, most patients can be revascularized emergently with use of the internal mammary artery instead of only vein grafts.

CARDIAC TRANSPLANTATION. The IABP is effective in treating patients with end-stage cardiomyopathy while they await cardiac transplantation, and the importance of the method has increased with a declining donor heart supply. IABP may provide sufficient afterload reduction for obviating the need for a more invasive left ventricular bridge or assist device. At the University of Pittsburgh, of patients requiring inotropic support before a cardiac transplant, 28 per cent required IABP therapy.

CONTRAINDICATIONS TO BALLOON PUMPING

With severe aortic insufficiency, balloon pumping enhances valvular regurgitation. However, patients with minor degrees of insufficiency tolerate balloon pumping well. Color echo-cardiography is helpful in determining the degree of regurgitation with balloon inflation. The presence of a thoracic or abdominal aneurysm may be a relative contraindication. Diffuse atherosclerosis may preclude femoral artery insertion in 10 to 25 per cent of patients. Newer guidewire methods as well as axillary artery and transthoracic introduction may now allow IABP therapy in patients with complicated aorto iliac disease or aneurysms.

INSERTION AND REMOVAL TECHNIQUES

The percutaneous method for IABP catheter insertion is used now for most patients. Currently, the smallest dual-lumen percutaneous catheter (70 cm. long) is 9 Fr. (outside diameter) and has a standard 40 ml. balloon. After pulsatile flow from a common femoral artery needle puncture is obtained, a guidewire is passed above the iliac bifurcation. A vessel dilator, larger dilator, and introducer sheath are passed sequentially. The catheter should be introduced over the wire until the tip is positioned just distal to the left subclavian artery. Extremity pulses, temperature, and color should be assessed frequently. In general, patients undergoing intra-aortic balloon pumping should be anticoagulated with heparin.

Although required infrequently, femoral surgical insertion techniques may become necessary. Catheters are inserted through a 10 mm. Dacron/polytetrafluoroethylene graft, sewn to the femoral artery. Some prefer to insert the balloon directly with suture hemostasis. For allowing patient mobility, balloon catheters can be inserted via the axillary artery and passed retrograde. When aorto-iliac disease precludes retrograde insertion during operation, the transthoracic approach has been helpful.

For balloon removal, heparin should be discontinued 6 hours in advance with a platelet count and coagulation factors assessed. Surgical balloons may be removed in the intensive care unit using appropriate sterile technique. Balloons must be evacuated completely before removal to reduce catheter size. Following withdrawal of percutaneous balloons, groin pressure should be applied constantly for 30 minutes with distal pulses monitored by either palpation or Doppler ultrasound. Transthoracic and axillary catheters usually are removed in the operating room.

COMPLICATIONS

Major complications with IABP include limb ischemia from primary thrombosis, emboli, or vascular dissection; intra-abdominal and intrathoracic hemorrhage from perforation and/or dissection; groin hematomas; lymph drainage; femoral artery false aneurysms; local wound infections; systemic sepsis; renal failure and bowel infarction from balloon malposition; device malfunction in dependent patients; and neurologic complications including paraplegia. Two to 10 per cent of patients require vascular repair including patch angioplasty or femorofemoral bypass grafting. The incidence of major IABP complications has been reported to be higher with percutaneous balloon catheters. In most situations, ischemic complications can be obviated by early removal or partial withdrawal of the introducer sheath. The period of counterpulsation and female sex appear to be the most significant determinants of complications. Smaller balloon catheters (8.5 Fr. and 9 Fr.) have helped to minimize distal ischemia in smaller patients.

TIMING OF COUNTERPULSATION AND WEANING

Balloon inflation can be timed from a peripheral electrocardiogram, a ventricular electrogram, a radial arterial catheter, or the IABP central pressure channel. Because inflation delays (50 to 120 msec.) may occur with use of peripheral catheters, central aortic pressure appears preferable. Malpositioned sensing electrodes, radial artery spasm, arrhythmias, pacing, and electrocautery interference can cause timing problems.

The IABP should inflate about 40 msec. before the dicrotic notch (ascending T wave) and deflate during early isovolumic contraction (after P wave). Total deflation must occur before ejection (R wave). Significant decreases in aortic systolic and end-diastolic pressures usually occur. Early inflation causes premature aortic valve closure with reduced stroke volume, and late inflation causes inadequate diastolic pressure augmentation. Early deflation causes poor afterload reduction, and late deflation impedes systole with increased cardiac work.

The author prefers to wean the majority of inotropic medications before withdrawal of the IABP. Inotropic and vasopressor drugs are minimal (i.e., dopamine less than 5 μg. per kg. per minute) before establishment of a 1:2 pumping ratio. The inflation ratio and remaining inotropes then are weaned simultaneously.

HELICOPTER AND AIR AMBULANCE IABP TRANSPORT

Portable IABP consoles are now available and are superb for air and ground ambulance transport (Datascope, Kontron, Mansfield). Evanston Hospital reported 50 IABP patients transported safely by helicopter. IABP catheters have been inserted in patients in cardiac shock at regional emergency rooms with effective air evacuation (University of Kentucky). Pump consoles probably will become even more compact, with improvement in transport of IABP-dependent patients.

XXVI

The Artificial Heart

Wayne E. Richenbacher, M.D., Don B. Olsen, D.V.M., and William A. Gay, Jr., M.D.

The pneumatic total artificial heart is a biventricular prosthetic device used to provide complete circulatory support in patients with end-stage cardiac failure. Each prosthetic ventricle contains inflow and outflow connectors and valves and is tethered to an external pneumatic drive unit. The pumping action is created by pulses of air that are generated by the drive unit, traverse the drive lines, enter the ventricles, and intermittently flex the air diaphragms.

The artificial heart is implanted through a median sternotomy with the patient on cardiopulmonary bypass. The patient's diseased heart is removed by dividing the atria along the atrioventricular grooves and the great vessels distal to the semilunar valves, in a manner identical to that employed in orthotopic cardiac transplantation. The artificial heart is positioned within the patient's pericardium; the percutaneous drive lines exit the skin on the patient's anterior abdominal wall.

Currently, artificial hearts are utilized in patients who are candidates for cardiac transplantation but who decompensate hemodynamically before the availability of a donor organ. Patients are considered to be suitable candidates for a mechanical "bridge to transplantation" when they fulfill cardiac transplantation selection criteria and develop cardiogenic shock that is unresponsive to maximal medical therapy consisting of inotropic support and intra-aortic balloon counterpulsation. The artificial heart is explanted and cardiac transplantation performed when the patient's condition stabilizes and a donor heart becomes available.

The results of artificial heart implantation in this severely ill patient population show that approximately 70 to 80 per cent of patients who receive an artificial heart undergo subsequent cardiac transplantation, whereas 50 to 60 per cent are discharged from the hospital. Complications of use of this device include sepsis, hemorrhage, and thromboembolism. Investigative efforts are currently directed toward the modification of blood pump and connector design, in an effort to reduce areas of stasis and potential thrombus formation, as well as the development of an ideal postimplantation anticoagulation regimen. Septic sequelae are often the result of ascending drive line infections. This source of sepsis will be eliminated with the development of electric motor artificial hearts. Electric artificial hearts possess implantable prosthetic ventricles and an electrically powered energy convertor. External battery packs are coupled to the intrathoracic blood pump with use of transcutaneous energy transmission,

See the corresponding chapter or part in the *Textbook of Surgery*, 14th edition, pp. 2126–2132, for a more detailed discussion of this topic, including a comprehensive list of references.

which obviates the need for any break in the integument. Electric artificial hearts will ultimately provide chronic circulatory support in patients who are excluded from cardiac transplant selection criteria. These devices have functioned well in experimental animals but have not, as yet, been approved for clinical use.

57

THE ROLE OF COMPUTERS IN SURGICAL PRACTICE

Peter K. Smith, M.D.

The application of all types of computers is becoming a common feature of surgical practice. It is incumbent upon all physicians, and especially surgeons, to be cognizant of both the role and the potential of such computer applications in order to be able to use them effectively and to ensure that their development proceeds in a manner that improves rather than interferes with patient care.

Continuing a trend that began in the early 1970s, most hospitals have installed a centralized mainframe computer for creation of a hospital information system (HIS). These systems were designed and developed in an era when the mainframe computer was the only alternative and when computer applications were principally designed by computer scientists under the direction of hospital administrators. Accordingly, these systems are not user-friendly, are designed principally as accounting and billing systems, and are difficult to modify because of their institutional character. Although they have the major benefits of being extremely powerful and have "squatter's rights" on terminal location and communication, they have many significant disadvantages. Minicomputers have been a second choice for hospital information systems because of their limited storage and computing capacity. Accordingly, most implementations using minicomputers revolved around computerization of intensive care units and the development of clinical databases representing subsets of hospitalized patients, usually composed of patients with specific problems.

Microcomputers initially became available in the late 1970s and were introduced when their computing ability was quite limited. Their initial impact was on individual surgeons and other physicians who use these devices as word processors and for constructing small clinical databases reflecting individual practice. A wide variety of specific applications were developed to perform advanced calculator functions such as repetitive physiologic calculations and the monitoring of individual devices. In the past decade, the microcomputer has been dramatically improved in terms of both computer power and storage capacity. At this time, it is difficult to distinguish an advanced microcomputer from a minicomputer. In addition, advances in networking have allowed the microcomputer to be a "smart" interface to both minicomputers and mainframe computers by allowing computational power to be placed in a distributed manner throughout a

See the corresponding chapter or part in the *Textbook of Surgery*, 14th edition, pp. 2133–2147, for a more detailed discussion of this topic, including a comprehensive list of references.

hospital. The presence of this distributed power, with access to increasing amounts of data routinely collected by hospitals, will permit the surgeon to view the data from essentially any location as well as permit the local development of computer software to serve the surgeon's special needs.

ESTABLISHED COMPUTER APPLICATIONS

Hospital information systems (HIS) have been successfully implemented in most large institutions. To a significant degree, the success of the HIS is primarily dependent on its ability to operate as an accounting and inventory maintenance system. Collection and dispersal of data related to patient care has been a secondary development and has been limited because of the architecture of the database and the need for institutional commitment for accomplishing change. In the latter case, changes that enhance activity related to patient care are often divergent from the original funding goals and may tend to interfere with the accounting processes of the database. A large number of *clinical databases* have been developed with the use of minicomputers or microcomputers. A clinical database can be described as a well-defined, discrete, and continuous series of data elements pertaining to patients. These computer applications have been designed to aid in patient management and have their primary emphasis placed on patient care assistance, data collection, report generation, and clinical research. The importance of using a *coding system* for data entry has been emphasized by the development of these databases. For maximal utility, data recall must be on-line, efficient, rapid, and addressable by use of common technology. The significant advantage of these databases, that of dealing with limited patient populations, has also revealed the major problem in the development of patient care–related computer applications. This problem is that biostatisticians and computer scientists who are necessary for the maintenance of data structure and quality have a paucity of common ground with clinicians, which often creates insurmountable communication problems.

As microcomputer power has expanded and easy-to-use commercial software has become available, comprehensive medical databasing on local devices has become attractive. A large number of such database applications have been developed and range in use from the maintenance of practice records to comprehensive operating room scheduling systems.

The principal advantage of a microcomputer database is the ease with which it can be created and eventually modified in an evolutionary manner. These systems, unlike minicomputers or mainframe systems, can be modified by the end-user without the need for extensive programming knowledge.

The National Library of Medicine represents a significant established bibliographic database consisting of the indexed medical literature. The majority of data is encoded by use of keywords and can be directly searched with use of a micro-computer and several available searching services. The use of a local microcomputer and commercially available software packages assists an individual surgeon (even with a limited computer background) in creating a relational database of bibliographic material in a specific area of interest. With a modest effort, it is then possible to fully utilize this vast reference library and to periodically update a locally stored, specially oriented, bibliographic database.

Computerization of intensive care units (ICUs), with either minicomputers or microcomputers, has been a significant feature of surgical interest and was pioneered by Sheppard and Kirklin at the University of Alabama. Computerized ICU systems will almost certainly become the practice in the near future because of the growing number of all types of ICUs and the increasing shortage of skilled personnel for managing the ICU patient population. These systems have also been shown to improve the quality of intensive care and to diminish the average length of stay in an ICU. The use of prospective data collection has made it possible to categorize patients and permit prediction of complications and outcome. In addition, the organization and storage of ICU information provide a superior environment for physician and nursing education. The networking of various data sources, including clinical input from surgeons and nurses, is the major task accomplished by these systems.

DEVELOPING COMPUTER APPLICATIONS

Developing applications are often microcomputer-based, and many are currently nearing the transition to broad application. These applications are primarily designed to coordinate the storage of much information (including the history and physical examination, laboratory values, proce-dural notes, pharmaceutical data, imaging results, and doc-tors' orders), all of which is, to some extent, quantifiable. The remainder of the salient features of such developments includes the impressions and thought processes of care pro-viders as they evolve throughout the patient's hospital stay.

In the development of these applications, the primary emphasis is the creation of an electronic medical record designed to replace current records that are now recognized as being poorly organized, incomplete, and "noisy" (that is, containing much material that is required for nonmedical, often legal, reasons). A secondary emphasis has been placed on assisting the physician in the diagnostic and therapeutic thought processes (often termed artificial intelligence, but probably more appropriately termed computer-aided instruc-tion).

Inhibitory Factors

Legal considerations have arisen in the application of computers to patient care problems. The broad issues of confidentiality and security have not only been difficult to ensure but, in many instances, have been the deciding factors against implementation in the current medical-legal climate. Although numerous legal decisions have been rendered regarding liability in software development, this question remains unanswered.

The language of medicine, which often appears to be elaborated to prevent the encoding of lexical medical information, is probably the single largest impediment to computerization. In fact, if the large work force that currently attempts to encode medical information were to be devoted to the problem of developing computer-based translating devices, the process of encoding would be greatly enhanced. The major difficulty in codification is the distance that separates the physician from the process. The development of a physician workstation with direct encoding by the physician would greatly simplify the process and make it a self-correcting one.

Academic credit for work in the field of medical informatics has been available since the early 1970s, although such credit for software development is not yet a reality. This goes hand in hand with physician and nurse attitudes, which have served as both an impetus and inhibitor in the development of computer applications. This situation can generally be expected to become more positive over time, as health care professionals are exposed to computer applications through their training. Coupled with the maintenance of the physician's role as the "chief architect" of patient management, increased exposure of health care practitioners to microcomputers will likely facilitate complete computerization of the medical record. This may enable the appropriate distribution of cost accountability across the variety of traditional funding lines in health care institutions.

Integration of Data Sources: Benefits of Computerization

It has been well demonstrated that hospital-wide applications can have a positive impact on the overall quality of care for all patients. The integration of many diverse applications with widely varying computer methods is imperative in order to structure data flow and provide universal sharing of data. Such integration is critical in that it provides the incentive for merging the goals of a number of financially responsible entities within the hospital as an institution. The impetus for this integration is from many sources. Efficient utilization of resources such as physician and nursing time, bed space, investigational space, and space for patient services is scarce and expensive. Efficiency of such utilization is paramount and requires the development of a centralized database that will serve as a communication hub for the use of these resources. In addition, such a communication network must become a reality in order to share patient-related data and minimize interpersonal contact currently required for the acquisition of such data. The ultimate goal is the computerization of the entire medical record, which supersedes the printing of a discharge summary by providing direct access for all physicians in the hospital and referring physicians. The increased emphasis provided by the Joint Commission for Accreditation of Hospitals and other accrediting or financial institutions demands that such a database be effected in order to provide quality assurance for hospital, nursing, and physician practice. This type of quality control requires an extensive database to normalize morbidity and mortality and to enable the identification of events that occur outside of established norms. In surgical patients, quality assurance is, in the main, an analysis of complications related to *patient selection* and to *patient outcome*. In such a well-defined area, these complications can be defined prospectively. The number of potential outcomes are limited and can be predicted from preoperative diagnostic information and from operative procedural information. The credentialling of fully trained surgeons and the assurance of quality training for house staff officers (as well as the various reports required in these areas) can be extracted from an integrated database containing procedural and outcome data maintained concurrently on in-hospital patients.

A number of administrative functions, including billing for services, can be accomplished with a well-designed computer system. Such information can be used to allocate scarce resources such as operating room facilities and, when combined with outcome data and length-of-stay data, can provide a positive feedback mechanism for improving the overall financial status of an institution.

Physician Workstations

The concept of distributed processing in local microcomputer workstations would promote the ability of the physician, nurse, or any health care provider to have immediate access to primary data regarding each patient. The workstations may be integrated by use of the HIS as a host. In this way, the integrated data functions described would supply the hospital accounting system, rather than be derived from it. Computer algorithms for addressing general problems would reside in the host computer, whereas algorithms related to specific groups of patients (i.e., general surgery patients) would reside at the workstation level. The patient database would reside in the host computer after data manipulation and entry at distributed stations. Local data manipulations (for example, processing and display of physiologic waveforms) can be performed without burdening the HIS with excessive amounts of information.

Microcomputers with faster response time, powerful local capabilities, superior "user-friendliness," and an increasing ability to be integrated into networks containing mini- and mainframe computers are likely to triumph as workstations in the fast-paced clinical environment. The alternative solution of enlarging the HIS and adding terminals will likely fail because of poor response time for data retrieval and an inability to effectively develop software.

INDEX

Prescribing Information

MEFOXIN®
(STERILE CEFOXITIN SODIUM)

DESCRIPTION

MEFOXIN* (Sterile Cefoxitin Sodium) is a semi-synthetic, broad-spectrum cepha antibiotic sealed under nitrogen for parenteral administration. It is derived from cephamycin C, which is produced by *Streptomyces lactamdurans*. It is the sodium salt of 3-(hydroxymethyl)-7α-methoxy-8-oxo-7-[2-(2-thienyl)acetamido]-5-thia-1-azabicyclo [4.2.0] oct-2-ene-2-carboxylate carbamate (ester). The empirical formula is $C_{16}H_{16}N_3NaO_7S_2$, and the structural formula is:

MEFOXIN contains approximately 53.8 mg (2.3 milliequivalents) of sodium per gram of cefoxitin activity. Solutions of MEFOXIN range from colorless to light amber in color. The pH of freshly constituted solutions usually ranges from 4.2 to 7.0.

CLINICAL PHARMACOLOGY

Clinical Pharmacology

After intramuscular administration of a 1 gram dose of MEFOXIN to normal volunteers, the mean peak serum concentration was 24 mcg/mL. The peak occurred at 20 to 30 minutes. Following an intravenous dose of 1 gram, serum concentrations were 110 mcg/mL at 5 minutes, declining to less than 1 mcg/mL at 4 hours. The half-life after an intravenous dose is 41 to 59 minutes; after intramuscular administration, the half-life is 64.8 minutes. Approximately 85 percent of cefoxitin is excreted unchanged by the kidneys over a 6-hour period, resulting in high urinary concentrations. Following an intramuscular dose of 1 gram, urinary concentrations greater than 3000 mcg/mL were observed. Probenecid slows tubular excretion and produces higher serum levels and increases the duration of measurable serum concentrations.

Cefoxitin passes into pleural and joint fluids and is detectable in antibacterial concentrations in bile.

Clinical experience has demonstrated that MEFOXIN can be administered to patients who are also receiving carbenicillin, kanamycin, gentamicin, tobramycin, or amikacin (see PRECAUTIONS and ADMINISTRATION).

Microbiology

The bactericidal action of cefoxitin results from inhibition of cell wall synthesis. Cefoxitin has *in vitro* activity against a wide range of gram-positive and gram-negative organisms. The methoxy group in the 7α position provides MEFOXIN with a high degree of stability in the presence of beta-lactamases, both penicillinases and cephalosporinases, of gram-negative bacteria. Cefoxitin is usually active against the following organisms *in vitro* and in clinical infections:

Gram-positive

Staphylococcus aureus, including penicillinase and non-penicillinase producing strains

Staphylococcus epidermidis

Beta-hemolytic and other streptococci (most strains of enterococci, e.g., *Streptococcus faecalis*, are resistant)

Streptococcus pneumoniae

Gram-negative

Escherichia coli

Klebsiella species (including *K. pneumoniae*)

Hemophilus influenzae

Neisseria gonorrhoeae, including penicillinase and non-penicillinase producing strains

Proteus mirabilis

Morganella morganii

Proteus vulgaris

Providencia species, including *Providencia rettgeri*

Anaerobic organisms

Peptococcus species

Peptostreptococcus species

Clostridium species

Bacteroides species, including the *B. fragilis* group (includes *B. fragilis*, *B. distasonis*, *B. ovatus*, *B. thetaiotaomicron*, *B. vulgatus*)

MEFOXIN is inactive *in vitro* against most strains of *Pseudomonas aeruginosa* and enterococci and many strains of *Enterobacter cloacae*.

Methicillin-resistant staphylococci are almost uniformly resistant to MEFOXIN.

Susceptibility Tests

For fast-growing aerobic organisms, quantitative methods that require measurements of zone diameters give the most precise estimates of antibiotic susceptibility. One such procedure* has been recommended for use with discs to test susceptibility to cefoxitin. Interpretation involves correlation of the diameters obtained in the disc test with minimal inhibitory concentration (MIC) values for cefoxitin.

Reports from the laboratory giving results of the standardized single disc susceptibility test* using a 30 mcg cefoxitin disc should be interpreted according to the following criteria:

Organisms producing zones of 18 mm or greater are considered susceptible, indicating that the tested organism is likely to respond to therapy.

Organisms of intermediate susceptibility produce zones of 15 to 17 mm, indicating that the tested organism would be susceptible if high dosage is used or if the infection is confined to tissues and fluids (e.g., urine) in which high antibiotic levels are attained.

Resistant organisms produce zones of 14 mm or less, indicating that other therapy should be selected.

The cefoxitin disc should be used for testing cefoxitin susceptibility.

Cefoxitin has been shown by *in vitro* tests to have activity against certain strains of *Enterobacteriaceae* found resistant when tested with the cephalosporin class disc. For this reason, the cefoxitin disc should not be used for testing susceptibility to cephalosporins, and cephalosporin discs should not be used for testing susceptibility to cefoxitin.

Dilution methods, preferably the agar plate dilution procedure, are most accurate for susceptibility testing of obligate anaerobes.

A bacterial isolate may be considered susceptible if the MIC value for cefoxitin** is not more than 16 mcg/mL. Organisms are considered resistant if the MIC is greater than 32 mcg/mL.

INDICATIONS AND USAGE

Treatment

MEFOXIN is indicated for the treatment of serious infections caused by susceptible strains of the designated microorganisms in the diseases listed below.

(1) **Lower respiratory tract infections,** including pneumonia and lung abscess, caused by *Streptococcus pneumoniae*, other streptococci (excluding enterococci, e.g., *Streptococcus faecalis*), *Staphylococcus aureus* (penicillinase and non-penicillinase producing), *Escherichia coli*, *Klebsiella* species, *Hemophilus influenzae*, and *Bacteroides* species.

(2) **Genitourinary infections.** Urinary tract infections caused by *Escherichia coli*, *Klebsiella* species, *Proteus mirabilis*, indole-positive Proteus (which include the organisms now called *Morganella morganii* and *Proteus vulgaris*), and *Providencia* species (including *Providencia rettgeri*). Uncomplicated gonorrhea due to *Neisseria gonorrhoeae* (penicillinase and non-penicillinase producing).

*Bauer, A. W.; Kirby, W. M. M.; Sherris, J. C.; Turck, M.: Antibiotic susceptibility testing by a standardized single disc method, Amer. J. Clin. Path. *45*: 493-496, Apr. 1966. Standardized disc susceptibility test, Federal Register *37*: 20527-20529, 1972. National Committee for Clinical Laboratory Standards: Approved Standard: ASM-2, Performance Standards for Antimicrobial Disc Susceptibility Tests, July 1975.

**Determined by the ICS agar dilution method (Ericsson and Sherris, Acta Path. Microbiol. Scand. [B] Suppl. No. 217, 1971) or any other method that has been shown to give equivalent results.

(3) **Intra-abdominal infections,** including peritonitis and intra-abdominal abscess, caused by *Escherichia coli, Klebsiella* species, *Bacteroides* species including the *Bacteroides fragilis* group*, and *Clostridium* species.

(4) **Gynecological infections,** including endometritis, pelvic cellulitis, and pelvic inflammatory disease caused by *Escherichia coli, Neisseria gonorrhoeae* (penicillinase and non-penicillinase producing), *Bacteroides* species including the *Bacteroides fragilis* group*, *Clostridium* species, *Peptococcus* species, *Peptostreptococcus* species, and Group B streptococci.

(5) **Septicemia** caused by *Streptococcus pneumoniae, Staphylococcus aureus* (penicillinase and non-penicillinase producing), *Escherichia coli, Klebsiella* species, and *Bacteroides* species including the *Bacteroides fragilis* group.*

(6) **Bone and joint infections** caused by *Staphylococcus aureus* (penicillinase and non-penicillinase producing).

(7) **Skin and skin structure infections** caused by *Staphylococcus aureus* (penicillinase and non-penicillinase producing), *Staphylococcus epidermidis,* streptococci (excluding enterococci e.g., *Streptococcus faecalis*), *Escherichia coli, Proteus mirabilis, Klebsiella* species, *Bacteroides* species including the *Bacteroides fragilis* group*, *Clostridium* species, *Peptococcus* species, and *Peptostreptococcus* species.

Appropriate culture and susceptibility studies should be performed to determine the susceptibility of the causative organisms to MEFOXIN. Therapy may be started while awaiting the results of these studies.

In randomized comparative studies, MEFOXIN and cephalothin were comparably safe and effective in the management of infections caused by gram-positive cocci and gram-negative rods susceptible to the cephalosporins. MEFOXIN has a high degree of stability in the presence of bacterial beta-lactamases, both penicillinases and cephalosporinases.

Many infections caused by aerobic and anaerobic gram-negative bacteria resistant to some cephalosporins respond to MEFOXIN. Similarly, many infections caused by aerobic and anaerobic bacteria resistant to some penicillin antibiotics (ampicillin, carbenicillin, penicillin G) respond to treatment with MEFOXIN. Many infections caused by mixtures of susceptible aerobic and anaerobic bacteria respond to treatment with MEFOXIN.

Prevention

When compared to placebo in randomized controlled studies in patients undergoing gastrointestinal surgery, vaginal hysterectomy, abdominal hysterectomy and cesarean section, the prophylactic use of MEFOXIN resulted in a significant reduction in the number of postoperative infections.

The prophylactic administration of MEFOXIN may reduce the incidence of certain postoperative infections in patients undergoing surgical procedures (e.g., hysterectomy, gastrointestinal surgery and transurethral prostatectomy) that are classified as contaminated or potentially contaminated.

The perioperative use of MEFOXIN may be effective in surgical patients in whom subsequent infection at the operative site would present a serious risk, e.g., prosthetic arthroplasty.

Effective prophylactic use depends on the time of administration. MEFOXIN usually should be given one-half to one hour before the operation, which is sufficient time to achieve effective levels in the wound during the procedure. Prophylactic administration should usually be stopped within 24 hours since continuing administration of any antibiotic increases the possibility of adverse reactions but, in the majority of surgical procedures, does not reduce the incidence of subsequent infection. However, in patients undergoing prosthetic arthroplasty, it is recommended that MEFOXIN be continued for 72 hours after the surgical procedure.

If there are signs of infection, specimens for culture should be obtained for identification of the causative organism so that appropriate treatment may be instituted.

CONTRAINDICATIONS

MEFOXIN is contraindicated in patients who have shown hypersensitivity to cefoxitin and the cephalosporin group of antibiotics.

WARNINGS

BEFORE THERAPY WITH 'MEFOXIN' IS INSTITUTED, CAREFUL INQUIRY SHOULD BE MADE TO DETERMINE WHETHER THE PATIENT HAS HAD PREVIOUS HYPERSENSITIVITY REACTIONS TO CEFOXITIN, CEPHALOSPORINS, PENICILLINS, OR OTHER DRUGS. THIS PRODUCT SHOULD BE GIVEN WITH CAUTION TO PENICILLIN-SENSITIVE PATIENTS. ANTIBIOTICS SHOULD BE ADMINISTERED WITH CAUTION TO ANY PATIENT WHO HAS DEMONSTRATED SOME FORM OF ALLERGY, PARTICULARLY TO DRUGS. IF AN ALLERGIC REACTION TO 'MEFOXIN' OCCURS, DISCONTINUE THE DRUG. SERIOUS HYPERSENSITIVITY REACTIONS MAY REQUIRE EPINEPHRINE AND OTHER EMERGENCY MEASURES.

Pseudomembranous colitis has been reported with virtually all antibiotics (including cephalosporins); therefore, it is important to consider its diagnosis in patients who develop diarrhea in association with antibiotic use. This colitis may range from mild to life threatening in severity.

Treatment with broad-spectrum antibiotics alters normal flora of the colon and may permit overgrowth of clostridia. Studies indicate a toxin produced by *clostridium difficile* is one primary cause of antibiotic-associated colitis.

Mild cases of pseudomembranous colitis may respond to drug discontinuance alone. In more severe cases, management may include sigmoidoscopy, appropriate bacteriological studies, fluid, electrolyte and protein supplementation, and the use of a drug such as oral vancomycin as indicated. Isolation of the patient may be advisable. Other causes of colitis should also be considered.

PRECAUTIONS

General

The total daily dose should be reduced when MEFOXIN is administered to patients with transient or persistent reduction of urinary output due to renal insufficiency (see DOSAGE), because high and prolonged serum antibiotic concentrations can occur in such individuals from usual doses.

Antibiotics (including cephalosporins) should be prescribed with caution in individuals with a history of gastrointestinal disease, particularly colitis.

As with other antibiotics, prolonged use of MEFOXIN may result in overgrowth of non-susceptible organisms. Repeated evaluation of the patient's condition is essential. If superinfection occurs during therapy, appropriate measures should be taken.

Drug Interactions

Increased nephrotoxicity has been reported following concomitant administration of cephalosporins and aminoglycoside antibiotics.

Drug/Laboratory Test Interactions

As with cephalothin, high concentrations of cefoxitin (>100 micrograms/mL) may interfere with measurement of serum and urine creatinine levels by the Jaffé reaction, and produce false increases of modest degree in the levels of creatinine reported. Serum samples from patients treated with cefoxitin should not be analyzed for creatinine if withdrawn within 2 hours of drug administration.

High concentrations of cefoxitin in the urine may interfere with measurement of urinary 17-hydroxy-corticosteroids by the Porter-Silber reaction, and produce false increases of modest degree in the levels reported.

A false-positive reaction for glucose in the urine may occur. This has been observed with CLINITEST* reagent tablets.

*B. fragilis, B. distasonis, B. ovatus, B. thetaiotaomicron, B. vulgatus.

*Registered trademark of Ames Company, Division of Miles Laboratories, Inc.

Carcinogenesis, Mutagenesis,
Impairment of Fertility

Long-term studies in animals have not been performed with cefoxitin to evaluate carcinogenic or mutagenic potential. Studies in rats treated intravenously with 400 mg/kg of cefoxitin (approximately three times the maximum recommended human dose) revealed no effects on fertility or mating ability.

Pregnancy

Pregnancy Category B. Reproduction studies performed in rats and mice at parenteral doses of approximately one to seven and one-half times the maximum recommended human dose did not reveal teratogenic or fetal toxic effects, although a slight decrease in fetal weight was observed.

There are, however, no adequate and well-controlled studies in pregnant women. Because animal reproduction studies are not always predictive of human response, this drug should be used during pregnancy only if clearly needed.

In the rabbit, cefoxitin was associated with a high incidence of abortion and maternal death. This was not considered to be a teratogenic effect but an expected consequence of the rabbit's unusual sensitivity to antibiotic-induced changes in the population of the microflora of the intestine.

Nursing Mothers

MEFOXIN is excreted in human milk in low concentrations. Caution should be exercised when MEFOXIN is administered to a nursing woman.

Pediatric Use

Safety and efficacy in infants from birth to three months of age have not yet been established. In children three months of age and older, higher doses of MEFOXIN have been associated with an increased incidence of eosinophilia and elevated SGOT.

ADVERSE REACTIONS

MEFOXIN is generally well tolerated. The most common adverse reactions have been local reactions following intravenous or intramuscular injection. Other adverse reactions have been encountered infrequently.

Local Reactions

Thrombophlebitis has occurred with intravenous administration. Pain, induration, and tenderness after intramuscular injections have been reported.

Allergic Reactions

Rash (including exfoliative dermatitis), pruritus, eosinophilia, fever, dyspnea, and other allergic reactions including anaphylaxis and angioedema have been noted.

Cardiovascular

Hypotension

Gastrointestinal

Diarrhea, including documented pseudomembranous colitis which can appear during or after antibiotic treatment. Nausea and vomiting have been reported rarely.

Blood

Eosinophilia, leukopenia including granulocytopenia, neutropenia, anemia, including hemolytic anemia, thrombocytopenia, and bone marrow depression. A positive direct Coombs test may develop in some individuals, especially those with azotemia.

Liver Function

Transient elevations in SGOT, SGPT, serum LDH, and serum alkaline phosphatase; and jaundice have been reported.

Renal Function

Elevations in serum creatinine and/or blood urea nitrogen levels have been observed. As with the cephalosporins, acute renal failure has been reported rarely. The role of MEFOXIN in changes in renal function tests is difficult to assess, since factors predisposing to prerenal azotemia or to impaired renal function usually have been present.

OVERDOSAGE

The acute intravenous LD_{50} in the adult female mouse and rabbit was about 8.0 g/kg and greater than 1.0 g/kg respectively. The acute intraperitoneal LD_{50} in the adult rat was greater than 10.0 g/kg.

DOSAGE

TREATMENT
Adults

The usual adult dosage range is 1 gram to 2 grams every six to eight hours. Dosage and route of administration should be determined by susceptibility of the causative organisms, severity of infection, and the condition of the patient (see Table 1 for dosage guidelines).

MEFOXIN may be used in patients with reduced renal function with the following dosage adjustments:

In adults with renal insufficiency, an initial loading dose of 1 gram to 2 grams may be given. After a loading dose, the recommendations for *maintenance dosage* (Table 2) may be used as a guide.

When only the serum creatinine level is available, the following formula (based on sex, weight, and age of the patient) may be used to convert this value into creatinine clearance. The serum creatinine should represent a steady state of renal function.

$$\text{Males:} \quad \frac{\text{Weight (kg)} \times (140 - \text{age})}{72 \times \text{serum creatinine (mg/100 mL)}}$$

Females: 0.85 × above value

In patients undergoing hemodialysis, the loading dose of 1 to 2 grams should be given after each hemodialysis, and the maintenance dose should be given as indicated in Table 2.

Antibiotic therapy for group A beta-hemolytic streptococcal infections should be maintained for at least 10 days to guard against the risk of rheumatic fever or glomerulonephritis. In staphylococcal and other infections involving a collection of pus, surgical drainage should be carried out where indicated.

The recommended dosage of MEFOXIN **for uncomplicated gonorrhea** is 2 grams intramuscularly, with 1 gram of BENEMID* (Probenecid) given by mouth at the same time or up to ½ hour before MEFOXIN.

Infants and Children

The recommended dosage in children three months of age and older is 80 to 160 mg/kg of body weight per day divided into four to six equal doses. The higher dosages should be used for more severe or serious infections. The total daily dosage should not exceed 12 grams.

At this time no recommendation is made for children from birth to three months of age (see PRECAUTIONS).

In children with renal insufficiency the dosage and frequency of dosage should be modified consistent with the recommendations for adults (see Table 2).

PREVENTION
General

For prophylactic use in surgery, the following doses are recommended:

Adults:

(1) 2 grams administered intravenously or intramuscularly just prior to surgery (approximately one-half to one hour before the initial incision).

(2) 2 grams every 6 hours after the first dose for no more than 24 hours (continued for 72 hours after prosthetic arthroplasty).

Children (3 months and older):

30 to 40 mg/kg doses may be given at the times designated above.

Obstetric-Gynecologic

For prophylactic use in vaginal hysterectomy, a single 2.0 gram dose administered intramuscularly one-half to one hour prior to surgery is recommended.

For patients undergoing cesarean section, a single 2.0 gram dose should be administered intravenously as soon as the umbilical cord is clamped. A 3-dose regimen may be more effective than a single dose regimen in preventing postoperative infection (esp. endometritis) following cesarean section. Such a regimen would consist of 2.0 grams given intravenously as soon as the umbilical cord is clamped, followed by 2.0 grams 4 and 8 hours after the initial dose.

Transurethral prostatectomy patients:

One gram administered just prior to surgery; 1 gram every 8 hours for up to five days.

*Registered trademark of MERCK & CO., INC.

Table 1 — Guidelines for Dosage of MEFOXIN		
Type of Infection	Daily Dosage	Frequency and Route
Uncomplicated forms+ of infections such as pneumonia, urinary tract infection, cutaneous infection	3 - 4 grams	1 gram every 6 - 8 hours IV or IM
Moderately severe or severe infections	6 - 8 grams	1 gram every 4 hours or 2 grams every 6 - 8 hours IV
Infections commonly needing antibiotics in higher dosage (e.g., gas gangrene)	12 grams	2 grams every 4 hours or 3 grams every 6 hours IV
+ Including patients in whom bacteremia is absent or unlikely.		

Table 2 — Maintenance Dosage of MEFOXIN in Adults with Reduced Renal Function			
Renal Function	Creatinine Clearance (mL/min)	Dose (grams)	Frequency
Mild impairment	50 - 30	1 - 2	every 8 - 12 hours
Moderate impairment	29 - 10	1 - 2	every 12 - 24 hours
Severe impairment	9 - 5	0.5 - 1	every 12 - 24 hours
Essentially no function	< 5	0.5 - 1	every 24 - 48 hours

Table 3 — Preparation of Solution			
Strength	Amount of Diluent to be Added (mL) + +	Approximate Withdrawable Volume (mL)	Approximate Average Concentration (mg/mL)
1 gram Vial	2 (Intramuscular)	2.5	400
2 gram Vial	4 (Intramuscular)	5	400
1 gram Vial	10 (IV)	10.5	95
2 gram Vial	10 or 20 (IV)	11.1 or 21.0	180 or 95
1 gram Infusion Bottle	50 or 100 (IV)	50 or 100	20 or 10
2 gram Infusion Bottle	50 or 100 (IV)	50 or 100	40 or 20
10 gram Bulk	43 or 93 (IV)	49 or 98.5	200 or 100
+ + Shake to dissolve and let stand until clear.			

PREPARATION OF SOLUTION

Table 3 is provided for convenience in constituting MEFOXIN for both intravenous and intramuscular administration.

For intravenous use, 1 gram should be constituted with at least 10 mL of Sterile Water for Injection, and 2 grams, with 10 or 20 mL. The 10 gram bulk package should be constituted with 43 or 93 mL of Sterile Water for Injection or any of the solutions listed under the *Intravenous* portion of the COMPATIBILITY AND STABILITY section. CAUTION: THE 10 GRAM BULK STOCK SOLUTION IS NOT FOR DIRECT INFUSION. One or 2 grams of MEFOXIN for infusion may be constituted with 50 or 100 mL of 0.9 percent Sodium Chloride Injection, 5 percent or 10 percent Dextrose Injection, or any of the solutions listed under the *Intravenous* portion of the COMPATIBILITY AND STABILITY section.

Benzyl alcohol as a preservative has been associated with toxicity in neonates. While toxicity has not been demonstrated in infants greater than three months of age, in whom use of MEFOXIN may be indicated, small infants in this age range may also be at risk for benzyl alcohol toxicity. Therefore, diluent containing benzyl alcohol should not be used when MEFOXIN is constituted for administration to infants.

For ADD-Vantage®* vials, see separate INSTRUCTIONS FOR USE OF MEFOXIN IN ADD-Vantage® VIALS. MEFOXIN in ADD-Vantage® vials should be constituted with ADD-Vantage® diluent containers containing 50 mL or 100 mL of either 0.9 percent Sodium Chloride Injection or 5 percent Dextrose Injection. MEFOXIN in ADD-Vantage® vials is for IV use only.

For intramuscular use, each gram of MEFOXIN may be constituted with 2 mL of Sterile Water for Injection, or—

For intramuscular use ONLY: each gram of MEFOXIN may be constituted with 2 mL of 0.5 percent lidocaine hydrochloride solution† (without epinephrine) to minimize the discomfort of intramuscular injection.

ADMINISTRATION

MEFOXIN may be administered intravenously or intramuscularly after constitution.

Parenteral drug products should be inspected visually for particulate matter and discoloration prior to administration whenever solution and container permit.

Intravenous Administration

The intravenous route is preferable for patients with bacteremia, bacterial septicemia, or other severe or life-threatening infections, or for patients who may be poor risks because of lowered resistance resulting from such debilitating conditions as malnutrition, trauma, surgery, diabetes, heart failure, or malignancy, particularly if shock is present or impending.

For intermittent intravenous administration, a solution containing 1 gram or 2 grams in 10 mL of Sterile Water for Injection can be injected over a period of three to five minutes. Using an infusion system, it may also be given over a longer period of time through the tubing system by which the patient may be receiving other intravenous solutions. However, during infusion of the solution containing MEFOXIN, it is advisable to temporarily discontinue administration of any other solutions at the same site.

For the administration of higher doses by continuous intravenous infusion, a solution of MEFOXIN may be added to an intravenous bottle containing 5 percent Dextrose Injection, 0.9 percent Sodium Chloride Injection, 5 percent Dextrose and 0.9 percent Sodium Chloride Injection, or 5 percent Dextrose Injection with 0.02 percent sodium bicarbonate solution. BUTTERFLY* or scalp vein-type needles are preferred for this type of infusion.

Solutions of MEFOXIN, like those of most beta-lactam antibiotics, should not be added to aminoglycoside solutions (e.g., gentamicin sulfate, tobramycin sulfate, amikacin sulfate) because of potential interaction. However, MEFOXIN and aminoglycosides may be administered separately to the same patient.

Intramuscular Administration

As with all intramuscular preparations, MEFOXIN should be injected well within the body of a relatively large muscle such as the upper outer quadrant of the buttock (i.e., gluteus maximus); aspiration is necessary to avoid inadvertent injection into a blood vessel.

COMPATIBILITY AND STABILITY

Intravenous

MEFOXIN, as supplied in vials or the bulk package and constituted to 1 gram/10 mL with Sterile Water for Injection, Bacteriostatic Water

---

*Registered trademark of Abbott Laboratories, Inc.
†See package circular of manufacturer for detailed information concerning contraindications, warnings, precautions, and adverse reactions.

*Registered trademark of Abbott Laboratories, Inc.

for Injection, (see PREPARATION OF SOLUTION), 0.9 percent Sodium Chloride Injection, or 5 percent Dextrose Injection, maintains satisfactory potency for 24 hours at room temperature, for one week under refrigeration (below 5°C), and for at least 30 weeks in the frozen state.

These primary solutions may be further diluted in 50 to 1000 mL of the following solutions and maintain potency for 24 hours at room temperature and at least 48 hours under refrigeration:

Sterile Water for Injection‡
0.9 percent Sodium Chloride Injection
5 percent or 10 percent Dextrose Injection‡
5 percent Dextrose and 0.9 percent Sodium Chloride Injection
5 percent Dextrose Injection with 0.02 percent Sodium Bicarbonate solution
5 percent Dextrose Injection with 0.2 percent or 0.45 percent saline solution
Ringer's Injection
Lactated Ringer's Injection‡
5 percent Dextrose in Lactated Ringer's Injection‡
5 percent or 10 percent invert sugar in water
10 percent invert sugar in saline solution
5 percent Sodium Bicarbonate Injection
Neut (sodium bicarbonate)*‡
M/6 sodium lactate solution
NORMOSOL-M in D5-W*‡
IONOSOL B w/Dextrose 5 percent*‡
POLYONIC M 56 in 5 percent Dextrose**
Mannitol 5% and 2.5%
Mannitol 10%‡
ISOLYTE*** E
ISOLYTE*** E with 5% Dextrose

MEFOXIN, as supplied in infusion bottles and constituted with 50 to 100 mL of 0.9 percent Sodium Chloride Injection, or 5 percent or 10 percent Dextrose Injection, maintains satisfactory potency for 24 hours at room temperature or for 1 week under refrigeration (below 5°C).

MEFOXIN is supplied in single dose ADD-Vantage® vials and should be prepared as directed in the accompanying INSTRUCTIONS FOR USE OF MEFOXIN IN ADD-Vantage® VIALS using ADD-Vantage® diluent containers containing 50 mL or 100 mL of either 0.9 percent Sodium Chloride Injection or 5 percent Dextrose Injection. When prepared with either of these diluents, MEFOXIN maintains satisfactory potency for 24 hours at room temperature.

Limited studies with solutions of MEFOXIN in 0.9 percent Sodium Chloride Injection, Lactated Ringer's Injection, and 5 percent Dextrose Injection in VIAFLEX† intravenous bags show stability for 24 hours at room temperature, 48 hours under refrigeration and 26 weeks in the frozen state and 24 hours at room temperature thereafter. Also, solutions of MEFOXIN in 0.9 percent Sodium Chloride Injection show similar stability in plastic tubing, drip chambers, and volume control devices of common intravenous infusion sets.

After constitution with Sterile Water for Injection and subsequent storage in disposable plastic syringes, MEFOXIN is stable for 24 hours at room temperature and 48 hours under refrigeration.

After the periods mentioned above, any unused solutions or frozen material should be discarded. Do not refreeze.

Intramuscular
MEFOXIN, as constituted with Sterile Water for Injection, Bacteriostatic Water for Injection, or 0.5 percent or 1 percent lidocaine hydrochloride solution (without epinephrine), maintains satisfactory potency for 24 hours at room temperature, for one week under refrigeration (below 5°C), and for at least 30 weeks in the frozen state.

*Registered trademark of Abbott Laboratories, Inc.
‡In these solutions, MEFOXIN has been found to be stable for a period of one week under refrigeration.
**Registered trademark of Cutter Laboratories, Inc.
***Registered trademark of American Hospital Supply Corporation.
†Registered trademark of Baxter International, Inc.

After the periods mentioned above, any unused solutions or frozen material should be discarded. Do not refreeze.

MEFOXIN has also been found compatible when admixed in intravenous infusions with the following:

Heparin 0.1 units/mL at room temperature — 8 hours

Heparin 100 units/mL at room temperature — 24 hours

M.V.I.†† concentrate at room temperature 24 hours; under refrigeration 48 hours

BEROCCA††† C-500 at room temperature 24 hours; under refrigeration 48 hours

Insulin in Normal Saline at room temperature 24 hours; under refrigeration 48 hours

Insulin in 10% invert sugar at room temperature 24 hours; under refrigeration 48 hours

HOW SUPPLIED

Sterile MEFOXIN is a dry white to off-white powder supplied in vials and infusion bottles containing cefoxitin sodium as follows:

No. 3356 — 1 gram cefoxitin equivalent
NDC 0006-3356-45 in trays of 25 vials
(6505-01-119-6005, 1 g 25's).

No. 3368 — 1 gram cefoxitin equivalent
NDC 0006-3368-71 in trays of 10 infusion bottles
(6505-01-195-0649, 1 g infusion bottle 10's).

No. 3357 — 2 gram cefoxitin equivalent
NDC 0006-3357-53 in trays of 25 vials
(6505-01-104-6393, 2 g 25's).

No. 3369 — 2 gram cefoxitin equivalent
NDC 0006-3369-73 in trays of 10 infusion bottles
(6505-01-185-2624, 2 g infusion bottle 10's).

No. 3388 — 10 gram cefoxitin equivalent
NDC 0006-3388-67 in trays of 6 bulk bottles
(6505-01-263-0730, 10 g 6's).

No. 3548 — 1 gram cefoxitin equivalent
NDC 0006-3548-45 in trays of 25 ADD-Vantage® vials
(6505-01-262-9509, 1 g ADD-Vantage® 25's).

No. 3549 — 2 gram cefoxitin equivalent
NDC 0006-3549-53 in trays of 25 ADD-Vantage® vials
(6505-01-263-4531, 2 g ADD-Vantage® 25's).

Special storage instructions
MEFOXIN in the dry state should be stored below 30°C. Avoid exposure to temperatures above 50°C. The dry material as well as solutions tend to darken, depending on storage conditions; product potency, however, is not adversely affected.

††Registered trademark of USV Pharmaceutical Corp.
†††Registered trademark of Roche Laboratories.

A.H.F.S. Category: 8:12.07

Issued January 1992   DC7057130

PRIMAXIN® I.V.
(IMIPENEM-CILASTATIN SODIUM FOR INJECTION, MSD)

DESCRIPTION

PRIMAXIN* I.V. (Imipenem-Cilastatin Sodium for Injection, MSD) is a sterile formulation of imipenem, a thienamycin antibiotic, and cilastatin sodium, the inhibitor of the renal dipeptidase, dehydropeptidase I, with sodium bicarbonate added as a buffer. PRIMAXIN I.V. is a potent broad spectrum antibacterial agent for intravenous administration.

Imipenem (N-formimidoylthienamycin monohydrate) is a crystalline derivative of thienamycin, which is produced by *Streptomyces cattleya*. Its chemical name is [5R-[5α, 6α (R*)]]-6-(1-hydroxyethyl)-3-[[2-[(iminomethyl)amino] ethyl]thio]-7-oxo-1-azabicyclo [3.2.0] hept-2-ene-2-carboxylic acid monohydrate. It is an off-white, nonhygroscopic crystalline compound with a molecular weight of 317.37. It is sparingly soluble in water, and slightly soluble in methanol. Its empirical formula is $C_{12}H_{17}N_3O_4S \cdot H_2O$, and its structural formula is:

Cilastatin sodium is the sodium salt of a derivatized heptenoic acid. Its chemical name is [R-[R*,S*-(Z)]]-7-[(2-amino-2-carboxyethyl)thio]-2-[[(2,2-dimethylcyclopropyl)carbonyl]amino]-2-heptenoic acid, monosodium salt. It is an off-white to yellowish-white, hygroscopic, amorphous compound with a molecular weight of 380.43. It is very soluble in water and in methanol. Its empirical formula is $C_{16}H_{25}N_2O_5S$ Na, and its structural formula is:

PRIMAXIN I.V. is buffered to provide solutions in the pH range of 6.5 to 7.5. There is no significant change in pH when solutions are prepared and used as directed. (See COMPATIBILITY AND STABILITY.) PRIMAXIN I.V. 250 contains 18.8 mg of sodium (0.8 mEq) and PRIMAXIN I.V. 500 contains 37.5 mg of sodium (1.6 mEq). Solutions of PRIMAXIN I.V. range from colorless to yellow. Variations of color within this range do not affect the potency of the product.

CLINICAL PHARMACOLOGY

Intravenous Administration

Intravenous infusion of PRIMAXIN I.V. over 20 minutes results in peak plasma levels of imipenem antimicrobial activity that range from 14 to 24 mcg/mL for the 250 mg dose, from 21 to 58 mcg/mL for the 500 mg dose and from 41 to 83 mcg/mL for the 1000 mg dose. At these doses, plasma levels of imipenem antimicrobial activity decline to below 1 mcg/mL or less in 4 to 6 hours. Peak plasma levels of cilastatin following a 20-minute intravenous infusion of PRIMAXIN I.V., range from 15 to 25 mcg/mL for the 250 mg dose, from 31 to 49 mcg/mL for the 500 mg dose and from 56 to 88 mcg/mL for the 1000 mg dose.

General

The plasma half-life of each component is approximately 1 hour. The binding of imipenem to human serum proteins is approximately 20%

and that of cilastatin is approximately 40%. Approximately 70% of the administered imipenem is recovered in the urine within 10 hours after which no further urinary excretion is detectable. Urine concentrations of imipenem in excess of 10 mcg/mL can be maintained for up to 8 hours with PRIMAXIN I.V. at the 500 mg dose. Approximately 70% of the cilastatin sodium dose is recovered in the urine within 10 hours of administration of PRIMAXIN I.V.

No accumulation of PRIMAXIN I.V. in plasma or urine is observed with regimens administered as frequently as every 6 hours in patients with normal renal function.

Imipenem, when administered alone, is metabolized in the kidneys by dehydropeptidase I resulting in relatively low levels in urine. Cilastatin sodium, an inhibitor of this enzyme, effectively prevents renal metabolism of imipenem so that when imipenem and cilastatin sodium are given concomitantly fully adequate antibacterial levels of imipenem are achieved in the urine.

After a 1 gram dose of PRIMAXIN I.V., the following average levels of imipenem were measured (usually at 1 hour post-dose except where indicated) in the tissues and fluids listed:

Tissue or Fluid	n	Imipenem Level mcg/mL or mcg/g	Range
Vitreous Humor	3	3.4 (3.5 hours post dose)	2.88-3.6
Aqueous Humor	5	2.99 (2 hours post dose)	2.4-3.9
Lung Tissue	8	5.6 (median)	3.5-15.5
Sputum	1	2.1	—
Pleural	1	22.0	—
Peritoneal	12	23.9 S.D. ±5.3 (2 hours post dose)	—
Bile	2	5.3 (2.25 hours post dose)	4.6 to 6.0
CSF (uninflamed)	5	1.0 (4 hours post dose)	0.26-2.0
CSF (inflamed)	7	2.6 (2 hours post dose)	0.5-5.5
Fallopian Tubes	1	13.6	—
Endometrium	1	11.1	—
Myometrium	1	5.0	—
Bone	10	2.6	0.4-5.4
Interstitial Fluid	12	16.4	10.0-22.6
Skin	12	4.4	NA
Fascia	12	4.4	NA

Microbiology

The bactericidal activity of imipenem results from the inhibition of cell wall synthesis. Its greatest affinity is for penicillin binding proteins (PBP) 1A, 1B, 2, 4, 5, and 6 of *Escherichia coli*, and 1A, 1B, 2, 4 and 5 of *Pseudomonas aeruginosa*. The lethal effect is related to binding to PBP 2 and PBP 1B. Imipenem has *in vitro* activity against a wide range of gram-positive and gram-negative organisms.

Imipenem has a high degree of stability in the presence of beta-lactamases, both penicillinases and cephalosporinases produced by gram-negative and gram-positive bacteria. It is a potent inhibitor of beta-lactamases from certain gram-negative bacteria which are inherently resistant to most beta-lactam antibiotics, e.g., *Pseudomonas aeruginosa*, *Serratia* spp., and *Enterobacter* spp.

In vitro, imipenem is active against most strains of clinical isolates of the following microorganisms:

Gram-positive:
Group D streptococci (including enterococci e.g., *Streptococcus faecalis*).
NOTE: Imipenem is inactive against *Streptococcus faecium*.
Streptococcus pyogenes (Group A streptococci)
Streptococcus agalactiae (Group B streptococci)
Group C streptococci
Group G streptococci
Viridans streptococci
Streptococcus pneumoniae (formerly *Diplococcus pneumoniae*)
Staphylococcus aureus including penicillinase producing strains
Staphylococcus epidermidis including penicillinase producing strains
NOTE: Many strains of methicillin-resistant staphylococci are resistant to imipenem.

Gram-negative:
Escherichia coli
Proteus mirabilis
Proteus vulgaris
Morganella morganii
Providencia rettgeri
Providencia stuartii
Citrobacter spp.

Klebsiella spp. including K. pneumoniae and K. oxytoca
  Enterobacter spp.
  Hafnia spp. including H. alvei
  Serratia marcescens
  Serratia spp. including S. liquefaciens
  Haemophilus parainfluenzae
  H. influenzae
  Gardnerella vaginalis
  Acinetobacter spp.
  Pseudomonas aeruginosa
    NOTE: Imipenem is inactive against P. maltophilia and some strains of P. cepacia.

Anaerobes:
  Bacteroides spp. including Bacteroides bivius, Bacteroides fragilis, Bacteroides melaninogenicus
  Clostridium spp. including C. perfringens
  Eubacterium spp.
  Fusobacterium spp.
  Peptococcus spp.
  Peptostreptococcus spp.
  Propionibacterium spp. including P. acnes
  Actinomyces spp.
  Veillonella spp.
  Imipenem has been shown to be active in vitro against the following microorganisms; however, clinical efficacy has not yet been established.

Gram-positive:
  Listeria monocytogenes
  Nocardia spp.

Gram-negative:
  Salmonella spp.
  Shigella spp.
  Yersinia spp. including Yersinia enterocolitica, Yersinia pseudotuberculosis
  Bordetella bronchiseptica
  Campylobacter spp.
  Achromobacter spp.
  Alcaligenes spp.
  Moraxella spp.
  Pasteurella multocida
  Aeromonas hydrophila
  Plesiomonas shigelloides
  Neisseria gonorrhoeae (including penicillinase-producing strains)

Anaerobes:
  Bacteroides asaccharolyticus
  Bacteroides disiens
  Bacteroides distasonis
  Bacteroides ovatus
  Bacteroides thetaiotaomicron
  Bacteroides vulgatus
  In vitro tests show imipenem to act synergistically with aminoglycoside antibiotics against some isolates of Pseudomonas aeruginosa.

Susceptibility Testing

Quantitative methods that require measurement of zone diameters give the most precise estimate of antibiotic susceptibility. One such procedure has been recommended for use with discs to test susceptibility to imipenem.

Reports from the laboratory giving results of the standard single-disc susceptibility test with a 10 mcg imipenem disc should be interpreted according to the following criteria:

Fully susceptible organisms produce zones of 16 mm or greater, indicating that the test organism is likely to respond to doses of 2 g per day or less (see DOSAGE AND ADMINISTRATION).

Moderately susceptible organisms produce zones of 14 to 15 mm and are expected to be susceptible if the maximum recommended dosage is used or if infection is confined to tissues and fluids in which high antibiotic levels are attained.

Resistant organisms produce zones of 13 mm or less, indicating that other therapy should be selected.

A bacterial isolate may be considered fully susceptible if the MIC value for imipenem is equal to or less than 4 mcg/mL. Organisms are considered moderately susceptible if the MIC value is 8 mcg/mL. Organisms are considered resistant if the MIC is equal to or greater than 16 mcg/mL.

The standardized quality control procedure requires the use of control organisms. The 10 mcg imipenem disc should give the zone diameters listed below for the quality control strains.

Organism	ATCC	Zone Size Range
E. coli	25922	26-32 mm
Ps. aeruginosa	27853	20-28 mm

Dilution susceptibility tests should give MICs between the ranges listed below for the quality control strains.

Organism	ATCC	MIC (mcg/mL)
E. coli	25922	0.06-0.25
S. aureus	29213	0.015-0.06
S. faecalis	29212	0.5-2.0
Ps. aeruginosa	27853	1.0-4.0

Based on blood levels of imipenem achieved in man, breakpoint criteria have been adopted for imipenem.

Category	Zone Diameter (mm)	Recommended MIC Breakpoint (mcg/mL)
Fully Susceptible	≥16	≤4
Moderately Susceptible	14-15	8
Resistant	≤13	≥16

INDICATIONS AND USAGE

PRIMAXIN I.V. is indicated for the treatment of serious infections caused by susceptible strains of the designated microorganisms in the diseases listed below:

(1) **Lower respiratory tract infections.** Staphylococcus aureus (penicillinase producing strains), Escherichia coli, Klebsiella species, Enterobacter species, Haemophilus influenzae, Haemophilus parainfluenzae*, Acinetobacter species, Serratia marcescens.

(2) **Urinary tract infections** (Complicated and uncomplicated). Staphylococcus aureus (penicillinase producing strains)*, Group D streptococci (enterococci), Escherichia coli, Klebsiella species, Enterobacter species, Proteus vulgaris*, Providencia rettgeri*, Morganella morganii*, Pseudomonas aeruginosa.

(3) **Intra-abdominal infections.** Staphylococcus aureus (penicillinase producing strains)*, Staphylococcus epidermidis, Group D streptococci (enterococci), Escherichia coli, Klebsiella species, Enterobacter species, Proteus species (indole positive and indole negative), Morganella morganii*, Pseudomonas aeruginosa, Citrobacter species, Clostridium species, Gram-positive anaerobes, including Peptococcus species, Peptostreptococcus species, Eubacterium species, Propionibacterium species*, Bifidobacterium species, Bacteroides species, including B. fragilis, Fusobacterium species.

(4) **Gynecologic infections.** Staphylococcus aureus (penicillinase producing strains)*, Staphylococcus epidermidis, Group B streptococci, Group D streptococci (enterococci), Escherichia coli, Klebsiella species*, Proteus species (indole positive and indole negative), Enterobacter species*, Gram-positive anaerobes, including Peptococcus species*, Peptostreptococcus species, Propionibacterium species*, Bifidobacterium species*, Bacteroides species, B. fragilis*, Gardnerella vaginalis.

(5) **Bacterial septicemia.** Staphylococcus aureus (penicillinase producing strains), Group D streptococci (enterococci), Escherichia coli, Klebsiella species, Pseudomonas aeruginosa, Serratia species*, Enterobacter species, Bacteroides species*, B. fragilis*.

(6) **Bone and joint infections.** Staphylococcus aureus (penicillinase producing strains), Staphylococcus epidermidis, Group D streptococci (enterococci), Enterobacter species, Pseudomonas aeruginosa.

(7) **Skin and skin structure infections.** Staphylococcus aureus (penicillinase producing strains), Staphylococcus epidermidis, Group D streptococci (enterococci), Escherichia coli, Klebsiella species, Enterobacter species, Proteus vulgaris, Providencia rettgeri*, Morganella morganii, Pseudomonas aeruginosa, Serratia species, Citrobacter species, Acinetobacter species, Gram-positive anaerobes, including Peptococcus species and Peptostreptococcus species, Bacteroides species, including B. fragilis, Fusobacterium species*.

(8) **Endocarditis.** Staphylococcus aureus (penicillinase producing strains).

*Efficacy for this organism in this organ system was studied in fewer than 10 infections.

(9) **Polymicrobic infections.** PRIMAXIN I.V. is indicated for polymicrobic infections including those in which *S. pneumoniae* (pneumonia, septicemia), Group A beta-hemolytic streptococcus (skin and skin structure), or nonpenicillinase-producing *S. aureus* is one of the causative organisms. However, monobacterial infections due to these organisms are usually treated with narrower spectrum antibiotics, such as penicillin G.

PRIMAXIN I.V. is not indicated in patients with meningitis because safety and efficacy have not been established.

Because of its broad spectrum of bactericidal activity against gram-positive and gram-negative aerobic and anaerobic bacteria, PRIMAXIN I.V. is useful for the treatment of mixed infections and as presumptive therapy prior to the identification of the causative organisms.

Although clinical improvement has been observed in patients with cystic fibrosis, chronic pulmonary disease, and lower respiratory tract infections caused by *Pseudomonas aeruginosa*, bacterial eradication may not necessarily be achieved.

As with other beta-lactam antibiotics, some strains of *Pseudomonas aeruginosa* may develop resistance fairly rapidly on treatment with PRIMAXIN I.V. When clinically appropriate during therapy of *Pseudomonas aeruginosa* infections, periodic susceptibility testing should be done.

Infections resistant to other antibiotics, for example, cephalosporins, penicillin, and aminoglycosides, have been shown to respond to treatment with PRIMAXIN I.V.

CONTRAINDICATIONS

PRIMAXIN I.V. is contraindicated in patients who have shown hypersensitivity to any component of this product.

WARNINGS

SERIOUS AND OCCASIONALLY FATAL HYPERSENSITIVITY (anaphylactic) REACTIONS HAVE BEEN REPORTED IN PATIENTS RECEIVING THERAPY WITH BETA-LACTAMS. THESE REACTIONS ARE MORE APT TO OCCUR IN PERSONS WITH A HISTORY OF SENSITIVITY TO MULTIPLE ALLERGENS.

THERE HAVE BEEN REPORTS OF PATIENTS WITH A HISTORY OF PENICILLIN HYPERSENSITIVITY WHO HAVE EXPERIENCED SEVERE HYPERSENSITIVITY REACTIONS WHEN TREATED WITH ANOTHER BETA-LACTAM. BEFORE INITIATING THERAPY WITH 'PRIMAXIN' I.V., CAREFUL INQUIRY SHOULD BE MADE CONCERNING PREVIOUS HYPERSENSITIVITY REACTIONS TO PENICILLINS, CEPHALOSPORINS, OTHER BETA-LACTAMS, AND OTHER ALLERGENS. IF AN ALLERGIC REACTION TO 'PRIMAXIN' I.V.' OCCURS, DISCONTINUE THE DRUG. SERIOUS HYPERSENSITIVITY REACTIONS MAY REQUIRE EPINEPHRINE AND OTHER EMERGENCY MEASURES.

Pseudomembranous colitis has been reported with virtually all antibiotics, including PRIMAXIN I.V.; therefore it is important to consider its diagnosis in patients who develop diarrhea in association with antibiotic use. This colitis may range in severity from mild to life threatening.

Mild cases of pseudomembranous colitis may respond to drug discontinuance alone. In more severe cases, management may include sigmoidoscopy, appropriate bacteriological studies, fluid, electrolyte and protein supplementation, and the use of a drug such as oral vancomycin, as indicated. Isolation of the patient may be advisable. Other causes of colitis should also be considered.

PRECAUTIONS

General
CNS adverse experiences such as confusional states, myoclonic activity, and seizures have been reported during treatment with PRIMAXIN I.V., especially when recommended dosages are exceeded. These experiences have occurred most commonly in patients with CNS disorders (e.g., brain lesions or history of seizures) and/or compromised renal function. However, there have been reports of CNS ad-

verse experiences in patients who had no recognized or documented underlying CNS disorder or compromised renal function.

Patients with severe or marked impairment of renal function, whether or not undergoing hemodialysis, had a higher risk of seizure activity when receiving maximum recommended doses than those with no impairment of renal function; therefore, maximum recommended doses should be used only where clearly indicated (see DOSAGE AND ADMINISTRATION).

Patients with creatinine clearances of ≤5 mL/min/1.73 m² should not receive PRIMAXIN I.V. unless hemodialysis is instituted within 48 hours.

For patients on hemodialysis, PRIMAXIN I.V. is recommended only when the benefit outweighs the potential risk of seizures.

Close adherence to the recommended dosage and dosage schedules is urged, especially in patients with known factors that predispose to convulsive activity. Anticonvulsant therapy should be continued in patients with known seizure disorders. If focal tremors, myoclonus, or seizures occur, patients should be evaluated neurologically, placed on anticonvulsant therapy if not already instituted, and the dosage of PRIMAXIN I.V. re-examined to determine whether it should be decreased or the antibiotic discontinued.

As with other antibiotics, prolonged use of PRIMAXIN I.V. may result in overgrowth of non-susceptible organisms. Repeated evaluation of the patient's condition is essential. If superinfection occurs during therapy, appropriate measures should be taken.

While PRIMAXIN I.V. possesses the characteristic low toxicity of the beta-lactam group of antibiotics, periodic assessment of organ system function during prolonged therapy is advisable.

Drug Interactions
Generalized seizures have been reported in patients who received ganciclovir and PRIMAXIN I.V. These drugs should not be used concomitantly unless the potential benefits outweigh the risks.

Since concomitant administration of PRIMAXIN I.V. and probenecid results in only minimal increases in plasma levels of imipenem and plasma half-life, it is not recommended that probenecid be given with PRIMAXIN I.V.

PRIMAXIN I.V. should not be mixed with or physically added to other antibiotics. However, PRIMAXIN I.V. may be administered concomitantly with other antibiotics, such as aminoglycosides.

Carcinogenesis, Mutagenesis,
Impairment of Fertility
Gene toxicity studies were performed in a variety of bacterial and mammalian tests *in vivo* and *in vitro*. The tests were: V79 mammalian cell mutation assay (PRIMAXIN I.V. alone and imipenem alone), Ames test (cilastatin sodium alone), unscheduled DNA synthesis assay (PRIMAXIN I.V.) and *in vivo* mouse cytogenicity test (PRIMAXIN I.V.). None of these tests showed any evidence of genetic damage.

Reproduction tests in male and female rats were performed with PRIMAXIN I.V. at dosage levels up to 8 times the usual human dose. Slight decreases in live fetal body weight were restricted to the highest dosage level. No other adverse effects were observed on fertility, reproductive performance, fetal viability, growth or postnatal development of pups. Similarly, no adverse effects on the fetus or on lactation were observed when PRIMAXIN I.V. was administered to rats late in gestation.

Pregnancy
Pregnancy Category C. Teratogenicity studies with cilastatin sodium in rabbits and rats at 10 and 33 times the usual human dose, respectively, showed no evidence of adverse effect on the fetus. No evidence of teratogenicity or adverse effect on postnatal growth or behavior was observed in rats given imipenem at dosage levels up to 30 times the usual human dose. Similarly, no evidence of adverse effect on the fetus was observed in teratology studies in rabbits with imipenem at doses up to 11 times the usual human dose.

Teratology studies with PRIMAXIN I.V. at doses up to 11 times the usual human dose in pregnant mice and rats during the period of major organogenesis revealed no evidence of teratogenicity.

Data from preliminary studies suggests an apparent intolerance to PRIMAXIN I.V. (including emesis, inappetence, body weight loss, diarrhea and death) at doses equivalent to the average human dose in pregnant rabbits and cynomolgus monkeys that is not seen in non-pregnant animals in these or other species. In other studies, PRIMAXIN I.V. was well tolerated in equivalent or higher doses (up to 11 times the average human dose) in pregnant rats and mice. Further studies are underway to evaluate these findings.

There are, however, no adequate and well-controlled studies in pregnant women. PRIMAXIN I.V. should be used during pregnancy only if the potential benefit justifies the potential risk to the fetus.

Nursing Mothers

It is not known whether this drug is excreted in human milk. Because many drugs are excreted in human milk, caution should be exercised when PRIMAXIN I.V. is administered to a nursing woman.

Pediatric Use

Safety and effectiveness in infants and children below 12 years of age have not yet been established.

ADVERSE REACTIONS

PRIMAXIN I.V. is generally well tolerated. Many of the 1,723 patients treated in clinical trials were severely ill and had multiple background diseases and physiological impairments, making it difficult to determine causal relationship of adverse experiences to therapy with PRIMAXIN I.V.

Local Adverse Reactions

Adverse local clinical reactions that were reported as possibly, probably or definitely related to therapy with PRIMAXIN I.V. were:

Phlebitis/thrombophlebitis—3.1%
Pain at the injection site—0.7%
Erythema at the injection site—0.4%
Vein induration—0.2%
Infused vein—0.1%

Systemic Adverse Reactions

The most frequently reported systemic adverse clinical reactions that were reported as possibly, probably, or definitely related to PRIMAXIN I.V. were nausea (2.0%), diarrhea (1.8%), vomiting (1.5%), rash (0.9%), fever (0.5%), hypotension (0.4%), seizures (0.4%) (see PRECAUTIONS), dizziness (0.3%), pruritus (0.3%), urticaria (0.2%), somnolence (0.2%).

Additional adverse systemic clinical reactions reported as possibly, probably or definitely drug related occurring in less than 0.2% of the patients or reported since the drug was marketed are listed within each body system in order of decreasing severity: *Gastrointestinal*—pseudomembranous colitis (see WARNINGS), hemorrhagic colitis, hepatitis (rarely), jaundice, gastroenteritis, abdominal pain, glossitis, tongue papillar hypertrophy, heartburn, pharyngeal pain, increased salivation; *Hematologic*—agranulocytosis, thrombocytopenia, neutropenia, leukopenia; *CNS* — encephalopathy, tremor, confusion, myoclonus, paresthesia, vertigo, headache, psychic disturbances; *Special Senses* — transient hearing loss in patients with impaired hearing, tinnitus, taste perversion; *Respiratory* — chest discomfort, dyspnea, hyperventilation, thoracic spine pain; *Cardiovascular* — palpitations, tachycardia; *Skin* — toxic epidermal necrolysis (rarely), erythema multiforme, angioneurotic edema, flushing, cyanosis, hyperhidrosis, skin texture changes, candidiasis, pruritus vulvae; *Body as a whole*—polyarthralgia, asthenia/weakness; *Renal*—acute renal failure (rarely), oliguria/anuria, polyuria. The role of PRIMAXIN I.V. in changes in renal function is difficult to assess, since factors predisposing to pre-renal azotemia or to impaired renal function usually have been present.

Adverse Laboratory Changes

Adverse laboratory changes without regard to drug relationship that were reported during clinical trials or reported since the drug was marketed were:

Hepatic: Increased SGPT, SGOT, alkaline phosphatase, bilirubin and LDH.

Hemic: Increased eosinophils, positive Coombs test, increased WBC, increased platelets, decreased hemoglobin and hematocrit, increased monocytes, abnormal prothrombin time, increased lymphocytes, increased basophils.

Electrolytes: Decreased serum sodium, increased potassium, increased chloride.

Renal: Increased BUN, creatinine.

Urinalysis: Presence of urine protein, urine red blood cells, urine white blood cells, urine casts, urine bilirubin, and urine urobilinogen.

OVERDOSAGE

The intravenous LD_{50} of imipenem is greater than 2000 mg/kg in the rat and approximately 1500 mg/kg in the mouse.

The intravenous LD_{50} of cilastatin sodium is approximately 5000 mg/kg in the rat and approximately 8700 mg/kg in the mouse.

The intravenous LD_{50} of PRIMAXIN I.V. is approximately 1000 mg/kg in the rat and approximately 1100 mg/kg in the mouse.

Information on overdosage in humans is not available.

DOSAGE AND ADMINISTRATION

The dosage recommendations for PRIMAXIN I.V. represent the quantity of imipenem to be administered. An equivalent amount of cilastatin is also present in the solution. Each 250 mg or 500 mg dose should be given by intravenous administration over 20 to 30 minutes. Each 1000 mg dose should be infused over 40 to 60 minutes. In patients who develop nausea during the infusion, the rate of infusion may be slowed.

The total daily dosage for PRIMAXIN I.V. should be based on the type or severity of infection and given in equally divided doses based on consideration of degree of susceptibility of the pathogen(s), renal function and body weight. Patients with impaired renal function, as judged by creatinine clearance $\leq$ 70 mL/min/1.73 m², require adjustment of dosage as described in the succeeding section of these guidelines.

Dosage regimens in column A in the Table for Adults with Normal Renal Function are recommended for infections caused by fully susceptible organisms which represent the majority of pathogenic species. Dosage regimens in column B of this Table are recommended for infections caused by organisms with moderate susceptibility to imipenem, primarily some strains of *Ps. aeruginosa*.

Doses cited in the Table below are based on a body weight of 70 kg. A further proportionate reduction in dose administered must be made for patients with a body weight less than 70 kg by multiplying the selected dose by the patient's weight in kg divided by 70.

INTRAVENOUS DOSAGE SCHEDULE FOR ADULTS WITH NORMAL RENAL FUNCTION

Type or Severity of Infection	A Fully susceptible organisms including gram-positive and gram-negative aerobes and anaerobes	B Moderately susceptible organisms, primarily some strains of *Ps. aeruginosa*
Mild	250 mg q6h	500 mg q6h
Moderate	500 mg q8h 500 mg q6h	500 mg q6h 1 g q8h
Severe, life threatening	500 mg q6h	1 g q8h 1 g q6h
Uncomplicated urinary tract infection	250 mg q6h	250 mg q6h
Complicated urinary tract infection	500 mg q6h	500 mg q6h

Due to the high antimicrobial activity of PRIMAXIN I.V., it is recommended that the maximum total daily dosage not exceed 50 mg/kg/day or 4.0 g/day, whichever is lower. There is no evidence that higher doses provide greater efficacy. However, patients over twelve years of age with cystic fibrosis and normal renal function have been treated with PRIMAXIN I.V. at doses up to 90 mg/kg/day in divided doses, not exceeding 4.0 g/day.

INTRAVENOUS DOSAGE SCHEDULE FOR ADULTS WITH IMPAIRED RENAL FUNCTION

Patients with creatinine clearance of ≤ 70 mL/min/1.73 m² require adjustment of the dosage of PRIMAXIN I.V. as indicated in the table below. Creatinine clearance may be calculated from serum creatinine concentration by the following equation:

$$T_{cc} \text{(Males)} = \frac{\text{(wt. in kg) (140 - age)}}{\text{(72) (creatinine in mg/dL)}}$$

T_{cc} (Females) = 0.85 x above value

Column A of the following Table shows maximum dosages recommended in each category of impaired renal function for infections caused by fully susceptible organisms which represent the majority of pathogenic species. The maximum dosages in column B are recommended only for infections caused by organisms with moderate susceptibility to imipenem, primarily some strains of *Ps. aeruginosa*. Doses cited are based on a body weight of 70 kg. A further proportionate reduction in dose administered must be made for patients with a body weight less than 70 kg by multiplying the selected dose by the patient's weight in kg divided by 70.

Patients with creatinine clearance ≤ 5 mL/min/1.73 m² should not receive PRIMAXIN I.V. unless hemodialysis is instituted within 48 hours. There is inadequate information to recommend usage of PRIMAXIN I.V. for patients undergoing peritoneal dialysis.

Maximum Recommended Intravenous Dosage of PRIMAXIN I.V. in Adults With Impaired Renal Function

Creatinine Clearance (mL/min/1.73 m²)	Renal Function	A Fully susceptible organisms including gram-positive and gram-negative aerobes and anaerobes	B Moderately susceptible organisms, primarily some strains of *Ps. aeruginosa*
31-70	Mild Impairment	500 mg q8h	500 mg q6h
21-30	Moderate Impairment	500 mg q12h	500 mg q8h
6-20	Severe to Marked Impairment	250 mg q12h See Text Below	500 mg q12h See Text Below
0-5	None, but on Hemodialysis		

Patients with creatinine clearances of 6 to 20 mL/min/1.73 m² should be treated with 250 mg (or 3.5 mg/kg whichever is lower) every 12 hours for most pathogens. When the 500 mg dose is used in these patients, there may be an increased risk of seizures.

Similar dosage and safety considerations apply in the treatment of patients with creatinine clearances of ≤ 5 mL/min/1.73 m² who are undergoing hemodialysis. Both imipenem and cilastatin are cleared from the circulation during hemodialysis. The patient should receive PRIMAXIN I.V. after hemodialysis and at 12 hour intervals timed from the end of that hemodialysis session. Dialysis patients, especially those with background CNS disease, should be carefully monitored; for patients on hemodialysis, PRIMAXIN I.V. is recommended only when the benefit outweighs the potential risk of seizures (see PRECAUTIONS).

PREPARATION OF SOLUTION

Infusion Bottles

Contents of the infusion bottles of PRIMAXIN I.V. Powder should be restored with 100 mL of diluent (see list of diluents under COMPATIBILITY AND STABILITY) and shaken until a clear solution is obtained.

Vials

Contents of the vials must be suspended and transferred to 100 mL of an appropriate infusion solution.

A suggested procedure is to add approximately 10 mL from the appropriate infusion solution (see list of diluents under COMPATIBILITY AND STABILITY) to the vial. Shake well and transfer the resulting suspension to the infusion solution container.

CAUTION: THE SUSPENSION IS NOT FOR DIRECT INFUSION.

Repeat with an additional 10 mL of infusion solution to ensure complete transfer of vial contents to the infusion solution. **The resulting mixture should be agitated until clear.**

ADD-Vantage®† Vials

See separate INSTRUCTIONS FOR USE OF 'PRIMAXIN I.V.' IN ADD-Vantage® VIALS. PRIMAXIN I.V. in ADD-Vantage® vials should be reconstituted with ADD-Vantage® diluent containers containing 100 mL of either 0.9% Sodium Chloride Injection or 100 mL 5% Dextrose Injection.

COMPATIBILITY AND STABILITY

Before reconstitution:

The dry powder should be stored at a temperature below 30°C.

Reconstituted solutions:

Solutions of PRIMAXIN I.V. range from colorless to yellow. Variations of color within this range do not affect the potency of the product.

PRIMAXIN I.V., as supplied in infusion bottles and vials and reconstituted as above with the following diluents, maintains satisfactory potency for four hours at room temperature or for 24 hours under refrigeration (5°C) (note exception below). Solutions of PRIMAXIN I.V. should not be frozen.

0.9% Sodium Chloride Injection*

5% or 10% Dextrose Injection

5% Dextrose Injection with 0.02% sodium bicarbonate solution

5% Dextrose and 0.9% Sodium Chloride Injection

5% Dextrose Injection with 0.225% or 0.45% saline solution

NORMOSOL† - M in D5-W

5% Dextrose Injection with 0.15% potassium chloride solution

Mannitol 2.5%, 5% and 10%

PRIMAXIN I.V. is supplied in single dose ADD-Vantage® vials and should be prepared as directed in the accompanying INSTRUCTIONS FOR USE OF 'PRIMAXIN I.V.' IN ADD-Vantage® VIALS using ADD-Vantage® diluent containers containing 100 mL of either 0.9% Sodium Chloride Injection or 5% Dextrose Injection. When prepared with either of these diluents, PRIMAXIN I.V. maintains satisfactory potency for 8 hours at room temperature.

PRIMAXIN I.V. should not be mixed with or physically added to other antibiotics. However, PRIMAXIN I.V. may be administered concomitantly with other antibiotics, such as aminoglycosides.

HOW SUPPLIED

PRIMAXIN I.V. is supplied as a sterile powder mixture in vials and infusion bottles containing imipenem (anhydrous equivalent) and cilastatin sodium as follows:

No. 3514—250 mg imipenem equivalent and 250 mg cilastatin equivalent and 10 mg sodium bicarbonate as a buffer
NDC 0006-3514-58 in trays of 25 vials (6505-01-332-4793 250 mg, 25's).

No. 3516—500 mg imipenem equivalent and 500 mg cilastatin equivalent and 20 mg sodium bicarbonate as a buffer
NDC 0006-3516-59 in trays of 25 vials (6505-01-332-4794 500 mg, 25's).

No. 3515—250 mg imipenem equivalent and 250 mg cilastatin equivalent and 10 mg sodium bicarbonate as a buffer
NDC 0006-3515-74 in trays of 10 infusion bottles
(6505-01-246-4126 infusion bottle, 10's).

No. 3517—500 mg imipenem equivalent and 500 mg cilastatin equivalent and 20 mg sodium bicarbonate as a buffer
NDC 0006-3517-75 in trays of 10 infusion bottles
(6505-01-234-0240 infusion bottle, 10's).

No. 3551—250 mg imipenem equivalent and 250 mg cilastatin equivalent and 10 mg sodium bicarbonate as a buffer

*PRIMAXIN I.V. has been found to be stable in 0.9% Sodium Chloride Injection for 10 hours at room temperature or 48 hours under refrigeration.
†Registered trademark of Abbott Laboratories, Inc.

NDC 0006-3551-58 in trays of 25 ADD-Vantage® vials.
No. 3552—500 mg imipenem equivalent and 500 mg cilastatin equivalent and 20 mg sodium bicarbonate as a buffer
NDC 0006-3552-59 in trays of 25 ADD-Vantage® vials
(6505-01-279-9627 500 mg ADD-Vantage®, 25's).

A.H.F.S. Category: 8:12.28

Issued August 1991   DC7362415

PRILOSEC®

(OMEPRAZOLE)

DELAYED-RELEASE CAPSULES

DESCRIPTION

The active ingredient in PRILOSEC* (Omeprazole) Delayed-Release Capsules is a substituted benzimidazole, 5-methoxy-2-[[(4-methoxy-3, 5-dimethyl-2-pyridinyl) methyl] sulfinyl]-1*H*-benzimidazole, a compound that inhibits gastric acid secretion. Its empirical formula is $C_{17}H_{19}N_3O_3S$, with a molecular weight of 345.42. The structural formula is:

Omeprazole is a white to off-white crystalline powder which melts with decomposition at about 155°C. It is a weak base, freely soluble in ethanol and methanol, and slightly soluble in acetone and isopropanol and very slightly soluble in water. The stability of omeprazole is a function of pH; it is rapidly degraded in acid media, but has acceptable stability under alkaline conditions.

PRILOSEC is supplied as delayed-release capsules for oral administration. Each delayed-release capsule contains 20 mg of omeprazole in the form of enteric-coated granules with the following inactive ingredients: cellulose, disodium hydrogen phosphate, hydroxypropyl cellulose, hydroxypropyl methylcellulose, lactose, mannitol, sodium lauryl sulfate and other ingredients. The capsule shell has the following inactive ingredients: gelatin, FD&C Blue #1, FD&C Red #40, titanium dioxide, synthetic black iron oxide, isopropanol, butyl alcohol, FD&C Blue #2, and D&C Red #7 Calcium Lake.

CLINICAL PHARMACOLOGY

Pharmacokinetics and Metabolism

PRILOSEC Delayed-Release Capsules contain an enteric-coated granule formulation of omeprazole (because omeprazole is acid-labile), so that absorption of omeprazole begins only after the granules leave the stomach. Absorption is rapid, with peak plasma levels of omeprazole occurring within 0.5 to 3.5 hours. Peak plasma concentrations of omeprazole and AUC are approximately proportional to doses up to 40 mg, but because of a saturable first-pass effect, a greater than linear response in peak plasma concentration and AUC occurs with doses greater than 40 mg. Absolute bioavailability (compared to intravenous administration) is about 30-40% at doses of 20-40 mg, due in large part to presystemic metabolism. In healthy subjects the plasma half-life is 0.5 to 1

hour, and the total body clearance is 500-600 mL/min. Protein binding is approximately 95%.

The bioavailability of omeprazole increases slightly upon repeated administration of PRILOSEC Delayed-Release Capsules.

Following single dose oral administration of a buffered solution of omeprazole, little if any unchanged drug was excreted in urine. The majority of the dose (about 77%) was eliminated in urine as at least six metabolites. Two were identified as hydroxyomeprazole and the corresponding carboxylic acid. The remainder of the dose was recoverable in feces. This implies a significant biliary excretion of the metabolites of omeprazole. Three metabolites have been identified in plasma—the sulfide and sulfone derivatives of omeprazole, and hydroxyomeprazole. These metabolites have very little or no antisecretory activity.

In patients with chronic hepatic disease, the bioavailability increased to approximately 100% compared to an I.V. dose, reflecting decreased first-pass effect, and the plasma half-life of the drug increased to nearly 3 hours compared to the half-life in normals of 0.5-1 hour. Plasma clearance averaged 70 mL/min, compared to a value of 500-600 mL/min in normal subjects.

In patients with chronic renal impairment, whose creatinine clearance ranged between 10 and 62 mL/min/1.73. m². the disposition of omeprazole was very similar to that in healthy volunteers, although there was a slight increase in bioavailability. Because urinary excretion is a primary route of excretion of omeprazole metabolites, their elimination slowed in proportion to the decreased creatinine clearance.

The elimination rate of omeprazole was somewhat decreased in the elderly, and bioavailability was increased. Omeprazole was 76% bioavailable when a single 40 mg oral dose of omeprazole (buffered solution) was administered to healthy elderly volunteers, versus 58% in young volunteers given the same dose. Nearly 70% of the dose was recovered in urine as metabolites of omeprazole and no unchanged drug was detected. The plasma clearance of omeprazole was 250 mL/min (about half that of young volunteers) and its plasma half-life averaged one hour, about twice that of young healthy volunteers.

Pharmacodynamics

Mechanism of Action

Omeprazole belongs to a new class of antisecretory compounds, the substituted benzimidazoles, that do not exhibit anticholinergic or H_2 histamine antagonistic properties, but that suppress gastric acid secretion by specific inhibition of the H^+/K^+ ATPase enzyme system at the secretory surface of the gastric parietal cell. Because this enzyme system is regarded as the acid (proton) pump within the gastric mucosa, omeprazole has been characterized as a gastric acid-pump inhibitor, in that it blocks the final step of acid production. This effect is dose-related and leads to inhibition of both basal and stimulated gastric acid secretion irrespective of the stimulus. Animal studies indicate that after rapid disappearance from plasma, omeprazole can be found within the gastric mucosa for a day or more.

Antisecretory Activity

After oral administration, the onset of the antisecretory effect of omeprazole occurs within one hour, with the maximum effect occurring within two hours. Inhibition of secretion is about 50% of maximum at 24 hours and the duration of inhibition lasts up to 72 hours. The antisecretory effect thus lasts far longer than would be expected from the very short (less than one hour) plasma half-life, apparently due to prolonged binding to the parietal H^+/K^+ ATPase enzyme. When the drug is discontinued, secretory activity returns gradually, over 3 to 5 days. The inhibitory effect of omeprazole on acid secretion increases with repeated once-daily dosing, reaching a plateau after four days.

Results from numerous studies of the antisecretory effect of multiple doses of 20 mg and 40 mg of omeprazole in normal volunteers and patients are shown below. The "max" value represents determinations at a time of maximum effect (2-6 hours after dosing), while "min" values are those 24 hours after the last dose of omeprazole.

Range of Mean Values from Multiple Studies
of the Mean Antisecretory Effects of Omeprazole
After Multiple Daily Dosing

Parameter	Omeprazole 20 mg		Omeprazole 40 mg	
	Max	Min	Max	Min
% Decrease in Basal Acid Output	78*	58-80	94*	80-93
% Decrease in Peak Acid Output	79*	50-59	88*	62-68
% Decrease in 24-hr. Intragastric Acidity		80-97		92-94

*Single Studies

Single daily oral doses of omeprazole ranging from a dose of 10 mg to 40 mg have produced 100% inhibition of 24-hour intragastric acidity in some patients.

Enterochromaffin-like (ECL) Cell Effects

In 24-month carcinogenicity studies in rats, a dose-related significant increase in gastric carcinoid tumors and ECL cell hyperplasia was observed in both male and female animals (see PRECAUTIONS, *Carcinogenesis, Mutagenesis, Impairment of Fertility*). Hypergastrinemia secondary to prolonged and sustained hypochlorhydria has been postulated to be the mechanism by which ECL cell hyperplasia and gastric carcinoid tumors develop. Omeprazole may also affect other cells in the gastrointestinal tract (e.g., G cells), either directly or by inducing sustained hypochlorhydria, but this possibility has not been extensively studied.

Human gastric biopsy specimens from about 200 patients treated continuously with omeprazole for an average of over 12 months have not detected ECL cell effects of omeprazole similar to those seen in rats. Longer term data are needed to rule out the possibility of an increased risk for the development of gastric tumors in patients receiving long-term therapy with omeprazole.

Serum Gastrin Effects

In studies involving more than 200 patients, serum gastrin levels increased during the first 1 to 2 weeks of once-daily administration of therapeutic doses of omeprazole in parallel with inhibition of acid secretion. No further increase in serum gastrin occurred with continued treatment. In comparison with histamine H_2-receptor antagonists, the median increases produced by 20 mg doses of omeprazole were higher (1.3 to 3.6 fold vs. 1.1 to 1.8 fold increase). Gastrin values returned to pretreatment levels, usually within 1 to 2 weeks after discontinuation of therapy.

Other Effects

Systemic effects of omeprazole in the CNS, cardiovascular and respiratory systems have not been found to date. Omeprazole, given in oral doses of 30 or 40 mg for 2 to 4 weeks, had no effect on thyroid function, carbohydrate metabolism, or circulating levels of parathyroid hormone, cortisol, estradiol, testosterone, prolactin, cholecystokinin or secretin.

No effect on gastric emptying of the solid and liquid components of a test meal was demonstrated after a single dose of omeprazole 90 mg. In healthy subjects, a single I.V. dose of omeprazole (0.35 mg/kg) had no effect on intrinsic factor secretion. No systematic dose-dependent effect has been observed on basal or stimulated pepsin output in humans.

However, when intragastric pH is maintained at 4.0 or above, basal pepsin output is low, and pepsin activity is decreased.

As do other agents that elevate intragastric pH, omeprazole administered for 14 days in healthy subjects produced a significant increase in the intragastric concentrations of viable bacteria. The pattern of the bacterial species was unchanged from that commonly found in saliva. All resolved within three days of stopping treatment.

Clinical Studies
Duodenal Ulcer Disease

Active Duodenal Ulcer: In a multicenter, double-blind, placebo-controlled study of 147 patients with endoscopically documented duodenal ulcer, the percentage of patients healed (per protocol) at 2 to 4 weeks was significantly higher with PRILOSEC 20 mg once a day than with placebo (p ≤ 0.01).

Treatment of Active Duodenal Ulcer
% of Patients Healed

	PRILOSEC 20 mg a.m. (n = 99)	Placebo a.m. (n = 48)
Week 2	*41	13
Week 4	*75	27

*(p ≤ 0.01)

Complete daytime and nighttime pain relief occurred significantly faster (p ≤ 0.01) in patients treated with PRILOSEC 20 mg than in patients treated with placebo. At the end of the study, significantly more patients who had received PRILOSEC had complete relief of daytime pain (p ≤ 0.05) and nighttime pain (p ≤ 0.01).

In a multicenter, double-blind study of 293 patients with endoscopically documented duodenal ulcer, the percentage of patients healed (per protocol) at 4 weeks was significantly higher with PRILOSEC 20 mg once a day than with ranitidine 150 mg b.i.d. (p < 0.01).

Treatment of Active Duodenal Ulcer
% of Patients Healed

	PRILOSEC 20 mg a.m. (n = 145)	Ranitidine 150 mg b.i.d. (n = 148)
Week 2	42	34
Week 4	*82	63

*(p < 0.01)

Healing occurred significantly faster in patients treated with PRILOSEC than in those treated with ranitidine 150 mg b.i.d. (p < 0.01).

In a foreign multinational randomized, double-blind study of 105 patients with endoscopically documented duodenal ulcer, 20 mg and 40 mg of PRILOSEC were compared to 150 mg b.i.d. of ranitidine at 2, 4 and 8 weeks. At 2 and 4 weeks both doses of PRILOSEC were statistically superior (per protocol) to ranitidine, but 40 mg was not superior to 20 mg of PRILOSEC, and at 8 weeks there was no significant difference between any of the active drugs.

Treatment of Active Duodenal Ulcer
% of Patients Healed

	PRILOSEC 20 mg (n = 34)	PRILOSEC 40 mg (n = 36)	Ranitidine 150 mg b.i.d. (n = 35)
Week 2	* 83	* 83	53
Week 4	* 97	*100	82
Week 8	100	100	94

*(p ≤ 0.01)

Gastroesophageal Reflux Disease (GERD)

In a U.S. multicenter double-blind placebo controlled study of 20 mg or 40 mg of PRILOSEC Delayed-Release Capsules in patients with symptomatic esophagitis and endoscopically diagnosed erosive esophagitis of grade 2 or above, the percentage healing rates (per protocol) were as follows:

Week	20 mg PRILOSEC (n = 83)	40 mg PRILOSEC (n = 87)	Placebo (n = 43)
4	39**	45**	7
8	74**	75**	14

**(p<0.01) PRILOSEC versus placebo.

In this study, the 40 mg dose was not superior to the 20 mg dose of PRILOSEC in the percentage healing rate. Other controlled clinical trials have also shown that PRILOSEC is effective in severe GERD. In comparisons with histamine H_2-receptor antagonists in patients with erosive esophagitis, grade 2 or above, PRILOSEC in a dose of 20 mg was significantly more effective than the active controls. Complete daytime and nighttime heartburn relief occurred significantly faster (p<0.01) in patients treated with PRILOSEC than in those taking placebo or histamine H_2-receptor antagonists.

Pathological Hypersecretory Conditions

In open studies of 136 patients with pathological hypersecretory conditions, such as Zollinger-Ellison (ZE) syndrome with or without multiple endocrine adenomas, PRILOSEC Delayed-Release Capsules significantly inhibited gastric acid secretion and controlled associated symptoms of diarrhea, anorexia, and pain. Doses ranging from 20 mg every other day to 360 mg per day maintained basal acid secretion below 10 mEq/hr in patients without prior gastric surgery, and below 5 mEq/hr in patients with prior gastric surgery.

Initial doses were titrated to the individual patient need, and adjustments were necessary with time in some patients (see DOSAGE AND ADMINISTRATION). PRILOSEC was well tolerated at these high dose levels for prolonged periods (>5 years in some patients). In most ZE patients, serum gastrin levels were not modified by PRILOSEC. However, in some patients serum gastrin increased to levels greater than those present prior to initiation of omeprazole therapy. At least 2 patients with ZE syndrome on long-term treatment with PRILOSEC developed gastric carcinoids. This finding was believed to be a manifestation of the underlying condition, which is known to be associated with such tumors, rather than the result of the administration of PRILOSEC.

INDICATIONS AND USAGE

Short-Term Treatment of Active Duodenal Ulcer
PRILOSEC Delayed-Release Capsules are indicated for short-term treatment of active duodenal ulcer. Most patients heal within four weeks. Some patients may require an additional four weeks of therapy.

PRILOSEC SHOULD NOT BE USED AS MAINTENANCE THERAPY FOR TREATMENT OF PATIENTS WITH DUODENAL ULCER DISEASE. (See boxed WARNING.)

Gastroesophageal Reflux Disease (GERD)
Severe Erosive Esophagitis
PRILOSEC Delayed-Release Capsules are indicated for the short-term treatment (4-8 weeks) of severe erosive esophagitis (grade 2 or above) which has been diagnosed by endoscopy (see CLINICAL PHARMACOLOGY, *Clinical Studies*).

Poorly Responsive Symptomatic GERD
PRILOSEC Delayed-Release Capsules are also indicated for the short-term treatment (4-8 weeks) of symptomatic gastroesophageal reflux disease (esophagitis) poorly responsive to customary medical treatment, usually including an adequate course of a histamine H_2-receptor antagonist.

The efficacy of PRILOSEC used for longer than 8 weeks in these patients has not been established. In the rare instance of a patient not responding to 8 weeks of treatment, it may be helpful to give up to an additional 4 weeks of treatment. If there is recurrence of severe or symptomatic GERD poorly responsive to customary medical treatment, additional 4-8 week courses of omeprazole may be considered. THE DRUG SHOULD NOT BE USED AS MAINTENANCE THERAPY. (See boxed WARNING.)

Pathological Hypersecretory Conditions
PRILOSEC Delayed-Release Capsules are indicated for the long-term treatment of pathological hypersecretory conditions (e.g., Zollinger-Ellison syndrome, multiple endocrine adenomas and systemic mastocytosis).

CONTRAINDICATIONS

PRILOSEC Delayed-Release Capsules are contraindicated in patients with known hypersensitivity to any component of the formulation.

WARNING

In long-term (2 year) studies in rats, omeprazole produced a dose-related increase in gastric carcinoid tumors (see PRECAUTIONS, *Carcinogenesis, Mutagenesis, Impairment of Fertility*). While available endoscopic evaluations and histologic examinations of biopsy specimens from human stomachs have not detected a risk from short-term exposure to PRILOSEC, further human data on the effect of sustained hypochlorhydria and hypergastrinemia are needed to rule out the possibility of an increased risk for the development of tumors in humans receiving long-term therapy with PRILOSEC. PRILOSEC should be prescribed only for the conditions, dosage and duration described (see INDICATIONS AND USAGE and DOSAGE AND ADMINISTRATION).

PRECAUTIONS

General
Symptomatic response to therapy with omeprazole does not preclude the presence of gastric malignancy.

Information for Patients
PRILOSEC Delayed-Release Capsules should be taken before eating. Patients should be cautioned that the PRILOSEC Delayed-Release Capsule should not be opened, chewed or crushed, and should be swallowed whole.

Drug Interactions
Omeprazole can prolong the elimination of diazepam, warfarin and phenytoin, drugs that are metabolized by oxidation in the liver. Although in normal subjects no interaction with theophylline or propranolol was found, there have been reports of interaction with other drugs metabolized via the cytochrome P-450 system (e.g., cyclosporine, disulfiram). Patients should be monitored to determine if it is necessary to adjust the dosage of these drugs when taken concomitantly with PRILOSEC.

Because of its profound and long lasting inhibition of gastric acid secretion, it is theoretically possible that omeprazole may interfere with absorption of drugs where gastric pH is an important determinant of their bioavailability (e.g., ketoconazole, ampicillin esters, and iron salts). In the clinical trials, antacids were used concomitantly with the administration of PRILOSEC.

Carcinogenesis, Mutagenesis,
Impairment of Fertility
In two 24-month carcinogenicity studies in rats, omeprazole at daily doses of 1.7, 3.4, 13.8, 44.0 and 140.8 mg/kg/day (approximately 4 to 352 times the human dose, based on a patient weight of 50 kg and a human dose of 20 mg) produced gastric ECL cell carcinoids in a dose-related manner in both male and female rats; the incidence of this effect was markedly higher in female rats, which had higher blood levels of omeprazole. Gastric carcinoids seldom occur in the untreated rat. In addition, ECL cell hyperplasia was present in all treated groups of both sexes. In one of these studies, female rats were treated with 13.8 mg omeprazole/kg/day (approximately 35 times the human dose) for one year, then followed for an additional year without the drug. No carcinoids were seen in these rats. An increased incidence of treatment-related ECL cell hyperplasia was observed at the end of one year (94% treated vs 10% controls). By the second year the difference between treated and control rats was much smaller (46% vs 26%) but still showed more hyperplasia in the treated group. An unusual primary malignant tumor in the stomach was seen in one rat (2%). No similar tumor was seen in male or female rats treated for two years. For this strain of rat no similar tumor has been noted historically, but a finding involving only one tumor is difficult to interpret. A 78-week mouse carcinogenicity study of omeprazole did not show increased tumor occurrence, but the study was not conclusive.

Omeprazole was not mutagenic in an *in vitro* Ames *Salmonella typhimurium* assay, an *in vitro* mouse lymphoma cell assay and an *in vivo* rat liver DNA damage assay. A mouse micronucleus test at 625 and 6250 times the human dose gave a borderline result, as did an *in vivo* bone marrow chromosome aberration test. A second mouse micronucleus study at 2000 times the human dose, but with different (suboptimal) sampling times, was negative.

In a rat fertility and general reproductive performance test, omeprazole in a dose range of 13.8 to 138.0 mg/kg/day (approximately 35 to 345 times the human dose) was not toxic or deleterious to the reproductive performance of parental animals.

Pregnancy
Pregnancy Category C
Teratology studies conducted in pregnant rats at doses up to 138 mg/kg/day (approximately 345 times the human dose) and in pregnant rabbits at doses up to 69 mg/kg/day (approximately 172 times the human dose) did not disclose any evidence for a teratogenic potential of omeprazole.

In rabbits, omeprazole in a dose range of 6.9 to 69.1 mg/kg/day (approximately 17 to 172 times the human dose) produced dose-related increases in embryo-lethality, fetal resorptions and pregnancy disruptions. In rats, dose-related embryo/fetal toxicity and postnatal developmental toxicity were observed in offspring resulting from parents treated with omeprazole 13.8 to 138.0 mg/kg/day (approximately 35 to 345 times the human dose). There are no adequate or well-controlled studies in pregnant women. Omeprazole should be used during pregnancy only if the potential benefit justifies the potential risk to the fetus.

Nursing Mothers

It is not known whether omeprazole is excreted in human milk. In rats, omeprazole administration during late gestation and lactation at doses of 13.8 to 138 mg/kg/day (35 to 345 times the human dose) resulted in decreased weight gain in pups. Because many drugs are excreted in human milk, because of the potential for serious adverse reactions in nursing infants from omeprazole, and because of the potential for tumorigenicity shown for omeprazole in rat carcinogenicity studies, a decision should be made whether to discontinue nursing or to discontinue the drug, taking into account the importance of the drug to the mother.

Pediatric Use

Safety and effectiveness in children have not been established.

ADVERSE REACTIONS

PRILOSEC Delayed-Release Capsules were generally well tolerated during domestic and international clinical trials in 3096 patients.

In the U.S. clinical trial population of 465 patients (including duodenal ulcer, Zollinger-Ellison syndrome and resistant ulcer patients), the following adverse experiences were reported to occur in 1% or more of patients on therapy with PRILOSEC. Numbers in parentheses indicate percentages of the adverse experiences considered by investigators as possibly, probably or definitely related to the drug:

	Omeprazole (n = 465)	Placebo (n = 64)	Ranitidine (n = 195)
Headache	6.9 (2.4)	6.3	7.7 (2.6)
Diarrhea	3.0 (1.9)	3.1 (1.6)	2.1 (0.5)
Abdominal Pain	2.4 (0.4)	3.1	2.1
Nausea	2.2 (0.9)	3.1	4.1 (0.5)
URI	1.9	1.6	2.6
Dizziness	1.5 (0.6)	0.0	2.6 (1.0)
Vomiting	1.5 (0.4)	4.7	1.5 (0.5)
Rash	1.5 (1.1)	0.0	0.0
Constipation	1.1 (0.9)	0.0	0.0
Cough	1.1	0.0	1.5
Asthenia	1.1 (0.2)	1.6 (1.6)	1.5 (1.0)
Back Pain	1.1	0.0	0.5

The following adverse reactions which occurred in 1% or more of omeprazole-treated patients have been reported in international double-blind, and open-label, clinical trials in which 2,631 patients and subjects received omeprazole.

	Incidence of Adverse Experiences ≥ 1% Causal Relationship not Assessed	
	Omeprazole (n = 2631)	Placebo (n = 120)
Body as a Whole, site unspecified		
Abdominal pain	5.2	3.3
Asthenia	1.3	0.8
Digestive System		
Constipation	1.5	0.8
Diarrhea	3.7	2.5
Flatulence	2.7	5.8
Nausea	4.0	6.7
Vomiting	3.2	10.0
Acid regurgitation	1.9	3.3
Nervous System/Psychiatric		
Headache	2.9	2.5

Additional adverse experiences occurring in < 1% of patients or subjects in domestic and/or international trials, or occurring since the drug was marketed, are shown below within each body system. In many instances, the relationship to PRILOSEC was unclear.

Body as a Whole: Fever, pain, fatigue, malaise, abdominal swelling

Cardiovascular: Chest pain or angina, tachycardia, bradycardia, palpitation, elevated blood pressure, peripheral edema

Digestive: Hepatitis including hepatic failure (rarely), elevated ALT (SGPT), elevated AST (SGOT), elevated γ-glutamyl transpeptidase, elevated alkaline phosphatase, elevated bilirubin (jaundice), anorexia, irritable colon, flatulence, fecal discoloration, esophageal candidiasis, mucosal atrophy of the tongue, dry mouth

Metabolic/Nutritional: Hypoglycemia, weight gain

Musculoskeletal: Muscle cramps, myalgia, joint pain, leg pain

Nervous System/Psychiatric: Psychic disturbances including depression, aggression, hallucinations, confusion, insomnia, nervousness, tremors, apathy, somnolence, anxiety, dream abnormalities; vertigo; paresthesia; hemifacial dysesthesia

Respiratory: Epistaxis, pharyngeal pain

Skin: Rash, skin inflammation, urticaria, angioedema, pruritus, alopecia, dry skin, hyperhidrosis

Special Senses: Tinnitus, taste perversion

Urogenital: Urinary tract infection, microscopic pyuria, urinary frequency, elevated serum creatinine, proteinuria, hematuria, glycosuria, testicular pain, gynecomastia

Hematologic: Agranulocytosis has been reported in a 65 year old diabetic male on several drugs in addition to omeprazole; the relationship of the agranulocytosis to omeprazole is uncertain. Pancytopenia, thrombocytopenia, neutropenia, anemia, leucocytosis, hemolytic anemia

The incidence of clinical adverse experiences in patients greater than 65 years of age was similar to that in patients 65 years of age or less.

OVERDOSAGE

There is no experience to date with deliberate overdosage. Dosages of up to 360 mg/day have been well tolerated. No specific antidote is known. Omeprazole is extensively protein bound and is, therefore, not readily dialyzable. In the event of overdosage, treatment should be symptomatic and supportive.

Lethal doses of omeprazole after single oral administration are about 1500 mg/kg in mice and greater than 4000 mg/kg in rats, and about 100 mg/kg in mice and greater than 40 mg/kg in rats given single intravenous injections. Animals given these doses showed sedation, ptosis, convulsions, and decreased activity, body temperature, and respiratory rate and increased depth of respiration.

DOSAGE AND ADMINISTRATION

Short-Term Treatment of Active Duodenal Ulcer

The recommended adult oral dose is 20 mg once daily. Most patients heal within four weeks. Some patients may require an additional four weeks of therapy. (See INDICATIONS AND USAGE.)

Severe Erosive Esophagitis or Poorly Responsive Gastroesophageal Reflux Disease (GERD)

The recommended adult oral dose is 20 mg daily for 4 to 8 weeks (see INDICATIONS AND USAGE).

Pathological Hypersecretory Conditions

The dosage of PRILOSEC in patients with pathological hypersecretory conditions varies with the individual patient. The recommended adult oral starting dose is 60 mg once a day. Doses should be adjusted to individual patient needs and should continue for as long as clinically indicated. Doses up to 120 mg t.i.d. have been administered. Daily dosages of greater than 80 mg should be administered in divided doses. Some patients with Zollinger-Ellison syndrome have been treated continuously with PRILOSEC for more than 5 years.

No dosage adjustment is necessary for patients with renal impairment, hepatic dysfunction or for the elderly.

PRILOSEC Delayed-Release Capsules should be taken before eating. In the clinical trials, antacids were used concomitantly with PRILOSEC.

Patients should be cautioned that the PRILOSEC Delayed-Release Capsule should not be opened, chewed or crushed, and should be swallowed whole.

HOW SUPPLIED

No. 3440 — PRILOSEC Delayed-Release Capsules, 20 mg, are opaque, hard gelatin, amethyst colored capsules, coded MSD 742. They are supplied as follows:

NDC 0006-0742-31 unit of use bottles of 30 (6505-01-314-2716, 20 mg 30's)

NDC 0006-0742-28 unit dose package of 100 (6505-01-314-2717, 20 mg individually sealed 100's).

PRILOSEC®
(Omeprazole)
Delayed-Release Capsules

Storage
Store PRILOSEC Delayed-Release Capsules in a tight container protected from light and moisture. Store between 59°F and 86°F (15°C and 30°C).

Jointly manufactured by:
MERCK SHARP & DOHME, Division of Merck & Co., Inc. West Point, Pa. 19486
and
AB ASTRA
Södertälje, Sweden

A.H.F.S. Category: 56:40

Issued January 1992   DC7685405

STERILE
INDOCIN® I.V.
(INDOMETHACIN SODIUM TRIHYDRATE, MSD)

DESCRIPTION

Sterile INDOCIN* I.V. (Indomethacin Sodium Trihydrate, MSD) for intravenous administration is lyophilized indomethacin sodium trihydrate. Each vial contains indomethacin sodium trihydrate equivalent to 1 mg indomethacin as a white to yellow lyophilized powder or plug. Variations in the size of the lyophilized plug and the intensity of color have no relationship to the quality or amount of indomethacin present in the vial.

Indomethacin sodium trihydrate is designated chemically as 1-(4-chlorobenzoyl)-5-methoxy-2-methyl-1*H*-indole-3-acetic acid, sodium salt, trihydrate. Its molecular weight is 433.82. Its empirical formula is $C_{19}H_{15}ClNNaO_4 \bullet 3H_2O$ and its structural formula is:

CLINICAL PHARMACOLOGY

Although the exact mechanism of action through which indomethacin causes closure of a patent ductus arteriosus is not known, it is believed to be through inhibition of prostaglandin synthesis. Indomethacin has been shown to be a potent inhibitor of prostaglandin synthesis, both *in vitro* and *in vivo*. In human newborns with certain congenital heart malformations, PGE 1 dilates the ductus arteriosus. In fetal and newborn lambs, E type prostaglandins have also been shown to maintain the patency of the ductus, and as in human newborns, indomethacin causes its constriction.

Studies in healthy young animals and in premature infants with patent ductus arteriosus indicated that, after the first dose of intravenous indomethacin, there was a transient reduction in cerebral blood flow velocity and cerebral blood flow. The clinical significance of this effect has not been established.

In double-blind placebo-controlled studies of INDOCIN I.V. in 460 small pre-term infants, weighing 1750 g or less, the infants treated with placebo had a ductus closure rate after 48 hours of 25 to 30 percent, whereas those treated with INDOCIN I.V. had a 75 to 80 percent closure rate. In one of these studies, a multicenter study, involving 405 pre-term infants, later re-opening of the ductus arteriosus occurred in 26 percent of infants treated with INDOCIN I.V., however, 70 percent of these closed subsequently without the need for surgery or additional indomethacin.

Pharmacokinetics and Metabolism
The disposition of indomethacin following intravenous administration (0.2 mg/kg) in preterm neonates with patent ductus arteriosus has not been extensively evaluated. Even though the plasma half-life of indomethacin was variable among premature infants, it was shown to vary inversely with postnatal age and weight. In one study, of 28 infants who could be evaluated, the plasma half-life in those infants less than 7 days old averaged 20 hours (range: 3-60 hours, n = 18). In infants older than 7 days, the mean plasma half-life of indomethacin was 12 hours (range: 4-38 hours, n = 10). Grouping the infants by weight, mean plasma half-life in those weighing less than 1000 g was 21 hours (range: 9-60 hours, n = 10); in those infants weighing more than 1000 g, the mean plasma half-life was 15 hours (range: 3-52 hours, n = 18).

Following intravenous administration in adults, indomethacin is eliminated via renal excretion, metabolism, and biliary excretion. Indomethacin undergoes appreciable enterohepatic circulation. The mean plasma half-life of indomethacin is 4.5 hours. In the absence of enterohepatic circulation, it is 90 minutes.

In adults, about 99 percent of indomethacin is bound to protein in plasma over the expected range of therapeutic plasma concentrations. The percent bound in neonates has not been studied. In controlled trials in premature infants, however, no evidence of bilirubin displacement has been observed as evidenced by increased incidence of bilirubin encephalopathy (kernicterus).

INDICATIONS AND USAGE

INDOCIN I.V. is indicated to close a hemodynamically significant patent ductus arteriosus in premature infants weighing between 500 and 1750 g when after 48 hours usual medical management (e.g., fluid restriction, diuretics, digitalis, respiratory support, etc.) is ineffective. Clear-cut clinical evidence of a hemodynamically significant patent ductus arteriosus should be present, such as respiratory distress, a continuous murmur, a hyperactive precordium, cardiomegaly and pulmonary plethora on chest x-ray.

CONTRAINDICATIONS

INDOCIN I.V. is contraindicated in: infants with proven or suspected infection that is untreated; infants who are bleeding, especially those with active intracranial hemorrhage or gastrointestinal bleeding; infants with thrombocytopenia; infants with coagulation defects; infants with or who are suspected of having necrotizing enterocolitis; infants with significant impairment of renal function; infants with congenital heart disease in whom patency of the ductus arteriosus is necessary for satisfactory pulmonary or systemic blood flow (e.g., pulmonary atresia, severe tetralogy of Fallot, severe coarctation of the aorta).

WARNINGS

Gastrointestinal Effects:
In the collaborative study, major gastrointestinal bleeding was no more common in those infants receiving indomethacin than in those infants on placebo. However, minor gastrointestinal bleeding (i.e., chemical detection of blood in the stool) was more commonly noted in those infants treated with indomethacin. Severe gastrointestinal effects have been reported in adults with various arthritic disorders treated chronically with oral indomethacin. [For further information, see package circular for Capsules INDOCIN* (Indomethacin, MSD)].
Central Nervous System Effects:
Prematurity per se, is associated with an increased incidence of spontaneous intraventricular hemorrhage. Because indomethacin may inhibit platelet aggregation, the potential for intraventricular bleeding may be increased. However, in the large multi-center study of INDOCIN

I.V. (see CLINICAL PHARMACOLOGY), the incidence of intraventricular hemorrhage in babies treated with INDOCIN I.V. was not significantly higher than in the control infants.

Renal Effects:

INDOCIN I.V. may cause significant reduction in urine output (50 percent or more) with concomitant elevations of blood urea nitrogen and creatinine, and reductions in glomerular filtration rate and creatinine clearance. These effects in most infants are transient, disappearing with cessation of therapy with INDOCIN I.V. However, because adequate renal function can depend upon renal prostaglandin synthesis, INDOCIN I.V. may precipitate renal insufficiency, including acute renal failure, especially in infants with other conditions that may adversely affect renal function (e.g., extracellular volume depletion from any cause, congestive heart failure, sepsis, concomitant use of any nephrotoxic drug, hepatic dysfunction). When significant suppression of urine volume occurs after a dose of INDOCIN I.V., no additional dose should be given until the urine output returns to normal levels.

INDOCIN I.V. in pre-term infants may suppress water excretion to a greater extent than sodium excretion. When this occurs, a significant reduction in serum sodium values (i.e., hyponatremia) may result. Infants should have serum electrolyte determinations done during therapy with INDOCIN I.V. Renal function and serum electrolytes should be monitored (see PRECAUTIONS, *Drug Interactions* and DOSAGE AND ADMINISTRATION).

PRECAUTIONS

General

INDOCIN (Indomethacin, MSD) may mask the usual signs and symptoms of infection. Therefore, the physician must be continually on the alert for this and should use the drug with extra care in the presence of existing controlled infection.

Severe hepatic reactions have been reported in adults treated chronically with oral indomethacin for arthritic disorders. [For further information, see package circular for Capsules INDOCIN (Indomethacin, MSD).] If clinical signs and symptoms consistent with liver disease develop in the neonate, or if systemic manifestations occur, INDOCIN I.V. should be discontinued.

INDOCIN I.V. may inhibit platelet aggregation. In one small study, platelet aggregation was grossly abnormal after indomethacin therapy (given orally to premature infants to close the ductus arteriosus). Platelet aggregation returned to normal by the tenth day. Premature infants should be observed for signs of bleeding.

The drug should be administered carefully to avoid extravascular injection or leakage as the solution may be irritating to tissue.

Drug Interactions

Since renal function may be reduced by INDOCIN I.V., consideration should be given to reduction in dosage of those medications that rely on adequate renal function for their elimination. Because the half-life of digitalis (given frequently to pre-term infants with patent ductus arteriosus and associated cardiac failure) may be prolonged when given concomitantly with indomethacin, the infant should be observed closely; frequent ECGs and serum digitalis levels may be required to prevent or detect digitalis toxicity early. In one study of premature infants treated with INDOCIN I.V. and also receiving either gentamicin or amikacin, both peak and trough levels of these aminoglycosides were significantly elevated.

Therapy with indomethacin may blunt the natriuretic effect of furosemide. This response has been attributed to inhibition of prostaglandin synthesis by non-steroidal anti-inflammatory drugs. In a study of 19 premature infants with patent ductus arteriosus treated with either INDOCIN I.V. alone or a combination of INDOCIN I.V. and furosemide, results showed that infants receiving both INDOCIN I.V. and furosemide had significantly higher urinary output, higher levels of sodium and chloride excretion, and higher glomerular filtration rates than did those infants receiving INDOCIN I.V. alone. In this study, the data suggested that therapy with furo-

semide helped to maintain renal function in the premature infant when INDOCIN I.V. was added to the treatment of patent ductus arteriosus.

Neonatal Effects

In rats and mice, oral indomethacin 4.0 mg/kg/day given during the last three days of gestation caused a decrease in maternal weight gain and some maternal and fetal deaths. An increased incidence of neuronal necrosis in the diencephalon in the live-born fetuses was observed. At 2.0 mg/kg/day, no increase in neuronal necrosis was observed as compared to the control groups. Administration of 0.5 or 4.0 mg/kg/day during the first three days of life did not cause an increase in neuronal necrosis at either dose level.

Pregnant rats, given 2.0 mg/kg/day and 4.0 mg/kg/day during the last trimester of gestation, delivered offspring whose pulmonary blood vessels were both reduced in number and excessively muscularized. These findings are similar to those observed in the syndrome of persistent pulmonary hypertension of the newborn.

ADVERSE REACTIONS

In a double-blind placebo-controlled trial of 405 premature infants weighing less than or equal to 1750 g with evidence of large ductal shunting, in those infants treated with indomethacin (n = 206), there was a statistically significantly greater incidence of bleeding problems, including gross or microscopic bleeding into the gastrointestinal tract, oozing from the skin after needle stick, pulmonary hemorrhage, and disseminated intravascular coagulopathy. There was no statistically significant difference between treatment groups with reference to intracranial hemorrhage.

The infants treated with indomethacin sodium trihydrate also had a significantly higher incidence of transient oliguria and elevations of serum creatinine (greater than or equal to 1.8 mg/dL) than did the infants treated with placebo.

The incidences of retrolental fibroplasia (grades III and IV) and pneumothorax in infants treated with INDOCIN I.V. were no greater than in placebo controls and were statistically significantly lower than in surgically-treated infants.

The following additional adverse reactions in infants have been reported from the collaborative study, anecdotal case reports, and from other studies using rectal, oral, or intravenous indomethacin for treatment of patent ductus arteriosus. The rates are based on the experience of 849 indomethacin-treated infants reported in the medical literature, regardless of the route of administration. One year follow-up is available on 175 infants and shows no long-term sequelae which could be attributed to indomethacin. In controlled clinical studies, only electrolyte imbalance and renal dysfunction (of the reactions listed below) occurred statistically significantly more frequently after INDOCIN I.V. than after placebo.

Renal: renal dysfunction in 41 percent of infants, including one or more of the following: reduced urinary output; reduced urine sodium, chloride, or potassium; urine osmolality, free water clearance, or glomerular filtration rate; elevated serum creatinine or BUN; uremia.

Cardiovascular: intracranial bleeding**, pulmonary hypertension.

Gastrointestinal: gastrointestinal bleeding*, vomiting, abdominal distention, transient ileus, localized perforation(s) of the small and/or large intestine.

Metabolic: hyponatremia*, elevated serum potassium*, reduction in blood sugar, including hypoglycemia, increased weight gain (fluid retention).

Coagulation: decreased platelet aggregation (see PRECAUTIONS).

The following adverse reactions have also been reported in infants treated with indomethacin, however, a causal relationship to therapy with INDOCIN I.V. has not been established:

---

*Incidence 3-9 percent. Those reactions which are unmarked occurred in 1-3 percent of patients.
**Incidence in both indomethacin and placebo-treated infants 3-9 percent. Those reactions which are unmarked occurred in less than 3 percent.

Cardiovascular: bradycardia.
Respiratory: apnea, exacerbation of pre-existing pulmonary infection.
Metabolic: acidosis/alkalosis.
Hematologic: disseminated intravascular coagulation.
Gastrointestinal: necrotizing enterocolitis.
Ophthalmic: retrolental fibroplasia.**

A variety of additional adverse experiences have been reported in adults treated with oral indomethacin for moderate to severe rheumatoid arthritis, osteoarthritis, ankylosing spondylitis, acute painful shoulder and acute gouty arthritis (see section ADDITIONAL ADVERSE REACTIONS—ADULTS). Their relevance to the pre-term neonate receiving indomethacin for patent ductus arteriosus is unknown, however, the possibility exists that these experiences may be associated with the use of INDOCIN I.V. in pre-term neonates.

DOSAGE AND ADMINISTRATION

FOR INTRAVENOUS ADMINISTRATION ONLY.

Dosage recommendations for closure of the ductus arteriosus depends on the age of the infant at the time of therapy. A course of therapy is defined as three intravenous doses of INDOCIN I.V. given at 12-24 hour intervals, with careful attention to urinary output. If anuria or marked oliguria (urinary output < 0.6 mL/kg/hr) is evident at the scheduled time of the second or third dose of INDOCIN I.V., no additional doses should be given until laboratory studies indicate that renal function has returned to normal (see WARNINGS, *Renal Effects*).

Dosage according to age is as follows:

AGE at 1st dose	DOSAGE (mg/kg)		
	1st	2nd	3rd
Less than 48 hours	0.2	0.1	0.1
2-7 days	0.2	0.2	0.2
over 7 days	0.2	0.25	0.25

If the ductus arteriosus closes or is significantly reduced in size after an interval of 48 hours or more from completion of the first course of INDOCIN I.V., no further doses are necessary. If the ductus arteriosus re-opens, a second course of 1-3 doses may be given, each dose separated by a 12-24 hour interval as described above.

If the infant remains unresponsive to therapy with INDOCIN I.V. after 2 courses, surgery may be necessary for closure of the ductus arteriosus. If severe adverse reactions occur, STOP THE DRUG.

Directions for Use
Parenteral drug products should be inspected visually for particulate matter and discoloration prior to administration whenever solution and container permit.

The solution should be prepared only with 1 to 2 mL of preservative-free sterile Sodium Chloride Injection, 0.9 percent or preservative-free Sterile Water for Injection. Benzyl alcohol as a preservative has been associated with toxicity in newborns. Therefore, all diluents should be preservative-free. If 1 mL of diluent is used, the concentration of indomethacin in the solution will equal approximately 0.1 mg/0.1 mL; if 2 mL of diluent are used, the concentration of the solution will equal approximately 0.05 mg/0.1 mL. Any unused portion of the solution should be discarded because there is no preservative contained in the vial. A fresh solution should be prepared just prior to each administration. Once reconstituted, the indomethacin solution may be injected intravenously over 5-10 seconds.

Further dilution with intravenous infusion solutions is not recommended. INDOCIN I.V. is not buffered, and reconstitution with solutions at pH values below 6.0 may result in precipitation of the insoluble indomethacin free acid moiety.

HOW SUPPLIED

No. 3406 — Sterile INDOCIN I.V. is a lyophilized white to yellow powder or plug supplied as single dose vials containing indomethacin sodium trihydrate, equivalent to 1 mg indomethacin.
NDC 0006-3406-17.

Storage
Store below 30°C (86°F). *Protect from light.* Store container in carton until contents have been used.

ADDITIONAL ADVERSE REACTIONS—ADULTS

The following adverse reactions have been reported in adults treated with oral indomethacin for moderate to severe rheumatoid arthritis, osteoarthritis, ankylosing spondylitis, acute painful shoulder and acute gouty arthritis. Complaints not of relevance in the treatment of the premature infant, such as anorexia, psychic disturbances, and blurred vision, are not listed.

Incidence 1% to 3%	Incidence less than 1%	
GASTROINTESTINAL		
diarrhea	bloating (includes distention)	gastrointestinal bleeding without obvious ulcer formation and perforation of pre-existing sigmoid lesions
constipation	flatulence	
	peptic ulcer	
	gastroenteritis	
	rectal bleeding	
	proctitis	
	single or multiple ulcerations, including perforation and hemorrhage of the esophagus, stomach, duodenum or small and large intestines	development of ulcerative stomatitis toxic hepatitis and jaundice (some fatal cases have been reported)
	intestinal ulceration associated with stenosis and obstruction	
CENTRAL NERVOUS SYSTEM		
none	involuntary muscle movements	aggravation of epilepsy coma peripheral neuropathy convulsions
SPECIAL SENSES		
none	hearing disturbances, deafness	
CARDIOVASCULAR		
none	hypertension hypotension tachycardia	arrhythmia congestive heart failure thrombophlebitis
METABOLIC		
none	edema weight gain flushing	hyperglycemia glycosuria hyperkalemia
INTEGUMENTARY		
none	rash; urticaria petechiae or ecchymosis	exfoliative dermatitis erythema nodosum loss of hair Stevens-Johnson syndrome erythema multiforme toxic epidermal necrolysis
HEMATOLOGIC		
none	leukopenia bone marrow depression anemia secondary to obvious or occult gastrointestinal bleeding	aplastic anemia hemolytic anemia agranulocytosis thrombocytopenic purpura
HYPERSENSITIVITY		
none	acute anaphylaxis acute respiratory distress rapid fall in blood pressure resembling a shock-like state	dyspnea asthma purpura angiitis pulmonary edema
GENITOURINARY		
none	hematuria vaginal bleeding	renal insufficiency, including renal failure
MISCELLANEOUS		
none	epistaxis breast changes, including enlargement and tenderness, or gynecomastia	

See package circular for Capsules INDOCIN (Indomethacin, MSD) for additional information concerning adverse reactions and other cautionary statements.

**Incidence in both indomethacin and placebo-treated infants 3-9 percent. Those reactions which are unmarked occurred in less than 3 percent.

A.H.F.S. Category: 28:08.04

Issued November 1991   DC7414812

TABLETS

DECADRON®

(DEXAMETHASONE, MSD)

DESCRIPTION

Glucocorticoids are adrenocortical steroids, both naturally occurring and synthetic, which are readily absorbed from the gastrointestinal tract.

Dexamethasone, a synthetic adrenocortical steroid, is a white to practically white, odorless, crystalline powder. It is stable in air. It is practically insoluble in water. The molecular weight is 392.47. It is designated chemically as 9-fluoro-11β,17,21-trihydroxy-16α-methyl-pregna-1,4-diene-3,20-dione. The empirical formula is $C_{22}H_{29}FO_5$ and the structural formula is:

DECADRON* (Dexamethasone, MSD) tablets are supplied in six potencies, 0.25 mg, 0.5 mg, 0.75 mg, 1.5 mg, 4 mg, and 6 mg. Inactive ingredients are calcium phosphate, lactose, magnesium stearate, and starch. Tablets DECADRON 0.25 mg also contain FD&C Yellow 6. Tablets DECADRON 0.5 mg also contain D&C Yellow 10 and FD&C Yellow 6. Tablets DECADRON 0.75 mg also contain FD&C Blue 1. Tablets DECADRON 1.5 mg also contain FD&C Red 40. Tablets DECADRON 6 mg also contain FD&C Blue 1 and iron oxide.

ACTIONS

Naturally occurring glucocorticoids (hydrocortisone and cortisone), which also have salt-retaining properties, are used as replacement therapy in adrenocortical deficiency states. Their synthetic analogs including dexamethasone are primarily used for their potent anti-inflammatory effects in disorders of many organ systems.

Glucocorticoids cause profound and varied metabolic effects. In addition, they modify the body's immune responses to diverse stimuli.

At equipotent anti-inflammatory doses, dexamethasone almost completely lacks the sodium-retaining property of hydrocortisone and closely related derivatives of hydrocortisone.

INDICATIONS

1. *Endocrine Disorders*
   Primary or secondary adrenocortical insufficiency (hydrocortisone or cortisone is the first choice; synthetic analogs may be used in conjunction with mineralocorticoids where applicable; in infancy mineralocorticoid supplementation is of particular importance)
   Congenital adrenal hyperplasia
   Nonsuppurative thyroiditis
   Hypercalcemia associated with cancer
2. *Rheumatic Disorders*
   As adjunctive therapy for short-term administration (to tide the patient over an acute episode or exacerbation) in:
   Psoriatic arthritis
   Rheumatoid arthritis, including juvenile rheumatoid arthritis (selected cases may require low-dose maintenance therapy)
   Ankylosing spondylitis
   Acute and subacute bursitis
   Acute nonspecific tenosynovitis
   Acute gouty arthritis
   Post-traumatic osteoarthritis
   Synovitis of osteoarthritis
   Epicondylitis
3. *Collagen Diseases*
   During an exacerbation or as maintenance therapy in selected cases of —
   Systemic lupus erythematosus
   Acute rheumatic carditis

Registered trademark of MERCK & CO., INC.

4. *Dermatologic Diseases*
   Pemphigus
   Bullous dermatitis herpetiformis
   Severe erythema multiforme (Stevens-Johnson syndrome)
   Exfoliative dermatitis
   Mycosis fungoides
   Severe psoriasis
   Severe seborrheic dermatitis
5. *Allergic States*
   Control of severe or incapacitating allergic conditions intractable to adequate trials of conventional treatment:
   Seasonal or perennial allergic rhinitis
   Bronchial asthma
   Contact dermatitis
   Atopic dermatitis
   Serum sickness
   Drug hypersensitivity reactions
6. *Ophthalmic Diseases*
   Severe acute and chronic allergic and inflammatory processes involving the eye and its adnexa, such as—
   Allergic conjunctivitis
   Keratitis
   Allergic corneal marginal ulcers
   Herpes zoster ophthalmicus
   Iritis and iridocyclitis
   Chorioretinitis
   Anterior segment inflammation
   Diffuse posterior uveitis and choroiditis
   Optic neuritis
   Sympathetic ophthalmia
7. *Respiratory Diseases*
   Symptomatic sarcoidosis
   Loeffler's syndrome not manageable by other means
   Berylliosis
   Fulminating or disseminated pulmonary tuberculosis when used concurrently with appropriate antituberculous chemotherapy
   Aspiration pneumonitis
8. *Hematologic Disorders*
   Idiopathic thrombocytopenic purpura in adults
   Secondary thrombocytopenia in adults
   Acquired (autoimmune) hemolytic anemia
   Erythroblastopenia (RBC anemia)
   Congenital (erythroid) hypoplastic anemia
9. *Neoplastic Diseases*
   For palliative management of:
   Leukemias and lymphomas in adults
   Acute leukemia of childhood
10. *Edematous States*
    To induce a diuresis or remission of proteinuria in the nephrotic syndrome, without uremia, of the idiopathic type or that due to lupus erythematosus
11. *Gastrointestinal Diseases*
    To tide the patient over a critical period of the disease in:
    Ulcerative colitis
    Regional enteritis
12. *Cerebral Edema* associated with primary or metastatic brain tumor, craniotomy, or head injury. Use in cerebral edema is not a substitute for careful neurosurgical evaluation and definitive management such as neurosurgery or other specific therapy.
13. *Miscellaneous*
    Tuberculous meningitis with subarachnoid block or impending block when used concurrently with appropriate antituberculous chemotherapy
    Trichinosis with neurologic or myocardial involvement
14. *Diagnostic testing of adrenocortical hyperfunction.*

CONTRAINDICATIONS

Systemic fungal infections
Hypersensitivity to this drug

WARNINGS

In patients on corticosteroid therapy subjected to unusual stress, increased dosage of rapidly acting corticosteroids before, during, and after the stressful situation is indicated.

Drug-induced secondary adrenocortical insufficiency may result from too rapid withdrawal of corticosteroids and may be minimized by gradual reduction of dosage. This type of relative insufficiency may persist for months after discontinuation of therapy; therefore, in any situation of stress occurring during that period,

18

hormone therapy should be reinstituted. If the patient is receiving steroids already, dosage may have to be increased. Since mineralocorticoid secretion may be impaired, salt and/or a mineralocorticoid should be administered concurrently.

Corticosteroids may mask some signs of infection, and new infections may appear during their use. There may be decreased resistance and inability to localize infection when corticosteroids are used. Moreover, corticosteroids may affect the nitroblue-tetrazolium test for bacterial infection and produce false negative results.

In cerebral malaria, a double-blind trial has shown that the use of corticosteroids is associated with prolongation of coma and a higher incidence of pneumonia and gastrointestinal bleeding.

Corticosteroids may activate latent amebiasis. Therefore, it is recommended that latent or active amebiasis be ruled out before initiating corticosteroid therapy in any patient who has spent time in the tropics or any patient with unexplained diarrhea.

Prolonged use of corticosteroids may produce posterior subcapsular cataracts, glaucoma with possible damage to the optic nerves, and may enhance the establishment of secondary ocular infections due to fungi or viruses.

Usage in pregnancy: Since adequate human reproduction studies have not been done with corticosteroids, use of these drugs in pregnancy or in women of childbearing potential requires that the anticipated benefits be weighed against the possible hazards to the mother and embryo or fetus. Infants born of mothers who have received substantial doses of corticosteroids during pregnancy should be carefully observed for signs of hypoadrenalism.

Corticosteroids appear in breast milk and could suppress growth, interfere with endogenous corticosteroid production, or cause other unwanted effects. Mothers taking pharmacologic doses of corticosteroids should be advised not to nurse.

Average and large doses of hydrocortisone or cortisone can cause elevation of blood pressure, salt and water retention, and increased excretion of potassium. These effects are less likely to occur with the synthetic derivatives except when used in large doses. Dietary salt restriction and potassium supplementation may be necessary. All corticosteroids increase calcium excretion.

Administration of live virus vaccines, including smallpox, is contraindicated in individuals receiving immunosuppressive doses of corticosteroids. If inactivated viral or bacterial vaccines are administered to individuals receiving immunosuppressive doses of corticosteroid the expected serum antibody response may not be obtained. However, immunization procedures may be undertaken in patients who are receiving corticosteroids as replacement therapy, e.g., for Addison's disease.

The use of DECADRON tablets in active tuberculosis should be restricted to those cases of fulminating or disseminated tuberculosis in which the corticosteroid is used for the management of the disease in conjunction with an appropriate antituberculous regimen.

If corticosteroids are indicated in patients with latent tuberculosis or tuberculin reactivity, close observation is necessary as reactivation of the disease may occur. During prolonged corticosteroid therapy, these patients should receive chemoprophylaxis.

Literature reports suggest an apparent association between use of corticosteroids and left ventricular free wall rupture after a recent myocardial infarction; therefore, therapy with corticosteroids should be used with great caution in these patients.

PRECAUTIONS

Following prolonged therapy, withdrawal of corticosteroids may result in symptoms of the corticosteroid withdrawal syndrome including fever, myalgia, arthralgia, and malaise. This may occur in patients even without evidence of adrenal insufficiency.

There is an enhanced effect of corticosteroids in patients with hypothyroidism and in those with cirrhosis.

Corticosteroids should be used cautiously in patients with ocular herpes simplex because of possible corneal perforation.

The lowest possible dose of corticosteroids should be used to control the condition under treatment, and when reduction in dosage is possible, the reduction should be gradual.

Psychic derangements may appear when corticosteroids are used, ranging from euphoria, insomnia, mood swings, personality changes, and severe depression, to frank psychotic manifestations. Also, existing emotional instability or psychotic tendencies may be aggravated by corticosteroids.

Aspirin should be used cautiously in conjunction with corticosteroids in hypoprothrombinemia.

Steroids should be used with caution in non-specific ulcerative colitis, if there is a probability of impending perforation, abscess, or other pyogenic infection, diverticulitis, fresh intestinal anastomoses, active or latent peptic ulcer, renal insufficiency, hypertension, osteoporosis, and myasthenia gravis. Signs of peritoneal irritation following gastrointestinal perforation in patients receiving large doses of corticosteroids may be minimal or absent. Fat embolism has been reported as a possible complication of hypercortisonism.

When large doses are given, some authorities advise that corticosteroids be taken with meals and antacids taken between meals to help to prevent peptic ulcer.

Growth and development of infants and children on prolonged corticosteroid therapy should be carefully observed.

Steroids may increase or decrease motility and number of spermatozoa in some patients.

Phenytoin, phenobarbital, ephedrine, and rifampin may enhance the metabolic clearance of corticosteroids, resulting in decreased blood levels and lessened physiologic activity, thus requiring adjustment in corticosteroid dosage. These interactions may interfere with dexamethasone suppression tests which should be interpreted with caution during administration of these drugs.

False-negative results in the dexamethasone suppression test (DST) in patients being treated with indomethacin have been reported. Thus, results of the DST should be interpreted with caution in these patients.

The prothrombin time should be checked frequently in patients who are receiving corticosteroids and coumarin anticoagulants at the same time because of reports that corticosteroids have altered the response to these anticoagulants. Studies have shown that the usual effect produced by adding corticosteroids is inhibition of response to coumarins, although there have been some conflicting reports of potentiation not substantiated by studies.

When corticosteroids are administered concomitantly with potassium-depleting diuretics, patients should be observed closely for development of hypokalemia.

ADVERSE REACTIONS

Fluid and Electrolyte Disturbances
  Sodium retention
  Fluid retention
  Congestive heart failure in susceptible patients
  Potassium loss
  Hypokalemic alkalosis
  Hypertension
Musculoskeletal
  Muscle weakness
  Steroid myopathy
  Loss of muscle mass
  Osteoporosis
  Vertebral compression fractures
  Aseptic necrosis of femoral and humeral heads
  Pathologic fracture of long bones
  Tendon rupture
Gastrointestinal
  Peptic ulcer with possible perforation and hemorrhage
  Perforation of the small and large bowel, particularly in patients with inflammatory bowel disease.

Pancreatitis
Abdominal distention
Ulcerative esophagitis
Dermatologic
Impaired wound healing
Thin fragile skin
Petechiae and ecchymoses
Erythema
Increased sweating
May suppress reactions to skin tests
Other cutaneous reactions, such as allergic dermatitis, urticaria, angioneurotic edema
Neurologic
Convulsions
Increased intracranial pressure with papilledema (pseudotumor cerebri) usually after treatment
Vertigo
Headache
Psychic disturbances
Endocrine
Menstrual irregularities
Development of cushingoid state
Suppression of growth in children
Secondary adrenocortical and pituitary unresponsiveness, particularly in times of stress, as in trauma, surgery, or illness
Decreased carbohydrate tolerance
Manifestations of latent diabetes mellitus
Increased requirements for insulin or oral hypoglycemic agents in diabetics
Hirsutism
Ophthalmic
Posterior subcapsular cataracts
Increased intraocular pressure
Glaucoma
Exophthalmos
Metabolic
Negative nitrogen balance due to protein catabolism
Cardiovascular
Myocardial rupture following recent myocardial infarction (see WARNINGS).
Other
Hypersensitivity
Thromboembolism
Weight gain
Increased appetite
Nausea
Malaise
Hiccups

OVERDOSAGE

Reports of acute toxicity and/or death following overdosage of glucocorticoids are rare. In the event of overdosage, no specific antidote is available; treatment is supportive and symptomatic.

The oral LD_{50} of dexamethasone in female mice was 6.5 g/kg.

DOSAGE AND ADMINISTRATION

For oral administration
DOSAGE REQUIREMENTS ARE VARIABLE AND MUST BE INDIVIDUALIZED ON THE BASIS OF THE DISEASE AND THE RESPONSE OF THE PATIENT.

The initial dosage varies from 0.75 to 9 mg a day depending on the disease being treated. In less severe diseases doses lower than 0.75 mg may suffice, while in severe diseases doses higher than 9 mg may be required. The initial dosage should be maintained or adjusted until the patient's response is satisfactory. If satisfactory clinical response does not occur after a reasonable period of time, discontinue DECADRON tablets and transfer the patient to other therapy.

After a favorable initial response, the proper maintenance dosage should be determined by decreasing the initial dosage in small amounts to the lowest dosage that maintains an adequate clinical response.

Patients should be observed closely for signs that might require dosage adjustment, including changes in clinical status resulting from remissions or exacerbations of the disease, individual drug responsiveness, and the effect of stress (e.g., surgery, infection, trauma). During stress it may be necessary to increase dosage temporarily.

If the drug is to be stopped after more than a few days of treatment, it usually should be withdrawn gradually.

The following milligram equivalents facilitate changing to DECADRON from other glucocorticoids:

DECADRON	Methyl-prednisolone Triamcinolone	Prednisolone and Prednisone	Hydrocortisone	Cortisone
0.75 mg =	4 mg =	5 mg =	20 mg =	25 mg

In *acute, self-limited allergic disorders or acute exacerbations of chronic allergic disorders,* the following dosage schedule combining parenteral and oral therapy is suggested: DECADRON Phosphate (Dexamethasone Sodium Phosphate, MSD) injection, 4 mg per mL:
First Day
1 or 2 mL, intramuscularly
DECADRON tablets, 0.75 mg:
Second Day
4 tablets in two divided doses
Third Day
4 tablets in two divided doses
Fourth Day
2 tablets in two divided doses
Fifth Day
1 tablet
Sixth Day
1 tablet
Seventh Day
No treatment
Eighth Day
Follow-up visit

This schedule is designed to ensure adequate therapy during acute episodes, while minimizing the risk of overdosage in chronic cases.

In *cerebral edema*, DECADRON Phosphate (Dexamethasone Sodium Phosphate, MSD) injection is generally administered initially in a dosage of 10 mg intravenously followed by 4 mg every six hours intramuscularly until the symptoms of cerebral edema subside. Response is usually noted within 12 to 24 hours and dosage may be reduced after two to four days and gradually discontinued over a period of five to seven days. For palliative management of patients with recurrent or inoperable brain tumors, maintenance therapy with either DECADRON Phosphate (Dexamethasone Sodium Phosphate, MSD) injection or DECADRON tablets in a dosage of two mg two or three times daily may be effective.

Dexamethasone suppression tests.
1. Tests for Cushing's syndrome
   Give 1.0 mg of DECADRON orally at 11:00 p.m. Blood is drawn for plasma cortisol determination at 8:00 a.m. the following morning. For greater accuracy, give 0.5 mg of DECADRON orally every 6 hours for 48 hours. Twenty-four hour urine collections are made for determination of 17-hydroxycorticosteroid excretion.
2. Test to distinguish Cushing's syndrome due to pituitary ACTH excess from Cushing's syndrome due to other causes.
   Give 2.0 mg of DECADRON orally every 6 hours for 48 hours. Twenty-four hour urine collections are made for determination of 17-hydroxycorticosteroid excretion.

HOW SUPPLIED

Tablets DECADRON are compressed, pentagonal-shaped tablets, colored to distinguish potency. They are scored and coded on one side and are available as follows:
No. 7648 — 6 mg, green in color and coded MSD 147.
NDC 0006-0147-50 bottles of 50
NDC 0006-0147-28 single unit packages of 100.
No. 7645 — 4 mg, white in color and coded MSD 97.
NDC 0006-0097-50 bottles of 50
NDC 0006-0097-28 single unit packages of 100.
No. 7638 — 1.5 mg, pink in color and coded MSD 95.

INJECTION

HYDROCORTONE®
Phosphate
(HYDROCORTISONE SODIUM PHOSPHATE, MSD)
STERILE

DESCRIPTION

Hydrocortisone sodium phosphate, a synthetic adrenocortical steroid, is a white to light yellow, odorless or practically odorless powder. It is freely soluble in water and is exceedingly hygroscopic. The molecular weight is 486.41. It is designated chemically as $11\beta,17$-dihydroxy-21-(phosphonooxy)pregn-4-ene-3,20-dione disodium salt. The empirical formula is $C_{21}H_{29}Na_2O_8P$ and the structural formula is:

HYDROCORTONE* Phosphate (Hydrocortisone Sodium Phosphate, MSD) injection is a sterile solution (pH 7.5 to 8.5), sealed under nitrogen, for intravenous, intramuscular, and subcutaneous administration.

Each milliliter contains hydrocortisone sodium phosphate equivalent to 50 mg hydrocortisone. Inactive ingredients per mL: 8 mg creatinine, 10 mg sodium citrate, sodium hydroxide to adjust pH, and Water for Injection, q.s. 1 mL, with 3.2 mg sodium bisulfite, 1.5 mg methylparaben, and 0.2 mg propylparaben added as preservatives.

ACTIONS

HYDROCORTONE Phosphate injection has a rapid onset but short duration of action when compared with less soluble preparations. Because of this, it is suitable for the treatment of acute disorders responsive to adrenocortical steroid therapy.

Naturally occurring glucocorticoids (hydrocortisone and cortisone) which also have salt-retaining properties, are used as replacement therapy in adrenocortical deficiency states. They are also used for their potent anti-inflammatory effects in disorders of many organ systems.

Glucocorticoids cause profound and varied metabolic effects. In addition, they modify the body's immune responses to diverse stimuli.

*Registered trademark of MERCK & CO., INC.

INDICATIONS

When oral therapy is not feasible:
1. *Endocrine disorders*
    Primary or secondary adrenocortical insufficiency (hydrocortisone or cortisone is the drug of choice; synthetic analogs may be used in conjunction with mineralocorticoids where applicable; in infancy, mineralocorticoid supplementation is of particular importance)
    Acute adrenocortical insufficiency (hydrocortisone or cortisone is the drug of choice; mineralocorticoid supplementation may be necessary, particularly when synthetic analogs are used)
    Preoperatively, and in the event of serious trauma or illness, in patients with known adrenal insufficiency or when adrenocortical reserve is doubtful.
    Shock unresponsive to conventional therapy if adrenocortical insufficiency exists or is suspected.
    Congenital adrenal hyperplasia
    Nonsuppurative thyroiditis
    Hypercalcemia associated with cancer

2. *Rheumatic disorders*
    As adjunctive therapy for short-term administration (to tide the patient over an acute episode or exacerbation) in:
    Post-traumatic osteoarthritis
    Synovitis of osteoarthritis
    Rheumatoid arthritis, including juvenile rheumatoid arthritis (selected cases may require low-dose maintenance therapy)
    Acute and subacute bursitis
    Epicondylitis
    Acute nonspecific tenosynovitis
    Acute gouty arthritis
    Psoriatic arthritis
    Ankylosing spondylitis

3. *Collagen diseases*
    During an exacerbation or as maintenance therapy in selected cases of:
    Systemic lupus erythematosus
    Acute rheumatic carditis
    Systemic dermatomyositis (polymyositis)

4. *Dermatologic diseases*
    Pemphigus
    Severe erythema multiforme (Stevens-Johnson syndrome)
    Exfoliative dermatitis
    Bullous dermatitis herpetiformis
    Severe seborrheic dermatitis
    Severe psoriasis
    Mycosis fungoides

5. *Allergic states*
    Control of severe or incapacitating allergic conditions intractable to adequate trials of conventional treatment in:
    Bronchial asthma
    Contact dermatitis
    Atopic dermatitis
    Serum sickness
    Seasonal or perennial allergic rhinitis
    Drug hypersensitivity reactions
    Urticarial transfusion reactions
    Acute noninfectious laryngeal edema (epinephrine is the drug of first choice)

6. *Ophthalmic diseases*
    Severe acute and chronic allergic and inflammatory processes involving the eye such as:
    Herpes zoster ophthalmicus
    Iritis, iridocyclitis
    Chorioretinitis
    Diffuse posterior uveitis and choroiditis
    Optic neuritis
    Sympathetic ophthalmia
    Anterior segment inflammation
    Allergic conjunctivitis
    Keratitis
    Allergic corneal marginal ulcers

7. *Gastrointestinal diseases*
    To tide the patient over a critical period of the disease in:
    Ulcerative colitis (Systemic therapy)
    Regional enteritis (Systemic therapy)

8. *Respiratory diseases*
    Symptomatic sarcoidosis
    Berylliosis

Fulminating or disseminated pulmonary tuberculosis when used concurrently with appropriate antituberculous chemotherapy

Loeffler's syndrome not manageable by other means

Aspiration pneumonitis

9. *Hematologic disorders*

Acquired (autoimmune) hemolytic anemia

Idiopathic thrombocytopenic purpura in adults (I.V. only; I.M. administration is contraindicated)

Secondary thrombocytopenia in adults

Erythroblastopenia (RBC anemia)

Congenital (erythroid) hypoplastic anemia

10. *Neoplastic diseases*

For palliative management of:

Leukemias and lymphomas in adults

Acute leukemia of childhood

11. *Edematous states*

To induce diuresis or remission of proteinuria in the nephrotic syndrome, without uremia, of the idiopathic type, or that due to lupus erythematosus

12. *Miscellaneous*

Tuberculous meningitis with subarachnoid block or impending block when used concurrently with appropriate antituberculous chemotherapy

Trichinosis with neurologic or myocardial involvement.

CONTRAINDICATIONS

Systemic fungal infections (see WARNINGS regarding amphotericin B)

Hypersensitivity to any component of this product, including sulfites (see WARNINGS).

WARNINGS

Because rare instances of anaphylactoid reactions have occurred in patients receiving parenteral corticosteroid therapy, appropriate precautionary measures should be taken prior to administration, especially when the patient has a history of allergy to any drug. Anaphylactoid and hypersensitivity reactions have been reported for Injection HYDROCORTONE Phosphate (see ADVERSE REACTIONS).

Injection HYDROCORTONE Phosphate contains sodium bisulfite, a sulfite that may cause allergic-type reactions including anaphylactic symptoms and life-threatening or less severe asthmatic episodes in certain susceptible people. The overall prevalence of sulfite sensitivity in the general population is unknown and probably low. Sulfite sensitivity is seen more frequently in asthmatic than in nonasthmatic people.

Corticosteroids may exacerbate systemic fungal infections and therefore should not be used in the presence of such infections unless they are needed to control drug reactions due to amphotericin B. Moreover, there have been cases reported in which concomitant use of amphotericin B and hydrocortisone was followed by cardiac enlargement and congestive failure.

In patients on corticosteroid therapy subjected to any unusual stress, increased dosage of rapidly acting corticosteroids before, during, and after the stressful situation is indicated.

Drug-induced secondary adrenocortical insufficiency may result from too rapid withdrawal of corticosteroids and may be minimized by gradual reduction of dosage. This type of relative insufficiency may persist for months after discontinuation of therapy; therefore, in any situation of stress occurring during that period, hormone therapy should be reinstituted. If the patient is receiving steroids already, dosage may have to be increased. Since mineralocorticoid secretion may be impaired, salt and/or a mineralocorticoid should be administered concurrently.

Corticosteroids may mask some signs of infection, and new infections may appear during their use. There may be decreased resistance and inability to localize infection when corticosteroids are used. Moreover, corticosteroids may affect the nitroblue-tetrazolium test for bacterial infection and produce false negative results.

In cerebral malaria, a double-blind trial has shown that the use of corticosteroids is associated with prolongation of coma and a higher incidence of pneumonia and gastrointestinal bleeding.

Corticosteroids may activate latent amebiasis. Therefore, it is recommended that latent or active amebiasis be ruled out before initiating corticosteroid therapy in any patient who has spent time in the tropics or any patient with unexplained diarrhea.

Prolonged use of corticosteroids may produce posterior subcapsular cataracts, glaucoma with possible damage to the optic nerves, and may enhance the establishment of secondary ocular infections due to fungi or viruses.

Usage in pregnancy. Since adequate human reproduction studies have not been done with corticosteroids, use of these drugs in pregnancy or in women of childbearing potential requires that the anticipated benefits be weighed against the possible hazards to the mother and embryo or fetus. Infants born of mothers who have received substantial doses of corticosteroids during pregnancy should be carefully observed for signs of hypoadrenalism.

Corticosteroids appear in breast milk and could suppress growth, interfere with endogenous corticosteroid production, or cause other unwanted effects. Mothers taking pharmacologic doses of corticosteroids should be advised not to nurse.

Average and large doses of cortisone or hydrocortisone can cause elevation of blood pressure, salt and water retention, and increased excretion of potassium. These effects are less likely to occur with the synthetic derivatives except when used in large doses. Dietary salt restriction and potassium supplementation may be necessary. All corticosteroids increase calcium excretion.

Administration of live virus vaccines, including smallpox, is contraindicated in individuals receiving immunosuppressive doses of corticosteroids. If inactivated viral or bacterial vaccines are administered to individuals receiving immunosuppressive doses of corticosteroids, the expected serum antibody response may not be obtained. However, immunization procedures may be undertaken in patients who are receiving corticosteroids as replacement therapy, e.g., for Addison's disease.

The use of HYDROCORTONE Phosphate injection in active tuberculosis should be restricted to those cases of fulminating or disseminated tuberculosis in which the corticosteroid is used for the management of the disease in conjunction with an appropriate antituberculous regimen.

If corticosteroids are indicated in patients with latent tuberculosis or tuberculin reactivity, close observation is necessary as reactivation of the disease may occur. During prolonged corticosteroid therapy, these patients should receive chemoprophylaxis.

Literature reports suggest an apparent association between use of corticosteroids and left ventricular free wall rupture after a recent myocardial infarction; therefore, therapy with corticosteroids should be used with great caution in these patients.

PRECAUTIONS

This product, like many other steroid formulations, is sensitive to heat. Therefore, it should not be autoclaved when it is desirable to sterilize the exterior of the vial.

Following prolonged therapy, withdrawal of corticosteroids may result in symptoms of the corticosteroid withdrawal syndrome including fever, myalgia, arthralgia, and malaise. This may occur in patients even without evidence of adrenal insufficiency.

There is an enhanced effect of corticosteroids in patients with hypothyroidism and in those with cirrhosis.

Corticosteroids should be used cautiously in patients with ocular herpes simplex for fear of corneal perforation.

The lowest possible dose of corticosteroid should be used to control the condition under treatment, and when reduction in dosage is possible, the reduction must be gradual.

Psychic derangements may appear when corticosteroids are used, ranging from euphoria, insomnia, mood swings, personality changes, and severe depression to frank psychotic manifestations. Also, existing emotional instability or psychotic tendencies may be aggravated by corticosteroids.

Aspirin should be used cautiously in conjunction with corticosteroids in hypoprothrombinemia.

Steroids should be used with caution in nonspecific ulcerative colitis, if there is a probability of impending perforation, abscess, or other pyogenic infection, also in diverticulitis, fresh intestinal anastomoses, active or latent peptic ulcer, renal insufficiency, hypertension, osteoporosis, and myasthenia gravis. Signs of peritoneal irritation following gastrointestinal perforation in patients receiving large doses of corticosteroids may be minimal or absent. Fat embolism has been reported as a possible complication of hypercortisonism.

When large doses are given, some authorities advise that antacids be administered between meals to help to prevent peptic ulcer.

Growth and development of infants and children on prolonged corticosteroid therapy should be carefully followed.

Steroids may increase or decrease motility and number of spermatozoa in some patients.

Phenytoin, phenobarbital, ephedrine, and rifampin may enhance the metabolic clearance of corticosteroids, resulting in decreased blood levels and lessened physiologic activity, thus requiring adjustment in corticosteroid dosage.

The prothrombin time should be checked frequently in patients who are receiving corticosteroids and coumarin anticoagulants at the same time because of reports that corticosteroids have altered the response to these anticoagulants. Studies have shown that the usual effect produced by adding corticosteroids is inhibition of response to coumarins, although there have been some conflicting reports of potentiation not substantiated by studies.

When corticosteroids are administered concomitantly with potassium-depleting diuretics, patients should be observed closely for development of hypokalemia.

Injection of a steroid into an infected site is to be avoided.

The slower rate of absorption by intramuscular administration should be recognized.

ADVERSE REACTIONS

Fluid and electrolyte disturbances
  Sodium retention
  Fluid retention
  Congestive heart failure in susceptible patients
  Potassium loss
  Hypokalemic alkalosis
  Hypertension
Musculoskeletal
  Muscle weakness
  Steroid myopathy
  Loss of muscle mass
  Osteoporosis
  Vertebral compression fractures
  Aseptic necrosis of femoral and humeral heads
  Pathologic fracture of long bones
  Tendon rupture
Gastrointestinal
  Peptic ulcer with possible subsequent perforation and hemorrhage
  Perforation of the small and large bowel, particularly in patients with inflammatory bowel disease
  Pancreatitis
  Abdominal distention
  Ulcerative esophagitis
Dermatologic
  Impaired wound healing
  Thin fragile skin
  Petechiae and ecchymoses
  Erythema
  Increased sweating
  May suppress reactions to skin tests
  Burning or tingling, especially in the perineal area (after I.V. injection)

Other cutaneous reactions, such as allergic dermatitis, urticaria, angioneurotic edema
Neurologic
  Convulsions
  Increased intracranial pressure with papilledema (pseudotumor cerebri) usually after treatment
  Vertigo
  Headache
  Psychic disturbances
Endocrine
  Menstrual irregularities
  Development of cushingoid state
  Suppression of growth in children
  Secondary adrenocortical and pituitary unresponsiveness, particularly in times of stress, as in trauma, surgery, or illness
  Decreased carbohydrate tolerance
  Manifestations of latent diabetes mellitus
  Increased requirements for insulin or oral hypoglycemic agents in diabetics
  Hirsutism
Ophthalmic
  Posterior subcapsular cataracts
  Increased intraocular pressure
  Glaucoma
  Exophthalmos
Metabolic
  Negative nitrogen balance due to protein catabolism
Cardiovascular
  Myocardial rupture following recent myocardial infarction (see WARNINGS).
Other
  Anaphylactoid or hypersensitivity reactions
  Thromboembolism
  Weight gain
  Increased appetite
  Nausea
  Malaise
  The following *additional* adverse reactions are related to parenteral corticosteroid therapy:
  Rare instances of blindness associated with intralesional therapy around the face and head
  Hyperpigmentation or hypopigmentation
  Subcutaneous and cutaneous atrophy
  Sterile abscess.

OVERDOSAGE

Reports of acute toxicity and/or death following overdosage of glucocorticoids are rare. In the event of overdosage, no specific antidote is available; treatment is supportive and symptomatic.

The intraperitoneal LD_{50} of hydrocortisone in female mice was 1740 mg/kg.

DOSAGE AND ADMINISTRATION

For intravenous, intramuscular, and subcutaneous injection.

HYDROCORTONE Phosphate injection can be given directly from the vial, or it can be added to Sodium Chloride Injection or Dextrose Injection and administered by intravenous drip.

Benzyl alcohol as a preservative has been associated with toxicity in premature infants. Solutions used for intravenous administration or further dilution of this product should be preservative-free when used in the neonate, especially the premature infant.

When it is mixed with an infusion solution, sterile precautions should be observed. Since infusion solutions generally do not contain preservatives, mixtures should be used within 24 hours.

DOSAGE REQUIREMENTS ARE VARIABLE AND MUST BE INDIVIDUALIZED ON THE BASIS OF THE DISEASE AND THE RESPONSE OF THE PATIENT.

The initial dosage varies from 15 to 240 mg a day depending on the disease being treated. In less severe diseases doses lower than 15 mg may suffice, while in severe diseases doses higher than 240 mg may be required. Usually the parenteral dosage ranges are one-third to one-half the oral dose given every 12 hours. However, in certain overwhelming, acute, life-threatening situations, administration in dosages exceeding the usual dosages may be justified and may be in multiples of the oral dosages.

The initial dosage should be maintained or adjusted until the patient's response is satis-

HYDROCORTONE® Phosphate
(Hydrocortisone Sodium Phosphate, MSD)

factory. If a satisfactory clinical response does not occur after a reasonable period of time, discontinue HYDROCORTONE Phosphate injection and transfer the patient to other therapy.

After a favorable initial response, the proper maintenance dosage should be determined by decreasing the initial dosage in small amounts to the lowest dosage that maintains an adequate clinical response.

Patients should be observed closely for signs that might require dosage adjustment, including changes in clinical status resulting from remissions or exacerbations of the disease, individual drug responsiveness, and the effect of stress (e.g., surgery, infection, trauma). During stress it may be necessary to increase dosage temporarily.

If the drug is to be stopped after more than a few days of treatment, it usually should be withdrawn gradually.

HOW SUPPLIED

No. 7633 — Injection HYDROCORTONE Phosphate, 50 mg hydrocortisone equivalent per mL, is a clear, light yellow solution, and is supplied as follows:

NDC 0006-7633-04 in 2 mL multiple dose vials
NDC 0006-7633-10 in 10 mL multiple dose vials.

Storage
Sensitive to heat. Do not autoclave.

MERCK SHARP & DOHME, Division of Merck & Co., Inc.
West Point, Pa. 19486

A.H.F.S. Category: 68:04

Issued March 1988   DC7349525